D1269170

j

CLINICAL
NEUROIMMUNOLOGY

CLINICAL NEUROIMMUNOLOGY

EDITED BY

JACK ANTEL, MD

NEUROLOGIST-IN-CHIEF, MONTREAL NEUROLOGICAL HOSPITAL
PROFESSOR AND CHAIRMAN, DEPARTMENT OF NEUROLOGY
  AND NEUROSURGERY, McGILL UNIVERSITY
MONTREAL, QUEBEC
CANADA

GARY BIRNBAUM, MD

PROFESSOR OF NEUROLOGY AND DIRECTOR, MULTIPLE SCLEROSIS
  RESEARCH AND TREATMENT CENTER
UNIVERSITY OF MINNESOTA MEDICAL SCHOOL
MINNEAPOLIS, MINNESOTA

HANS-PETER HARTUNG, MD

PROFESSOR AND CHAIRMAN, DEPARTMENT OF NEUROLOGY
KARL-FRANZENS-UNIVERSITÄT GRAZ
GRAZ, AUSTRIA

Blackwell Science

© 1998 BY BLACKWELL SCIENCE, INC.

EDITORIAL OFFICES:

350 Main Street, Malden, MA 02148-5018, USA
Osney Mead, Oxford OX2 0EL, England
25 John Street, London WC1N 2BL, England
23 Ainslie Place, Edinburgh EH3 6AJ, Scotland
54 University Street, Carlton, Victoria 3053, Australia

OTHER EDITORIAL OFFICES:

Blackwell Wissenschafts-Verlag GmbH
Kurfürstendamm 57
10707 Berlin, Germany

Blackwell Science KK
MG Kodenmacho Building
7–10 Kodenmacho Nihombashi
Chuo-ku, Tokyo 104, Japan

DISTRIBUTORS

Marston Book Services Ltd
PO Box 269
Abingdon, Oxon OX14 4YN, England
(Orders: Tel: 44-01235-465500
Fax: 44-01235-465555)

USA
Blackwell Science, Inc.
Commerce Place
350 Main Street
Malden, MA 02148-5018
(Orders: Tel: 800-759-6102
617-388-8250
Fax: 617-388-8255)

Canada
Copp Clark Professional
200 Adelaide Street, West, 3rd Floor
Toronto, Ontario M5H 1W7
(Orders: Tel: 800-815-9417
416-597-1616
Fax: 416-597-1617)

Australia
Blackwell Science Pty Ltd
54 University Street
Carlton, Victoria 3053
(Orders: Tel: 3-9347-0300
Fax: 3-9349-3016)

FIRST PUBLISHED 1998

ACQUISITIONS: CHRIS DAVIS

PRODUCTION: KEVIN SULLIVAN

MANUFACTURING: LISA FLANAGAN

TYPESET BY THE COMPOSING ROOM OF MICHIGAN, INC.

PRINTED AND BOUND BY BRAUN-BRUMFIELD, INC.

PRINTED IN THE UNITED STATES OF AMERICA

97 98 99 00 5 4 3 2 1

The Blackwell Science logo is a trade mark of Blackwell Science Ltd, registered at the United Kingdom Trade Marks Registry

LIBRARY OF CONGRESS CATALOGING-IN-PUBLICATION DATA

Clinical Neuroimmunology / edited by Jack P. Antel, Gary Birnbaum,
  and Hans-Peter Hartung.
      p.   cm.
    Includes bibliographical references and index.
    ISBN 0-86542-411-X (c)
    1. Nervous system—Diseases—Immunological aspects.
    2. Neuroimmunology. I. Antel, Jack P. II. Birnbaum, Gary.
  III. Hartung, Hans-Peter.
    [DNLM: 1. Nervous System Diseases—immunology. WL 140 N4913
  1997]
  RC346.5.N478 1997
  616.8'0479—dc21
  DNLM/DLC
  for Library of Congress   97-2678
                                                     CIP

Contents

CONTRIBUTORS   vii

PREFACE   ix

1. Introduction to Immunology   1
   GARY BIRNBAUM

2. Fundamentals in Autoimmunity   13
   TREVOR OWENS

3. Central Nervous System–Immune
   Interactions: Contribution to Neurologic
   Disease and Recovery   26
   JACK ANTEL AND BURKHARD BECHER

4. Local Immune Responses in the Peripheral
   Nervous System   40
   HANS-PETER HARTUNG, RALF GOLD,
   AND STEFAN JUNG

5. Neural Regulation of the Immune System   55
   ANTHONY T. REDER

6. Viral-Immune Interactions   72
   M. KARIUKI NJENGA AND MOSES RODRIGUEZ

7. Principles of Immunotherapy   92
   DEREK R. SMITH, MICHAEL J. OLEK,
   KONSTANTINE E. BALASHOV, SAMIA J. KHOURY,
   DAVID A. HAFLER, AND HOWARD L. WEINER

8. The Immunology of Multiple Sclerosis   105
   GARY BIRNBAUM AND JACK ANTEL

9. Acute Disseminated Encephalomyelitis   116
   ALEX C. TSELIS AND ROBERT P. LISAK

10. Paraneoplastic Neurologic Disorders   148
    JAN VERSCHUUREN AND JOSEP DALMAU

11. Involvement of Inflammation and
    Complement in Alzheimer's Disease   172
    DOUGLAS G. WALKER, EDITH G. MCGEER,
    AND PATRICK L. MCGEER

12. HIV-1 Infection and Its Related
    Neurologic Diseases   189
    LESLIE P. WEINER, RODRIGO RODRIGUEZ,
    AND DAVID HINTON

13. Infectious Immune Disorders: HTLV-I   204
    STEVEN JACOBSON, MICHAEL LEVIN,
    URSULA UTZ, AND PAUL DREW

14. Lyme Disease   218
    JOHN J. HALPERIN

15. Central Nervous System Tumors
    and the Immune System   228
    PIERRE-YVES DIETRICH, PAUL R. WALKER,
    PHILIPPE SAAS, AND NICOLAS DE TRIBOLET

16. Neurologic Manifestations of CNS
    Vasculitides   254
    PATRICIA M. MOORE

17. Inflammatory Cytokines, Astrocytes,
    and the Regeneration of the Central
    Nervous System   271
    VOON WEE YONG, ABBAS F. SADIKOT,
    AND GORDON H. BALTUCH

18. Immunology of the Central Nervous
    System Grafts   281
    ABBAS F. SADIKOT AND VOON WEE YONG

19. Guillain-Barré Syndrome and Chronic
    Inflammatory Demyelinating
    Polyradiculoneuropathy   294
    HANS-PETER HARTUNG, KLAUS V. TOYKA,
    AND JOHN W. GRIFFIN

20. Dysglobulinemic Neuropathies   307
    G. C. MIESCHER, N. LATOV, AND A. J. STECK

21. Vasculitic Neuropathies   316
    MICHAEL P. COLLINS, JOHN T. KISSEL,
    AND JERRY R. MENDELL

22. Antibody-Mediated Disorders
    of the Neuromuscular Junction
    and Myasthenia Gravis   340
    ANGELA VINCENT

23. Antibody-Mediated Disorders of the
    Neuromuscular Junction: The Lambert-
    Eaton Myasthenic Syndrome, Acquired
    Neuromyotonia, and Conditions Associated
    with Antiglycolipid Antibodies   360
    ANGELA VINCENT

24. Immunopathogenesis of Inflammatory
    Myopathies   374
    MARINOS C. DALAKAS

25. Neural-Immune Interactions During Axonal
    Degeneration and Regeneration   385
    JOHN W. GRIFFIN AND HSING-FEI CHIEN

26. Historical Perspective and Overview   391
    BYRON H. WAKSMAN

BRIEF DICTIONARY OF IMMUNOLOGIC
TERMS   405

INDEX   411

Contributors

KONSTANTINE E. BALASHOV, MD
Harvard Medical School; Multiple Sclerosis Unit, Brigham and Women's Hospital, Boston, Massachusetts

GORDON H. BALTUCH, PhD
Division of Neurosurgery, University of Pennsylvania School of Medicine, Philadelphia, Pennsylvania

BURKHARD BECHER, MD
Neuroimmunology Unit, Montreal Neurological Hospital; Department of Neurology and Neurosurgery, McGill University, Montreal, Quebec, Canada

HSING-FEI CHIEN, MD
Visiting Scientist, Department of Neurology, Johns Hopkins University School of Medicine, Baltimore, Maryland

MICHAEL P. COLLINS, MD
Major, United States Air Force, Medical Corps; Director, Neuromuscular Services Division, Neurology Department, Wilford Hall Medical Center, Lackland Air Force Base, Texas

MARINOS C. DALAKAS, MD
Chief, Neuromuscular Diseases Section, National Institutes of Neurological Disorders and Stroke, National Institutes of Health, Bethesda, Maryland

JOSEP DALMAU, MD, PhD
Department of Neurology, Memorial Sloan-Kettering Cancer Center, New York, New York

NICOLAS DE TRIBOLET, MD
Division of Oncology, Laboratory of Tumor Immunology and Division of Neurosurgery, Hopitaux Universitaires de Geneve, Geneva, Switzerland

PIERRE-YVES DIETRICH, MD
Division of Oncology, Laboratory of Tumor Immunology and Division of Neurosurgery, Hopitaux Universitaires de Geneve, Geneva, Switzerland

PAUL DREW, PhD
Neuroimmunology Branch, National Institutes of Neurological Disorders and Stroke, National Institutes of Health, Bethesda, Maryland

RALF GOLD, MD
Assistant Professor, Department of Neurology, Julius-Maximilians-Universität Würzburg, Würzburg, Germany

JOHN W. GRIFFIN, MD
Professor and Chairman, Department of Neurology, Johns Hopkins University School of Medicine, Baltimore, Maryland

DAVID A. HAFLER, MD
Harvard Medical School; Multiple Sclerosis Unit, Brigham and Women's Hospital, Boston, Massachusetts

JOHN J. HALPERIN, MD
Professor of Neurology, New York University School of Medicine, New York, New York; Chairman, Department of Neurology, North Shore University Hospital, Manhasset, New York

DAVID HINTON, MD
Department of Neurology, University of Southern California School of Medicine, Los Angeles, California

STEVEN JACOBSON, PhD
Neuroimmunology Branch, National Institutes of Neurological Disorders and Stroke, National Institutes of Health, Bethesda, Maryland

STEFAN JUNG, MD
Department of Neurology, Julius-Maximilians-Universität Würzburg, Würzburg, Germany

SAMIA J. KHOURY, MD
Harvard Medical School; Multiple Sclerosis Unit, Brigham and Women's Hospital, Boston, Massachusetts

JOHN T. KISSEL, MD
Associate Professor, Department of Neurology, Ohio State University College of Medicine, Columbus, Ohio

NORMAN LATOV, MD, PhD
Department of Neurology, Columbia University College of Physicians and Surgeons, New York, New York

MICHAEL LEVIN, MD
Neuroimmunology Branch, National Institutes of Neurological Disorders and Stroke, National Institutes of Health, Bethesda, Maryland

ROBERT P. LISAK, MD
Department of Neurology, Wayne State University School of Medicine; Detroit Medical Center, Detroit, Michigan

EDITH G. MCGEER, PhD
Kinsmen Laboratory of Neurological Research, Department of Psychiatry, University of British Columbia, Vancouver, British Columbia, Canada

PATRICK L. MCGEER, PhD, FRCP(c)
Kinsmen Laboratory of Neurological Research, Department of Psychiatry, University of British Columbia, Vancouver, British Columbia, Canada

JERRY R. MENDELL, MD
Professor and Chairman, Department of Neurology, Ohio State University College of Medicine, Columbus, Ohio

G. C. MIESCHER, MD
Departments of Neurology and Research, University Hospitals, Basle, Switzerland

PATRICIA M. MOORE, MD
Associate Professor of Neurology, Wayne State University School of Medicine, Detroit, Michigan

M. KARIUKI NJENGA, PhD
Departments of Immunology and Neurology, Mayo Clinic, Rochester, Minnesota

MICHAEL J. OLEK, DO
Harvard Medical School; Multiple Sclerosis Unit, Brigham and Women's Hospital, Boston, Massachusetts

TREVOR OWENS, PhD
Neuroimmunology Unit, Montreal Neurological Hospital; Department of Neurology and Neurosurgery, McGill University, Montreal, Quebec, Canada

ANTHONY T. REDER, MD
Associate Professor, Department of Neurology, University of Chicago, Chicago, Illinois

MOSES RODRIGUEZ, MD
Departments of Immunology and Neurology, Mayo Clinic, Rochester, Minnesota

RODRIGO RODRIGUEZ, MD
Fellow in Neuropsychiatry, Department of Neurology, University of Southern California School of Medicine, Los Angeles, California

PHILIPPE SAAS, PhD
Division of Oncology, Laboratory of Tumor Immunology and Division of Neurosurgery, Hopitaux Universitaires de Geneve, Geneva, Switzerland

ABBAS F. SADIKOT, MDCM, PhD, FRCS(c)
Montreal Neurological Hospital; Department of Neurology and Neurosurgery, McGill University, Montreal, Quebec, Canada

DEREK R. SMITH, MD
Harvard Medical School; Multiple Sclerosis Unit, Brigham and Women's Hospital, Boston, Massachusetts

ANDREAS J. STECK, MD
Departments of Neurology and Research, University Hospitals, Basle, Switzerland

KLAUS V. TOYKA, MD
Professor and Chairman, Department of Neurology, Julius-Maximilians-Universität Würzburg, Würzburg, Germany

ALEX C. TSELIS, MD, PhD
Department of Neurology, Wayne State University School of Medicine; Detroit Medical Center, Detroit, Michigan

URSULA UTZ, PhD
Neuroimmunology Branch, National Institutes of Neurological Disorders and Stroke, National Institutes of Health, Bethesda, Maryland

JAN VERSCHUUREN, MD, PhD
Department of Neurology, Leiden University Hospital, Leiden, The Netherlands

ANGELA VINCENT, MD, MSc, FRCPath
Neurosciences Group, Institute of Molecular Medicine, John Radcliffe Hospital, Headington, Oxford, England

BYRON H. WAKSMAN, MD
Adjunct Professor, Department of Pathology, New York University School of Medicine, New York, New York; Visiting Scientist, Center for Neurologic Diseases, Brigham and Women's Hospital, Boston, Massachusetts

DOUGLAS G. WALKER, PhD
Kinsmen Laboratory of Neurological Research, Department of Psychiatry, University of British Columbia, Vancouver, British Columbia, Canada

PAUL R. WALKER, PhD
Division of Oncology, Laboratory of Tumor Immunology and Division of Neurosurgery, Hopitaux Universitaires de Geneve, Geneva, Switzerland

HOWARD L. WEINER, MD
Robert L. Kroc Chair in Neurologic Diseases, Harvard Medical School; Director, Multiple Sclerosis Unit, Brigham and Women's Hospital, Boston, Massachusetts

LESLIE P. WEINER, MD
Chairman, Department of Neurology, University of Southern California School of Medicine, Los Angeles, California

VOON WEE YONG, PhD
Departments of Oncology and Clinical Neurosciences, University of Calgary, Calgary, Alberta, Canada

Preface

Neuroimmunology has traditionally been regarded as the study of the interactions of the immune and nervous systems under both physiologic and pathologic conditions. In the normal state, the immune system is involved in surveillance of the nervous system and in informing the nervous system of ongoing systemic immune responses. Conversely, the nervous system regulates activity of the immune system. Disease-related issues include how the immune system recognizes and responds to disease or injury within the nervous system and the basis whereby the usually "immunologically privileged" nervous system becomes a target of immune attack.

The cellular and molecular mediators underlying communication between the immune system and the nervous system continue to be identified. Many of the inter-system active molecules, such as immune system–produced cytokines and nervous system–produced neurotrophins, were initially considered to be active within rather than between specific systems. The nervous system is now known to be capable of producing many of the same molecules used by the immune system for cell–cell signaling. The availability of virtually unlimited amounts of recombinant forms of many of these molecules and of pharmacologic or biologic reagents that can modulate their expression, coupled with novel means to deliver such reagents to a target site, has initiated a new era of therapy for an array of neurologic disorders.

This book is intended to present emerging concepts regarding interactions of the immune and nervous systems, specifically in the context of their contribution to disease and injury of the nervous system. The initial chapters present basic principles regarding the cellular and molecular organization of the immune system, the basis for development of autoimmunity, the events involved in promoting immune system interaction with the central and peripheral nervous systems, the means whereby the nervous system regulates the immune system, how virus–immune system interactions can impact on the nervous system, and strategies for immunotherapy. These chapters emphasize the diverse actions of the immune system on the nervous system, a diversity that is dependent on both the nature of the inducing event and the individual properties of the host.

The second portion of the book presents the application of the above principles in the context of disease or injury of the nervous system. We have divided these disorders into those affecting the central nervous system (CNS) and those affecting the peripheral nervous system (PNS). As expected there can be overlapping involvement, and many of the basic pathogenic principles are shared. In our CNS section, we have included disorders in which the immune-mediated mechanisms are considered the primary mediators of disease. Multiple sclerosis (MS) and acute disseminated encephalomyelitis (ADEM) are diseases dependent on myelin-directed cellular immune responses. The paraneoplastic syndromes feature humoral immune responses that are often reactive with neuronal antigens, which may also be expressed in the underlying tumor. Constituents of the blood vessels are the presumed prime targets of aberrant immune reactions resulting in the CNS vasculitides.

We also present neurologic disorders in which an immune response, or lack thereof, contributes to the ultimate disease outcome. The detection of immune system–associated molecules in brain regions affected by Alzheimer's disease raises the possibility of a secondary contribution of immune-mediated mechanisms to the degenerative tissue injury. In cases of neurologic disorders resulting from infection with the retroviruses HIV-1 and HTLV-I, and of Lyme disease resulting from infection with the tic-associated spirochaete *Borrelia burgdoferi*, the molecular mediators derived from either infiltrating immune cells or endogenous activated glial cells may be the major contributors to tissue injury. Similar considerations would apply to an array of parasitic disorders. Malignant brain tumors represent a situation in which there is usually evidence of an immune response. Although this response seems ineffective in controlling tumor growth, there is hope that a more effective response could be engineered. The immune response to CNS trauma illustrates that the immune system can play a role not only in tissue injury, but also in tissue remodeling and regeneration. The advent of tissue grafting as a therapeutic modality further raises the challenge to understand the basis of the CNS-directed immune response. These cited examples are but a few of the many instances in which there are opportunities to manipulate the immune response for the benefit of the host.

The section on PNS-directed disorders focuses on entities in which the immune system is considered a principal mediator. We consider diseases of the peripheral nerves associated with acute and chronic inflammation and with aberrant autoantibodies (dysimmune neuropathies), as well as those that result secondarily from immune-mediated vascular disease (vasculitic neuropathies). We then consider disorders of the neuromuscular junction in which the role of specific antibodies in disease pathogenesis is firmly established. Finally, we consider the inflammatory disorders of muscle, whose pathologic phenotype implicates immune mechanisms as central disease mediators. As with the CNS, we again take into account how immune response can contribute to remodeling and regeneration of tissues.

The field of neuroimmunology as a basic science and clinical discipline is expanding rapidly, benefiting from the work of individuals with an array of backgrounds and insights. This book hopefully will provide significant information regarding concepts and applications of neuroimmunology to both basic scientists and clinicians. Since serendipity is often the nucleus of discovery, we hope that by fostering interactions amongst a diverse community we will increase the chances for such occurrences. The importance of synthesis of information, as viewed from a historical perspective, is presented by Byron H. Waksman, whom the editors are honored to consider as a mentor, advisor, and friend.

Jack Antel
Gary Birnbaum
Hans-Peter Hartung

Notice: The indications and dosages of all drugs in this book have been recommended in the medical literature and conform to the practices of the general medical community. The medications described do not necessarily have specific approval by the U.S. Food and Drug Administration for use in the diseases and dosages for which they are recommended. The package insert for each drug should be consulted for use and dosage as approved by the FDA. Because standards for usage change, it is advisable to keep abreast of revised recommendations, particularly those concerning new drugs.

Chapter 1
Introduction to Immunology

Gary Birnbaum

Any chapter claiming to be an introduction to a field as large as immunology must, of necessity, be abridged and skewed. For the purposes of this book, I emphasize three things. First, I present an overview of the basic mechanisms of the immune system. Second, I discuss how the immune system is regulated. Finally, because autoimmune phenomena are an important component of many diseases of the nervous system, I briefly discuss some mechanisms for the development of autoimmune phenomena. Autoimmune paradigms and their control are presented in greater detail in Chapter 2.

Categories of Immune Response

The primary role of the immune system is to protect the organism from external agents, usually infectious but also toxic. In addition to this primary function, the immune system plays an important role in maintaining antigenic homeostasis in the body. It does this by eliminating cells perceived by the immune system to be foreign. To meet these demands, the immune system has evolved into two parts: one responsible for immediate, relatively generic, action against external agents, and the other a system that responds specifically to an external threat. The immediately responding system is called the *innate immune system*. The one responding specifically is called the *adaptive or acquired immune system*. Within the last 5 years it has become clear that these two systems are not separate, but are functionally intertwined such that the actions of one have a profound effect on the actions of the other. Some details of these interactions are discussed later in the sections on regulation of immune responsiveness.

The Innate Immune System

While most of this chapter is devoted to a discussion of the adaptive immune system, it is important to understand some differences between innate and adaptive immunity. The innate immune system recognizes particular carbohydrate structures, especially those present on the surfaces of bacteria. These carbohydrate moieties are different from those present on host cell surfaces and are recognized by proteins encoded in the germline. Some of these proteins are found on cell surfaces. Some are soluble. Since the genes responsible for

producing these protein receptors are stable, responses of the innate immune system are stereotyped. Upon interaction with these carbohydrate moieties, a variety of responses can ensue, ranging from the secretion of immunologically active substances such as cytokines, to the activation of the major soluble effector protein of the innate immune system, complement.

There is overlap between the cellular components of the innate immune system and those of the adaptive immune system. Cells that participate in the innate immune system are polymorphonuclear leukocytes (PMLs), macrophages, dendritic cells, natural killer (NK) cells, and T cells. PMLs and NK cells are drawn to sites of acute injury by attractant substances released by macrophages and dendritic cells. These in turn release additional substances such as cytokines and chemokines that are important in attracting lymphocytes, the main cellular effectors of the adaptive immune system. The spectra of cytokines and chemokines released during the initial phases of the innate immune response affect the patterns of the subsequent adaptive responses.

The Adaptive Immune Response

Cells of the Adaptive Immune System

Lymphocytes

There are two main categories of lymphocytes: T lymphocytes and B lymphocytes. Both are derived from primary lymphoid tissues such as the bone marrow, fetal liver, and spleen.

T Lymphocytes

The great majority of cells destined to become T lymphocytes (called *prothymocytes*) migrate to the thymus. A much smaller number of T cells mature completely or partially at other anatomic sites such as the liver and gut (1). Here I focus on the thymus. This organ consists of a combination of ectodermally and mesodermally derived cells such as thymic epithelial cells, macrophages, and interdigitating or dendritic cells (2). Within the microenvironments created by these cells, two processes occur. The first is the induction of genes leading to the expression of each T cell's unique antigen receptor, as well as other T lymphocyte–specific proteins. The second involves a complex process of both negative and positive selection of T cells, based on their antigen specificities. This latter phenomenon is discussed in greater detail later in this chapter. All T-cell receptors (TCRs) are dimers, composed of either an α and a β chain or a γ and a δ chain. There are also very small populations of T cells with TCRs composed of two α chains. This population may play a role in certain autoimmune diseases (3). Each TCR chain is made up of several different peptides, joined together as a result of genetic recombination. Sets of genes arranged longitudinally on the chromosome recombine with one another in a stochastic fashion (see Figure 15-4, P. 232). There are V-region genes, D-region genes (found only in β chains), J-region genes, and C (for constant)-region genes. Each category of genes is divided into families, with varying numbers of genes in each family. One of the group of V-region genes will combine with one of the group of D-region genes and these two will then recombine with one of the group of J-region genes. Finally these V-D-J genes will combine with one of a limited number of C-region genes. At that point, synthesis of the TCR chain proceeds. Additional diversity of the TCR repertoire results from the addition, during α-chain transcription, of varying numbers of amino acids to the V-J junction (called the *N-region*).

The antigenic specificity of TCRs is determined by the tertiary structures, or complementarity regions, of the V-D-J regions of the chain. No further recombination or diversification of the TCR repertoire occurs once T cells mature. This is in contrast to the situation in B cells where there is continuous somatic mutation of antibody genes during antigenic stimulation and B-cell proliferation. The roles each chain plays in antigen recognition and histocompatibility complex recognition are still not fully elucidated, but it is becoming clear that different TCRs can recognize the same peptide. Thus, one cannot predict antigen specificity on the basis of TCR protein sequence alone.

Once immature T cells in the thymus express TCRs on their cell surface, they undergo a rigorous process of selection. The selection process involves intrinsically contradictory paradigms. On the one hand, the selection process must eliminate cells that recognize autologous antigens or self-antigens, and thus prevent "horror autotoxicus." On the other hand, cells that have the capacity to recognize peptides in the context of autologous histocompatibility complex proteins must be selected. As a result, both negative and positive selection occurs. Negative selection of T cells occurs in the populations of cells that have TCRs on their surfaces binding autologous antigens with high affinity. Cells also are destroyed if they express receptors that do not interact at all with autologous proteins. The mechanisms for these phenomena are incompletely understood. Positive selection occurs in the populations of T cells with antigen receptors that have "just the right amount" of affinity for self- or autologous antigens. Upon interaction of these cells' TCRs with endogenous thymic cells, they are stimulated and allowed to emigrate from the thymus. As a result of the selective processes, more than 90% of T cells in the thymus die, usually through apop-

tosis. In addition to acquisition of TCRs, T cells in the thymus acquire other cell surface proteins. Three of the most important are the CD3 protein complex, CD4, and CD8. These proteins are important in signal transduction, or the transmission of signals from the cell surface to the cells interior (CD3) and in stabilizing the TCR-antigen interaction (CD4 and CD8). They are discussed in more detail later in this chapter.

TCRs can be subdivided into different *families* based on the amino acid sequences of their V, D, and J regions. The potential diversity is illustrated by the β chains of TCRs, where there are 20 different families of V regions, two different families of D regions, and seven different families of J regions in humans. There are only two C regions. The association of different V-, D-, and J-region genes is not entirely random. Rather, certain V, D, and J regions preferentially associate with one another. This is especially notable in T cells expressing γ/δ TCRs. In addition, proportions of T cells bearing receptors coded by the different gene families are not equal but vary from individual to individual and are similar, though not identical, in related individuals. The repertoire of TCR gene expression also varies during the immune system's maturation and continues to change as an individual ages (4).

The antigenic specificity of the TCR is determined by certain key amino acids in the antigen-binding cleft of the TCR in the third complementarity-determining region. The locations of these critical anchor points have been determined for several families of TCRs. In many instances, antigen binding is "degenerate" in that several different peptides can bind to a TCR. In addition, different TCRs, produced by different genes, can have similar peptide-binding capabilities. In other words, one *cannot* predict antigen specificity on the bases of gene family expression. In inbred strains of rodents, immune responses to particular antigens involve activation of particular populations of T lymphocytes expressing particular families of V- and J-region genes. The occurrence of restricted, or oligoclonal, TCR utilization in response to antigenic stimulation, especially in response to self-, or autologous, antigen stimulation, forms the basis for a potentially important therapeutic approach, namely, the elimination of restricted, pathogenic populations of T cells either by immunization with TCR peptides or by administration of monoclonal antibodies directed against TCR proteins recognizing the autoantigens. This approach is very successful in the treatment of experimental autoimmune diseases such as experimental autoimmune encephalomyelitis (EAE) and experimental autoimmune myasthenia gravis. In outbred populations, such as in humans, utilization of restricted populations of TCRs in response to antigenic stimulation is not so clear. Some data suggest that persons with autoimmune disease such as multiple sclerosis (MS) respond to autoantigens such as myelin basic protein (MBP) (5) with a limited number of TCRs. Other data suggest that the response is heterogeneous, with utilization of large numbers of different TCRs (6–8). Nevertheless, clinical trials are studying whether TCR peptide "vaccination" or administration of monoclonal antibodies to certain TCRs can modulate the course of MS (1) (see Chapter 8).

B Lymphocytes

Immature B lymphocytes originate in primary lymphoid organs (bone marrow, fetal liver) and then migrate to secondary lymphoid organs (spleen, lymph nodes, gut-associated lymphoid tissues). There they come into contact with antigens and if their immunoglobulin receptors are able to interact with specific antigens, the immature B cells proliferate and differentiate further. Proliferation and differentiation require both contact with antigen and a series of additional stimulatory signals. Some antigens are able to stimulate B cells directly (so-called T cell–independent antigens). An example of such an antigen would be bacterial lipopolysaccharide. Other antigens stimulate B cells only when additional signals are provided to the cell by helper T cells. Such antigens are called *T cell–dependent antigens* and include most proteins and peptides.

The unique feature of B cells is their ability to express and secrete antibodies or immunoglobulins. These proteins are heterodimers composed of four peptide chains, that is, two light chains (of either the κ or the λ type) and two heavy chains. These chains also arise as a result of genetic recombination. Similar to the phenomenon observed during the maturation of TCRs, V-region genes are combined with D-region and J-region genes and finally C-region genes to result in the final heavy- or light-chain product. Diversity is further increased by the addition of nongermline nucleotides onto the ends of recombining genes to give rise to N-residues. However, unlike the situation with TCRs, where the final product is fixed upon maturation of the T cell, antibody genes continually change as B cells encounter antigen and proliferate. Certain portions of the V regions of genes, called *hypervariable regions*, are active sites of mutation. As a result, there is a continually changing repertoire of antibody molecules on the surfaces of B cells as the immune response to a particular antigen or antigens progresses. This continuing evolution of response also results in changes in the populations of secreted or circulating antibody molecules. Not only are there increases in antibody concentrations with time but the affinities of antibodies for the stimulating antigens continually increase, as B cells expressing higher-affinity antibodies on their cell surfaces are selectively activated. This "maturation" of antibodies greatly increases both the efficiency and the specificity of the immune response. There are also changes in the constant or C regions of the heavy chains of the antibody molecules as B cells differentiate. Heavy chains are categorized into five classes, depending on their C regions. They are IgD, IgM, IgG, IgA, and IgE. Most resting B cells and pre-B cells express IgD and IgM antibodies on their surfaces. After contact with antigen, class switching occurs and most B cells will begin to synthesize IgG antibodies. Populations of B cells in secretory organs such as the gut will synthesize and secrete IgA antibodies, whereas B cells in such organs as skin and lung will express IgE antibodies. The antigen specificity of an antibody molecule is determined by the variable or V regions of the heavy and light chains. However, the general biologic activity of the antibody (Does it form dimers or pentamers? Does it readily activate the complement cascade? Does it bind to particular cell surface receptors?) is determined by the C region of the heavy chain and does not affect antigen specificity. The determinants of class switching are not completely defined, but cytokines, secreted by T cells as well as costimulatory signals, provided to these cells in the microenvironment of differentiating B cells are important, as is the genetic background of the individual.

By virtue of their membrane-expressed immunoglobulins, B cells are able to capture and concentrate proteins in an antigen-specific fashion. Thus they have the ability to function as highly efficient antigen-presenting cells (APCs). That is, they have the capacity to bind antigen, internalize it, digest it, and re-express the digested protein's peptides on their cell surfaces in the context of major histocompatibility complex (MHC) proteins. This is in contrast to other APCs such as macrophages and dendritic cells that capture antigens in a non-antigen-specific fashion.

Natural Killer Cells

NK cells are bone marrow–derived cells of special lineage. They appear to arise from the same lineage precursors as T cells and share several characteristics of T cells (9,10). They are called *natural killers* because they occur in the absence of any immune challenge and remain relatively unchanged after antigenic stimulation. They are part of the innate immune system. NK cells have the capacity to recognize certain targets and to kill cells, such as tumor cells, bearing these targets. Recent work defined several NK receptors in mice and humans (11). Requirements for antigen recognition are not well defined at this time. Recent data suggest that expression of class I MHC proteins (see below) on the cell surface inhibits NK cell activity (11). Since many neoplastic cells do not display class I MHC proteins, this may explain in part their susceptibility to NK cell lysis.

Macrophages and Dendritic Cells

Macrophages are bone marrow–derived cells that have multiple functions in the immune system. They are not antigen specific in the sense that they do not express receptors on their surfaces that are able to recognize individual peptides. However, they do express, especially when activated, cell surface proteins coded for by genes in the MHC. These MHC proteins have grooves into which peptides can fit. The shapes of the grooves are determined by certain critical amino acid sites in the α helices and β pleated sheets of these proteins. Thus, there is a certain specificity in terms of which peptides can nestle in these grooves. However, binding to MHC peptide-binding grooves is far less discriminatory than the antigen-specific receptors of T cells and B cells. In addition to expressing MHC proteins, macrophages have the capacity to ingest proteins and digest them via distinct proteolytic pathways. The peptides that result from these digestive processes attach to the binding groves of newly synthesized MHC proteins and these peptide-MHC complexes are transported to the cell surface. This process of protein ingestion, proteolysis, association of the resulting peptides with MHC proteins, and expression of peptide-MHC complex on the cells surface is called *antigen processing*. It requires metabolic activity, and while it is not unique to macrophages, these cells are among the most ubiquitous and efficient cells of the body for this function. In fact, macrophages and dendritic cells are true professionals in this regard, for not only do they process and present peptides to T cells, but they also can provide the additional costimulatory (described below) signals necessary for a successful T-cell response to antigen. Macrophages are also able to secrete biologically active materials called *cytokines*. Again, this is especially pronounced when macrophages are activated. Cytokines are able to modulate T-cell, B-cell, and macrophage function within the microenvironment of the tissue. Important cytokines secreted by macrophages are interleukin (IL)-1, tumor necrosis factor (TNF)-α, and prostaglandins.

Dendritic cells are pleomorphic populations of cells that originate in the bone marrow. The lineages of these cells continue to be debated but some are most closely related to macrophages (12) while others may be derived from T cells (13). The morphology of dendritic cells varies with their anatomic location. Characteristically they have multiple, long processes, or a "veiled" appearance (14). They are present in at least two functional states. Immature dendritic cells in lymph node follicles have the capacity to strongly bind antigens. Mature dendritic cells are highly efficient APCs.

Dendritic cells are found on many body surfaces, for example, in the skin, where they are called *Langerhans' cells*. By virtue of their anatomic location, they are often the first cells of the immune system to encounter foreign substances. Following antigen exposure, dendritic cells migrate to areas of lymphoid cell accumulation and differentiation, such as the thymus gland, lymph nodes (15), and Peyer's patches. There they play an essential role in T-lymphocyte selection (thymus), and in stimulating T cells and B cells with their captured antigens (16). Indeed, dendritic cells are believed to serve as a reservoir of processed antigens that may be important in maintaining immunologic memory.

Major Histocompatibility Complex

The MHC is a complex of genes, present in humans on chromosome 6. MHC genes are found in all vertebrates and play essential roles, not only in the immune system, but also in somatic cell differentiation (17). A large number of different genes are present in the MHC, many of them not directly involved in immune activities (18). However, since there are major differences in MHCs among different geographic and ethnic groups, and since certain MHC phenotypes are associated with autoimmune disease (19), it is possible that these MHC-associated genes play a role in disease susceptibility.

There are three major classes of MHC genes, class I, class II, and class III genes. There are also a number of minor, or nonclassic MHC genes. Their roles in the immune response are not well defined. Class I and class II MHC proteins are required for antigen recognition by T cells. Class III proteins are part of the complement system and are not directly involved in antigen presentation. The MHC genes are among the most pleiomorphic of gene complexes, with large numbers of different alleles in each class. Because of this great polymorphism, it is extremely rare for two individuals, other than identical twins, to have identical MHC alleles.

There are major differences in the patterns of expression of class I and class II genes. Class I MHC gene products are expressed on almost all somatic cells of an individual. In contrast, under normal conditions the products of class II genes are expressed almost exclusively on the surfaces of bone marrow–derived cells such as macrophages, dendritic cells, and B cells. In areas of inflammation, where there are increased concentrations of inflammatory cytokines such as interferon (IFN)-γ and TNF-α, cells other than those derived from bone marrow can be induced to express class II MHC proteins. This phenomenon may be important for the development of autoimmune diseases (see below and Chapter 2).

Class I and class II MHC proteins have peptide-binding grooves into which potential antigens nestle (20). The shapes of these peptide-binding sites vary between class I and class II proteins and also between alleles of the different classes. Variations are the result of differences in the primary and secondary sequences of these proteins. Peptides lodge within these grooves after the proteins from which they are derived undergo proteolysis. Binding results from a combination of hydrogen bonding and van der Waals interactions between residues of the peptide and two to three "anchoring" amino acids within the MHC groove. Given the allelic variations in class I and class II proteins, peptide-binding sites within MHC proteins will differ greatly, resulting in differences in the abilities of different MHC proteins to interact with peptides. If a particular MHC protein is unable to bind and present a particular peptide, that peptide will be "invisible" to that individual's immune system. This phenomenon in which the nature of the MHC binding region determines which peptides are recognized by the immune system is called *determinant selection*. Since the characteristics of the peptide-binding grooves of MHC proteins are genetically determined, and since each individuals MHC is different, there will be major differences in the kinds of peptides recognized by different individuals. Such differences are believed to be important in the determining susceptibility to autoimmune disease (19).

There are important differences in the sources of the peptides that bind to class I and class II grooves. Class I–bound peptides are derived from cytosolic proteins degraded in proteosomes (see Figure 15-2, P. 230) (21,22). An example would be proteins synthesized within infected cells by viral genes. In contrast, Class II–bound peptides are derived from exogenous proteins that have undergone endocytosis and proteolysis in endosomes (22). The reasons for these differences in the categories of proteins binding to different MHC proteins are related to the sites of synthesis and assembly of the class I and class II molecules as well as the accessory molecules involved in transporting the peptides to the MHC proteins (23,24). There are also differences in the sizes of peptides bound within class I and class II binding sites. Class I binding sites are closed at both ends and so peptides of 8 to 10 residues are bound. Class II binding sites are more open, so peptides of 10 to 34 residues can be presented (25).

Requirements for the Initiation of an Adaptive Immune Response

TCRs cannot interact with intact proteins. The antigen-binding site of the TCR can only recognize peptides 9 to 15 amino acids long. Thus, proteins must undergo antigen processing, a metabolically active process that requires digestion of proteins in the antigen-processing cell (26). Even that is not sufficient. The peptide also must be nestled in the antigen-binding groove of an MHC molecule. Only this combination of peptide-MHC is recognized by the TCR. This implies at least three things. First, the TCR must have two recognition sites, one for peptide and the other for a nonpolymorphic region of the MHC molecule. Since T cells were selected in the thymus on the basis of a modest degree of responsiveness to self proteins, most T cells respond to peptide presented by their own constellation of MHC molecules. In other words, T-cells are restricted in their responses to peptides presented by autologous (i.e., self) MHC proteins. Second, in the absence of the appropriate MHC molecule, there will be no antigen recognition and therefore no immune response. Finally, if there is inappropriate expression of MHC molecules by cells that normally do not express them, inappropriate and possibly pathogenic immune responses may occur.

Still other requirements must be met. There must be stabilization of the TCR-peptide-MHC complex (the trimolecular complex) to allow the transmission of signals from the T-cell membrane to the cytosol (27). This occurs by interaction of other proteins on the T-cell surface with those of the APC (see Figure 15-6, P. 239). The major proteins involved in these interactions are the CD3 protein, present on all T cells, and the CD4 and CD8 proteins, present on subpopulations of T cells. As noted already, mature T cells express either CD4 or CD8 proteins. CD4 proteins interact with class II MHC molecules. CD8 proteins interact with class I MHC proteins. T cells that are CD4+ recognize antigen presented by class II molecules. Such cells are usually helper cells because they are involved in the initial stages of an immune response and are required to assist B cells in responding to thymic-dependent antigens. They also are needed to assist in the differentiation of precytolytic T cells into cytolytic or killer cells. T cells that are CD8+

recognize antigen in the context of class I MHC molecules and often are cytotoxic cells. Some CD4+ cells can also manifest cytotoxicity even though antigen recognition occurred in the context of class II.

Even more requirements must be met before a T-cell response can occur. In addition to interaction of the TCR with peptide presented in the context of the MHC, and of interaction of either CD4 or CD8 with class II or class I MHC, respectively, T cells must receive at least one more stimulatory signal. This costimulatory signal is provided by "professional" APCs such as macrophages, dendritic cells, and activated B cells (28). The T cell receives this costimulatory signal via two receptors, CD28 and CTLA-4. The APC ligands for these receptors are B7-1 and B7-2. Different intracellular signal pathways result from interaction of these receptors (29) and cells expressing them are present in different anatomic locations within lymph nodes (30). If T cells are exposed to a potentially stimulating peptide in the absence of costimulation, as occurs when antigen is presented by nonprofessional cells such as astrocytes, T cells become unresponsive or anergic (see Figure 15-7, P. 240) (31). Anergy is a long-lasting state of unresponsiveness in which T cells are unable to produce the cytokine IL-2. Induction of anergy is one of the major regulatory or controlling mechanisms of the immune system.

Cytokines

Cytokines are biologically active polypeptides released at sites of inflammation by a variety of cell types ranging from fibroblasts, to astrocytes, to macrophages, to T cells. Cytokines have a wide variety of effects on the immune system, ranging from activation to suppression. Thus, some cytokines are considered *proinflammatory*, whereas others are considered *anti-inflammatory*. As expected, cytokines can either synergize with one another or act antagonistically. In many instances, there is a cascade of cytokine secretion within the microenvironment of the responding T cell, such that one cytokine triggers the release of another cytokine. Often, antagonistic cytokines will be released at the same site. Thus, responses of T cells within that microenvironment will be the result of the net effects of these competing molecules. Following secretion of proinflammatory cytokines, an additional group of inflammatory mediators, called *chemokines*, are released (32). These function as chemoattractants for lymphocytes but differ in their attractant specificities. Thus, the secretion of different chemokines will result in the recruitment of different lymphocyte subpopulations to the site of inflammation. Since a review of cytokines is beyond the scope of this chapter, the reader is referred to recent reviews (33–35). One interesting aspect of cytokine biology is that receptors for cytokines exist within the nervous system and thus have the potential to affect nervous system function (36–38). Details of immune-nervous system interactions are described in greater detail in Chapter 3.

When all necessary TCRs are stimulated, and appropriate signals are transduced into the T cell's interior, the T cell begins to produce a series of cytokines necessary for proliferation. Most important is IL-2. This acts both on the cell producing the cytokine (autocrine function) and on adjacent cells (paracrine function). Other cytokines also are produced and these will vary according to the subtype of T cell. For CD4+ cells there are two broad categories, defined by the patterns of cytokines they secrete. At one end of the spectrum are Th1 cells. When stimulated, they secrete IFN-γ and IL-2. Th1 cells are involved in delayed-type hypersensitivity responses that involve the recruitment of other inflammatory cells to the site of stimulation and the differentiation of CD8+ cells into mature cytotoxic cells. They have been implicated as effectors in autoimmune diseases in general (39,40), and in central nervous system diseases such as EAE and MS in particular (41,42). At the other end of the spectrum are Th2 cells. They secrete, in addition to IL-2, the cytokines IL-4, IL-5, IL-6, IL-10, and IL-13. Th2 cells and their cytokines are necessary for the stimulation and differentiation of B cells into mature antibody-secreting cells, or plasma cells. Th2 cells also secrete a cytokine called *transforming growth factor (TGF)-β*. In general, the cytokines produced by Th2 cells have effects antagonistic to those of Th1 cells. Th2 cytokines are being studied as possible therapies for autoimmune diseases such as MS (43–45) (see Chapter 8). The classification of CD4+ cells into discrete Th1 and Th2 subpopulations may be simplistic. More recent data suggest that there is a spectrum of cells between the extremes of Th1 and Th2, with large numbers of cells producing cytokines of both types. The determinants for inducing a particular pattern of cytokine secretion are not fully known but important factors may be the nature of the costimulatory signal provided by the APC (i.e., B7-1 versus B7-2) as well as the concentrations of other cytokines in the microenvironment of the stimulated cell (46–48). For example, if an uncommitted T cell is stimulated in the presence of IFN-γ, it differentiates into a Th1 cell. If it differentiates in the presence of IL-4, it becomes a Th2 cell. Since cytokines produced by the innate immune system are secreted first in the course of an inflammatory response, the nature of these cytokines will be of critical importance in determining the subsequent patterns of adaptive immune responses at that site.

In contrast to TCRs, secreted antibody molecules can interact with their specific ligands without the need for antigen processing or presentation. All that is necessary is that the antigenic site be exposed to the antibody molecule. Interaction with antibody results in the formation of an antigen-antibody complex and this in turn evokes a wide variety of different biologic effects, many of which depend on the heavy-chain class of the antibody bound to the antigen. For example, antibodies with IgM heavy chains tend to form pentamers and these are especially efficient in triggering the complement cascade, activating a series of proteolytic enzymes that form pores in cell membranes, resulting in cell lysis. Many cells, especially macrophages, have cell surface receptors, called *Fc receptors*, that bind to the C regions of antibody molecules. Binding of antibody

molecules to Fc receptors on macrophages activates them, resulting in increased phagocytic activity and the secretion of cytokines such as IL-1. Activated macrophages can ingest and destroy antigen-antibody complexes (e.g., on the surface of harmful bacterium) or can result in the lysis of a cell that has antibody bound to its surface (antibody-dependent cell-mediated lysis (ADCC)). IgE heavy chains bind to Fc receptors on basophils and mast cells, resulting in the release of these cells' granules, which contain, among other substances, vasoactive amines such as histamine.

Prior to the release of antibody into the circulation, B cells must be stimulated to secrete antibodies. This can occur in one of two ways. Some antigens, the T cell–independent antigens, have the capacity to stimulate B cells directly. Example of such antigens are the polysaccharides. Other antigens require a complex series of cell-cell interactions as well as the secretion of particular cytokines in order for B cells to be stimulated. These are usually protein antigens and are the T cell–dependent antigens. Especially important sites of B-cell differentiation to T cell–dependent antigens are in germinal centers of secondary lymphoid tissue follicles. Such regions contain large numbers of follicular dendritic cells, a specialized population of APCs that is especially efficient in antigen processing and presentation and also has the capacity to retain captured antigens for prolonged periods of time. This results in the continued recruitment, stimulation, and expansion of populations of immunocompetent cells with particular specificities. To these antigen-rich regions come a constant stream of T cells as well as B cells of varying specificities, drawn there by chemoattractant cytokines. When a B cell comes into contact with its ligand in a germinal center, it does so in a microenvironment consisting of activated T cells, expressing on their cell surfaces ligands for stimulating receptors on B cells (such as CD40), as well as secreted cytokines, such as IL-4 and IL-5, that are necessary for B-cell differentiation. In contrast to T cells, whose TCRs remain immutable during proliferation, the immunoglobulin genes of B cells undergo rapid somatic mutation with the creation of ever-changing repertoires of antibody molecules. The B cells expressing antibody molecules of especially high affinity for the antigen are preferentially activated. Over time there is a gradual shift in the fine specificity and affinity of secreted antibodies toward those of greater specificity and higher affinity. In addition, there is a shift in antibody class from IgM antibodies to IgG antibodies. Different isotypes of IgG antibodies are produced in different cytokine microenvironments. In mice, B cells stimulated in the presence of IL-4 produce antibodies of the IgG1 isotype. Those stimulated in the presence of IFN-γ produce IgG2a. Isotypes vary in their abilities to bind to Fc receptors of different cells and in their abilities to activate the complement cascade.

Stimulated B cells differentiate into antibody-secreting factories called *plasma cells*. These are terminally differentiated cells that die without further proliferation. However, one of the important features of the immune system is its immunologic memory, that is, its capacity to respond quickly to antigens with which it has had previous contact. This trait is the foundation of vaccination therapy. The exact mechanisms for maintaining immunologic memory are not known but it probably results from a combination of such phenomena as retention of antigens in regions of lymphocyte concentration such as germinal centers, the continuous recruitment and expansion of cells specific for a particular antigen, as well as the persistence of committed, but not terminally differentiated T cells and B cells.

Lymphocyte Circulation

One of the essential functions of the immune system is to protect its host from perceived "foreignness," be it internal or external. While some areas of the organism, such as the skin and mucosal surfaces, are populated by resident populations of immunocompetent cells, other areas do not have such defenses. For immunologic surveillance, they are dependent on the constant recirculation of immunocompetent cells through them. There are two general patterns of lymphocyte circulation. Naive T cells that have yet to encounter their specific ligand continuously circulate to and through lymphoid organs (49). Memory T cells circulate through both lymphoid organs and nonlymphoid tissues. Not only do they have the capacity to enter nonlymphoid organs, but also subpopulations of T cells go to particular organs such as the gut, skin, and joints. They have this additional capacity because of the expression of particular receptors that they are able to rapidly acquire as they come into contact with endothelial cells expressing the appropriate ligands. Examples of such receptors are the L-selectin and integrin families of proteins. Tissue specificity of homing is dependent not only on the expression of particular receptors and ligands, but also on the sequence of ligand-receptor interactions as the T cell encounters activated endothelial cells (see Figure 16-1, P. 255, and Figure 21-1, P. 326).

Under normal conditions, ligands for these receptors are present only on specialized endothelial cells called *high endothelium* (because of their shape). These are present in the venules of secondary lymphoid tissues (lymph nodes, spleen, gut-associated lymphoid tissues). Examples of such ligands are vascular cell adhesion molecule (VCAM)-1, intercellular adhesion molecule (ICAM)-1, and P-selectin. Expression of these ligands on the surfaces of high endothelial cells results in a constant adhesion of circulating lymphocytes to these cells. Following adhesion, the lymphocytes flatten, traverse the capillary, and enter the tissue. Once inside the secondary lymphoid tissues, lymphocytes are exposed to captured and processed antigens, which can lead to their stimulation and expansion. Since endothelial cells in nonlymphoid tissues do not normally express ligands, circulating lymphocytes roll on by. However, endothelial cells in nonlymphoid tissues can acquire the characteristics of high endothelium; that is, they can become "activated" to express cell surface proteins that are ligands for receptors on circulating lymphocytes. The stimuli for such activation are multiple, but im-

munologic cytokines such as IFN-γ and certain chemokines are especially important. Thus, if an endothelial cell is exposed to IFN-γ secreted by a Th1 T cell, it will express proteins able to interact with lymphocyte selectins and integrins. Circulating lymphocytes then will adhere to such endothelial cells and begin the process of entering the tissue, analogous to that seen in lymphoid tissues. Once in the organ, lymphocytes will interact with the microenvironment and ideally function in their role of protecting the host.

While the initial secretion of cytokine almost certainly results from an immunologically specific action, recruitment of circulating lymphocytes into an area of inflammation is not antigen specific. Thus, the overwhelming majority (>95%) of the inflammatory cells present at such a site have no specificity for the inciting agent. Their role is to amplify the immune response and provide the necessary backup to defend the host. Of course, a key question in the phenomenon of lymphocyte circulation, homing, adhesion, and organ entry is, What initiates the primary process? That is, what draws the first antigen-specific T cell to the site in question? Perhaps antigens are expressed on the surfaces of endothelial cells and these draw antigen-specific cells to that region. Another important issue, as yet unresolved, is whether there are homing receptors specific for particular organs. While some may exist for certain organs, such as skin, no nervous system–specific ligands have been found. This is especially important if one wishes to prevent the entry of inflammatory cells into organs that are the target of an autoimmune attack such as the brain in persons with MS. Antibodies to homing receptors can prevent the entry of pathogenic lymphocytes into the central nervous systems of animals with EAE and even reverse active disease (50,51).

The Role of Genes in Immune Reactivity

While environmental influences play a major role in shaping the patterns of immune responses to a particular antigen, the genetic background of an individual also plays an essential role in this process. A multitude of different genes are involved. Especially important are the genes encoding for TCRs, the genes of the MHC, genes involved in regulating the secretion of cytokines, and genes associated with proteins involved in antigen processing. For example, individuals of different genetic backgrounds will utilize different families of TCRs in responding to the same antigen (7,52,53). This has been demonstrated convincingly in inbred strains of mice responding to autoantigens such as myelin (54). In other systems, investigators found that limited or oligoclonal populations of T cells respond to an autoantigen such as MBP (55,56). These observations led to a potentially useful treatment approach. By immunization with TCR peptides, or administration of antibodies to the TCRs expressed on these pathogenic T cells, the course of an autoimmune disease such as EAE was ameliorated (55,57). Much work has been done to determine whether persons with autoimmune diseases such as MS utilize certain families of TCRs in their responses to myelin proteins. The data are conflicting, but to date a simple pattern has not been observed. Nevertheless, as described in Chapter 8, clinical trials are in progress in which patients are being immunized with TCR peptides believed to be involved in the responses to myelin antigens, in hopes of modulating the course of this disease. In some experimental animals such as mice, there are strains in which whole families of TCRs are absent (58). In spite of the polymorphism and flexibility of the immune system, such deletions give rise to a complete lack of responsiveness to particular antigens (59). While such "holes" in the repertoire have not been described in humans, they may exist and could play a role in determining susceptibility to autoimmune diseases.

There are major differences in MHC proteins in regards to the molecular configuration of their antigen-binding pockets (60,61). As a result, a particular peptide may be able to nestle in the antigen-binding groove of one person's MHC molecule but will not "fit" into the groove of another person's MHC molecule. If peptide binding to MHC does not occur, T-cell immune recognition of the peptide will not occur and no immune response will be evoked. (Sloan-Lancaster and Allen (62) have reviewed this altered peptide ligand concept.) Conversely, recognition of certain potentially pathogenic peptides may only occur in individuals with particular MHC phenotypes. Such persons may be especially susceptible to autoimmune diseases such as MS. This is discussed in greater detail in Chapter 8. As discussed previously under the MHC heading, the phenomenon whereby the MHC molds the pattern of immune response is called *determinant selection*.

In species such as mice and rats, genetic susceptibility to autoimmune disease is associated with differences in the expression of inflammatory cytokines (63–66). For example, susceptibility to EAE is associated with an increased secretion of TNF-α in Lewis rats (67). Differences in alleles of genes involved with antigen processing, such as the transporter associated with antigen processing (TAP), are also linked to differences in susceptibility to certain autoimmune diseases (68–71), but not MS (72,73). Whether similar paradigms exist in other immune-mediated neurologic diseases in humans remains to be determined. The subject of genetic susceptibility to autoimmune diseases is discussed in greater detail in Chapter 2.

Mechanisms of Immune Tolerance

The workings of the immune system are, in many ways, paradoxical. For example, one of the most important characteristics of the immune response is its exquisite specificity, that is, its ability to recognize hundreds of thousands of different peptides, polysaccharides, and lipoglycans. Yet in the process of an immune response, cytokines and chemokines are released and are able to recruit immunocompetent cells to sites of inflammation without regard to their antigen specificity. It is these cells that contribute to an immune and inflammatory reaction by greatly amplifying a response that may have been initiated by a small number of specific antigen-activated cells. The combination of highly specific immune system activation followed by a more generalized, non-antigen-specific recruitment of immunocompetent cells explains both the power of the immune system to respond quickly to a wide variety of antigenic challenges and the potentially toxicity that may occur as a result of such a broad-spectrum response. A number of different mechanisms have evolved to prevent that most damaging potential of the immune system, a destructive response to self-antigens. Some of the most important ones related to T-cell regulation are described here.

1. Intrathymic clonal deletion: As noted previously, strong positive and negative selective forces work in the thymus eliminating cells with TCRs that have too high or too low an affinity for self-antigens. If this process is impaired or suppressed during the immune systems ontogeny, either by exposure to immune modulating drugs, such as cyclosporine (74,75), or because of metabolic disturbances, such as deficiencies of certain minerals or vitamins (76), selective processes may be altered, with the result that cells with autoimmune potential are allowed to leave the thymus.

2. Peripheral clonal deletion: Since not all autologous antigens are expressed in the thymus, there must be a means to eliminate such autoreactive cells in the periphery. One mechanism for deletion of potentially harmful T cells occurs when antigen-specific cells are exposed to high doses of antigen (77,78). This results in apoptosis of the stimulated cells, deletion of the pathogenic populations, and recovery from disease, in this case, EAE. A similar paradigm of "clonal exhaustion" is observed with foreign antigens such as viral proteins (79,80).

3. Peripheral clonal unresponsiveness: As described previously, when T cells encounter antigen in the absence of necessary costimulatory signals, the cells become unresponsive or anergic (31). This can occur when antigen is presented by nonprofessional APCs. Thus, the site of antigen presentation, for example, in organs without cells able to provide costimulation, is critical to inducing this regulatory phenomenon.

However, in the presence of increased concentrations of IL-2, and in the presence of professional APCs, or tissue cells that have acquired professional properties by virtue of exposure to certain cytokines, such as IFN-γ, anergy can be reversed. This can occur in tissues that are injured or infected. Macrophages and populations of T cells and B cells with specificity for the antigens of the infectious agent are recruited to that site where they become activated and secrete large amounts of cytokines and other chemoattractants. This results in the non-antigen-specific recruitment of large numbers of additional inflammatory cells to the tissue, some of which may have autoimmune potential but failed to respond because they were anergic. In the cytokine-rich microenvironment of the inflammatory locus, anergy is reversed and previously unresponsive autoimmune cells respond to tissue-specific antigens. These cells then can become self-perpetuating as long as exposure to antigens continues. This sequence of events may explain the association between infections, and traumas such as surgery, with the development or recrudescence of autoimmune processes.

4. Clonal ignorance: If antigen is "sequestered" from autoreactive T cells, they will not respond. But in some instances, via mechanisms that are not well understood, expression of antigens by cells that are not immunologically competent results in the inactivation of potentially reactive T cells. This was first demonstrated in transgenic mice expressing a viral protein in pancreatic beta cells (81). Nonresponsiveness was not due to anergy, as vigorous immune responses were obtained when animals were infected with live virus. Activation of cytotoxic CD8+ T cells required the presence of CD4+ T cells, suggesting that lack of responsiveness was the result of deficient T-cell activation separate from the costimulation provided by professional APCs.

5. Regulatory networks: As proteins can be potent antigens, it is not unexpected that the proteins of TCRs or antibodies can function as stimulators of immune responses. If responses are directed against the antigen-binding portions of these receptors (the idiotypes), they are called *anti-idiotypic* and have the capability of suppressing or augmenting the effects of idiotype-expressing T cells and antibodies (82–88). Anti-idiotypic responses occur normally, but can also be induced. Induction of anti-idiotypic T-cell responses was used successfully to protect against and modulate the course of EAE (86,89).

Naturally occurring regulatory cells were demonstrated in a transgenic mouse model in which the majority of T cells expressed a receptor for an encephalitogenic epitope of MBP (90). In the group of mice in which a majority of T cells expressed this receptor, but a portion of "normal" T cells also existed, few animals became ill with EAE. When animals were manipulated such that 100% of the T cells expressed anti-MBP TCRs, all animals eventually became ill. Thus, even a small population of "normal," nonautoimmune cells can regulate the responsiveness of autologously reactive lymphocytes. The mechanism of this regulation is not known.

6. Immune deviation: From the previous discussions, it is apparent that the site of antigen expression and presentation is an important variable in determining the pattern of immune responses. For example, exposure of antigen to the immune system via gut-associated lymphoid tissue results in suppression of T cell–mediated immune responses; that is, the phenomenon of oral tolerance. If high doses of antigen are fed, reactive cells become anergic, whereas low doses of ingested antigen result in the induction of anti-inflammatory cytokines by Th2 cells (91–95). Inducing changes in patterns of immune responses has therapeutic potential, with amelioration of experimental autoimmune arthritis, uveitis, and EAE (95).

Similar mechanisms as those for T cells exist for the immune regulation of B lymphocytes. Some of these mechanisms are bone marrow clonal deletion, peripheral clonal unresponsiveness, and peripheral clonal deletion. In addition, there are additional, unique, B cell–specific mechanisms of regulation.

1. Maturational arrest: Normal expression of autoantigens can prevent the maturation of autoreactive B cells. This was demonstrated in B-cell receptor transgenic mice expressing receptors for a cell membrane–expressed protein (reviewed elsewhere (76)). Autoreactive precursor B cells were found in the marrow, but no mature cells were detectable in the periphery. When precursor cells were cultured in vitro, in the absence of antigen, normal development was noted.

2. Follicular exclusion: Autoreactive B cells, especially those that have captured antigen on their surfaces, are excluded from entering secondary lymphoid follicles. As a result, such cells undergo apoptosis (97,98). The mechanism for this phenomenon is not known, but exclusion from follicles may also prevent autoreactive B cells from becoming tolerant, and thus may actually promote the development of autoimmune responses.

References

1. Medaer R, Stinissen P, Truyen L, et al. Depletion of myelin-basic-protein autoreactive T cells by T-cell vaccination: pilot trial in multiple sclerosis. *Lancet* 1995; 346:807–808.
2. Martin-Fontecha A, Schuurman HJ, Zapata A. Role of thymic stromal cells in thymocyte education: a comparative analysis of different models. *Thymus* 1994;22: 201–213.
3. Elliott JI, Altmann DM. Dual T cell receptor alpha chain T cells in autoimmunity. *J Exp Med* 1995;182:953–959.
4. Posnett DN. Environmental and genetic factors shape the human T-cell receptor repertoire. *Ann NY Acad Sci* 1995;756:71–80.
5. Oksenberg JR, Stuart S, Begovich AB, et al. Limited heterogeneity of rearranged T-cell receptor V alpha transcripts in brains of multiple sclerosis patients. *Nature* 1990;345:344–346.
6. Hvas J, Oksenberg JR, Fernando R, et al. Gamma delta T cell receptor repertoire in brain lesions of patients with multiple sclerosis. *J Neuroimmunol* 1993;46:225–234.
7. Martin R, Utz U, Coligan JE, et al. Diversity in fine specificity and T cell receptor usage of the human CD4+ cytotoxic T cell response specific for the immunodominant myelin basic protein peptide 87-106. *J Immunol* 1992;148:1359–1366.
8. Utz U, Brooks JA, McFarland HF, et al. Heterogeneity of T-cell receptor alpha-chain complementarity-determining region 3 in myelin basic protein-specific T cells increases with severity of multiple sclerosis. *Proc Natl Acad Sci USA* 1994;91:5567–5571.
9. Poggi A, Mingari MC. Development of human NK cells from the immature cell precursors. *Semin Immunol* 1995;7:61–66.
10. Versteeg R. NK cells and T cells: mirror images? *Immunol Today* 1992;13:244–247.
11. Lanier LL, Phillips JH. NK cell recognition of major histocompatibility complex class I molecules. *Semin Immunol* 1995;7:75–82.
12. Knight SC, Stagg A, Hill S, et al. Development and function of dendritic cells in health and disease. *J Invest Dermatol* 1992;99:33S–38S.

13. O'Neill HC. The lineage relationship of dendritic cells with other haematopoietic cells. *Scand J Immunol* 1994;39:513–516.

14. Romani N, Schuler G. The immunologic properties of epidermal Langerhans cells as a part of the dendritic cell system. *Springer Semin Immunopathol* 1992;13:265–279.

15. Steinman R, Hoffman L, Pope M. Maturation and migration of cutaneous dendritic cells. *J Invest Dermatol* 1995;105(suppl):2S–7S.

16. Szakal AK, Tew JG. Follicular dendritic cells: B-cell proliferation and maturation. *Cancer Res* 1992;52(suppl):5554s–5556s.

17. Salter-Cid L, Flajnik MF. Evolution and developmental regulation of the major histocompatibility complex. *Crit Rev Immunol* 1995;15:31–75.

18. Milner CM, Campbell RD. Genes, genes and more genes in the human major histocompatibility complex. *Bioessays* 1992;14:565–571.

19. Nepom BS. The role of the major histocompatibility complex in autoimmunity. *Clin Immunol Immunopathol* 1993;67:S50–S55.

20. Young AC, Nathenson SG, Sacchettini JC. Structural studies of class I major histocompatibility complex proteins: insights into antigen presentation. *FASEB J* 1995;9:26–36.

21. Gaczynska M, Rock KL, Goldberg AL. Role of proteasomes in antigen presentation. *Enzyme Protein* 1993;47:354–369. Review.

22. Neefjes JJ, Momburg F. Cell biology of antigen presentation. *Curr Opin Immunol* 1993;5:27–34. Review.

23. Monaco JJ. Major histocompatibility complex-linked transport proteins and antigen processing. *Immunol Res* 1992;11:125–132.

24. Teyton L. Assembly and transport of major histocompatibility complex molecules. *Nouv Rev Fr Hematol* 1994;36(suppl 1):S33–S36.

25. Appella E, Padlan EA, Hunt DF. Analysis of the structure of naturally processed peptides bound by class I and class II major histocompatibility complex molecules. *EXS* 1995;73:105–119.

26. Germain RN. The biochemistry and cell biology of antigen presentation by MHC class I and class II molecules. Implications for development of combination vaccines. *Ann NY Acad Sci* 1995;754:114–125.

27. Griesser H, Mak TW. The T-cell receptor—structure, function, and clinical application. *Hematol Pathol* 1994;8:1–23. Review.

28. Finkelman FD, Lees A, Morris SC. Antigen presentation by B lymphocytes to CD4+ T lymphocytes in vivo: importance for B lymphocyte and T lymphocyte activation. *Semin Immunol* 1992;4:247–255. Review.

29. Ghiotto-Ragueneau M, Battifora M, Truneh A, et al. Comparison of CD28-B7.1 and B7.2 functional interaction in resting human T cells: phosphatidylinositol 3-kinase association to CD28 and cytokine production. *Eur J Immunol* 1996;26:34–41.

30. Vyth-Dreese FA, Dellemijn TA, Majoor D, de JD. Localization in situ of the co-stimulatory molecules B7.1, B7.2, CD40 and their ligands in normal human lymphoid tissue. *Eur J Immunol* 1995;25:3023–3029.

31. Johnson JG, Jenkins MK. The role of anergy in peripheral T cell unresponsiveness. *Life Sci* 1994;55:1767–1780.

32. Graves DT, Jiang Y. Chemokines, a family of chemotactic cytokines. *Crit Rev Oral Biol Med* 1995;6:109–118.

33. Belardelli F. Role of interferons and other cytokines in the regulation of the immune response. *APMIS* 1995;103:161–179. Review.

34. Karnitz LM, Abraham RT. Cytokine receptor signaling mechanisms. *Curr Opin Immunol* 1995;7:320–326. Review.

35. Liles WC, Van VWC. Review: nomenclature and biologic significance of cytokines involved in inflammation and the host immune response. *J Infect Dis* 1995;172:1573–1580.

36. Chao CC, Hu S, Peterson PK. Glia, cytokines, and neurotoxicity. *Cri Rev Neurobiol* 1995;9:189–205.

37. Hopkins SJ, Rothwell NJ. Cytokines and the nervous system. I: expression and recognition [see comments]. *Trends Neurosci* 1995;18:83–88.

38. Watkins LR, Maier SF, Goehler LE. Cytokine-to-brain communication: a review and analysis of alternative mechanisms. *Life Sci* 1995;57:1011–1026. Review.

39. Liblau RS, Singer SM, McDevitt HO. Th1 and Th2 CD4+ T cells in the pathogenesis of organ-specific autoimmune diseases [see comments]. *Immunol Today* 1995;16:34–38.

40. Romagnani S, Olsson T. Biology of human TH1 and TH2 cells. *J Clin Immunol* 1995;15:121–129.

41. Olsson T. Critical influences of the cytokine orchestration on the outcome of myelin antigen-specific T-cell autoimmunity in experimental autoimmune encephalomyelitis and multiple sclerosis. *Immunol Rev* 1995;144:245–268.

42. Olsson T. Cytokine-producing cells in experimental autoimmune encephalomyelitis and multiple sclerosis. *Neurology* 1995;45(suppl 6):S11–S15.

43. Johns LD, Flanders KC, Ranges GE, Sriram S. Successful treatment of experimental allergic encephalomyelitis with transforming growth factor-beta 1. *J Immunol* 1991;147:1792–1796.

44. Racke MK, Dhib Jalbut S, Cannella B, et al. Prevention and treatment of chronic relapsing experimental allergic encephalomyelitis by transforming growth factor-beta 1. *J Immunol* 1991;146:3012–3017.

45. Racke MK, Sriram S, Carlino J, et al. Long-term treatment of chronic relapsing experimental allergic encephalomyelitis by transforming growth factor-beta 2. *J Neuroimmunol* 1993;46:175–183.

46. De Carli M, D'Elios MM, Zancuoghi G, et al. Human Th1 and Th2 cells: functional properties, regulation of development and role in autoimmunity. *Autoimmunity* 1994;18:301–308.

47. Romagnani S. Human TH1 and TH2 subsets: regulation of differentiation and role in protection and immunopathology. *Int Arch Allergy Immunol* 1992;98:279–285. Review.

48. Romagnani S. Induction of TH1 and TH2 responses: a key role for the 'natural' immune response? [see comments]. *Immunol Today* 1992;13:379–381. Review.

49. Butcher EC, Picker LJ. Lymphocyte homing and homeostasis. *Science* 1996;272:60–66.

50. Kent SJ, Karlik SJ, Cannon C, et al. A monoclonal antibody to alpha 4 integrin suppresses and reverses active experimental allergic encephalomyelitis. *J Neuroimmunol* 1995;58:1–10.

51. Yednock TA, Cannon C, Fritz LC, et al. Prevention of experimental autoimmune encephalomyelitis by antibodies against alpha 4 beta 1 integrin. *Nature* 1992;356:63–66.

52. Ben-Nun A, Liblau RS, Cohen L, et al. Restricted T-cell receptor V beta gene usage by myelin basic protein-specific T-cell clones in multiple sclerosis: predominant genes vary in individuals. *Proc Natl Acad Sci USA* 1991;88:2466–2470.

53. Boitel B, Ermonval M, Panina-Bordignon P, et al. Preferential V beta gene usage and lack of junctional sequence conservation among human T cell receptors specific for a tetanus toxin-derived peptide: evidence for a dominant role of a germline-encoded V region in antigen/major his-

tocompatibility complex recognition. *J Exp Med* 1992;175:765–777.

54. Sakai K, Sinha AA, Mitchell DJ, et al. Involvement of distinct murine T-cell receptors in the autoimmune encephalitogenic response to nested epitopes of myelin basic protein. *Proc Natl Acad Sci USA* 1988;85:8608–8612.

55. Acha-Orbea H, Mitchell DJ, Timmermann L, et al. Limited heterogeneity of T cell receptors from lymphocytes mediating autoimmune encephalomyelitis allows specific immune intervention. *Cell* 1988;54:263–273.

56. Zamvil SS, Mitchell DJ, Lee NE, et al. Predominant expression of a T cell receptor V beta gene subfamily in autoimmune encephalomyelitis. *J Exp Med* 1988;167:1586–1596.

57. Vandenbark AA, Hashim G, Offner H. Immunization with a synthetic T-cell receptor V-region peptide protects against experimental autoimmune encephalomyelitis. *Nature* 1989;341:541–544.

58. Behlke MA, Chou HS, Huppi K, Loh DY. Murine T-cell receptor mutants with deletions of beta-chain variable region genes. *Proc Natl Acad Sci USA* 1986;83:767–771.

59. Haqqi TM, Banerjee S, Jones WL, et al. Identification of T-cell receptor V beta deletion mutant mouse strain AU/ssJ (H-2q) which is resistant to collagen-induced arthritis. *Immunogenetics* 1989;29:180–185.

60. Madden DR. The three-dimensional structure of peptide-MHC complexes. *Annu Rev Immunol* 1995;13:587–622.

61. Parker KC, Shields M, DiBrino M, et al. Peptide binding to MHC class I molecules: implications for antigenic peptide prediction. *Immunol Res* 1995;14:34–57.

62. Sloan-Lancaster J, Allen PM. Altered peptide ligand-induced partial T cell activation: molecular mechanism and role in T cell biologys. *Annu Rev Immunol* 1996;14:1–27.

63. de Kozak Y, Naud MC, Bellot J, et al. A role for non-MHC genetic polymorphism in susceptibility to spontaneous autoimmunity. *Immunity* 1994;1:73–83.

64. Mustafa M, Vingsbo C, Olsson T, et al. The major histocompatibility complex influences myelin basic protein 63-88-induced T cell cytokine profile and experimental autoimmune encephalomyelitis. *Eur J Immunol* 1993;23:3089–3095.

65. Mustafa M, Vingsbo C, Olsson T, et al. Differential tumor necrosis factor expression by resident retinal cells from experimental uveitis-susceptible and -resistant rat strains. *J Neuroimmunol* 1994;55:1–9.

66. Takacs K, Douek DC, Altmann DM, et al. Exacerbated autoimmunity associated with a T helper-1 cytokine profile shift in H-2E-transgenic mice. *Eur J Immunol* 1995;25:3134–3141.

67. Chung IY, Norris JG, Benveniste EN. Differential tumor necrosis factor alpha expression by astrocytes from experimental allergic encephalomyelitis-susceptible and -resistant rat strains. *J Exp Med* 1991;173:801–811.

68. Barron KS, Reveille JD, Carrington M, et al. Susceptibility to Reiter's syndrome is associated with alleles of TAP genes. *Arthritis Rheum* 1995;38:684–689.

69. Gonzalez-Escribano MF, Morales J, Garcia-Lozano JR, et al. TAP polymorphism in patients with Behçet's disease. *Ann Rheum Dis* 1995;54:386–388.

70. Ploski R, Undlien DE, Vinje O, et al. Polymorphism of human major histocompatibility complex-encoded transporter associated with antigen processing (TAP) genes and susceptibility to juvenile rheumatoid arthritis. *Hum Immunol* 1994;39:54–60.

71. Singal DP, Ye M, Qiu X, D'Souza M. Polymorphisms in the TAP2 gene and their association with rheumatoid arthritis. *Clin Exp Rheumatol* 1994;12:29–33.

72. Bell RB, Ramachandran S. The relationship of TAP1 and TAP2 dimorphisms to multiple sclerosis susceptibility. *J Neuroimmunol* 1995;59:201–204.

73. Liblau R, van EPM, Sandberg-Wollheim M, et al. Antigen processing gene polymorphisms in HLA-DR2 multiple sclerosis. *Neurology* 1993;43:1192–1197.

74. Sakaguchi N, Sakaguchi S. Causes and mechanism of autoimmune disease: cyclosporin A as a probe for the investigation. *J Invest Dermatol* 1992;98(suppl):70S–76S.

75. Schuurman HJ, Van LH, Rozing J, Vos JG. Chemicals trophic for the thymus: risk for immunodeficiency and autoimmunity. *Int J Immunopharmacol* 1992;14: 369–375.

76. Revillard JP, Cozon G. Experimental models and mechanisms of immune deficiencies of nutritional origin. *Food Addit Contam* 1990;7(suppl 1):S82–S86.

77. Critchfield JM, Racke MK, Zuniga-Pflucker JC, et al. T cell deletion in high antigen dose therapy of autoimmune encephalomyelitis. *Science* 1994;263:1139–1143.

78. Critchfield JM, Zuniga-Pflucker JC, Lenardo MJ. Parameters controlling the programmed death of mature mouse T lymphocytes in high-dose suppression. *Cell Immunol* 1995;160:71–78.

79. Moskophidis D, Laine E, Zinkernagel RM. Peripheral clonal deletion of antiviral memory CD8+ T cells. *Eur J Immunol* 1993;23:3306–3311.

80. Moskophidis D, Lechner F, Pircher H, Zinkernagel RM. Virus persistence in acutely infected immunocompetent mice by exhaustion of antiviral cytotoxic effector T cells [see comments]. *Nature* 1993;362:758–761. Published erratum appears in *Nature* 1993;364:262.

81. Ohashi PS, Oehen S, Buerki K, et al. Ablation of "tolerance" and induction of diabetes by virus infection in viral antigen transgenic mice. *Cell* 1991;65:305–317.

82. Beraud E. T cell vaccination in autoimmune diseases. *Ann NY Acad Sci* 1991;636:124–134.

83. Calvanico NJ. The humoral immune response in autoimmunity. *Dermatol Clin* 1993;11:379–389. Review.

84. Cerny J, Smith JS, Webb C, Tucker PW. Properties of anti-idiotypic T cell lines propagated with syngeneic B lymphocytes. I. T cells bind intact idiotypes and discriminate between the somatic idiotypic variants in a manner similar to the anti-idiotopic antibodies. *J Immunol* 1988; 141:3718–3725.

85. Lider O, Beraud E, Reshef T, et al. Vaccination against experimental autoimmune encephalomyelitis using a subencephalitogenic dose of autoimmune effector T cells. (2). Induction of a protective anti-idiotypic response. *J Autoimmun* 1989;2:87–99.

86. Offner H, Vainiene M, Gold DP, et al. Protection against experimental encephalomyelitis. Idiotypic autoregulation induced by a nonencephalitogenic T cell clone expressing a cross-reactive T cell receptor V gene. *J Immunol* 1991;146:4165–4172.

87. Shoenfeld Y, Amital H, Ferrone S, Kennedy RC. Anti-idiotypes and their application under autoimmune, neoplastic, and infectious conditions. *Int Arch Allergy Immunol* 1994;105:211–223. Review.

88. Zaghouani H, Fidanza V, Bona CA. The significance of idiotype-anti-idiotype interactions in the activation of self-reactive clones. *Clin Exp Rheumatol* 1989;7(suppl 3): S19–S25.

89. Lider O, Reshef T, Beraud E, et al. Anti-idiotypic network induced by T cell vaccination against experimental autoimmune encephalomyelitis. *Science* 1988;239:181–183.

90. Lafaille JJ, Nagashima K, Katsuki M, Tonegawa S. High incidence of spontaneous autoimmune encephalomyelitis in immunodeficient anti-myelin basic protein T cell receptor transgenic mice. *Cell* 1994;78:399–408.

91. Friedman A, al-Sabbagh A, Santos LM, et al. Oral tolerance: a biologically relevant pathway to generate peripheral tolerance against external and self antigens. *Chem Immunol* 1994;58:259–290.

92. Keren DF. Antigen processing in the mucosal immune system. *Semin Immunol* 1992;4:217–226.

93. Mitchison A, Sieper J. Immunological basis of oral tolerance. *Z Rheumatol* 1995;54:141–144.

94. Staines NA, Harper N. Oral tolerance in the control of experimental models of autoimmune disease. *Z Rheumatol* 1995;54:145–154.

95. Weiner HL, Friedman A, Miller A, et al. Oral tolerance: immunologic mechanisms and treatment of animal and human organ-specific autoimmune diseases by oral administration of autoantigens. *Annu Rev Immunol* 1994; 12:809–837.

96. Goodnow CC, Cyster JG, Hartley SB, et al. Self-tolerance checkpoints in B lymphocyte development. *Adv Immunol* 1995;59:279–368.

97. Cyster JG, Goodnow CC. Pertussis toxin inhibits migration of B and T lymphocytes into splenic white pulp cords. *J Exp Med* 1995;182:581–586.

98. Cyster JG, Hartley SB, Goodnow CC. Competition for follicular niches excludes self-reactive cells from the recirculating B-cell repertoire [see comments]. *Nature* 1994; 371:389–395.

Chapter 2
Fundamentals in Autoimmunity

Trevor Owens

The immune system's major role is to protect the organism in its constant war against pathogens. To fulfill this role in the setting of continually evolving viruses, parasites with a capacity to alter their antigenic makeup, and a host species whose success stems in part from the ability to migrate to and colonize new environments, the immune system has evolved receptors with the capability to recognize a broad universe of antigenic determinants, and an arsenal of cytopathic mechanisms. It is probably inevitable, as in many wars, that a system with such recognitive scope and cytopathic power as this would occasionally become misdirected and cause damage to its host. *Autoimmunity* is the response of the immune system to components of the host organism, or self. Strictly speaking, this would be of little interest in itself but for its pathologic sequela, autoimmune disease, which represents persistent or dysregulated autoimmunity. In fact, during development, cells of the immune system focus on recognition of self, and self, in the form of major histocompatibility complex (MHC)–encoded molecules, plays a central role in guiding and inducing immune responses. Thus, in seeking to understand autoimmunity, we are addressing a specific instance of more general questions: How does the immune system recognize antigen, and how is this controlled? Or, can we understand the immune dysregulation that leads to autoimmunity?

In the context of neuroimmunology, autoimmunity necessarily involves recognition by the immune system of neural components, and infiltration of immune cells and mediators into nervous tissues, including across the blood-brain barrier. Therefore, we must consider how tolerance against neural antigens is induced, maintained, and broken; how and where such antigens are recognized to induce an immune response; how immune cells cross the blood-brain barrier; and the mechanism of immune pathology in neuroautoimmune disease.

Components of the Immune System

The immune system is described in the preceding chapter. Nevertheless, there are a few points of perspective that should be mentioned. The cellular components of the immune system (leukocytes) derive from the bone marrow. Those with specific receptors are the lympho-

cytes. These contain two distinct lineages. T lymphocytes develop in the thymus, and do not secrete their antigen receptor, whereas B lymphocytes (in mammals) develop in the bone marrow and can secrete their immunoglobulin antigen receptor in the form of antibody. T and B lymphocytes differ also in their recognition of antigen, although there is homology at the primary and secondary structure levels, and in the genetics of rearrangement and expression of their antigen receptors (1).

Major Histocompatibility Complex

T cells are guided in their functions by molecules encoded by the MHC. The highly polymorphic class I and II MHC genes (e.g., the immunoglobulin gene superfamily) encode proteins that are homologous in their domain structure and organization to immunoglobulin (2). They serve to "present" small peptides that are recognized as a complex with MHC by T-cell receptors. The origin of these peptides varies with the class of MHC molecule, class I presenting endogenously synthesized peptides (e.g., those encoded by viruses as well as cellular genes) and class II molecules presenting peptides that derive from proteolytic processing of proteins that originate in the extracellular milieu. These include components of phagocytosed particles such as bacteria, as well as serum and other self-proteins (3).

MHC Linkage of Autoimmune Diseases

Many autoimmune diseases show linkage with MHC type (4). This is strongest for the MHC class I locus HLA-B27 and arthritis, but is more commonly seen for MHC class II, for example, HLA-DR2 with multiple sclerosis and HLA-DR4 for type I diabetes. It is assumed that these linkages reflect preferential presentation of self-antigenic peptides by these MHC molecules, or predisposition to molecular mimicry consequent to this presentation (vide infra). Another way in which MHC might influence autoimmune susceptibility is through its influence on the developing T-cell receptor repertoire. As discussed in Chapter 1, some strains of rodents delete whole subpopulations of T cells in ontogeny on the basis of MHC-directed negative selection in the thymus (vide infra), and this can influence the ability of these animals to mount immune responses against certain antigens, including autoantigens. Analogous processes may influence MHC-associated autoimmune disease susceptibility in humans, although, as discussed in Chapter 1, the degree to which this influences disease susceptibility is modulated significantly by the outbred nature of the human population, and there is no consensus yet as to the prevalence of any T-cell receptor usage in autoimmune disease in humans. It is probable that other MHC-linked genes, such as peptide transporters, complement, or cytokines, also influence autoimmunity (e.g., tumor necrosis factor (TNF) is encoded in the MHC) (2). The fact that autoimmune diseases are often more prevalent in females than in males is considered to reflect hormonal influences on immune function (5).

Macrophages/Monocytes

Leukocytes without specific receptors include cells of the myeloid lineage. Macrophages/monocytes, which concern us most here, are phagocytic cells that also secrete an array of cytotoxic and inflammatory mediators. These secretory characteristics are shared by neutrophils and other granular leukocytes, which feature inflammatory infiltrates associated with certain autoimmune responses. Therefore, such cells represent a major component of the immune system's weaponry (4,6). Table 2-1 summarizes the major components of the autoimmune response; these are discussed in subsequent sections.

Tolerance

One of the most fundamental aspects of the immune system and the one that is most directly relevant to the issue of autoimmunity is tolerance. During T- and B-cell ontogeny, antigen receptors are expressed as a consequence of random rearrangement of immunoglobulin and T-cell receptor variable-, joining-, diversity-, and constant-region genes, which generates a repertoire that potentially contains 10^{12} to 10^{15} specificities. This randomly generated repertoire has enormous potential for antigen recognition, including self-antigens (1,6).

Table 2-1.
Immune Components and Interactions in Autoimmune Responses

Immune cells	Cellular interactions
CD4+ T cells	MHC class II restricted
Macrophages	Costimulation
CD8+ T cells	Antigen directed
Inflammatory cytokines	Regulatory cytokines
Interferon-γ	Interleukin-4
Tumor necrosis factor-α	Interleukin-10
Interleukin-12	Transforming growth factor-β
Nitric oxide, reactive oxygen species	Interferon-β

Systems have evolved to purge the repertoire of potentially destructive specificities during lymphocyte ontogeny. Therefore, the lymphocytes that emerge from bone marrow and thymus comprise a repertoire of antigen specificities that has been pruned from the original potential, to exclude receptors that do not interact with self-MHC and do not react with high avidity to MHC that is expressed in the thymus (6,7). This is considered a self-restricted and self-tolerant repertoire. However, if that were truly the case, there would be no discussion of autoimmune disease.

B-Cell Tolerance: Deletion Versus Anergy

Both B and T lymphocytes are made tolerant against high-avidity self-recognition during ontogeny. Thus, B cells that transgenically express an immunoglobulin receptor for self-MHC or for a membrane-bound form of lysozyme are deleted during ontogeny (7–9). If the transgene encodes an immunoglobulin that is specific for a soluble self-antigen, then developing B cells are not deleted, but are functionally inactivated and remain unresponsive in the continued presence of the antigen (7,8). This state of unresponsiveness is referred to as *anergy* (10). It can be assumed that B cells with specificity for many self-antigens in normal animals and humans exist in a similarly anergic state. This state of anergy can be overcome if B cells encounter antigen at the same time that they interact with an activated helper T cell (8). This observation shifts the burden for maintenance of self-tolerance to the T cell, and requires that we examine both the T cell–B cell interaction that induces a B-cell response and the process of T-cell tolerance induction.

T-Cell Tolerance

T-cell precursors migrate from the bone marrow to the thymus, where they mature. During this process thymocytes express the T-cell receptor and its associated CD3 signaling complex, and both CD4 and CD8, cell surface molecules that bind to MHC class II and class I, respectively, and so play a coreceptor role in T-cell receptor recognition of antigen-MHC complexes (6,7,11). The final outcome is generation of "single-positive" CD4+ or CD8+ T lymphocytes that have been selected during maturation. These emigrate from the thymic medulla to populate peripheral lymphoid tissue.

Selection Processes in the Thymus

The process of positive selection selects the T cells that are signaled through encounter with MHC presented by cells in the thymus. Lack of such a signal condemns a T cell to programmed cell death. It is of particular relevance to autoimmunity that only those T cells that productively interact with self-MHC are selected to survive in the thymus. Therefore, recognition of self-MHC is not so much an anathema as a fundamental component of T-cell function. However, for this to be meaningful, the peptides associated with thymic MHC molecules should be representative of those encountered in the periphery. Conventional wisdom suggests that there is at least some overlap (11).

Those T cells that recognize MHC plus peptide complexes with a high avidity are also condemned to die, by the process of negative selection (6). In this case, recognition of self-MHC also forms the basis for maturational decision making on the part of the T cell. Thus, expression of a self-antigen in the thymus functionally deletes autoreactive T cells. This was demonstrated in an autoimmune diabetes disease model in rats. Intrathymic injection of pancreatic beta-islet insulin-producing cells prevented diabetes (12). Similarly, intrathymic injection of glutamic acid decarboxylase (GAD), a pancreatic autoantigen that is implicated as a target for autoimmune induction, tolerized nonobese diabetic mice and prevented the onset of diabetes at 6 to 10 weeks that normally occurs in these mice (13). In the experimental allergic encephalomyelitis (EAE) model, intrathymic injection of myelin antigens likewise prevented disease (14,15).

Presentation of Antigen in the Thymus

Which self-antigens are presented in the thymus? Being able to induce autoimmune disease in mature animals, and being able to tolerize via intrathymic administration of autoantigen, might indicate that autoreactive T cells are not deleted during ontogeny, and that those particular self-antigens are not presented in the thymus. Thymic expression of an MHC class I transgene was invoked to account for the lack of T-cell reactivity in the work of Morahan et al (16) and Heath et al (17). Interestingly, in a complementary transgenic system a soluble form of MHC class I was expressed and did not induce tolerance, despite the fact that the soluble antigen must have distributed to the thymus at some level (18). Whether this can be extrapolated to other soluble, serum proteins is not known, but could have implications for putative autoantigens such as insulin and myelin proteins. Sequestration of autoantigens has been invoked to explain the lack of tolerization of peripheral T cells (19), although the soluble MHC class I transgenic experiment introduces a note of caution about this interpretation. In any event, even the tissues that may be considered as "sequestered" in mature animals are usually accessible at some point during development (e.g., myelin antigens in neonates). A defined neural autoantigen, S100-β, is expressed in rat thymus, in seeming contradiction to the logic that if an antigen is expressed in the thymus, then potentially reactive T cells will be tolerized (20). There is also evidence from chimera experiments that the thymic microenvironment shapes the eventual T-cell repertoire, in the case of the Lewis rat toward a T-cell receptor Vβ8-dominated and potentially autoimmune specificity (21). The role of the thymus is thus not confined to removal of self-reactive specificities, but extends to other influences on the eventual T-cell repertoire.

Autoimmune T-Cell Activation: General Principles

To understand aberrant or autoimmune antigen recognition, it is necessary to understand the requirements for lymphocyte activation generally. The activation of CD4+ T lymphocytes is fundamental to the generation of an immune response. These cells are the principal cytokine secretors and their activation is synonymous with "help" for T- and B-cell responses. It states the obvious to say that autoimmune T cells are nontolerant of self. Thymic selection deletes only high-avidity self-reactive T cells, which explains why autoreactive T cells can be isolated from many normal healthy individuals, with frequencies not strikingly different from those in the circulation of patients with autoimmune disease (4,22,23). It becomes important to differentiate whether such T cells are normally tolerant, and this state is "broken" to induce autoreactivity or to assess reactivity in culture, or whether such T cells are not tolerant but have never encountered autoantigen. In the former case, the T cells by definition have previously encountered antigen, and our interest is in the mechanism of maintaining tolerance. In the latter case, there is interest in controlling release of autoantigen, as well as in imposing tolerance. Both situations require understanding of the mechanisms underlying autoimmune T-cell activation. A number of animal models have addressed the linked questions of maintenance of tolerance versus activation of autoreactive T cells. In established viral models, lymphocytic choriomeningitis virus (LCMV) glycoproteins were expressed under control of the rat insulin promoter in mouse pancreas. Animals were functionally tolerant of the transgene until they were infected with immunogenic virus, whereupon a vigorous T-cell response was induced and led to infiltration and destruction of pancreatic islet cells, and diabetes (24,25). Clearly, the protective immune response–associated processing and presentation of viral antigens were sufficient for response, whereas transgenic expression in pancreas was not.

In a complementary series of experiments, Miller and colleagues (16) expressed MHC class I transgenically in the pancreas, and as for the LCMV glycoprotein, potentially reactive T cells were functionally tolerant. Tolerance was broken by intercrossing the mice with transgenic mice that expressed a high frequency of T-cell receptors specific for MHC class I (17). This alone had no effect, and did not cause an autoimmune response, but when a further intertransgenic cross was done to generate mice that also expressed the T cell–activating cytokine interleukin (IL)-2, the pancreata became inflamed and infiltrated with lymphocytes, and were destroyed (17). Two general principles were identified by these experiments. The first is that for autoimmune T-cell activation, antigen must somehow be appropriately presented. When it is expressed in healthy tissue, no response ensues, but presentation via viral infection or in the context of T cell–activating cytokine induces disease. The second is the concept of costimulation, which arose from studies of antigen presentation and requirements for CD4+ T-lymphocyte induction (3). Costimulation (or its absence) determines the induction of tolerance in the periphery (peripheral tolerance), which has emerged as an important mode of autoimmune regulation.

Costimulation for Lymphocyte Activation

CD4+ T cells are MHC class II restricted, so their activation depends on the recognition of MHC class II–associated antigen (3). This means that antigen-presenting cells (APCs) that induce primary T-cell responses must express MHC class II. MHC class II is not widely expressed in the body, and is constitutively expressed only by B cells and macrophages and dendritic cells (3,6). Resting B cells do not induce T-cell responses (26). Whether activated B cells can induce a primary T-cell response is currently a controversial topic. That primary T-cell responses can be induced by dendritic cells and macrophages is not disputed. Among the features that characterize these cells is their constitutive expression of B7-2 (CD86), a ligand for CD28 and CTLA4, which are homologous molecules expressed by T cells (3,27,28). Signaling through CD28 is required for induction of most T-cell responses; this signaling must accompany TCR/CD3 signals, for example, antigen recognition (3,27,28). The B7-2 homologue B7-1 (CD80) also functions as a CD28/CTLA4 ligand on APCs. Reagents that block costimulation, especially a fusion protein of CTLA4 and human IgG1 (CTLA4-Ig) abrogate or strongly inhibit T-cell responses. Both B7-1 and B7-2 are upregulated on APCs consequent to interaction with T cells. B7-1 is expressed later than B7-2, and indeed is difficult to detect in many instances. Recent data show that another costimulator ligand on T cells, CD40L, induces expression of B7 molecules on APCs, suggesting that T cells control the costimulation that regulates their activation (29–31). A further point of interest, to be dealt with in a later section, is that B7-1 and B7-2 may differentially induce cytokine production, B7-1 being associated with Th1 or inflammatory responses (32,33).

Of interest is the fact that autoimmune T-cell responses are also inhibited by CTLA4-Ig, for example, progression of autoimmune diabetes in nonobese diabetic mice (34), or of murine lupus in (NZB×NZW)F1 mice (35). The role of costimulation in inducing autoimmune diabetes was addressed in a transgenic model by Flavell and colleagues (36–38), by expressing B7 with or without TNF-α in the pancreas. Expression of TNF-α alone induced MHC expression, which led to peri-islet infiltration but no islet cell destruction or overt diabetes (36,37). However, when these mice were crossed with mice that expressed B7 in pancreas, then diabetes ensued (38). The point of this experiment is similar to that made by Heath et al (17), that both MHC presentation of autoantigen and costimulation are required to induce a T-cell response.

Thus, to activate a naive T cell, an APC must express MHC class II, B7, and perhaps other costimulators. It becomes instructive to consider where such cells are found, in particular with reference to autoimmune diseases and their animal models. Prevention of macrophage infiltration to autoimmune target tissues did inhibit the induction of diabetes and autoimmune encephalomyelitis in animal models (39,40). One role that these macrophages may play is as APCs for the T-cell response—they may also mediate cytopathology, as discussed later.

Peripheral Tolerance

It is also important to consider how and whether T cells with autoimmune specificity are available in the peripheral pool in order to become activated. Despite defects in thymic negative selection, the frequency of potentially autoreactive T cells (identified by their T-cell receptor Vβ expression) in peripheral lymphoid tissue does not significantly increase in many models (41). Such extrathymic regulation is ascribed to the operation of peripheral tolerance. The mechanisms underlying peripheral tolerance are linked to the issue of costimulation. A seminal observation that has guided much of our thinking was that not only did transgenic expression of class II MHC in pancreatic islet cells not induce an immune response against the allo-MHC, but also T cells from these animals were unresponsive in vitro, and indeed addition of isolated pancreatic beta-islet cells to in vitro cultures downregulated T-cell responses to the MHC class II in question (42). These results were supported by other transgenic systems, and interpreted as showing that in the absence of appropriate costimulator activity (i.e., expression of B7 molecules by APCs), potentially responsive T cells are anergized. This interpretation can be extended to all self-reactive T cells in normal animals, as one basis for lack of self-reactivity. Given that expression of MHC class II and costimulator ligands is restricted to professional APCs, self-antigen is normally "presented" by costimulator-negative cells that anergize potentially responsive T cells. The transgenic experiment of Guerder et al (38), in which B7-1 was expressed in the pancreas of mice, illustrated the consequence of removal of such negative regulation. Pancreata of B7 transgenic mice were infiltrated with lymphocytes, indicating functional recognition, although without clinical consequences.

The functional consequences of peripheral tolerance range from anergy to physical deletion of cells via apoptosis. Apoptotic death is the means by which thymocytes die during negative selection, and is often the consequence of inadequate (e.g., non-costimulated) signals in in vitro experiments (43). Loss of T cells through apoptosis is more difficult to demonstrate in vivo, owing to the low frequency of most populations, but has been shown in responses to superantigens in mice (44) and in more recent systems involving adoptive transfer of T cells from T-cell receptor transgenic mice, whose fate can be monitored by staining with monoclonal antibodies (MAbs) (45). Obviously, whether a potentially autoreactive T cell is anergized or dies by apoptosis has important implications for the host and for our understanding of autoimmunity. If the former occurs, then the potential for an autoimmune response must always exist (through costimulator ligand upregulation). If the latter occurs, then autoimmunity either cannot occur or does so because the potential deleting self-antigen is only expressed in association with costimulatory ligands.

B cells also require costimulation for their activation. This is provided in the context of B cell–T cell interactions that form the basis for T help. CD40 on B cells is ligated by CD40L, a transiently expressed ligand on CD4+ T cells that recognize antigen presented with MHC class II by B cells (46). In vitro experiments showed that ligation of CD40 or of MHC class II without accompanying surface immunoglobulin ligation (e.g., antigen recognition) can induce B-cell apoptosis (47,48). Thus, both T and B lymphocytes require not only an antigen-derived signal but also at least one if not many accompanying costimulatory signals in order for productive activation; absence of the latter signals leads to inactivation.

Molecular Mimicry

Molecular mimicry provides a mechanism by which functional tolerance can be broken, through cross-reactivity between self and pathogen-derived antigens. This cross-reactivity between autoreactive and host-protective T cells occurs as follows. If a T cell recognizes viral epitope A on MHC B, and the resultant determinant is conformationally, or in its T-cell receptor contact residues, similar to an epitope formed by autoantigen X with MHC Y, then in an animal with MHC A + Y that is infected with virus A, the virus-reactive T-cell population will include those with specificity for autoantigen X (49). Thus, even though the autoantigen in its native tissue may not be presented in a form that induces a T-cell response, viral infection can override that and lead to an autoimmune response. Such a scenario is envisaged for the development of multiple sclerosis, and Wucherpfennig and Strominger (50) identified regions of homology, or mimicry, between viral and myelin proteins that allow identification of those viruses as candidate inducers of autoimmune cross-reactive T-cell responses in multiple sclerosis. The LCMV glycoprotein transgenic experiments referred to previously illustrate how mimicry might induce an autoimmune response (24,25). Given a potent primary immune response to virus presented by professional APCs, any cross-reactively recognized antigen would then evade the necessity for costimulation and become a target for immune attack. Molecular mimicry has been invoked to explain the frequent association of reactive arthritis with infections, especially those involving enteric bacteria. Cross-reactivity between enteric bacterial antigens and HLA-B27 (an MHC locus that confers strong disease susceptibility), and shared peptide sequences between bacterial proteins and human collagen predictive of degenerate T-cell recognition, have been demonstrated (51).

This establishes the principle that if an autoantigenic

mimic is appropriately expressed to induce a T-cell response, then autoreactivity ensues. Can autoantigens themselves induce a primary response? This question can be restated: Do APCs that can induce a T-cell response exist in autoimmune target tissues? The question has been addressed in relation to the central nervous system (CNS) by examination of glial cells as potential APCs. The majority of experiments reported assessed astrocytes or microglia as APCs for secondary T-cell activation (e.g., that of lines or clones). Both glial populations are identified as competent for such activation (52,53). However, primary T-cell responses were not induced by astroglial cells (54–56). One report claimed that microglia are inferior as APCs to either macrophages or astrocytes, even for activation of T-cell lines (57), but this is open to debate. It has been shown that microglia and astrocytes can be induced to express B7 costimulator molecules by IL-1, which is produced by microglia (56), and also that autocrine responses to TNF-α might influence both B7 expression and further cytokine production (58), both of which must contribute to the potential of these cells to induce a T-cell response.

Access to Autoantigen Versus Sequestration

It is particularly pertinent to CNS autoimmunity to consider whether the immune system has access to autoantigens. A related issue is whether MHC-associated antigenic peptide presentation actually occurs in potential target tissues, and lack of MHC expression in tissues such as CNS may protect these tissues from the emergence of autoimmune responses (59). Thus, aberrant MHC expression, as can be induced by cytokines (vide infra), may contribute to autoimmune reactivity through making autoantigens "visible" to T cells, although one must also keep in mind the constraints imposed on this by requirements for costimulation, as already discussed.

The issue also arises in consideration of autoantibody recognition of intracellular antigens, which are not normally presented to the cell's exterior. Thus, for induction of response against a sequestered antigen, either antigen release to the periphery or facilitation of immune entry to the tissue would be required. An interpretative difficulty with any model that invokes antigen release as a triggering event in autoimmunity is that release of antigen presupposes tissue damage or trauma, and is more usually identified as a consequence of immune attack. A difficulty that is specific to neuroautoimmune disease is that despite perceptions to the contrary, the brain may be accessible to the immune system.

Entry of T Cells to Tissues

The T-cell surface may be regarded as being designed for crossing endothelia and infiltrating tissues. This is especially true of the activated T cell, on which many adhesion ligands and receptors are upregulated, or expressed with elevated affinity for their counterligands

(60). Although the normal, uninfected, or manipulated CNS is devoid of leukocytic infiltrates, many groups have detected labeled, activated T cells of irrelevant specificities in the brains of experimental animals (61,62). It is proposed that when sufficiently activated, any T cell might cross the blood-brain barrier (63). The mechanism of such extravasation is probably the same as that described for extravasation generally. The rolling adhesion model proposes that T cells normally roll along endothelia, and when they encounter adhesion ligands or chemokines, the rolling is slowed and converted into adhesion, followed by extravasation (64,65). The optimal site for extravasation is first where the endothelium is inflamed, therefore expressing high levels of adhesion ligands and either endothelial cell– or leukocyte-derived chemokines that attract leukocytes in circulation to the locale, and second where the lymphocytes are themselves activated.

Adhesion Ligands

Adhesion ligands on endothelia include intercellular adhesion molecule (ICAM)-1 and vascular cell adhesion molecules (VCAMs), both members of the Ig gene superfamily. Their corresponding ligands on T lymphocytes and leukocytes are leukocyte function–associated antigen (LFA)-1 (an $\alpha_1\beta_2$ integrin) and very late activation antigen (VLA)-4. Other adhesion ligands whose expression or isoform is modified on activated leukocytes and endothelia include the selectins, which share an N-terminal lectin domain that binds carbohydrate determinants on cell surfaces and on extracellular matrix (65). The CNS autoimmune disease EAE was inhibited in rats by in vivo administration of anti–VLA-4 MAbs, and the ability of CD4+ T lymphocytes to transfer disease correlated with their expression of VLA-4 (66,67). Such observations indicate the central role of endothelial interactions in autoimmune infiltration to tissues.

The paradigmatic site for adhesion and extravasation is the high endothelial venule, which describes the morphology of endothelial cells (columnar or raised, rather than cuboid) at that site, and reflects specialized sites for leukocyte extravasation such as those found in lymph nodes, where they were first defined. Such structures are induced in inflamed endothelia, for instance, in multiple sclerosis (68). It can be assumed that fulfillment of only one side of the lymphocyte-endothelial bargain may be sufficient for extravasation, so that activation of T cells would allow them to cross even uninflamed endothelia. Activated or memory (recently activated) T cells are in fact defined by their levels of expression of adhesion ligands such as L-selectin and CD44 (hyaluronate receptor) as well as isoforms of CD45, the common leukocyte antigen (60). This is the most likely explanation for the finding of labeled ovalbumin-specific T cells in uninflamed mouse or rat CNS (61,62), as these expressed CD44 levels consistent with activation and therefore an ability to cross endothelia.

Given that only activated T cells can cross endothelia, then the issue of whether primary T-cell activation can be induced in a tissue such as CNS may be less critical.

This would shift the discussion to the nature of the antigenic stimulus for autoreactive T-cell activation in the periphery, and the nature of the APC that reactivates these T cells in the target organ. Molecular mimicry models can be extended in this way to encompass induction of autoimmunity via activation of cross-reactive T cells in the periphery (e.g., "normal" or host-protective response), followed by infiltration of some T cells into the CNS, in a stochastic manner, and their secondary activation in the target organ via autoantigen (cross-reactive) recognition.

Chemokines

Chemokines are low-molecular-weight chemoattractant molecules implicated in leukocyte extravasation and infiltration into tissues (69). Three aspects of chemokine biology are relevant to our understanding of autoimmunity. They are produced by activated cells (e.g., in response to inflammatory stimuli), their action is cell type specific, and they may be presented by the extracellular matrix, and so act remote from the producing cell. Migration inhibitory protein (MIP)-1α and MIP-1β, both Cys-Cys (C-C) β-family chemokines, selectively induce extravasation of CD4+ and CD8+ T lymphocytes, via presentation by the hyaluronate receptor CD44 on extracellular matrix (70,71). Hulkower et al (72) directly showed that the C-C chemokine macrophage chemotactic protein (MCP)-1 is upregulated, coincident with symptoms of EAE in rats. Ransohoff et al (73) showed that astrocytes are the principal source of MCP-1 in a similar model. Karpus et al (74) inhibited EAE in mice by in vivo administration of anti–MIP-1α. Ransohoff et al (75) also showed that upregulation of MCP-1 production is coincident with relapses in murine EAE. Chemokine production is probably initiated consequent to infiltration and activation of early waves of T cells or macrophages, or to virus or trauma, and represents a target tissue response to damage or infection. In either scenario, leukocyte infiltration is promoted and amplified, so the majority of cellular infiltration that is characteristic of inflammatory autoimmune disease is conceived of as being induced in this way. This speaks to a role for chemokines in neuroautoimmune disease such as multiple sclerosis, and in autoimmune diseases generally.

Cytokines

Cytokine production is tightly linked to antigen recognition and costimulation. Thus, cytokine-mediated cytotoxicity would be at the same time dependent on MHC-restricted interaction for induction, and MHC independent for effect. Cytotoxic cytokines are also secreted by monocytes/macrophages, and rodent macrophages can produce other cytopathic mediators such as nitric oxide and reactive oxygen intermediates (76). Human counterparts to these potent antiviral and antiparasitic mechanisms likely also exist. Where macrophage activation is itself induced by T cells, the net effect is again one of T cell–dependent cytokine release. Although many cytokines are undetectable in fluids such as serum, effective concentrations at their site of production may be high because they operate over a short range, often in the context of cell-cell apposition. Polymerase chain reaction (PCR) and enzyme-linked immunosorbent assay (ELISA) technologies allow analysis of cytokine production by infiltrating and activated cells isolated from target tissues. An aspect of cytokine biology that arouses current interest is the distinction between cytokines that cause or exacerbate inflammation, and those that downregulate inflammatory responses.

Cytokines and the Quality of an Immune Response

The outcome of a T-cell response depends not only on the MHC restriction pattern of the T cells that are activated (e.g., CD8+ versus CD4+), but also on the cytokines that the T cells secrete. Thus, secretion of a Th1 pattern of cytokines (typified by interferon (IFN)-γ is synonymous with an inflammatory response and IgG2a production, as seen in delayed-type hypersensitivity. This is in comparison to a Th2 pattern of cytokines, typified by IL-4, which is biased toward production of IgG1 and IgE antibodies (77). It should be stressed from the outset that autoimmunity is not generally associated with either pattern, but that specific autoimmune diseases are. Because these cytokine subsets counteract each other, and especially because IL-4 inhibits the production of IFN-γ and the action of Th1 CD4+ T cells (77), the outcome of an autoimmune T-cell response is critically dependent on the quality of cytokine production. This has stimulated interest in the regulation of cytokine production.

Inflammatory or Disease-Inducing Cytokines

TNF-α is an inflammatory cytokine that is cytotoxic for many cell types (78). Expression of TNF-α and the related T-cell cytokine lymphotoxin (TNF-β) has been directly demonstrated in autoimmune target tissues such as pancreas, arthritic synovium, and CNS by in situ hybridization and immunostaining (79–83). Anti-TNF antibodies can modulate autoimmune disease, although whether they prevent or exacerbate disease depends on the specific disease and aspects of administration (84–86). A clinical trial of anti–TNF-α MAb showed promising effects in rheumatoid arthritis (83). The encephalitogenicity of T-cell clones was correlated with TNF-α production (84), and levels of TNF-α messenger RNA (mRNA) correlated directly with EAE progression (87). TNF-α is produced by infiltrating macrophages and by resident macrophage-like cells (Kupffer cells in liver, microglia and astrocytes in CNS) (78,87). TNF-α induces murine oligodendrocyte death through apoptosis in vitro (88), so there is considerable interest in this cytokine as a possible effector molecule in EAE and multiple sclerosis. TNF-α also regulates MHC expression, macrophage activation, and leukocyte extravasation (78).

IFN-γ is involved in antiviral immune responses, macrophage activation, and the upregulation of MHC expression on the surface of APCs and other cells (89). This cytokine is implicated in inflammatory immune responses generally, and in many autoimmune responses, including multiple sclerosis (63,78,89). In a clinical trial, administration of IFN-γ to multiple sclerosis patients exacerbated disease (90). In other studies, T cells isolated from the cerebrospinal fluid (CSF) and blood of multiple sclerosis patients showed elevated IFN-γ production in vitro both constitutively (linked to attacks) and following restimulation with mitogens or with myelin basic protein (MBP) or proteolipid protein (PLP), compared to normal and other neurologic disease control subjects (91). Immunostaining has demonstrated the presence of IFN-γ in astrocytes and inflammatory cells in multiple sclerosis and EAE lesions (82,92). Because IFN-γ is also a regulatory cytokine (6,77), it may have more complex effects, as evidenced by conflicting reports of its proinflammatory activity in EAE models (reviewed elsewhere (63,89)). The ability of both TNF-α and IFN-γ to induce MHC expression on a variety of cell types implicates these cytokines in aberrant MHC expression on potential autoimmune target tissues, which is one precondition for autoimmune attack.

IL-1 is implicated in costimulation of T-cell activation, and as a proinflammatory cytokine owing to its wide ranging effects on leukocytes, endothelial cells, and glial cells (93). IL-1 induces production of IL-6 and TNF-α by cells of the macrophage/monocyte lineage, and is itself induced by a variety of stimuli, including bacterial lipopolysaccharide and viral infections (6,93). IL-2 is the major growth factor for T lymphocytes, and is chiefly produced by them (6). Its detection at the lesion edge in multiple sclerosis plaques correlates with the presence of IL-2 receptor–positive T cells (68,94). As for IFN-γ and TNF-α, levels of IL-2 mRNA correlate with severity of EAE (87).

Cytokines in Autoimmune Disease

A number of inflammatory and proinflammatory cytokines can be detected in target tissues of autoimmune responses. These include IFN-γ, TNF-α, IL-1, and IL-6 (63,95). The in vitro and experimental activities of these cytokines are consistent with their playing a role in promoting demyelination, either directly via cytotoxicity or indirectly via their stimulatory effects on cytopathic cells such as macrophages and microglia. A number of transgenic models have been established to test whether these cytokines induce or regulate autoimmunity. Transgenic expression of IFN-γ in the pancreas, eye, and neuromuscular junction induced autoimmune diabetes, retinitis, and a myasthenia gravis–like disease, respectively (96–98). Also, IL-6 induced profound neural degeneration when expressed in CNS, as did overexpression of TNF-α or IFN-γ (99–101). Perhaps more pertinent to the disease situation, some transgenic models show that low-level expression of cytokines (TNF-α, IFN-γ) does not induce spontaneous degeneration or inflammation, but promotes or maintains responses that are otherwise induced (81). In either case, the observation is of a central role for cytokines in disease. Other models include expression of chemokines in transgenic animals, where again the evidence is that these mediators exert a powerful influence on immune responsiveness in the tissue in which they are expressed (102).

Regulation of Autoimmunity by Cytokines

Regulatory cytokines can be considered in two classes. The first are those whose production is induced via feedback from the action of inflammatory cytokines. Chief among these are the type I IFNs, whose production is induced by TNF-α and IL-6. Type I IFNs (IFN-α and IFN-β) are principally implicated in antiviral responses, and their production is also induced by viral infection (89,103). Principal sources of type I IFNs are fibroblasts and leukocytes, in contrast to IFN-γ which is produced by T lymphocytes and natural killer (NK) cells. IFN-α and IFN-β have antiproliferative effects on activated cells, including lymphocytes, and also can inhibit cytokine secretion. They inhibit the extravasation of lymphocytes, and so their combined effect on an autoimmune response is inhibitory. IFN beta is the first drug specifically approved for use in multiple sclerosis, and its action in preliminary trials fits with predictions for a type I IFN in an inflammatory autoimmune response (103–105).

Regulatory Cytokines

Certain cytokines have been implicated in the downregulation of immune responses generally, and are thought to play a role in regulating autoimmune disease. These include IL-4, transforming growth factor (TGF)-β, and IL-10. All three fall into the broad category of Th2 cytokines, and their role as inhibitors of autoimmunity corresponds to the general predominance of Th1-driven inflammatory responses in autoimmune disease. In autoimmune responses that are driven by Th2 cytokines (e.g., IgG1 or IgE mediated), one would not expect these cytokines to downregulate. In vivo administration of IL-4 prevents the onset of diabetes in nonobese diabetic mice (106), and production of IL-10 and IL-4 in CNS correlates temporally with remission from EAE (107,108). However, cotransfer of IL-4–producing, islet-reactive T cells, and IFN-γ–producing diabetogenic T-cell receptor–positive T cells in various ratios did not affect the ability to transfer disease (109), suggesting that once an inflammatory autoreactive T cell is initiated, the response is less susceptible to cytokine immunoregulation. Also, although transgenic expression of IL-10 in the pancreas did not induce diabetes, leukocytic infiltration of the pancreas was induced, likely indicating pleiotropy of this cytokine's functions (110).

Animals can be made tolerant by experimental manipulation, and some of these tolerance-inducing regimens can influence ongoing autoimmune disease, and involve downregulatory cytokines. One of the best-described systems is that of oral tolerance, whereby feed-ing an animal a protein antigen induces gut-associated T cells that are specific for the antigen and that secrete TGF-β (108,111–113). Such a pattern of cytokine secretion is characteristic of gut-associated T cells, as TGF-β regulates the IgA isotype switch. TGF-β–secreting myelin-specific T cells are implicated in the suppression of EAE in rats orally tolerized by MBP (108,111–113). Oral autoantigen therapy is now under trial for rheumatoid arthritis (114) and multiple sclerosis (115).

Switch Cytokines

Whether a T cell produces IFN-γ or IL-4 when activated is influenced by a number of factors, probably not all of them defined. One regulatory mechanism is the production by APCs or accessory cells of so-called switch cytokines, which themselves control cytokine gene transcription by T cells. Curiously, the best-defined switch cytokine for an IL-4 response is IL-4 itself (116). Although this creates conceptual problems in understanding the initiation of responses, it should be remembered that not only T cells produce IL-4, and it is assumed that cells of the nonlymphoid stroma, such as mast cells, are responsible for the IL-4 production that initiates a Th2 response. This raises questions about the role of such cells more generally, but these are beyond the scope of this chapter. Certainly, it can be appreciated that once IL-4 production has been initiated, it can serve a self-amplifying role. Other Th2 cytokines, including IL-10 and TGF-β, also influence Th2 responses (Fig 2-1) (116). IL-12 is produced by activated macrophages and is implicated in the induction of IFN-γ production (117). A growing number of reports described associations between IL-12 and Th1 responses, including those implicated in autoimmunity (118). The stimuli that induce an activated macrophage to produce IL-12 have not been sufficiently defined to allow detailed understanding of how a Th1 response is preferentially induced, but they include certain bacterial infections and autocrine action of TNF-α (58,119).

Cytokine Switch via Differential Costimulation

Recent reports identified an intriguing mechanism for regulating Th1 versus Th2 choices by activated T cells. Differential expression of B7-1 versus B7-2 by APCs influences whether CD4+ T-cell populations preferentially produce IFN-γ (B7-1) or IL-4 (B7-2) (32,33). This implication of costimulatory ligands in the quality of a cytokine response emphasizes the rapidly growing interest in mechanisms of costimulation as intrinsic regulators of T-cell responses generally, and autoimmune responses in particular.

Mechanisms of Cytopathology

T-Cell Cytotoxicity

CD8+ T cells lyse targets in an MHC class I and antigen-specific manner. The mechanism of killing includes re-

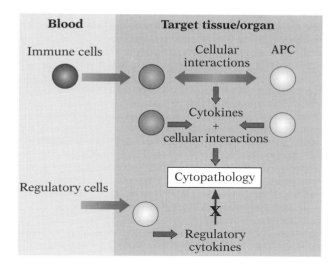

Blood **Target tissue/organ**

Immune cells Cellular APC
interactions

Cytokines
+
cellular interactions

Cytopathology

Regulatory cells

Regulatory
cytokines

Figure 2-1. Immune entry to target tissue and interactions that lead to cytopathology. This schematic demonstrates the extravasation of immune cells from the blood (at left) into target tissues or organs. Autoantigen recognition on tissue resident or infiltrating antigen-presenting cells (APCs) induces cytokine production, by both infiltrating T cells and macrophages and resident APCs. The combination of cytokines and cellular interactions then leads to cytopathology and autoimmune sequelae. Regulatory cytokines counteract the inflammatory sequence.

lease from cytotoxic T lymphocyte granules of perforin and granzymes, proteolytic enzymes, and membrane-disrupting mediators (120). NK cells (CD3-, CD4-, CD8-cells that are spontaneously cytotoxic for a variety of targets in vitro) may use similar means to kill their targets, which usually express low levels of or no MHC (121). In the case of target cell killing in the absence of MHC class I and class II expression (e.g., oligodendrocytes), and where NK cells are not indicated, the ability of antigen-specific CD4+ and CD8+ T cells to kill cells in the absence of MHC recognition becomes of interest. This process is termed *promiscuous killing* (122). Such cytotoxicity in vitro in many (but not all) cases is due to the action of membrane-associated TNF (123), and so may be considered as cytokine-mediated killing.

γ/δ T Cells

γ/δ T cells express a T-cell receptor comprising γ/δ chains, rather than the more abundant α/β T cells. γ/δ T cells are a minority in most animals, have cytotoxic potential, are often sessile in tissues, and have been proposed to play a sentinel role in countering pathogens (124). These T cells can recognize a family of proteins called *heat shock proteins* (HSPs). HSPs are expressed by autoimmune target tissues and cells (such as oligodendrocytes) under conditions of stress in vitro, and γ/δ T cells are cytopathic for oligodendrocytes in vitro (125). Whether this reflected HSP recognition is un-

known, but HSPs are expressed on oligodendrocytes in multiple sclerosis lesions (126), and γ/δ T cells colocalize to these sites (127).

Antibody/Complement-Mediated Cytopathology

Antibody-directed, complement-mediated cytotoxicity plays a role in cytopathology in some autoimmune responses. Possibly the most enduring immunologic parameter in multiple sclerosis and EAE is the elevation of IgG to abnormal levels in the CSF (128,129). The B-cell clones that secrete CSF IgG enter the CNS via similar routes as activated T cells (see above) (130). The simultaneous administration of an antimyelin antibody with T-cell passive transfer markedly enhances demyelination in EAE, suggesting a role for antibody in oligodendrocyte cytopathology (131). Activated macrophages may effect pathology via an antibody-dependent cell cytotoxicity (ADCC) mechanism, whereby immunoglobulin molecules link macrophages to specific myelin antigens through attachment by Fc receptors (132). This is consistent with a general mechanism for autoimmune disease involving activated macrophages whose infiltration is required for induction of disease (39,40).

Overview and Conclusions

Autoimmune disease can thus be understood as a consequence of dysregulated immunity. The normal, protective immune response is directed toward pathogen-derived peptides and determinants that become apparent to the immune system via inflammatory processes that lead to upregulation of MHC, costimulator ligands, cytokines, and adhesion molecules in infected cells and tissues. The lack of autoimmunity in normal situations reflects functional tolerance (deletion or unresponsiveness) of potential autoimmune effector cells, and lack of access to or recognition of autoantigens. This functional tolerance is broken whenever autoantigenic peptides or determinants enter the conventional processing and presentation pathway; that is, they are perceived in the same context as pathogens. The immune response that ensues is innately "normal," but is misdirected.

Therefore, it may seem reasonable that current efforts are directed at regulating autoimmune responses rather than preventing autoimmunity. The goal of immunotherapy is to design interventions that do not compromise aspects of the immune response that are not directly focused on autoantigen recognition or accompanying pathology. Directions under consideration or trial include use of peptide antagonists to block autoreactive T-cell recognition of antigen (133), use of T-cell receptor peptides and immunization with T cells to induce responses against selected, autoreactive clones of T cells (134–136), intervention at the level of costimulation, and use or induction of cytokine and anticytokine therapy to inhibit regulatory and cytopathologic cytokines (137–139). These approaches complement the more general use of systemic immunosuppressants such as steroids. As our understanding of autoimmune processes and the diseases they mediate increases, our ability to intervene selectively and ameliorate them must also increase. This is the principal goal of current research in autoimmunity.

References

1. Jorgensen JL, Reay PA, Ehrich EW, Davis MM. Molecular components of T-cell recognition. *Annu Rev Immunol* 1992;10:835–873.
2. Germain RN. MHC-dependent antigen processing and peptide presentation: providing ligands for T lymphocyte activation. *Cell* 1994;76:287–299.
3. Janeway CA Jr, Bottomly K. Signals and signs for lymphocyte responses. *Cell* 1994;76:275–285.
4. Sriram S, Owens T. Neuroimmunology. In: Bradley WG, Daroff RB, Fenichel GM, Marsden CD, eds. *Neurology in clinical practice.* Newton, MA:Butterworth-Heinemann, 1996:709–722.
5. Fox HS. Androgen treatment prevents diabetes in nonobese diabetic mice. *J Exp Med* 1992;175:1409–1412.
6. Janeway CA, Travers P. Immunobiology: the immune system in health and disease. New York: Current Biology/Garland, 1994.
7. Nossal GJV. Negative selection of lymphocytes. *Cell* 1994;76:229–239.
8. Goodnow CC. Transgenic mice and analysis of B-cell tolerance. *Annu Rev Immunol* 1992;10:489–518.
9. Nemazee D, Russell D, Arnold B, et al. Clonal deletion of autospecific B lymphocytes. *Immunol Rev* 1991;122:117–132.
10. Pike BL, Boyd AW, Nossal GJ. Clonal anergy: the universally anergic B lymphocyte. *Proc Natl Acad Sci USA* 1982;79:2013–2017.
11. Jameson SC, Hogquist KA, Bevan MJ. Positive selection of thymocytes. *Annu Rev Immunol* 1995;13:93–126.
12. Posselt AM, Barker CF, Friedman AL, Naji A. Prevention of autoimmune diabetes in the BB rat by intrathymic islet transplantation at birth. *Science* 1992;256:1321–1324.
13. Tisch R, Yang XD, Singer SM, et al. Immune response to glutamic acid decarboxylase correlates with insulitis in non-obese diabetic mice. *Nature* 1993;366:72–75.
14. Khoury SJ, Sayegh MH, Hancock WW, et al. Acquired tolerance to experimental autoimmune encephalomyelitis by intrathymic injection of myelin basic protein or its major encephalitogenic peptide. *J Exp Med* 1993;178:559–566.
15. Goss JA, Nakafusa Y, Roland CR, et al. Immunological tolerance to a defined myelin basic protein antigen administered intrathymically. *J Immunol* 1994;153:3890–3898.
16. Morahan G, Allison J, Miller JF. Tolerance of class I histocompatibility antigens expressed extrathymically. *Nature* 1989;339:622–624.
17. Heath WR, Allison J, Hoffmann MW, et al. Autoimmune diabetes as a consequence of locally produced interleukin-2. *Nature* 1992;359:547–549.
18. Arnold B, Dill O, Kublbeck G, et al. Alloreactive immune responses of transgenic mice expressing a foreign transplantation antigen in a soluble form. *Proc Natl Acad Sci USA* 1988;85:2269–2273.
19. Miller JF, Morahan G. Peripheral T cell tolerance. *Annu Rev Immunol* 1992;10:51–69.
20. Wekerle H, Bradl M, Linington C, et al. The shaping of the brain-specific T lymphocyte repertoire in the thymus. *Immunol Rev* 1996;149:231–243.
21. Kääb G, Brandl G, Marx A, et al. The myelin basic protein specific T cell repertoire in (transgenic) Lewis rat/SCID mouse chimeras: preferential Vβ8.2 T cell receptor usage depends on an intact Lewis thymic microenvironment. *Eur J Immunol* 1996;26:360–365.
22. Hafler DA, Benjamin DS, Burks J, Weiner HL. Myelin basic protein and proteolipid protein reactivity of brain- and cerebrospinal fluid-derived T cell clones in multiple sclerosis and postinfectious encephalomyelitis. *J Immunol* 1987;139:68–72.
23. Pette M, Fujita K, Kitze B, et al. Myelin basic protein-specific T lymphocyte lines from MS patients and from healthy individuals. *Neurology* 1990;40:1770–1776.
24. Oldstone MB, Nerenberg M, Southern P, et al. Virus infection triggers insulin-dependent diabetes mellitus in a transgenic model: role of anti-self (virus) immune response. *Cell* 1991;65:319–331.
25. Ohashi PS, Oehen S, Buerki K, et al. Ablation of "tolerance" and induction of diabetes by virus infection in viral antigen transgenic mice. *Cell* 1991;65:305–317.
26. Matzinger P. Tolerance, danger and the extended family. *Annu Rev Immunol* 1994;12:991–1045.
27. Bluestone JA. New perspectives of CD28-B7-mediated T cell costimulation. *Immunity* 1995;2:555–559.
28. Thompson CB. Distinct roles for the costimulatory ligands B7-1 and B7-2 in T helper cell differentiation? *Cell* 1995;81:979–982.
29. Wu Y, Xu J, Shinde S, et al. Rapid induction of a novel costimulatory activity on B cells by CD40 ligand. *Curr Biol* 1995;5:1303–1311.
30. Grewal IS, Xu J, Flavell RA. Impairment of antigen specific T cell priming in mice lacking CD40 ligand. *Nature* 1995;378:617–620.
31. Owens T. Co-stimulation—T cells themselves call the shots. *Curr Biol* 1996;6:32–35.
32. Kuchroo VK, Das MP, Brown JA, et al. B7-1 and B7-2 costimulatory molecules activate differentially the Th1/Th2 developmental pathways: application to autoimmune disease therapy. *Cell* 1995;80:707–718.
33. Freeman GJ, Boussiotis VA, Anumanthan A, et al. B7-1 and B7-2 do not deliver identical costimulatory signals, since B7-2 but not B7-1 preferentially costimulates the initial production of IL-4. *Immunity* 1995;2:523–532.
34. Lenschow DJ, Zeng Y, Thistlethwaite JR, et al. Long-term survival of xenogeneic pancreatic islet grafts induced by CTLA4Ig. *Science* 1992;257:789–792.
35. Finck BK, Linsley PS, Wofsy D. Treatment of murine lupus with CTLA4Ig. *Science* 1994;265:1225–1227.
36. Picarella DE, Kratz A, Li C, et al. Transgenic tumor necrosis factor (TNF)-alpha production in pancreatic islets leads to insulitis, not diabetes. Distinct patterns of inflammation in TNF-alpha and TNF-beta transgenic mice. *J Immunol* 1993;150:4136–4150.
37. Higuchi Y, Herrera P, Muniesa P, et al. Expression of a tumor necrosis factor alpha transgene in murine pancreatic beta cells results in severe and permanent insulitis without evolution towards diabetes. *J Exp Med* 1992;176:1719–1731.
38. Guerder S, Picarella DE, Linsley PS, Flavell RA. Costimulator B7-1 confers antigen-presenting-cell function to parenchymal tissue and in conjunction with tumor necrosis factor alpha leads to autoimmunity in transgenic mice. *Proc Natl Acad Sci USA* 1994;91:5138–5142.
39. Huitinga I, van Rooijen N, de Groot CJA, et al. Suppres-

sion of experimental allergic encephalomyelitis in Lewis rats after elimination of macrophages. *J Exp Med* 1990; 172:1025–1033.

40. Hutchings P, Rosen H, O'Reilly L, et al. Transfer of diabetes in mice prevented by blockade of adhesion-promoting receptor on macrophages. *Nature* 1990;348: 639–642.

41. Foy TM, Page DM, Waldschmidt TJ, et al. An essential role for gp39, the ligand for CD40, in thymic selection. *J Exp Med* 1995;182:1377–1388.

42. Lo D, Burkly LC, Widera G, et al.Diabetes and tolerance in transgenic mice expressing class II MHC molecules in pancreatic beta cells. *Cell* 1988;53:159–168.

43. Cohen JJ. Exponential growth in apoptosis. *Immunol Today* 1995;16:346–348.

44. Kawabe Y, Ochi A. Programmed cell death and extrathymic reduction of Vbeta8+ CD4+ T cells in mice tolerant to *Staphylococcus aureus* enterotoxin B. *Nature* 1991;349:245–248.

45. Kearney ER, Pape KA, Loh DY, Jenkins MK. Visualization of peptide-specific T cell immunity and peripheral tolerance induction in vivo. *Immunity* 1994;1:327–339.

46. Foy TM, Durie FH, Noelle RJ. The expansive role of CD40 and its ligand in immunity. *Semin Immunol* 1994;6:259–266.

47. Rothstein TL, Wang JK, Panka DJ, et al. Protection against Fas-dependent Th1-mediated apoptosis by antigen receptor engagement in B cells. *Nature* 1995;374: 163–165.

48. Newell MK, VanderWall J, Beard KS, Freed JH. Ligation of major histocompatibility complex class II molecules mediates apoptotic cell death in resting B lymphocytes. *Proc Natl Acad Sci USA* 1993;90:10459–10463.

49. Moudgil KD, Sercarz EE. The T cell repertoire against cryptic self determinants and its involvement in autoimmunity and cancer. *Clin Immunol Immunopathol* 1994;73:283–289.

50. Wucherpfennig KW, Strominger JL. Molecular mimicry in T cell-mediated autoimmunity: viral peptides activate human T cell clones specific for myelin basic protein. *Cell* 1995;80:695–705.

51. Inman RD, Scofield RH. Etiopathogenesis of ankylosing spondylitis and reactive arthritis. *Curr Opin Rheumatol* 1994;6:360–370.

52. Fontana A, Fierz W, Wekerle H. Astrocytes present myelin basic protein to encephalitogenic T cell lines. *Nature* 1984;307:273–276.

53. Hickey WF, Kimura H. Perivascular microglial cells of the CNS are bone marrow-derived and present antigen in vivo. *Science* 1988;239:290–292.

54. Sedgwick JD, Mosner R, Schwender S, ter Meulen V. Major histocompatibility complex-expressing nonhaematopoietic astroglial cells prime only CD8+ T lymphocytes: astroglial cells as perpetuators but not initiators of CD4+ T cell responses in the central nervous system. *J Exp Med* 1991;173:1235–1246.

55. Matsumoto Y, Ohmori K, Fujiwara M. Immune regulation by brain cells in the central nervous system: microglia but not astrocytes present myelin basic protein to encephalitogenic T cells under in vivo-mimicking conditions. *Immunology* 1992;76:209–216.

56. Williams K, Bar-Or A, Ulvestad E, et al. Biology of adult human microglia in culture: comparisons with peripheral blood monocytes and astrocytes. *J Neuropathol Exp Neurol* 1992;51:538–549.

57. Ford AL, Goodsall AL, Hickey WF, Sedgwick JD. Normal adult ramified microglia separated from other central nervous system macrophages by flow cytometric sorting. Phenotypic differences defined and direct ex vivo antigen presentation to myelin basic protein-reactive CD4+ T cells compared. *J Immunol* 1995;154: 4309–4321.

58. Becher B, et al. Soluble TNF-receptor inhibits IL-12 production by stimulated human adult microglial cells in vitro. *J Clin Invest* 1996;98:1539–1543.

59. Bottazzo GF, Pujol-Borrell R, Hanafusa T, Feldmann M. Role of aberrant HLA-DR expression and antigen presentation in induction of endocrine autoimmunity. *Lancet* 1983;2:1115–1119.

60. Gray D. Immunological memory. *Annu Rev Immunol* 1993;11:49–77.

61. Wekerle H, Linington C, Lassmann H, Meyermann R. Cellular immune reactivity within the CNS. *Trends Neurosci* 1986;9:271–277.

62. Zeine R, Owens T. Direct demonstration of the infiltration of murine CNS by Pgp-1/CD44[high] CD45RB[low] CD4+ T cells that induce experimental allergic encephalomyelitis. *J Neuroimmunol* 1992;40:57–70.

63. Owens T, Renno T, Taupin V, Krakowski M. Inflammatory cytokines in the brain: does the CNS shape immune responses? *Immunol Today* 1994;15:566–571.

64. Shimizu Y, Newman W, Tanaka Y, Shaw S. Lymphocyte interaction with endothelial cells. *Immunol Today* 1992; 13:106–112.

65. Antel JP, Owens T. The attraction of adhesion molecules. *Ann Neurol* 1993;34:123–124.

66. Yednock TA, Cannon C, Fritz LC, et al. Prevention of experimental allergic encephalomyelitis by antibodies against α4β1 integrin. *Nature* 1992;356:63–66.

67. Baron JL, Madri JA, Ruddle NH, et al. Surface expression of alpha 4 integrin by CD4 T cells is required for their entry into brain parenchyma. *J Exp Med* 1993; 177:57–68.

68. Sobel RA. The pathology of multiple sclerosis. *Neurol Clin* 1995;13:1–21.

69. Oppenheim JJ, Zachariae COC, Mukaida N, Matsushima K. Properties of the novel proinflammatory supergene "intercrine" cytokine family. *Annu Rev Immunol* 1991;9:617–648.

70. Taub DD, Conlon K, Oppenheim JJ, Kelvin DJ. Preferential migration of activated CD4+ and CD8+ T cells in response to MIP-1 alpha and MIP-1 beta. *Science* 1993; 260:355–358.

71. Tanaka Y, Adams DH, Hubscher S, et al. T-cell adhesion induced by proteoglycan-immobilized cytokine MIP-1 beta. *Nature* 1993;361:79–82.

72. Hulkower K, Brosnan CF, Aquino DA, et al. Expression of CSF-1, c-fms, and MCP-1 in the central nervous system of rats with experimental allergic encephalomyelitis. *J Immunol* 1993;150:2525–2533.

73. Ransohoff RM, Hamilton TA, Tani M, et al. Astrocyte expression of mRNA encoding cytokines IP-10 and JF/MCP-1 in experimental autoimmune encephalomyelitis. *FASEB J* 1993;7:592–600.

74. Karpus WJ, Lukacs NW, McRae BL, et al. Treatment of mice with anti-MIP-1 alpha prevents PLP peptide-induced experimental autoimmune encephalomyelitis. *FASEB J* 1994;8:A199.

75. Ransohoff RM, Tuohy VK, Hamilton TA, et al. Chemokines in CNS inflammation. Genetic models for multiple sclerosis and related disorders. Presented at a Multiple Sclerosis Society meeting, Quebec City, August 23–26, 1995.

76. Moncada S, Palmer RMJ, Higgs EA. Nitric oxide: phys-

iology, pathophysiology and pharmacology. *Pharmacol Rev* 1991;43:109–142.

77. Mosmann TR, Coffman RL. TH1 and TH2 cells: different patterns of cytokine secretion lead to different functional properties. *Annu Rev Immunol* 1989;7:145–173.

78. Vassalli P. The pathophysiology of tumour necrosis factors. *Annu Rev Immunol* 1993;10:411–520.

79. Hofman FM, Hinton DR, Johnson K, Merrill JE. Tumor necrosis factor identified in multiple sclerosis brain. *J Exp Med* 1989;170:607–612.

80. Selmaj K, Raine CS, Cannella B, Brosnan CF. Identification of lymphotoxin and tumor necrosis factor in multiple sclerosis. *J Clin Invest* 1991;87:949–954.

81. Jiang Z, Woda BA. Cytokine gene expression in the islets of the diabetic Biobreeding/Worcester rat. *J Immunol* 1991;146:2990–2994.

82. Merrill JE, Kono DH, Clayton J, et al. Inflammatory leukocytes and cytokines in the peptide-induced disease of experimental allergic encephalomyelitis in SJL and B10.PL mice. *Proc Natl Acad Sci USA* 1992;89:574–578.

83. Brennan FM, Maini RN, Feldman M. TNF alpha—a pivotal role in rheumatoid arthritis? *Br J Rheumatol* 1992;31:293–298.

84. Ruddle NH, Bergman CM, McGrath KM, et al. An antibody to lymphotoxin and tumor necrosis factor prevents transfer of experimental allergic encephalomyelitis. *J Exp Med* 1990;172:1193–1200.

85. Selmaj K, Raine CS, Cross AH. Anti-tumor necrosis factor therapy abrogates autoimmune demyelination. *Ann Neurol* 1991;30:694–700.

86. Campbell IL, Oxbrow L, Harrison LC. Reduction in insulitis following administration of IFN-gamma and TNF-alpha in the NOD mouse. *J Autoimmun* 1991;4:249–262.

87. Renno T, Krakowski M, Piccirillo C, et al. TNFα production by resident microglial cells and infiltrating leukocytes in experimental allergic encephalomyelitis: regulation by Th1 cytokines. *J Immunol* 1995;154:944–953.

88. Selmaj KW, Raine CS. Tumour necrosis factor mediates myelin and oligodendrocyte damage in vitro. *Ann Neurol* 1988;23:339–346.

89. Panitch HS, Bever CT. Clinical trials of interferons in multiple sclerosis: what have we learned? *J Neuroimmunol* 1993;46:155–164.

90. Panitch HS, Hirsch RL, Schindler J, Johnson KP. Treatment of multiple sclerosis with gamma interferon: exacerbations associated with activation of the immune system. *Neurology* 1987;37:1097–1102.

91. Olsson T, Wang W-Z, Höjeberg B, et al. Autoreactive T lymphocytes in multiple sclerosis determined by antigen-induced secretion of interferon-γ. *J Clin Invest* 1990;86:981–985.

92. Renno T, Zeine R, Girard JM, et al. Selective enrichment of Th1 CD45RB^low CD4+ T cells in autoimmune infiltrates in experimental allergic encephalomyelitis. *Int Immunol* 1994;6:347–354.

93. Romagnani S. Lymphokine production by human T cells in disease states. *Annu Rev Immunol* 1994;12:227–257.

94. Hofman FM, von Hanwehr RI, Dinarello CA, et al. Immunoregulatory molecules and IL 2 receptors identified in multiple sclerosis brain. *J Immunol* 1986;136:3239–3245.

95. Owens T, Sriram S. The immunology of MS and of its animal model, EAE. *Neurol Clin* 1995;13:51–73.

96. Sarvetnick N, Shizuru J, Liggitt D, et al. Loss of pancreatic islet tolerance induced by beta-cell expression of interferon-gamma. *Nature* 1990;346:844–847.

97. Geiger K, Howes E, Gallina M, et al. Transgenic mice expressing IFN-gamma in the retina develop inflammation of the eye and photoreceptor loss. *Invest Ophthalmol Vis Sci* 1994;35:2667–2681.

98. Gu D, Wogensen L, Calcutt NA, et al. Myasthenia gravis-like syndrome induced by expression of interferon gamma in the neuromuscular junction. *J Exp Med* 1995;181:547–557.

99. Campbell IL, Abraham CR, Masliah E, et al. Neurologic disease induced in transgenic mice by cerebral overexpression of interleukin 6. *Proc Natl Acad Sci USA* 1993;90:10061–10065.

100. Probert L, Akassoglou K, Pasparakis M, et al. Spontaneous inflammatory demyelinating disease in transgenic mice showing central nervous system-specific expression of tumor necrosis factor alpha. *Proc Natl Acad Sci USA* 1995;92:11294–11298.

101. Taupin V, et al. Increased severity of EAE, chronic macrophage microglial reactivity and demyelination in transgenic mice producing tumor necrosis factor-alpha in central nervous system. *Eur J Immunol* 1997;27.

102. Lira SA, Zalamea P, Heinrich JN, et al. Expression of the chemokine N51/KC in the thymus and epidermis of transgenic mice results in marked infiltration of a single class of inflammatory cells. *J Exp Med* 1994;180:2039–2048.

103. Arnason BG. Interferon beta in multiple sclerosis. *Neurology* 1993;43:641–643.

104. The IFNβ Multiple Sclerosis Study Group. Interferon beta-1b is effective in relapsing-remitting multiple sclerosis. I. Clinical results of a multicenter, randomized, double-blind, placebo-controlled trial. *Neurology* 1993;43:655–661.

105. Paty DB, Li DKB, UBC Study Group, IFNB Multiple Sclerosis Study Group. Interferon-1β is effective in relapsing-remitting multiple sclerosis: II. MRI analysis results of a multicenter, randomized, double-blind, placebo-controlled trial. *Neurology* 1993;43:662–667.

106. Rapoport MJ, Jaramillo A, Zipris D, et al. Interleukin 4 reverses T cell proliferative unresponsiveness and prevents the onset of diabetes in nonobese diabetic mice. *J Exp Med* 1993;178:87–99.

107. Kennedy MK, Torrance DS, Picha KS, Mohler KM. Analysis of cytokine mRNA expression in the central nervous system of mice with experimental allergic encephalomyelitis reveals that IL-10 mRNA expression correlates with recovery. *J Immunol* 1992;149:2496–2505.

108. Khoury SJ, Hancock WW, Weiner HL. Oral tolerance to myelin basic protein and natural recovery from experimental autoimmune encephalomyelitis are associated with downregulation of inflammatory cytokines and differential upregulation of transforming growth factor β, interleukin 4, and prostaglandin E expression in the brain. *J Exp Med* 1992;176:1355–1364.

109. Katz JD, Benoist C, Mathis D. T helper cell subsets in insulin-dependent diabetes. *Science* 1995;268:1185–1188.

110. Wogensen L, Huang X, Sarvetnick N. Leukocyte extravasation into the pancreatic tissue in transgenic mice expressing interleukin 10 in the islets of Langerhans. *J Exp Med* 1993;178:175–185.

111. Bitar DM, Whitacre CC. Suppression of experimental autoimmune encephalomyelitis by the oral administration of myelin basic protein. *Cell Immunol* 1988;112:364–370.

112. Lider O, Santos LMB, Lee CSY, et al. Suppression of experimental autoimmune encephalomyelitis by oral administration of myelin basic protein. II. Suppression of disease and in vitro immune responses is mediated by

antigen-specific CD8+ T lymphocytes. *J Immunol* 1989; 142:748–752.

113. Miller A, Lider O, Roberts AB, et al. Suppressor T cells generated by oral tolerization to myelin basic protein suppress both in vitro and in vivo immune responses by the release of TGF-β following antigenic specific triggering. *Proc Natl Acad Sci USA* 1992;89:421–425.

114. Trentham DE, Dynesius-Trentham RA, Orav EJ, et al. Effects of oral administration of type II collagen on rheumatoid arthritis. *Science* 1993;261:1727–1730.

115. Weiner HL, Mackin GA, Matsui M, et al. Double-blind pilot trial of oral tolerization with myelin antigens in multiple sclerosis. *Science* 1993;259:1321–1324.

116. Paul WE, Seder RA. Lymphocyte responses and cytokines. *Cell* 1994;76:241–251.

117. Scott P. IL-12: initiation cytokine for cell-mediated immunity. *Science* 1993;260:496–497.

118. Leonard JP, Waldburger KE, Goldman SJ. Prevention of experimental autoimmune encephalomyelitis by antibodies against interleukin 12. *J Exp Med* 1995;181: 381–386.

119. Flesch IE, Hess JH, Huang S, et al. Early interleukin 12 production by macrophages in response to mycobacterial infection depends on interferon gamma and tumor necrosis factor alpha. *J Exp Med* 1995;181:1615–1621.

120. Berke G. Unlocking the secrets of CTL and NK cells. *Immunol Today* 1995;16:343–346.

121. Leibson PJ. MHC-recognizing receptors: they're not just for T cells anymore. *Immunity* 1995;3:5–8.

122. Thiele DL, Lipsky PE. The role of cell surface recognition structures in the initiation of MHC-unrestricted "promiscuous" killing by T cells. *Immunol Today* 1989; 10:375–381.

123. D'Souza S, Alinauskas K, McCrea E, et al. Differential susceptibility of human CNS-derived cell populations to TNF-dependent and independent immune-mediated injury. *J Neurosci* 1995;15:7293–7300.

124. Haas W, Pereira P, Tonegawa S. Gamma delta T cells. *Annu Rev Immunol* 1993;11: 637–685.

125. Freedman MS, Ruijs TCG, Selin LK, Antel JP. Peripheral blood γ/δ T cells lyse fresh human brain-derived oligodendrocytes. *Ann Neurol* 1991;30:794–800.

126. Selmaj K, Brosnan CF, Raine CS. Expression of heat shock protein-65 by oligodendrocytes in vivo and in vitro: implications for multiple sclerosis. *Neurology* 1992; 42:795–800.

127. Selmaj K, Brosnan CF, Raine CS. Colocalization of lymphocytes bearing γ/δ T-cell receptor and heat shock protein HSP65+ oligodendrocytes in multiple sclerosis. *Proc Natl Acad Sci USA* 1991;88:5452–5456.

128. Moulin D, Paty DW, Ebers G. The predictive value of cerebrospinal fluid electrophoresis in possible multiple sclerosis. *Brain* 1983;106:809–816.

129. Whitacre CC, Mattson DH, Paterson PY, et al. Cerebrospinal fluid and serum oligoclonal IgG bands in rabbits with experimental allergic encephalomyelitis. *Neurochem Res* 1981;6:87–96.

130. Cserr HF, Knopf PM. Cervical lymphatics, the blood-brain barrier and the immunoreactivity of the brain: a new view. *Immunol Today* 1992;13:507–512.

131. Schluesener HJ, Sobel RA, Linington C, Weiner H. A monoclonal antibody against a myelin oligodendrocyte glycoprotein induces relapses and demyelination in central nervous system autoimmune disease. *J Immunol* 1987;139:4016–4021.

132. Looney RJ. Structure and function of human and mouse Fc gamma RII. *Blood Cells* 1993;19:353–359.

133. Gaur A, Wiers B, Liu A, et al. Amelioration of autoimmune encephalomyelitis by myelin basic protein synthetic peptide-induced anergy. *Science* 1992;258: 1491–1494.

134. Vandenbark AA, Bourdette DN, Whitham R, et al. T-cell receptor peptide therapy in EAE and MS. *Clin Exp Rheumatol* 1993;11(suppl 8):51–53.

135. Zhang J, Medaer R, Stinissen P, et al. MHC-restricted depletion of human myelin basic protein-reactive T cells by T cell vaccination. *Science* 1993;261:1451–1454.

136. Utz U, Biddison WE, McFarland HF, et al. Skewed T-cell receptor repertoire in genetically identical twins correlates with multiple sclerosis. *Nature* 1993;364:243–247.

137. Johns LD, Flanders KC, Ranges GE, Sriram S. Successful treatment of experimental allergic encephalomyelitis with transforming growth factor-β1. *J Immunol* 1991; 147:1792–1796.

138. Racke MK, Bonomo A, Scott DE, et al. Cytokine-induced immune deviation as a therapy for inflammatory autoimmune disease. *J Exp Med* 1994;180:1961–1966.

139. Kuruvilla AP, Shah R, Hockwald GM, et al. Protective effect of transforming growth factor β1 in experimental autoimmune diseases in mice. *Proc Natl Acad Sci USA* 1991;88:2918–2922.

Chapter 3

Central Nervous System–Immune Interactions: Contribution to Neurologic Disease and Recovery

Jack Antel and Burkhard Becher

Although in the past the central nervous system (CNS) has been regarded as a site of immunologic privilege, it is also the site of the most intensively studied experimental autoimmune-mediated disorder, experimental allergic encephalomyelitis (EAE). This chapter describes the properties of the CNS that contribute to the variable susceptibility or resistance of this compartment to immune-mediated injury. Such variability is considered in terms of the following properties of the CNS:

1. Those that effect entry of immune mediators into the CNS
2. The capacity of endogenous CNS cells, particularly the astroglia and microglia, to regulate reactivity of immune mediators within the CNS
3. The differing susceptibility of specific neural cell populations, particularly neurons and oligodendroglia, to each of the multiple mediators of immune injury

A recurrent theme is to define the molecular basis whereby cells of the immune system and those of the nervous system interact and modulate the functional properties of one another. Such interactions, resultant from direct cell-cell interactions or mediated by soluble factors, comprise a neuroimmune network within the CNS. This network of interactions can also contribute to recovery following disease or injury within the CNS. A neuroimmune network also exists outside the CNS, with neural signals mediated via neuroendocrine or autonomic nervous system pathways (see Chapter 5).

Immune Mediator Entry into the CNS

Cell-Mediated Immunity

Since the cell mediators of immune responses occurring in the CNS are recruited from the systemic lymphoid organs, one needs to consider how these cells reach the CNS parenchyma and what attracts them to it. Transit from the circulation into the CNS occurs at the microvascular level and requires passage through a blood-brain barrier, which is composed of endothelial cells, smooth muscle cells, perivascular microglia, and astroglia foot processes. In the autoimmune CNS diseases multiple sclerosis (MS) and EAE, disruption of the blood-brain barrier is an early event in the process of lesion formation (1,2).

The molecular events underlying leukocyte migration from the systemic circulation into the CNS continue to be clarified (3,4). A current general concept regarding lymphocyte trafficking indicates that intravascular cells moving slowly (rolling) through the microvasculature initially become loosely bound to the endothelium via the selectin family of adhesion molecules (5). Firmer adhesion then occurs via the integrin family of molecules (6). Transendothelial passage then follows, dependent on additional adhesion molecules. Individual members of the adhesion molecule families favor passage of different leukocyte cell populations (T cells, monocytes, neutrophils) (reviewed elsewhere (3) and summarized in Fig 3-1).

The precise role of adhesion molecules in regulating the development of an immune response within the CNS remains under active study (7–9). Normal-appearing white matter does not constitutively express these adhesion molecules. Such molecules are upregulated on blood vessels, as well as on microglia and macrophages, in MS lesions (10). However, expression levels do not appear to correlate closely with the duration or activity of the lesion; most prominent expression is found in chronic active lesions. There is also upregulation of these molecules in noninflammatory neurologic diseases, raising the issue of what the inducing stimulus is. Analysis of microvessels isolated from lesion sites in the CNS of patients dying of MS further documents expression of vascular cell adhesion molecule (VCAM)-1, E-selectin, and intercellular adhesion molecule (ICAM)-1 (11). These microvessels show evidence of activation, based on upregulation of the urokinase plasminogen activator receptor (11). In the EAE model, antibodies reactive with very late activation (VLA)-4 selectin prevent disease development (12); anti–ICAM-1–directed antibodies have produced less consistent results (13–16).

Expression of both ligand and receptor molecules involved in cell adhesion is induced by cytokines that can

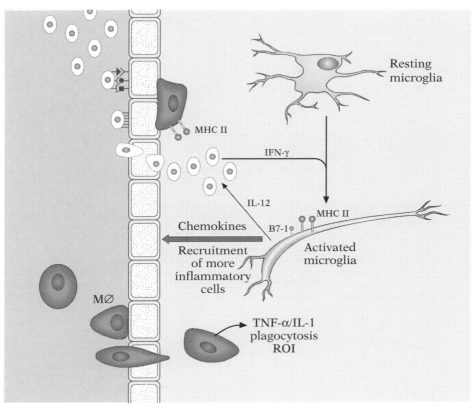

Figure 3-1. Immune-mediator entry into the CNS. Chemokine signals, adhesion molecules, and perivascular cell expression of MHC molecules play roles in the migration of neural antigen-specific and nonspecific T cells and monocytes across the blood-brain barrier. MØ = monocyte; ROI = reactive oxygen intermediate.

be released from either circulating leukocytes or endogenous CNS cells (17,18). Levels of cytokines released by leukocytes are increased in concert with cell activation, consistent with the observations that activated T cells more readily transit from the circulation into tissues (19–21). Levels of an array of adhesion molecules are increased in the serum of MS patients (22,23); highest levels of VCAM-1 and L-selectin are found in patients with lesions showing gadolinium enhancement on magnetic resonance images (MRIs) (6). Increased levels of soluble adhesion molecules in the cerebrospinal fluid (CSF) of patients with inflammatory diseases of the CNS suggest that these molecules are also upregulated within the CNS (22,24–26). Lymphoid cells derived from the CSF of MS patients bind more avidly to endothelium in vitro than do blood-derived cells (27), consistent with findings that lymphoid cells within the CNS are in a relatively more activated state than are such cells in the systemic circulation (28–30). However, this enhanced binding is not selective for CNS endothelium (27). Under inflammatory conditions, cerebral endothelial cells assume the morphology of high endothelial venules, with deposition of proteins

such as fibronectin, which further enhance leukocyte-endothelial interactions (31).

Although the process of T cell–microvessel adhesion apparently does not depend on major histocompatibility complex (MHC) antigen interactions (19,20), MHC class II expression is important in the process of antigen presentation and may be involved in the selection of specific T cells that will persist in the CNS (see below). CNS microvessels express MHC class II molecules in situ under pathologic conditions associated with inflammation and in vitro in response to interferon (IFN)-γ (11,31). Initially, expression was ascribed to the endothelial cells (32). Many in situ studies now identify the perivascular microglial cell as the major cell type expressing these molecules (33,34). Direct analysis of microvessels isolated from MS lesions shows MHC class II molecule upregulation (11). Although only a small proportion (2%) of the T cells in EAE lesions are antigen specific, these cells are considered to arrive early in the immune response (35). The antigen-specific T cells, concentrated in the perivascular region rather than the parenchyma, would be a source of cytokines acting on the cells comprising the blood-brain barrier, and thus contribute to enhanced recruitment of a large number of non-antigen-specific cells that need not even be in an activated state (36).

Other molecules derived from the CNS or the immune cells can also contribute to disruption of the blood-brain barrier during the course of CNS inflammatory disease. The metalloproteases are produced by endogenous CNS cells, including capillary endothelial cells, astroglia and microglia, and leukocytes (37,38). Blocking their activity can inhibit the EAE disease process (39). Such molecules could also disrupt the extracellular matrix to permit T-cell migration to selective lesion sites. Levels of an array of proteases are increased in the CSF of persons with inflammatory disorders (40–42). Vasoactive molecules, such as histamine, can modulate the permeability of the blood-brain barrier; strain-related differences in sensitivity to this agent correlate with susceptibility to murine EAE (43).

Signals from within the CNS actively attract the components of the systemic hematopoietic system to the CNS. Specific molecules, termed *chemokines*, are now delineated and have been shown to serve as concentration gradient–dependent chemoattractants for leukocytes (43–47). Individual chemoattractants can select for lymphocytes and monocytes, as well as for polymorphonuclear cells. These molecules are upregulated during inflammatory disorders; blocking their activity can abrogate EAE (48).

Humoral Immunity

Antibody-mediated immunity within the CNS can involve either antibodies reaching the CNS from the systemic circulation or intrathecal production by B-cell lineage cells that have entered this compartment as part of an inflammatory response. The normal blood-brain barrier excludes most circulating immunoglobulin (Ig) (reviewed elsewhere (49)), so that the concentration of IgG in normal CSF (5–10 mg/dL) is only a fraction of that contained in serum. The potential mechanisms whereby antibody can contribute to CNS injury is described in a later section.

Regulation of Immune Reactivity Within the CNS

From an immunologic viewpoint, the microenvironment of the CNS is primarily shaped by microglial and astroglial cells. The environment encountered by leukocytes entering into the CNS determines whether the cells will or will not persist within this compartment. Results of studies in which the myelin antigen– and non-CNS antigen–sensitized T-cell lines are passively transferred into the systemic circulation indicate that a proportion of both cell populations access the CNS. The myelin-reactive cells, which presumably encounter their antigen, persist, whereas the cells that do not encounter their antigen remain only transiently (19,20,50). As discussed later, the functional consequences of T-cell interaction with antigen (i.e., whether

the T cells will undergo further stimulation or whether they will become anergic or undergo apoptosis) depends on the capacity of the antigen-presenting cell (APC) to deliver critical costimulatory signals. Most of the T cells found in inflammatory lesions are not reactive to CNS antigens. To be considered is whether putative APCs, whether located in perivascular or parenchymal regions of the CNS, can present antigen with sufficient competence to result in generating a novel cellular immune response.

Within the perivascular regions, the perivascular "microglia" are demonstrated to be fully functional APCs (51). Within the CNS parenchyma, the resident microglia and astroglia are implicated as the cells with immune regulatory potential. Rio Hortega (52) first identified parenchymal microglia as a distinct cell type, and most current opinion holds them to be of bone marrow origin (53,54). The parenchymal microglia, in contrast to the perivascular "microglia," do not undergo rapid turnover and are not replaced by systemic monocytes (51). Immunocytochemical studies indicate that microglia express many of the same surface molecules characteristic of monocytes and tissue macrophages (55). Qualitative differences do exist, as, for example, the low expression of CD45 observed on both rodent and human parenchymal microglia compared to monocytes and perivascular microglia (56,57).

The state of activation of the microglia cells is a crucial variable determining their immune regulatory and effector functions. Such activation states were initially defined by comparing morphologic features observed in situ under normal and pathologic conditions (58). Resting microglia are referred to as *ramified cells*. Under conditions of CNS injury, the cells assume a rounded or bipolar ameboid profile. To some extent, these properties can be reproduced in vitro (59–61). Although *microglia proliferation* is a frequently used term in the description of pathologic responses in the adult human CNS, in contrast to rodent and fetal human microglia, little evidence for human adult microglia proliferation in situ or in vitro is available (62). As discussed later, microglial activation is now increasingly being defined on the basis of the surface molecules expressed or the soluble molecules produced.

Astroglia are derived from neuroectoderm and share a developmental lineage with oligodendroglia. These cells are recognized by their expression of the intermediate filament protein, glial fibrillary acidic protein (GFAP). The extent of GFAP expression and detectability by immunocytochemical assay can be used as an index of astroglial reactivity (63) (see Chapter 17). Reactive astroglia are a hallmark of most CNS inflammatory, traumatic, and ischemic lesions. Reactive astroglia also surround sites of abnormal neurons in neuronal degenerative diseases (see Chapter 11). Astroglia within the adult human CNS can undergo cell cycling, although to a much lower extent than that seen in fetal human tissue and in newborn rodents (64).

The potential of the parenchymal microglia and astroglia to regulate immune reactivity within the CNS can be viewed in terms of their function as APCs and

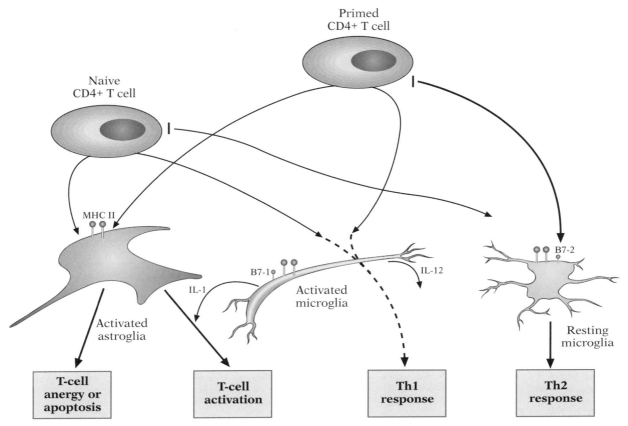

Figure 3-2.   Glial cell regulation of immune reactivity within the CNS. Microglia and astrocytes interact with T cells, leading to activation, anergy, or apoptosis of the T cells.

production of soluble molecules (cytokines), which can act in an autocrine or paracrine fashion to amplify or suppress immune response–related functions of cells (Fig 3-2).

Antigen-Presenting Capacity of Glial Cells

CD4+ T cells recognize antigens in the context of an MHC class II molecule expressed by an APC. The two CNS resident cells that are suspected of having antigen-presenting capacity are the microglia and the astroglia.

Microglia

The role of parenchymal microglial cell as APCs has been examined by in situ and in vitro studies aimed at detecting surface molecules required for the process of antigen presentation to lead to T-cell activation and in vitro studies designed to show functional responses. Although the results of most studies of rodent CNS tissue indicate that microglia, under resting conditions, do not express MHC class II molecules, Sedgwick et al (65), analyzing immediately ex vivo cells, demonstrated that

strain differences exist. They found expression on microglia isolated from the spinal cord of the EAE-resistant Brown Norway rat, but not on cells isolated from Lewis rats. Based on in vitro functional studies using immediately ex vivo microglia to present myelin basic protein (MBP) to CD4 T cells sensitized to this antigen, they concluded that such microglia are not fully competent APCs (66). On the contrary, Krakowski and Owens (67), using similar in vitro paradigms applied to SJL mice, did consider such microglia as competent APCs. Microglia that have been maintained in culture upregulate MHC class II expression and are functionally competent APCs (68). As regards human microglia, Peudenier et al (69) did not detect MHC class II molecules on microglia isolated from fetal human material. Several groups including our own (70–72) detected MHC class II expression in apparently normal tissues in the human adult CNS. We also detected expression in immediately ex vivo cells isolated from tissue without detectable pathology (57). Whether these findings in the normal human adult CNS reflect intrinsic species- or age-related differences, or reflect recurrent exposure of the CNS of most humans over time to potentially activating factors such as viruses, remains speculative. At sites of injury, inflammation, or degenerating neurons in the adult human CNS, MHC class II expression on microglia is readily detected and exceeds that reported for normal tissue (73). Expression is also upregulated on human adult microglia during tissue culture and, even more so, on exposure to IFN-γ (57). Under both immediately ex vivo and sustained tissue culture conditions, we found, using a mixed leukocyte response assay, that these adult human CNS-derived microglia can function as competent APCs (57).

Expression of MHC class II molecules alone is insufficient for competent antigen presentation. Other surface molecules that serve as crucial costimulatory molecules are now identified (74). CD80 (B7/B7-1) and CD86 (B70/B7-2) expression has been demonstrated on rodent and human microglia in situ and in vitro (75,76). The in situ expression is most readily detected in microglia and macrophages participating in the inflammatory lesions of EAE and MS, respectively. In vitro studies indicate that blocking interaction of these molecules with their CD28 ligands on T cells will impair the APC capacity of the microglia (75). The relative expression of B7-1 versus B7-2 on microglia and macrophages may influence the cytokine profile (Th1 versus Th2) of the T cells to which they present antigen (77,78).

Astroglia

Astroglia were implicated initially as cells with potential antigen-presenting capability, based on the detection of MHC class II molecules on the surface of newborn murine–derived astroglia in vitro, particularly after activation of these with IFN-γ (79,80). Susceptibility to CNS autoimmunity (EAE) of different mouse strains was correlated with the extent to which these MHC molecules could be induced with IFN-γ on astroglia in vitro (81). However, these observations have not been consistently confirmed (82). Results of in vitro studies of human CNS-derived astroglia indicate that an increased proportion of such cells, compared to rodent astroglia, express MHC class II molecules under the same basal culture conditions (83). These observations indicate that species and age variables need to be considered in studies of regulation of expression of MHC and other immune accessory molecules.

Functional studies of astroglia as APCs have been limited by the technical capacity to obtain purified populations of these cells. Concern remains that any degree of microglia contamination could account for "positive" results. Newborn mouse–derived astroglia, induced to express MHC class II molecules, do not support proliferation of naive CD4 T cells but could support the continued proliferation of previously activated antigen (MBP)-specific T cells (84). Using human fetal astroglia, we found that these cells also did not support a proliferative response by allogenic CD4 T cells freshly isolated from the peripheral blood, but did support a secondary mixed lymphocyte reaction (MLR) (85). Addition either of microglia (in numbers that themselves were insufficient to support an MLR) or of exogenous interleukin (IL)-1 permits the astroglia to support a primary MLR. The astroglia did not express the crucial CD80 and CD86 costimulatory molecules (75). In the CD28 knockout mouse, IL-1 can replace the stimulatory signal provided by CD80 acting on its CD28 receptor (86).

The above-cited data suggest that within the CNS, cells comprising the blood-brain barrier, and specifically the perivascular microglia, can serve as competent APCs. Within the parenchyma of the CNS, the microglia, rather than the astroglia, are the cells with the most competent antigen-presenting capability. The incomplete antigen-presenting capacity of the astroglia, apparently even under conditions of activation, may result in dampening any immune response (87). Whether there is a state in which microglia lose antigen-presenting capacity remains to be established. In this regard, CD4 T cells encountering noncompetent MHC class II–expressing APCs may either become anergic or undergo apoptosis. Apoptotic T cells are a feature found in the CNS of the acute EAE model (88,89). Matsumoto et al (90) proposed the concept that microglia favor turning on the immune response, whereas astroglia favor turning it off. Note, however, that astroglia and microglia coexist within the CNS and their interactions could modulate their respective APC functions. Thus, the dynamic nature of the glial cell microenvironment is an important variable that determines the state of immune reactivity within the CNS.

Cytokines and Glial Cell Immune Regulation

Microglia

Results of in vitro studies of purified microglia cultures indicate that these cells can be a source of an array of cytokines that may either amplify (proinflammatory) or inhibit immune responses. The cytokines can act in a paracrine manner to regulate the functional responses of T cells or, potentially, in an autocrine manner to regulate the function of the microglial cell itself (reviewed elsewhere (3)). Among the proinflammatory cytokines produced by microglia are IL-1, which, as mentioned previously, serves as a T-cell costimulatory factor and exacerbates EAE (91), and IL-6, which induces Ig production by activated B cells and stimulates T-cell proliferation.

IL-12 produced by activated microglia (92) is an important molecule that promotes expression of Th1 cytokines (IFN-γ, IL-2) by CD4 T cells (93). A Th1 response is characteristic of the cellular immune response encountered in the CNS during the acute inflammatory phase of EAE (94,95). Only Th1 cytokine–producing cells are recovered from the CNS of animals injected systemically with myelin-reactive CD4 T cells producing Th1 and Th2 cytokines (95). The precise molecular signals from within the CNS that determine selective T-cell entry or that modulate their cytokine profiles, an occurrence referred to as *cytokine switching*, remain to be identified (96). Anti–IL-12 antibody can inhibit the development of EAE (97).

IL-10 and transforming growth factor (TGF)-β are examples of inhibitory cytokines produced by microglia, as well as by Th2 CD4 T cells. IL-10 downregulates MHC class II expression on microglia and inhibits their antigen-presenting capacity (98,99). TGF-β is a potent suppressor of T-cell responses and is implicated in the process of bystander suppression underlying oral tolerance (see Chapter 1). Both IL-10 and TGF-β are expressed in the CNS of animals recovering from EAE (100). Systemic administration of either IL-10 or TGF-β blocks the development of EAE (101,102).

Analysis of cytokines in human CSF has been limited by the lack of sensitivity of available assays to detect such proteins and by the paucity of cells that can be recovered for messenger RNA (mRNA) analysis. The rather constant finding in MS of intrathecal IgG production would implicate a contribution by Th2 cytokines. Both Th1 (IFN-β) and Th2 (IL-4 and TGF-β) cytokine mRNAs are found in CSF cells derived from patients with noninflammatory disorders, as well as from those with MS and other inflammatory disorders, using in situ hybridization (103). In the MS group, Th2 cytokines are most prominent in those with early or nondisabling disease. Our data from patients with noninflammatory disorders, using semiquantitative polymerase chain reaction (PCR) analysis of total cell RNA, show a predominance of Th1 cells, as defined by expression of IFN-γ and absence of IL-4 mRNA (104).

Astroglia

The extent to which astroglia can produce regulatory cytokines is not resolved. Malignant astroglia are a demonstrated source of an array of these molecules, including IL-1, IL-6, and TGF-β (see Chapter 15). IL-6 and TGF-β have been detected in cultures of astroglia derived from the immature rodent and from human CNS following activation with IL-1β, IFN-γ, or lipopolysaccharide (LPS) (105–107). In a recent analysis using in situ hybridization, we compared expression of IL-6 mRNA by human adult astroglia with that detected in adult microglia and fetal astroglia maintained under the same culture conditions (108). We detected IL-6 transcripts only in a minority of the adult astroglia, even after stimulation with LPS and IFN-γ. Under these conditions, the large majority of microglia and fetal astroglia were positive for these transcripts. These results emphasize the differences between astroglia as a function of maturity. The data further implicate microglia, rather than astroglia, as being the prime endogenous cell source of regulatory cytokines in the adult human CNS.

The cytokine molecules involved in regulating immune reactivity within the CNS also have important functional effects on other properties of the endogenous neural cell populations. IL-1 and IL-6 can induce astrogliosis, at least in the immature rodent CNS (109), and enhance production of β amyloid (110,111). TGF-β suppresses astroglia proliferation while promoting new-vessel formation (see Chapter 17). Cytokines may also regulate the production of neuroprotective molecules, such as ciliary neurotrophic factor (CNTF), by glial cells (see later section). Conversely, both neurons and oligodendroglia also are capable of producing cytokine molecules, using them to signal to the glial cells in their microenvironment (112,113) (see Chapter 17).

Although this discussion has focused on immune regulation within the CNS, increasing evidence indicates that CNS-derived antigens can reach the systemic compartment, and thus interact with the systemic immune system. Although the CNS is regarded as lacking a lymphatic system, repeated studies show that intracerebral injection of antigen does result in systemic immune sensitization (114). Such antigens can be recovered from deep cervical lymph nodes, confirming that transport of antigen out of the CNS does occur. Thus, recurrent or progressive immune reactivity directed at a CNS antigen could reflect systemic rather than intra-CNS events.

Susceptibility of Neural Cells to Immune-Mediated Injury

Variables that need to be considered in this regard are:

- What potential mechanisms of immune-mediated injury are likely to be operative within the CNS under conditions of disease or injury?
- Are specific neural populations susceptible or resistant to particular immune effector mechanisms?
- What is the nature of the injury response by neural cells subjected to immune-mediated injury?

Potential effector mechanisms could derive both from immune constituents gaining entry into the CNS from the systemic compartment and from endogenous CNS components. Specific target cell populations to be considered are the neurons and the oligodendroglia. Differential susceptibility of particular cell targets to a common effector mechanism could just as readily account for the apparent selective involvement of a particular cell type in a given disease state, as could the presence of an immune effector that is restricted by its capacity to recognize a unique target. Injury response can be classified either as primary cell membrane directed (lysis) or as dependent on intracellular signaling events leading to nuclear or DNA fragmentation (apoptosis) (115–117). All these variables (Fig 3-3) contribute to the design of therapeutic strategies aimed at protecting cells from injury.

Humoral Immune-Mediated Injury

Antibodies specific for neurons and oligodendroglia have been implicated as primary mediators of tissue injury or as factors that amplify such injury. The classic means whereby antibodies induce cell injury is via cell membrane injury that occurs subsequent to the anti-

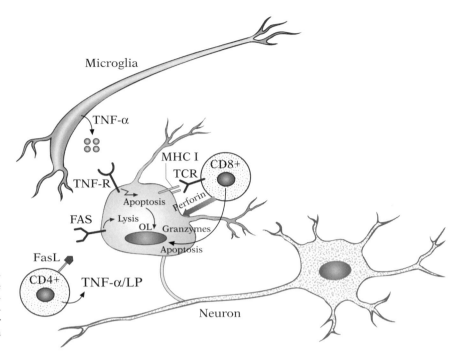

Figure 3-3. Mechanisms of immune-mediated neural cell injury within the CNS. The multiple cell contact– and soluble factor–dependent immune effector mechanisms can induce selective or nonselective target cell injury within the CNS. OL = oligodendrocyte.

body binding to a cell surface determinant, followed by fixation and activation of complement (118). Microglial cells and macrophages provide an endogenous CNS source for many complement components (119).

Antibody-independent complement-mediated injury of oligodendroglia is well demonstrated in rodents but not in humans, a finding explained by the presence of the complement inhibitory protein CD59 on human oligodendroglia (120). Results of studies of complement-mediated injury in rodent oligodendroglia indicate that such injury need not be irreversible and that sublethal injury could occur (121). Such sublethal injury could phenotypically appear as a breakdown of the cells' myelin processes, even though the primary target is cell body directed. Such a process would be analogous to distal axon disruption secondary to disease of the neuronal cell soma (122).

A novel complement-independent mechanism whereby antibody can contribute to disease pathogenesis involves antibody binding to functional receptors on the target cells. Examples of this mechanism include the excitotoxicity that occurs consequent to glutamate receptor binding by antibody in Rasmussen's encephalitis and γ-aminobutyric acid (GABA) receptor binding in stiff-man syndrome (123). In a number of disease states, high-titer antibody responses are directed against intracellular rather than cell surface constituents. An example is the anti–Purkinje cell antibody found in the serum of patients with ovarian cancer who develop cerebellar degeneration (see Chapter 10). The Purkinje neurons do not have extra-CNS projections. Such findings raise the issue of how target recognition

occurs and whether and how these antibodies induce tissue injury.

Cell-Mediated Immune Injury

Potential mediators to be considered are T cells or macrophages derived from the systemic compartment or endogenous CNS cells, microglia, and astroglia. Mechanisms used to effect injury would include those involving cell-cell contact and those mediated via soluble factors.

Cell Contact–Dependent Mechanisms

α/β T Cells

Antigen-specific α/β T-cell effector cytotoxic responses classically require T cells to recognize their target antigen in association with MHC molecules, either class I for CD8 T cells or class II for CD4 T cells. Whether neurons or oligodendroglia can express MHC molecules, and under what conditions, remain under study. Recent findings suggest that neurons in situ can express MHC class I molecules and do so when their electrical activity is interrupted (124). Such expression is also described for neuronal cell in vitro (125–127). MHC class I–restricted cytotoxicity remains to be shown for neurons. MHC class I expression and MHC class I–restricted cytotoxicity have been demonstrated for human adult CNS-derived oligodendroglia in vitro (128). MHC class I–restricted CD8 T cells specific for human T-cell lymphotropic virus type I (HTLV-I) antigens are a hallmark of HTLV-I myelopathy, but specific cytotoxicity of a neural target has not yet been shown (see Chapter 13). These findings raise the question of whether lack of MHC class I expression reflects active inhibitory mechanisms within the CNS and whether these can be perturbed by disease or injury.

For neither neurons nor oligodendroglia are there consistent reports of MHC class II expression (129). Such findings are particularly relevant to the immune-mediated demyelinating diseases EAE and MS, in which myelin-reactive MHC class II–restricted CD4 α/β T cells are implicated as the initiators of the disease process. The absence of the MHC recognition molecule raises the issue as to whether the CD4 T cells can induce injury via MHC nonrestricted mechanisms or whether additional effector mediators contained within the inflammatory response are the mediators of actual tissue injury. Currently, no evidence exists to indicate that only one mechanism may be operative.

The α/β T-cell cytotoxic responses involving non-MHC-restricted mechanisms are described (129). Antigen- or mitogen-activated CD4 or CD8 α/β T cells maintained in culture in the presence of IL-2 acquire the capacity to function as "promiscuous" killers (130). This function, measured in long-term cytotoxicity assays, is not mediated by soluble factors. Although the results of most studies of CD4 T-cell cytotoxicity using non-CNS-derived proliferating cells as targets suggest that such injury is mediated via an apoptotic mechanism, our data, showing cell membrane injury preceding any nuclear injury of nonproliferating oligodendroglia as targets, suggest that these principles may not apply to at least some terminally differentiated neural cells (131,132). The ligand required for such non-MHC-restricted effector-target interaction is not yet identified, but adhesion molecules are prime candidates.

The mechanisms whereby cytotoxic cells deliver their lethal signal are increasingly being defined (133); one cautions, however, that these are mainly defined using nonneural cells as targets. CD8 T cells are considered to function via the calcium-dependent release of perforin and granzyme molecules (134–136). The former punch initial holes in cell membranes; the latter initiate intracellular events leading to apoptosis. CD4 T cells seem to favor a calcium-independent cytotoxicity mechanism mediated by binding of a surface molecule termed *ligand* to the Fas molecule on the target, with subsequent initiation of apoptosis (137). Nonproliferating cells may, however, undergo lysis without apoptosis (138). Fas expression was initially considered not to occur in the normal CNS. Expression is now reported in pathologic conditions such as ischemia and Alzheimer's disease and in vitro on cultured human adult CNS-derived oligodendroglia (139,140). Fas and tumor necrosis factor (TNF) receptors belong to the same receptor superfamily and have significant homology (141).

γ/δ T Cells
These cells are a distinct T-cell lineage with potent cytotoxic capability. They are not restricted by MHC molecules for target recognition. Neural cells, particularly

glial cells, are susceptible targets (142). Candidate recognition molecules for these cells include the heat shock family of proteins (143–146). Some of these molecules are constitutively expressed, whereas others are induced. Among glial cells, induction seems to occur most readily in oligodendroglia (147,148). IL-1 is a potent inducer of heat shock proteins in oligodendroglia (149).

Natural Killer (CD56+) Cells
Natural killer (NK) cells, defined on the basis of expression of CD56 and lack of CD3, are potent killers of target cells that fail to express MHC class I molecules (150). NK cells are identified in some pathologic lesions in the CNS, such as in tumor infiltrates (see Chapter 15). Oligodendroglia are reported to be NK cell resistant (151); few data exist regarding neurons.

Soluble Factor-Dependent Mechanisms

Cytokines

TNF-α and -β, molecules that share a 70% homology, are the cytokines most implicated as potential immune effectors (152). Both soluble and cell-bound forms exist and are used to effect target cell injury (153). TNF-α is produced by T cells, but even more so by macrophages. Studies of fetal human microglia in culture indicate expression of TNF-α transcripts in these cells; results regarding secretion of TNF-α protein have been inconsistent (154). Adult human microglia in vitro are demonstrated to secrete TNF-α (155). Astroglia also are implicated as sources of TNF-α (156–158), although our in situ hybridization data of human adult glial cells indicate greater mRNA expression in microglia than astroglia (108). TNF-β production is largely restricted to T cells. TNF-α and -β utilize the same receptors and both are implicated to induce apoptosis in their cell targets (152,153). In the CNS, oligodendroglia appear particularly susceptible to TNF-α–mediated injury, whereas neurons are relatively resistant (131,159). This observation provides an example whereby a single molecule could produce selective injury to a particular cell type.

Noncytokine Soluble Molecules

In situ techniques such as microdialysis, performed under conditions of experimental disease or injury, and in vitro studies of neural cell–directed injury indicate that multiple noncytokine soluble mediators found in the CNS under conditions of inflammation or glial cell activation have the potential to effect tissue injury. Giulian et al (160) implicated a low-molecular-weight factor, whose activity can be blocked by N-methyl-D-aspartate (NMDA) antagonists, as being the microglia-derived factor that is toxic to neurons but not to oligodendroglia. Nitric oxide has been implicated as a microglia-derived injury mediator of oligodendroglia and neurons (161,162). Eitan and Schwarz (163) found that in the goldfish, IL-2 can be converted by a transglutaminase expressed in the transected optic nerve into a dimeric form that is toxic to oligodendroglia. Other potential mediators include the proteases and free radicals released by microglia (164).

Combined Humoral and Cellular Effector Mechanisms

Microglia/macrophages are cells with classic phagocytic capacity, usually directed at small particles such as bacteria and cell debris rather than whole cells. Such activity is increased when the cells are activated and, even more so, when specific cell surface receptors are involved in their interactions with the target. Microglia and macrophages express receptors for the Fc portion of the Ig molecule (165). Binding through this receptor to opsonized antigen markedly enhances phagocytosis. As we showed using opsonized MBP, the enhanced phagocytosis is associated with a marked increase in proinflammatory cytokine secretion by microglia (166). Antibody recognizing a specific neural target through the Fab portion of the IgG molecule and binding via its Fc portion to microglia or macrophages could call into action an antibody-dependent cell cytotoxicity (ADCC) response (167). Although microglia do not phagocytose normal cell targets, a specific phagocytic mechanism is now demonstrated for cells undergoing apoptosis (168). Microglia-target cell binding can also be promoted by complement components (169).

Contribution of Immune Mediators to CNS Recovery

Although the above discussion focuses on immune-mediated injury within the CNS, one need also consider the role of the immune system and its mediators on positive physiologic functions. The cytokine molecules produced in high amounts during pathologic conditions may, under physiologic conditions, be produced in low amounts and play roles in modeling the CNS as, for example, during development. Cytokine signaling on hypothalamic neurons, a region not protected from the systemic compartment by the blood-brain barrier, may be a means to regulate autonomic nervous system responses to systemic events such as infection.

A number of paradigms indicate a role for glia in either protecting the CNS from injury or promoting recovery. Astroglia are shown to protect oligodendroglia from free radical–mediated injury, as might be effected via microglia or macrophages (170). A series of related molecules (CNTF, leukocyte inhibitory factor (LIF), and IL-6) are shown to protect oligodendroglia from TNF-α–mediated injury (171–173). Astroglia are a source of CNTF, microglia can produce LIF, and both cell types can produce IL-6. CNTF does not, however, protect the oligodendroglia from promiscuous CD4 T cell–mediated injury (173). Supernatants of cultures of microglia and macrophage contain molecules that promote neurite extension (174,175). The array of surface molecules that these cells express also needs to be considered. A current hypothesis implicates inhibitory molecules expressed by oligodendroglia as retarding axonal re-

growth following injury. Selective toxicity of oligodendroglia, such as mediated by TNF-α or dimeric IL-2, could provide a means to remove this negative regulator of regeneration.

Conclusions

The dynamic molecular events underlying the interactions between immune mediators and the endogenous cells of the CNS are increasingly being identified as central to the observations that the CNS can be either susceptible or resistant to immune-mediated responses. Manipulation of the events involved in the recruitment and persistence of immune mediators to the CNS has already been carried out to interrupt autoimmune disease. With further insights into the properties of the endogenous glial cells that determine their participation as regulators or effectors of the immune response within the CNS, opportunities will arise either to amplify or to suppress immune reactivity within the CNS for therapeutic purposes. Strategies for protecting cells from injury will require further understanding of the nature of the injury response and how the CNS might be manipulated to provide essential neuroprotective molecules. The findings that endogenous CNS cells differ in their susceptibility to specific immune mediators provide a potential explanation as to how nonspecific immune mediators may induce rather selective target injury within the CNS.

References

1. Kermode A, Tompson A, Tofts P, et al. Breakdown of the blood-brain barrier precedes symptoms and other MRI signs of new lesions in multiple sclerosis. *Brain* 1990;113:1477–1489.
2. Stone LA, Smith ME, Albert PS, et al. Blood-brain barrier disruption on contrast-enhanced MRI in patients with mild relapsing-remitting multiple sclerosis. *Neurology* 1995;45:1122–1126.
3. Fabry A, Raine CS, Hart MN. Nervous tissue as an immune compartment: the dialect of immune responses in the CNS. *Immunol Today* 1994;15:218–224.
4. Cross AH. Immune cell traffic control and the central nervous system. *Semin Neurosci* 1992;4:213–219.
5. Springer T. Traffic signals for lymphocyte recirculation and leukocyte emigration: the multistep paradigm. *Cell* 1994;76:301–314.
6. Baron JL, Madri JA, Ruddle NH, et al. Surface expression of alpha 4 integrin by CD4 T cells is required for their entry into brain parenchyma. *J Exp Med* 1993;177:57–68.
7. McFarland HF. The multiple sclerosis lesion. *Ann Neurol* 1995;37:419–420.
8. Dopp JM, Breneman SM, Olschowka JA. Expression of ICAM-1, VCAM-1 L-selectin and leukosialin in the mouse central nervous system during the induction and remission stages of experimental allergic encephalomyelitis. *J Neuroimmunol* 1994;54:129–144.
9. Rieckmann P, Michel U, Albrecht M, et al. Soluble forms of intercellular adhesion molecule-1 (ICAM-1) block lymphocyte attachment to cerebral endothelial cells. *J Neuroimmunol* 1995;60:9–15.
10. Cannella B, Raine CS. The adhesion molecule and cy-

tokine profile of multiple sclerosis lesions. *Ann Neurol* 1995;37:424–435.

11. Washington R, Burton J, Todd RF, et al. Expression of immunologically relevant endothelial cell activation antigens on isolated central nervous system microvessels from patients with multiple sclerosis. *Ann Neurol* 1994;35:89–97.

12. Yednock T, Cannon C, Fritz LC, et al. Prevention of experimental autoimmune encephalomyelitis by antibodies against α4β1 integrin. *Nature* 1993;356:63–66.

13. Archelos JJ, Jung S, Maurer M, et al. Inhibition of experimental autoimmune encephalomyelitis by an antibody to the intercellular adhesion molecule ICAM-1. *Ann Neurol* 1993;34:145–154.

14. Welsh CT, Rose JW, Hill JE, Townsend JJ. Augumentation of adoptively-transferred experimental allergic encephalomyelitis by administration of a monoclonal antibody specific for LFA-1α. *J Neuroimmunol* 1993;43:161–168.

15. Willenbord DO, Simmons RD, Tamati T, Miyasaka M. ICAM-1 dependent pathway is not critically involved in the inflammatory process of autoimmune encephalomyelitis or in cytokine-induced inflammation of the central nervous system. *J Neuroimmunol* 1993;45:147–154.

16. Cannella B, Cross A, Raine C. Upregulation and expression of adhesion molecules correlate with relapsing autoimmune demyelination in the central nervous system. *J Exp Med* 1994;172:1521–1524.

17. Pober JS. Cytokine-mediated activation of vascular endothelium: physiology and pathology. *Am J Pathol* 1988;133:426–436.

18. Wong D, Dorovni-Zis K. Upregulation of intercellular adhesion molecule-1 (ICAM-1) expression in primary cultures of human brain microvessel endothelial cells by cytokines and lipopolysaccharide. *J Neuroimmunol* 1992;39:11–22.

19. Hickey WF, Hsu BL, Kimura H. T-lymphocyte entry into the central nervous system. *J Neurosci Res* 1991;20:254–260.

20. Hickey WF. Migration of hematogenous cells through the blood-brain barrier and the initiation of CNS inflammation. *Brain Pathol* 1991;1:97–105.

21. Sloan DJ, Wood MJ, Charlton HM. Leucocyte recruitment and inflammation in the CNS (news). *Trends Neurosci* 1992;15:276–278.

22. Dore-Duffy P, Newman W, Balabanov R, et al. Circulating, soluble adhesion proteins in cerebrospinal fluid and serum of patients with multiple sclerosis: correlation with clinical activity. *Ann Neurol* 1995;37:55–62.

23. Hartung HP, Reiners K, Archelos JJ, et al. Circulating adhesion molecules and tumor necrosis factor receptor in multiple sclerosis: correlation with magnetic resonance imaging. *Ann Neurol* 1995;38:186–193.

24. Svenningsson A, Hansson G, Andersson R, et al. Adhesion molecule expression on cerebrospinal fluid T lymphocytes: evidence for common recruitment mechanisms in multiple sclerosis, aseptic meningitis and normal controls. *Ann Neurol* 1993;34:155–161.

25. Jander S, Heidenreich F, Stoll G. Serum and CSF levels of soluble intercellular adhesion molecule-1 (ICAM-1) in inflammatory neurologic disease. *Neurology* 1993;43:1809–1813.

26. Riechmann P, Nunke K, Burchardt M, et al. Soluble intercellular adhesion molecule-1 in cerebrospinal fluid: an indicator for the inflammatory impairment of the blood-cerebrospinal fluid barrier. *J Neuroimmunol* 1993;47:133–140.

27. Elfont RM, Griffin DE, Goldstein GW. Enhanced endothelial cell adhesion of human cerebrospinal fluid lymphocytes. *Ann Neurol* 1995;38:405–413.

28. Hafler DA, Fox DA, Manning ME, et al. In vivo activated T lymphocytes in the peripheral blood and cerebrospinal fluid of patients with multiple sclerosis. *N Engl J Med* 1985;312:1405–1411.

29. Spencer J, Hall JG. Studies on the lymphocytes of sheep. IV. Migration patterns of lung-associated lymphocytes efferent from the caudal mediastinal lymph node. *Immunology* 1984;51:1–5.

30. Hedlund G, Sandberg WM, Sjogren HO. Increased proportion of CD4+CDw29+CD45R-UCHL-1+ lymphocytes in the cerebrospinal fluid of both MS patients and healthy individuals. *Cell Immunol* 1989;118:406–412.

31. Sobel RA. The pathology of multiple sclerosis. In: Antel JP, ed. *Neurologic clinics: multiple sclerosis.* Vol. 13. Philadelphia: WB Saunders, 1995:1–22.

32. McCarron RM, Wang L, Cowan EP, Spatz M. Class II MHC antigen expression by cultured human cerebral vascular endothelial cells. *Brain Res* 1991;556:325.

33. Lassmann H, Rossler K, Zimprich F, Vass K. Expression of adhesion molecules and histocompatibility antigens at the blood-brain barrier. *Brain Pathol* 1990;1:115–123.

34. Bö L, Mörk S, Kong PA, et al. Dectection of MHC class II macrophages and microglia, but not on astrocytes and endothelia in active MS lesions. *J Neuroimmunol* 1994;51:135–146.

35. Cross AH, O'Mara T, Raine CS. Chronologic localization of myelin-reactive cells in the lesions of relapsing EAE. *Neurology* 1993;43:1028–1033.

36. Oksranta O, Tarvone S, Ilonen J, et al. Influx of non-activated T lymphocytes into the cerebrospinal fluid during relapse of multiple sclerosis. *Ann Neurol* 1995;38:465–468.

37. Apodaca G, Rutka JT, Bouhana K, et al. Expression of metalloproteinases and metalloproteinase inhibitors by fetal astrocytes and glioma cells. *Cancer Res* 1990;50:2322–2329.

38. Herron GS, Werb Z, Dwyer K, Banda MJ. Secretion of metalloproteinases by stimulated capillary endothelial cells. I. Production of procollagenase and prostromyelysin exceeds expression of proteolytic activity. *J Biol Chem* 1986;261:2810–2813.

39. Gijbels K, Masure S, Carton H, Opdenakker G. Gelatinase in the cerebrospinal fluid of patients with multiple sclerosis and other inflammatory neurological disorders. *J Neuroimmunol* 1992;44:29–34.

40. Cuzner ML, Davison AN, Rudge P. Proteolytic enzyme activity of blood leukocytes and cerebrospinal fluid in multiple sclerosis. *Ann Neurol* 1978;4:337–344.

41. Gijbels K, Galardy RE, Steinman L. Reversal of experimental autoimmune encephalomyelitis with a hydroxamate inhibitor of matrix metalloproteases. *J Clin Invest* 1994;94:2177–2182.

42. Roznieckie JJ, Hauser SL, Stein M, et al. Elevated mast cell tryptase in cerebrospinal fluid of multiple sclerosis patients. *Ann Neurol* 1995;37:63–66.

43. Linthicum DS, Frelinger JA. Acute autoimmune encephalomyelitis in mice. Susceptibility is controlled by the combination of H-2 and histamine sensitization genes. *J Exp Med* 1982;156:31–40.

44. Rollins BJ, Yoshimura T, Leonard EJ, Pober JS. Cytokine-activated human endothelial cells synthesize and secrete a monocyte chemoattractant, MCP-1/JE. *Am J Pathol* 1990;136:1229–1233.

45. Rovin BH, Yoshimura T, Tan L. Cytokine-induced production of monocyte chemoattractant protein-1 by cul-

tured human mesangial cells. *J Immunol* 1992;148:2148–2153.

46. Hayashi M, Luo Y, Laning J, et al. Production and function of monocyte chemoattractant protein-1 and other β-chemokines in murine glial cells. *J Neuroimmunol* 1995;60:143–150.

47. Ransohoff RM, Hamilton TA, Tani M, et al. Astrocyte expression of mRNA encoding cytokines IP-10 and JE/MCP-1 in experimental autoimmune encephalomyelitis. *FASEB J* 1993;7:592–600.

48. Karpus WJ, Lukas NW, McRae BL, et al. Treatment of mice with anti-MIP-1α prevents PLP peptide-induced experimental autoimmune encephalomyelitis. *FASEB J* 1994;8:A199.

49. Tourtellotte WW, Walsh MJ. Cerebrospinal fluid profile in multiple sclerosis. In: Posner CM, et al. eds. *Diagnosis of MS*. Stuttgart: Georg Thieme, 1994:165–178.

50. Skundric DS, Kim C, Tse HY, Raine CS. Homing of T cells to the central nervous system throughout the course of relapsing experimental autoimmune encephalomyelitis in Thy-1 congenic mice. *J Neuroimmunol* 1993;46:113–121.

51. Hickey WF, Kimura H. Perivascular microglial cells of the CNS are bone marrow-derived and present antigen in vivo. *Science* 1988;239:290–292.

52. Rio Hortega P. Microglia. In: Penfield W, ed. *Cytology and cellular pathology of the nervous system*. New York: Paul P. Hocker, 1932:481–584.

53. Ling EA, Wong WC. The origin and nature of ramified and amoeboid microglia: a historical review and current concepts. *Glia* 1993;7:9–18.

54. Theele DP, Streit WJ. A chronicle of microglial ontogeny. *Glia* 1993;7:5–8.

55. Ulvestad E, Williams K, Mork S, et al. Phenotypic differences between human monocytes/macrophages and microglial cells studied in situ and in vitro. *J Neuropathol Exp Neurol* 1994;53:492–501.

56. Sedgwick JD, Schwender S, Imrich H, et al. Isolation and direct characterization of resident microglial cells from the normal and inflamed central nervous system. *Proc Natl Acad Sci USA* 1991;88:7438–7442.

57. Becher B, Antel JP. Comparison of phenotypic and functional properties of immediately *ex vivo* and cultured human adult microglia. *Glia* 1996;18:1–10.

58. Rio Hortega P, Penfield W. Cerebral cicatrix: the reaction of neuroglia and microglia to brain wounds. *John Hopkins Hosp Bull* 1927;41:278–303.

59. Guilian D. Ameboeid microglia as effectors of inflammation in the central nervous system. *J Neurosci Res* 1987;18:155–171.

60. Davis EJ, Foster TD, Thomas WE. Cellular forms and functions of brain microglia. *Brain Res Bull* 1994;34:73–78.

61. Suzumura A, Marunouchi T, Yamamoto H. Morphological transformation of microglia in vitro. *Brain Res* 1991;545:301–306.

62. Whittemore SR, Sanon HR, Wood PM. Concurrent isolation and characterization of oligodendrocytes, microglia and astrocytes from adult human spinal cord. *J Dev Neurosci* 1993;11:755–764.

63. Norton WT, Aquino DA, Hozumi I, et al. Quantitative aspects of reactive gliosis: a review. *Neurochem Res* 1992;17:877–885.

64. Yong VW, Tejada-Berges T, Goodyer CG, et al. Differential proliferative response of human and mouse astrocytes to γ-interferon. *Glia* 1992;6:269–290.

65. Sedgwick JD, Schwender S, Gregersen R, et al. Resident macrophages (ramified microglia) of the adult Brown Norway rat central nervous system are constitutively major histocompatibility complex class II positive. *J Exp Med* 1993;177:1145–1152.

66. Ford AL, Goodsall AL, Hickey F, Sedgwick JD. Normal adult ramified microglia separated from other central nervous system macrophages by flow cytometric sorting. Phenotypic differences defined and direct ex vivo antigen presentation to myelin basic protein-reactive CD4⁺ T cells compared. *J Immunol* 1995;154:4309–4321.

67. Krakowski M, Owens T. The CNS environment controls CD4⁺ T cell cytokine profile in EAE (abstract). *J Cell Biochem* 1995;21A:445.

68. Frei K, Siepl C, Groscurth P, et al. Antigen presentation and tumor cytotoxicity by interferon-gamma-treated microglial cells. *Eur J Immunol* 1987;17:1271–1278.

69. Peudenier S, Hery C, Montagnier L, Tardieu M. Human microglial cells: characterization in cerebral tissue and in primary cultures and study of their susceptibility to HIV-1 infection. *Ann Neurol* 1991;29:152–181.

70. Sasaki A, Nakazato Y. The identity of cells expressing MHC class II antigens in normal and pathological human brain. *Neuropathol Appl Neurobiol* 1992;18:13–36.

71. Graeber MB, Streit WJ, Bueringer D, et al. Ultrastructural location of major histocompatibility complex (MHC) class II positive perivascular cells in histologically normal human brain. *J Neuropathol Exp Neurol* 1992;51:303–311.

72. Ulvestad E, Williams K, Bo L, et al. HLA class II molecules (HLA-DR,-DP,-DQ) on cells in the human CNS studies in situ and in vitro. *Immunology* 1994;82:533–541.

73. McGeer PL, Kawamata T, Walter DG, et al. Microglia in degenerative neurological disease. *Glia* 1993;7:84–92.

74. Lanier LL, O'Fallon S, Somoza C, et al. CD80 (B7) and CD86 (B70) provide similar costimulatory signals for T cell proliferation, cytokine production, and generation of CTL. *J Immunol* 1995;154:97–105.

75. Williams K, Ulvestad E, Antel JP. B7/BB-1 antigen expression on adult human microglia studies in vitro and in situ. *Eur J Immunol* 1994;24:3031–3037.

76. Windhagen A, Newcombe J, Dangond F, et al. Expression of co-stimulatory molecules B7-1 (CD80), B7-2 (CD86), and interleukin 12 cytokine in multiple sclerosis lesions. *J Exp Med* 1995;182:1985–1996.

77. Kuchroo VK, Das MP, Brown JA, et al. B7-1 and B7-2 costimulatory molecules activate differentially the Th1/Th2 developmental pathways: application to autoimmune disease therapy. *Cell* 1995;60:707–718.

78. Mosmann TR, Coffman RL. TH1 and TH2 cells: different patterns of cytokine secretion lead to different functional properties. *Annu Rev Immunol* 1989;7:145–173.

79. Fontana A, Fierz F, Wekerle H. Astrocytes present myelin basic protein to encephalitogenic T-cell lines. *Nature* 1994;307:273–276.

80. Fierz W, Endler B, Reske K, et al. Astrocytes as antigen-presenting cells. I. Induction of Ia antigen expression on astrocytes by T cells via immune interferon and its effect on antigen presentation. *J Immunol* 1985;134:3785–3793.

81. Massa PT, ter Meulen V, Fontana A. Hyperinductability of Ia antigens on astrocytes correlates with strain-specific susceptibility to experimental autoimmune encephalomyelitis. *Proc Natl Acad Sci USA* 1987;84:4219–4223.

82. Birnbaum G, Kitilinek L. Immunologic differences in

murine glial cells and their association with susceptibility to experimental allergic encephalomyelitis. *J Neuroimmunol* 1990;26:119–129.

83. Yong VW, Yong FP, Ruijis TCG, et al. Expression and modulation of HLA-DR on cultured human adult astrocytes. *J Neuropathol Exp Neurol* 1991;50:16–28.

84. Sedgwick JD, Mossner R, Schwender S, ter Meulen V. Major histocompatibility complex-expressing nonhematopoietic astroglial cells prime only CD8$^+$ T lymphocytes: astroglial cells as perpetuators but not initiators of CD8$^+$ cell responses in the central nervous system. *J Exp Med* 1991;173:1235–1246.

85. Williams K, Dooley N, Ulvestad E, et al. Antigen presentation by astrocytes: correction of the inability of astrocytes to initiate immune responses by the addition of microglia or the microglia-derived cytokine IL-1. *J Neurosci* 1995;15:1869–1875.

86. Kawai K, Shainian A, Mak TW, Ohashi PS. Skin allograft rejection in CD28-deficient mice. *Transplantation* 1996;61:352–355.

87. Weber F, Meinl E, Aloisi F, et al. Human astrocytes are only partially competent antigen presenting cells. Possible implications for lesion development in multiple sclerosis. *Brain* 1994;117:59–69.

88. Pender MP, McCombe PA, Yoong G, Nguyen KB. Apoptosis of alpha beta T lymphocytes in the nervous system in experimental autoimmune encephalomyelitis: its possible implications for recovery and acquired tolerance. J *Autoimmun* 1992;5:401–410.

89. Ohmori K, Hong Y, Fujiwara M, Matsumoto Y. In situ demonstration of proliferating cells in the rat central nervous system during experimental autoimmune encephalomyelitis. Evidence suggesting that most infiltrating T cells do not proliferate in the target organ. *Lab Invest* 1992;66:54–62.

90. Matsumoto Y, Ohmori K, Fujiwara M. Immune regulatory brain cells in the central nervous system: microglia but not astrocytes present myelin basic protein to encephalitogenic T cells under in vivo mimicking conditions. *Immunology* 1992;76:209–216.

91. Jacobs CA, Baker PE, Roux ER, et al. Experimental autoimmune encephalomyelitis is exacerbated by IL-1 alpha and suppressed by soluble IL-1 receptor. *J Immunol* 1991;146:2983–2989.

92. Becher B, Lafortune L, Antel JP. Resting and activated human microglia ex vivo: relation with cytokine production. *J Neuroimmunol* 1995;61(suppl 1):11.

93. Scott P. IL-12: initiation cytokine for cell-mediated immunity (comment). *Science* 1993;260:496–497. Review.

94. Renno T, Zeine R, Girard JM, et al. Selective enrichment of Th1 CD45RB^{low} CD4$^+$ T cells in autoimmune infiltrates in experimental allergic encephalomyelitis. *Int Immunol* 1994;6:347–354.

95. Nicholson LB, Greer JM, Sobel RA, et al. An altered peptide ligand mediates deviation and prevents autoimmune encephalomyelitis. *Immunity* 1995;3:397–405.

96. Owens T, Renno T, Taupin V, Krakowski M. Inflammatory cytokines in the brain: does the CNS shape immune responses? *Immunol Today* 1995;15:566–571.

97. Leonard JP, Waldburger KE, Goldman SJ. Prevention of experimental autoimmune encephalomyelitis by antibodies against interleukin 12. *J Exp Med* 1995;181:381–386.

98. Frei K, Lin SH, Schwerdel C, Fontana A. Antigen presentation in the central nervous system. The inhibitory effect of IL-10 on MHC class II expression and production of cytokines depends on the inducing signals and type of cell analyzed. *J Immunol* 1994;152:2720–2708.

99. Williams K, Dooley N, Ulvestad E, et al. IL-10 production by adult human derived microglial cells. *Neurochem Int* 1996;29:55–64.

100. Kennedy MK, Torrance DS, Picha KS, Mohler KM. Analysis of cytokine mRNA expression in the central nervous system of mice with experimental autoimmune encephalomyelitis reveals that IL-10 mRNA expression correlates with recovery. *J Immunol* 1992;149:2496–2505.

101. Rott O, Fleishcer B, Cash E. Interleukin-10 prevents experimental allergic encephalomyelitis in rats. *Eur J Immunol* 1994;24:1434–1440.

102. Racke MK, Dhib-Jalbut S, Cannella B, et al. Prevention and treatment of chronic relapsing experimental allergic encephalomyelitis by transforming growth factor-β1. *J Immunol* 1991;146:3012–3017.

103. Link J, Soderstrom M, Olsson T, et al. Increased transforming growth factor-beta, interleukin-4, and interferon-gamma in multiple sclerosis. *Ann Neurol* 1994;36:379–386.

104. Blain M, Nalbantoglu J, Antel JP. Interferon-γ mRNA expression in immediately ex-vivo CSR T cells. *J Neuroimmunol* 1994;54:149.

105. Norris JG, Tang L-P, Sparacio SM, Benveniste EN. Signal transduction pathways mediating astrocyte IL-6 induction by IL-1β and tumor necrosis factor-α. *J Immunol* 1994;152:841–850.

106. Lee SC, Liu W, Dickson DW, et al. Cytokine production by human fetal microglia and astrocytes. Differential induction by lipopolysaccharide and IL-1β. *J Immunol* 1993;150:2659–2667.

107. Aloisi F, Caré A, Borsellino G, et al. Production of hemolymphopoietic cytokines (IL-6, IL-8, colony-stimulating factors) by normal human astrocytes in response to IL-1β and tumor necrosis factor-α. *J Immunol* 1992;149:2358–2366.

108. Lafortune L, Nalbantoglu J, Antel JP. Expression of tumor necrosis factor α (TNFα) and interleukin 6 (IL-6) mRNA in adult human astrocytes: comparison with adult microglia and fetal astrocytes. *J Neuropathol Exp Neurol* 1996;55:515–521.

109. Chiang CS, Stalder A, Samimi A, Campbell IL. Reactive gliosis as a consequence of interleukin-6 expression in the brain: studies in transgenic mice. *Dev Neurosci* 1994;16:212–221.

110. Leveugle B, Ding W, Buee L, Fillit HM. Interleukin-1 and nerve growth factor induce hypersecretion and hypersulfation of neuroblastoma proteoglycans which bind beta-amyloid. *J Neuroimmunol* 1995;60:151–160.

111. Dickson DW, Lee SC, Mattiace LA, et al. Microglia and cytokines in neurological disease, with special reference to AIDS and Alzheimer's disease. *Glia* 1993;7:75–83.

112. Yamabe T, Dhir G, Cowan EP, et al. Cytokine-gene expression in measles-infected adult human glial cells. *J Neuroimmunol* 1994;49:171–179.

113. Olsson T, Kristensson K, Ljugdahl A, et al. Gamma-interferon-like immunoreactivity in axotomized rat motor neurons. *J Neurosci* 1989;9:3870–3875.

114. Cserr HF, Knopf PM. Cervical lymphatics, the blood-brain barrier and the immunoreactivity of the brain: a new view. *Immunol Today* 1992;13:507–512.

115. Cohen JJ. Apoptosis. *Immunol Today* 1993;14:126–130.

116. Ju S-T, Ruddle NH, Strack P, et al. Expression of two distinct cytolytic mechanisms among murine CD4 subsets. *J Immunol* 1990;144:23–31.

117. Schwartz LM, Smith SW, Jones MEE, Osborne BA. Do

all programmed cell deaths occur via apoptosis? *Proc Natl Acad Sci USA* 1993;90:980–984.

118. Zajicek JP, Wing M, Scolding NJ, Compston DAS. Interactions between oligodendrocytes and microglia. A major role for complement and tumor necrosis factor in oligodendrocyte adherence and killing. *Brain* 1992;115:1611–1631.

119. Gasque P, Fontaine M, Morgan BP. Complement expression in human brain: biosynthesis of terminal pathway components and regulators in human glial cells and cell lines. *J Immunol* 1995;154:4726–4733.

120. Wing MG, Zajicek J, Seilly DJ, et al. Oligodendrocytes lack glycolipid anchored proteins which protect them against complement lysis. Restoration of resistance to lysis by incorporation of CD59. *Immunology* 1992;76:140–145.

121. Scolding NJ, Morgan BP, Houston WAJ, et al. Vesicular removal by oligodendrocytes of membrane attack complexes formed by activated complement. *Nature* 1989;339:620–622.

122. Rodriguez M, Scheihauer BW, Forbes G, Kelly PJ. Oligodendrocyte injury is an early event in lesions of multiple sclerosis. *Mayo Clin Proc* 1993;68:627–636.

123. Antel JP, Rasmussen T. Rasmussen's encephalitis and the new hat. *Neurology* 1996;46:9–11. Editorial.

124. Neumann N, Cavalle A, Jenne DE, Wekerle H. Induction of MHC class I genes in neurons. *Science* 1995;269:549–552.

125. Drew PD, Lonergan M, Goldstein ME, et al. Regulation of MHC class I and beta 2-microglobulin gene expression in human neuronal cells. Factor binding to conserved cis-acting regulatory sequences correlates with expression of the genes. *J Immunol* 1993;50:3300–3310.

126. Lehky TJ, Cowan EP, Lampson LA, Jacobson S. Induction of HLA class I and class II expression in human T-lymphotropic virus type I-infected neuroblastoma cells. *J Virol* 1994;68:1854–1863.

127. Lee SC, Raine CS. Multiple sclerosis: oligodendrocytes in active lesions do not express class II major histocompatibility complex molecules. *J Neuroimmunol* 1989;25:261–266.

128. Ruijs TCG, Freedman MS, Grenier YG, et al. Human oligodendrocytes are susceptible to cytolysis by major histocompatibility complex class I-restricted lymphocytes. *J Neuroimmunol* 1990;27:89–97.

129. Patel SS, Thiele DL, Lipsky PE. Major histocompatibility complex-unrestricted cytolytic activity of human T cells. Analysis of precursor frequency and effector phenotype. *J Immunol* 1987;139:3886–3895.

130. Nishioka WK, Welsh RM. Susceptibility to cytotoxic T lymphocyte-induced apoptosis is a function of the proliferative status of the target. *J Exp Med* 1994;179:769–774.

131. D'Souza S, Alinauskas K, McCrea E, et al. Differential susceptibility of human CNS-derived cell populations to TNF-dependent and independent immune-mediated injury. *J Neurosci* 1995;15:7293–7300.

132. Carter LL, Dutton RW. Relative perforin- and Fas-mediated lysis in T1 and T2 CD8 effector populations. *J Immunol* 1995;155:1713–1724.

133. Berke G. The binding and lysis of target cells by cytotoxic lymphocytes: molecular and cellular aspects. *Annu Rev Immunol* 1994;12:735–773.

134. Duke RC. Apoptosis in cytotoxic T lymphocytes and their targets. *Semin Immunol* 1992;4:497–512.

135. Taylor MK, Cohen JJ. Cell-mediated cytotoxicity. *Curr Opin Immunol* 1992;4:338–343.

136. Stalder T, Hahn S, Erb P. Fas antigen is the major target molecule for CD4+ T cell-mediated cytotoxicity. *J Immunol* 1994;152:1127–1133.

137. Matsuyama T, Hata R, Tagaya M, et al. Fas antigen mRNA induction in postischemic murine brain. *Brain Res* 1994;657:342–346.

138. D'Souza S, Balasingam V, Cashman N, et al. Susceptibility of human oligodendrocytes to fas-mediated injury. *Neurology* 1996;46(suppl):A466.

139. Nishimura T, Akiyama H, Yonehara S, et al. Fas antigen expression in brains of patients with Alzheimer-type dementia. *Brain Res* 1995;695:137–145.

140. Aggarwal BB, Singh S, LaPushin R, Totpal K. Fas antigen signals proliferation of normal human diploid fibroblasts and its mechanism is different from tumor necrosis factor receptor. *FEBS Lett* 1995;364:5–8.

141. Smith CA, Farrah T, Goodwin RG. The TNF receptor superfamily of cellular and viral proteins: activation, costimulation, and death. *Cell* 1994;78:959–962.

142. Freedman MS, Ruijs TCG, Selin LK, Antel JP. Peripheral blood γδ-T cells lyse fresh human brain-derived oligodendrocytes. *Ann Neurol* 1991;30:794–800.

143. Haregewoin A, Soman G, Hom RC, Finberg RW. Human γδ+ T cells respond to mycobacterial heat shock protein. *Nature* 1989;340:309–312.

144. Selmaj K, Brosnan CF, Raine CS. Colocalization of lymphocytes bearing γδ-T cell receptor and heat shock protein hsp65+ oligodendrocytes in multiple sclerosis. *Proc Natl Acad Sci USA* 1991;88:6452–6456.

145. Wucherpfennig KW, Newcombe J, Li H, et al. γδ-T cell receptor repertoire in acute multiple sclerosis lesions. *Proc Natl Acad Sci USA* 1992;89:4588–4592.

146. Freedman MS, Ruijs TCG, Antel JP. The role of heat shock proteins in oligodendrocyte γδ-T cell interaction. *J Neuroimmunol* 1991;33(suppl 1):112.

147. Freedman MS, Buu NN, Ruijs TCG, et al. Differential expression of heat shock proteins by human glial cells. *J Neuroimmunol* 1992;41:231–237.

148. Satoh J, Yamamura T, Kunishita T, Tabira T. Heterogeneous induction of 72-kDa heat shock protein (HSP72) in cultured mouse oligodendrocytes and astrocytes. *Brain Res* 1992;573:37–43.

149. D'Souza S, Antel JP, Freedman MS. Cytokine induction of heat shock protein expression in human oligodendrocytes: an IL-1-mediated mechanism. *J Neuroimmunol* 1994;50:17–24.

150. Versteeg R. NK cells and T cells: mirror images? *Immunol Today* 1992;13:244–247.

151. Satoh J, Kim SU, Kastrukoff LF. Absence of natural killer (NK) cell activity against oligodendrocytes in multiple sclerosis. *J Neuroimmunol* 1990;26:75–80.

152. Heller RA, Kronke M. TNF receptor-mediated signaling pathways. *J Cell Biol* 1994;126:5–9.

153. Wilt SG, Milward E, Zhou JM, et al. In vitro evidence for a dual role of tumor necrosis factor-α in human immunodeficiency virus type I encephalopathy. *Ann Neurol* 1995;37:381–394.

154. Sébire G, Emilie D, Wallon C, et al. In vitro production of IL-6, IL-8, and tumor necrosis factor-α by human embryonic microglial and neural cells. *J Immunol* 1993;150:1517–1523.

155. Williams L, Ulvestad E, Waage A, et al. Activation of adult human derived microglia by myelin phagocytosis in vitro. *J Neurosci Res* 1994;38:433–443.

156. Lieberman AP, Pitha PM, Shin HS, Shin ML. Production of tumor necrosis factor and other cytokines by astrocytes stimulated with lipopolysaccharide or a neu-

rotropic virus. *Proc Natl Acad Sci USA* 1989;86:6348–6352.

157. Chung IY, Benveniste EN. Tumor necrosis factor-α production by astrocytes: induction by lipopolysaccharide, IFN-γ and IL-1. *J Immunol* 1990;144:2999–3007.

158. Bethea JR, Gillespie GY, Chung IY, Beneviste EN. TNF production and receptor expression by a human malignant glioma cell line, D54-MG. *J Neuroimmunol* 1990; 30:1–13.

159. Giulian D, Vaca K, Corpuz M. Brain glia release factors with opposing actions upon neuronal survival. *J Neurosci* 1993;13:229–237.

160. Giulian D, Li J, Lears B, Keenen C. Phagocytic microglia release cytokines and cytotoxins that regulate the survival of astrocytes and neurons in culture. *Neurochem Int* 1994;25:227–233.

161. Merril JE, Ignarro LJ, Sherman MP, et al. Microglial cell cytotoxicity of oligodendrocytes is mediated through nitric oxide. *J Immunol* 1993;151:2132–2141.

162. Boje KM, Arora PK. Microglial-produced nitric oxide and reactive nitrogen oxide mediate neuronal cell death. *Brain Res* 1992;587:250–256.

163. Eitan S, Schwartz M. A transglutaminase that converts interleukin-2 into a factor cytotoxic to oligodendrocytes. *Science* 1993;261:106–108.

164. Griot C, Vandevelde M, Richard A, et al. Selective degeneration of oligodendrocytes mediated by reactive oxygen species. *Free Radic Res Commun* 1990;11: 181–193.

165. Ulvestad E, Williams K, Matre R, et al. Fc receptors for IgG on cultured human microglia mediate cytotoxicity and phagocytosis of antibody-coated targets. *J Neuropathol Exp Neurol* 1994;53:27–36.

166. Williams K, Ulvestad E, Waage A, et al. Activation of adult human derived microglia by myelin phagocytosis in vitro. *J Neurosci Res* 1994;38:433–443.

167. Scolding NJ, Compston DA. Oligodendrocyte-macrophage interactions in vitro triggered by specific antibodies. *Immunology* 1991;72:127–132.

168. Ren Y, Silverstein RL, Allen J, Savill J. CD36 gene transfer confers capacity for phagocytosis of cells undergoing apoptosis. *J Exp Med* 1995;181:1857–1862.

169. Zajicek JP, Wing M, Scolding NJ, Compston DA. Interactions between oligodendrocytes and microglia. A major role for complement and tumor necrosis factor in oligodendrocyte adherence and killing. *Brain* 1992;115: 1611–1631.

170. Noble PG, Antel JP, Yong VW. Astrocytes and catalase prevent the toxicity of catecholamines to oligodendrocytes. *Brain Res* 1994;633:83–90.

171. Louis JC, Magal E, Takayama S, Varon S. CNTF protection of oligodendrocytes against natural and tumor necrosis factor-induced death. *Science* 1993;259:698–692.

172. Kahn MA, de Vellis J. Regulation of an oligodendrocyte progenitor cell line by the interleukin-6 family of cytokines. *Glia* 1994;12:87–98.

173. D'Souza S, Alinauskas K, Antel JP. Ciliary neurotrophic factor selectively protects human oligodendrocytes from tumor necrosis factor-mediated injury. *J Neurosci Res* 1996;43:289–298.

174. David S, Bouchard C, Tsatas O, Giftochristos N. Macrophages can modify the nonpermissive nature of the adult mammalian central nervous system. *Neuron* 1990;5:463–469.

175. Fagan AM, Gage FH. Cholinergic sprouting in the hippocampus: a proposed role for IL-1. *Exp Neurol* 1990; 110:105–120.

Chapter 4
Local Immune Responses in the Peripheral Nervous System

Hans-Peter Hartung, Ralf Gold, and Stefan Jung

Local immune activation requires presentation of antigens (or autoantigens) by specialized cells in the context of major histocompatibility complex (MHC) class II antigens to reactive (autoreactive) CD4+ T lymphocytes. In detail, particular MHC class II molecules on antigen-presenting cells interact with immunogenic epitopes of processed antigen (autoantigen) that in liaison are bound by antigen-specific T-cell receptors.

The peripheral nervous system (PNS) has long been considered an immunologically privileged site. This notion was based on the assumptions that 1) there is a more or less strict anatomic separation between the systemic immune compartment (blood) and the neural tissue, 2) MHC molecules required for antigen presentation are absent, 3) there is no lymphatic drainage, and 4) immune surveillance by T cells is lacking. It has become clear that most of these tenets do not hold up. While the blood-nerve barrier does restrict access of immune cells and solutes to a certain degree, this is not complete either in anatomic terms (absent or relatively deficient at the roots, in the ganglia, and at the motor terminals) or functionally (1). Activated T cells can penetrate the intact blood-nerve barrier irrespective of antigen specificity, and under certain circumstances (e.g., infections) release cytokines that upregulate the expression of MHC class II molecules in the PNS (2,3). Professional and nonprofessional antigen-presenting cells are abundant in peripheral nerve tissue (resident endoneurial and perivascular macrophages, Schwann cells).

Normal nerves contain macrophages near the endoneurial vessels. These cells usually lie outside the basal lamina of the blood vessels and have a dendritic appearance (4–9). Their perivascular distribution at the blood-nerve interface makes them uniquely suited to act as antigen-presenting cells in the PNS. Many of these resident macrophages constitutively express MHC class II molecules, complement receptor type 3 (CR3), and CD4, but the level of expression of these molecules can be greatly enhanced in inflammatory conditions (4,5,8,10–13).

Human and rat Schwann cells in culture express little if any MHC class II antigen, but can be induced to do so by coculture with T lymphoblasts, T lymphoblasts and mycobacterial antigen, or interferon (IFN)-γ and possibly tumor necrosis factor (TNF) (14–18) (Fig 4-1). Pharmacologic inhibitors of IFN-γ synthesis greatly diminish MHC class II antigen expression on cultured rat Schwann cells (19). IFN-γ also induces expression of intercellular adhesion molecule (ICAM)-1 on rat Schwann cells and TNF-α synergizes with IFN-γ in this respect (14, 15). The interaction of T cells with antigen-presenting cells is greatly strengthened by the expression of ICAM-1, suggesting that Schwann cells can acquire the role of a facultative antigen presenter (Fig 4-2). When exposed to IFN-γ or IFN-γ plus TNF-α, they are able to present exogenous P2 protein to P2-specific neuritogenic T-cell lines (14). Schwann cells also can present endogenous antigens to autoreactive T-cell lines (14, 20, 21). Furthermore, some reports (22–25) showed that HLA-DR immunoreactivity is associated with Schwann cells in human sural nerve biopsy specimens. Whether Schwann cells can act as antigen-presenting cells in vivo is still debated (4,12,26).

Schwann cells also constitutively express low levels of MHC class I molecules, which are markedly increased following incubation with IFN-γ (17,19). This would mark Schwann cells as targets for T cell–mediated cytotoxicity. In fact, Schwann cells primed with *Mycobacterium leprae* could be lysed in the presence of IFN-γ through an antigen-specific interaction with *M. leprae*–reactive CD8+ T lymphocytes (27). Activated P2 CD4+ T cells have also been shown to destroy rat Schwann cells in vitro (28).

Rat Schwann cells are endowed with a cytokine-inducible nitric oxide synthase (iNOS). IFN-γ and TNF-α upregulate iNOS-specific messenger RNA (mRNA) in Schwann cells and precipitate the release of nitrite in a dose-dependent manner (29). Nitric oxide (NO) production may account in part for the strong suppressive effect on T-cell activation by thymic antigen-presenting cells seen in a coculture model where Schwann cells were present. These observations raise the possibility that Schwann cells exert potent immunoregulatory functions beyond their role as antigen presenters. They may terminate immunoinflammatory reactions in the PNS by releasing NO (30). Whether some constitutive expression of mRNA for the downregulatory cytokine

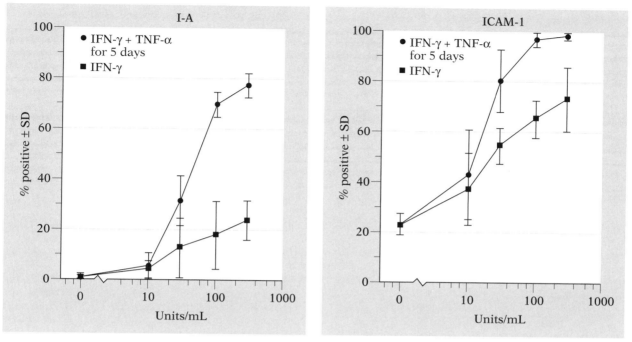

Figure 4-1. Dose-response studies of I-A and ICAM-1 expression on neonatal Schwann cells. Cultures were treated either with IFN-γ alone or in combination with TNF-α at the indicated concentrations for 5 days. Expression was quantified by FACS analysis. Values are given as mean ± SD of three experiments.

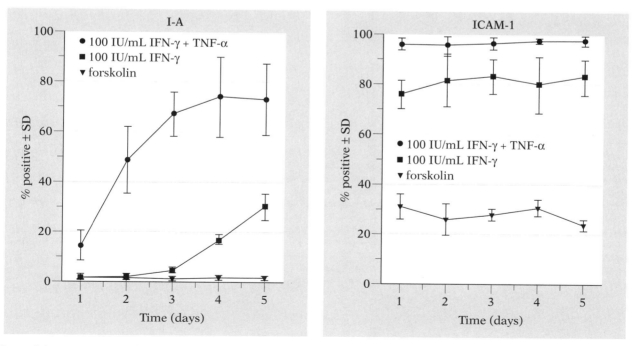

Figure 4-2. Time course of I-A and ICAM-1 expression on neonatal Schwann cells. Cultures were treated with cytokines of forskolin on day 0. Upregulation of I-A and ICAM-1 was assessed by daily FACS analysis. Values are given as mean ± SD of three experiments.

transforming growth factor (TGF)-β1 observable in Schwann cells may be sufficient to contribute to these control mechanisms is unclear at present (31). When challenged with lipopolysaccharide (LPS) or cytokines, rat Schwann cells release another possibly immuno-suppressive molecule, prostaglandin E (32). LPS, TNF-α, and interleukin (IL)-1α are able to stimulate rat Schwann cells to produce the cytokine IL-6. Interest-ingly, Schwann cells respond to exogenous IL-6 by in-duction of IL-6 mRNA and expression of the IL-6 receptor and the signal transduction component glyco-protein (gp) 130 (33). Moreover, IFN-γ can stimulate TNF-α and IL-6 mRNA in primary rat Schwann cells and an SV40 transfected Schwann cell line (34). Mouse Schwann cells can locally produce neurosteroids, but their role in immune regulation presently remains elusive (35). Local steroid generation may also bear on intraneural apoptosis of autoreactive T cells, an impor-tant mechanism of terminating an immunoinflamma-tory response.

Schwann cells express the complement receptor type 1 (CR1, CD35), which recognizes C3b and C4b and the immunoglobulin Fc receptor (FcγR) in vivo. The latter is present only when Schwann cells have contact with axons. CR1 and FcγR act as immune adherence recep-tors mediating the uptake of immune complexes. Schwann cells are known to be capable of phagocyto-sis. In addition, CR1 may function as a cofactor for fac-tor I–mediated C3b cleavage and dissociation of the al-ternative pathway convertase C3b,Bb. Thereby, it could serve to downregulate complement activation occur-ring in the vicinity of Schwann cells (36). Expression of the complement regulatory factor CD59 may also be crucial in limiting serum-induced Schwann cell lysis (37,38).

Schwann cells respond to stimulation with macro-phage-derived IL-1 by synthesizing nerve growth factor (39). Peripheral nerve regeneration in vitro is impeded by an IL-1 receptor antagonist released from a poly-meric tube surrounding regenerating nerve segments (40). Furthermore, Schwann cells proliferate when challenged with conditioned media from macrophages that have taken up and processed myelin constituents (41,42).

Systemic Immune Activation

Evidence of systemic immune activation is available in a number of experimental models of immunoinflam-matory PNS disorders as well as in human diseases. Thus, it is possible to detect circulating activated T cells by their enhanced expression of HLA-DR, the transfer-rin receptor (43), and the IL-2 receptor, both in its mem-brane bound and shed forms (43–45); by increased fre-quencies of mutant T cells (46); and by the presence in increased amounts of soluble products of activated T cells such as IL-2 (47), IFN-γ (48), and TFN-α in serum (49,50). Monocytes/macrophages are activated and re-lease ex vivo increased amounts of inflammatory medi-ators (48). Moreover, it appears that within the im-mune repertoire, there is a small population of autore-active T cells that under specific conditions may turn into autoaggressive T lymphocytes and damage the host's PNS (51, 52).

Peripheral Nerve Antigens

Protein Antigens

The myelin sheath is composed of three major proteins (P0, P1, and P2) with molecular sizes of 14 to 30 kd that make up more than 70% of the total protein content (53). In human PNS myelin, P0 accounts for more than half of the total membrane protein; it is not found in central nervous system (CNS) myelin. P0 is a 29-kd, 219–amino acid transmembrane glycoprotein with a larger extracellular domain, a highly hydrophobic membrane-spanning portion, and a basic cytoplasmic domain. It belongs to the immunoglobulin gene super-family and acts as a homophilic cell adhesion molecule (54). P0 is thought to be involved in starting and sta-bilizing the compaction of the extracellular apposition of the myelin membrane in the PNS. P1 is identical to myelin basic protein (MBP) in the CNS. The 14-kd P2 protein containing 131 amino acids is common to both CNS and PNS but predominates in the latter. It is con-centrated in the paranodal loops and in Schmidt-Lanterman incisures rather than in compact internodal myelin. The conformation of P0 is highly dependent on its association with lipids. Circulating antibodies to P0 and P2 have been detected in Lewis rats with experi-mental autoimmune neuritis (EAN) (55,56) and in a mi-nority of patients with Guillain-Barré syndrome (GBS), but also in other disease and healthy control subjects (57,58). Similarly, T cells reactive with P0 or P2 and pep-tides thereof are retrieved infrequently from GBS pa-tients, but also from healthy donors (51,52,59).

Lipid and Glycoconjugate Antigens

Lipids make up about 75% of the total nerve dry weight. Major myelin lipids are cholesterol, galactosylceramide (galactocerebroside), and galactosylceramide-3-O-sul-fate (sulfatide), and in smaller amounts gangliosides and complex neutral glycolipids (GD_{1a}, N-acetylgalac-tosaminyl GD_{1a}, GD_{1b}, GT_{1b}, GM_1, GM_{1b}, GM_2, GM_3, GD_2, GD_3, LM_1) (53,60–63). Carbohydrate structures are shared extensively with glycolipids and glycopro-teins. They appear to be major targets of humoral im-mune responses in GBS.

Myelin-Associated Glycoprotein

Myelin-associated glycoprotein (MAG) is a glycosylated transmembrane glycoprotein and member of the im-munoglobulin gene superfamily. It shares homologies with a number of cell adhesion molecules, P0, a gly-coprotein originally described on natural killer (NK) cells that is recognized by the monoclonal antibody HNK-1, and peripheral myelin protein (PMP)-22. MAG occurs in two isoforms of 76 and 62 kd (53). A very minor component of peripheral myelin (<1% of all myelin protein), it is concentrated in membranes adjacent to Schwann cells' cytoplasm such as the Schmidt-Lanterman incisures and paranodes. MAG is a target antigen for IgM antibodies in a clinically characteristic chronic immune-mediated neuropathy (see Chapter 20).

Experimental Autoimmune Neuritis

EAN is an acute demyelinating inflammatory polyradiculoneuropathy that can be induced in susceptible species by active immunization with whole peripheral nerve homogenate, myelin, or the myelin proteins P2 (64–69) and P0 (70), cyanogen bromide fragments of P2, and synthetic peptides from P2, in particular those comprising the amino acid sequences P2 53–78 and P2 61–70 (minimal neuritogenic epitopes) (65,69,71,72). Immunization efficacy can be enhanced by adding cerebroside to the inoculum (68) but not by gangliosides (73,74), although both are potential antigens of peripheral nerve. EAN can also be produced by adoptive transfer (AT-EAN) of P2, P2 peptide–specific, P0, and P0 peptide–specific T-cell lines (75–82). Rabbits, monkeys (83), rats, and mice are susceptible to one or another form of disease induction (69). As recently reported, EAN can be produced by adoptive transfer of MBP-specific CD4+ helper T-cell clones in BALB/c mice (84). MBP is present in peripheral myelin where it is designated P1, making up for approximately 2% to 16% of all myelin proteins. Two T-cell clones recognizing epitopes contained in the 21- and 18.5-kd isoforms induce changes predominantly in the peripheral but not the central nervous system. EAN mirrors many of the immunologic, electrophysiologic, and morphologic aspects of GBS and hence has been widely used as a model to investigate disease mechanisms.

Immunopathology of Experimental Autoimmune Neuritis

EAN is characterized by infiltration of the PNS by lymphocytes and macrophages (85), which leads to focal demyelination of nerves predominantly around venules (Fig 4-3). Electron microscopic studies revealed that macrophages actively strip off myelin lamellae from axons, induce vesicular disruption of the myelin sheath, and phagocytose both intact and damaged myelin (86). Depending on the amount of myelin or neuritogenic P2 peptides used for immunization, demyelinative changes and admixed axonal degeneration occur (69,87,88). Similarly, depending on the number of autoreactive cells transferred, T-cell line–mediated EAN can take the form of a predominantly demyelinating condition (low cell dose) or of a fulminant neuritis morphologically characterized by prominent endoneurial edema and axonal degeneration when a higher cell dose is injected to produce disease. This axonal degeneration is reflected in the profound functional deficit resulting from the higher cell dose injection (76,77,89,90).

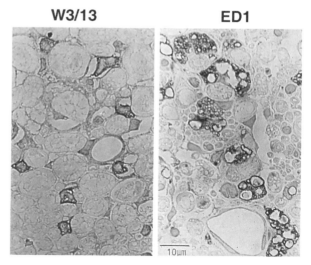

W3/13   **ED1**

Figure 4-3. Immunocytochemical demonstration of T-cell and macrophage invasion in actively induced EAN. Micrometer sections were taken from ventral roots of sciatic nerves from animals with peripheral myelin-induced EAN at day 12 (left) and day 16 (right) after immunization. T cells, labeled with the monoclonal antibody W3/13, are prominent during the early stages of the disease whereas macrophages, labeled by ED1, predominate beyond day 13.

The Role of T Cells

Sensitization of T lymphocytes to PNS myelin or isolated P2 and its neuritogenic peptide sequences was demonstrated in rats, with skin testing and lymphocyte transformation assays (75,91–93). The capacity to mount a cell-mediated response to P2 differed between high-responder Lewis and low-responder Sprague-Dawley and Brown-Norway (BN) rats (82,92). However, while BN rats are not very susceptible to actively induced EAN, T-cell lines specifically reactive to bovine P2 can be isolated from these rats, and upon transfer to syngeneic BN recipients, these cell lines are capable of evoking EAN (82). This indicates that autoreactive T-cell clones are contained in the T-cell repertoire of these animals.

An important role for T cells in the initiation of EAN was suggested by transfer of the disease to naive Lewis rats, using lymph node cells obtained from animals that had been actively immunized with myelin or P2 (93). Formal proof was presented by two groups who showed that injection of P2-reactive CD4+ T cells into Lewis rats produces EAN (75,89). Conversely, rats rendered T-cell deficient by adult thymectomy and lethal irradiation or treated with anti–T cell antibodies are much less susceptible to disease induction by active immunization (94,95). Indirect evidence was also advanced by showing that administration of high-dose cyclosporine or a monoclonal antibody directed to the IL-2 receptor on activated T cells, to the surface antigen CD2, or to the α and β chains of the T-cell receptor (TCR) prevents the development of transfer EAN (96–98). It is also possible to transfer disease with CD4+ T cells specifically reactive to bovine P0 (81). Epitope specificity of neuritogenic T-cell lines resides primarily in the amino acid sequence 61–70 in P2, and in amino acid sequence 180–199 of the P0 protein. These are amphipathic peptide fragments with an α-helical configuration (71,72, 77–82).

Usage of TCR V gene families has been analyzed in EAN. Clark et al (99,100) reported that T-cell lines and hybridomas generated with a neuritogenic peptide, SP26, use exclusively the same TCR V gene families, Vα2 and Vβ8, for their TCR as T cells that cause experimental allergic encephalomyelitis (EAE). Subsequent studies from our group showed a more heterogeneous expression of TCR Vα and Vβ gene usage (101).

Early invasion of the PNS by T lymphocytes has been documented immunocytochemically. Before the onset of clinical signs, most T cells express the CD4+ helper/inducer phenotype, whereas CD8+ cells prevail after the disease has peaked and during recovery. However, macrophages greatly outnumber lymphocytes in affected peripheral nervous tissue, particularly beyond day 13–17 p.i. (post immunization) when only few T cells continue to be present in the active EAN model (26,102–106).

T-Cell Homing and Migration

Crucial to the genesis of an inflammatory lesion is the transendothelial migration of blood-borne leukocytes. Circulating autoreactive T lymphocytes need to be activated in the periphery in order to cross the blood-brain or blood-nerve barrier and to initiate a local immune response in the nervous tissue (2,3).

The process of homing and transmigration is governed by an ensemble of adhesion molecules that are reciprocally expressed on endothelial cells and leukocytes. This is a multistep process occurring in an ordered sequential fashion (107,108). First, slow-flowing leukocytes in blood roll along the vascular wall and weakly attach to endothelium via the selectin family of adhesion molecules (109). This allows them to sample the local environment. When the leukocytes encounter specific activating or chemoattractant factors, the potentially transient and unstable interaction of leukocytes with endothelium is strengthened. This second step of activation and adhesion is accomplished through the interaction of β_2 integrins such as leukocyte function–associated antigen (LFA)-1 on lymphocytes and their counterparts ICAM-1 and ICAM-2, both members of the immunoglobulin superfamily (110). The second ligand-receptor pair is represented by very late activation antigen (VLA)-4 present on T cells and vascular cell adhesion molecule (VCAM)-1 expressed on the surface of vascular endothelium. Finally, T cells flatten and migrate across the endothelium following chemotactic signals such as activated complement component C5a, platelet-activating factor (PAF), and members of the chemokine family of cytokines (111).

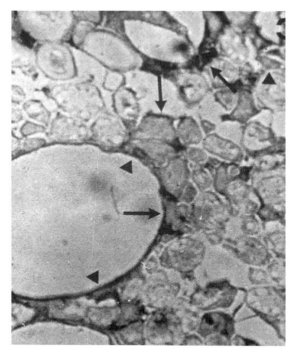

Figure 4-4. ICAM-1 expression in EAN. One micrometer cryosection of a ventral root from a Lewis rat with actively-induced EAN. ICAM-1 is immunolabeled and detectable on endothelial cells (arrows) and invading leukocytes (triangles) in nerve lesions before onset of clinical disease (day 12 after immunization).

The mechanisms by which circulating autoreactive CD4+ T cells home in on the PNS have recently been investigated in EAN. Shortly before disease manifestation, invading T cells, macrophages, and endoneurial endothelial cells upregulate their expression of ICAM-1 (112) (Fig 4-4). VCAM-1 mRNA is maximal at sites of T-cell infiltration (113). Expression of the counter-receptor for ICAM-1, LFA-1, is likewise greatly enhanced on infiltrating mononuclear cells (114). We and others recently reported increased serum concentrations of the endothelial cell adhesion molecule E-selectin early in the course of GBS that returned to normal when patients recovered (115,116). Breakdown of the blood-nerve barrier is one of the earliest morphologically demonstrable events in lesion development in EAN (76,86,117,118). Local reactivation of immigrated neuritogenic T cells initiates a cascade of inflammatory responses involving cytokines, additional effector cells, and a host of inflammatory effector molecules both inside and outside the blood-nerve barrier.

Proinflammatory Cytokines

Among the cytokines that orchestrate cellular interactions during immune responses, IFN-γ is of major importance (119). IFN-γ is released by CD4+ T cells of the Th1 inflammatory phenotype. It can 1) induce MHC class II antigens on macrophages and their production of toxic oxygen free radicals and other proinflammatory mediators (26,120); 2) induce adhesion molecules on endothelial cells, macrophages, T cells, and Schwann cells (14); and 3) enhance vascular permeability. Therefore, IFN-γ might be instrumental in allowing an influx of antibodies, soluble mediators, and inflammatory cells into the endoneurium.

IFN-γ immunoreactivity is expressed by T cells, some macrophages, and polymorphonuclear cells that, concomitantly with the invasion of T lymphocytes, enter the nerve early in EAN (121). However, IFN-γ–positive cells are present only transiently from day 11 to day 13 after active immunization before the onset of overt disease (see Plate I). The presence of IFN-γ–positive cells in nerve roots correlates with the number of Ia-positive macrophages during the course of EAN. In the early phase of the disease, many lean (prephagocytic) macrophages are present and carry MHC class II gene products, whereas most of the postphagocytic macrophages with large ED1-positive vacuoles no longer express Ia at later stages of EAN (11,26). Lymph nodes taken from animals with EAN contain increased numbers of T cells that on exposure to P2 secrete IFN-γ as early as 7 days after immunization with peripheral myelin (122). Similarly there is augmented mRNA expression of IFN-γ by mononuclear cells stimulated with P2 (123). The functional role of IFN-γ in the pathogenesis of EAN was established by in vivo administration of recombinant IFN gamma, which markedly augmented disease severity in actively induced EAN as well as in EAN induced by P2 T-cell lines. Conversely, in vivo application of a monoclonal antibody to IFN-γ suppressed the disease (120).

The other important activator of macrophages is TNF-α. In EAN, TNF-α is found in nerve lesions around the time of the first clinical symptoms. As animals recover, TNF-α immunoreactivity is no longer detectable. Neutralization of endogenously generated TNF-α ameliorates the experimental disease (124). Furthermore, direct injection of TNF-α into the sciatic nerve of mice produced predominantly axonal damage in one study, and a mixture of vascular damage, demyelination, and degeneration in another (125,126). Finally 20% to 50% of GBS patients have raised serum levels of TNF-α (49,50). These observations may be particularly important because TNF-α exerts multiple phlogistic effects and apparently possesses myelinotoxic properties (127–129).

The Role of Macrophages

Macrophages are the predominant cell population in affected nerves of animals with EAN. They have been identified both in spinal roots and in more distal segments of nerves by immunocytochemistry with the monoclonal antibody ED1 (130,131). Most ED1-positive macrophages also express MHC class II antigen (OX6) and hence could function as antigen presenters (11,26).

In EAN, macrophages adhere to normally appearing nerve fibers, a feature never observed with wallerian degeneration, where macrophages selectively attack degenerating fibers (4). They strip off myelin lamellae from the axons causing demyelination.

Local complement activation may play a role in this process by providing the ligand for the adhesion molecule and complement type 3 receptor CR3/Mac1. Thereby macrophages may be attracted to the myelin sheath. A monoclonal antibody to CR3 inhibits phagocytosis by macrophages and prevents nerve regeneration (132).

Detailed immunopharmacologic investigations have elucidated the role of macrophages in the amplification and effector phase of the disease. The essential requirement of macrophages for disease expression was highlighted by depletion experiments using either silica or the macrophage-specific toxin dichlormethylene disphosphonate encapsulated in liposomes. Macrophage depletion prevented all clinical, electrophysiologic, and histologic signs of EAN and AT-EAN (131,133–135).

There is evidence for macrophage activation at the time of infiltrate formation in nerve roots. Shortly before the onset of clinical symptoms, blood monocytes exhibit a significant increase in spontaneous chemiluminescence. Likewise, superoxide anion release and chemiluminescence, both indices of heightened oxidative burst activity in macrophages, are enhanced in peritoneal macrophages collected from animals with EAN (136,137).

Treatment with inhibitors of arachidonic acid conversion such as dexamethasone, indomethacin, and BW755c (Fig 4-5) or with physiologically occurring

EAN

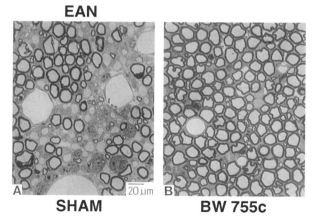

Figure 4-5. Blockade of arachidonic acid conversion to prostaglandins and leukotrienes inhibits EAN. Lewis rats, following immunization with peripheral nerve myelin, were either sham-treated with saline or treated with the joint cyclooxygenase and lipoxygenase inhibitor BW755c intraperitoneally. The latter treatment almost completely abrogated clinical disease and prevented development of pathologic changes in the nerve.

oxygen radical scavengers such as superoxide dismutase and catalase prevents myelin-induced EAN when the treatment is initiated early, or greatly attenuates disease expression when it is administered after the onset of clinical signs (131). Arachidonic acid metabolites, possibly synergizing with activated complement, could function as chemoattractants and secretagogues for inflammatory cells or enhance the permeability of the blood-nerve barrier. Reactive oxygen species such as superoxide anion, hydrogen peroxide, and hydroxyl radicals could inflict peroxidation injury on myelin but may also act by generating chemotactic signals and by exerting cytotoxic effects on endothelial cells (138–141). Rodent macrophages are endowed with a cytokine-inducible form of NO synthase and hence are capable upon appropriate stimulation to generate toxic NO metabolites. A role for these compounds is suggested by our recent demonstration that competitive NO synthase inhibitors can mitigate Lewis rat EAN (142).

Increased lysosomal enzyme activities closely correspond to the histologic distribution of EAN lesions (143). Macrophage-derived neutral proteases and phospholipases have been implicated in myelin damage in vitro (144,145). In vivo microinjection of proteinases into the sciatic nerve of rats produces inflammatory demyelination (146,147). Finally, treatment of EAN rats with proteinase inhibitors delays development of the disease (150).

The Role of Mast Cells

The number of endoneurial mast cells decreases in the course of EAN (149). Electron microscopically they can be shown to degranulate, possibly as a consequence of T cell–mediated delayed-type hypersensitivity (150). These cells may release vasoactive amines (5-hydroxytryptamine, histamine) and arachidonic acid–derived metabolites that could augment vascular permeability. Blood-nerve barrier integrity and nerve conduction in rat tibial nerve are greatly disturbed when mast cell degranulation is induced by intraneural injection of compound 48/80 (151). A contributory pathogenic role of mast cell degranulation is supported by pharmacologic experiments in which mast cell–stabilizing drugs like reserpine and nedocromil prevented or attenuated the disease (152).

Termination of the Immunoinflammatory Response

Several different mechanisms may operate to terminate the acute immunoinflammatory attack in this monophasic disease model. In EAN, increased production of the downregulatory cytokine TGF-β1 has been recorded (31,153) (see Plate II). TGF-β1 and mRNA might be localized mainly to macrophages and to a lesser extent to T lymphocytes invading the PNS during the course of EAN in Lewis rats (31). Importantly, systemic administration of recombinant TGF-β1 markedly inhibits the clinical signs and histologic changes of actively induced EAN in the Lewis rat (153,154). Zhu et al (123) demonstrated augmented mRNA expression of the downregulatory cytokine IL-4 in lymph node and spleen cells from EAN rats cultured with peripheral myelin, P2, or P0, peaking late in the course of the disease. IL-10 mRNA is upregulated, mostly in macrophages, in sciatic nerve in EAN when recovery is about to start (155). Administration of human IL-10 mitigates EAN (156).

Apoptosis (i.e., programmed cell death) of activated T cells accumulating in peripheral nerve may be another mechanism to terminate the ongoing immune response and limit tissue damage (157,158). Apoptotic T cells in sciatic nerve can be identified by their condensed nuclear chromatin and the labeling of fragmented DNA in their nuclei in EAN. This process is greatly enhanced after administration of high-dose glucocorticosteroids (159,160) (Fig 4-6).

The Pathogenic Role of Antibodies

Humoral immune factors include circulating and locally produced antibodies and components of the complement system. Antibodies can conceivably induce myelin damage by three mechanisms. First, upon binding to macrophages via the Fc receptor, they can direct these to the putative antigenic (autoantigenic) structures on the myelin sheath, which become the target of so-called antibody-dependent cellular cytotoxicity. Second, they can bind to the antigenic epitopes via their Fab portion and activate the classic complement pathway with subsequent formation of the terminal complement complex (TCC) (see below). Third, by opsonizing target structures, they can promote their internalization by macrophages.

Figure 4-6. Immunocytochemical characterization of apoptotic cells in Lewis rat EAN. (A) T cells in the sciatic nerve positive for B115-1, a rat T-cell marker, show nuclear morphology characteristic of apoptosis (arrows). An open arrow denotes the advanced stage of apoptosis with loss of membrane immunoreactivity. (B) Double labeling for DNA fragmentation versus expression of ED-1, a macrophage marker antigen. After antigen therapy with P2 protein, there is abundant T-cell apoptosis and macrophages engulf apoptotic DNA. (C, E, G) Double labeling for DNA fragmentation versus expression of B115-1, a T-cell marker antigen in control animals receiving an irrelevant myelin protein (C), after antigen therapy with IV administration of recombinant P2 protein (E), and after IV administration of glucocorticosteroids (G). Parts D, F, and H are higher magnifications of C, E, and G, respectively. A reduction of inflammatory T cells and an increase in apoptotic fragments are visible after antigen therapy and glucocorticosteroid treatment. At higher magnification, cells double-stained for T-cell antigen and DNS fragmentation are visible (arrows in D and H). Terminal stages of apoptosis have lost membrane immunoreactivity (arrowheads in D and H).

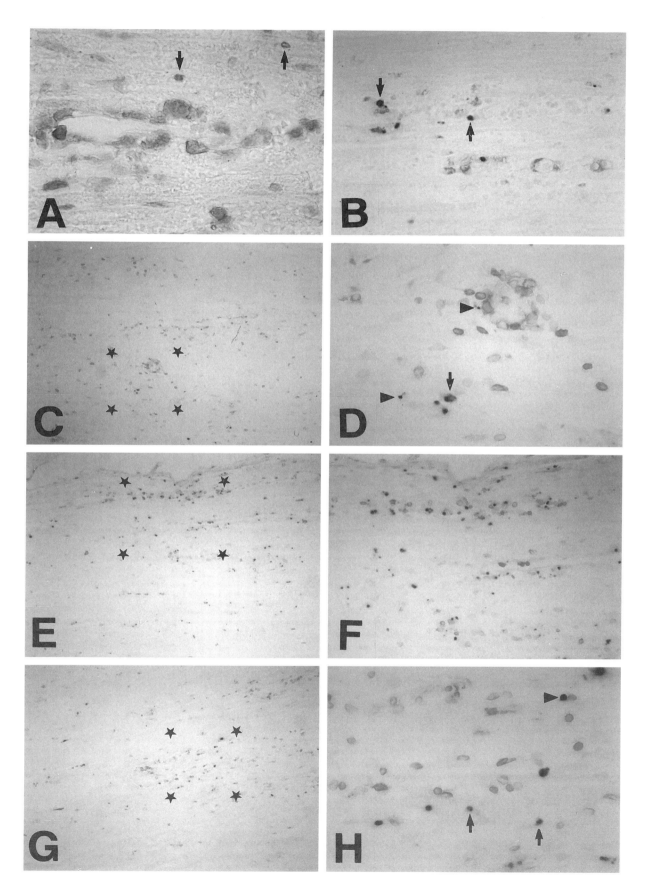

47

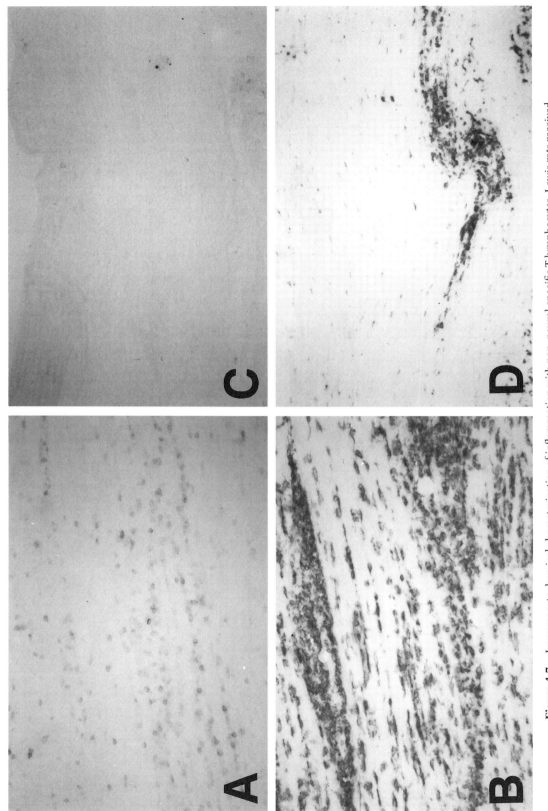

Figure 4-7. Immunocytochemical characterization of inflammation with non-neural-specific T lymphocytes. Lewis rats received a single 10 μL sterile injection of sterile ovalbumin into proximal tibial nerves on the lefthand side, in addition to similar control injections of sterile casein on the right side. Then a single IV tail vein injection of freshly activated ovalbumin-specific T cells was given. Four days later, the rats were sacrificed. Parts A and B show staining for T cells and macrophages on the ovalbumin-injected side using mAb R73 (α/β T-cell receptor) (A) and ED1 (macrophage marker antigen) (B). Parts C and D show the control sides of A and B, respectively. In D there is accumulation of macrophages around the injection site, but no T-cell inflammation.

Antibodies to the P2 protein have been detected in the circulation of animals with EAN (56,93). However, their titers and kinetics did not correlate with disease activity, casting doubts on an essential causative function. With enzyme-linked immunosorbent assay (ELISA) spot technique, IgG and IgM antibodies to P2 were demonstrated in lymph nodes and spleens from rats with EAN. Yet again there was no correlation to stage or activity of the disease (161). Similar observations were made regarding P0 (161). Using ELISA and Western blot analysis, we found circulating high-titer antibodies to the extracellular domain of P0 in the blood and cerebrospinal fluid (CSF) of Lewis rats on day 13 after immunization with purified bovine myelin. Titers were maintained for approximately 2 weeks and then declined, which was in sharp contrast to the antibody response to P2. This came on later and persisted for several weeks despite complete clinical recovery. When EAN was induced by immunization with P2, no significant antibody reactivity against P0 or its extracellular domain was detectable (55). Evidence arguing against an exclusive role for antibodies in the pathogenesis of EAN stems from studies in which the disease was pro-duced by adoptive transfer of P2 autoreactive T-lymphocyte cell lines. Disease developed in recipient rats within 4 to 5 days of T-cell transfer, an interval too short for a significant antibody response to be elicited. In fact, circulating antibodies to P2 could not be measured in the sera of these recipient animals (72,89). Screening the B-cell repertoire in EAN induced by peripheral nerve myelin, Zhu et al (161) detected increased numbers of B cells in lymph nodes and spleen cells that synthesized antibodies to ganglioside GM_1 and MAG peptides.

The Role of Complement

Complement involvement in lesion pathogenesis is highlighted by the immunocytochemical demonstration of TCC (C5b-9) deposition on Schwann cells and along the myelin sheath prior to demyelination (162). Decomplementation of animals with cobra venom factor partly suppresses EAN (163,164) and injection in rats of soluble CR1, a regulatory glycoprotein of the complement cascade, mitigates disease (165).

In myelin-induced EAN, macrophages concentrate in

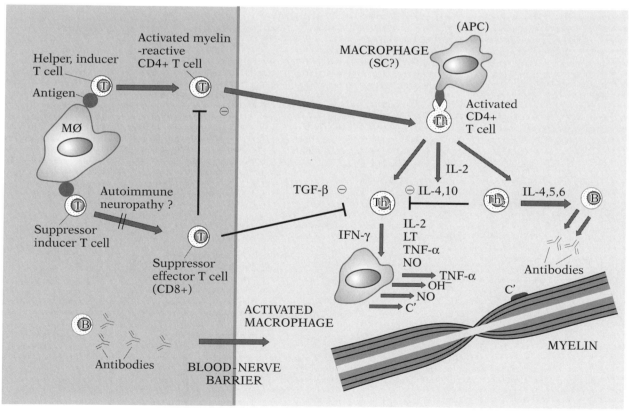

Figure 4-8.   Synoptic view of immune responses in the peripheral nervous system. Systemic immune responses (blood, left panel) are focused into the nerve (right panel) where, after in situ reactivation of invading T cells, a cascade of immunopathogenic events is set in motion. APC=antigen presenting cell; SC=Schwann cell; C'=activated complement.

areas of strong TCC staining (162). Strikingly similar observations recently were made in acute inflammatory demyelinating polyneuropathy (166). TCC deposition on the surface of Schwann cells and myelin sheaths may promote an influx of calcium, which is considered an important initial step in myelin breakdown. Alternatively, TCC formation in myelin membranes may cause the activation of myelin-associated neutral proteases, with subsequent hydrolysis of myelin proteins. It is conceivable that TCC-targeted myelin is selectively attacked by macrophages. Macrophages in culture respond to TCC by liberating chemotactically active and proinflammatory eicosanoids that contribute to the pathogenesis of EAN (131). Myelin degeneration after nerve transection did not give rise to the formation of TCC in rats, which excludes a nonspecific activation process in EAN (162). Collectively, available evidence suggests that complement may be important in recruiting macrophages into the endoneurium, in opsonizing myelin for phagocytosis, and in amplifying ongoing inflammatory reactions.

Synergy of T- and B-Cell Responses

The apparent dichotomy of the cell-mediated and humorally mediated immune responses considered pathogenic, as reviewed, may be resolved by envisaging a cooperative action of T cells and antibodies in effecting nerve damage. Experimental evidence to corroborate this notion has recently become available (3,167–169) (Fig 4-7). Injection of Lewis rats with an antibody to myelin or to galactocerebroside enhanced disease in P2 peptide T-cell transfer EAN (167,169). Local breach of the blood-nerve barrier by neuritogenic T cells would facilitate the influx of demyelinating antibodies from the circulation (168). Most importantly, this permissive action of activated T lymphocytes appears not to be related to their antigenic specificity. When ovalbumin-specific T cells accumulated in the nerve of Lewis rats at sites of ovalbumin injection, intraperitoneal administration of a galactocerebroside antiserum produced local conduction block and demyelination (2,3).

Summary

Figure 4-8 provides a schematic synopsis of local immune circuitry in peripheral nerve, summarizing evidence gathered from in vitro works, analysis of experimental autoimmunity, and studies of the immune-mediated neuropathies.

References

1. Olsson Y. Microenvironment of the peripheral nervous system under normal and pathological conditions. *Crit Rev Neurobiol* 1990;5:265–311.
2. Harvey GK, Gold R, Hartung H-P, Toyka KV. Nonneural-specific T lymphocytes can orchestrate inflammatory peripheral neuropathy. *Brain* 1995;118:1263–1272.
3. Pollard JD, Westland KW, Harvey GK, et al. Activated T cells of nonneural specificity open the blood-nerve bar-
rier to circulating antibody. *Ann Neurol* 1995;37: 467–475.
4. Griffin JW, Stoll G, Li CY, et al. Macrophage responses in inflammatory demyelinating neuropathies. *Ann Neurol* 1990;27(suppl):S64–S68.
5. Griffin JW, George R, Lobato C, et al. Macrophage responses and myelin clearance during wallerian degeneration: relevance to immune-mediated demyelination. *J Neuroimmunol* 1992;40:153–165.
6. Griffin JW, George R, Ho T. Macrophage systems in peripheral nerves. A review. *J Exp Neurol* 1993;52:553–560.
7. Oldfors A. Macrophages in peripheral nerves. *Acta Neuropathol(Berl)* 1980;49:43–49.
8. Monaco S, Gehrmann J, Raivich G, Kreutzberg GW. MHC-positive, ramified macrophages in the normal and injured rat peripheral nervous system. *J Neurocytol* 1992;21:623–634.
9. Arvidson B. Cellular uptake of exogenous horseradish peroxidase in mouse peripheral nerve. *Acta Neuropathol(Berl)* 1977;37:35–41.
10. Stevens A, Schabet M, Schott K, Wietholter H. Role of endoneural cells in experimental allergic neuritis and characterisation of a resident phagocytic cell. *Acta Neuropathol(Berl)* 1989;77:412–419.
11. Olsson T, Holmdahl R, Klareskog L, Forsum U. Ia-expressing cells and T lymphocytes of different subsets in peripheral nerve tissue during experimental allergic neuritis in Lewis rats. *Scand J Immunol* 1983;18: 339–343.
12. Cowley SA, Butter C, Gschmeissner SE, et al. An immunoelectronmicroscopical study of the expression of major histocompatibility complex (MHC) class II antigens in guinea pig sciatic nerves following induction of intraneural mycobacterial granulomas. *J Neuroimmunol* 1989;23:223–231.
13. Bonetti B, Monaco S, Ciannini C, et al. Human peripheral nerve macrophages in normal and pathological conditions. *J Neurol Sci* 1993;118:158–168.
14. Gold R, Toyka KV, Hartung H-P. Synergistic effect of IFN gamma and TNF alpha on expression of immune molecules and antigen presentation by Schwann cells. *Cell Immunol* 1995;165:65–70.
15. Lilje O, Armati PJ. The distribution and abundance of MHC and ICAM-1 on Schwann cells in vitro. *J Neuroimmunol* 1997;77:75–84.
16. Samuel NM, Jessen KR, Grange JM, Mirsky R. Gamma interferon, but not *Mycobacterium leprae*, induces major histocompatibility class II antigens on cultured rat Schwann cells. *J Neurocytol* 1987;16:281–287.
17. Samuel NM, Mirsky R, Grange JM, Jessen KR. Expression of major histocompatibility complex class I and class II antigens in human Schwann cell cultures and effects of infection with *Mycobacterium leprae*. *Clin Exp Immunol* 1987;68:500–509.
18. Armati PJ, Pollard JD, Gatenby P. Rat and human Schwann cells in vitro can synthesize and express MHC molecules. *Muscle Nerve* 1990;13:106–116.
19. Tsai CP, Pollard JD, Armati PJ. Interferon-gamma inhibition suppresses experimental allergic neuritis: modulation of major histocompatibility complex expression of Schwann cells in vitro. *J Neuroimmunol* 1991;31: 133–145.
20. Wekerle H, Schwab M, Linington C, Meyermann R. Antigen presentation in the peripheral nervous system: Schwann cells present endogenous myelin autoantigens to lymphocytes. *Eur J Immunol* 1986;16:1551–1557.
21. Argall KG, Armati PJ, Pollard JD, Bonner J. Interactions between CD4+ T-cells and rat Schwann cells in vitro. 2.

Cytotoxic effects of P2-specific CD4+ T-cell lines on Lewis rat Schwann cells. *J Neuroimmunol* 1992;40:19–29.

22. Pollard JD, Baverstock J, McLeod JG. Class II antigen expression and inflammatory cells in the Guillain-Barré syndrome. *Ann Neurol* 1987;21:337–341.

23. Pollard JD, McCombe PA, Baverstock J, et al. Class II antigen expression and T lymphocyte subsets in chronic inflammatory demyelinating polyneuropathy. *J Neuroimmunol* 1986;13:123–134.

24. Mitchell GW, Williams GS, Bosch EP, Hart MN. Class II antigen expression in peripheral neuropathies. *J Neurol Sci* 1991;102:170–176.

25. Mancardi GL, Cadoni A, Zicca A, et al. HLA-DR Schwann cell reactivity in peripheral neuropathies of different origins. *Neurology* 1988;38:848–851.

26. Schmidt B, Stoll G, Hartung HP, et al. Macrophages but not Schwann cells express Ia antigen in experimental autoimmune neuritis. *Ann Neurol* 1990;28:70–77.

27. Steinhoff U, Kaufmann SHE. Specific lysis by CD8+ T cells of Schwann cells expressing *Mycobacterium leprae* antigens. *Eur J Immunol* 1988;18:969.

28. Argall KG, Armati PJ, Pollard JD, et al. Interactions between CD4+ T-cells and rat Schwann cells in vitro. 1. Antigen presentation by Lewis rat Schwann cells to P2-specific CD4+ T-cell lines. *J Neuroimmunol* 1992;40:1–18.

29. Gold R, Zielasek J, Kiefer R, et al. Secretion of nitrite by Schwann cells and its effect on T-cell activation in vitro. *Cell Immunol* 1996;168:69–77.

30. Liew FY. Regulation of lymphocyte functions by nitric oxide. *Curr Opin Immunol* 1995;7:396–399.

31. Kiefer R, Funa K, Schweitzer T, et al. Transforming growth factor beta1 in experimental autoimmune neuritis: cellular localization and time course. *Am J Pathol* 1996;148:211–223.

32. Constable AL, Armati PJ, Toyka KV, Hartung HP. Production of prostanoids by Lewis rat Schwann cells in vitro. *Brain Res* 1994;635:75–80.

33. Bolin LM, Verity N, Silver JE, et al. Interleukin-6 production by Schwann cells and induction in sciatic nerve injury. *J Neurochem* 1995;64:850–858.

34. Murwani R, Hodgkinson S, Armati P. Tumor necrosis factor alpha and interleukin-6 mRNA expression in neonatal Lewis rat Schwann cells and a neonatal rat Schwann cell line following interferon gamma stimulation. *J Neuroimmunol* 1996;71:65–71.

35. Koenig HL, Schumacher M, Ferzaz B, et al. Progesterone synthesis and myelin formation by Schwann cells. *Science* 1995;268:1500–1503.

36. Vedeler CA, Matre R. Peripheral nerve CR1 express in situ cofactor activity for degradation in C3b. *J Neuroimmunol* 1990;26:51–56.

37. Koski CL, et al. Complement regulatory molecules on human myelin and glial cells: differential expression affects the deposition of activated complement proteins. *J Neurochem* 1996;66:303–312.

38. Sawant-Mane S, et al. CD59 homologue regulates complement-dependent cytolysis of rat Schwann cells. *J Neuroimmunol* 1996;69:63–71.

39. Lindholm D, Heumann R, Meyer M, Thoenen H. Interleukin-1 regulates synthesis of nerve growth factor in non-neuronal cells of rat sciatic nerve. *Nature* 1987;330:658–659.

40. Guenard V, Dinarello CA, Weston PJ, Aebischer P. Peripheral nerve regeneration is impeded by interleukin-1 receptor antagonist released from a polymeric guidance channel. *J Neurosci Res* 1991;29:396–400.

41. Bigbee JW, Yoshino JE, Devries GH. Morphological and proliferative responses of cultured Schwann cells following rapid phagocytosis of a myelin-enriched fraction. *J Neurocytol* 1987;16:487–496.

42. Baichwal RR, DeVries GH. A mitogen for Schwann cells is derived from myelin basic protein. *Biochem Biophys Res Commun* 1989;164:883–888.

43. Taylor WA, Hughes RAC. T lymphocyte activation antigens in Guillain-Barré syndrome and chronic idiopathic demyelinating polyradiculoneuropathy. *J Neuroimmunol* 1989;24:33–39.

44. Hartung HP, Hughes RAC, Taylor WA, et al. T cell activation in Guillain-Barré syndrome and in MS: elevated serum levels of soluble IL-2 receptors. *Neurology* 1990;40:215–218.

45. Bansil S, Mithen FA, Cook SD, et al. Clinical correlation with serum-soluble interleukin-2 receptor levels in Guillain-Barré syndrome. *Neurology* 1991;41:1302–1305.

46. Van Den Berg LH, Mollee I, Wokke JH, Logtenberg T. Increased frequencies of HPRT mutant T lymphocytes in patients with Guillain-Barré syndrome and chronic inflammatory demyelinating polyneuropathy: further evidence for a role of T cells in the etiopathogenesis of peripheral demyelinating diseases. *J Neuroimmunol* 1995;58:37–42.

47. Hartung HP, Reiners K, Schmidt B, et al. Serum interleukin-2 concentrations in Guillain-Barré syndrome and chronic idiopathic demyelinating polyradiculoneuropathy: comparison with other neurological diseases of presumed immunopathogenesis. *Ann Neurol* 1991;30:48–53.

48. Hartung HP, Toyka KV. T-cell and macrophage activation in experimental autoimmune neuritis and Guillain-Barré syndrome. *Ann Neurol* 1990;27(suppl):S57–S63.

49. Exley AR, Smith N, Winer JB. Tumour necrosis factor-alpha and other cytokines in Guillain-Barré syndrome. *J Neurol Neurosurg Psychiatry* 1994;57:1118–1120.

50. Sharief MK, McLean B, Thompson EJ. Elevated serum levels of tumor necrosis factor-alpha in Guillain-Barré syndrome. *Ann Neurol* 1993;33:591–596.

51. Pette M, Gengaroli C, Hartung HP, et al. Human T lymphocytes distinguish bovine from human P2 peripheral nyelin protein: implications for immunological studies on inflammatory demyelinating neuropathies. *J Neuroimmunol* 1994;52:47–52.

52. Burns J, Krasner LJ, Rostami A, Pleasure D. Isolation of P2 protein-reactive T-cell lines from human blood. *Ann Neurol* 1986;19:391–393.

53. Linington C, Brostoff SW. Peripheral nerve antigens. In: Dyck PJ, Thomas PK, Griffin JW, et al, eds. *Peripheral neuropathy*. 3rd ed. Philadelphia: WB Saunders, 1993: 404–417.

54. Filbin MT, Walsh FS, Trapp BD, et al. Role of myelin P0 protein as a homophilic adhesion molecule. *Nature* 1990;344:871–872.

55. Archelos JJ, Roggenbruck K, Schneider-Schaulies J, et al. Detection and quantification of antibodies to the extracellular domain of P0 during experimental allergic neuritis. *J Neurol Sci* 1993;117:197–205.

56. Rostami A, Brown MJ, Lisak RP, et al. The role of myelin P2 protein in the production of experimental allergic neuritis. *Ann Neurol* 1984;16:680–685.

57. Quarles RH, Ilyas AA, Willison HJ. Antibodies to gangliosides and myelin proteins in Guillain-Barré syndrome. *Ann Neurol* 27(suppl):S48–S52.

58. Khalili-Shirazi A, Atkinson P, Gregson N, Hughes RA. Antibody responses to P0 and P2 myelin proteins in Guillain-Barré syndrome and chronic idiopathic demyelinating polyradiculoneuropathy. *J Neuroimmunol* 1993;46:245–251.

59. Pette M, Linington C, Gengaroli C, et al. T lymphocyte recognition sites on peripheral nerve myelin P0 protein. *J Neuroimmunol* 1994;54:29–34.

60. Svennerholm L, Boström K, Fredman P, et al. Gangliosides and allied glycosphingolipids in human peripheral nerve and spinal cord. *Biochim Biophys Acta* 1994; 1214:115–123.

61. Kusunoki S, Chiba A, Kon K, et al. *N*-Acetylgalactosaminyl CD1a is a target molecule for serum antibody in Guillain-Barré syndrome. *Ann Neurol* 1994;35: 570–576.

62. Yu RK, Saito M. Structure and localization of gangliosides. In: Margolis RU, Margolis RK, eds. *Neurobiology of glycoconjugates*. New York: Plenum, 1989:1–42.

63. Svennerholm L, Fredman P. Antibody detection in Guillain-Barré syndrome. *Ann Neurol* 27(suppl):S36–S40.

64. Suzuki M, Kitamura K, Uyemura K, et al. Neuritogenic activity of peripheral nerve myelin proteins in Lewis rats. *Neurosci Lett* 1980;19:353–358.

65. Shin HC, McFarlane EF, Pollard JD, Watson EG. Induction of experimental allergic neuritis with synthetic peptides from myelin P2 protein. *Neurosci Lett* 1989; 102:309–312.

66. Mizisin AP, Wiley CA, Hughes RA, Powell HC. Peripheral nerve demyelination in rabbits after inoculation with Freund's complete adjuvant alone or in combination with lipid haptens. *J Neuroimmunol* 1987;16:381–395.

67. Kadlubowski M, Hughes RA. Identification of the neuritogen for experimental allergic neuritis. *Nature* 1979; 277:140–141.

68. Hughes RA, Powell HC. Experimental allergic neuritis: demyelination induced by P2 alone and non-specific enhancement by cerebroside. *J Neuropathol Exp Neurol* 1984;43:154–161.

69. Hartung HP, Heininger K, Schäfer B, et al. Immune mechanisms in inflammatory polyneuropathy. *Ann NY Acad Sci* 1988;540:122–161.

70. Milner P, Lovelidge CA, Taylor WA, Hughes RAC. P0 myelin protein produces experimental allergic neuritis in Lewis rats. *J Neurol Sci* 1987;79:275–285.

71. Rostami A, Gregorian SK. Peptide 53-78 of myelin P2 protein is a T cell epitope for the induction of experimental autoimmune neuritis. *Cell Immunol* 1991;132: 433–441.

72. Rostami A, Gregorian SK, Brown MJ, Pleasure DE. Induction of severe experimental autoimmune neuritis with a synthetic peptide corresponding to the 53-78 amino acid sequence of the myelin P2 protein. *J Neuroimmunol* 1990;30:145–151.

73. Zielasek J, Jung S, Schmidt B, et al. Effects of ganglioside administration on experimental autoimmune neuritis induced by peripheral nerve myelin or P2-specific T cell lines. *J Neuroimmunol* 1993;43:103–111.

74. Ponzin D, Meneggus AM, Kirschner G, et al. Effects of gangliosides upon the expression of autoimmune demyelination in the peripheral nervous system. *Ann Neurol* 1992;30:678–685.

75. Rostami A, Burns JB, Brown MJ, et al. Transfer of experimental allergic neuritis with P2-reactive T-cell lines. *Cell Immunol* 1985;91:354–361.

76. Powell HC, Myers RR, Mizisin AP, et al. Response of the axon and barrier endothelium to experimental allergic neuritis induced by autoreactive T cell lines. *Acta Neuropathol(Berl)* 1991;82:364–377.

77. Olee T, Powell HC, Brostoff SW. New minimum length requirement for a T cell epitope for experimental allergic neuritis. *J Neuroimmunol* 1990;27:187–190.

78. Powell HC, Olee T, Brostoff SW, Mizisin AP. Comparative histology of experimental allergic neuritis induced with minimum length neuritogenic peptides by adoptive transfer with sensitized cells or direct sensitization. *J Neuropathol Exp Neurol* 1991;50:658–674.

79. Olee T, Weise M, Powers J, Brostoff S. A T cell epitope for experimental allergic neuritis is an amphipathic alpha-helical structure. *J Neuroimmunol* 1989;21: 235–240.

80. Olee T, Powers JM, Brostoff SW. A T cell epitope for experimental allergic neuritis. *J Neuroimmunol* 1988;19: 167–173.

81. Linington C, Lassmann H, Ozawa K, et al. Cell adhesion molecules of the immunoglobulin supergene family as tissue-specific antoantigens: induction of experimental allergic neuritis (EAN) by P0 protein-specific T cell lines. *Eur J Immunol* 1992;22:1813–1817.

82. Linington C, Mann A, Izumo S, et al. Induction of experimental allergic neuritis in the BN rat: P2 protein-specific T cells overcome resistance to actively induced disease. *J Immunol* 1986;137:3826–3831.

83. Eylar EH, Toro Goyco E, Kessler MJ, Szymanska I. Induction of allergic neuritis in rhesus monkeys. *J Neuroimmunol* 1982;3:91–98.

84. Abromson-Leeman S, Bronson R, Dorf ME. Experimental autoimmune peripheral neuritis induced in BALB/c mice by myelin basic protein-specific T cell clones. *J Exp Med* 1995;182:587–592.

85. Lampert PW. Mechanism of demyelination in experimental allergic neuritis. Electron microscopic studies. *Lab Invest* 1969;20:127–138.

86. Rosen JL, Brown MJ, Hickey WF, Rostami A. Early myelin lesions in experimental allergic neuritis. *Muscle Nerve* 1990;13:629–636.

87. Hahn AF, Feasby TE, Wilkie L, Lovgren D. P2-peptide induced experimental allergic neuritis: a model to study axonal degeneration. *Acta Neuropathol (Berl)* 1991; 82:60–65.

88. Hahn AF, Feasby TE, Steele A, et al. Demyelination and axonal degeneration in Lewis rat experimental allergic neuritis depend on the myelin dosage. *Lab Invest* 1988;59:115–125.

89. Linington C, Izumo S, Suzuki M, et al. A permanent rat T cell line that mediates experimental allergic neuritis in the Lewis rat in vivo. *J Immunol* 1984;133: 1946–1950.

90. Heininger K, Stoll G, Linington C, et al. Conduction failure and nerve conduction slowing in experimental allergic neuritis induced by P2-specific T-cell lines. *Ann Neurol* 1986;19:44–49.

91. Taylor WA, Hughes RA. Responsiveness to P2 of blood- and cauda equina-derived lymphocytes in experimental allergic neuritis in the Lewis rat: preliminary characterisation of a P2-specific cauda equina-derived T cell line. *J Neuroimmunol* 1988;19:279–289.

92. Steinman L, Smith ME, Forno LS. Genetic control of susceptibility to experimental allergic neuritis and the immune response to P2 protein. *Neurology* 1981;31: 950–954.

93. Hughes RA, Kadlubowski M, Gray IA, Leibowitz S. Immune responses in experimental allergic neuritis. *J Neurol Neurosurg Psychiatry* 1981;44:565–569.

94. Holmdahl R, Olsson T, Moran T, Klareskog L. In vivo treatment of rats with monoclonal anti-T-cell antibodies. Immunohistochemical and functional analysis in normal rats and in experimental allergic neuritis. *Scand J Immunol* 1985;22:157–169.

95. Brosnan JV, Craggs RI, King RH, Thomas PK. Reduced susceptibility of T cell-deficient rats to induction of experimental allergic neuritis. *J Neuroimmunol* 1987;14: 267–282.

96. Jung S, Kramer S, Schluesener HJ, et al. Prevention and therapy of experimental autoimmune neuritis by an antibody against T cell receptors-alpha/beta. *J Immunol* 1992;148:3768–3775.

97. Hartung HP, Schäfer B, Fierz W, et al. Cyclosporin A prevents P2 T cell line-mediated experimental autoimmune neuritis (AT-EAN) in rat. *Neurosci Lett* 1987;83: 195–200.

98. Jung S, Toyka KV, Hartung H-P. T cell directed immunotherapy of inflammatory demyelination in the peripheral nervous system. Potent suppression of the effector phase of experimental autoimmune neuritis by anti-CD2 antibodies. *Brain* 1996;119:1079–1090.

99. Zhang XM, Esch TR, Clark L, et al. Neuritogenic Lewis rat T cells use Tcrb chains that include a new Tcrb-V8 family member. *Immunogenetics* 1994;40:266–270.

100. Clark L, Heber-Katz E, Rostami A. Shared T-cell receptor gene usage in experimental allergic neuritis and encephalomyelitis. *Ann Neurol* 1992;31:587–592.

101. Jung S, Hartung HP, Toyka KV. Shared T-cell receptor gene usage in experimental allergic neuritis and encephalomyelitis. *Ann Neurol* 1993;34:113–114.

102. Ota K, Irie H, Takahashi K. T cell subsets and Ia-positive cells in the sciatic nerve during the course of experimental allergic neuritis. *J Neuroimmunol* 1987;13: 283–292.

103. Strigard K, Brismar T, Olsson T, et al. T-lymphocyte subsets, functional deficits, and morphology in sciatic nerves during experimental allergic neuritis. *Muscle Nerve* 1987;10:329–337.

104. Olsson T, Holmdahl R, Klareskog L, et al. Dynamics of Ia-expressing cells and T lymphocytes of different subsets during experimental allergic neuritis in Lewis rats. *J Neurol Sci* 1984;66:141–149.

105. Hughes RAC, Atkinson PF, Gray IA, Taylor WA. Major histocompatibility antigens and lymphocyte subsets during experimental allergic neuritis in the Lewis rat. *J Neurol* 1987;234:390–395.

106. Brosnan JV, Fellowes R, Craggs RI, et al. Changes in lymphocyte subsets during the course of experimental allergic neuritis. *Brain* 1985;108:315–334.

107. Bevilacqua MP. Endothelial-leukocyte adhesion molecules. *Annu Rev Immunol* 1993;91:379–387.

108. Springer TA. Traffic signals for lymphocyte recirculation and leukocyte emigration: the multiple step paradigm. *Cell* 1994;76:301–314.

109. Bevilacqua MP, Nelson RM. Selectins. *J Clin Invest* 1993;91:379–387.

110. Hynes RO. Integrins: versatility, modulation, and signaling in cell adhesion. *Cell* 1992;69:11–25.

111. Schall TJ, Bacon KB. Chemokines, leukocyte trafficking and inflammation. *Curr Opin Immunol* 1994;6:865–873.

112. Stoll G, Jander S, Jung S, et al. Macrophages and endothelial cells express intercellular adhesion molecule-1 in immune-mediated demyelination but not in wallerian degeneration of the rat peripheral nervous system. *Lab Invest* 1993;68:637–644.

113. Jander S, et al. Vascular cell adhesion molecule-1 mRNA is expressed in immune-mediated and ischemic injury of the rat nervous system. *J Neuroimmunol* 1996;70: 75–80.

114. Archelos JJ, Mäurer M, Jung S, et al. Inhibition of experimental autoimmune neuritis by an antibody to the lymphocyte function-associated antigen-1. *Lab Invest* 1994;70:667–675.

115. Hartung HP, Reiners K, Michels M, et al. Serum levels of soluble E-selectin (ELAM-1) in immune-mediated neuropathies. *Neurology* 1994;44:1153–1158.

116. Oka N, Akiguchi I, Kawasaki T, et al. Elevated serum levels of endothelial leukocyte adhesion molecules in Guillain-Barré syndrome and chronic inflammatory demyelinating polyneuropathy. *Ann Neurol* 1994;35: 621–624.

117. Powell HC, Braheny SL, Myers RR, et al. Early changes in experimental allergic neuritis. *Lab Invest* 1983; 48:332–338.

118. Hahn AF, Feasby TE, Gilbert JJ. Blood-nerve barrier studies in experimental allergic neuritis. *Acta Neuropathol(Berl)* 1985;68:101–109.

119. Paul WE, Seder RA. Lymphocyte responses and cytokines. *Cell* 1994;76:241–251.

120. Hartung HP, Schäfer B, Van Der Meide P, et al. The role of interferon-gamma in the pathogenesis of experimental autoimmune disease of the peripheral nervous system. *Ann Neurol* 1990;27:247–257.

121. Schmidt B, Stoll G, Van Der Meide P, et al. Transient cellular expression of gamma-interferon in myelin-induced and T-cell line-mediated experimental autoimmune neuritis. *Brain* 1992;115:1633–1646.

122. Zhu J, Link H, Mix E, et al. Th1-like cell responses to peripheral nerve myelin components over the course of experimental allergic neuritis in Lewis rats. *Acta Neurol Scand* 1994;90:19–25.

123. Zhu J, Mix E, Olsson T, Link H. Cellular mRNA expression of interferon-gamma, IL-4 and transforming growth factor beta (TGF-beta) by rat mononuclear cells stimulated with peripheral nerve myelin antigens in experimental allergic neuritis. *Clin Exp Immunol* 1994; 98:306–312.

124. Stoll G, Jung S, Jander S, et al. Tumor necrosis factor-alpha in immune-mediated demyelination and wallerian degeneration of the rat peripheral nervous system. *J Neuroimmunol* 1993;45:175–182.

125. Redford EJ, Hall SM, Smith KJ. Vascular changes and demyelination induced by the intraneural injection of tumour necrosis factor. *Brain* 1995;118:869–878.

126. Said G, Hontebeyrie-Joskowicz M. Nerve lesions induced by macrophage activation. *Res Immunol* 1992; 143:589–599.

127. Selmaj K, Raine CS. Tumor necrosis factor mediates myelin and oligodendrocyte damage in vitro. *Ann Neurol* 1988;23:339–346.

128. Hartung HP. Immune-mediated demyelination. *Ann Neurol* 1993;33:563–567.

129. Hartung HP, Jung S, Stoll G, et al. Inflammatory mediators in demyelinating disorders of the CNS and PNS. *J Neuroimmunol* 1992;40:197–210.

130. Stoll G, Hartung HP. The role of macrophages in degeneration and immune-mediated demyelinating of the peripheral nervous system. *Adv Neuroimmunol* 1992;2: 163–179.

131. Hartung HP, Schäfer B, Heininger K, et al. The role of macrophages and eicosanoids in the pathogenesis of experimental allergic neuritis. Serial clinical, electrophysiological, biochemical and morphological observations. *Brain* 1988;111:1039–1059.

132. Brück W, Friede RL. Anti-macrophage CR3 antibody blocks myelin phagocytosis by macrophages in vitro. *Acta Neuropathol (Berl)* 1990;80:415–418.

133. Jung S, Huitinga I, Schmidt B, et al. Selective elimina-

tion of macrophages by dichlormethylene disphospho-nate-containing liposomes suppresses experimental autoimmune neuritis. *J Neurol Sci* 1993;119:195–202.

134. Tansey FA, Brosnan CF. Protection against experimental allergic neuritis with silica quartz dust. *J. Neuroimmunol* 1982;3:169–179.
135. Heininger K, Schäfer B, Hartung HP, et al. The role of macrophages in experimental autoimmune neuritis induced by a P2-specific T-cell line. *Ann Neurol* 1988;23:326–331.
136. Hartung HP, Schäfer B, Heininger K, Toyka KV. Suppression of experimental autoimmune neuritis by the oxygen radical scavengers superoxide dismutase and catalase. *Ann Neurol* 1988;23:453–460.
137. Stevens A, Lang R, Schabet M, et al. Spontaneous chemiluminescence activity of peripheral blood cells during experimental allergic neuritis (EAN). *J Neuroimmunol* 1990;27:33–40.
138. Halliwell B. Reactive oxygen species and the central nervous system. *J Neurochem* 1992;59:1609–1623.
139. Halliwell B, Gutteridge JM, Cross CE. Free radicals, antioxidants, and human disease: where are we now? *J Lab Clin Med* 1992;119:598–620.
140. Konat GW, Wiggins RC. Effect of reactive oxygen species on myelin membrane proteins. *J Neurochem* 1985;45:1113–1118.
141. Chia LS, Thompson JE, Moscarello MA. Disorder in human myelin induced by superoxide radical: an in vitro investigation. *Biochem Biophys Res Commun* 1983;117:141–146.
142. Zielasek J, Jung S, Gold R, et al. Administration of nitric oxide synthase inhibitors in experimental autoimmune neuritis and experimental autoimmune encephalomyelitis. *J Neuroimmunol* 1995;58:81–88.
143. Sobue G, Yamoto S, Hirayama M, et al. The role of macrophages in demyelination in experimental allergic neuritis. *J Neurol Sci* 1982;56:75–87.
144. Cammer W, Brosnan CF, Basile C, et al. Complement potentiates the degradation of myelin proteins by plasmin: implications for a mechanism of inflammatory demyelination. *Brain Res* 1986;364:91–101.
145. Cammer W, Brosnan CF, Bloom BR, Norton WT. Degradation of the P0, P1, and Pr proteins in peripheral nervous system myelin by plasmin: implications regarding the role of macrophages in demyelinating diseases. *J Neurochem* 1981;36:1506–1514.
146. Watson SL, Westland K, Pollard JD. An electrophysiological and histological study of trypsin induced demyelination. *J Neurol Sci* 1994;126:116–125.
147. Westland K, Pollard JD. Proteinase induced demyelination. An electrophysiological and histological study. *J Neurol Sci* 1987;82:41–53.
148. Schabet M, Whitaker JN, Schott K, et al. The use of protease inhibitors in experimental allergic neuritis. *J Neuroimmunol* 1991;31:265–272.
149. Brosnan CF, Lyman WD, Tansey FA, Carter TH. Quantitation of mast cells in experimental allergic neuritis. *J Neuropathol Exp Neurol* 1985;44:196–203.
150. Izumo S, Linington C, Wekerle H, Meyermann R. Morphologic study on experimental allergic neuritis mediated by T cell line specific for bovine P2 protein in Lewis rats. *Lab Invest* 1985;53:209–218.
151. Harvey GK, Toyka KV, Hartung HP. Effects of mast cell degranulation on blood-nerve barrier permeability and nerve conduction in vivo. *J Neurol Sci* 1994;125:102–109.

152. Brosnan CF, Tansey FA. Delayed onset of experimental allergic neuritis in rats treated with reserpine. *J Neuropathol Exp Neurol* 1984;43:84–93.
153. Gregorian SK, Lee WP, Beck LS, et al. Regulation of experimental autoimmune neuritis by transforming growth factor-beta 1. *Cell Immunol* 1994;156:102–112.
154. Jung S, Schluesener HJ, Schmidt B, et al. Therapeutic effect of transforming growth factor-beta 2 on actively induced EAN but not adoptive transfer EAN. *Immunology* 1994;83:545–551.
155. Jander S, Pohl J, Gillen C, Stoll G. Differential expression of interleukin-10 mRNA in Wallerian degeneration and immune-mediated inflammation of the rat peripheral nervous system. *J Neurosci Res* 1996;43:254–259.
156. Bai X-U, et al. IL-10 suppresses experimental autoimmune neuritis and down-regulates Th1-type immune responses. *Clin Immunol Immunopathol* 1997;83:117–126.
157. Kabelitz D, Pohl T, Pechhold K. Activation-induced cell death (apoptosis) of mature peripheral T lymphocytes. *Immunol Today* 1993;14:338–339.
158. Gold R, Hartung H-P, Lassmann H. T cell apoptosis in autoimmune diseases: termination of inflammation in the nervous system and other sites with specialized immune-defense mechanisms. *Trends Neurosci* 1997 (in press).
159. Zettl UK, Gold R, Toyka KV, Hartung H-P. Intravenous glucocorticosteroid treatment augments apoptosis of inflammatory T cells in experimental autoimmune neuritis (EAN) of the Lewis rat. *J Neuropathol Exp Neurol* 1995;54:540–547.
160. Zettl UK, Gold R, Hartung HP, Toyka KV. Apoptotic cell death of T lymphocytes in experimental autoimmune neuritis. *Neurosci Lett* 1994;176:75–79.
161. Zhu J, Link H, Weerth S, et al. The B cell repertoire in experimental allergic neuritis involves multiple myelin proteins and GM1. *J Neurol Sci* 1994;125:132–137.
162. Stoll G, Schmidt B, Jander S, et al. Presence of the terminal complement complex (C5b-9) precedes myelin degradation in immune-mediated demyelination of the rat peripheral nervous system. *Ann Neurol* 1991;30:147–155.
163. Vriesendorp FJ, Flynn RE, Pappolla MA, Koski CL. Complement depletion affects demyelination and inflammation in experimental allergic neuritis. *J Neuroimmunol* 1995;58:157–165.
164. Feasby TE, Gilbert JJ, Hahn AF, Neilson M. Complement depletion suppresses Lewis rat experimental allergic neuritis. *Brain Res* 1987;419:97–103.
165. Jung S, Toyka KV, Hartung H-P. Soluble complement receptor type 1 inhibits experimental autoimmune neuritis in Lewis rats. *Neurosci Lett* 1995;200:167–170.
166. Hafer-Macko CE, Sheikh KA, Li CY, et al. Immune attack on the Schwann cell surface in acute inflammatory demyelinating polyneuropathy. *Ann Neurol* 1996;39:625–635.
167. Spies JM, Pollard JD, Bonner JG, et al. Synergy between antibody and P2-reactive T cells in experimental allergic neuritis. *J Neuroimmunol* 1995;57:77–84.
168. Spies JM, Westland KW, Bonner JG, Pollard JD. Intraneural activated T cells cause focal breakdown of the blood-nerve barrier. *Brain* 1995;118:857–868.
169. Hahn AF, Feasby TE, Wilkie L, Lovgren D. Antigalactocerebroside antibody increases demyelination in adoptive transfer experimental allergic neuritis. *Muscle Nerve* 1993;16:1174–1180.

Chapter 5
Neural Regulation of the Immune System

Anthony T. Reder

The brain controls motor and sensory functions, endocrine hormone levels, and body temperature. The brain also affects the immune system in a number of ways:

1. During *development*, the brain exerts trophic effects on bones, muscles, and the immune system.
2. Even in the *adult, brain lesions* affect immunity.
3. *Cytokines and neurotransmitters are shared* between the brain and the immune system. The endocrine hormones and cytokines found in the periphery are frequently used as messengers in the central nervous system (CNS), often in the very neural pathways that regulate the relevant peripheral endocrine and immune responses.
4. The *autonomic nervous system* (*ANS*) controls the blood supply to the immune organs. It also releases neurotransmitters that cause demargination of immune cells from blood vessel walls, control vascular permeability, and promote inflammation. ANS lesions change the rate of development of the immune system and modify autoimmune diseases.
5. The *brain has relative immune privilege* compared to most of the rest of the body. In addition to the immune privilege within the brain, the CNS alters peripheral immunity by secreting immunoregulators and by modifying immune cells as they pass through the CNS parenchyma.
6. *Circadian rhythms*, generated in the CNS, affect immunity. There are daily fluctuations in responses to antigens and other immune activators, and also changes in responses to immunosuppressive therapy.

Common terms and concepts link the brain and the immune system. During the development of these two complex systems, many cell precursors are weeded out through apoptosis (programmed cell death). Positive selection of both immune cells and neurons requires a combination of adhesion molecules and cell-specific signals.

The two systems also share operational patterns after development. The mature immune system is a type of sensory organ that responds to noncognitive stimuli such as viruses and exogenous antigens (1). Memory of past events is stored and determines future responses to

similar situations. Networks of cells communicate with each other, often using the same messengers. Only a few cells respond to a stimulus—responses are specific because of convergence onto specialized areas in the CNS, or focusing of immune responses through highly specific subsets of immune cells. Inhibition of fellow cells is often the rule; many pathologic states—seizures and spasticity or autoimmune disease—are caused by loss of inhibition.

Finally, the two systems interact through analogous patterns. Neural-immune interactions are bidirectional, with positive and negative feedback loops. Crosstalk exists because of shared cytokines and neurotransmitters (2). This chapter focuses on several ways in which the brain affects immunity.

Brain Development and Immune Function

Affects of Early Brain Damage

Damage to one side of the brain at birth causes contralateral spasticity and weakness. As these children grow, they also typically have smaller hands, feet, and nail beds on the affected side. Early brain damage, especially to the parietal lobes (3), disrupts the contralateral outflow of trophic factors to developing limbs. Structural brain damage can also modify the immune system.

In utero, systemic insults to the developing brain alter immune regulation. In humans, prenatal insults may engender development of schizophrenia and modify adult behavior patterns by altering levels of neurotransmitters and glucocorticoid (GCC) receptors (GCCRs). These changes may be immune mediated, and can also affect immunity in the adult.

Viral infection and malnutrition in the second trimester of pregnancy increased the frequency of schizophrenia in England, Wales, Finland, and Denmark (4) though the effect was not seen in other series (5). During the fifth month, neurons migrate from the ventricular walls to the cortical plate. In schizophrenia, localization of neurons in the frontal and temporal lobes and the entorhinal parahippocampal region is distorted, with high numbers in the subcortical white matter and low numbers in the superficial white matter and overlying cortex (4). These NADPH diaphorase neurons are resistant to neurodegenerative effects, making them good markers for this type of histologic study. They also contain nitrous oxide synthase, somatostatin, and neuropeptide Y (NPY) and most are γ-amino butyric acid (GABA)-ergic, and migration defects can affect their control of behavior. A defect in neuronal migration through the cortical subplate could cause a lack of inhibitory GABAergic neurons in the overlying cortex. There is also a superabundance of glutaminergic associative inputs to the upper portion of layer IIIa of the cingulate cortex, possibly from a disturbance in neuronal migration or differentiation during the perinatal period (6). Loss of inhibitory neurons could allow a flooding or overflow of associations. A link between virus induction of a CNS immune response, microglial activation, and interference with neuronal migration is logical (5), but not proved. Microglia secrete multiple cytokines, and this ability changes during development. For instance, nitrous oxide is secreted by fetal, but not adult, human microglia (7).

In utero, immune stimuli alter behavior, and endocrine and immune function. Perinatal exposure to interleukin (IL)-1β causes decreased stress responses (increased motor activity, less of an increase in GCCs), a change in learning (increased locomotion and speed, but less able to learn complex tasks), and more female lordosis behavior by male rats (8).

Secondly, in rodents, primates, and humans, prenatal stress elevates maternal GCC levels and affects brain development and social behavior (9,10). Even a stimulus that is relatively inconsequential (to the animal husband), such as neonatal handling, results in elevated numbers of type II GCCRs in the hippocampus. This makes animals more sensitive to the negative feedback effects of stress into adulthood (11). Because CNS neurotransmitter levels and neuronal pathways are altered in utero, offspring have increased stress responses and behavioral changes throughout life. Offspring of a mother stressed during pregnancy are more susceptible to stress. Transfer of these traits from generation to generation is possible, reminiscent of Lamarck's 200-year-old theory that acquired characteristics can be transmitted.

Finally, in an extensive speculative essay, Geschwind and Galaburda (9) described how in utero and perinatal insults might modify both the brain and the immune system. Left-handedness, viewed throughout history and across cultures as abnormal or even evidence of demonic influence, was postulated to issue from prenatal disruption of CNS development, possibly a result of a "male-related factor." Strong left-handedness (actually "anomalous dominance") is statistically associated with autoimmune disorders ($p < 0.005$, n = 506), including atopy, asthma, thyroiditis, myasthenia gravis, inflammatory bowel disease, and migraine (and with the likelihood of being mathematically gifted or an architect). In addition, asthmatic mothers are more likely to have left-handed children (12), again suggesting that immune function affects brain development. More

rigidly defined experimental conditions reveal that certain manipulations of the CNS during development have a clear effect on immunity (see below).

The above-mentioned diseases link toxic or immune-mediated perinatal events to alterations in behavior and immune responses. However, the strongest association between an immunoregulatory molecule and the brain lies in a disorder with no obvious immune abnormalities.

Narcolepsy

This neurobehavioral disorder is genetically linked to major histocompatibility complex (MHC) DR and DQ; however, there are no evident immune abnormalities in narcolepsy. The linkage to HLA loci is stronger than in any known immune-mediated disease: 95% for HLA-DR2 and approximately 99% for HLA-DQw1 (13). (Specifically, the links are DR15/DRB1*1501, DQA1*0102, DQ6/DQB1*0602.) Concordance for monozygotic twins is only 15%, indicating that unknown environmental factors are important (14). Possibly related, HLA-DQw1 is linked to rapid-eye-movement (REM) sleep behavior disorder (15). Two explanations are possible: 1) There is a gene very near HLA-DQ that controls sleep, or 2) HLA-D itself affects sleep patterns, narcolepsy, cataplexy, hypnogogic hallucinations, and sleep paralysis. First, genes near these HLA loci include *TNF* (tumor necrosis factor, a cytokine involved in cell death and lymphocyte activation); *TAP* (transporter in antigen processing) and *LMP* (low molecular weight proteosome component), both involved in intracellular transport and processing of antigenic peptides; and *Bf* (properdin factor B, alternate complement pathway) (Fig. 5-1). These genes are normal in narcolepsy and are not obviously connected to sleep or behavior. In addition, there are no associated autoimmune diseases, and there is no increase of narcolepsy in women.

HLA is not expressed on normal neurons, and HLA expression in glial cells of the brain of adult narcoleptic humans and dogs is normal—class I MHC expression is minimal and class II expression is essentially absent (14). However, it is possible that HLA-D or a linked molecule could be expressed transiently in specific neuronal pathways during development, and modify neural adhesion molecules or act as a target for trophic or death factors. This presupposes that the function of HLA-D, or the promoter for the gene, somehow has an additional character that differs from other MHC molecules. Of interest, peripheral lymphocytes of narcoleptics express more HLA class II protein (14). In addition, there is almost no binding of muramyl dipeptide (MDP) to lymphocytes from narcoleptics or in DR2-positive controls (16). MDP is derived from bacterial cell walls and triggers the release of IL-1 from glia and monocytes. (The human gut contains 2 kg of feces and bacteria—bacterial products include useful vitamins and IL-1. Germ-free mice sleep less than normal, possibly because they have low levels of IL-1 or other bacterially derived sleep factors (17). However, a decrease in MDP receptors as a cause for narcolepsy is counterintuitive because a lack of MDP receptors would reduce

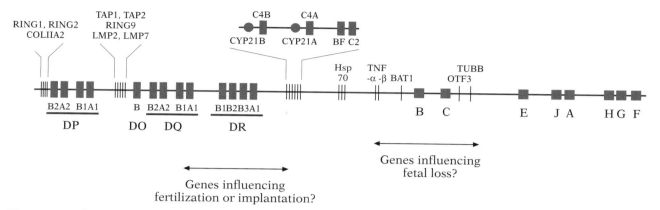

Figure 5-1. The human MHC and associated genes. HLA genes are labeled below the line and non-HLA genes are labeled above the line. The approximate locations are shown for a gene(s) hypothesized to influence fertilization or implantation (HLA-DR linked) and a gene(s) hypothesized to influence fetal loss (HLA-B linked). Class I genes: HLA-A, HLA-B, HLA-C, HLA-E, HLA-F, HLA-G, HLA-H, and HLA-J; class II genes: DRA1, HLA-DRB1, HLA-DRB2, HLA-DRB3, HLA-DQA1, HLA-DQA2, HLA-DQB1, HLA-DQB2, HLA-DOB, HLA-DPA1, HLA-DPA2, HLA-DPB1, and HLA-DPB2; complement component genes: C2, BF, C4A, and C4B; steroid 21-hydroxylase genes: CYP21A and CYP21B; proteosome-like genes: LMP2 and LMP7; ABC transporter genes: TAP1 and TAP2; collagen gene: COLIIA2; tumor necrosis factor genes: TNF-α and TNF-β; heat shock protein genes: Hsp70; transcription factor gene: OTF3; tubulin gene: TUBB; and genes of unknown function: RING1, RING2, RING9, and BAT1. (Modified from Ober C. Current topic: HLA and reproduction: lessons from studies in the Hutterites. *Placenta* 1995;16:569–577.)

IL-1 and sleep. This may suggest that MDP receptors in narcolepsy are defective or downregulated by an endogenous ligand—MDP or a related protein.

Immune and Endocrine Effects on Brain Cells, Autoimmune Disease, and Mate Selection

The immune system has potential developmental effects on schizophrenia and stress responses (as discussed above), and on other diseases and behaviors. Sapolsky demonstrated that neonatal and perinatal stress causes lifelong changes in hippocampal and amygdalar mineralocorticoid receptors (cortisol receptors; low-affinity, high-capacity, type I GCCRs) and in regulation of the hypothalamus-pituitary-adrenal (HPA) axis (10,18). Cautioning that bodies and psyches differ tremendously in their vulnerability to stress, he showed that social stress induces hypersecretion of adrenocorticotropin hormone (ACTH) and cortisol. High levels of GCC result in insensitivity to corticotropin-releasing hormone (CRF) and to dexamethasone feedback. Similar steroid resistance follows cerebral infarcts and characterizes depression. In addition, multiple sclerosis (MS), experimental autoimmune encephalomyelitis (EAE), and adjuvant arthritis are all linked to dysregulation of the HPA axis (see below). Finally, hypercortisolism synergizes with excitatory amino acids and stress to cause loss of hippocampal neurons and atrophy, and might exacerbate various neurodegenerative diseases (19).

Changes in CNS immune regulation during development and in adult brains can potentially affect neurons and glial cells. Neuronal survival and growth can be directly modified by electrical activity affecting adhesion molecule expression (20), by virus infection, and by cytokines. Neuronal growth is supported by IL-1 (induces nerve growth factor (NGF)), IL-2 (neurons of hippocampal dentate gyrus), IL-3 (cholinergic neurons), IL-4, IL-6 (catecholaminergic and cholinergic), TNF-α (hippocampus, septum, cortex), and transforming growth factor (TGF)-β (through anti-inflammatory effects) (21). These cytokines are produced by glial cells. Neuronal migration and function are also affected by the glial milieu. Substance P (SP), produced by neurons, also appears at certain stages of development and affects glial migration and function (22) as well as neuronal function (23). Microglial IL-1 modifies astrocyte shape, induces gliosis, and inhibits the growth of neonatal oligodendroglia; mature oligodendroglia are not affected by IL-1 (22,24).

Immune makeup also controls fertility and mate selection, an indirect effect of brain and behavior on immune regulation by future generations: HLA-disparate human mates have a much lower rate of miscarriages than do closely matched couples (25). This suggests there is selection against fetuses homozygous for HLA alleles, or homozygous for non-HLA genes linked to HLA. Rodents choose MHC-disparate mates (i.e., nonassortive mating). The selection is based on smell, possibly through characteristic MHC aroma in urine. In humans, the olfactory sense is certainly less keen, but human aromas or perfumes may be potent enough to influence behavior. MHC-based mate choice appears to occur in humans as well (26). Not all gentlemen prefer blonds, and women find male body odors more pleasant when the men's MHC makeup differs (27).

Brain Lesions

Brain lesions affect immunity. Bilateral anterior hypothalamic lesions reduce the number of thymus and spleen cells, and markedly decrease the mitogenic response to concanavalin A (ConA) 4 days after the lesion occurs (28,29). Lesions in the spinal cord, lateral reticular formation, and central amygdala are also immunosuppressive (30). Not all brain lesions are immunosuppressive; lesions of the hippocampus, raphe, basilar amygdala, mamillary bodies, and medial frontal lobe facilitate mitogenic responses (28–30). Note that the immune responses investigated were often chosen not for relevance to an immune-mediated neurologic disease, but because there were only a limited number of readouts available to measure immune function. More specific effects of CNS regions on immunity may be found in the future.

Patients with hemiplegia from unilateral CNS lesions or with peripheral nerve damage do not develop inflammation in the paretic limb (see later section on sympathetic nervous system (SNS) lesions).

Increased corticosteroid release is not solely responsible for brain lesions affecting immune regulation. Both frontal and anterior hypothalamic lesions induce the same temporary rise in corticosterone levels, but only the hypothalamic lesions are immunosuppressive (29). Pituitary hormones, however, have some additional influence on brain lesions. Hypophysectomy abrogates many of the inhibitory effects of anterior hypothalamic lesions (29). (Neuroendocrine regulation of immunity is discussed below.)

CNS areas with high local concentrations of cytokines often are specialized for functions related to those cytokines. For instance, in fever (31) a neurotransmitter that regulates thermoregulation in the hypothalamus (IL-1) is the same as the cytokine evoked in the periphery for control of temperature. There is also *regional* brain variation in nonneuronal cells. Mast cells are most numerous in the thalamus, astrocyte and microglial responses to cytokines vary at different sites, and levels of chemokines and cytokines such as the interferons (IFNs), IL-1, IL-6, TNF, cyclo-oxygenase, prostaglandin (PG)E, and PGD show wide regional differences (32). Astrocyte responses to adrenergic agonists, such as isoproterenol, α-melanocyte-stimulating hormone (MSH), and vasoactive intestinal peptide, (VIP) vary as much as 20-fold between different brain regions, and TGF-β_1 causes growth of brainstem astrocytes but not forebrain glia (33). Regional differences in the control of CNS cell growth and in cytokine responses could affect brain development and modify inflammatory brain disease.

Certain genetic disorders affect both the brain and the immune system. In *Down syndrome*, trisomy of chromosome 21 causes 50% higher expression of the (chromosome 21) IFN-α/β receptor gene. The extra receptors increase responses to interferons. Chromosome 16 in mice is homologous, and encodes the IFN receptor. Mice with trisomy 16 are supersensitive to IFNs, and have abnormalities related to Down syndrome—growth retardation, abnormal eye opening, and abnormal back curvature. These abnormalities are largely reversed when anti-IFN antibodies are given to pregnant females (34). This demonstrates that environment and genetic predisposition interact, and raises the question of whether similar molecular variation affects schizophrenia and narcolepsy. In *ataxia telangiectasia*, there is a defect in the recombinase needed to generate T-cell receptors and immunoglobulins. This causes an underdeveloped thymus, T-cell defects, and low levels of IgA and IgG, which are responsible for immunosuppression and frequent infections (which are associated with this neurologic disease).

Cytokines, Hormones, and Receptors Shared Between the Nervous and Immune Systems

The body is conservative in how it uses biologic technology for growth and homeostasis. Many signaling systems are present in both neurons and immune cells, and some couple the two systems (Tables 5-1 and 5-2) (35–71). Cytokines regulate the phenotype and function of specific, sometimes very small populations of neurons. This implies complex wiring and precise regulation of target neurons (32). Just as with CNS cells, white blood cells are a complex mixture of cell types in different states of differentiation or activation. Cytokines and neuropeptides, and their receptors, often are specific for immune cell subsets, just as certain neurotransmitters characterize neuronal subpopulations.

Trophic Factors Affecting Brain and Immune Cells

NGF, neurotrophins, cholinergic differentiation factor/leukemia inhibitory factor (CDF/LIF), ciliary neurotrophic factor (CNTF), and possibly IL-1, epidermal growth factor (EGF), fibroblast growth factor (FGF), insulin, insulin-like growth factor (IGF), platelet-derived growth factor (PDGF), and TGF-α and -β are needed for the survival and growth of neurons (32). These trophic factors also affect the function of immune cells. NGF is the most extensively studied.

In the CNS, forebrain cholinergic neurons are responsive to NGF. NGF also causes a widespread increase in the size and number of CNS mast cells, and induces histamine release from them. Mast cells appear late in MS plaques (72); their function and the inducing stimulus are unknown in MS.

NGF supports the survival of dorsal root ganglion (DRG) neurons, but withdrawal or lower levels of NGF induce programmed cell death. Fifty percent of fetal DRG cells have NGF receptors, but only 20% of adult DRG express them (71). These DRG neurons are small sensory unmyelinated C fibers. Their products, SP and somatostatin, modify immune responses. NGF also supports long adrenergic sympathetic neurons that densely innervate immune organs and have marked effects on immune regulation (see the section on sympathectomy below).

Table 5-1.
Neuropeptides Produced by Immune Cells

	Stimulus	*Inhibitor*	*Cells*	*References*
CRH	IL-2, PMA/PHA, lipoxygenation inhibition, inflamed tissue	CsA; substance P, dopamine, α-MSH (pit)	Thymic epithelial, lymphocytes, T cells, monocytes, PMN	35–39
ACTH	CRH, IL-1 pIC, viruses mitogens	GCC	Lymphocytes, monocytes, testes	40
α-MSH	IL-1, PMA, UV light	SST	Lymphocytes, keratinocytes	41
β-endorphin	5-HT, CRH; IL-1		T cells	36, 42
PreproENK A	ConA for T cells; LPS for B cells; IL-1 10^{-14-13} M, NF-κB, AP-1	IL-1 10^{-11-10} M	Th, mast, Mø, B cells, thymus	43–46
Growth hormone	GHRH, ConA, media (↓ tonic suppression)		T cells + B cells	47
PRL	?LHRH, ConA	TNF-α and IFN-γ → ↓PRL (in anterior pituitary)	Lymphocytes	
HCG	MLR		Spleen	?48 in 42
Luteinizing hormone	LHRH		Spleen, MNC	49
Oxytocin			Thymic epithelial	in 42
NGF				
Substance P	Granuloma		Eosinophil, monocytes, microglia	in 50
SST	Granuloma		Mø	in 50
TSH	TRH SEA (T cells); LPS (Mø)	T_3, T_4	T cells	51
VIP	Granuloma		Eosinophil, mast cell, PMN, thymic epithelial	in 42, 50, 52

CRH = corticotropin-releasing hormone; ACTH = adrenocorticotropic hormone; MSH = melanocyte-stimulating hormone; preproENK = preproenkephalin; PRL = prolactin; HCG = human chorionic gonadotropin; NGF = nerve growth factor; SST = somatostatin; TSH = thyroid-stimulating hormone; VIP = vasoactive intestinal peptide; IL- interleukin; PMA = phorbol myristate acetate; PHA = phytohemagglutinin; pIC = polyinosinic:polycytidylic acid; UV = ultraviolet; 5-HT = serotonin; LPS = lipopolysaccharide; NF = nuclear factor; AP = activator protein; GHRH = growth hormone–releasing hormone; LHRH = luteinizing hormone–releasing hormone; MLR = mixed lymphocyte reaction; TRH = thyroid-releasing hormone; SEA = staphylococcal entertoxin A; Mø = macrophage; CsA = cyclosporine; GCC = glucocorticoids; TNF = tumor necrosis factor; IFN = interferon; T_3 = triiodothyronine; T_4 = thyroxine; PMN = polymorphonuclear cells; Th = helper T lymphocytes; MNC = mononuclear cells.

NGF is synthesized by lymphocytes and macrophages. It directly enhances lymphocyte proliferation and differentiation, and is probably important in the development of the thymus and spleen (71).

Products of the HPA Axis Regulate Brain and Immune Function

The HPA axis illustrates the overlap between neurotransmitters, endocrine hormones, and cytokines (Fig. 5-2). Corticotropin-releasing hormone (CRH/CRF) is secreted by neurons in the paraventricular nucleus of the hypothalamus. CRH release is under the control of stimulators; such as serotonin, acetylcholine, and IL-1; and inhibitors, such as catelcholamines, GABA, and GCCs (cortisol in humans, corticosterone in rodents). CRH induces the release of ACTH from the pituitary; this release is also under feedback control by GCCs and cytokines. ACTH secretion is inhibited by feedback through GCCRs located in the hippocampi and possibly the pituitary (73). Of interest, these hippocampal GCCRs

are sensitive to prenatal and postnatal stress (10,18). Finally, ACTH induces the secretion of cortisol by the adrenal gland and the cortisol has inhibitory effects on upstream sites of the HPA.

Extrapituitary tissues also secrete ACTH (see Table 5-1), and do so in quantities significant enough to stimulate the adrenal secretion of GCCs. These tissues include the lungs, testes, and immune cells. In mice lacking pituitaries, Newcastle disease virus infection causes ACTH production by spleen cells, and in turn elevation of corticosterone levels (58). Mimicking the regulation of the HPA axis, CRF/arginine vasopressin (AVP) and IL-1β induce ACTH protein and messenger RNA (mRNA) in human mononuclear cells; dexamethasone inhibits secretion (40,74). In addition, peripheral immune activation feeds back onto the HPA axis. Newcastle disease virus infection elevates IL-1 levels and increases pituitary ACTH levels in intact mice and rats; peripheral immune responses also trigger firing of hypothalamic neurons (75).

CRF secretion from the hypothalamus is under

Table 5-2.
Neurotransmitter and Neuropeptide Receptors on Immune Cells

	Receptor on	Affinity or Subtype	Second Messenger	Effect	References
ACh	L, Mo, PMN, RBC, thymocytes	M1, M2 ligand binding; m3, m4, m5 mRNA	M1, 3, 5: PI M2, 4: cGMP	↑CTL, ↑ERFC, ↑Ig	53, 54
Dopamine	Thymus, spleen	D3	↑cAMP		55
Epinephrine	β2-adrR: B ≫ CD8 ≥ Mo > CD4	α ≤ β	β2→↑cAMP	↓T prolif.	56
NE		α ≫ β			
5-HT					
CRF	Mø > Th > B		cAMP	↓EAA, ↑ACTH, ↑IL-1, ↑IL-2, ↑IL-2R, ↓IFN-γ, ↓MHC induction, ↓Ab, ↑B prolif.	36, 57
ACTH	MNC, B, T, Mo	High and low CNS→PNS	cAMP	↓MHC II on Mø, ↓CTL, ↓Mø tumoricidal, ↓Ig	40, 58–60
α-MSH	Melanocytes			↓EAE, IFN-γ, ↓MHC I; antagonist of IL-1, IL-6, TNF-α, LPS	61
α-Endorphin	B, thymoma	ε, (μ,δ) R on L; 3000 R/Mo, 4000 R/granulocyte		↓Ig, ↓ConA, PHA prolif.; ↑CTL, ↓AMLR, ↓class II	62
β-Endorphin	T, Mo			↑monokines; ↑IFN-γ, ↑IL-2, ↑NK, ↑CTL, ↑↓T mitogen response (↑in rat, ↓in man), ↑hAMLR, ↓Ig Primes Mø as well as IFN-γ does	42, 62
γ-Endorphin	L	δR	↓cAMP	↑IFN-γ, ↑NK, ↑CTL	62
Enkephalin	?B, Mø > T	δ-2 R	↓Ig, ↑IL-2, ↑NK, ↑CTL	↓Ig, ↑IL-2, ↑NK, ↑CTL	62
CGRP	Mø, T		cAMP	↑Monokines (IL-1β, TNF-α, PGE2), not Mo prolif., ↑eos, ↓T prolif., ↓IL-2, ↓Ig	50, 52, 63
GH	T + ?B			Reverses thymic involution in aged rats, ↑CTL	64, 65
IGF-1	T	↓cAMP	Supports GH action		64, 65
PRL	B, Mø, thymus T	>360R/L (GH/PRL R superfamily)	PKC?, IRF-1	↑Prolif., ↑IL-2R, ↑IFN-γ, permits immune response/ reverses GCC, CsA effects (bromocriptine→ ↓Ig, ↓DTH, ?↓IFNα)	42, 65–67
HCG				?↑Thymocyte prolif.	42
Oxytocin	Thymus			↑Mitogen prolif., ↑IL-1, ↑IL-2, ↑IgG, M	68
Luteinizing hormone	T, Mø			↑Thymus size, T prolif.	69
LHRH	Thymocytes				
NPY				↓↑L prolif.	52
SP	B, T		Non-NK$_1$R, protein kinase	↑Mitogen-induced T prolif., ↑B, ↑mast cell activation, ↑IgA, ↑monokines and PG, ↑IFN-γ, ↑IL-2, ↑neurogenic inflammation	50, 52, 70
SST	T, B, ?Mø, thymocytes		↓cAMP	Low [SST] →↓mitogen-induced T prolif., high [SST] →↑; ↓Ig, ↓IFN-γ, ↓NK	50, 52, 70
TSH	T		PKC?	↓Mitogen-induced T prolif., ↑, ↓Ig, ↓NK	42, 58
VIP	MNC, T, B, CD4 > CD8		cAMP	↑IL-5, ↓IL-2, ↓IL-4, ↑Ig; replaces IL-2, alters mucosal migration of L	50, 52, 70

Table 5-2. *Continued*

	Receptor on	*Affinity or Subtype*	*Second Messenger*	*Effect*	*References*
NGF	L, Mø, thymus, mast, ?dendritic cells		cAMP	Replaces IL-2, ↑IL-2, ↑Ig, L prolif., mast cell hyperplasia and degranulation, activates PMN, basophils	52, 71

NE = norepinephrine; 5-HT serotonin; CRF = corticotropin-releasing factor; ACTH = adrenocorticotropin hormone; MSH = melanocyte-stimulating hormone; CGRP = calcitonin gene–related peptide; GH = growth hormone; IGF = insulin-like growth factor; PRL = prolactin; HCG = human chorionic gonadotropin; LHRH = luteinizing hormone–releasing hormone; NPY = neuropeptide Y; SP = substance P; SST = somatostatin; TSH = thyroid-stimulating hormone; VIP = vasoactive intestinal peptide; NGF = nerve growth factor; L = lymphocyte; Mo = monocyte; PMN = polymorphonuclear cells; RBC = red blood cells; β2-adrR = β$_2$-adrenergic receptor; B = B cells; Mø = macrophages; Th = helper T lymphocyte; MNC = mononuclear cells; T = T cells; CNS = central nervous system; PNS = peripheral nervous system; R = receptor; PI = phosphatidyl inositol; cGMP = cyclic guanosine monophosphate; cAMP = cycle adenosine monophosphate; Ig = immunoglobulin; IL = interleukin; NK = natural killer cells; CTL = cytolytic T lymphocytes; PKC = protein kinase C; IRF = interferon regulatory factor; ERFC = erythrocyte rosette-forming cells; EAA = experimental allergic arthritis; IFN = interferon; MHC = major histocompatibility complex; Ab = antibody; EAE = experimental autoimmune encephalomyelitis; TNF = tumor necrosis factor; LPS = lipopolysaccharide; PHA = phytohemagglutinin; AMLR = autologous mixed lymphocyte reaction; hAMLR = human autologous mixed lymphocyte reaction; PGE2 = prostaglandin E$_2$; eos = eosinophils; GCC = glucocorticoids; CsA = cyclosporine; DTH = delayed-type hypersensitivity; PG = prostaglandin; prolif. = proliferation.

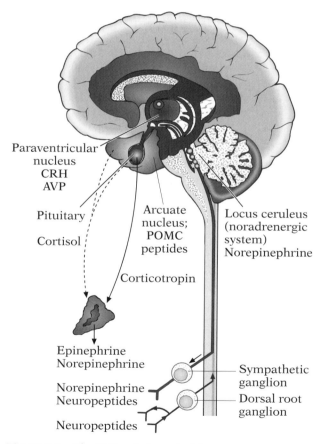

Figure 5-2. The HPA axis is central in responses to stress. CRH = corticotropin-releasing hormone; AVP = arginine vasopressin; POMC = proopiomelanocortin; GABA = γ-aminobutyric acid. (Modified from Flier JS, Underhill LH. The hypothalamic-pituitary-adrenal axis and immune-mediated information. *N Engl J Med* 1995;332:1351–1362.)

genetic control. This has profound implications for immune function and for behavior. Adjuvant arthritis can be experimentally induced in the Lewis strain of rats, but not in Fischer rats (76). Reduced GCC levels predispose to adjuvant arthritis and EAE in Lewis rats (77,78). On the flip side, Lewis rats are more resistant to infection and Fischer rats are more likely to develop cancer (79). The adjuvant arthritis–susceptible Lewis rats secrete lower levels of GCCs as arthritis develops—one reason they are unable to shut down the inflammatory response. Lewis rats have CRF-secreting neurons that are hyporesponsive to all stimulatory neurotransmitters (e.g., serotonin and IL-1), so feedback from peripheral inflammation is reduced and the immune response is not controlled by GCCs (80). The ACTH response to AVP, however, is normal (81). Finally, Lewis rats are more docile, explore more and produce fewer fecal boli in novel situations, and have increased benzodiazepine receptors in their paraventricular nuclei—all linked to the decrease in CRF secretion and low levels of corticosterone (82).

MS patients have subnormal HPA-axis feedback responses to dexamethasone during active disease (83), even though they have high resting cortisol levels (83,84), enlarged adrenal glands (85), and threefold increased numbers of CRF- and CRF/AVP-positive cells in the paraventricular nuclei (86,87). Indeed, subnormal feedback responses to dexamethasone are also present in cultured MS lymphocytes (83), indicating that higher steroid levels than normal are necessary to inhibit inflammation in MS. Even though many of these study findings seem to indicate that the HPA axis is overactive in MS, the cortisol produced is not sufficient to prevent exacerbations.

CRF has direct and indirect effects on immunity. CRF levels are high in inflammatory sites (38), and CRF mRNA and protein are produced in the thymus (thymic epithelial cells) and spleen (lymphocytes) (34,35). (Thymic epithelial cells also produce pregnenolone and deoxycorticosterone, which prevent apoptosis of immature thymocytes, and may be under CRH control. This may be important in thymic education and possibly autoimmune disease (88).) Unlike in hypothalamic neurons, IL-1 does not induce CRF secretion by immune cells (35).

CRF receptors are present on macrophages and helper T cells (see Table 5-2). CRF induces cyclic adenosine monophosphate (cAMP) in mononuclear cells, but appears to have stimulatory as well as inhibitory effects on immune function (56). Centrally administered CRF is immunosuppressive; effects are independent of circulating levels (56). This immunosuppression parallels CRF's activation of the SNS, which causes increased arousal, and inhibited feeding and sexual activity. Central effects of CRH are blocked by sympathectomy and β-adrenergic blockade.

Surprisingly, hypothalamic CRF mRNA levels fall during the peak of EAE severity, even though proopiomelanocortin (POMC) (ACTH) mRNA and corticosterone levels are high (89). This suggests 1) there is an extrahypothalamic source of CRF such as lymphocytes, or 2) that another mediator, such as AVP or a cytokine, is inducing POMC. Although CRF is the main inducer of POMC in acute stress, a more pronounced role for AVP is seen with chronic inflammatory stress, and possibly in MS (84,87).

POMC is cut into α-MSH, ACTH, and endorphins in the pituitary by a posttranslational process (Fig. 5-3). Lymphocytes also produce POMC mRNA and protein, but the processing can differ (40,58).

Regulation of POMC-derived peptides in lymphocytes is under some of the same control as in the pituitary. CRF and AVP, as well as viruses, polyinosinic:polycytidylic acid, and mitogens, induce ACTH and β-endorphin in lymphocytes (40,58,74). Splenic macrophages have low basal levels of ACTH; thioglycollate induces strong fluorescence in 80% of peritoneal macrophages (58). IL-1 is a more potent stimulus than CRF for production of POMC mRNA or ACTH in mononuclear cells; the situation is reversed in pituitary cells (40) (Blalock

JE, personal communication, 1993). The pathway is sometimes not direct; CRF and AVP induce IL-1 secretion by monocytes, and IL-1 in turn induces B cells (but not T cells) to secrete POMC-derived proteins (90).

POMC processing varies between the anterior and posterior pituitary as well as immune cell subsets. The anterior pituitary secretes $ACTH_{1-24 \text{ and } 1-39}$, whereas the posterior pituitary secretes $ACTH_{1-13}$ (α-MSH) and β-endorphin (processing is similar in the brain). Extrapituitary POMC mRNA is shorter than the pituitary form (91). Human mononuclear cells stimulated with CRF of Newcastle disease virus release $ACTH_{1-39}$ (Fig. 5-4) and β-endorphin; lipopolysaccharide induces secretion of $ACTH_{1-24}$ and α- or γ-endorphin (92). Immune cells also produce a novel form of ACTH ($ACTH_{1-25}$ instead of $ACTH_{1-24}$) (92). Thus, the HPA axis and the immune system exhibit cell-specific processing of large precursor molecules. The lymphocyte products might have different effects on immune function than do the pituitary products.

Intracellular "neuropeptides" in immune cells are often not located in neurosecretory granules, as in pituitary cells. Surprisingly, much of the CRF-like material is in the nuclear fraction of phytohemagglutinin (PHA)/phorbol myristate acetate (PMA)–stimulated mononuclear cells and T cells (36). ACTH-immunoreactive material appears in a small region of the nucleus of mononuclear cells 4 hours after stimulation with CRF or PMA (40). Prolactin, as well as FGF, IL-1, PDGF, and insulin, also translocate to the nucleus (93). This suggests that these peptides have direct intracellular feedback to the nucleus—the function is unknown. Finally, ACTH-immunoreactive material is localized in different areas of subtypes of T-cell clones.

ACTH, 10^{-10} to 10^{-5} M, elevates cAMP levels in lymphocytes (94). Elevated cAMP levels usually have an immunosuppressive effect on T cells and monocytes, and most of the ACTH effects listed in Table 5-2 are immunoinhibitory. ACTH processing further adds to the spectrum of immune regulation. $ACTH_{1-39}$ inhibits IFN-γ secretion and macrophage function (95,96), and

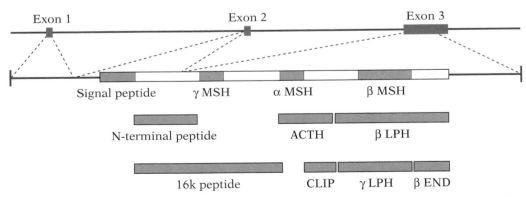

Figure 5-3.   Organization of pro-opiomelanocortin gene, RNA, and peptide products. MSH = melanocyte-stimulating hormone; ACTH = adrenocorticotropin hormone; LPH = lipotropic hormone; CLIP = corticotropin-like intermediate peptide; END = endorphin.

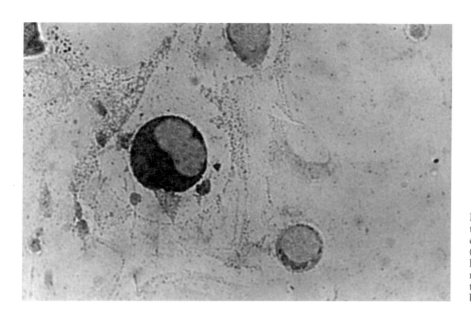

Figure 5-4. ACTH-like immunoreactive material in human mononuclear cells stimulated with $10-7$ M dbcAMP (dbc AMP = dibutyl cyclic AMP) for 18 hours. In this representative stain, a monocyte shows intense immunoreactivity and a lymphocyte is stained less brightly.

suppresses MHC class II expression, but $ACTH_{1-24}$ and α-MSH are ineffective (59). Of interest, a 2.1-kd peptide related to α-MSH copurified with ACTH from pituitary extracts; it was also a potent IFN-γ inhibitor. It is possible that this peptide is present in commercial porcine ACTH preparations used to treat MS exacerbations.

ACTH, especially $ACTH_{4-9 \text{ and } 4-10}$, and α-MSH also directly enhance nerve development and regeneration (97). In developing rodents, ACTH or its components accelerate development of the neuromuscular junction, accelerate eye opening, and increase spontaneous motor activity.

α-MSH ($ACTH_{1-13}$) has multiple effects on immunity. It elevates cAMP and profoundly inhibits IL-1– and TNF-inducible responses such as fever, acute-phase protein synthesis, PG secretion, increased capillary permeability, neutrophilia, and contact hypersensitivity (98,99). It is produced in the brain and pituitary, and also by lymphocytes and keratinocytes after stimulation by IL-1, PMA, or ultraviolet light (40). (Keratinocyte-derived α-MSH binds to melanocytes in the epidermis and causes skin pigmentation.) α-MSH inhibits lymphocyte IFN-γ secretion, possibly leading to a Th2 bias (100). It also induces IL-10 secretion by monocytes and promotes hapten-specific tolerance (101). These effects are particularly important in the "immunologically privileged" eye and brain where α-MSH acts along with TGF-β, calcitonin gene–related peptide (CGRP), and VIP to suppress inflammation. α-MSH and IL-10 inhibit the clinical and histologic signs of adjuvant-induced arthritis (60) and EAE (102,103). α-MSH, along with IL-1 receptor antagonist and soluble TNF receptor, may counterbalance the inflammation in the joints of patients with rheumatoid arthritis (104).

Endorphins bind to specific opiate receptors on immune cells, but they also work through nonopiate mechanisms. Endorphins bind to immune cells and decrease cAMP levels by inhibiting adenylate cyclase. These effects are usually inhibited by naloxone. α-Endorphin blocks T- and B-cell generation of antigen-specific IgM secretion (105). β-Endorphin, acting through a nonopiate receptor mechanism (not by blockable naloxone) doubles lymphocyte proliferation to T-cell mitogens, but has no effect on lipopoly-saccharide-stimulated spleen cells (106). Another group found that endorphins inhibit T-cell proliferation (not reversible by naloxone) and immunoglobulin synthesis, but increase IFN production and generation of cytolytic T lymphocytes (61).

Three precursors give rise to peptides that bind to opiate receptors—POMC (processed to ACTH, MSH, α-endorphin, β-endorphin, γ-endorphin, and β-lipotropic hormone), preproenkephalin A (met- and leu-enkephalin), and preproenkephalin B (dynorphin). Preproenkephalin is 0.4% of mRNA in activated T-cell clones (42). This approximates the amount of immunoglobulin mRNA produced by activated plasma cells, and suggests preproenkephalin has an important function. Enkephalins enhance T-cell immunity, but decrease immunoglobulin secretion (see Table 5-2).

Prolactin Regulates Immune Function

Prolactin (PRL) has a permissive or stimulatory role in immune regulation. It induces expression of the IFN regulatory factor-1 (IRF-1) transcription factor to allow entry of cells into S phase (107). PRL is taken up from fetal bovine serum and internalized in murine cells (108), but PRL mRNA is also synthesized in murine T cells (109) and human immune cells (108). PRL is required for IL-2–stimulated proliferation of lymphocytes (93), and enhanced mixed lymphocyte reactions, macrophage function, and IFN-γ secretion in some studies, but not others (96). Its absence, however, causes profound defects—anemia, shrunken immune organs, and nearly absent immune responses (110). These immune deficits are reversed when PRL is administered. PRL translocates directly to the nucleus during IL-2–stimulated mitogenesis (see above).

Dopamine from the arcuate nucleus and surrounding tuberoinfundibular system inhibits PRL secretion. Reduction of serum PRL levels with dopamine agonists such as bromocriptine can decrease cellular and humoral immunity, tumoricidal activity of macrophages, and secretion of IFN-γ (111,112). Bromocriptine (which decreases PRL) has some additive immunosuppressive effect with cyclosporine in uveitis (113), but immunosuppression is not obvious in Parkinson's disease patients treated with bromocriptine (109).

Conversely, breast-feeding and dopamine antagonists such as neuroleptics stimulate PRL release. The possibility that breast-feeding could activate immune cells and exacerbate inflammatory diseases has been investigated. There is a postpartum increase in exacerbations in MS, but the increase with breast-feeding is not statistically significant (114). Moreover, baseline PRL levels are normal in MS, and cyclosporine, which blocks the binding of PRL to its receptor, does not elevate PRL levels in MS patients (111). This makes a role for PRL in MS unlikely, in keeping with the permissive nature of PRL for immune function.

Second Messengers Shared Between the Brain and the Immune System

Finally, neuropeptides usually trigger the same second messengers in the brain and immune systems (see Table 5-2). In general, cAMP inhibits immune cells, and cyclic guanosine monophosphate is stimulatory. β$_2$-Adrenergic agonists elevate cAMP levels, but as a single signal they have only a modest effect on resting immune cells (2) (see below). Activation by mitogens allows immune cells to move through the cell cycle, and cAMP agonists then synergize with mitogens to raise cAMP levels. cAMP activation is also dependent on the activation state of the receptor/G protein complex. Although PGE$_2$ and isoproterenol elevate cAMP levels to the same extent, PGE$_2$ is 100-fold more potent in regulating some immune functions (115).

The Autonomic Nervous System Controls Peripheral Immune Responses

The thymus, spleen, lymph nodes, and gut-associated lymphoid tissue (GALT—Peyer's patches, immunocytes within the lamina propria) are richly innervated by the ANS (116) (Fig. 5-5). This innervation is not coincidence. Cells in peripheral immune organs are bathed in norepinephrine and neuropeptides (thymus—VIP, NPY, SP, CGRP; spleen—cholecystokinin, NPY, metenkephalin, CGRP, SP, neurotensin; GALT—NPY, SP,

leu-enkephalin, cholecystokinin) (117). Local concentrations of norepinephrine reach 10^{-6} M in the spleen. Endocrine organs are also densely innervated, which suggests that immune cells in endocrine organs would be subjected to similar influences.

During spleen development, tyrosine hydroxylase (TH)–positive nerve fibers mature in parallel with the immune architecture. By day 14, norepinephrine concentrations and β-adrenergic receptors on lymphocytes reach adult levels, and TH-positive nerves are densely distributed throughout the periarteriolar lymphatic sheath in the white pulp. β-Adrenergic receptor–positive cells also increase in the thymic medulla during development (118). Innervation of lymphoid tissue is usually regional and specific—zones of T cells and plasma cells, but not developing B cells, are "innervated" (117).

In addition to the "hard wiring" from peripheral nerves impinging on immune cells, cytokines and circulating hormones such as pituitary ACTH and α-MSH, and adrenal cortisol and epinephrine, are likely to interact with ANS products. The ANS can potentially modify the function of these peripheral immune organs by affecting development of immunity, immune activation, immune tolerance (including oral tolerance), or anergy.

Generalized Effects on Immune Regulation; Destruction Modifies Immunity

6-Hydroxydopamine (6-OHDA) or antibodies to NGF ablate central catecholaminergic and peripheral sympathetic pathways. In adults, 6-OHDA acutely destroys the ANS, causing a surge of catecholamines from dying nerves. These catecholamines transiently inhibit immune functions.

In the fetus, anti-NGF and 6-OHDA are able to penetrate the blood-brain barrier, so that central noradrenergic and dopaminergic pathways are also destroyed. In fetal or newborn animals, this permanently reduces SNS release of norepinephrine and colocalized peptides such as NPY. These animals are half the normal size, lethargic, and hypothermic. They have ptosis from ciliary nerve damage, small sclerotic sympathetic ganglia, atrophic thymuses, and hyperactive immune systems from SNS damage. In addition, vascular changes occur after sympathectomy; tumor metastases spread easily through alterations in the blood supply or an enhanced ability to extravasate through blood vessels (119).

When the SNS is ablated in newborns, spleen norepinephrine levels drop dramatically, and the tonic inhibitory effect of norepinephrine on immune responses is removed (a situation opposite that seen in acute SNS ablation in adult animals). The number of β-adrenergic receptors on lymphocytes doubles (120). The increase in β-adrenergic receptors on lymphocytes is a form of denervation supersensitivity, and the lymphocytes are hyperresponsive to adrenergic agonists. After sympathectomy, NK cells appear earlier in development, and the number of CD8+ T cells is halved.

With the low levels of (immunoinhibitory) catecholamines after neonatal sympathectomy, there are

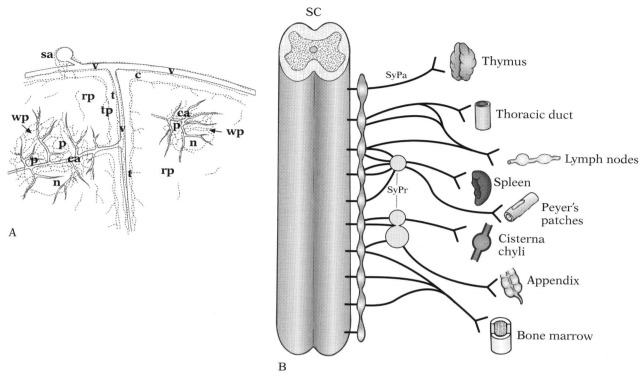

Figure 5-5. Noradrenergic innervation of the spleen. Noradrenergic fibers enter the spleen around the splenic artery (sa), travel with the vasculature in plexuses (v), and continue into the spleen along the trabeculae (t) in trabecular plexuses (tp). Fibers from both the vascular and trabecular plexuses enter the white pulp (wp), continuing mainly along the central artery (ca) and its branches. Noradrenergic varicosities radiate from these plexuses into the periarterial lymphatic sheath (p), but avoid the nodular areas (n). These parenchymal fibers end among fields of lymphocyte and other cell types. rp = red pulp. (Modified from Felten DL, et al. Noradrenergic and peptidergic innervation of lymphoid tissue. *J Immunol* 1985;135:755s–765s.)

increased mitogen responses, immunoglobulin secretion (reviewed elsewhere (121)), and cytokine production (122). Autoimmune diseases are worse, including EAE (123) and experimental autoimmune myasthenia gravis (124). As a corollary, β-adrenergic agonists would be expected to inhibit autoimmune disease.

Multiple Sclerosis as a Model of Denervation Supersensitivity

In progressive MS, the numbers of β-adrenergic receptors are elevated on lymphocytes, especially on suppressor T cells (125). Baseline cAMP levels and the stimulated increase in cAMP are also greater in the CD8 population. There is also a modest increase in the numbers of β-adrenergic receptors on T cells (126). Since Th1 cells respond to cAMP agonists much more vigorously than do Th2 cells (78), the modest increase in the numbers of β-adrenergic receptors in the helper T-cell population in MS is probably from a selective change on Th1 cells. Ordinarily, baseline cAMP levels are higher in normal CD8 than CD4 cells, but both T-cell subsets show a 10-fold increase after stimulation with isopro-

terenol (55). The β-adrenergic receptors in MS are supersensitive, and in a high-affinity state. Elevation of cAMP levels caused by more numerous, more responsive β-adrenergic receptors may inhibit suppressor cells (55), but also may inhibit Th1 cells.

Beta-adrenergic drugs affect immune responses in normal cells, and are likely to do so in MS. Catecholamines (such as epinephrine and norepinephrine, which raise intracellular cAMP levels) affect immunity. cAMP inhibits the function of Th cells and monocytes (78), but is essential for immunoglobulin secretion (127). Therapy with terbutaline, a β$_2$-adrenergic agonist, increases ConA suppressor function (Reder AT, et al., unpublished data, 1989). Whether terbutaline acts through downregulation of β-adrenergic receptors on immune cells or through an effect of Th1 cells is unknown.

In parallel with the changes in β-adrenergic receptors, M2 muscarinic receptors are increased on CD4 T cells in active MS. Elevation of cyclic guanosine monophosphate levels through the M2 receptors could activate helper T cells (52).

Several mechanisms can alter receptor levels. One indication is that the SNS is abnormal in progressive MS. The amplitudes of sympathetic skin responses, triggered by a mild electrical shock, are absent or reduced in these patients. R-R variation on electrocardiograms and bowel motility are also abnormal, again reflecting ANS dysfunction. The parallel between these SNS changes and experimental sympathectomy is obvious, but again, several mechanisms could account for peripheral SNS changes in MS, a CNS disease. One possibility is that plaques in the spinal cord disrupt CNS sympathetic pathways, and in parallel, cause the leg spasticity so commonly seen in progressive MS (Arnason BGW, personal communication, 1988). This would induce long-term changes in lymphocyte function from chronic loss of SNS input to immune organs. Induction of β-adrenergic receptors on immune cells by an unknown stimulus is also possible.

We reasoned that if the SNS were disrupted in MS, then patients would have subnormal orthostatic responses. Upon standing, the SNS releases norepinephrine and neuropeptides. NPY is cosecreted with norepinephrine by sympathetic nerves and is relatively specific for SNS fibers innervating immune organs. It also acts as a vasopressor at nanomolar amounts by increasing the intracellular concentrations of Ca^{2+} in blood vessels and potentiates the effects of norepinephrine, which acts through G proteins (128). Surprisingly, resting and orthostatic release of epinephrine, norepinephrine, and NPY in MS was equivalent or above levels of that in normal controls (55) (Reder AT, unpublished data, 1988). This suggests that most SNS fibers, including the norepinephrine/NPY fiber subset, are spared in MS patients with progressive disease. However, there is a conjunction of high resting serum norepinephrine along with high levels of β-adrenergic receptors in progressive MS. Feedback theory suggests this is an unstable situation, and that fluctuations in serum catecholamines might have a pronounced effect in MS.

Arthritis as a Model of Profound Local Effects of the SNS

Occasionally patients who have unilateral paralyzing CNS or peripheral nervous system damage will develop rheumatoid arthritis (129). The paralyzed limb is not affected by rheumatoid arthritis. Gout and osteoarthritis are also less severe in the denervated limb. This phenomenon has also been seen in 1) Heberden's nodes in osteoarthritis, 2) tophaceous deposits in gout, and 3) experimental adjuvant arthritis after sciatic nerve transection. In humans, regional sympathetic block with sympatholytic agents such as guanethidine reduces inflammation in reflex sympathetic dystrophy and in rheumatoid arthritis. In (bilateral) adjuvant-induced arthritis in the rat, sciatic nerve section prevents inflammation and joint injury in the treated limb; sympathectomy (destruction of SNS efferents) and capsaicin (nociceptive afferents) also prevent arthritis. Furthermore, spontaneously hypertensive rats have increased sympathetic tone and have more severe adjuvant-

induced arthritis. The severity of arthritis is proportional to the density of SNS innervation and SP content; distal more than proximal joints are richly innervated and most severely affected.

SP is present in 20% of the small bipolar dorsal root ganglia cells. These cells send impulses and SP to laminae I and II of the spinal cord. Surprisingly, 90% of a dorsal root ganglion cell's SP is antidromically released in the periphery by nociceptive C-fibers (130). These fibers, plus a feedback loop between local inflammation and SNS efferents (axon reflex), control inflammation. There is a symmetric inflammatory response on the contralateral side after (antidromic) stimulation of one hindlimb through spinal cord interconnections (130). SP, somatostatin, VIP, and CGRP released by peripheral nervous system fibers help trigger the classic weal-and-flare response after skin irritation. SP induces vasodilatation, increases vascular permeability and polymorphonuclear cell adhesion and activation, and causes mast cells to release histamine (131) and possibly IL-1, IL-3, IL-4, IL-5, IL-6, IFN-γ, and granulocyte-macrophage colony-stimulating factor (132). These lymphokines are all capable of amplifying immune responses. When SP is absent, as in transgenic mice with antibodies to SP expressed by neurons, pain in not affected but neurogenic skin inflammation is markedly reduced (23). Thus, SP has profound effects on immune function as well as on the sensation of pain.

SNS Neuropeptides Have Direct Effects on Immune Cells

VIP, somatostatin, and SP are released by SNS fibers in the gut lamina propria, in apposition to immune cells (lymphocytes, plasma cells, macrophages, mast cells, and eosinophils). As its name indicates, this lamina is very close to the gut lumen. VIP and somatostatin inhibit immunoglobulin secretion and T-cell proliferation to mitogens; SP stimulates proliferation and IgA secretion (69) (see Tables 5-1 and 5-2). Opioids are also produced by the SNS and immune cells. They include α-, β-, and γ-endorphins and met- and leu-enkephalins, and have been discussed already.

NPY, as well as cosecreted β-adrenergic agonists, affect immune cell function. NPY, at levels seen in serum (2–20 pM), enhances mitogen-induced T-cell proliferation (133). This stimulation is not mediated through an intracellular influx of Ca^{2+}, so a G protein is suspect. The effects of NPY in the splenic microenvironment are unknown.

Immune Privilege of the Brain

The immune privilege of the brain sometimes extends outside the CNS. The brain is an immunologically privileged site because of 1) minimal MHC and costimulatory molecule expression on brain cells or on capillary endothelial cells (induction of anergy, lack of activation), 2) the blood-brain barrier (reduced white blood cell trafficking), and 3) endogenous immunosuppressive cytokines secreted by glial cells (PG, TGF-β). The eyes and testes are also immunologically privileged. The eye, an extension of the CNS, also induces anterior chamber-associated immune deviation (ACAID)—a switch from Th1 and Th2 responses (discussed in detail in Chapter 3).

Circulating immune cells in normal people are sometimes reactive to CNS antigens, but normal people have no autoimmune disease. Relatives of MS patients have the same number of myelin basic protein–reactive cells as do the patients, yet the relatives do not develop MS (134). Several factors induce suppression of autoimmune responses. Most autoreactive cells are deleted in the thymus during early development, but many brain antigens are presumably not presented to thymic cells. Postnatally, there is some penetration of the normal blood-brain barrier by T cells. Even if these T cells recognize brain antigens, they do not react—likely a consequence of locally produced anergy and immunosuppressive cytokines. Anergy is induced when antigen is seen without costimulation (i.e., when there are no B7 molecules on antigen-presenting or endothelial cells, and no IL-2 is present). The normal CNS lacks these costimulatory molecules. These anergized/tolerized cells do not react against brain antigens and moreover could prevent other CNS-reactive cells from attacking the brain (135).

Brain tumors secrete immunosuppressive compounds that reach the periphery. The invasiveness of gliomas is correlated with TGF-β and PDGF secretion (136). These immunosuppressive cytokines prevent cytolytic cells from destroying the tumors in the brain, and also dramatically reduce peripheral immune responses (see also Chapters 10, 15, 18).

Circadian Rhythms, Controlled by the CNS, Affect Immune Responses

All eukaryotic organisms have diurnal physiologic rhythms. These rhythms have marked effects on normal regulation of body physiology. The rhythms are derived from endogenous oscillators sensitive to periodic environmental stimuli (*zeitgebers*, such as light). In mammals, the pacemaker for circadian changes is located in the suprachiasmatic nuclei of the anterior hypothalamus immediately above the optic chiasm. Circadian rhythms are impaired in some brain diseases, including general paresis of the insane, Wernicke's encephalopathy, Alzheimer's disease, and localized hypothalamic disorders.

Circadian changes in catecholamines and endocrine hormones modify immune responses. Maximal immune responses occur at night in humans (137). Plasma epinephrine and cAMP levels reach a nadir at 4 AM (138), and cortisol levels fall throughout the day and do not begin to rise until the early morning hours. (Cortisol levels are lowest at midnight and reach their maximum at 6 AM.) Catecholamines and GCCs inhibit inflammation, but there is a several-hour lag in cortisol effects. It is no coincidence that asthma attacks are much more frequent between midnight and 5 AM, and that pulmonary function is worst at 4 AM (139). Around

midnight or the early morning hours, the number of circulating lymphocytes peaks (140), and dermal weal-and-flare reactions and hay fever symptoms are most pronounced (141).

Rheumatoid hands are weaker and joints are more swollen at 6 AM; nonsteroidal anti-inflammatory drugs are most effective when given before bedtime (137). Levels of circulating white blood cells, including lymphocytes, monocytes, and polymorphonuclear cells, are lowest at 8 AM and highest at midnight (140), owing to redistribution from other compartments. Maximum proliferation to mitogens (at 6 AM) lags 6 hours after the lymphocyte peak. All of these phenomena indicate that immune responsiveness is heightened in the early morning.

Cytokine levels show circadian variability and modify CNS control of behavior and metabolic homeostasis. Serum IL-1 concentrations correlate with sleep; IL-1 (endogenous pyrogen) is a major factor in the lethargy engendered by bacterial infection. The highest IL-1 levels occur at the beginning of sleep; levels of growth hormone-releasing hormone, nitric oxide, and PGD_2 also rise at this time (142). IL-1 and these other agents all induce sleep. Other factors regulate this periodic behavior. (Sleep is opposed by anti-IL-1 antibodies, and by α-MSH, CRH, ACTH, GCCs, PGE$_2$, IL-10, and arginine analogues (nitrous oxide synthase inhibitors); it is stimulated by IFN-α and IFN-β, acidic FGF, TNF-α, TNF-β, IGF, PRL, and VIP.) In addition, levels of β-endorphin, a pituitary product, are inversely correlated with fever; although GCC levels are likely to be the most potent circadian temperature regulators (143). α-MSH, from the same POMC precursor as β-endorphin, is also an inhibitor of IL-1. Other cytokines such as IL-6, IL-2, TNF-α, and granulocyte-macrophage colony-stimulating factor have circadian rhythms (144,145). It follows that immune responses, as well as sleep and body temperature, would vary during the course of the day.

Circadian changes affect the symptoms of immune-mediated diseases, even without directly affecting immunity. The symptoms of MS are affected by circadian *temperature* changes. One of the most common symptoms of MS is fatigue. It presumably stems from a combination of cytokines and temperature effects that disturb impulse conduction. Body temperature rises as cortisol levels fall in the afternoon. Fatigue in MS patients is frequently most severe in the afternoon; demyelinated axons have a reduced safety factor and do not conduct impulses when the body temperature rises. This is the basis for the "hot-bath test," which amplifies clinical and subclinical MS symptoms. Fortunately, ice water can dramatically reverse heat-induced deficits (146).

Chronotherapy takes into account the normal daily rhythms in hormone levels and how circadian rhythms affect drug treatments. For asthma therapy, β$_2$-adrenergic agonists and theophylline can be given in the evening to compensate for the fall in epinephrine levels at 4 AM. Oral GCCs are most potent if given in the evening. Unfortunately, evening GCC administration is most likely to suppress the HPA axis. GCCs should be administered in the morning daily or every other day to alleviate side effects. Administration of two thirds of a dose in the morning and one third in the afternoon allows carryover into the night without markedly suppressing the HPA axis (141). Circadian immune responses have not been studied in MS and other inflammatory neurologic diseases. Based on the clear circadian effects in asthma and rheumatoid arthritis, circadian effects may be potent.

References

1. Blalock JE. The immune system as a sensory organ. *J Immunol* 1984;132:1067–1070.
2. Roszman TL, Carlson SL. Neural-immune interactions: circuits and networks. *Prog Neuroendocrinimmunol* 1991;4:69–78.
3. Menkes JH. *Textbook of child neurology.* Philadelphia: Lea & Febiger, 1985.
4. Akbarian S, Bunney WE, Potkin SG. Altered distribution of nicotinamide-adenine dinucleotide phosphate-diaphorase cells in frontal lobe of schizophrenics implies disturbances of cortical development. *Arch Gen Pyschiatry* 1993;50:169–177.
5. Fricchione GL, Bilfinger TV, Stefano GB. The macrophage and neuropsychiatric disorders. *Neuropsychiatry Neuropsychol Behav Neurol* 1996;9:16–29.
6. Benes RM. Neurobiological investigations in cingulate cortex of schizophrenic brain. *Schizophr Bull* 1993;19:537–539.
7. Lee SC, Liu W, Dickson DW, et al. Cytokine production by human fetal microglia and astrocytes. *J Immunol* 1993;150:2659–2667.
8. Götz F, Dörner G, Malz U, et al. Short- and long-term effects of perinatal interleukin-1β-application in rats. *Neuroendocrinology* 1993;58:344–351.
9. Geschwind N, Galaburda AM. Cerebral lateralization. *Arch Neurol* 1985;42:428–459, 521–552, 634–654.
10. Sapolsky RM. Individual differences and the stress response. *Semin Neurosci* 1994;6:261–269.
11. Meaney MJ, Aitken DH, Viau V, et al. Neonatal handling alters adrenocortical negative feedback sensitivity and hippocampal type II glucocorticoid receptor binding in the rat. *Neuroendocrinology* 1989;50:597–604.
12. Weinstein RE, Gurvitz M, Greenberg D, et al. Altered cerebral dominance in atopy and in children of asthmatic mothers. *Ann NY Acad Sci* 1992;650:25–29.
13. Aldrich MS. The neurobiology of narcolepsy-cataplexy. *Prog Neurobiol* 1993;41:533–541.
14. Mignot E, Tafti M, Dement WC, Grumet FC. Narcolepsy and immunity. *Adv Neuroimmunol* 1995;5:23–37.
15. Schenck CH, Garcia-Rill E, Segall M, et al. HLA class II genes associated with REM sleep behavior disorder. *Ann Neurol* 1996;39:261–263.
16. Silverman DH, Sayegh MH, Alvarez CE, et al. HLA class II-restricted binding of muramyl peptides to B lymphocytes of normal and narcoleptic subjects. *Hum Immunol* 1990;27:145–154.
17. Krueger JM, Karnovsky ML. Sleep as a neuroimmune phenomenon: a brief historical perspective. *Adv Neuroimmunol* 1995;5:5–12.
18. Sapolsky RM, Krey LC, McEwen BS. Stress down-regulates corticosterone receptors in a site-specific manner in the brain. *Endocrinology* 1984;114:287–292.
19. Sapolsky RM. Glucocorticoids, stress and exacerbation of excitotoxic neuron death. *Semin Neurosci* 1994;6:323–331.
20. Itoh K, Stevens B, Schachner M, Fields RD. Regulated expression of the neural cell adhesion molecule L1 by specific patterns of neural impulses. *Science* 1995;270:1369–1372.
21. Sei Y, Vitkovic L, Yokoyama MM. Cytokines in the central nervous system: regulatory roles in neuronal function, cell death and repair. *Neuroimmunomodulation* 1995;2:121–133.
22. Merrill JE. Tumor necrosis factor alpha, interleukin 1 and related cytokines in brain development: normal and pathological. *Dev Neurosci* 1992;14:1–10.
23. Piccioli P, Di Luzio A, Amann R, et al. Neuroantibodies: ectopic expression of a recombinant anti-substance P antibody in the central nervous system of transgenic mice. *Neuron* 1995;15:373–384.
24. Giulian D, Lachman LB. Interleukin-1 stimulation of astroglial proliferation after brain injury. *Science* 1985;228:497–499.
25. Ober C, Elias S, Kostyu DD, Hauck WW. Decreased fecundability in Hutterite couples sharing HLA-DR. *Am J Hum Genet* 1992;50:6–14.
26. Ober C. Current topic: HLA and reproduction: lesions from studies in the Hutterites. *Placenta* 1995;16:569–577.
27. Wedekind C, Seebeck T, Bettens F, Paepke AJ. MHC-dependent mate preferences in humans. *Proc R Soc Med* 1995;260:245–249.
28. Cross RJ, Markesbery WR, Brooks WH, Roszman TL. Hypothalamic-immune interactions. I. The acute effect of anterior hypothalamic lesions on the immune response. *Brain Res* 1980;196:79–87.
29. Roszman TL, Jackson JC, Cross RJ, et al. Neuroanatomic and neurotransmitter influences on immune function. *J Immunol* 1985;135:769s–772s.
30. Petrovicky P, Masek K, Seifert J. Brain regulatory system for the immune response: immunopharmacology and morphology. *Neuroimmunomodulation* 1994;1:165–173.
31. Breder CD, Dinarello CA, Saper CB. Interleukin-1 immunoreactive innervation of the human hypothalamus. *Science* 1988;240:321–323.
32. Patterson PH, Nawa H. Neuronal differentiation factors/cytokines and synaptic plasticity. *Neuron* 1993;10:123–137.
33. Johns LD, Babcock G, Green D, et al. Transforming growth factor-β₁ differentially regulates proliferation and MHC class-II antigen expression in forebrain and brainstem astrocyte primary cultures. *Brain Res* 1992;585:229–236.
34. Maroun LE. Anti-interferon immunoglobulins can improve the trisomy 16 mouse phenotype. *Teratology* 1995;51:329–335.
35. Stephanou A, Jessop DS, Knight RA, Lightman SL. Corticotrophin-releasing factor-like immunoreactivity and mRNA in human leukocytes. *Brain Behav Immun* 1990;4:67–73.
36. Aird F, Clevenger CV, Prystowskky MB, Redei E. Corticotropin-releasing factor mRNA in rat thymus and spleen. *Proc Natl Acad Sci USA* 1993;90:7104–7108.
37. Ekman R, Servenius B, Castro MG, et al. Biosynthesis of corticotropin-releasing hormone in human T-lymphocytes. *J Neuroimmunol* 1993;44:7–14.
38. Karanth S, Lyson K, McCann SM. Cyclosporin A inhibits interleukin-2-induced release of corticotropin-releasing hormone. *Neuroimmunomodulation* 1994;1:82–85.
39. Chrousos GP. The hypothalamic-pituitary-adrenal axis and immune-mediated inflammation. *N Engl J Med* 1995;332:1351–1362.
40. Reder AT. Regulation of production of adrenocorticotropin-like proteins in humans mononuclear cells.

Immunology 1992;77:436–442.

41. Schauer E, Trautinger F, Kock A, et al. Proopiome-lanocortin-derived peptides are synthesized and released by human keratinocytes. *J Clin Invest* 1994;93:2258–2262.

42. Brown SL, Blalock JE. Neuroendocrine immune inter-actions. In: Oppenheim JJ, Shevach EM, eds. *Immuno-physiology.* New York: Oxford University, 1990:306–319.

43. Zurawski G, Benedik M, Kamb BJ, et al. Activation of mouse T-helper cells induces abundant preproenkephalin mRNA synthesis. *Science* 1986;232:772–775.

44. Martin J, Prystowsky MB, Angeletti RH. Preproenke-phalin mRNA in T-cells, macrophages, and mast cells. *J Neurosci Res* 1987;18:82–87.

45. Rosen H, Behar O, Abramsky O, Ovadia H. Regulated ex-pression of proenkephalin A in normal lymphocytes. *J Immunol* 1989;143:3703–3707.

46. Linner KM, Quist HE, Sharp BM. Met-enkephalin-con-taining peptides encoded by proenkephalin A mRNA ex-pressed in activated murine thymocytes inhibit thymo-cyte proliferation. *J Immunol* 1995;154:5049–5060.

47. Blalock JE. Neuroendocrine peptide hormones in the immune system. *Prog Neuroendocrinimmunol* 1988; 1:9–12.

48. Walton PE, Cronin MJ. Tumor necrosis factor-α and in-terferon-γ reduce prolactin release in vitro. *Am J Physi-ol* 1990;259:E672–E676.

49. Costa O, Mulchahey JJ, Blalock JE. Structure and func-tion of luteinizing hormone-releasing hormone (LHRH) receptors on lymphocytes. *J Neuroendocrinimmunol* 1990;3:55–60.

50. Fabry Z, Raine CS, Hart MN. Nervous tissue as an im-mune compartment: the dialect of the immune response in the CNS. *Immunol Today* 1994;15:218–224.

51. Smith EM, Phan M, Kruger TE, et al. Human lympho-cyte production of immunoreactive thyrotropin. *Proc Natl Acad Sci USA* 1983;80:6010–6013.

52. Stanisz AM. Neuronal factors modulating immunity. *Neuroimmunomodulation* 1994;1:217–230.

53. Anlar B, Karaszewski JW, Reder AT, Arnason BG. In-creased muscarinic cholinergic receptor density on CD4+ lymphocytes in progressive multiple sclerosis. *J Neuroimmunol* 1992;36:171–177.

54. Costa P, Auger CB, Traver DJ, Costa LG. Identification of m3, m4 and m5 subtypes of muscarinic receptor mRNA in human blood mononuclear cells. *J Neuroimmunol* 1995;60:45–51.

55. Ovadia H, Abramsky O. Dopamine receptors on isolated membranes of rat lymphocytes. *J Neurosci Res* 1987;18:70–74.

56. Karaszewski JW, Reder AT, Anlar B, Arnason BGW. In-creased high affinity beta-adrenergic receptor densities and cyclic AMP responses of CD8 cells in mutiple scle-rosis. *J Neuroimmunol* 1993;43:1–7.

57. Tsagarakis S, Grossman A. Corticotropin-releasing hor-mone: interactions with the immune system. *Neuroim-munomodulation* 1994;1:329–334.

58. Smith EM, Meyer WJ, Blalock JE. Virus-induced corti-costerone in hypophysectomized mice: a possible lym-phoid adrenal axis. *Science* 1982;218:1311–1314.

59. Lyons PD, Blalock JE. The kinetics of ACTH expression in rat leukocyte subpopulations. *J Neuroimmunol* 1995;63:103–112.

60. Zwilling BS, Lafuse WP, Brown D, Pearl D. Characteri-zation of ACTH mediated suppression of MHC class II expression by murine peritoneal macrophages. *J Neu-roimmunol* 1992;39:133–138.

61. Ceriani G, Diaz J, Murphree S, et al. The neuropeptide alpha-melanocyte-stimulating hormone inhibits experi-mental arthritis in rats. *Neuroimmunomodulation* 1994;1:28–32.

62. Carr DJJ. Opioid receptors on cells of the immune sys-tem. *Prog Neuroendocrinimmunol* 1998;1:8–14.

63. Bulloch K, Radojcic T, Yu R, et al. The distribution and function of calcitonin gene-related peptide in the mouse thymus and spleen. *Prog Neuroendocrinimmunol* 1991; 4:186–194.

64. Kelley KW, Arkins S, Li YM. Growth hormone, pro-lactin, and insulin-like growth factors: new jobs for old players. *Brain Behav Immun* 1992;6:317–326.

65. Berczi I. The role of the growth and lactogenic hormone family in immune function. *Neuroimmunomodulation* 1994;1:201–216.

66. Bernton EW. Prolactin and immune host defenses. *Prog Neuroendocrinimmunol* 1989;2:21–29.

67. Gagnerault M, Touraine P, Savino W, et al. Expression of prolactin receptors in murine lymphoid cells in nor-mal and autoimmune situations. *J Immunol* 1993; 150:5673–5681.

68. Rouabhia M, Chakir J, Deschaux P. Interaction between the immune and endocrine systems: immunomodulato-ry effects of luteinizing hormone. *Prog Neuroendocrin-immunol* 1991;4:86–91.

69. Azad N, Jurgens J, Young MR, et al. Presence of luteiniz-ing hormone-releasing hormone in rat thymus. *Prog Neuroendocrinimmunol* 1991;4:113–120.

70. Roche JK. Immune response modulation by intesti-nal neuropeptides. *Prog Neuroendocrinimmunol* 1988; 1:4–7.

71. Levi-Montalcini R, Aloe L, Alleva E. A role for nerve growth factor in nervous, endocrine and immune sys-tems. *Prog Neuroendocrinimmunol* 1990;3:1–10.

72. Ibrahim MZM, Reder AT. The mast cells of the multiple sclerosis brain. *J Neuroimmunol* 1996;70:131–138.

73. Martin JB, Reichlin S. *Clinical neuroendocrinology.* Philadelphia: FA Davis, 1987.

74. Smith EM, Morrill AC, Meyer WJ, Blalock JE. Corti-cotropin releasing factor induction of leukocyte-derived immunoreactive ACTH and endorphins. *Nature* 1986; 321:881–882.

75. Besedovsky HO, Del Ray A. Mechanism of virus-induced stimulation of the hypothalamus-pituitary-adrenal axis. *J Steroid Biochem* 1989;34:235–239.

76. Sternberg EM, Hill JM, Chrousos GP, et al. Inflammato-ry mediator-induced hypothalamic-pituitary-adrenal axis activation is defective in streptococcal cell wall arthritis-susceptible Lewis rats. *Proc Natl Acad Sci USA* 1989;86:2374–2378.

77. Mason D. Genetic variation in the stress response: sus-ceptibility to experimental allergic encephalomyelitis and implications for human inflammatory disease. *Im-munol Today* 1991;12:57–60.

78. Reder AT, Thapar M, Sapugay AM, Jensen MA. Prostaglandins and inhibitors of arachidonate metab-olism suppress experimental allergic encephalomyelitis. *J Neuroimmunol* 1994;54:117–127.

79. Dhabhar FS, Miller AH, McEwen BS, Spencer RL. Dif-ferential activation of adrenal steroid receptors in neur-al and immune tissues of Sprague Dawley, Fischer 344, and Lewis rats. *J Neuroimmunol* 1995;56:77–90.

80. Sternberg EM, Young WS, Bernardini R, et al. A central nervous system defect in biosynthesis of corticotropin-releasing hormone is associated with susceptibility to streptococcal cell wall-induced arthritis in Lewis rats. *Proc Natl Acad Sci USA* 1989;86:4771–4775.

81. Spinedi E, Salas M, Chisari A, et al. Sex differences in the hypothalamo-pituitary-adrenal axis response to in-

flammatory and neuroendocrine stressors. *Neuroendocrinology* 1994;60:609–617.

82. Sternberg EM, Glowa JR, Smith MA, et al. Corticotropin releasing hormone related behavioral and neuroendocrine responses to stress in Lewis and Fischer rats. *Brain Res* 1992;570:54–60.

83. Reder AT, Lowy MT, Meltzer HY, Antel JP. Dexamethasone suppression test abnormalities in multiple sclerosis: relation to ACTH therapy. *Neurology* 1987;37:849–853.

84. Michelson D, Stone L, Galliven E, et al. Multiple sclerosis is associated with alterations in hypothalamic-pituitary-adrenal axis function. *J Clin Endocrinol Metab* 1994;79:848–853.

85. Reder AT, Makowiec RL, Lowy M. Adrenal size is increased in multiple sclerosis. *Arch Neurol* 1993; 51:151–154.

86. Purba JS, Raadsheer FC, Hofman MA, et al. Increased number of corticotropin-releasing hormone expressing neurons in the hypothalamic paraventricular nucleus of patients with multiple sclerosis. *Neuroendocrinology* 1995;62:62–70.

87. Erkut ZA, Hofman MA, Ravid R, Swaab DF. Increased activity of hypothalamic corticotropin-releasing hormone neurons in multiple sclerosis. *J Neuroimmunol* 1995;62:27–33.

88. Vacchio MS, Papadopoulos V, Ashwell JD. Steroid production in the thymus: implications for thymocyte selection. *J Exp Med* 1994;179:1835–1846.

89. Harbuz MS, Leonard JP, Lightman SL, Cuzner ML. Changes in hypothalamic corticotrophin-releasing factor and anterior pituitary pro-opiomelanocortin mRNA during the course of experimental allergic encephalomyelitis. *J Neuroimmunol* 1993;45:127–132.

90. Kavelaars A, Ballieux RE, Heijnen CJ. The role of IL-1 in the corticotropin-releasing factor and arginine-vasopressin-induced secretion of immunoreactive β-endorphin by human peripheral blood mononuclear cells. *J Immunol* 1989;142:2338–2342.

91. Lacaze-Masmonteil T, de Keyzer Y, Luton J, et al. Characterization of proopiomelanocortin transcripts in human nonpituitary tissues. *Proc Natl Acad Sci USA* 1987;84:7261–7265.

92. Harbour-McMenamin D, Smith EM, Blalock JE. Bacterial lipopolysaccharide induction of leukocyte-derived corticotropin and endorphins. *Infect Immun* 1985; 48:813–817.

93. Clevenger CV, Altmann SW, Prystowsky MB. Requirement of nuclear prolactin for interleukin-2-stimulated proliferation of T lymphocytes. *Science* 1991;253:77–79.

94. Johnson EW, Blalock JE, Smith EM. ACTH receptor-mediated induction of leukocyte cyclic AMP. *Biochem Biophys Res Commun* 1988;157:1205–1211.

95. Johnson HM, Torres BA, Smith EM, et al. Regulation of lymphokine (γ-interferon) production by corticotropin. *J Immunol* 1984;132:246–250.

96. Reder AT. Neuroendocrine regulation and the immune response in MS. *Res Immunol* 1989;140:239–245.

97. Strand FL, Rose KJ, King JA, et al. ACTH modulation of nerve development and regeneration. *Prog Neurobiol* 1989;33:45–85.

98. Robertson B, Dostal K, Daynes RA. Neuropeptide regulation of inflammatory and immunologic responses. The capacity of α-melanocyte-stimulating hormone to inhibit tumor necrosis factor and IL-1 inducible biologic responses. *J Immunol* 1988;140:4300–4307.

99. Lipton JM. Neuropeptide α-melanocyte-stimulating hormone in control of fever, the acute phase response, and inflammation. In: Goetzl EJ, Spector NH, eds. *Neu-*

roimmune networks: physiology and diseases. New York: Alan R. Liss, 1989:243–250.

100. Taylor AW, Streilein JW, Cousins SW. Identification of alpha-melanocyte stimulating hormone as a potential immunosuppressive factor in aqueous humor. *Curr Eye Res* 1992;11:1199–1206.

101. Grabbe S, Bhardwaj RS, Mahnke K, et al. α-Melanocyte-stimulating hormone induces hapten-specific tolerance in mice. *J Immunol* 1996;156:473–478.

102. Rott O, Fleischer B, Cash E. Interleukin-10 prevents experimental allergic encephalomyelitis in rats. *Eur J Immunol* 1994;24:1434–1440.

103. Skias DD, Reder AT. IL-10 inhibits EAE. *Neurology* 1995;45(suppl 4):A349.

104. Catania A, Gerloni V, Procaccia S, et al. The anticytokine neuropeptide α-melanocyte-stimulating hormone in synovial fluid of patients with rheumatic diseases: comparisons with other anticytokine molecules. *Neuroimmunomodulation* 1994;1:321–328.

105. Heijnen CJ, Bevers C, Kavelaars A, Ballieux RE. Effect of α-endorphin on the antigen-induced primary antibody response of human blood B cells in vitro. *J Immunol* 1986;136:213–216.

106. Gilman SC, Schwartz JM, Milner RJ, et al. β-Endorphin enhances lymphocyte proliferative responses. *Proc Natl Acad Sci USA* 1982;79:4226–4230.

107. Clevenger CV, Sillman AL, Hanley-Hyde J, Prystowsky MB. Requirement for prolactin during cell cycle regulated gene expression in cloned T-lymphocytes. *Endocrinology* 1992;130:3216–3222.

108. Clevenger CV. Regulation of interleukin 2-driven T-lymphocyte proliferation by prolactin. *Proc Natl Acad Sci USA* 1990;87:6460–6464.

109. Bernton EW. Prolactin and immune host defenses. *Prog Neuroendocrinimmunol* 1989;2:21–29.

110. Nagy E, Berczi I. Hypophysectomized rats depend on residual prolactin for survival. *Endocrinology* 1991; 128:2776–2784.

111. Reder AT, Lowy MT. Serum prolactin in active multiple sclerosis. *J Neurosci* 1993;117:192–196.

112. Cross RJ, Roszman TL. Neuroendocrine modulation of immune function: the role of prolactin. *Prog Neuroendocrinimmunol* 1989;2:17–20.

113. Palestine AG, Nussenblatt RB. The effect of bromocriptine on anterior uveitis. *Am J Ophthalmol* 1988;106:488–489.

114. Nelson LM, Franklin GM, Jones MC, Group TMSS. Risk of multiple sclerosis exacerbation during pregnancy and breast-feeding. *JAMA* 1988;259:3441–3443.

115. Bartik MM, Brooks WH, Roszman TL. Modulation of T cell proliferation by stimulation of β-adrenergic receptor: lack of correlation between inhibition of T cell proliferation and cAMP accumulation. *Cell Immunol* 1993;148:408–421.

116. Felten DL, Felten SY, Bellinger DL, et al. Noradrenergic sympathetic neural interactions with the immune system: structure and function. *Immunol Rev* 1987;100:225–267.

117. Felten DL, Felten SY, Carlson SL, et al. Noradrenergic and peptidergic innervation of lymphoid tissue. *J Immunol* 1985;135:755s–765s.

118. Marchetti B, Morale MC, Pelletier G. Sympathetic nervous system control of rat thymus gland maturation: autoradiographic localization of the β$_2$-adrenergic receptor in the thymus and presence of sexual dimorphism during ontogeny. *Prog Neuroendocrinimmunol* 1990;3:103–115.

119. Brenner GJ, Felten SY, Felten DL, Moynihan JA. Sympathetic nervous system modulation of tumor metastases and host defense mechanisms. *J Neuroimmunol* 1992;37:191–202.

120. Miles K, Chelmicka-Schorr E, Atweh S, et al. Sympathetic ablation alters lymphocyte membrane properties. *J Immunol* 1985;135:797s–801s.

121. Reder AT, Karaszewski J, Arnason BGW. Sympathetic nervous system involvement in immune responses of mice and in patients with multiple sclerosis. In: Goetzl EJ, Spector NH, eds. *Neuroimmune networks: physiology and diseases.* New York: Alan R. Liss, 1989:137–147.

122. Kruszewska B, Felten SY, Moynihan JA. Alterations in cytokine and antibody production following chemical sympathectomy in two strains of mice. *J Immunol* 1995;155:4613–4620.

123. Chelmicka-Schorr E, Checinski M, Arnason BGW. Chemical sympathectomy augments the severity of experimental allergic encephalomyelitis. *J Neuroimmunol* 1988;17:347–350.

124. Agius MA, Checinski ME, Richman DP, Chelmicka-Schorr E. Sympathectomy enhances the severity of experimental autoimmune myasthenia gravis (EAMG). *J Clin Invest* 1987;16:11–12.

125. Karaszewski JW, Reder AT, Anlar B, et al. Increased lymphocyte beta-adrenergic receptor density in progressive multiple sclerosis is specific for the CD8+, CD28− suppressor cell. *Ann Neurol* 1991;30:42–47.

126. Karaszewski JW, Reder AT, Maselli R, et al. Sympathetic skin responses are decreased and lymphocyte beta-adrenergic receptors are increased in progressive multiple sclerosis. *Ann Neurol* 1990;27:366–372.

127. Gilbert KM, Hoffmann MK. cAMP is an essential signal in the induction of antibody production by B cells but inhibits helper function of T cells. *J Immunol* 1985;135:2084–2089.

128. Shine J, Potter EK, Biden T, et al. Neuropeptide Y and regulation of the cardiovascular system. *J Hypertens* 1994;12:S41–S45.

129. Levine JD, Dardick SJ, Roizen MF, et al. Contribution of sensory afferents and sympathetic efferents to joint injury in experimental arthritis. *J Neurosci* 1986;6:3423–3429.

130. Levine JD, Moskowitz MA, Basbaum AI. The contribution of neurogenic inflammation in experimental arthritis. *J Immunol* 1985;135:843s–847s.

131. Pernow B. Role of tachykinins in neurogenic inflammation. *J Immunol* 1985;135:812s–815s.

132. Burd PR, Rogers HW, Gordon JR, et al. Interleukin 3-dependent and -independent mast cells stimulated with IgE and antigen express multiple cytokines. *J Exp Med* 1989;170:245–257.

133. Zwolinski R, Lee P, Rohwer-Nutter D, Reder AT. NPY effects on human mononuclear cell function. *FASEB J* 1989;3:A481.

134. Fredrikson S, Soderstrom M, Hillert J, et al. Multiple sclerosis: occurrence of myelin basic protein peptide-reactive T cells in healthy family members. *Acta Neurol Scand* 1994;89:184–189.

135. Brocke S, Gijbels K, Allegretta M, et al. Treatment of experimental encephalomyelitis with a peptide analogue of myelin basic protein. *Nature* 1996;379:343–346.

136. Whelan HT, Pledger WJ, Maciunas RJ, et al. Growth factors in the tumorigenicity of a brain tumor cell line. *Pediatr Neurol* 1989;5:271–279.

137. Kowanko IC, Pownall R, Knapp MS, et al. Circadian variations in the signs and symptoms of rheumatoid arthritis and in the therapeutic effectiveness of flurbiprofen at different time of day. *Br J Clin Pharmacol* 1981;11:477–484.

138. Barnes P, FitzGerald G, Brown M, Dollery C. Nocturnal asthma and changes in circulating epinephrine, histamine, and cortisol. *N Engl J Med* 1990;303:263–267.

139. Martin RJ. Nocturnal asthma: circadian rhythms and therapeutic interventions. *Am Rev Respir Dis* 1993;147:S25–S28.

140. Haus E, Lakatua DJ, Swoyer J, Sackett-Lundeen L. Chronobiology in hematology and immunology. *Am J Anat* 1983;168:467–517.

141. Smolensky MH, D'Alonzo GE. Medical chronobiology: concepts and applications. *Am Rev Respir Dis* 1993;147:S2–S19.

142. Krueger JM, Toth LA. Cytokines as regulators of sleep. *Ann NY Acad Sci* 1994;739:299–310.

143. Covelli V, Massari F, Fallacara C, et al. Interleukin-1 beta and beta-endorphin circadian rhythms are inversely related in normal and stress-altered sleep. *Int J Neurosci* 1992;63:299–305.

144. Sothern RB, Roitman-Johnson B, Kanabrocki EL, et al. Circadian characteristics of circulating interleukin-6 in men. *J Allergy Clin Immunol* 1995;95:1029–1035.

145. Young MR, Matthews JP, Kanabrocki EL, et al. Circadian rhythmometry of serum interleukin-2, interleukin-10, tumor necrosis factor-alpha, and granulocyte-macrophage colony-stimulating factor in men. *Chronobiol Int* 1995;12:19–27.

146. Namerow NS. Circadian temperature rhythm and vision in multiple sclerosis. *Neurology* 1968;18:417–422.

Chapter 6
Viral-Immune Interactions

M. Kariuki Njenga and Moses Rodriguez

Anatomic and Physiologic Considerations

The central nervous system (CNS), based on its unique anatomy, is relatively isolated from the immune system, giving it immunologic privileges unmatched by any other organ. First, there is the blood-brain barrier, which consists of cerebral capillaries and the associated astrocyte foot processes found in close apposition with endothelial cells to the abluminal side. The cerebral endothelial cells are tightly packed, form tight junctions, lack fenestrations, and are surrounded by a dense basement membrane. On the other hand, the choroid plexus forms a barrier between the blood and the cerebrospinal fluid (CSF). Whereas its vascular endothelium, where CSF is produced, is easily permeable, the epithelium has tight junctions and denies particles access to the CSF. The blood-brain barrier plays an important protective role in inhibiting viral invasion of the CNS, but it may also deter viral clearance from the CNS. The barrier denies access to nonactivated leukocytes and soluble immune mediators that may be important components of the host primary immune response against viral infection. Access to the CNS is restricted to activated T cells. Proteins, including immunoglobulins and complement effector molecules, are also relatively excluded from the CSF under normal circumstances.

The CNS also lacks an organized lymphoid system. In most other organs, regional draining lymph nodes are important in isolating an infecting virus, recruiting and cloning T and B lymphocytes, and enhancing the effect of cytokines. Microglial cells in the CNS have the potential of functioning as phagocytic cells. However, there is no constitutive expression of major histocompatibility complex (MHC) class I and class II genes in neurons or glial cells, obviating the CD8+ and CD4+ T cell–mediated immune mechanisms of viral clearance. For example, neurons, even when cultured in vitro and exposed to high levels of cytokines, do not express MHC genes. Studies have demonstrated that astrocytes, oligodendrocytes, and microglial cells can upregulate MHC antigens on their surfaces following viral infection, allowing for T cell–mediated clearance of the pathogen. The main antigen-presenting cells in the CNS are probably the perivascular microglial cells; thus, early inflammatory reactions are focused primarily at the perivascular areas. This preserves the delicate CNS parenchyma, allowing minimal infiltration. Finally, most CNS neurons are fully differentiated, nondividing cells that cannot be replaced. While this negates infection by viruses that require active cellular replication mechanisms, it may also inhibit antiviral mechanisms that are most effective in replicating cells.

Pathogenesis of Neurotropic Viruses

Any basic virology textbook elaborates on the stages of viral pathogenesis in a susceptible host. The steps include entry into the host, primary replication, spread in the body, invasion of the organs (cell and tissue tropism), virus shedding, host immune response, and viral clearance or persistence. The viral replication cycle within the target cells includes attachment and penetration into cells, uncoating, transcription and translation, replication of the genome, viral particle assembly, and release from the cell. In this section, we deal with the aspects of viral pathogenesis that are important to the CNS. There is no evidence that the viral replication cycle in CNS cells is different from that of other cells.

Route of Entry

Viruses enter the host through the skin, conjunctiva, respiratory tract, gastrointestinal tract, and genitourinary system. While intact and healthy, the skin provides an impermeable barrier against most viral infections. However, injuries and bites from arthropod vectors allow viruses to enter the host via this route. Most viruses, if introduced past the skin barrier to the underlying vascularized tissues, can cause infection. Viruses can also enter through the conjunctiva, resulting in local infection. Examples of neurotropic viruses that enter through the conjunctiva are enteroviruses and adenoviruses.

The respiratory tract serves as the most important portal of entry for many viruses. Neurotropic viruses that use this route include varicella-zoster, Epstein-Barr (EBV), cytomegalovirus, lymphocytic choriomeningitis (LCMV), rabies, Lassa, measles, rubella, and influenza A viruses. To initiate an infection via the respiratory system, a virus must overcome local defense mechanisms designed to protect the seemingly vulnerable epithelial cells. The epithelial cell surface is covered by mucus that traps viral particles, and ciliated cells that sweep the particles along the surface to the pharynx, where they are either swallowed or coughed out. Very small particles (≤5 µm) are inhaled directly into the lungs where they are susceptible to destruction by alveolar macrophages. However, viruses are capable of overcoming these defenses to initiate a localized infection (e.g., rhinoviruses and parainfluenza viruses) or to spread to the regional lymph nodes and the circulation to cause a systemic disease (e.g., varicella-zoster, mumps, measles, and rubella viruses and polyomaviruses).

The gastrointestinal tract provides the second most important route of viral entry. Neurotropic viruses that gain entry in this manner include EBV, poliovirus, and adenovirus. The gastrointestinal tract presents a formidable defense against viral infection that includes tough stratified squamous epithelium in the esophagus and mucus cover, secretory IgA, low pH, bile salts, and proteases in the stomach and intestines. Therefore, viruses that invade through this route must be acid stable, withstand local antibodies and high bile salt concentration, and resist inactivation by proteases. These conditions are prohibitive for most of the enveloped viruses. The enveloped viruses that use this route, such as EBV, must infect the upper oropharyngeal regions of the tract before they encounter the harsh conditions in the stomach and intestines. Recently, the rectum has gained attention as a portal of entry, due to the threat posed by acquired immunodeficiency syndrome (AIDS) among the human population, and an increasing awareness of the diversity of human sexual habits. Human immunodeficiency virus (HIV) type 1, the virus that causes AIDS, and essentially any other sexually transmitted agents can gain access to the body via this route. The mucosal surface of the genitourinary tract also provides access to sexually transmitted viruses, including HIV, human T-lymphotropic virus (HTLV) type I, and herpes simplex virus (HSV).

Mechanism of Spread to the CNS

Most neurotropic viruses spread to the CNS via the blood. Following primary replication at the site of entry and the regional lymph nodes, the viruses spread through the efferent lymphatics and thoracic duct to reach the systemic circulation. The first entry of virus in blood is referred to as the *primary viremia*. This low-titer viremia spreads the virus to distant organs, but not necessarily to every organ where the virus ultimately establishes infection. Further replication occurs in these secondary sites, leading to the secretion of higher titers of virus in blood in a *secondary viremia*. Secondary viremia can lead to the establishment of infections in other organs of the body.

In the bloodstream, viral particles are either free in plasma (e.g., enteroviruses, togaviruses, and flaviviruses) or associated with leukocytes, platelets, and erythrocytes (e.g., measles virus in lymphocytes, and HIV in CD4+ T cells). Free-flowing viruses have to contend with macrophages, which continuously remove viral particles from the circulation. Viruses carried in leukocytes, mainly lymphocytes and monocytes, enjoy a certain degree of immune protection from antibodies and other plasma components. Neurotropic viruses must maintain an adequate level and duration of viremia to invade the CNS.

The other important route of infection of the CNS is via peripheral nerves. Examples of viruses that spread through this route include rabies virus, pseudorabies virus, poliovirus, varicella-zoster virus, and HSV. Viruses infect the nerves innervating the primary replication site and then travel through the neuron via intra-axonal transport. The rate of migration is quite slow, ranging from 3 mm/day for rabies virus up to 16 mm/day for HSV (1,2).

Invasion of the CNS

The blood-brain barrier and lack of lymphatic system limit access to the parenchyma of the CNS. Some viruses in the systemic circulation can damage the blood-brain barrier and compromise its integrity. For example, some strains of HIV-1 infect the endothelial cells of the blood-brain barrier in a noncytolytic manner, perhaps inducing dysfunctions that permit entry of viral particles (3). Neurotropic viruses that migrate via the hematogenous route enter the CNS after they localize in the blood vessels of either the meninges and choroid plexus, or the brain and spinal cord. From the meninges and choroid plexus, the virus is shed into the CSF, from where direct neuronal infection can occur. From the brain and spinal cord, the virus can enter the parenchyma by infecting the endothelial cells, being transported passively across normal endothelium and basement membrane, or being transported passively within infected leukocytes or macrophages by diapedesis (Trojan horse mechanism). Once in the CNS parenchyma, the virus spreads via the CSF or by sequential infection of neural cells.

Cell Tropism

Many host factors influence the tissue and cell tropism of viruses. These include the immune status, age, genetic constitution, species, and presence of viral receptors. The results of recent studies suggest that most viruses do not induce expression of novel receptor molecules on the cell surface for their attachment, but use normal cellular molecules to initiate infection. For example, HIV uses the CD4 molecule on T cells (4); EBV binds CD21, a type 2 complement receptor on T lymphocytes (5); polioviruses use an immunoglobulin superfamily protein found on human chromosome 19 (6); and rhinoviruses bind intercellular adhesion molecule (ICAM)-1 (7). However, few virus receptors have been identified and most remain unknown.

The viral tropism of cells also depends on the location of a particular cell type within the CNS, and the stage of infection. A classic example of a virus with differential infection of the same cell type in different areas of the CNS is poliovirus, which infects neurons. Neurons of the cerebral motor cortex and the brainstem are always infected, whereas those in the hippocampus and striate cortex are never infected. This differential infection appears to be associated with an inherent resistance of some nerve centers to infection, and restricted movement of the virus in certain fiber pathways. In experimental infection with Theiler's murine encephalomyelitis virus (TMEV), a picornavirus, a temporal pattern of viral nucleic acid antigen distribution is observed following intracerebral infection (8,9). Viral particles, antigen, and RNA can be localized mainly in neurons 12 to 72 hours after inoculation, with few oligodendrocytes infected. An electron micrograph of a large number of TMEV particles in neurons is shown in Figure 6-1. In contrast, viral antigens and RNA are observed in oligodendrocytes and astrocytes but not neurons in the chronic stages of the infection. The reasons for this shift in cytotropism in the chronic stages of disease are unknown.

Under normal circumstances, immune effector cells, including CD4+ and CD8+ T cells, are not found in the CNS. However, during disease these cells are present in varying proportions, and may become infected with viruses. These infected immune cells not only can demonstrate altered physiologic functions, but also can serve as a virus reservoir in the CNS. Examples of this are HTLV-I and LCMV, which persist in lymphocytes within the CNS.

Host Immune Response to CNS Virus Infection

In response to CNS viral infection, both humoral and cellular responses are involved. Antiviral antibodies may prevent initial CNS invasion during the viremia, as well as prevent virus spread through the CSF. Once CNS cells are infected by the virus, however, cell-mediated immune (CMI) responses become most important. In addition to virus-specific CD4+ and CD8+ T cells, other immune effector cells, such as macrophages and natural killer (NK) cells, help to isolate and clear infected cells to minimize spread of the infection. This "division of labor" is only a generalization: In most in vivo situations, both humoral and CMI responses are involved throughout the disease process. For example, macrophages are involved in removing virus particles from the circulation throughout the course of the infection, and antibodies may be involved in eliminating virus from infected cells (10,11).

Humoral Immune Response

The antiviral antibody response may have three somewhat conflicting results. Antibodies may neutralize the virus, thus preventing extracellular spread. Paradoxically, antibodies may also enhance viral infection by facilitating its replication in otherwise nonpermissive cells. The third potential role of antiviral antibodies in the CNS is to induce immunopathology.

Neutralizing antiviral antibodies bind the virus, thereby preventing attachment on the cell surface. For antibodies to prevent attachment, they must bind the receptor binding sites on the viral particle. Antibodies may also neutralize the virus after it has attached by preventing penetration or uncoating of the virus. Once the viral genome has been released into the cell and replication has begun, antibodies are no longer effective. Some persistent viruses undergo antigenic variation to escape neutralization by circulating antibodies. This occurs mainly by point mutations in the viral gene sequences that encode the neutralizing epitopes. Lentiviruses, including HIV in humans and visna virus in sheep, provide the best examples of antigenic variation.

Complement-mediated lysis of virus-infected cells also requires antibodies, perhaps because antiviral antibodies alter the surface distribution of viral antigen, providing sites for complement activation. However, since normal CSF is deficient of complement, this mechanism may be of little biologic significance in clearance of the virus from the CNS. Antiviral antibodies may also act through antibody-dependent cell-mediated cytotoxicity (ADCC). ADCC kills virus-infected cells precoated with virus-specific immunoglobulin, and is mediated by NK cells. Theoretically, ADCC can occur in the absence of antiviral antibodies, but is more efficient when the target is precoated with antibody. The antiviral IgG serves two functions in ADCC, a cognitive function that allows coated cells to be preferentially killed over infected cells not coated with the antibody, and an activation function that stimulates NK cells to secrete the granules responsible for cell lysis. Despite these in vitro experimental data, there is little evidence that ADCC plays a role in controlling viral infections in vivo.

Antiviral antibodies in the CNS may also enhance viral replication. This enhanced viral replication requires an infectious immune complex (virus-IgG or virus-IgM-complement complex) and a target cell with either an Fc receptor or a complement receptor. The Fc or complement receptor acts as a virus receptor in cells that are otherwise nonpermissive for the virus. Fc receptors are present in immune cells involved in ADCC. Herpesviruses can also induce Fc receptors in infected cells, creating the possibility of superinfection or coinfection through the antibody-dependent enhancement of the viral replication mechanism.

Antiviral antibodies can also mediate immunopathologic processes in the host. Viral alteration of or cross-reactivity (molecular mimicry) with host cell proteins can lead to the production of autoantibodies. Autoantibodies can then react directly with the host cell antigen, which can lead to an autoimmune disease. In addition, immune complexes can form in persistent infection in the presence of antiviral antibodies. Deposition of these complexes in blood vessel walls results in immunopathology.

Cell-Mediated Immune Response

The CMI response in the CNS viruses mimics what is seen in other organs. Virus-specific CD8+ T cells attempt

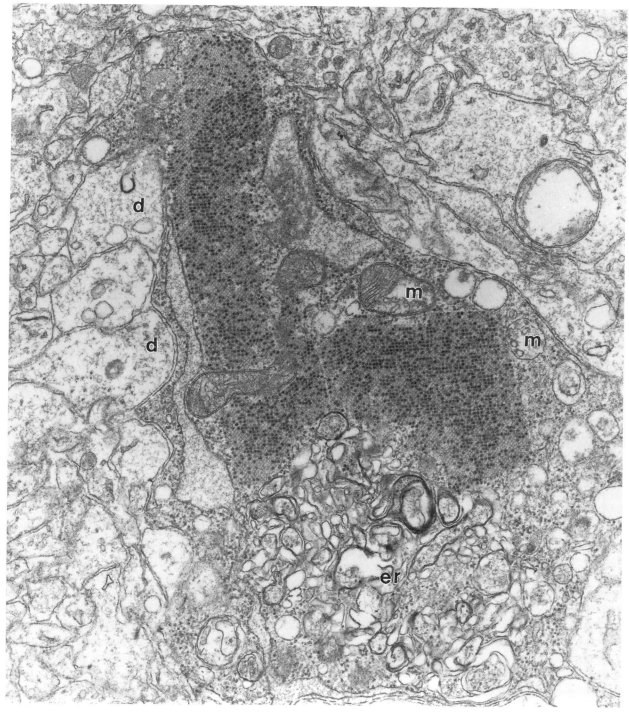

Figure 6-1.   Theiler's murine encephalomyelitis virus particles in the neurons of neonates. This electron micrograph shows a large non-membrane-bound paracrystalline array of picornavirus particles freely within the cytoplasm, consisting of both dense and hollow-cored virions. m = mitochondria; d = dendritic cell; er = endoplasmic reticulum.

to eliminate the virus-supporting cells early in the infection by targeting the infected cells through the interaction of the αβ T-cell receptor with viral peptides presented in the context of MHC class I glycoproteins. To ensure CD8+ T-cell surveillance, most glial cells can be induced to express MHC class I. Under normal circumstances, virus is cleared within 7 to 10 days after the onset of primary CNS infection unless a persistent infection develops. NK cells and macrophages are also involved in this process, as evidenced by viral clearance in athymic nu/nu and severe combined immunodeficient (SCID) mice. TMEV-infected mice treated with anti–NK cell antibodies have more severe encephalitis (Fig 6-2) than do untreated infected mice. However, the CNS presents two problems to the immune system.

First, infected neurons may not express MHC class I and class II molecules to act as targets for class I–re-

stricted CD8+ and class II–restricted CD4+ T cells. Therefore, viruses can persist in neurons despite the presence of a strong CMI response. The lack of MHC expression on neurons, which are irreplaceable, may be designed to prevent their destruction by the immune system cells. The second problem is that the CNS parenchyma is structurally delicate with extensive cell-to-cell signaling that is easily damaged by edema attributed to infiltration by immune effector cells and subsequent cytolysis. Despite these constraints, most viral infections of the CNS are cleared and recovery ensues with minimal or no deleterious effects on nervous system functions.

The precise contributions of CD4+ and CD8+ T cells in controlling persistent CNS infection are only now beginning to emerge. In experimental LCMV infection, mice depleted of CD4+ T cells by monoclonal antibody

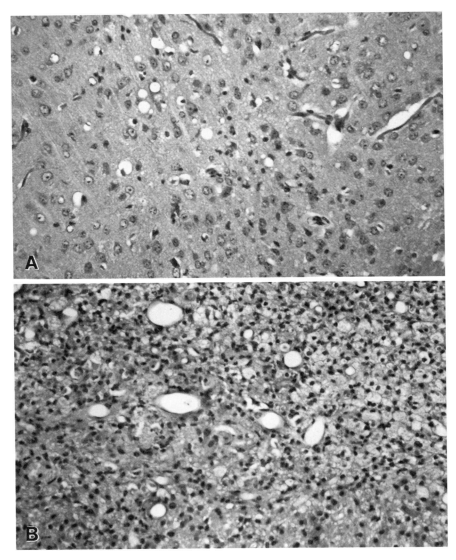

Figure 6-2. The role of natural killer (NK) cells in clearing virus from the CNS. (A) Mild inflammation and mild vacuolar changes in the brain of C57BL/10 mouse infected with Theiler's virus for 7 days. (B) Intense inflammation and neuronal necrosis in C57BL/10 mouse depleted of NK cells by treatment with anti–asialoGM₁ antibodies.

treatment were able to generate LCMV-specific CD8+ cytotoxic T-cell responses and eliminate the virus with normal kinetics following inoculation with a strain that causes acute infection (12). In contrast, CD4+ T cell–depleted mice infected with variant strains of LCMV that cause a chronic infection had no LCMV-specific CD8+ T-cell responses, resulting in the development of high titers of virus in most of their tissues throughout life. These results suggest that CD4+ T cells are not necessary for controlling acute infection, but are required for sustaining the function of CD8+ T cells in chronic infection. The failure of CD8+ T cells to clear virus in the absence of CD4+ T cells in chronic infections has also been observed in mice infected with Theiler's virus (13).

Cytokines in CNS Viral Infection

Many viruses infect a large number of cells in the CNS within a few days after exposure. Because the extent of tissue destruction associated with viral clearance is much less than the extent of cellular infectivity, it has become apparent that the immune system may clear virus through noncytolytic mechanisms. The most likely candidates are cytokines.

Interferon (IFN) types I (IFN-α and IFN-β) and II (IFN-γ) are known to establish an antiviral state following virus infection. Type I IFNs are thought to impair various steps in the viral replication cycle, including penetration and uncoating, transcription, translation, and assembly of the progeny viruses (14,15). Type I IFNs may target one or several steps of virus replication. In vivo studies have identified various IFN-induced gene products responsible for inhibiting the replication of different viruses (15,16). For example, the antiviral action in picornavirus infection is mediated by 2'-5'-oligoadenylate synthetase, whereas in influenza virus it is mediated by matrix (Mx) protein (14,15). The 2'-5'-oligoadenylate synthetase acts by activating a latent ribonuclease, RNase L, present in every cell, which in turn cleaves viral single-stranded RNAs. The mechanism of action of Mx protein in anti-influenza virus defense is not known. Some researchers have speculated that Mx protein interferes with the intracellular transport system in infected cells by diverting viral particles into lysosomes, where they are destroyed (17). Another IFN-induced protein, double-stranded RNA–dependent protein kinase (also known as *P68 kinase*), is implicated in antiviral functions. Once activated, the kinase phosphorylates other proteins, especially the eukaryotic initiation factor-2, resulting in inhibition of protein synthesis (18).

IFNs of all types, particularly IFN-γ, are involved in CD8+ T cell–mediated cytolysis of virus-infected cells, by enhancing the expression of class I MHC molecules on the target cells (19). A recent study using transgenic mice lacking type I and II IFN receptors confirmed the role of IFNs in antiviral defense (20). Following infection with vesicular stomatitis, vaccinia, Semliki Forest, and lymphocytic choriomeningitis viruses, these transgenic mice were extremely susceptible to low viral doses, despite their otherwise normal immune responses. In addition, treatment of Theiler's virus–infected mice with neutralizing antibodies to IFN-γ converted resistant C57BL/10 mice to susceptibility manifested by virus persistence and demyelination (21). Viruses have developed mechanisms to counter these IFN-associated antiviral effects by evolving IFN-resistant viral strains (22), and blocking steps in the IFN gene activation pathway (16,23).

The role of the other cytokines in the regulation of CNS viral infection is not known. Experimental infection of mice with a neurotropic strain of mouse hepatitis virus (MHV) results in upregulation of messenger RNA (mRNA) for interleukin (IL)-1α, IL-1β, tumor necrosis factor (TNF)-α, and IFN-γ in the olfactory bulb (24). In HIV-1 infection, IL-2, IL-6, transforming growth factor (TGF)-α, TGF-β, and TNF-α and -β can modulate viral replication (25,26). Cytokines in HIV infection are believed to also interrupt viral latency and increase spread of the virus through activation of viral gene expression and replication. Furthermore, treatment of TMEV-infected mice with TNF-α (27) or IL-6 (28) inhibits the chronic demyelination associated with virus persistence in susceptible strains of mice.

A bystander mechanism for the development of cytokine-mediated immunopathology has been proposed. This mechanism assumes that viral infection results in the release of lymphokines by virus-specific T cells (either Th1 or Th2 subtype), which in turn can result in further clonal expansion and differentiation of T cells in a nonspecific manner. Lymphokines produced by these T cells lead to recruitment, accumulation, and activation of monocytes and macrophages in the tissue, causing a nonspecific bystander tissue damage. The bystander hypothesis has particularly been advanced in TMEV-induced demyelination in mice following observation of enhanced MHC class II–restricted, delayed-type hypersensitivity responses in susceptible mice during chronic infection (29,30). This mechanism probably plays only a secondary, not a primary, role in tissue damage in chronic viral diseases. Evidence that argues against this hypothesis includes the fact that in TMEV-induced demyelinating disease in mice, the presence of virus in the CNS white matter, and particularly in glial cells, is an absolute requirement for the development of demyelination. In addition, viruses from different families result in a clearly delineated pathologic pattern and not in a nonspecific sequence of tissue damage. What the hypothesis has done, however, is take a first step in attempting to understand what must be a "common pathway" of many chronic infections, that is, a classic inflammatory response characterized by mononuclear cell infiltration that is associated with tissue damage.

Role of MHC Class I and II Genes in Resistance to CNS Viral Diseases

Most cells of the CNS do not express MHC class I molecules under normal circumstances. However, infection with some viruses, such as MHV and TMEV, results in class I glycoprotein expression in the CNS (Fig 6-3)

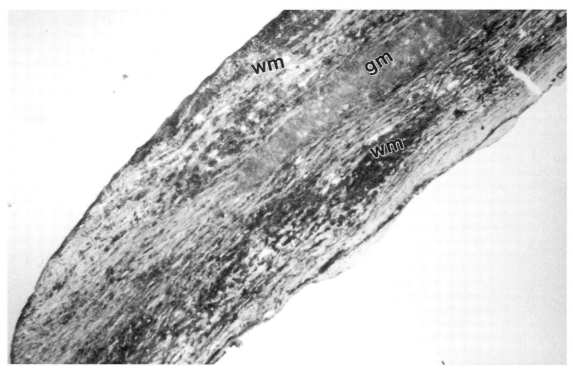

Figure 6-3. Upregulation of MHC class I expression in Theiler's murine encephalomyelitis virus infection, as shown by immunoperoxidase staining for H-2D antigens in a spinal cord section of a B10.Q mouse chronically infected with the virus. Increased expression is observed in both the white (wm) and the gray (gm) matter.

(24,31). While the mechanism of this upregulation remains to be clarified, this phenomenon suggests that class I components may play a critical role in CNS viral disease.

Evidence for the importance of MHC class I in the resistance to CNS disease has been demonstrated in experimental TMEV-induced demyelination in mice. Viral inoculation of recombinant inbred strains of mice demonstrated that MHC class I genes are critical in determining resistance or susceptibility to viral infection, which is associated with demyelinating disease (32,33). Mice with b, k, and d haplotypes of H-2, mouse MHC class I genes, on a C57BL/10 background are resistant to TMEV-induced demyelinating disease. Following intracerebral infection, these mice clear the virus within 21 days without evidence of clinical disease. In contrast, mice with s, f, p, r, v, and q haplotypes in an identical background allow TMEV to persist in the CNS, leading to chronic inflammatory demyelinating disease with clinical deficits. Within the H-2 genes, the D and not the K region appears to be primarily responsible for deter-

mining susceptibility or resistance to TMEV (34,35). The significance of H-2D over H-2K may be based on differences in D and K locus gene expression in response to TMEV infection. Such a mechanism is supported by a study that demonstrated higher expression of H-2D relative to H-2K antigens in the brain and spinal cord of susceptible mice chronically infected by TMEV (31). Back crossing congenic mice of resistant background to those of susceptible strains indicates that MHC-associated resistance is inherited as a dominant trait (36).

TMEV causes a chronic demyelinating disease in susceptible strains of mice, and the immune system is thought to play a role in the disease pathogenesis. Mice with disrupted β_2-microglobulin gene (β_2m(-/-)) do not express significant levels of MHC class I genes or functional CD8+ T cells. When such β_2m(-/-) "knockout" mice from a resistant haplotype (H-2^b) are infected with TMEV, there is abrogation of resistance that results in viral persistence and demyelination in the CNS (Fig 6-4), but without the development of neurologic signs (37).

Figure 6-4. Abrogation of resistance to Theiler's murine encephalomyelitis virus–induced demyelination in MHC class I–deficient mice. Electron micrographs show demyelination in the spinal cord of a β_2-microglobulin–disrupted mouse of a resistant H-2^b haplotype. (A) Completely demyelinated axons (a). To the left is a normal myelinated axon and below is a macrophage (M) with ingested myelin debris. (B) Early stages of demyelination with dissolution of myelin and preservation of the axon (a). Nu = nucleus.

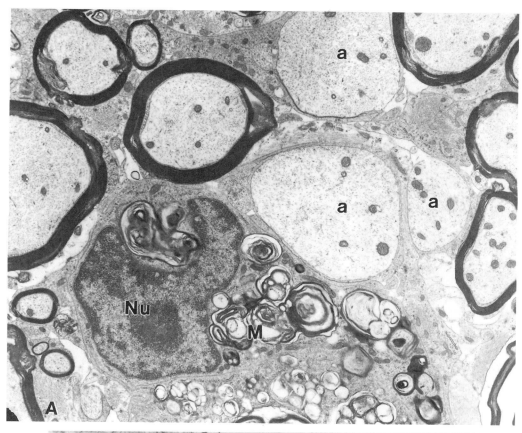

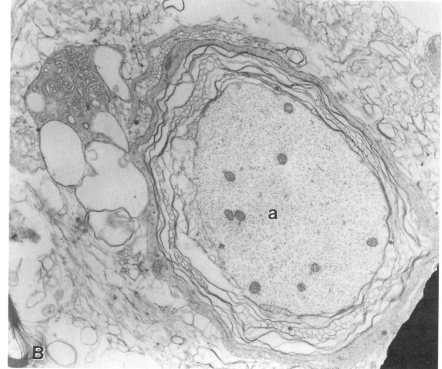

Under normal circumstances, mice of H-2^b haplotype clear TMEV from the CNS within 21 days and therefore do not develop demyelinating disease. The results of the β_2m(-/-) mice indicate that MHC class I components are required for viral clearance and clinical manifestations of the disease, but not for demyelination. In contrast, class II "knockout" mice that lack functional CD4+ T cells, from the same H-2^b haplotype, and are infected with TMEV show viral persistence, demyelination, and neurologic signs (13). Taken together, these results in β_2m(-/-) and class II "knockout" mice indicate that class I–restricted CD8+ T cells require the help of class II–restricted CD4+ T cells to clear virus from the CNS. Clearly, both MHC class I and II gene products are not required for the development of TMEV-induced demyelinating lesions. However, MHC class I determinants (possibly CD8+ T cells) but not class II determinants appear to be necessary for the development of clinical demyelinating disease in the TMEV model.

Mechanism of Evading Host Immune Response/Establishment of Persistent Infection

Most viruses cause acute infection that usually results in recovery and elimination of the virus from the host. Some viruses, however, establish persistent infections that can last for a lifetime (e.g., measles virus and herpesviruses). The definition of *persistence* as it applies to viral infection is controversial. In some cases, *persistent infection* has been defined to embrace latent, chronic, and slow infections, whereas in other cases *persistent infection* has been regarded as an independent condition. The main cause of confusion arises from the various states of the virus during such prolonged intracellular existence. Some viruses such as herpesviruses persist as nucleic acids with no detectable viral particles, while others persist as infectious viral particles. For the purposes of this chapter, we use the term *persistent infection* to broadly refer to any viral infection that is not completely cleared from the host in the normal viral clearance kinetics. Therefore, the term includes latent, chronic, and slow infections.

To establish and maintain a persistent infection, the virus must avoid elimination by the immune system, and sometimes limit expression of the genome. Studies have shown that in persistent LCMV infection, there is decreased production of viral glycoproteins by up to 50 times (38). Figure 6-5 shows the presence of nucleocapsid proteins in the neurons of mice persistently infected with LCMV. For cytolytic viruses, limited genome expression is especially important as a means to avoid destroying host cells, but it may also serve as a mechanism for evading the immune system. Persistent infections that do not result in host death are advantageous to the virus in an evolutionary manner, in that the virus can propagate and be transmitted to another host. Various mechanisms through which viruses can establish a persistent infection have been identified:

1. Antigenic variation (e.g., lentiviruses)
2. Restricted expression of viral genes (latency, e.g., herpesviruses)
3. Altered regulation of cell adhesion molecules (e.g., HIV-1)
4. Suppression of MHC antigen expression (e.g., adenoviruses)
5. Induction of nonneutralizing antibodies (e.g., measles virus)
6. Immunosuppression by infection of immune effector cells (e.g., HIV in CD4+ T cells and macrophages, and EBV in B lymphocytes)
7. Induction of immunologic tolerance (e.g., LCMV)

These mechanisms are discussed in further detail in the following sections. Some viruses that cause persistent CNS infections are listed in Table 6-1.

Antigenic Variation

Antigenic variation represents alterations in the surface antigens of the virus, allowing it to escape attack by the immune system. In vivo virus antigenic variation results in persistence of the virus with a normal replication cycle and within a functionally competent immune system. Antigenic variation is caused by either point mutation or recombination. Point mutation is the more common method and is especially frequent in RNA viruses because the replication apparatus lacks an efficient 3'-5' exonucleolytic "proofreading" mechanism. The high number of replication cycles viruses undergo also contributes to point mutation. Viruses that undergo antigenic variation in vivo include influenza viruses, which experience most of their changes on hemagglutinin or neuraminidase glycoproteins; measles virus; rabies virus; and most of the lentiviruses (visna, equine infectious anemia virus, HIV) (39–42).

Retroviruses, especially the lentivirus subfamily, are perhaps the most proficient in antigenic variation due to the infidelity of reverse transcriptase. Studies on visna virus and HIV-1 illustrate antigenic variation the best. In a 3-year study of experimental visna virus infection in sheep, animals were inoculated with plaque-purified virus and assays of neutralizing antibodies from blood were performed (43). The earliest antibodies neutralized the parental strain of the virus used for inoculation, but did not neutralize later viral isolates from the blood leukocytes of infected sheep. However, sera obtained later neutralized the variant strains. Sera obtained at the end of the study recognized the parental and variant strains. Using RNase T1-resistant oligonucleotide fingerprinting on the visna virus isolates, investigators found the antigenic variants to be closely related to the parental strain, differing by only a few changes in the envelope (*env*) region of the viral genome (44,45). Further analysis showed that many of the changes were common to the variants, suggesting an organized pattern of antigenic drift (43).

The retroviral reverse transcriptase has been estimated to have an incorporation error of between 3×10^{-3}

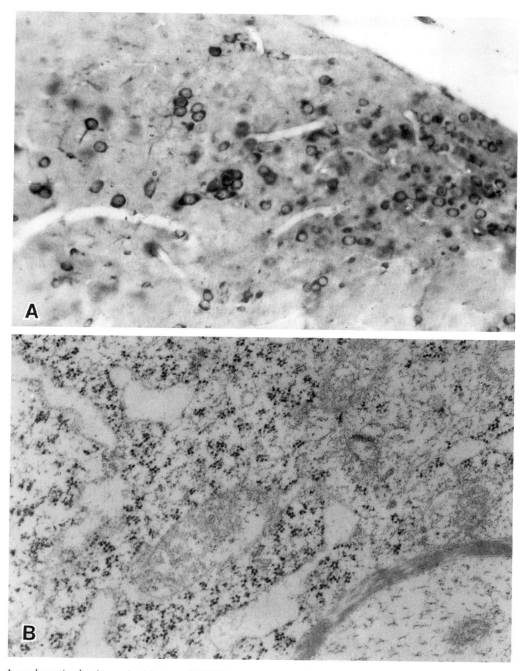

Figure 6-5. Lymphocytic choriomeningitis virus (LCMV) persistence in the CNS of mice. (A) Immunoperoxidase staining of a Vibratome section from the brain shows neurons expressing LCMV nucleocapsid proteins in a mouse persistently infected with the virus. Similar brain sections stained for glycoproteins were negative during the chronic stage of disease but positive during acute infection. (B) Electron microscopy of one of the neurons shown in A demonstrates ultrastructural immunoperoxidase staining within the polyribosomes that express LCMV nucleocapsid protein.

Table 6-1.
Some Viruses That Establish Persistent Nervous System Infection

Virus	Cytotropism	Mechanism of Persistence*	Nervous System Disease
Herpes simplex	Neurons	1	Encephalitis
Varicella-zoster	Neurons	1	Shingles
Epstein-Barr	Lymphocytes	1, 2	Meningitis, transverse myelitis
Theiler's murine encephalomyelitis	Oligodendrocytes, astrocytes, macrophages	Unknown	Encephalitis, chronic demyelination
JC (papovavirus)	Oligodendrocytes, lymphocytes	1, 2	PML
Canine distemper	Astrocytes, oligodendrocytes	Unknown	Demyelination
Measles	Monocytes, neurons, oligodendrocytes	2, 4, 5	SSPE
Mouse hepatitis	Microglia, neurons, glia	Unknown	Encephalitis, demyelination
Semliki Forest	Neurons, glia	Unknown	Demyelination
Ross River	Ependymal cells, oligodendrocytes	Unknown	Demyelination, hydrocephalus
Rabies	Neurons	Unknown	Encephalomyelitis
HIV	Lymphocytes, microglia	2, 3, 5	Encephalitis, white matter disease
Visna	Microglia	3	Encephalitis, demyelination
HTLV-1	Lymphocytes, microglia	2	Encephalomyelitis
LCMV	Lymphocytes, neurons	2, 6	Meningitis
Reovirus	Neurons, astrocytes, ependymal cells	Unknown	Hydrocephalus
Adenovirus	Unknown	7	Meningitis, encephalitis

*Identified mechanism of establishing persistence: 1 = latency; 2 = immunosuppression by infection of immmune effector cells; 3 = antigenic variation; 4 = defective transcription and/or translation; 5 = escape neutralizing antibodies; 6 = immunologic tolerance; 7 = suppression of MHC expression.
HIV = human immunodeficiency virus; HTLV = human T-lymphotropic virus; LCMV = lymphocytic choriomeningitis virus; PML = progressive multifocal leukoencephalopathy; SSPE = subacute sclerosing panencephalitis.

and 15.8×10^{-3} nucleotides per site per year on the envelope protein of the virus, based on the sequence comparison of sequentially isolated viruses (46). The rate of nucleotide misincorporation depends on the A-G mismatches (47–49). Like visna virus, variations on HIV-1 have been localized mostly in the *env* region, and rarely in the *gag* and *pol* regions (46). Within the HIV-1 *env* region, most errors occur on the receptor-binding V3 loop, which is the major neutralizing domain, thus allowing the virus to escape neutralizing antibody. Antigenic variation of HIV-1 was confirmed by experimental infection of chimpanzees, which resulted in neutralization-resistant variants within 16 weeks after inoculation (50). Strains isolated 32 weeks or earlier post-infection were neutralized by early and late (after 32 weeks post-infection) sera collected from the chimpanzees, while those isolated later in the infection were not neutralized by early sera. There is extensive diversity among HIV-1 isolates either from the same human patient or from different patients. The number of variant HIV isolates assayed by sensitive techniques like polymerase chain reaction (PCR) are extensive, leading to the reference of HIV-1 viruses within a host as a "quasispecies" (51). Within an individual infected with HIV-

1, there are different frequencies and distributions of sequence variants from different organs, that is, variants from brain tissue compared to those from blood cells, which suggests a tissue-specific evolution of the HIV-1 isolates (52). Interestingly, when the isolates are cultured, the diversity seen in vivo is lost by selective outgrowth of HIV-1 isolates capable of rapid replication.

A second mechanism of antigenic variation is homologous recombination. Homologous recombination is the exchange of nucleic acid sequences between related viruses that occurs mostly during viral replication. Recombination occurs in all DNA viruses and is attributed to strand switching by DNA polymerase; it has also been demonstrated in RNA viruses.

Restricted Expression of Viral Genes (Latency)

Latency is defined as a persistent infection in which the infectious virus is not demonstrable and disease is absent until after reactivation. During latency, the virus exists in a nonreplicative state within the tissue, but has the capacity to resume replication. Herpesviruses, which establish latency in a wide range of organisms, have been extensively studied, particularly HSV. Some herpesviruses, such as HSV and varicella-zoster virus, persist in neurons that are nondividing and long-lived cells, whereas others such as cytomegalovirus and EBV persist in the rapidly dividing, short-lived lymphocytes. During latency, the viral genome is integrated in the cellular chromosome in some viruses, whereas it survives as a free plasmid in the cytoplasm or nucleus in others. Viral replication is not necessary for the development of latency, because thymidine kinase–negative HSV-1 strains, which do not replicate in neurons, can establish latency in the sensory ganglia.

HSV persists in both the peripheral nervous system (sensory ganglia) and the CNS, although most studies have been performed in the sensory ganglia (53,54). Under normal circumstances, HSV-infected neurons experience a complete replication cycle of the virus, which is initiated by transcription of the immediate early (IE) genes (ICP0, ICP4, ICP22, ICP27, ICP47). The IE genes then activate the early genes, leading to DNA replication and late gene expression (55). In some neurons, however, there are inadequate levels or a complete lack of IE gene expression, resulting in stagnation of the viral replication cycle and the development of latency (56–58). This is supported by experimental evidence showing low levels of IE genes during the establishment and maintenance of latency (59).

Viral, cellular, and immune factors regulate the establishment and maintenance of latency, and reactivation in HSV.

Latency-Associated Transcripts

The latency-associated transcripts (LATs) are a group of overlapping nonpolyadenylated antisense viral RNA transcripts that are produced in large numbers by latently infected neurons. LATs are the only detectable viral transcripts during latency, even though no LAT-specific proteins have been identified. LATs are not required for the establishment of latency, but they enhance the efficiency of HSV-1 to establish latency (60,61). Ironically, they are also suspected of increasing the speed and efficacy of reactivation from latency. The mechanism of action of LATs is not known. There are suggestions that LATs inhibit some IE gene expression in an antisense manner.

Loss of Viral Protein Important in Upregulation of Immediate Early Gene Expression

As indicated earlier, IE gene expression is activated by the interaction of viral and cellular factors. For example, VP16, a HSV tegument protein, interacts with a host cell factor, Oct-1, to induce transcription of the IE genes. Ocular infection of mice with a mutant HSV-1 strain that carries VP16 molecules lacking IE gene–transinducing activity results in a higher frequency of latency established in infected neurons, compared to wild-type HSV-1 infection (59).

Cellular Factors

Some cellular transcription factors interact with the binding sites of the IE promoter of HSV-1 and induce IE gene expression. These factors include c-Jun, c-Fos, and Oct-1. Levels of these transcription factors are normal in adult sensory neurons, but data suggest that local stress, such as axotomy, axonal transport block, or noxious stimulation, can upregulate expression of these factors in the nerves (62). Induction and maintenance of HSV-1 latency are associated with low expression of c-Jun, c-Fos, and Oct-1, whereas reactivation is associated with increased expression of these factors in sensory neurons. One transcription factor, Oct-2, appears to serve as a repressor of HSV IE gene expression during the maintenance of the latency stage (63).

Immunologic Factors

Another possible mechanism to enhance latency development is the prevention of IE gene expression by inhibitory antibody activity or CD8+ T-cell activity. Neither of these immune functions appear to be required for the establishment of HSV latency because latency can occur in mice lacking T and B cells (64,65). However, these factors may influence the efficiency and maintenance of latency by suppressing viral replication, which results in latent infection rather than cytolytic infection. The role of immunologic factors in latency or reactivation is supported by experiments demonstrating that immunosuppression of latently infected animals leads to HSV reactivation. During acute HSV infections, latency occurs in the neurons where IE gene expression does not occur or is at minimal levels owing to a lack of viral and cellular transactivators. Decreased IE gene expression may also result from inhibitory antibodies and CD8+ T-cell activity. In addition, antibodies or cytokines released by latently infected lymphocytes at the early reactivation process may suppress HSV gene expression, resulting in re-establishment of latency.

In subacute sclerosing panencephalitis (SSPE), a complication of measles virus infection, measles virus persistence in the CNS associated with an accumulation of large numbers of viral nucleocapsids plays a central role in the disease pathogenesis. Unlike in latency where viral proteins and transcripts (excepts LATs) are not detectable, in SSPE, measles virus proteins accumulate (Fig 6-6) but without infectious virus or cytopathic change because of a defective replication cycle. The lack of mature viral particles is associated with transcriptional or translational abnormalities observed in the fusion, matrix, or hemagglutinin proteins of the envelope (66–69).

Altered Expression of Cell Adhesion Molecules

Adhesion molecules play an important role in the recruitment of immune-inflammatory cells from the

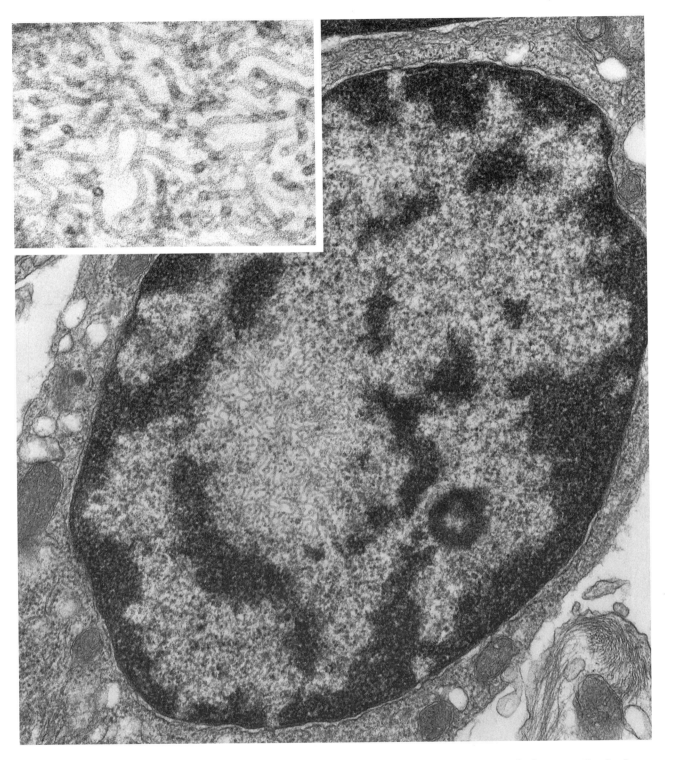

Figure 6-6.   Measles virus in subacute sclerosing panencephalitis (SSPE). This electron micrograph shows an oligodendrocyte from a cerebral biopsy specimen of a patient with clinical features of SSPE. Note the measles virus nucleocapsids in the nucleus. The inset shows the paramyxovirus at higher magnification.

circulation. Adherence of circulating lymphocytes on endothelial cells, and subsequent extravasation depend on the expression of appropriate adhesion molecules on vascular endothelial cells. In regards to viral infection, interaction with adhesion molecules presents several possible scenarios. First, some viruses may use adhesion molecules as surface receptors for gaining entry into cells (e.g., rhinoviruses use ICAM-1) (7). Second, enhanced extravasation of inflammatory cells as a result of upregulation of adhesion molecules may provide a mechanism for a virus to invade tissue (e.g., HIV is transported into the CNS through lymphocytes) (70). Third, infiltration of mononuclear cells within a virus-infected organ may serve as an immune effector and contribute to immunopathology.

The data on the alteration of adhesion molecule expression in virus-infected cells are confounding. Whereas ICAM-1 is upregulated in cytomegalovirus-infected endothelial cells (71), hepatitis B virus–infected hepatocytes (72), and HTLV-I–transformed T cells (73), it is downregulated in HIV-1–infected T-cell lines (74). Leukocyte function–associated antigen (LFA)-1 is increased in HIV-1– but decreased in HTLV-1–infected T cells (74), whereas extracellular leukocyte adhesion molecule (ELAM)-1 and vascular cell adhesion molecule (VCAM)-1 are not affected by cytomegalovirus infection of endothelial cells (71). Within the CNS, ICAM-1 upregulation is observed in multiple sclerosis and human viral encephalitis patients (75). It is expressed mainly on the endothelial cells but also on parenchymal mononuclear cells and glia.

Suppression of MHC Gene Expression

Viruses can evade the immune system by suppressing expression of MHC genes. This mechanism may be of minor importance in neurotropic viruses, as there is very low constitutive expression of the MHC genes in the nervous tissues. Normally, the main line of defense of the host against viral persistence is through cytotoxic T lymphocytes (CTLs) that destroy virus-infected cells. The absence of MHC class I impairs antigen recognition by CTLs, allowing the cell to survive and the virus to persist.

The importance of class I antigens in viral clearance is demonstrated by LCMV, which persists in lymphocytes/monocytes and neurons. Adoptive transfer of LCMV-specific CTLs into LCMV-infected mice leads to destruction of infected lymphocytes/monocytes but not neurons, because they did not express MHC class I on their surface (76). In vitro studies using a neuronal cell line (OBL-21), which is permissive to LCMV infection and expresses viral antigens on the plasma membrane, confirm these findings (76). Minimal levels of MHC class I glycoproteins are found on the surface of OBL-21 cells as they are unable to transcribe the class I heavy chain. Therefore, these cells are resistant to LCMV-specific CTL lysis. Transfection of OBL-21 cells with retroviral vector expressing the MHC class I, followed by infection with LCMV, results in lysis by LCMV-specific CTLs (77). Transgenic mice expressing MHC class I in

neurons and persistently infected with LCMV demonstrate high neuronal morbidity following adoptive transfer of LCMV-specific CTLs (77). This conclusively demonstrates that lack of MHC class I expression in LCMV-infected neurons in vivo helps them evade CTL surveillance.

Viral infection can downregulate surface expression or induce defective expression of MHC class I molecules on the surface of infected cells. The best example is provided by human adenovirus type 12, which decreases class I glycoprotein expression in infected cells either by blocking transcription or by viral proteins complexing with the class I molecules to prevent travel to the surface (78,79). For example, rat kidney cells transformed with adenovirus type 12 E1 protein demonstrate impaired processing of NFκB and KBF1, transcription factors important in the regulation of MHC expression (79). In SSPE, defective class II–restricted, measles virus–specific CTLs have been demonstrated (80). An intriguing aspect derives from studies demonstrating that viral infection can also induce MHC class expression in the CNS (24,31). This is counterintuitive from the virus standpoint, as it allows the infected cells to be targeted by cytotoxic CD8+ T cells. However, the virus-associated MHC upregulation may be associated with the induction of tissue pathology.

Apart from down regulating MHC class I molecules, virus-infected cells may escape immunologic surveillance by their disabling transportation of the appropriate antigen peptides from the cytosol to endoplasmic reticulum, where they are conjugated with the MHC molecule. Studies with the OBL-21 cells failed to detect transcripts of the peptide transporters HAM (histocompatibility antigen modifier) 1 and HAM 2, which translocate peptides from the cytosol to endoplasmic reticulum (81).

Nonneutralizing Antibodies

Anti–measles virus antibodies are suspected of fostering viral persistence in SSPE. Rat and mice treated with monoclonal antibodies against hemagglutinin envelope protein develop subacute measles encephalitis with transcriptional restriction of viral mRNA (82,83). Possibly, the nonneutralizing antibodies contribute to persistence by stripping viral antigens from the surface of infected cells, reducing their susceptibility to lysis by complement.

Immunosuppression

Downregulation or upregulation of immune mediators including cytokines and MHC glycoproteins, and replication in immune cells such as lymphocytes and macrophages are some of the virus-associated processes that alter host immune response. LCMV in the mouse and HIV and measles virus in the human are examples of viruses that replicate in immune effector cells (84–88). The most devastating is HIV infection, which leads to a depletion of CD4+ T cells (86–88). In HIV-infected patients, there is a gradual decrease in peripheral blood CD4+ T cells, leading to generalized immunosuppression. The CD4+ T-cell depletion is associated with excessive viral production, cytolysis of infected CD4+ T cells by cytotoxic cells (86), and apoptosis (87). Mice persistently infected with LCMV have undetectable or limited cytotoxic T-cell or delayed-type hypersensitivity responses to the virus. T cells recovered from infected mice show limited or no proliferation when stimulated with the virus in vitro. One study separated different lymphocyte subpopulations in LCMV-infected mice and examined for viral infection (85). LCMV infection was found primarily in helper T cells with minimal involvement of cytotoxic T cells and B cells, suggesting that infected helper T cells are responsible for the LCMV-specific T-cell unresponsiveness observed in the persistently infected mice. Temporal studies monitoring the replication cycle of measles virus–infected B lymphocytes demonstrated that virus-induced immunosuppression was a result of arresting clonal expansion of lymphocytes (84). Infected lymphocytes were activated early but replication was arrested at the G_1 phase of the cell cycle. Measles virus infection also induces immunosuppression by decreasing T-cell proliferation and immunoglobulin secretion by B lymphocytes, and probably suppressing CTL activity (89). Viral replication is required for immunosuppression as viral inactivation by heat, ultraviolet light, or neutralizing antibodies impairs induction of immunosuppression.

Induction of Immunologic Tolerance

Immunologic tolerance is associated with an unresponsiveness to viral antigen, resulting in no detectable virus-specific CTLs and antibodies. If the host is infected either in utero or early in life, then the infection is retained throughout life. The mechanism of induction of tolerance is considered to be clonal deletion of virus-specific CTLs. However, one study using LCMV infection showed that persistently infected mice, including those infected in utero, do not undergo clonal elimination of the LCMV-specific CTLs (90). In this study, mice containing Thy1.2 MHC-restricted CTLs were persistently infected with LCMV, and then LCMV-specific Thy 1.1 MHC-restricted immune CTLs were adoptively transferred (90). After viral clearance, recipient mice generated their own Thy1.2 LCMV-specific CTLs. This suggested that the presence of overwhelming viral infection suppresses host virus–specific CTL and antibody production, or that the CTLs and antibodies are made but are functionally suppressed by the virus, making them undetectable. The study questioned the clonal deletion hypothesis, but did not address the issue of viral antigen presentation in the thymus.

Elegant studies using transgenic mice that express a T-cell receptor for LCMV glycoprotein presented by a class I H-2D^b molecule demonstrated tolerance resulting from clonal deletion following viral antigen presentation in the thymus early in life (91). Transgenic expression of LCMV antigen in the thymus readily caused clonal elimination of antigen-specific CTLs whereas expression in the periphery (pancreatic islet cells) caused neither clonal deletion nor inactivation of virus-specific CTLs. Further transgenic mice experiments showed that unlike T cells, autoreactive B cells are neither clonally eliminated nor unresponsive to an antigen presented in various organs (91). The studies attributed the unresponsiveness of B cells to antigens in tolerant mice is associated with the deletion of helper T cells.

Alterations of Host Immune Response

Autoimmunity

Several genetic and environmental factors have associated the development of autoimmune diseases with viral infection. Autoimmune responses are enhanced by infection with a wide range of both DNA and RNA viruses. In experimental mice, the rapidity of appearance, as well as the level of anti-DNA and anti–red blood cell antibodies, are enhanced by infection with polyomavirus and LCMV (92). Viruses can enhance or induce autoimmunity in several ways. They may act directly with the cells of the immune system to alter function or direct the release of various cytokines that subsequently modulate the immune response. Viruses can also act indirectly by inducing new antigens, altering self-antigens, or exposing immunologically inactive self-antigens. An example of this is measles virus, which is suspected to induce autoimmune reactions against normally resident brain antigens (93). The last potential mechanism is molecular mimicry, which involves cross-reactive epitopes shared by the virus and the host. In studies of infectious mononucleosis in humans, there is accumulation of EBV-associated IgM and IgG autoantibodies against two autoantigens, p542, which cross-reacts with EBV antigen, and p554, which is not cross-reactive (94,95). The molecular mimicry mechanism is discussed in detail below. However, it must be emphasized that there are no substantial data on virus-associated autoimmune diseases in humans, and that most of the evidence is circumstantial.

Molecular Mimicry

Molecular mimicry is the phenomenon whereby a viral protein shares antigenic epitopes with a host protein. This results in a B or T cell–mediated immune response against the virus that might cross-react with the host protein. Due to the presence of introns and GC sequences that are spliced prior to translation, meaningful molecular mimicry is analyzed at a protein level using either immunologic reactants or matching protein structures in computer storage banks. The concept of viral molecular mimicry as a mechanism of autoimmune diseases in the CNS assumes that there are activated T cells specific for a CNS antigen in the peripheral immune system, as only activated T cells can cross the blood-brain barrier. These activated T cells then undergo clonal expansion after migrating to the CNS.

There is a wide body of data demonstrating that both RNA and DNA viruses share antigenic determinants with host proteins. For example, there is cross-reactivity between the measles virus phosphoprotein of 72 kd and a 54-kd component of cytoskeletal protein keratin (96); HSV glycoprotein D and the human acetylcholine receptor that is the target autoantigen in myasthenia gravis (97); and vaccinia virus hemagglutinin and the cytoskeletal protein vimentin (98). In one study to determine the frequency of cross-reactive epitopes, 24 (4%) of 600 monoclonal antibodies raised against viral peptides were cross-reactive with host proteins expressed in normal tissues (99). The monoclonal antibodies were raised from 14 different RNA and DNA viruses, including herpesviruses, myxoviruses, coronaviruses, flaviviruses, rhabdoviruses, and retroviruses. Some antibodies did cross-react with potentially interesting host tissues, including the coxsackie B virus VP1 protein with myocardium, measles viral hemagglutinin with a subset of human T cells, Theiler's VP1 protein with galactocerebroside, and HIV-1 gp41 with astrocytes.

In the only study that attempted to demonstrate autoimmune disease associated with molecular mimicry, the amino acid sequences of the encephalitogenic site (8–10 amino acids) of myelin basic protein (MBP) were mapped in several species and then fitted with various viral proteins (100). MBP is an important target antigen in the immunopathogenesis of experimental autoimmune encephalomyelitis and possibly multiple sclerosis. The best fit occurred between the rabbit MBP and hepatitis B virus polymerase. Inoculation of rabbits with hepatitis B polymerase peptides resulted in small perivascular infiltrates localized to the CNS without parenchymal disease or demyelination. A recent study provided some evidence that certain pathogens can activate T cells specific for MBP (101). A protein data base was searched for viral and bacterial peptides that could fit the structural motif of residues 85 to 99 of MBP that contained the MHC and T-cell receptor contacts important in the activation of the three T-cell clones used. The T-cell clones were isolated from two patients with relapsing-remitting multiple sclerosis (102,103). Several contrived epidemiologic criteria were used to narrow down the initial field of more than 600 candidate sequences. A total of 129 peptides were synthesized and tested for activation of human MBP [85–99]–specific T-cell clones. Viral peptides from HSV, adenovirus type 12, human papillomavirus, EBV, influenza virus, and reovirus, and one bacterial peptide from *Pseudomonas aeruginosa*, activated the T cells. MHC class II subtype HLA-DR2, associated with a susceptibility to multiple sclerosis, was a better presenter of the viral mimicry peptides compared to other class II subtypes. The results suggest that childhood immunization against viral pathogens carrying the mimicry epitope, while avoiding the cross-reactive epitopes in vaccine design, may reduce the risk of multiple sclerosis. However, the paucity of data on experimentally induced autoimmune disease in animals, based on the molecular mimicry hypothesis casts doubt as to whether this phenomenon occurs in human or animal diseases.

Viral open reading frames also code for proteins homologous to cellular proteins. Most of the virally encoded proteins thus far identified have the ability to modify the host immune response, to the benefit of the virus. The proteins include MHC class I and II glycoproteins, IFN, TNF, IL-1, IL-10, and complement. A recent surprise is the finding that immunization of macaques with human MHC class II proteins (HLA-DR) can protect against simian immunodeficiency virus (104).

Superantigen Stimulation of T Cells

Superantigens are a class of homologous disease-associated proteins that stimulate a large number of T cells. Members of the superantigen family include toxins from streptococcal and staphylococcal infections, and antigens from *Mycoplasma arthritidis* which causes arthritis in rats, mouse mammary tumor virus (MMTV), and a mouse reovirus (reviewed elsewhere (105)). The mechanism by which superantigens stimulate T cells differs from that of normal antigens. Conventional T-cell antigens are short proteolytic peptides from foreign proteins, bound in the peptide-binding groove of class I or class II MHC molecules. These MHC-bound peptides are part of the molecule displayed by antigen-presenting cells to specific T cells, resulting in an immune response. In contrast, superantigens are not processed into smaller peptides but rather the entire molecule interacts with the MHC class II molecule outside of the peptide-binding groove, resulting in nonspecific T-cell stimulation. A three-dimensional structure of *Staphylococcus aureus* enterotoxin B superantigen bound to HLA-DR, a human MHC class II molecule, has been documented by x-ray crystallography (106). Binding of superantigens to MHC class II glycoproteins is of high affinity, resulting in activation of as many as 20% of all peripheral T cells.

Like conventional antigenic peptides, superantigens must bind to an MHC molecule before they can be recognized by the T-cell receptor. Normally, antigen specificity on T cells is determined by the T-cell receptor, which forms a binding site for the peptide-MHC complex. Superantigens bypass this specificity requirement of T-cell receptors by binding at a site outside of the peptide-MHC binding site on the V_β domain. In the *S. aureus* enterotoxin B–HLA-DR complexes, the enterotoxin residues that are important for interaction with the T-cell receptor are positioned to the inside, suggesting that superantigen-MHC complexes with T-cell receptors result in blocking of the conventional T-cell receptor–MHC site (106).

Mouse mammary tumor virus, a retrovirus, is the only virus shown to produce superantigens (107,108), although HIV and rabies virus are also known to make proteins with the characteristics of superantigens (109,110). Unlike the bacterial superantigens, which are soluble globular proteins, mouse mammary tumor virus superantigens are membrane proteins that can undergo cleavage before activating T cells. Superantigenic proteins are closely related based on amino acid sequences except for the C terminal 20 to 30 residues

(105). Only a small number of class II MHC–superantigen complexes are formed, and superantigens appear to have preference for class II isotypes. Bacterial superantigens seem to bind the DR molecule of MHC class II better than DQ and DP in humans, while in mice the I-E molecule is a better ligand than I-A regardless of the allele (105).

Conclusions

Viruses can use a variety of methods to stay one step ahead of the host immune system. These can involve altering the host immune system or undergoing structural and physiologic changes. In most cases, the virus uses more than one mechanism to realize persistence. Many factors play an important role in the immune response to viruses; these include age and genetics of the host, magnitude of the infection, state of virus replication, immunogenicity of viral proteins, and immune status of the host. This interplay determines whether there is asymptomatic infection, rapid viral clearance without clinical sequela, or chronic infection with neurologic disabilities. Studying the detailed interactions between viruses and the immune system should provide important insights for disease prevention and therapy.

References

1. Iwasaki Y, Liu D, Yamamoto T, Kono H. On the replication and spread of rabies virus in the human central nervous system. *J Neuropathol Exp Neurol* 1985;44:185–195.
2. Tyler K, McPhee D, Fields B. Distinct pathway of viral spread in the host determined by reovirus S1 gene segment. *Science* 1986;233:770–774.
3. Moses AV, Nelson JA. HIV infection of human brain capillary endothelial cells–implications for AIDS dementia. *Adv Neuroimmunol* 1994;4:239–246.
4. Dagleish AG, Beverly PCL, Clapham PR, et al. The CD4 (T4) antigen is an essential component of the receptor for the AIDS retrovirus. *Nature* 1985;312:763–767.
5. Fingeroth JD, Clabby ML, Strominger JL. Characterization of a T lymphocyte Epstein-Barr virus/CD3 (CD21). *J Virol* 1988;62:1442–1447.
6. Ren R, Kostanini F, Gorga ZJ, et al. Transgenic mice expressing a human poliovirus receptor: a new model for poliomyelitis. *Cell* 1990;63:353–362.
7. Greve J, Davis G, Meyer A, et al. The major human rhinovirus receptor is ICAM-1. *Cell* 1989;56:839–847.
8. Graves MC, Bologa L, Siegel L, Londe H. Theiler's virus in brain cell cultures: lysis of neurons and oligodendrocytes and persistence in astrocytes and macrophages. *J Neurosci Res* 1986;15:491–501.
9. Rodriguez M. Virus-induced demyelination in mice: "dying back" of oligodendrocytes. *Mayo Clin Proc* 1985; 60:433–438.
10. Levine B, Hardick JM, Trapp BD, et al. Antibody-mediated clearance of alphavirus infection from neurons. *Science* 1991;254:856–860.
11. Mazanec MB, Kaetzel CS, Lamm ME, et al. Intracellular neutralization of virus by immunoglobulin A antibodies. *Proc Natl Acad Sci USA* 1992;89:6901–6905.
12. Matloubian M, Concepcion RJ, Ahmed R. CD4+ T cells are required to sustain CD8+ T cell responses during chronic viral infection. *J Virol* 1994;68:8056–8063.
13. Kariuki Njenga M, Pavelko KD, Baisch J, et al. Theiler's virus persistence and demyelination in MHC class II-deficient mice. *J Virol* 1996;70:1729–1737.
14. Samuel CE. Mechanism of antiviral action of interferons. *Prog Nucleic Acid Res Mol Biol* 1988;35:27–72.
15. Staeheli P. Interferon-induced proteins and the antiviral state. *Adv Virus Res* 1990;38:147–200.
16. Samuel CE. Antiviral action of interferon. Interferon-regulated cellular proteins and their surprisingly selective antiviral activities. *Virology* 1991;183:1–11.
17. Arnheiter H, Meier E. Mx proteins: antiviral proteins by chance or necessity? *New Biologist* 1990;2:851–857.
18. Honavessian AG. The double stranded RNA-activated protein kinase induced by interferon: dsRNA-PK. *J Interferon Res* 1989;9:641–647.
19. Blanar MA, Baldwin AS Jr, Flavell RA, Sharp PA. A gamma-interferon-induced factor that binds the interferon response sequence of the MHC class I gene, H-2K^b. *EMBO J* 1989;8:1139–1144.
20. Müller U, Steinhoff U, Reis LFL, et al. Functional role of type I and II interferons in antiviral defense. *Science* 1994;264:1918–1921.
21. Rodriguez M, Pavelko K, Coffman RL. Gamma interferon is critical for resistance to Theiler's virus-induced demyelination (in press).
22. Carrigan DR, Knox KK. Identification of interferon-resistant subpopulations in several strains of measles virus: positive selection by growth of the virus in brain tissue. *J Virol* 1990;64:1606–1615.
23. Ackrill A, Foster G, Laxton C, et al. Inhibition of the cellular response to interferons by products of the adenovirus type 5 E1A. *Nucleic Acids Res* 1991;19:4387–4393.
24. Pearce BD, Hubbs MV, McGraw TS, Buchmeier MJ. Cytokine induction during T-cell-mediated clearance of mouse hepatitis virus from neurons in vivo. *J Virol* 1994;68:5483–5495.
25. Poli G, Fauci AS. Cytokine modulation of HIV expression. *Semin Immunol* 1993;5:165–173.
26. Wesselingh SL, Glass J, McArthur JC, et al. Cytokine dysregulation in HIV-associated neurological disease. *Adv Neuroimmunol* 1994;4:199–206.
27. Paya CV, Leibson PJ, Patick AK, Rodriguez M. Inhibition of Theiler's virus-induced demyelination in vivo by tumor necrosis factor alpha. *Int Immunol* 1990;2:909–913.
28. Rodriguez M, Pavelko KD, McKinny CW, Leibowitz JL. Recombinant human IL-6 suppresses demyelination in a viral model of multiple sclerosis. *J Immunol* 1994;153:3811–3821.
29. Clatch RJ, Lipton HL, Miller SD. Characterization of Theiler's murine encephalomyelitis virus (TMEV)-specific delayed type hypersensitivity responses in TMEV-induced demyelinating disease: correlation with clinical signs. *J Immunol* 1986;136:920–927.
30. Miller SD, Clatch RJ, Pevear DC, et al. Class II-restricted T cell responses in Theiler's murine encephalomyelitis virus (TMEV)-induced demyelinating disease. I. Cross-specificity among TMEV substrains and related picornaviruses, but not myelin proteins. *J Immunol* 1987; 138:3776–3784.
31. Altintas A, Cai Z, Pease LR, Rodriguez M. Differential expression of H-2K and H-2D in the central nervous system of mice infected with Theiler's virus. *J Immunol* 1993;151:2803–2812.
32. Rodriguez M, David CS. Demyelination induced by Theiler's virus: influence of the H-2 haplotype. *J Immunol* 1985;135:2145–2148.
33. Rodriguez M, David CS, Pease LR. The contribution of MHC gene products to demyelination by Theiler's virus.

In: David CS, ed. *H-2 antigens*. New York: Plenum, 1987:747–756.

34. Rodriguez M, Leibowitz J, Davis CS. Susceptibility to Theiler's virus-induced demyelination: mapping of genes within the H-2D region. *J Exp Med* 1986;163:620–621.

35. Clatch RJ, Melvold RW, Dal Canto MC, et al. The Theiler's murine encephalomyelitis virus (TMEV) model for multiple sclerosis shows a strong influence of the murine equivalents of HLA-A, B, C. *J Neuroimmunol* 1987;15:121–135.

36. Patick AK, Pease LP, David CS, Rodriguez M. Major histocompatibility complex-conferred resistance to Theiler's virus-induced demyelinating disease is inherited as a dominant trait in B10 congenic mice. *J Virol* 1990;64:5570–5576.

37. Rodriguez M, Dunkel AJ, Thiemann RL, et al. Abrogation of resistance to Theiler's virus-induced demyelination in H-2^b mice deficient in β2-microglobulin. *J Immunol* 1993;151:266–276.

38. Francis SJ, Southern PJ. Deleted viral RNAs and lymphocytic choriomeningitis virus persistence in vitro. *J Gen Virol* 1988;69:1893–1902.

39. Webster RG, Laver WG, Air GM, Schild GC. Molecular mechanisms of variation in influenza virus. *Nature* 1982;296:115–121.

40. Ter Muelen V, Loffler S, Carter MJ, Stephenson JR. Antigenic characterization of measles and SSPE virus hemagglutinin by monoclonal antibodies. *J Gen Virol* 1981;57:357–364.

41. Wiktor TJ, Koprowski H. Antigenic variants of rabies virus. *J Exp Med* 1980;152:99–112.

42. Montelaro RC, Parekh B, Orrego A, Issel CJ. Antigenic variation during persistent infection by equine infectious anemia virus, a retrovirus. *J Biol Chem* 1984;259: 10539–10544.

43. Clements JE, Gdovin SL, Montelaro RC, Narayan O. Antigenic variation in lentiviral diseases. *Annu Rev Immunol* 1988;6:139–159.

44. Clements JE, D'Antonio N, Narayan O. Genomic changes associated with antigenic variation of visna virus. II. Common nucleotide changes detected in variants from independent isolations. *J Mol Biol* 1982;158:415–434.

45. Dubois-Dalcq M, Narayan O, Griffin DE. Cell surface changes associated with mutation of visna virus in antibody treated cell cultures. *Virology* 1979;92:353–366.

46. Hahn BH, Shaw GM, Taylor ME, et al. Genetic variation in HTLV-III/LAV over time in patients with AIDS or at risk for AIDS. *Science* 1986;232:1548–1553.

47. Roberts JD, Preston BD, Johnston LA, et al. Fidelity of two retroviral reverse transcriptases during DNA-dependent DNA synthesis in vitro. *Mol Cell Biol* 1989;9:469–476.

48. Preston BD, Poisz BJ, Loeb LA. Fidelity of HIV-1 reverse transcriptase. *Science* 1988;242:1168–1171.

49. Weber J, Grosse F. Fidelity of human immunodeficiency virus type 1 reverse transcriptase in copying natural DNA. *Nucleic Acids Res* 1989;17:1379–1393.

50. Nara PL, Smit SL, Dunlop N, et al. Emergence of viruses resistant to neutralization by V3-specific antibodies in experimental human immunodeficiency virus type 1 IIIB infection of chimpanzees. *J Virol* 1990;64:3779–3791.

51. Epstein LG, Kuiken C, Blumberg BM, et al. HIV-1 V3 domain variation in brain and spleen of children with AIDS: tissue specific evolution within host-quasispecies. *Virology* 1991;180:583–590.

52. Goodenow M, Huet T, Saurin W, et al. HIV-1 isolates are rapidly evolving quasispecies: evidence for viral mixtures and preferred nucleotide substitutions. *J Acquir Immune Defic Syndr* 1989;2:344–352.

53. Steiner I, Kennedy PGE. Herpes simplex virus latency in the nervous system–a new model. *Neuropathol Appl Neurobiol* 1991;17:433–440.

54. Stevens JG. Human herpesvirus. A consideration of the latent state. *Microbiol Rev* 1989;53:318–332.

55. Honess RW, Roizman B. Regulation of herpesvirus macromolecular synthesis. I. Cascade regulation of the synthesis of three groups of viral proteins. *J Virol* 1974;14:8–19.

56. Margolis TP, Sederati F, Dobson AT, et al. Pathways of viral gene expression during acute neuronal infection with HSV-1. *Virology* 1992;189:150–160.

57. Steiner I, Spivak JG, Deshmane SL, et al. A herpes simplex virus type mutant containing a non-transducing Vmw65 protein establishes latent infection in vivo in the absence of viral replication and reactivates efficiently from explanted trigeminal ganglia. *J Virol* 1990;64:1630–1638.

58. Speck PG, Simmons A. Synchronous appearance of antigen-positive and latently infected neurons in spinal ganglia of mice infected with a virulent strain of herpes simplex virus. *J Gen Virol* 1992;73:1281–1285.

59. Valyi-Nagy T, Deshmane SL, Spivak JG, et al. Investigation of herpes simplex virus type 1 (HSV-1) gene expression and DNA synthesis during the establishment of latent infection by an HSV-1 mutant, *in 1819*, that does not replicate in mouse trigeminal ganglia. *J Gen Virol* 1991;72:641–649.

60. Steiner I, Spivak JG, Lirrete RP, et al. Herpes simplex virus type 1 latency-associated transcripts are evidently not essential for latent infection. *EMBO J* 1989;8:505–511.

61. Stevens JG, Wagner EK, Devi-Rao GB, et al. RNA complementary to a herpesvirus alpha gene mRNA is prominent in latently infected neurons. *Science* 1987;235:1056–1059.

62. Leah JD, Herdegen T, Bravo R. Selective expression of Jun proteins following axotomy and axonal transport block in peripheral nerves in rat: evidence for a role in the regeneration process. *Brain Res* 1991;566:198–207.

63. Lillycrop KA, Latchman DS. Alternative splicing of the Oct-2 transcription factor RNA is differentially regulated in neuronal cells and B cells and results in protein isoforms with opposite effect on the activity of octamer/TAATGARAT-containing promoters. *J Biol Chem* 1992; 267:24960–24965.

64. Valyi-Nagy T, Deshmane SL, Raengsakulrach B, et al. Herpes simplex virus type 1 mutant strain *in 1819* establishes a unique, slow progressing infection in SCID mice. *J Virol* 1992;66:7336–7345.

65. Moriyama K, Mohri S, Watanabe T, Mori R. Latent infection of SCID mice with herpes simplex virus 1 and lethal cutaneous lesions in pregnancy. *Microbiol Immunol* 1992;36:841–853.

66. Cattaneo R, Schmid A, Spielhofer P, et al. Mutated and hypermutated genes of persistent measles viruses which caused lethal human brain diseases. *Virology* 1989; 173:415–425.

67. Hirano A, Wang AH, Gombart AF, Wong TC. The matrix proteins of neurovirulent subacute sclerosing panencephalitis virus and its acute measles virus progenitor are functionally different. *Proc Natl Acad Sci USA* 1992;89:8745–8749.

68. Hirano A, Ayata M, Wang AH, Wong TC. Functional analysis of matrix proteins expressed from cloned genes of measles virus variants that cause subacute sclerosing panencephalitis reveal a common defect in nucleocapsid binding. *J Virol* 1993;67:1848–1853.

69. Hummel KB, Vanchiere JA, Bellini WJ. Restriction of fusion protein mRNA as a mechanism of measles virus persistence. *Virology* 1994;202:665–672.

70. Hurwitz AA, Berman JW, Lyman WD. The role of the blood brain barrier in HIV infection of the central nervous system. *Adv Neuroimmunol* 1994;4:249–256.

71. Sedmak DD, Knight DA, Vook NC, Waldman JW. Divergent patterns of ELAM-1, ICAM-1, and VCAM-1 expression on cytomegalovirus-infected endothelial cells. *Transplantation* 1994;58:1379–1385.

72. Chu CM, Liaw YT. Coexpression of intercellular adhesion molecule-1 and class I major histocompatibility complex antigen on hepatocyte membrane in chronic viral hepatitis. *J Clin Pathol* 1993;46:1004–1008.

73. Fukudome K, Furuse M, Fukuhara N, et al. Strong induction of ICAM-1 in human T cells transformed by human T-cell leukemia virus type 1 and depression of ICAM-1 or LFA-1 in adult T cell leukemia-derived cell lines. *Int J Cancer* 1992;52:418–427.

74. Noraz N, Verrier B, Fraiser C, Desgranges C. Cell surface phenotypic changes induced in H9 T cells chronically infected with HTLV type I or HIV type I or coinfected with the two viruses. *AIDS Res Human Retroviruses* 1995;11:145–154.

75. Sobel RA, Mitchell ME, Fondren G. Intercellular adhesion molecule-1 (ICAM-1) in cellular immune reactions in the human central nervous system. *Am J Pathol* 1990;136:1309–1316.

76. Joly E, Mucke L, Oldstone MBA. Virus persistence in neurons explained by lack of major histocompatibility class I expression. *Science* 1991;253:1283–1285.

77. Oldstone MBA, Rall GF. Mechanism and consequence of viral persistence in cells of the immune system and neurons. *Intervirology* 1993;35:116–121.

78. Burgert HG, Maryanski JL, Kvist S. "E3/19K" protein of adenovirus type 2 inhibits lysis of cytolytic T lymphocytes by blocking cell-surface expression of histocompatibility class I antigens. *Proc Natl Acad Sci USA* 1987;84:1356–1360.

79. Schouten GJ, van der Eb AJ, Zantema A. Downregulation of MHC class I expression due to interference with p105-NFκB1 processing by Ad12E1A. *EMBO J* 1995;14:1498–1507.

80. Dhib-Jalbut S, Jacobson S, McFarlin DE, McFarland HF. Impaired HLA-restricted measles virus specific cytotoxic T-cell response in SSPE. *Ann Neurol* 1989;25:272–280.

81. Joly E, Oldstone MBA. Neuronal cells are deficient in loading peptides onto MHC class I molecules. *Neuron* 1992;8:1185–1190.

82. Rammohan KW, McFarland HF, McFarlin DE. Induction of subacute murine measles encephalitis by monoclonal antibodies to virus hemagglutinin. *Nature* 1981;290:588–589.

83. Liebert UG, Schneider-Schanlies S, Buczko K, тer Muelen V. Antibody-induced restriction of viral antigen expression measles encephalopathy in rat. *J Virol* 1990;64:706–713.

84. McChesney MB, Kehrl JH, Valsamakis A, et al. Measles virus infection of B lymphocytes permits cellular activation but blocks progression through the cell cycle. *J Virol* 1987;61:3441–3447.

85. Ahmed R, King C-C, Oldstone MBA. Virus lymphocyte interaction: T cells of the helper subset are infected with lymphocytic choriomeningitis virus during persistent infection in vivo. *J Virol* 1987;61:1571–1576.

86. Leonard R, Zagury D, Desportes I, et al. Cytopathic effect of human immunodeficiency virus in T4 cells is linked to the last stage of virus infection. *Proc Natl Acad Sci USA* 1988;85:3570–3574.

87. Siliciano RF, Lawton T, Knall C, et al. Analysis of host-virus interactions in AIDS with anti-gp120 T cell clones: effect of HIV sequence variation and a mechanism for CD4+ T cell depletion. *Cell* 1988;54:561–575.

88. Laurent-Crawford AG, Krust B, Muller S, et al. The cytopathic effects of HIV is associated with apoptosis. *Virology* 1991;185:829–839.

89. McChesney MB, Fujinami RS, Lampert PW, Oldstone MBA. Viruses disrupt functions of human lymphocytes. II. Measles virus suppresses antibody production by acting on B lymphocytes. *J Exp Med* 1986;163:1331–1336.

90. Jamieson BD, Ahmed R. T-cell tolerance: exposure to virus in utero does not cause a permanent deletion of specific T cells. *Proc Natl Acad Sci USA* 1988;85:2265–2268.

91. Zinkernagel RM, Pircher HP, Ohashi P, et al. T and B cell tolerance and responses to viral antigens in transgenic mice: implications for the pathogenesis of autoimmune versus immunopathologic disease. *Immunol Rev* 1991;122:133–171.

92. Tonietti G, Oldstone MBA, Dixon FJ. The effect of induced chronic viral infections on the immunologic diseases of new Zealand mice. *J Exp Med* 1970;132:89–109.

93. тer Muelen V, Liebert UG. Measles virus-induced autoimmune reaction against brain antigen. *Intervirology* 1993;35:86–94.

94. Vaughan JH, Nguyen M-D, Valbracht JR, et al. Epstein-Barr virus-induced autoimmune responses. I: immunoglobulin M autoantibodies to proteins mimicking and not mimicking Epstein-Barr virus nuclear antigen-1. *J Clin Invest* 1995;95:1306–1315.

95. Vaughan JH, Nguyen M-D, Valbracht JR, et al. Epstein-Barr virus-induced autoimmune responses. II: immunoglobulin G autoantibodies to mimicry and mimicking epitope presence in autoimmune disease. *J Clin Invest* 1995;95:1316–1327.

96. Fujinami RS, Oldstone MBA, Wroblewska Z, et al. Molecular mimicry in virus infection: cross reaction of measles phosphoprotein or of herpes simplex virus with human intermediate filaments. *Proc Natl Acad Sci USA* 1983;80:2346–2350.

97. Smimmbeck PL, Dyrberg T, Drachman DB, Oldstone MBA. Molecular mimicry and myasthenia gravis: an autoantigenic site of the acetylcholine receptor α-subunit that has biologic activity and reacts immunochemically with herpes simplex virus. *J Clin Invest* 1989;84:1174–1180.

98. Dales S, Fujinami RS, Oldstone MBA. Serologic relatedness between Thy1.2 and actin revealed by monoclonal antibody. *J Immunol* 1983;131:1332–1338.

99. Srinivasappa J, Saegusa J, Prabhakar BS, et al. Molecular mimicry: frequency of reactivity of monoclonal antiviral antibodies with normal tissues. *J Virol* 1986;57:397–401.

100. Oldstone MBA. Virus-induced autoimmunity: molecular mimicry as a route to autoimmune disease. *J Autoimmun* 1989;2(suppl):187–194.

101. Wucherpfennig KW, Strominger JL. Molecular mimicry in T cell mediated autoimmunity: viral peptides activate human T cell clones specific for myelin basic protein. *Cell* 1995;80:695–705.

102. Wucherpfennig KW, Sette A, Southwood S, et al. Structural requirements for binding of an immunodominant myelin basic protein peptide to DR2 isotypes and for its recognition by human T cell clones. *J Exp Med* 1994;179:279–290.

103. Wucherpfennig KW, Zhang J, Witek C, et al. Clonal expansion and persistence of human T cells specific for an immunodominant myelin basic protein peptide. *J Immunol* 1994;150:5581–5592.

104. Arthur LO, Bess JW Jr, Urban RG, et al. Macaques immunized with HLA-DR are protected from challenge

with simian immunodeficiency virus. *J Virol* 1995; 69:3117–3124.

105. Marrack P, Winslow GM, Choi Y, et al. The bacterial and mouse tumor virus antigens; two different families of proteins with the same functions. *Immunol Rev* 1993;131:79–92.

106. Jardetzky TS, Brown JH, Gorga JC, et al. Three-dimensional structure of a human class II histocompatibility molecule complexed with superantigen. *Nature* 1994;368:711–718.

107. Marrack P, Kappler JW, Choi Y. A superantigen encoded in the open reading frame of the 3′ terminal repeat of mouse mammary tumor virus. *Nature* 1991;350:203–206.

108. Acha-Orbea H, Sharhov AN, Scarpellino L, et al. Clonal deletion of Vβ 14-bearing T cells in mice transgenic for mammary tumor virus. *Nature* 1991;350:207–211.

109. Laurence J, Hodtser AS, Posnett D. Superantigen implicated in dependence of HIV-1 replication in T cells on TCR V beta expression. *Nature* 1992;358:255–259.

110. Lafon M, Lafage M, Martinez-Arends A, et al. Evidence for a superantigen in humans. *Nature* 1992;358:507.

Chapter 7
Principles of Immunotherapy

Derek R. Smith, Michael J. Olek, Konstantine E. Balashov,
Samia J. Khoury, David A. Hafler, and Howard L. Weiner

Immunotherapy for immune-mediated neurologic diseases is in a state of rapid development. The current therapeutic arsenal consists of a mixture of older and new agents whose uses are actively being redefined. In the first part of this chapter, our current understanding of the mechanisms of action of established medications and developing approaches is discussed in relation to disease pathogenesis models. In the second part a framework for incorporating current and future therapies into rational treatment strategies is addressed together with a review of relevant clinical studies. Mechanisms of immunotherapy and clinical strategies are discussed primarily in the context of multiple sclerosis (MS) as well as other common immune-mediated neurologic diseases including myasthenia gravis (MG), chronic inflammatory demyelinating polyneuropathy (CIDP), and idiopathic polymyositis (IPM). More monophasic inflammatory diseases such as Guillain-Barré syndrome (GBS) and transverse myelitis are also covered. This discussion does not specifically address immunotherapy of diseases with clear etiologic factors such as paraneoplastic syndromes or human T-cell lymphotropic virus type I (HTLV-I)–associated myelopathy, or of neurologic manifestations of systemic autoimmunity.

Mechanistic Strategies for Immune Intervention

Most researchers would now agree that a T cell–mediated cellular immune response is central to the pathogenesis of MS as well as CIDP and IPM. The therapeutic efficacy of thymectomy together with other data argue strongly for a role for T cells in MG also. Although MS has not been formally proved to be a cell-mediated autoimmune disease directed against central nervous system (CNS) myelin, it is this hypothesis on which most investigators base their therapeutic strategies. Animal models for these more common neurologic immune-mediated diseases have been developed. The approaches of immunotherapy or immunomodulation that are being applied to MS derive from treatment of experimental autoimmune encephalomyelitis (EAE), which has become the primary animal model for MS, and from the application to MS of immunosuppressant

or immunomodulatory drugs used for cancer, transplantation, and other organ-specific inflammatory conditions. Whether EAE is a true model for MS remains an open question, but the application of immunotherapeutic strategies to MS has often stemmed from their success in EAE (1). Furthermore, independent of its relationship to MS, EAE has become one of the prime immunologic paradigms used by immunologists for studying the cellular mechanisms of experimental autoimmune disease. Animal models for the other neurologic immune-mediated diseases will likely also serve a useful purpose in understanding the role of new therapeutic approaches in these diseases. There are a number of ways in which immune intervention can affect T-cell biology. Our current understanding of T-cell activation is that T cells recognize antigen in the context of the major histocompatibility complex (MHC). Activation requires appropriate costimulatory signals by an antigen-presenting cell. In MS, activated T cells then migrate to the nervous system where they recognize the myelin antigen to which they were sensitized, release inflammatory cytokines, and initiate the destruction of the myelin sheath. Figure 7-1 depicts mechanisms by which immunotherapy may affect the autoimmune process in MS.

Anergy and Apoptosis

If disease is initiated by an antigen-reactive T cell, then one strategy is to block the activation of such a cell by inducing anergy. As shown in Figure 7-1, the triggering of a myelin-reactive cell in MS may involve antigen presentation of a cross-reactive antigen such as a virus or stimulation of the autoreactive T cell by other mechanisms such as a superantigen (2). The induction of anergy implies that the myelin-reactive cell is paralyzed so that it is not functional and cannot be activated to cause damage in the nervous system. Anergy can be induced if the myelin-reactive cells encounter free antigen or an antigen is presented by a cell that does not have costimulatory properties such as B7. Of note is that orally administered antigens can induce anergy if free antigen enters the bloodstream (3). The B7-CD28 interaction is required for a disease-inducing T cell (Th1 type, discussed below) to be activated. Alternately, some con-

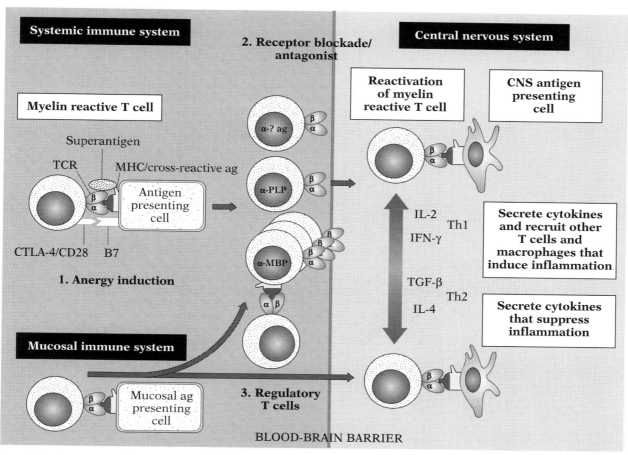

Figure 7-1.   Immune mechanisms and strategies of immunotherapy in multiple sclerosis. Myelin-reactive T cells are activated in the periphery and migrate to the central nervous system (CNS) where they initiate an autoimmune response against CNS myelin. Strategies of immunotherapy include 1) induction of anergy, or paralyzing myelin reactive cells; 2) receptor blockade to interfere with the function or migration of myelin-reactive cells; and 3) generation of regulatory cells to inactivate myelin-reactive cells or secrete cytokines that suppress inflammation at the target organs. TCR = T-cell receptor; MHC = major histocompatibility complex; ag = antigen; PLP = proteolipid protein; MBP = myelin basic protein; IL = interleukin; IFN = interferon; TGF = transforming growth factor.

ditions, for example, repeated exposure of activated cells to high doses of antigen, to agonists of some tumor necrosis factor (TNF) superfamily receptors (4), or to superantigen, can result in programmed cell death or apoptosis (5).

Receptor Blockade

Three classes of receptor can be targeted for blockade: adhesion molecules, the T-cell receptor (TCR)–MHC complex, and costimulatory molecules. In MS, myelin-reactive T cells include those with reactivity against proteolipid protein (PLP), myelin basic protein (MBP), other myelin antigens such as myelin oligodendrocyte glycoprotein (MOG) and myelin-associated glycoprotein (MAG), or other undefined antigens (6). These cells can be blocked with compounds that affect their abil-

ity to migrate into the nervous systems by interfering with their adhesion to endothelial cell surfaces. In addition, receptor blockade by antagonists for components of the MHC-TCR complex or costimulatory molecules could prevent myelin-specific cells from being activated. In MG, peptides designed to block the binding of antibodies to immunodominant epitopes of the acetylcholine receptor (AChR) could also be designed (7). Receptor blockage could occur in the systemic immune system or in the CNS.

Regulatory T Cells and Immune Deviation

Although the biology of regulatory or suppressor T cells is not completely understood, two types of regulatory T cells have been characterized and found effective in the EAE model and can be applied for the treatment of neurologic immune-mediated diseases. One is an anti-clonotypic or an anti-idiotypic T cell that reacts with antigen-specific autoreactive T cells (8). These cells may be generated during T-cell vaccination (discussed below). The second is an antigen-specific regulatory T cell. These regulatory T cells can migrate to the CNS or cervical lymphatics where they encounter antigen and secrete anti-inflammatory cytokines that suppress inflammation such as interleukin (IL)-4, IL-10, and transforming growth factor (TGF)-β (9,10). These cells can be generated by oral tolerization. As more is learned about the immune mechanisms of inflammation and regulation, it appears there is a balance between Th1- and Th2-type responses. Disease-inducing cells, or Th1-type cells, can secrete inflammatory cytokines such as IL-2, TNF, and interferon-γ, which recruit other T cells and macrophages that induce inflammation. Regulatory Th2-type cells secrete cytokines that suppress inflammation. Strategies to block Th1-type cytokines or administer or enhance Th2-type cytokines are being developed. Similarly, anticlonotypic T cells may also function by secreting anti-inflammatory cytokines.

It must be emphasized that although it is possible to interrupt an immune response in the EAE model with the aforementioned strategies of immune manipulation, not all of these strategies are easily translated for use in humans. For example, not all compounds cross the blood-brain barrier and some compounds need to be administered by intravenous or subcutaneous injection over prolonged periods of time. In animal models, the time of immunization and disease induction is known so that therapeutic agents can be given at critical points in the immune response. In MS, the intermittent chronic activation of the immune system makes such time-dependent targeted therapy difficult. Furthermore, one of the difficulties with immune-specific therapies is that although the specific therapy may suppress animal models of disease in which inbred strains are used, patients represent an outbred population. Thus, in individual patients, different portions of an autoantigen may be recognized and a relatively nonrestricted set of TCRs used.

In the following sections, mechanistic treatment approaches are reviewed. Some are established or being tested in clinical trials, whereas others have been shown to be effective in animal models or have been used in other conditions and may be applied to neurologic immune-mediated diseases.

Antigen-Specific Immunotherapy

Antigen-specific modulation of the immune response is an attractive approach for treating an autoimmune disease. The difficulty with any antigen-specific therapy, however, is the presumption that one knows the autoantigen that pathogenic T cells attack and that there is only one autoantigen being attacked. Furthermore, once a tissue is inflamed, multiple reactivities may develop and inflammatory cells that are not specific for myelin antigens could play an important role in the on-

going disease process. The spreading of autoimmune responses has been shown in EAE and diabetes models. In rheumatoid arthritis, even though it is initiated by T cells, joint inflammation and destruction may then become a T cell–independent process. In addition, γ/δ T cells reactive to heat shock proteins may be secondarily generated and participate in CNS inflammation and damage.

Copolymer 1

Copolymer 1 is a random polymer of a design initially based on the amino acid composition of MBP. The mechanism by which copolymer 1 may work in humans is unknown. It could function by generating regulatory cells, as this has been observed in animals treated with altered myelin peptides (11,12). Altered myelin peptides will likely also reach clinical trials. Proliferation of MBP-specific T-cell clones also is suppressed by copolymer 1 and it theoretically could interfere with binding of MBP or other peptides to the MHC cleft (13,14) .

T-Cell Vaccination and T-Cell Receptor Therapy

In animal models, restricted TCR usage by MBP-reactive cells has been demonstrated and it is possible to suppress EAE by vaccination or immunization with MBP-reactive clones or TCR peptides (8,15,16). This approach induces regulatory cells that interact with the injected clones or peptides. The mechanism for this protection involves both an "antiactivated T-cell" response, which is short-lived, and anticlonotypic T-cell responses, which are longer-lived. Moreover, results of animal experiments suggest the safety of T-cell vaccination using either fixed or irradiated T-cell clones. Two phase I studies of T-cell vaccination have been performed in MS patients. In the first, four subjects with progressive MS were given a total of seven inoculations of attenuated, autologous T-cell clones isolated from the cerebrospinal fluid (CSF) (17). Theses cells were not antigen specific. The patients showed no untoward side effects and immunologic studies suggested that the inoculation of autologous T cell–activated clones was associated with partial, short-term immunosuppression as evidenced by the downregulation of subsequent stimulation via the CD2 pathway of activation. In addition, the autologous mixed lymphocyte response, which is reduced in about half of the patients with MS, was enhanced for a short period of time after the T-cell vaccination. In a second study, six patients were inoculated with MBP-specific T cells (18). T-cell responses to the inoculants developed and there was a depletion of MBP-reactive cells in the recipients. Furthermore, CD8+ anticlonotypic T-cell lines that recognized the CD4+ MBP-specific T cells were isolated from treated patients. In addition to using T-cell clones for vaccination, in a phase I trial investigators inoculated MS patients with immunogenic regions of the TCR that recognize immunodominant regions of MBP, and changes in MBP-reactive cells were observed. The conceptual problem with T-cell vaccination and TCR therapy is that in MS, TCR usage of MBP-reactive cells is not likely to be as restricted as in animals. Furthermore, there are reactivities to other myelin antigens such as PLP in MS (19). Thus, T-cell vaccination or TCR therapy may be too specific, downregulating only a small proportion of autoreactive cells. Although a subcategory of patients could theoretically benefit from such an approach, administration very early in the disease course may be required and may not be effective over time in a chronic disease such as MS.

Anergy Induction

An alternative approach to inactivating autoreactive T cells is to use free antigen, antigen coupled to autologous cells, or antigen-MHC complexes. This approach induces anergy and has been used successfully in the EAE model. It is well known that intravenous administration of soluble antigen can lead to tolerogenic signals to the immune system. Investigators attempted phase I trials to induce tolerance to MBP by injecting MBP into MS patients, but the attempts were unsuccessful and in some instances the patients became sensitized. Although less specific than TCR therapy, as one is suppressing all cells reacting to a particular antigen, anergy induction does not address the issue that there is reactivity to more than one myelin antigen in MS. However, it is theoretically possible to anergize against a number of different myelin antigens. Important issues for clinical use are how often the treatment would need to be given, by what route, and whether sensitization might occur with repeated treatment. Similar issues are raised by approaches that attempt to induce apoptosis of autoreactive cells and are as yet less developed.

Oral Tolerance

Oral tolerance refers to the long-recognized observation that proteins that pass through the gastrointestinal tract generate systemic hyporesponsiveness. Thus, if one feeds animals a protein such as ovalbumin or MBP and then immunizes the animals, the immune response against the fed antigen is reduced. Oral tolerance evolved to allow the mucosal immune system (gut-associated lymphoid tissue (GALT)) to absorb proteins without becoming sensitized to them. In recent years, a great deal has been learned about the mechanism of oral tolerance and the use of oral tolerance has been successfully applied to several animal models of autoimmune diseases including MS, arthritis, uveitis, diabetes, thyroiditis, and myasthenia, and in transplantation (20). Oral tolerance is also being tested clinically in the human diseases MS, rheumatoid arthritis, uveitis, and juvenile diabetes. Depending on the amount of antigen fed, orally administered antigens result in the generation of active suppression or anergy. Low doses favor active suppression whereas higher doses favor anergy or apoptosis (3,21). The doses and strategy being used in clinical trials are to generate regulatory T cells that suppress inflammation at the target organ. Antigens that pass through the gut preferentially generate Th2-type cells that secrete IL-4, IL-10, and TGF-β. Such cells leave the gut and migrate to the organ that contains the fed antigen. The regulatory cells are then stimulated to release anti-inflammatory cytokines. Oral tolerance can be conceptualized as a natural drug delivery system in which physiologic anti-inflammatory cytokines are delivered to the target organ by one's own cells depending on the protein fed. Thus, one need not know what the autoantigen is in an autoimmune disease in order for oral tolerization to be effective. In this regard, MBP- or PLP-induced EAE in the mouse can be suppressed by feeding MBP (22). Similarly, adjuvant- or antigen-induced arthritis can be suppressed by feeding collagen (19). Oral tolerance also has the advantage of involving oral administration of a medication with no apparent side effects. An initial trial in relapsing-remitting MS demonstrated a decrease in the number of MBP-reactive cells in patients fed bovine myelin and suggested a clinical effect on the number of attacks (23). However, a phase II/III pivotal multicenter clinical trial in relapsing-remitting MS patients with prospective randomization for different subgroups failed to show any benefit over placebo. Recombinant human proteins and the use of compounds that enhance the generation of Th2-type regulatory cells may enhance the biologic effects of oral tolerance. Of note is that in animals interferon beta enhances the protection of orally administered myelin antigens (24).

Non–Antigen-Specific Immunomodulation

A number of approaches of non–antigen-specific immunotherapy have been successful in animal models and are being considered for clinical trials. They are designed to affect the immune system in a number of different ways. The therapies are listed as having minimal to moderate systemic toxicity.

Interferon Beta

The interferons alpha, beta, and tau act through the same receptor. It is not yet clear whether there are immunologically significant differences in the way they activate this receptor. The intracellular events following receptor binding are being rapidly elucidated. Activated receptors turn on Janus kinase enzymes termed *Jaks* and *MAP kinase*, which then phosphorylate proteins termed *STAT*, which then form intranuclear complexes that bind to DNA regulatory regions controlling gene expression (25). While interferon beta affects the course of relapsing-remitting MS (see below), its mechanism of action at the level of cellular interactions is currently unknown (26). The possibilities are as follows: 1) Interferon-γ augments immune responses and increases MS attacks (27). Interferon beta decreases interferon-γ production by activated lymphocytes (28). 2) Interferon beta may help reverse a suppressor cell defect that has been observed in MS (29), although the defect is more common in patients with progressive MS (30). 3) Viral infections have been associated with increased MS attacks (31) and interferon beta could be working through its antiviral effects, although there is no evidence from one trial that interferon beta worked by this mechanism (26). 4) As described in Figure 7-1, a balance between Th1- and Th2-type immune responses may be important in MS and interferon beta may favor the generation of Th2-type responses (32). 5) Interferon beta downregulates the IL-2 receptor on the lymphocytes of treated MS patients, and thus may act to block the expansion phase of an immune response (33). 6) Interferon beta can stimulate IL-10 production by macrophages, which can suppress immune responses (34).

Drugs To Alter Lymphocyte Traffic

It is known that there is rapid trafficking of cells from the peripheral immune system into the CNS in MS (35). In this regard, total lymphoid irradiation (TLI) has an ameliorating effect on progressive MS and only involves manipulation of the peripheral immune system. EAE can be suppressed by monoclonal antibodies and other drugs that alter the traffic of the cells into the nervous system (36,37) and such compounds are being considered for treatment of MS. Such treatment has the advantage of not being dependent on the antigen specificity of the migrating cells. However, one potential difficulty with this treatment is that it is given at a specific point in time when the disease is active in animals and such time-dependent therapy is difficult in MS. The degree to which it could be applied to the chronic progressive type of MS remains to be seen.

Monoclonal Antibodies

Phase I studies of anti–T-cell monoclonal antibody infusions have been undertaken in MS. Our group studied the immunologic effects of three anti–T-cell monoclonal antibodies: anti-CD2, anti-CD4, and anti-T12 (38,39). Other investigators reported that anti–T-cell monoclonal antibody infusions suppressed in vitro measures of the human immune response. Specifically, an anti-CD2 monoclonal antibody decreased T-cell activation by phytohemagglutinin, and anti-CD4 monoclonal antibody infusions abolished pokeweed mitogen–induced immunoglobulin synthesis without lysis of the CD4+ T-cell populations. With repeated infusions, human antimouse antibodies were found in the circulation. Although most of the human antimouse antibodies were not immunoglobulin isotype specific, significant anti-idiotypic activity was observed after repeated infusions. Other investigators reported that anti-CD3 infusions were associated with significant toxic effects in MS patients (40).

Although the clinical usefulness of currently available anti–T-cell murine monoclonal antibodies in chronic disease such as MS is hampered by the presence of hu-

man antimouse antibodies, there are a number of potential approaches to solve the problem. First is the use of humanized monoclonal antibodies with a human Fc and mouse Fab region. A second approach is to attach a toxin to the murine monoclonal antibody, which would result in a greater elimination of the targeted T-cell population in addition to potentially preventing human antimouse antibodies. More extensive studies with anti-CD4 were carried out by Steinman et al at Stanford University using a humanized anti-CD4 monoclonal antibody, and a larger trial was undertaken at the Institutes of Neurology at Queen's Square, London. At Stanford, patients with chronic progressive MS were treated with a chimeric anti-CD4 antibody with a humanized Fc region (1). Results of the large trial were essentially negative despite the finding of a very marked reduction in the number of CD4+ cells (41,42). Possible explanations are that MS becomes a T cell–independent disease late in its course, or that regulatory T cells are also removed by this therapy.

Interleukin-2 Toxin

IL-2 toxin targets activated cells and is effective in some animal models. It is being tried in diseases such as rheumatoid arthritis and MS.

Transforming Growth Factor-β

This naturally suppressive cytokine suppresses animal models of autoimmune diseases including EAE and arthritis (43). As discussed previously, it mediates the effect of regulatory cells generated by oral tolerance. Trials of injectable TGF-β have been initiated in MS patients. There has been some interest in trying IL-4 or IL-10 similarly.

Tumor Necrosis Factor Antagonists

As TNF may be a mediator of tissue damage in MS, investigators have tried treatment with TNF antagonists for MS. This includes the use of pentoxifylline, a drug that favors Th2-type responses and downregulates TNF production (44), and the use of anti-TNF monoclonal antibodies. Such antibodies have shown some usefulness in rheumatoid arthritis (45), but appear to exacerbate MS (46).

Immunoglobulin

The mechanism of action of immunoglobulin is unclear but may relate to anti-idiotypic effects (47). One hypothesis based on animal work that serves as a basis for a trial of intravenous immunoglobulin in MS is that it can promote remyelination (48).

Psoralen Ultraviolet Light Treatment

Psoralen ultraviolet light treatment given extracorporally can benefit patients with certain skin conditions and is being tested in MS. The mechanism of action is unclear but may relate to an alteration of cytokine patterns (49).

Linomide

Linomide is an anticancer compound that has been shown to be effective in both the chronic and acute EAE models with minimal side effects (50). However, linomide trials in MS have been canceled due to cardiotoxic side effects.

Plasmapheresis

Plasmapheresis removes plasma proteins and replaces them with colloid. The benefits in MG relate to the removal of anti-AChR antibodies. The mechanism of action in GBS is unclear but could be related to the removal of antibodies or circulating proinflammatory proteins.

Thymectomy

The reasons for the benefit of thymectomy in MG are unclear but it may involve removal of an antigenic stimulus, alteration of cytokine patterns, or an alteration of lymphocyte subsets.

Non–Antigen-Specific Immunosuppression

Table 7-1 lists immunosuppressive agents that have been used in neurologic immune-mediated diseases. Clinical studies of the specific agents in these diseases are discussed later. The mechanisms of immunosuppression of these agents are likely multiple. One shared component is probably a direct cytotoxic effect on pathogenic leukocytes. However, this cannot explain the entire effect, as severely leukopenic treated patients with very active autoimmune disease have been reported. Therefore, other mechanisms should be involved. We have data suggesting that in some chronic progressive MS patients receiving pulse cyclophosphamide treatment, the Th1-type cytokine production shifts to Th2-type production (32). On the other hand, in diseases characterized by hypergammaglobulinemia and exaggerated B-cell responses, these functions seem to be selectively reduced by cyclophosphamide therapy (51). An explanation for these findings is that proliferating cells are selectively vulnerable to the cytotoxic effects of cyclophosphamide, as is the case in in vitro studies. In addition, monocyte functions and cytokine production are inhibited and this may impact both antigen presentation and effector mechanisms. Azathioprine has similar effects to cyclophosphamide except that cytokine production seems to be unchanged. The main effects of cyclosporine seem to be due to a downregulation of IL-2 and IL-2 receptor and thus lymphocyte activation. Other agents in this group are being tested. FK 506 is a medication used in transplantation and is in the same

Table 7-1.
Non–Antigen-Specific Immunosuppression

Azathioprine
Cyclophosphamide
Deoxyspergualin
Cyclosporine
FK 506
Methotrexate
Mitoxantrone
Sulfasalazine
Total lymphoid irradiation
Cladribine

family as cyclosporine. It is being considered for use in MS and is associated with neurotoxicity. Sulfasalazine is an antirheumatoid drug that is currently being tried in MS. Mitoxantrone is an anticancer drug that can be effective in MS, although its use may be limited by cardiac toxicity. Specific trials of these agents are discussed below.

Corticosteroids

Corticosteroids have been used in autoimmune disease since the 1940s but their mechanism of action remains poorly understood. Similarly to type I interferons, the intracellular events following glucocorticoid receptor binding are being elucidated. The principal immunomodulatory effects seem to involve binding of the activated glucocorticoid receptor to immunoregulatory transcription factors, preventing them from activating genes, and also increasing expression of the inhibitors of these transcription factors (52). At the level of cellular interaction there are effects on leukocyte circulatory kinetics, functional capabilities, and cytokine production, all of which probably play a role in their therapeutic benefit. Intravenous corticosteroids probably are of benefit in acute inflammation in MS by decreasing the entry of cells into the brain and by preventing proliferation and perhaps inducing apoptosis of activated cells. These agents deplete CD4+ cells, decrease the release of cytokines including TNF and interferon-γ, and decrease class II expression (53). In animal models, glucocorticoids cause a shift from Th1 to Th2 cytokine production (54). In humans delayed-type hypersensitivity responses are suppressed only after 2 weeks of therapy. In MS steroids also decrease IgG synthesis in the CNS and reduce CSF antibodies to MBP and oligoclonal bands. The factors underlying the difference in response to oral versus intravenous glucocorticoids brought out in the optic neuritis trial are unknown (55,56).

Principles for Clinical Application of Therapies

We believe the following principles are important for immunotherapy and can serve as a framework from which to view the various treatment modalities that are currently being used and tested. In essence, there is a hierarchy of treatments, with the least toxic therapy given first. Some of the new therapies now available to MS patients are beginning to make an impact on immunotherapy of other neurologic immune-mediated diseases. Advances in magnetic resonance imaging (MRI) and a clearer understanding of how the immune system functions have made an impact on developing therapy for MS.

First-Line Therapy

Agents in this group are not currently approved for neurologic immune-mediated diseases other than MS. In patients with relapsing-remitting MS receiving 8 MIU of recombinant interferon beta, the frequency of relapses decreased from 1.27/yr to 0.84/yr after 2 years (57). The drug has been approved by the Food and Drug Administration (FDA) for use in MS. It did not affect clinical disability in patients followed over the 3-year period, but it did significantly affect the accumulation of lesions on MRIs (58), suggesting that the underlying disease process was affected. It is administered every other day by self injection. Side effects include flulike symptoms and reactions at the injection site, but these tend to diminish with time. Recent 5-year follow-up data (59) indicate that disease progression was less in the interferon beta–treated group (35%) compared with the placebo group (46%). Not all patients respond to the drug, and with time all patients have additional attacks. There is no evidence that interferon beta is of benefit in patients with progressive disease. This question is being addressed in a current study. The potential mechanisms of action of interferon beta are discussed above. A second major study investigating the efficacy of weekly injections of a glycosylated recombinant interferon beta in 301 relapsing-remitting MS patients found a one third decrease in the exacerbation rate and a delay in the progression of disability over 2 years (60). There also appeared to be fewer side effects with this preparation. The FDA has approved it. Encouraging results have also been reported for a preliminary trial of interferon alfa-2 (61). Case reports of patients with CIDP improving with interferon alfa or beta treatment have begun to appear in the literature. Copolymer 1 is an injectable synthetic polymer that recently underwent a large double-blind trial involving 251 relapsing-remitting MS patients (62). The copolymer-treated patients had a 2-year relapse rate of 1.19, versus 1.68 for placebo-treated patients, a 29% reduction. A similar percentage of the copolymer-treated patients also experienced injection site reactions, and a few systemic reactions including chest pain, flushing, dyspnea, palpitations, and anxiety were reported.

The success of these drugs in MS does provide some hope for other neurologic immune-mediated diseases. It seems probable that interferon beta will eventually reach trials on other neurologic immune-mediated diseases, and copolymer 1 conceivably could be tested as treatment for peripheral nervous system demyelination

as well. The oral tolerization approach is being tried in a broad range of autoimmune diseases including experimental myasthenia (20). Interferon beta and copolymer are the first drugs that can be classified in this category of therapy even though they are not free from toxicity. In addition to the side effects of injectable interferon, interferon beta causes abortion and thus cannot be given to women planning pregnancy. Furthermore, although there are positive clinical effects, it does not halt the disease process in most patients. Orally administered drugs are preferable to those given by frequent injection or intravenous infusion. As discussed previously, some forms of antigen-specific therapy such as T-cell or TCR vaccination could also represent first-line therapy. Ultimately, drugs such as copolymer 1 and oral myelin must be compared to interferon beta in terms of efficacy, ease of administration, and side-effect profile. In addition, the cost of treatment will be an important factor in therapy if there are no major differences in the efficacy or toxicity profile of these first-line drugs. With interferon beta an approved therapy for MS, the question arises of how additional therapies will be tested, whether in small phase I/II trials or in pivotal phase III trials. Possibilities include treating patients who did not respond to interferon beta treatment, comparing the new drug against interferon beta, or administering the drug to be tested to patients taking interferon beta. Identifying nonresponding subgroups of patients, such as patients who make neutralizing antibodies to interferon beta (59), will be an important component of future trials. The resolution of these issues will depend on the efficacy of interferon beta as determined when larger populations are treated, the specifics of the drugs to be tested, and FDA requirements.

Appropriate Use of Steroids

For Relapses or Acute Attacks

Based on what is currently known about interferon beta and other relatively nontoxic drugs that could be given early in the course of MS, it is expected that patients will continue to have relapses. While relapsing forms of MG and CIDP do exist, corticosteroids are typically used in a more chronic manner for these diseases. Their use is accepted for the treatment of relapse or attack in these diseases, with the caveat that there is no accepted use for corticosteroids in GBS (63). Thus, short courses of intravenous methylprednisolone are given to speed recovery when a significant relapse occurs. Given what was reported in the optic neuritis study, intravenous methylprednisolone may have a prolonged salutary effect on the course of MS. Acute attacks are either not treated or treated with a short course of corticosteroids. Indications for treatment of an MS relapse include functionally disabling symptoms with objective evidence of neurologic impairment. Thus, mild sensory attacks are typically not treated. In the past, adrenocorticotropin (ACTH) and oral prednisone were primarily used. More recently, physicians have been treating with short courses of intravenous methylprednisolone, 500 to 1000 mg daily for 3 to 7 days, with or without a short prednisone taper (53). Optic neuritis may occur during the course of MS or be one of the initial symptoms. A recent trial of optic neuritis demonstrated that patients treated with oral prednisone alone were more likely to have recurrent episodes of optic neuritis as compared to those treated with methylprednisolone followed by oral prednisone (55,56). These results now make intravenous methylprednisolone the primary treatment used for optic neuritis and further support its use for major attacks. Furthermore, the optic neuritis study found that treatment with a 3-day course of high-dose methylprednisolone reduced the rate of development of MS over a 2-year period (64). The protective effect was most apparent in patients at highest risk for MS, those with multiple focal brain MRI abnormalities. Although these results need to be confirmed in a larger series of patients, they support the use of high-dose intravenous methylprednisolone for acute MS attacks. Postinfectious encephalitis and transverse myelitis can also be managed with this approach. High-dose intravenous methylprednisolone appears to have relatively few side effects in most patients, although a number of side effects have been reported and include mental changes, unmasking of infections, gastric disturbances, and an increased incidence of fractures. Anaphylactoid reactions and arrhythmias may also occur.

Chronic Steroid Therapy

Maintenance therapy on oral corticosteroids has been the mainstay of immunotherapy for CIDP, IPM, and MG resistant to anticholinesterase medications and thymectomy. The goal is to achieve the lowest possible dose that will maintain quiescence of disease to avoid the long-term side effects of these medications. Many strategies have been employed to achieve this goal, including alternate-day dosing and combination therapy with immunosuppressive agents (discussed below). Because steroids can cause an initial weakening of muscle strength, the dose should be gradually increased in MG patients unless the disease is very mild or the patients are being artificially maintained; the dose should begin at 15 to 20 mg/day and be increased by 5 mg/day until a clinical response occurs or the dose of 50 mg/day is achieved. Weakening is a signal to proceed with greater caution. In CIDP and IPM, beginning at a dose of 1 mg/kg is usual, tapering at a rate of 10 mg/mo or less thereafter. This gradual decrement is recommended because the clinical effect of a given dose is believed to lag by several months. While up to 90% of MG patients respond to steroid therapy, it is rare that they can be tapered completely off the drugs. Alternate-day dosing should be gradually introduced and is especially recommended in IPM patients because it can significantly reduce the incidence of steroid myopathy. Our center and others have begun to investigate the effect of monthly pulses of intravenous methylprednisolone for the treatment of relapsing-remitting progressive and progressive MS. Long-term side effects of corticosteroids

include cataracts, osteoporosis, aseptic bone necrosis, Cushing's syndrome, hypertension, and exacerbation of diabetes. Thus, patients on these regimens should be preventively managed for these problems, though frequently the side effects cannot be avoided.

Second-Line Immunotherapy To Halt Refractory or Progressive Disease

Although some patients may respond to first-line treatments, it is expected that others will be refractory to therapy or the disease will enter a progressive stage. In these instances, immunotherapy or immunosuppression with stronger medication may be warranted, depending on the individual case. Drugs in this category would be classified as second- or third-line treatment depending on the risk-benefit ratio of the therapy. Second- or third-line therapy could find utility, even if it is only given effectively on a short-term basis, if such treatment allowed reinstitution of first-line therapy. The neurologic immune-mediated diseases being discussed all have progressive forms, and experienced clinicians' preferences for which agents to use vary. Treatment directed at the progressive phase is the most difficult, as the immune-mediated diseases may be harder to affect once a progressive stage has been initiated. For this reason, there is a trend toward using these agents either before or earlier in the progressive stage of some autoimmune diseases such as rheumatoid arthritis.

Immunosuppressive Agents

Cyclophosphamide, TLI, methotrexate, azathioprine, cladribine, and cyclosporine have some positive clinical effects in neurologic immune-mediated diseases. Most of these agents have been tried as treatment for several of the diseases. The present discussion of the agents focuses on controlled studies, which have been done mainly in MS patients, in part because of its higher incidence.

At our center over the past decade we investigated the use of cyclophosphamide to treat progressive MS. The initial study demonstrated a positive effect in patients treated with a 2-week course of cyclophosphamide with ACTH as compared to patients who received ACTH alone (65). However, within 1 to 3 years, the disease in most patients began to progress again (66). These findings led to the study of the Northeast Cooperative Treatment Group, a randomized single-blind trial that tested the efficacy of cyclophosphamide boosters given every 2 months on an outpatient basis in 236 patients who received an initial induction of cyclophosphamide with ACTH (67). The results demonstrated a modest positive clinical effect in the patients receiving boosters as opposed to those who did not. Most striking was the finding that younger patients (<40 years) with short duration of progression tended to respond to therapy whereas older patients did not. Our current regimen involves intravenous administration of methylprednisolone for 5 days followed by monthly pulses of cyclophosphamide and methylprednisolone designed to produce a leukopenia (68). If there is a clinical response at 6 months, pulses are given monthly for a year, every 6 months in the second year, and every 2 months in the third year. Not all investigators found positive clinical effects treating patients with only a 2-week course of cyclophosphamide (69). Smaller studies of pulse therapy found positive clinical effects (reviewed elsewhere (70)). The side effects of intravenous cyclophosphamide include infertility, cystitis, alopecia, and gastrointestinal disturbance. The results to date and the toxicities of cyclophosphamide make the use of the drug only appropriate for carefully selected patients with actively progressive disease that has not responded to other treatment regimens. For patients with progressive disease who have not had an adequate trial of steroids, we use methylprednisolone induction followed by monthly methylprednisolone boosters before we initiate cyclophosphamide therapy. Pulse cyclophosphamide is not widely used in the treatment of other autoimmune diseases other than lupus nephritis. More acute vasculitic syndromes such as Wegener's granulomatosis and primary angiitis of the CNS are treated with a combination of high-dose cyclophosphamide and glucocorticoids followed by a prednisone taper, with the option of pulse cyclophosphamide therapy.

TLI has potent immunosuppressive effects and a double-blind study of lymphoid irradiation reported benefit in patients with progressive MS (reviewed elsewhere (71)). The absolute lymphocyte count appeared to be a crude indication of therapeutic efficacy, with greater efficacy found in patients with lower counts. In many patients the disease began progressing again after initial therapy and a major limitation of the use of TLI is whether it or other treatments that similarly affect the immune system can be given to those who re-enter the progressive phase of disease despite therapy.

A large multicenter trial of cyclosporine in the United States (72) and a trial in London (73) suggest that cyclosporine has a beneficial, albeit modest effect in ameliorating progressive MS, but it has not found clinical use because of the narrow benefit-risk ratio. Cyclosporine has found limited use in the treatment of MG (74) and IPM and may be easier to use than azathioprine.

Azathioprine has been the subject of a large number of studies in MS (reviewed elsewhere (75)) and meta-analysis of the results of all published blind, randomized, controlled trials showed a statistically significant benefit in reducing the frequency of relapses over a 3-year period, but minimal effect on disability (76). Azathioprine, as a substitute or sparing agent for corticosteroids, has been used to treat MG, CIDP, and IPM. A test dose of 50 mg is given daily for a week. If well tolerated, the dose can be escalated to 2 to 3 mg/kg/day. Beneficial effects may be delayed by 6 or more months. The target is to maintain white blood cell counts at approximately 3000 cells/μL. Side effects include fever, myalgias, hepatotoxicity, and gastrointestinal distress.

Methotrexate has found widespread use in the treatment of autoimmune diseases such as rheumatoid arthritis, which has led to its use in neurologic immune-mediated disease. A recent double-blind trial of oral methotrexate at 7.5 mg/wk in 60 patients with chronic progressive MS showed a significant beneficial effect on measures of upper extremity disability (77). It has also been used with some success in IPM. Further experience may help clinicians to avoid a drawback to the use of methotrexate, which is its ability to induce an irreversible hepatotoxicity.

Cladribine, an immunosuppressive agent approved for the treatment of hairy cell leukemia, showed positive effects in a recent trial wherein 7 of 23 placebo-treated patients versus 1 of 24 cladribine-treated patients had a worsening of 1 point or more on the Expanded Disability Status Scale (EDSS) at 1 year (78). A large multicenter trial is under way.

Plasmapheresis and Intravenous Immunoglobulin

These approaches have been used in fulminant neurologic immune-mediated diseases with variable success, which has led to some extension of their use into more chronic diseases. A considerable literature has accumulated regarding the use of plasmapheresis for GBS within the first 2 weeks after the onset of symptoms (79,80). There is also evidence supporting the use of plasmapheresis in CIDP and MG (81). Several studies are addressing the question of plasmapheresis versus intravenous immunoglobulin in the treatment of GBS, with the results of at least one completed study favoring the use of intravenous immunoglobulin (82). Intravenous immunoglobulin is easier and generally safer to use than plasmapheresis, but both remain expensive. Intravenous immunoglobulin may also be beneficial in the treatment of dermatomyositis and CIDP (83,84) and has been tried in initial MS trials (85).

Thymectomy for Myasthenia Gravis

Thymectomy is recommended for adult generalized MG patients with an enlarged thymus for whom medical treatment does not control the disease. Remission or improvement occurs in more than 80% of patients but is usually gradual and delayed (86). About 15% of these patients will have had thymomas. Perioperative and operative management require expertise and should be done in centers with experience.

Reinstitution of First-Line Therapy

The principle of second- or third-line therapy is to induce remission of disease activity, following which one would reinstitute first-line, nontoxic therapy to maintain quiescence. The degree to which subsequent first-line therapy will be effective is unknown. Furthermore, a major problem that confronts clinicians is determining when a remission has indeed occurred (discussed below).

Combination and Pulse Therapy

Until the pathogeneses of neurologic immune-mediated diseases are precisely understood, it is unlikely that a single treatment will be effective in all patients. The principle of combination therapy has found utility in cancer treatment and is becoming an important principle for the therapy of MS and other neurologic immune-mediated diseases. Rationales for combining different mechanistic approaches exist. Combining therapies involving systemic immune deviation with those involving immune deviation of antigen-specific cells or molecular blockades provides interesting possibilities. In this respect, studies of the EAE animal model demonstrated that interferon beta and oral myelin have synergistic effects when given together (24). Pulse steroids or relatively nontoxic immunomodulation may find utility in conjunction with other antigen-specific forms of therapy. As it becomes clear which mechanistic strategies work best, more rational combinations can be designed. The use of immunosuppressive agents as steroid-sparing agents has been discussed already. Furthermore, because some forms of chronic therapy cannot be given safely, intermittent pulse administration of drugs that affect the immune system may become an important mode of therapy. This is currently being tested in our center using pulse steroids and pulse cyclophosphamide.

Disease Monitoring

The major problems confronting therapy of neurologic immune-mediated diseases are unpredictable courses and the length of time over which disability accumulates. Even for treatments that have proven efficacy, it may be difficult to determine in an individual patient whether the treatment is having a therapeutic effect unless the disease becomes truly quiescent clinically or the patient improves during therapy. In some instances, it is clear that a patient is either a responder or a nonresponder to a particular treatment. We have occasionally seen such positive clinical effects in younger patients with rapidly progressive, steroid-unresponsive MS treated with pulse cyclophosphamide. The hope is that surrogate markers that are linked to the underlying disease process will allow a more rational approach to assessing therapy apart from clinical assessment. MRI has provided such a surrogate marker in MS and was one of the major factors in the approval of interferon beta for the treatment of relapsing-remitting MS (87). Even though MRI does not provide a perfect correlate of disease activity, it may ultimately serve as the best objective tool for measuring ongoing disease in the nervous system since it is now known that MS is chronically active even when clinical activity is not present (88,89). However, apart from formal clinical trials, MRI is costly and impractical to perform on a frequent basis in a general neurology practice.

There is a large body of evidence showing abnormalities of immune function in MS including activated T cells, loss of suppressor influences, the presence of activated myelin-reactive T cells in the peripheral blood, and abnormal cytokine patterns. One intriguing recent observation is that measures of the cytokine TNF-α may correlate with disease activity and disease disability

(90,91). TNF-α can be measured in whole peripheral blood following stimulation with phytohemagglutinin, and TNF-α message can be measured in frozen blood samples. TNF-α may play a role in the disease process as it is an important inflammatory cytokine that can result in damage of CNS myelin. Ultimately, however, immune parameters such as TNF must be correlated with response to therapy as measured by clinical and MRI criteria.

In a disease such as IPM, muscle enzymes such as creatine phosphokinase (CPK) have been used for monitoring, with the goal being to maintain normal levels. However, serum CPK values do not always accurately reflect disease activity. This may be due to circulating inhibitors of enzyme activity, the focal nature of the inflammation, development of weakness due to accumulated disease damage or drug effects, and delay between disease activity and clinical effects (92). This latter reason is especially prominent in CIDP where recovery of function can take months. Even the measurement of anti-AChR antibodies, which are the pathogenic agents in MG patients, remains an imperfect marker, presumably because of the diversity of epitopes and auto-anti-idiotype antibodies (93).

Apart from formal studies, the treating neurologist must decide on therapy based on clinical assessment and accumulation of disability. Furthermore, a decision must be made as to whether a person has responded to therapy or whether additional treatment should be given. These decisions are generally based on the frequency with which the patient is having attacks and the level of disease progression.

References

1. Steinman L, Lindsey JW, et al. From treatment of experimental allergic encephalomyelitis to clinical trials in multiple sclerosis. In: Bach JF, ed. *Monoclonal antibodies and peptide therapy in autoimmune diseases*. New York: Marcel Dekker, 1993:253–260.
2. Brocke S, Gaur A, et al. Induction of relapsing paralysis in experimental autoimmune encephalomyelitis by bacterial superantigen. *Nature* 1993;365:642–644.
3. Friedman A, Weiner HL. Induction of anergy or active suppression following oral tolerance is determined by frequency of feeding and antigen dosage. *Proc Natl Acad Sci USA* 1994;91:6688–6692.
4. Abbas A. Die and let live: eliminating dangerous lymphocytes. *Cell* 1996;84:655–657.
5. Webb S, Morris C, et al. Extrathymic tolerance of mature T cells: clonal elimination as a consequence of immunity. *Cell* 1990;63:1249–1256.
6. Kerlero de Rosbo N, Milo R, et al. Reactivity to myelin antigens in multiple sclerosis. *J Clin Immunol* 1993; 92:2602–2610.
7. Sela M, Kirshner S, et al. Dominant epitopes and synthetic peptides in myasthenia gravis. *Israel J Med Sci* 1995;31:10–20.
8. Ben-Nun A, Wekerle H, et al. Vaccination against autoimmune encephalomyelitis using attenuated cells of a T lymphocyte line reactive against myelin basic protein. *Nature* 1981;292:60–61.
9. Khoury SJ, Hancock WW, et al. Oral tolerance to myelin basic protein and natural recovery from experimental au-

toimmune encephalomyelitis are associated with down-regulation of inflammatory cytokines and differential up-regulation of TGF-β, IL-4 and PGE expression in the brain. *J Exp Med* 1992;46:1355–1364.

10. Chen Y, Kuchroo VK, et al. Regulatory T cell clones induced by oral tolerance: suppression of autoimmune encephalomyelitis. *Science* 1994;265:1237–1240.

11. Nicholsen L, Greer J, et al. An altered peptide ligand mediates immune deviation and prevents EAE. *Immunity* 1995;3:397–405.

12. Brocke S, Gijbels K, et al. Treatment of EAE with a peptide analogue of MBP. *Nature* 1996;379:343–346.

13. Racke MK, Martin R, et al. Copolymer-1-induced inhibition of antigen-specific T-cell activation: interference with antigen presentation. *J Neuroimmunol* 1992;37:75–84.

14. Teitelbaum D, Milo R, et al. Synthetic copolymer-1 inhibits human T-cell lines specific for myelin basic protein. *Proc Natl Acad Sci USA* 1992;89:137–141.

15. Howell MD, Winters ST, et al. Vaccination against experimental allergic encephalomyelitis with T cell receptor peptides. *Science* 1989;246:668–670.

16. Vandenbark AA, Hashim G, et al. Immunization with a synthetic T-cell receptor V-region peptide protects against experimental autoimmune encephalomyelitis. *Nature* 1989;341:541–544.

17. Hafler DA. T cell vaccination in multiple sclerosis: a preliminary report. *Clin Immunol Immunopathol* 1992; 62:307–313.

18. Zhang J, Medaer R, et al. MHC-restricted depletion of human myelin basic protein-reactive T cells by T cell vaccination. *Science* 1993;261:1451–1454.

19. Zhang J, Markovic S, et al. Increased frequency of IL-2 responsive T cells specific for myelin basic protein and proteolipid protein in peripheral blood and cerebrospinal fluid of patients with multiple sclerosis. *J Exp Med* 1994;179:973–977.

20. Weiner HL, Friedman A, et al. Oral tolerance: immunologic mechanisms and treatment of murine and human organ specific autoimmune diseases by oral administration of autoantigens. *Annu Rev Immunol* 1994;12:809–837.

21. Chen Y, Inobe J, et al. Peripheral deletion of antigen reactive T cells in oral tolerance. *Nature* 1995;376:177–180.

22. Al-Sabbagh A, Miller A, et al. Suppression of PLP induced EAE in the SJL mouse by oral administration of MBP. *Neurology* 1992;42(suppl 3):346.

23. Weiner HL, Mackin GA, et al. Double-blind pilot trial of oral tolerization with myelin antigens in multiple sclerosis. *Science* 1993;259:1321–1324.

24. Al-Sabbagh A, Nelson PA, et al. Beta interferon enhances oral tolerance to MBP and PLP in experimental autoimmune encephalomyelitis [abstract]. *Neurology* 1994; 44(suppl 2):A242.

25. David M, Petricoin EI, et al. Requirement of MAP kinase (ERK2) activity in interferon alpha and interferon beta stimulated gene expression through STAT proteins. *Science* 1995;269:1721–1724.

26. Arnason BGW. Interferon beta in multiple sclerosis. *Neurology* 1993;43:641–643.

27. Hirsch RL, Panitch HS, et al. Lymphocytes from multiple sclerosis patients produce elevated levels of gamma interferon in vitro. *J Clin Immunol* 1987;22:139–144.

28. Noronha A, Toscas A, et al. IFN-β downregulates T cell activation and IFN-γ production: implications for MS. *J Neuroimmunol* 1993;46:145–153.

29. Antel JP, Brown-Bania M, et al. Activated suppressor cell dysfunction in multiple sclerosis. *J Immunol* 1986;137: 137–141.

30. Noronha A, Toscas A, et al. Interferon beta augments sup-

pressor cell function in multiple sclerosis. *Ann Neurol* 1990;27:207–210.

31. Sibley WA, Bamford CR, et al. Clinical viral infections and multiple sclerosis. *Lancet* 1985;1:1313–1315.

32. Smith D, Balshov K, et al. Increased IL-4 secretion and decreased gamma-IFN secretion in multiple sclerosis patients treated with cyclophosphamide or beta-interferon. Presented at the 9th International Congress of Immunology, San Francisco, CA, 1995.

33. Rudick R, et al. In vitro and in vivo inhibition of mitogen driven T cell activation by recombinant interferon beta. *Neurology* 1993;43:2080–2087.

34. Porrini A, Gambi D, et al. Interferon effects on IL-10 secretion; mononuclear cell response to IL-10 is normal in multiple sclerosis patients. *J Neuroimmunol* 1995;61:27–34.

35. Hafler DA, Weiner HL. In vivo labeling of peripheral blood T-cells using monoclonal antibodies: rapid traffic into cerebrospinal fluid in multiple sclerosis. *Ann Neurol* 1987;22:90–93.

36. Yednock TA, Cannon C, et al. Prevention of experimental autoimmune encephalomyelitis by antibodies against α4β1 integrin. *Nature* 1992;356:63–66.

37. Archelos JJ, Jung S, et al. Inhibition of experimental autoimmune encephalomyelitis by an antibody to the intercellular adhesion molecule ICAM-1. *Ann Neurol* 1993; 34:145–154.

38. Hafler DA, Fallis RJ, et al. Immunologic responses of progressive multiple sclerosis patients treated with anti-T-cell monoclonal antibody. *Neurology* 1986;36:777–784.

39. Hafler DA, Ritz J, et al. Anti-CD4 and anti-CD2 monoclonal antibodies infusions in humans: immunosuppressive effects and human anti-mouse responses. *J Immunol* 1988;141:131–138.

40. Weinshenker BG, Bass B, et al. An open trial of OKT3 in patients with multiple sclerosis. *Neurology* 1991;41: 1047–1052.

41. Lindsey J, Hodgkinson S, et al. Repeated treatment with chimeric anti-CD4 antibody in multiple sclerosis. *Ann Neurol* 1994;36:183.

42. Barkhof F, Thompson A, et al. Double-blind, placebo-controlled, MR monitored exploratory trial of chimeric anti-CD4 antibodies in MS. Presented at the 11th European Congress on Multiple Sclerosis, Jerusalem, Israel, September 1995.

43. Santambrogio L, Hochwald GM, et al. Studies on the mechanisms by which transforming growth factor-β (TGF-β) protects against allergic encephalomyelitis. *J Immunol* 1993;151:1116–1127.

44. Rott O, Cash E, et al. Phosphodiesterase inhibitor pentoxifylline, a selective suppressor of T helper type 1- but not type 2-associated lymphokine production, prevents induction of experimental autoimmune encephalomyelitis in Lewis rats. *Eur J Immunol* 1993;23:1745–1751.

45. Elliot M, Maini R, et al. Treatment of rheumatoid arthritis with chimeric monoclonal antibodies to TNF alpha. *Arthritis Rheum* 1993;36:1681–1686.

46. van Oosten BW, et al. Increased MRI activity and immune activation in two MS patients treated with monoclonal anti-TNF antibody A2. *Neurology* 1996;47:1531–1534.

47. Dwyer JM. Manipulating the immune system with immune globulin. *N Engl J Med* 1992;326:107–116.

48. Noseworthy J, O'Brien P, et al. Intravenous immunoglobulin therapy in MS: progress from remyelination in the Theiler's virus model to a randomized double blind placebo controlled clinical trial. *J Neurol Neurosurg Psychiatry* 1994;57(suppl):11.

49. Araneo B, et al. Ultraviolet radiation exposure depresses IL-2 and enhances IL-4 production by T cells through an

IL-1 independent mechanism. *J Immunol* 1989;143: 1734–1744.

50. Karussis DM, Lehmann D, et al. Inhibition of acute, experimental autoimmune encephalomyelitis by the synthetic immunomodulator linomide. *Ann Neurol* 1993; 34:654–660.
51. Cupps T, Edgar L, et al. Suppression of human B lymphocyte function by cyclophosphamide. *J Immunol* 1985; 128:2453–2461.
52. Scheinman R, Cogswell P, et al. Role of transcriptional activation of IKB alpha in mediation of immunosuppression by glucocorticoids. *Science* 1995;270:283–287.
53. Kupersmith MJ, Kaufman D, et al. Megadose corticosteroids in multiple sclerosis. *Neurology* 1994;44:1–4.
54. Daynes R, Araneo B. Contrasting effects of glucocorticoids on the capacity of T cells to produce the growth factors interleukin 2 and interleukin 4. *Eur J Immunol* 1989;19:2319–2327.
55. Beck RW, Cleary PA, et al. A randomized, controlled trial of corticosteroids in the treatment of acute optic neuritis. *N Engl J Med* 1992;326:581–588.
56. Beck RW, Cleary PA. Optic neuritis treatment trial: one-year follow-up results. *Arch Ophthalmol* 1993;111: 773–775.
57. Group TIMSS. Interferon beta-1b is effective in relapsing-remitting multiple sclerosis: clinical results of a multicenter, randomized, double-blind, placebo-controlled trial. *Neurology* 1993;43:655–661.
58. Paty DW, Li DKB, et al. Interferon beta-1β is effective in relapsing-remitting multiple sclerosis: MRI results of a multicenter, randomized, double-blind, placebo-controlled trial. *Neurology* 1993;43:662–667.
59. The IFN-β MS Study Group and The University of British Columbia MS MRI Analysis Group. Interferon beta-1β in the treatment of multiple sclerosis: final outcome of the randomized controlled trial. *Neurology* 1995;45:1277–1285.
60. Jacobs L, et al. Intramuscular interferon beta-1α for disease progression in relapsing multiple sclerosis. *Ann Neurol* 1996;39:285–294.
61. Durelli L, Bongioanni M, et al. Interferon alpha treatment of relapsing remitting multiple sclerosis: long term study of the correlations between clinical and magnetic imaging results and effects on immune function. *MS Clin Lab Res* 1995;1:S32.
62. Johnson K, Brooks B, et al. Copolymer 1 reduces relapse rate and improves disability in relapsing remitting multiple sclerosis: results of a phase III multicenter, double-blind, placebo-controlled trial. *Neurology* 1995;45:1268–1276.
63. Hughes R. Ineffectiveness of high dose methylprednisolone in Guillain-Barré syndrome. *Lancet* 1991;338:1142.
64. Beck RW, Cleary PA, et al. The effect of corticosteroids for acute optic neuritis on the subsequent development of multiple sclerosis. *N Engl J Med* 1993;239:1764–1769.
65. Hauser SL, Dawson DM, et al. Intensive immunosuppression in progressive multiple sclerosis: a randomized, three-arm study of high dose intravenous cyclophosphamide, plasma exchange and ACTH. *N Engl J Med* 1983;308:173–180.
66. Carter JL, Hafler DA, et al. Immunosuppression with high-dose IV cyclophosphamide and ACTH in progressive multiple sclerosis: cumulative 6-year experience in 164 patients. *Neurology* 1988;38:9–14.
67. Weiner HL, Mackin GA, et al. Intermittent cyclophosphamide pulse therapy in progressive multiple sclerosis: final report of the Northeast Cooperative Multiple Sclerosis Treatment Group. *Neurology* 1993;43:910–918.
68. Hohol MJ, Mackin GA, et al. Pilot study of three year intermittent pulse cyclophosphamide/methylprednisolone

therapy in multiple sclerosis therapy. *Ann Neurol* 1992;32:256–257. Abstract.
69. The Canadian Cooperative MS Study Group. The Canadian cooperative trial of cyclophosphamide and plasma exchange in progressive multiple sclerosis. *Lancet* 1991;337:442–446.
70. Mackin GA, Dawson DM, et al. Treatment of multiple sclerosis with cyclophosphamide. In: Rudick RA, Goodkin DE, eds. *Treatment of multiple sclerosis: trial design, results, and future perspectives*. New York: Springer, 1992:199–216.
71. Cook SD, Devereux C, et al. Total lymphoid irradiation in multiple sclerosis. In: Rudick RA, Goodkin DE, eds. *Treatment of multiple sclerosis: trial design, results, and future perspectives*. New York: Springer, 1992:267–280.
72. The Multiple Sclerosis Study Group. Efficacy and toxicity of cyclosporine in chronic progressive multiple sclerosis: a randomized, double-blinded, placebo-controlled clinical trial. *Ann Neurol* 1990;27:591–605.
73. Rudge P, Koetsier JC, et al. Randomized double blind controlled trial of cyclosporin in multiple sclerosis. *J Neurol Neurosurg Psychiatry* 1989;52:559–565.
74. Tindall R, et al. Preliminary results of a double blind placebo controlled trial of cyclosporine in myasthenia gravis. *N Engl J Med* 1987;316:719–724.
75. Hughes RA. Treatment of multiple sclerosis with azathioprine. In: Rudick RA, Goodkin DE, eds. *Treatment of multiple sclerosis: trial designs, results, and future perspectives*. New York: Springer, 1992:157–172.
76. Yudkin PL, Ellison GW, et al. Overview of azathioprine treatment in multiple sclerosis. *Lancet* 1991;338: 1051–1055.
77. Goodkin D, Rudick RA, et al. Low-dose (7.5 mg) oral methotrexate reduces the rate of progression in chronic progressive multiple sclerosis. *Ann Neurol* 1995;37:30–40.
78. Sipe JD, Romine J, et al. Cladribine in the treatment of chronic progressive multiple sclerosis. *Lancet* 1994;344: 9–13.
79. The Guillain Barré Syndrome Study Group. Plasmapheresis and acute Guillain-Barré syndrome. *Neurology* 1984;35:1096–1105.
80. The French Cooperative Group on Plasma Exchange. Efficiency of plasma exchange in Guillain-Barré syndrome: role of replacement fluids. *Ann Neurol* 1987;22:753–761.
81. Shumack K, Rock G. Therapeutic plasma exchange. *N Engl J Med* 1984;301:763.
82. van der Meche F, Schmitz P, et al. A randomized trial comparing intravenous immune globulin to and plasma exchange in Guillain-Barré syndrome. *N Engl J Med* 1992;326:1123–1127.
83. van Doorn P, et al. High dose intravenous immune globulin treatment in chronic inflammatory demyelinating polyneuropathy: a double blind placebo controlled crossover study. *Neurology* 1990;40:209.
84. Dalakas MC, Illa I, et al. A controlled trial of high-dose intravenous immune globulin infusions as treatment of dermatomyositis. *N Engl J Med* 1993;329:1993–2000.
85. Achiron A, Pras E, et al. Open controlled therapeutic trial of intravenous immune globulin in relapsing-remitting multiple sclerosis. *Arch Neurol* 1992;49:1233–1236.
86. Durelli I, et al. Actuarial analysis of the occurrence of remission following thymectomy for myasthenia gravis in 400 patients. *J Neurol Neurosurg Psychiatry* 1991; 54:406–412.
87. Paty DW. Magnetic resonance imaging in the assessment of disease activity in multiple sclerosis. *Can J Neurol Sci* 1988;15:266–272.
88. McFarland HF, Frank JA, et al. Using gadolinium-en-

hanced magnetic resonance imaging lesions to monitor disease activity in multiple sclerosis. *Ann Neurol* 1992;32:758–766.

89. Khoury SJ, Guttmann CRG, et al. Longitudinal MR imaging in multiple sclerosis: correlation between disability and lesion burden. *Neurology* 1994;44:2120–2124.

90. Sharief MK, Hentges R. Association between tumor necrosis factor-α and disease progression in patients with multiple sclerosis. *N Engl J Med* 1991;325:467–472.

91. Chofflon M, Juillard C, et al. Tumor necrosis factor α production as a possible predictor of relapse in patients with multiple sclerosis. *Eur Cytokine Netw* 1992;3:523–531.

92. Kagan L, Aram S. Creatine kinase activity inhibitor in sera from patients with muscle disease. *Arthritis Rheum* 1991;34:1580–1585.

93. Qing Y, Levfert A. Idiotypic and antiidiotypic T and B cells in myasthenia gravis. *J Immunol* 1992;149:3423–3430.

Chapter 8
The Immunology of Multiple Sclerosis

Gary Birnbaum and Jack Antel

This chapter is not a comprehensive review of all immunologic aspects of multiple sclerosis (MS). Rather it focuses on newer data obtained within the past 5 years. Because vast amounts of information related to immune changes in MS have been accumulated even in this time frame, only the observations we believe are of particular relevance to understanding the pathogenesis of MS or its treatment are included. For a complete overview of this area, readers are referred to the encyclopedic descriptions provided in the excellent review by Reder and Arnason (1).

Neuropathology

Among the earliest and most persistent abnormalities found in the brains of persons with MS are perivenular accumulations of lymphocytes and changes in the blood-brain barrier (BBB) (see Figure 2-1, P. 21, and Figure 7-1, P. 93) (2–5). The BBB changes are believed to result from alterations not only in endothelial cells but also to astrocytic pericytes whose processes abut the capillary basement membrane (6). The mechanisms responsible for such a breakdown are not known but most likely are related to cytokines released by activated inflammatory cells. These consist predominantly of T cells and macrophages. Among the cytokines implicated in the breakdown of the BBB are tumor necrosis factor (TNF)-α, interleukin (IL)-1β (7,8), and matrix metalloproteinases (9) (see Figure 3-1, P. 27). Changes in the breakdown of the BBB are believed to underlie the gadolinium enhancement of MS lesions observed on persons with acute, relapsing, or secondary progressive disease (10,11) and the numbers of enhancing lesions correlate with the disease activity. Persistent alteration in the BBB may make areas of previous demyelination especially susceptible to systemic changes in circulating cytokines and antibodies. This may explain why areas of acute disease activity are often seen at the edges of otherwise quiescent plaques (2,3). However, while breakdown of the BBB may be an early and constant event in MS, its role in the disease process, whether primary to it or merely a consequence of tissue damage, is not known. Against changes in the BBB being of primary importance are the pathologic observations that changes in the BBB are detectable in old, inactive MS plaques (2,3); that disease progression can occur in the absence of gadolinium enhancement (11,12); and that

high-dose steroids, while decreasing gadolinium enhancement acutely, continue to have a beneficial effect on disease activity, even after enhancement is again noted on repeat brain MRIs (13). A major difficulty in defining the role of BBB breakdown in the pathophysiology of MS pertains to the various parameters used for its measurement and their variable sensitivity to detecting changes of function. Clearly, allowing greater egress of immunologically active materials from the blood into the central nervous system (CNS) has the potential to amplify, if not necessarily initiate, disease processes.

The extent of lymphocyte accumulation has been used as an index of lesion activity, and MRI-pathologic correlations indicate that the earliest lesions feature inflammation. Yet lesion resolution is frequently seen with MRI, suggesting that inflammation can occur without tissue destruction. Conversely, more chronic lesions can expand in the apparent absence of inflammatory cells. The potential role of glial cells as mediators of tissue injury is discussed in Chapter 3. Because lymphocytes play a major role in the initiation of MS lesions, much recent work has attempted to define the populations of lymphocytes in these regions using a variety of markers. Some laboratories defined the populations on the basis of their cell surface antigens, attempting to determine whether these were cytotoxic or helper T cells (14–16). Other investigators defined populations of lymphocytes on the basis of their classes of antigen T-cell receptor (TCR) (17–21). As described in Chapter 1, there are two classes of T cells, those that express TCR consisting of α/β dimers and those that express TCR composed of γ/δ dimers. While the majority of T cells around areas of plaques are of the α/β phenotype, several groups of investigators noted the presence of γ/δ T cells around oligodendrocytes at the edges of plaques (18,19,21). These oligodendrocytes were also noted to express increased levels of heat shock proteins (HSPs), especially HSP60 and HSP70. It is not possible to determine the antigen specificity of T cells on the basis of their class of TCR. However, a high percentage of γ/δ T cells respond to these HSPs (vide infra). In view of this fact, these investigators hypothesized that immune responses to HSP may be important in the formation of plaques. What still is uncertain is the role of γ/δ T cells: Are they protective or cytotoxic? There is evidence in favor of both possibilities (22,23). Additional data to support a role for γ/δ cells in MS are provided by Shimonkevitz et al (24) and Birnbaum et al (25). Shimonkevitz et al (24) described the presence of activated, clonally expanded γ/δ T cells in the spinal fluids of patients with recent-onset MS, whereas Birnbaum et al (25) noted that spinal fluid lymphocytes from a subgroup of patients with recent-onset MS exhibited strong proliferative responses to mycobacterial proteins, most probably HSP. Oksenberg et al (17) isolated TCR RNA from the brains of persons with MS and control subjects, prepared complementary DNA (cDNA), and analyzed the sequences of these TCR messages. They noted a preferential accumulation of T cells expressing the Vβ5.2 chain of TCR in the brains of MS patients with the HLA DRB1*1501, DQA1*0102, DQB1*0602, DPB1*0401 genotype and that the V-D-J regions of these receptors were very similar to those used in an MS patient's peripheral T-cell clone specific for an epitope of the encephalitogenic protein, myelin basic protein (MBP). A similar sequence was also found in MBP-reactive T-cell clones from rats with experimental autoimmune encephalomyelitis (EAE). The investigators interpreted these data to indicate that T-cell responses to MBP occur in the brains of persons with MS and that they may contribute to its pathogenesis. Needless to say, such interpretations are controversial because responses to other myelin proteins such as proteolipid protein (PLP) (26), myelin-associated glycoprotein (MAG) (27,28), and myelin oligodendrocyte glycoprotein (MOG) (29) are also significantly increased in persons with MS (vide infra).

In parallel with studies on populations of T cells in areas of demyelination, other groups studied the patterns of cytokines in these regions. Cytokine sources in the inflamed CNS include macrophages and endogenous glial cells, microglia, and astrocytes in addition to lymphocytes. As expected from areas in which there are large numbers of activated immunocompetent cells, many different cytokines are found. Some are "proinflammatory" in that they have the potential to enhance tissue destruction. These include TNF-α (8,30–33) and interferon (IFN)-γ (31,34,35). Other cytokines such as transforming growth factor (TGF)-β have "anti-inflammatory" properties (36–39). Additional cytokines found in areas of demyelination and inflammation are IL-1 and IL-2, IL-4, and IL-10 (40) and a relatively new class of compounds called *chemokines* that have leukocyte attractant properties (41–43). What role cytokines play in the MS disease process is not clear but it is reasonable to assume they are contributory. For example, several laboratories showed that TNF-α and lymphotoxin are directly toxic to oligodendrocytes (44) and that administration of TGF-β protects animals from EAE (36,37,45). Chemokine levels are also increased in the brains of animals with EAE (46,47) and in the cerebrospinal fluid (CSF) of MS patients (48). The patterns of cytokines found in MS plaques suggest that many, if not most, of the T cells in these areas are of the Th1 phenotype (see Chapter 1); that is, they secrete proinflammatory cytokines. However, on a quantitative basis, most cytokine-producing cells are microglia, macrophages, and astrocytes. Modulation of these cells so they

secrete a preponderance of Th2 cytokines may provide a new treatment approach to the disease (vide infra).

As discussed in Chapter 1, circulating lymphyocytes enter target organs by adhering to endothelial cells that express ligands for receptors expressed on the surfaces of activated T cells (see Figure 16-1, P. 255, and Figure 21-1, P. 326). Examples of endothelial cell ligands are vascular adhesion molecule (VCAM)-1 and intercellular adhesion molecule (ICAM)-1. Examples of TCRs for these ligands are very late activation antigen (VLA)-4 and leukocyte function–associated antigen (LFA)-1. Expression of these cell adhesion molecules by endothelial cells requires that they be exposed to a variety of inflammatory cytokines (49). Several groups of investigators studied endothelial cells and the expression of cell adhesion molecules in and around regions of inflammation and demyelination in MS. Increased concentrations of several cell molecules, such as ICAM and VCAM, were found not only in the brains of persons with MS but also in the brains of persons with other inflammatory and noninflammatory CNS diseases (40,50). No unique patterns of adhesion molecule expression were seen in MS brains nor were there clear correlations with other parameters used to measure the activity of lesions, such as extent of inflammation. Isolated MS brain microvessels expressed much higher levels of adhesion molecules than did microvessels from control brains (51) but findings in inflammatory, non-MS control brains were not described. These data indicate that endothelial cells in lesions of active demyelination are activated by the large amounts of cytokines present in these regions, and that these activated endothelial cells probably play an important role in the recruitment of circulating, activated T cells into the brain. However, since any activated T cell has the potential to enter the brain (52,53), perivenular and periplaque T cells in the brain probably represent populations of cells specific for both brain antigens and non-CNS antigens. The "nonspecific" recruitment of cells to areas of demyelination may play an important role in amplifying and perpetuating the disease process in MS, as such cells are able to secrete cytokines and participate in cytotoxic responses. Remaining to be explained is how "nonspecific" effectors can induce apparently selective tissue injury to myelin and oligodendrocytes. Whether the latter targets are particularly susceptible to such effector mechanisms is discussed in Chapter 3. Related to the findings in the CNS are observations that levels of circulating cell adhesion molecules in both serum and CSF are increased in persons with active MS, and these increased levels correlate with both relapses of disease (54) and numbers of enhancing lesions on MRIs (55). A new therapeutic approach may result from clinical trials with agents that alter the trafficking of activated cells into the brain during exacerbations of disease. Such an approach has succeeded in ameliorating EAE (56), though not in all experimental paradigms (57).

Characteristic of the brains and spinal fluids of persons with MS are increased concentrations of immunoglobulins, especially oligoclonal antibodies present in spinal fluids and not in paired sera. The synthesis of antibodies in the CNS of persons with MS is increased but such findings are not unique to MS, also being present in the brains of individuals with a number of different chronic inflammatory CNS diseases (58). Much work has attempted to demonstrate the antigen specificities of the oligoclonal bands in MS CSF but none have been demonstrated to date. Some data suggest that oligoclonal antibodies are "nonsense" antibodies with specificities unrelated to the disease process (59). However, whereas the antigen specificities of oligoclonal antibodies remain unknown, there are increased concentrations of antibodies to a variety of different viruses (60) as well as antibodies to myelin proteins (61,62) in the nonoligoclonal fraction of immunoglobulins, and some of these may play a role in demyelination. For example, in a murine and a primate model of EAE, sensitization of T cells to MBP results in encephalitis but little demyelination. When antibodies to MOG are present, demyelination is greatly enhanced (63,64). In MS, degenerating myelin can have a swollen appearance, characteristic of antibody-mediated demyelination (65), with final removal of injured myelin by phagocytic macrophages, a process also enhanced by antibodies (66). In addition, there is evidence of complement activation in the spinal fluids and brains of persons with MS (67,68), suggesting that this cytotoxic arm of the immune system may participate in the disease process. Indirect support for the role of antibodies in the demyelinating process comes from the observation that plasmapheresis can shorten the duration of an attack of MS (69). Whether the effects of plasmapheresis are related to removal of antibodies or cytotoxic cytokines (70) is not clear.

Immune System

While MS is believed to be an autoimmune disease, there is little evidence that the immune system per se is abnormal in this illness. There are few other autoimmune diseases associated with MS (the exception being inflammatory bowel diseases (71,72)), and immune responses of MS patients to antigens other than myelin antigens are normal. These data suggest that MS does not result from an intrinsic disorder of immune regulation or control, but rather from a normal response to an inappropriate antigen. Indeed, given the epidemiologic and clinical evidence cited below, the initiating event of MS and those involved in perpetuating the disease may be different. In this regard the human disease that follows exposure to myelin, acute disseminated encephalomyelitis (ADEM), is characterized by its monophasic rather than recurrent course. Whether an intrinsic or acquired deficit in immune regulation contributes to the recurrent or chronic course of MS or whether perpetuation is the result of recurring immune responses to antigens expressed in regions of myelin injury is not known. Functional deficits in systemic immune regulation in MS have been identified most consistently in patients in the progressive phase of the disease (73,74). Such observations suggest that these changes are acquired, perhaps secondary to the disease process.

The issue of whether MS is exclusively an autoimmune illness is not settled. Some investigators believe that a persistent viral infection of oligodendrocytes is the initiating event of MS and that immune responses subsequent to this infection either cause or contribute to the demyelination. An enormous amount of effort has been expended trying to find viruses in MS brains (e.g., the recent work with herpes virus (75,76)), and viruses have been isolated. However, their role in the pathogenesis of MS is uncertain because latent virus is present in the brains of normal persons (76). Yet the demyelination associated with Theiler's virus infection is an example of a condition in which there is viral infection of oligodendrocytes with superimposed immune responses to the infected cells and myelin (77–80). Suppression of the immune response reduces the intensity of the disease but does not eliminate it, indicating that both infection and inflammation contribute to the pathogenesis. Whether a similar constellation of events occurs in MS is not known.

One of the important unanswered questions in MS is, where does the presumed immune abnormality originate? Is the demyelination the result of changes in the peripheral immune system or does the disease begin because of changes in the brain itself (81,82)? There is clear evidence that persons with MS have alterations in the peripheral immune system. The numbers of activated lymphocytes undergoing DNA synthesis are increased in the blood of persons with MS (83) and subpopulations of T cells, such as memory cells and suppressor cells, are altered (73,74). In addition, the numbers of activated cells responding to myelin proteins such as MBP (84), as well as the precursor frequencies of cells responding to myelin proteins (26), are increased in peripheral blood. It can be argued that all these phenomena are secondary to the inflammatory changes in the brain, and indeed, changes in peripheral blood do not accurately reflect what is happening within the CNS. Nevertheless, an established clinical observation strongly suggests that peripheral immune events are primary to the perpetuation, if not the initiation, of the disease process in MS. That is the observation that antecedent non-CNS infections, especially viral infections, are associated with relapses of disease (85,86).

Activation of the peripheral immune system is a constant feature of infections and it is possible to propose several mechanisms for how activation of the peripheral immune system could result in an exacerbation of an organ-restricted inflammatory disease.

1.   Exacerbation could be the result of non-antigen-specific factors. For example, infection-related activation of the peripheral immune system results in increased concentrations of circulating cytokines such as IFN-γ and TNF. In the presence of an altered BBB, ingress of these materials into the CNS is facilitated, resulting in activation of antimyelin cytotoxic cells resident in the brain. In support of this mechanism are the observations that there are increased blood and spinal fluid concentrations of TNF in persons with MS and such increases are associated with increased disease ac-

tivity (87). In addition, administration of IFN gamma, as described by Panitch et al (34,35), significantly increases disease activity. Activation of lymphocytes also results in the expression of ligands on their surfaces that enable them to bind to activated endothelial cells (88–90). Such expression would facilitate the entry of activated cells into the CNS, even without the need for specificity to myelin antigens (53,91,92). Once inside the CNS, such nonspecifically recruited cells would be drawn to areas of increased cytokine and chemokine gradients, where they could become additionally activated and begin secreting their own tissue-destructive cytokines.

2.   Alternatively, or perhaps additionally, an increase in disease activity could be the result of specific responses to myelin antigens. For example, as a result of an immune response to an infectious agent, T cells that cross-react with particular myelin proteins may be generated. This has been observed in responses to viral proteins (93) as well as bacterial proteins (94). In both instances there was molecular mimicry such that peptides present in the infectious agents induced cross-reactive responses with peptides of myelin proteins, such as MBP and 2′,3′ cyclic nucleotide 3′ phosphodiesterase (CNP), respectively. Immune responses to proteins other than those of the infectious agent may also play a role in disease exacerbation. An example would be immune responses to HSPs. HSPs are families of proteins expressed both constitutively and in response to a variety of stresses, including heat shock, cytokines such as TNF, ischemia, and oxidative radicals (reviewed elsewhere (95,96)). HSPs are also the immunodominant proteins for a variety of infectious agents, in that immune responses to these organisms are mainly directed against their HSP. The proteins are categorized by their molecular sizes, ranging from small HSPs of 15 to 27 kd to large HSPs of more than 100 kd. One characteristic of HSPs that greatly increases their potential to act as autoantigens is their remarkable phylogenetic conservation. Amino acid sequence homologies between human and bacterial HSPs are more than 50%. Thus, there is potential for significant immunologic cross-reactivity between mammalian and nonmammalian HSPs. Several laboratories described increased amounts of HSP in areas of demyelination in MS brains, in particular in oligodendrocytes (18,19,97,98). In addition, immune responses to HSP are present in the spinal fluids of a subpopulation of persons with MS, and while this is not disease specific, it is present predominantly in persons with MS of recent onset (25). Finally, very recent data indicate that the course of both acute and relapsing EAE, an animal model of MS, can be modified by changing patterns of the immune response to HSP, in particular to a peptide of HSP60 that has sequence homology with the myelin protein CNP (94). Immune responses to HSPs, induced during the course of an infection, could therefore serve as a final common pathway for perpetuating a demyelinating disease process that may have been initiated by a myelin-specific reaction.

An equally important, and unresolved question, re-volves around which myelin antigen is responsible for the pathogenic immune response in MS. Recent data suggest that more than one antigen may be important and that these may vary over time. It has been known for many years that immune responses to a variety of myelin proteins are increased in both the blood and spinal fluids of persons with MS. These include immune responses to MBP, PLP, and MOG. Methods for determining these immune responses have varied greatly, and have ranged from determining frequencies of reactive cells (29), to determining the frequency of mutations in MBP-responsive cells (99), to showing that a high proportion of activated, IL-2–responsive lymphocytes isolated from peripheral blood and spinal fluids of MS patients are specific for myelin proteins (26), to claiming that anti-MBP–responsive T cells are present in the brains of persons with MS based on the similarity of the patterns of TCRs expressed by these cells compared to MBP-responsive cells found in human peripheral blood and in mice (100). The difficulty with these studies are several. First is that normal individuals contain large numbers of anti–myelin protein–responsive T cells, making the differences between MS patients and normal control subjects more quantitative than qualitative. Second is the difficulty in establishing whether these responses are directly involved in the disease process, or whether they result secondarily to myelin destruction. Perhaps most importantly is that immune responses, even to well-defined peptides, change over time such that the diversity of the immune response broadens (101,102). This phenomenon is called *epitope spreading* and is described in more detail in Chapter 1. While there are limits to this diversification (103), the fact remains that a multitude of different antigens may be responsible for continuing the presumed autoimmune destruction in MS and it is unlikely that a single, dominant epitope will be found. Rather, because of the effects of determinant selection (see Chapter 1), the dominance of particular myelin protein epitopes appears related more to the MHC phenotype of the individual rather than to the disease state (104,105).

Genes and Susceptibility

Numerous data indicate the important role genetic factors play in determining susceptibility to MS. For example, about 10% of patients with MS also have first- and second-degree relatives with MS (106). In addition, the disease concordance rate for MS among monozygotic twins is more than 25%, a value much higher than the 1% concordance rate in dizygotic twins (107). MHC gene phenotyping of persons with MS reveals the frequency of certain class II MHC genes to be much higher in the patient population than in the population from which these individuals are derived (108,109). While clustering of particular class II phenotypes with MS has been observed in several different population bases, the genes associated with disease vary between different geographic groups. For example, in MS patients of northern European extraction, the incidence of HLA-Dw2 and -DR2 phenotypes is much higher than that of the general population. With genomic typing techniques, the phenotype has been additionally characterized as being DRw15, DQw6, Dw2, or the DRB1*1501-DQA1*0102-DQB1*0602 haplotype (108). MS patients from Mediterranean countries have no such increased incidence (110–112). While initial studies of HLA typing in multiplex families with MS did not indicate any association between particular MHC phenotypes and the disease, with new techniques of microsatellite mapping and two-stage, multianalytical genomic screening to establish linkage disequilibria, an association of MS with the class II MHC locus was found (113–115) along with weaker linkages to other sites (116). The data make it highly unlikely that a single MS susceptibility gene exists, but rather that there are epistatic interactions between a number of different genes (up to five or six), one of which may reside in or near the MHC. The picture may be more complex in that persons wth primary progressive disease, comprising about 10% of MS patients, may have different susceptibility genes than do persons with the more common relapsing-remitting disease (117,118).

In addition to the above-mentioned work involving total genome analyses, a great deal of effort has gone into identifying genes other than those of the MHC that are associated with susceptibility to MS. Some investigators found an association between certain TCR genes and MS (119–121), but these findings were not universally confirmed (104,122,123). Other studies indicated an association between particular immunoglobulin heavy-chain variable-region polymorphisms and MS (124). As noted in the previous paragraph, studies involving linkage analyses of the entire genome did not detect significant linkages to any of these genes (113–116).

Environmental Factors and Susceptibility

The data just presented on MS concordance in monozygotic twins establish that genetic identity alone is insufficient for the development of disease. Another critical factor is the environment. Numerous observations support this hypothesis. For example, there is a striking North-South gradient in disease incidence in Europe, Australia, and North America, as well as a West-East gradient in the United States, independent of genetic or ethnic factors (125). Persons from the same genetic groups have different rates of disease in different geographic locations (126). Studies of populations migrating to and from zones of different risk suggested that the environmental event triggering the disease occurs prior to the ages of 13 to 15 years (126). Epidemics of MS, such as those in the Faroe Islands (127,128) and Iceland (129), occurred following the introduction of new infectious agents into a sheltered geographic location. Looking at patterns of immune responses in monozygotic twins concordant or discordant for MS, Utz et al (130) showed that the repertoire of TCRs used to respond to nonmyelin antigens was similar in all twin sets. In contrast, the repertoire of TCR genes used in responses to myelin antigens differed in discordant twin

sets yet was the same in condordant sets. The authors interpreted these data as showing that either an environmental factor changed the patterns of immune response in these genetically identical individuals or the disease process itself engendered these differences. Studies of birth order in siblings with MS (131) indicated that there is no contemporaneous exposure to an environmental factor that leads to the development of disease. Indeed, environmental exposure alone also is insufficient to cause disease, as shown by the studies of resistant populations living in high-risk areas (132,133). In addition, a study of adopted relatives, with or without MS, living with other first-degree nonbiologic relatives demonstrated that exposure to a common environment is insufficient for the development of disease (134).

What remains elusive is the nature of the environmental factors that appear to be associated with the initiation of the MS disease process. A clue can perhaps be extrapolated from experimental models of autoimmune diseases such as EAE. In recent years, several laboratories produced transgenic animals in which most, and even all, of the T cells express receptors specific for encephalitogenic peptides of the autoantigen MBP (135,136). Contrary to expectations, animals did not develop rampant spontaneous EAE. In animals in which more than 80% of the T cells were specific for a peptide of MBP, induction of disease usually required immunization with MBP in complete Freund's adjuvant with injection of pertussis toxin or injection of pertussis toxin alone. Only a fraction developed spontaneous EAE (14%–44%), and this occurred exclusively in animals reared in a non-pathogen-free environment. Genetically identical animals reared in specific pathogen-free environments did not develop EAE. Thus, environmental exposure, probably to an infectious agent, triggered this organ-restricted, autoimmune disease. Preliminary data from our laboratory suggest that immune responses to HSP may be involved in this process (137).

Treatments

While there is no cure for MS, the disease does respond in modest ways to treatment with anti-inflammatory and immune-modulating drugs. The degrees of responsiveness vary among individuals and some physicians in the field continue to be therapeutic nihilists regarding all treatments. Nevertheless, the fact that improvement is observed in some treated individuals indicates that inflammation in the brains of persons with MS contributes to the disease process. A broad discussion of immunomodulatory treatments is presented in Chapter 7. Here we briefly discuss some of the newer approaches to MS therapy.

The key to truly successful therapy in MS requires the identification of the inciting antigen or antigens, or identification of the components of the immune system most directly responsible for the tissue damage. Until now, most immune-directed therapies in MS involved a variety of nonspecific immune suppressants or immune modifiers (e.g., steroids, azathioprine, methotrexate, cyclophosphamide, IFN beta). The success of the IFN betas in altering both clinical and MRI parameters in patients with relapsing MS provides supportive evidence for the role of immune mechanisms in the pathogenesis of MS. Based on the assumption that immune responses to myelin, in particular MBP, are important in the pathogenesis of MS, a large clinical trial was recently completed in which individuals with MS injected themselves with a mixture of random polymers made up of the amino acids comprising MBP. This material (copolymer 1 or Copaxone) reduced exacerbation rates by about one third. Interestingly, it had little effect on MS-related changes noted on MRIs of the brains of study participants. While the mechanism of action of copolymer 1 is not known, it is known that administration of antigen in high doses can eliminate antigen-responsive cells via a mechanism involving apoptosis (138). In addition, administration of soluble antigen can result in a change in the pattern of immune responses to that antigen such that there is a shift away from the production of Th1 cytokine to a protective Th2 pattern of cytokine secretion (see Chapter 1). While we do not believe that immune responses to MBP are exclusively involved in the pathogenesis of MS, they may contribute to this process. Modifying the response to this antigen could have a salutary effect. Indeed, if modification of anti-MBP immune responses results in the induction of Th2 cytokines, such as TGF-β, a non-antigen-specific anti-inflammatory effect on adjacent pathogenic T cells responding to myelin antigens other than MBP (the so-called bystander effect) could be observed (139,140). In any case, the fact that copolymer 1 did modify MS is strong evidence in favor of the hypothesis that immune responses to myelin antigens are important in MS.

In a similar context, another clinical trial, currently not completed, is studying the effects of feeding bovine myelin to persons with MS. Again, the hypothetical foundation of this trial is the assumption that immune responses to myelin are important in MS. As described in Chapter 1, when antigens are introduced to the immune system via the gut-associated lymphoid tissues (GALTs), Th2 patterns of immune response are engendered. This results in the secretion of anti-inflammatory cytokines such as TGF-β and is responsible for the phenomenon called *oral tolerance*. In a preliminary study, oral myelin not only reduced the numbers of exacerbations in persons with relapsing-remitting MS, but also appeared to reduce disability (141). However, subgroup analysis of the data indicated that only males who were HLA-DR2 negative benefited from therapy. The reasons for this are not clear. If oral tolerance to myelin is effective in treating MS, it would be another piece of evidence in favor of the importance of antimyelin immune responses in the pathogenesis of this disease. Results of the trial will be available in 1997.

Approaching the question of disease-specific therapy in a different fashion have been studies in which immune responses to subpopulations of T cells are induced in persons with MS. There are several reasons for believing that such an approach may be of benefit. Inbred strains of mice and rats that are susceptible to EAE respond to immunization with encephalitogenic peptides using very restricted populations of T cells expressing a restricted repertoire of TCRs (142,143). Administration of antibodies to these TCRs prevents the development of EAE as well as relapses of disease (144). This indicates that in these animals, alternative populations of T cells are not able to mount a pathogenic response. However, such observations are not universal in EAE (145) and in an outbred species such as humans the results are even less uniform. Whereas some investigators described immunodominant epitopes of MBP peptides related to the HLA phenotype of the responders (146), as well as restricted use of TCRs in responding to these epitopes (147), other researchers did not note such restrictions (104,123). Rather they described immune responses to an array of MBP peptides in persons with MS as well as a diversity of TCR utilization that increases with disease severity (148). Nevertheless, several groups are immunizing MS patients with TCR proteins or whole T cells, choosing those TCRs and T cells that are utilized by these individuals in their in vitro responses to stimulation with MBP peptides (149–152). Preliminary data from these groups show that immune responses to TCR proteins can be detected, along with a decrease in T-cell populations expressing these TCRs (149,151,153,154). Encouragingly, two publications cited beneficial effects after "vaccination" of small numbers of MS patients with MBP-reactive T cells or TCR peptides (150,152). Both papers noted either stabilization of disease or improvement in subgroups of persons receiving vaccines and one paper reported an association of clinical responsiveness with a decrease in MRI-noted lesions, compared to increases noted in control MS patients (150). While much more work needs to be done, these results are encouraging as they indicate that it may be technically feasible to decrease, at least temporarily, potentially pathogenic populations of T cells in a disease-specific fashion. There are several caveats to extrapolating the use of such techniques for MS patients in general. Studies in animal models show sufficient adaptability of immune systems such that over time other populations of T cells can "take over" for depleted, initially responding T cells and successfully mount immune responses to the stimulating antigen (155). Second, and perhaps more important, is the observation of Lodge et al (156) that in patients with MS, unique, activated T lymphocytes responding to specific epitopes of MBP utilize multiple families of TCRs. However, as suggested by the work of Vandenbark et al (152), vaccination with a single TCR peptide could result in "bystander suppression" of other antigen-responsive T cells by secretion of immunomodulatory cytokines such as IL-10 or TGF-β (see Chapter 1).

References

1. Reder AT, Arnason BGW. Immunology of multiple sclerosis. In: Vinken PJ, Bruyn GW, Klawans HL, eds. *Hand-*

book of clinical neurology. Vol. 3. Amsterdam: Elsevier Science, 1985:337–395.

2. Kermode AG, Thompson AJ, Tofts P, et al. Blood-brain barrier abnormalities in longstanding multiple sclerosis lesions. An immunohistochemical study. *J Neuropathol Exp Neurol* 1994;53:625–636.

3. Kwon EE, Prineas JW. Evidence of persistent blood-brain barrier abnormalities in chronic-progressive multiple sclerosis. *Acta Neuropathol (Berl)* 1995;90:228–238.

4. Gay D, Esiri M. Breakdown of the blood-brain barrier precedes symptoms and other MRI signs of new lesions in multiple sclerosis. Pathogenetic and clinical implications. *Brain* 1990;113:1477–1489.

5. Kermode AG, Thompson AJ, Tofts P, et al. Breakdown of the blood-brain barrier precedes symptoms and other MRI signs of new lesions in multiple sclerosis. Pathogenetic and clinical implications. *Brain* 1990;113:1477–1489.

6. Rafalowska J, Krajewski S, Dolinska E, Dziewulska D. Does damage of perivascular astrocytes in multiple sclerosis plaques participate in blood-brain barrier permeability? *Neuropatol Polska* 1992;30:73–80.

7. Claudio L, Martiney JA, Brosnan CF. Ultrastructural studies of the blood-retina barrier after exposure to interleukin-1 beta or tumor necrosis factor-alpha. *Lab Invest* 1994;70:850–861.

8. Sharief MK, Thompson EJ. In vivo relationship of tumor necrosis factor-alpha to blood-brain barrier damage in patients with active multiple sclerosis. *J Neuroimmunol* 1992;38:27–33.

9. Rosenberg GA, Dencoff JE, Correa N Jr, et al. Effect of steroids on CSF matrix metalloproteinases in multiple sclerosis: relation to blood-brain barrier injury. *Neurology* 1996;46:1626–1632.

10. Lai M, Hodgson T, Gawne-Cain M, et al. A preliminary study into the sensitivity of disease activity detection by serial weekly magnetic resonance imaging in multiple sclerosis. *J Neurol Neurosurg Psychiatry* 1996;60:339–341.

11. McLean BN, Zeman AZ, Barnes D, Thompson EJ. Patterns of blood-brain barrier impairment and clinical features in multiple sclerosis. *J Neurol Neurosurg Psychiatry* 1993;56:356–360.

12. Revesz T, Kidd D, Thompson AJ, et al. A comparison of the pathology of primary and secondary progressive multiple sclerosis. *Brain* 1994;117:759–765.

13. Miller DH, Thompson AJ, Morrissey SP, et al. High dose steroids in acute relapses of multiple sclerosis: MRI evidence for a possible mechanism of therapeutic effect. *J Neurol Neurosurg Psychiatry* 1992;55:450–453.

14. Traugott U, Reinherz EL, Raine CS. Multiple sclerosis. Distribution of T cells, T cell subsets and Ia-positive macrophages in lesions of different ages. *J Neuroimmunol* 1983;4:201–221.

15. Traugott U, Reinherz EL, Raine CS. Multiple sclerosis: distribution of T cell subsets within active chronic lesions. *Science* 1983;219:308–310.

16. Hauser SL, Bhan AK, Gilles F, et al. Immunohistochemical analysis of the cellular infiltrate in multiple sclerosis lesions. *Ann Neurol* 1986;19:578–587.

17. Oksenberg JR, Stuart S, Begovich AB, et al. Limited heterogeneity of rearranged T-cell receptor V alpha transcripts in brains of multiple sclerosis patients. *Nature* 1990;345:344–346.

18. Selmaj K, Brosnan CF, Raine CS. Colocalization of lymphocytes bearing gamma delta T-cell receptor and heat shock protein hsp65+ oligodendrocytes in multiple sclerosis. *Proc Natl Acad Sci USA* 1991;88:6452–6456.

19. Wucherpfennig KW, Newcombe J, Li H, et al. Gamma delta T-cell receptor repertoire in acute multiple sclero-

sis lesions. *Proc Natl Acad Sci USA* 1992;89:4588–4592.

20. Wucherpfennig KW, Newcombe J, Li H, et al. T cell receptor V alpha-V beta repertoire and cytokine gene expression in active multiple sclerosis lesions. *J Exp Med* 1992;175:993–1002.

21. Hvas J, Oksenberg JR, Fernando R, et al. Gamma delta T cell receptor repertoire in brain lesions of patients with multiple sclerosis. *J Neuroimmunol* 1993;46:225–234.

22. Rajan AJ, Gao Y-L, Raine CS, Brosnan CF. A pathogenic role for γ/δ T cells in relapsing-remitting experimental allergic encephalomyelitis in the SJL mouse. *J Immunol* 1996;157:941–949.

23. McMenamin C, McKersey M, Kuhnlein P, et al. Gamma delta T cells down-regulate primary IgE responses in rats to inhaled soluble protein antigens. *J Immunol* 1995;154:4390–4394.

24. Shimonkevitz R, Colburn C, Burnham JA, et al. Clonal expansions of activated gamma/delta T cells in recent-onset multiple sclerosis. *Proc Natl Acad Sci USA* 1993;90:923–927.

25. Birnbaum G, Kotilinek L, Albrecht L. Spinal fluid lymphocytes from a subgroup of multiple sclerosis patients respond to mycobacterial antigens. *Ann Neurol* 1993;34:18–24.

26. Zhang J, Markovic-Plese S, Lacet B, et al. Increased frequency of interleukin 2-responsive T cells specific for myelin basic protein and proteolipid protein in peripheral blood and cerebrospinal fluid of patients with multiple sclerosis. *J Exp Med* 1994;179:973–984.

27. Johnson D, Hafler DA, Fallis RJ, et al. Cell-mediated immunity to myelin-associated glycoprotein, proteolipid protein, and myelin basic protein in multiple sclerosis. *J Neuroimmunol* 1986;13:99–108.

28. Link H, Sun JB, Wang Z, et al. Virus-reactive and autoreactive T cells are accumulated in cerebrospinal fluid in multiple sclerosis. *J Neuroimmunol* 1992;38:63–73.

29. Kerlero de Rosbo N, Milo R, Lees MB, et al. Reactivity to myelin antigens in multiple sclerosis. Peripheral blood lymphocytes respond predominantly to myelin oligodendrocyte glycoprotein. *J Clin Invest* 1993;92:2602–2608.

30. Brosnan CF, Selmaj K, Raine CS. Hypothesis: a role for tumor necrosis factor in immune-mediated demyelination and its relevance to multiple sclerosis. *J Neuroimmunol* 1988;18:87–94.

31. Esparza I, Mannel D, Ruppel A, et al. Interferon gamma and lymphotoxin or tumor necrosis factor act synergistically to induce macrophage killing of tumor cells and schistosomula of *Schistosoma mansoni*. *J Exp Med* 1987;166:589–594.

32. Hofman FM, Hinton DR, Johnson K, Merrill JE. Tumor necrosis factor identified in multiple sclerosis brain. *J Exp Med* 1989;170:607–612.

33. Selmaj K, Raine CS, Cannella B, Brosnan CF. Identification of lymphotoxin and tumor necrosis factor in multiple sclerosis lesions. *J Clin Invest* 1991;87:949–954.

34. Panitch HS, Hirsch RL, Haley AS, Johnson KP. Exacerbations of multiple sclerosis in patients treated with gamma interferon. *Lancet* 1987;1:893–895.

35. Panitch HS, Hirsch RL, Schindler J, Johnson KP. Treatment of multiple sclerosis with gamma interferon: exacerbations associated with activation of the immune system. *Neurology* 1987;37:1097–1102.

36. Johns LD, Flanders KC, Ranges GE, Sriram S. Successful treatment of experimental allergic encephalomyelitis with transforming growth factor-beta 1. *J Immunol* 1991;147:1792–1796.

37. Racke MK, Dhib Jalbut S, Cannella B, et al. Prevention and treatment of chronic relapsing experimental aller-

gic encephalomyelitis by transforming growth factor-beta 1. *J Immunol* 1991;146:3012–3017.

38. Racke MK, Sriram S, Carlino J, et al. Long-term treatment of chronic relapsing experimental allergic encephalomyelitis by transforming growth factor-beta 2. *J Neuroimmunol* 1993;46:175–183.

39. Stevens DB, Gould KE, Swanborg RH. Transforming growth factor-beta 1 inhibits tumor necrosis factor-alpha/lymphotoxin production and adoptive transfer of disease by effector cells of autoimmune encephalomyelitis. *J Neuroimmunol* 1994;51:77–83.

40. Cannella B, Raine CS. The adhesion molecule and cytokine profile of multiple sclerosis lesions [see comments]. *Ann Neurol* 1995;37:424–435.

41. Taub DD, Oppenheim JJ. Chemokines, inflammation and the immune system. *Ther Immunol* 1994;1:229–246.

42. Graves DT, Jiang Y. Chemokines, a family of chemotactic cytokines. *Crit Rev Oral Biol Med* 1995;6:109–118.

43. Glabinski AR, Tani M, Aras S, et al. Regulation and function of central nervous system chemokines. *Int J Dev Neurosci* 1995;13:153–165.

44. Selmaj K, Raine CS, Farooq M, et al. Cytokine cytotoxicity against oligodendrocytes. Apoptosis induced by lymphotoxin. *J Immunol* 1991;147:1522–1529.

45. Santambrogio L, Hochwald GM, Saxena B, et al. Studies on the mechanisms by which transforming growth factor-beta (TGF-beta) protects against allergic encephalomyelitis. Antagonism between TGF-beta and tumor necrosis factor. *J Immunol* 1993;151:1116–1127.

46. Godiska R, Chantry D, Dietsch GN, Gray PW. Chemokine expression in murine experimental allergic encephalomyelitis. *J Neuroimmunol* 1995;58:167–176.

47. Karpus WJ, Lukacs NW, McRae BL, et al. An important role for the chemokine macrophage inflammatory protein-1 alpha in the pathogenesis of the T cell-mediated autoimmune disease, experimental autoimmune encephalomyelitis. *J Immunol* 1995;155:5003–5010.

48. Miyagishi R, Kikuchi S, Fukazawa T, Tashiro K. Macrophage inflammatory protein-1 alpha in the cerebrospinal fluid of patients with multiple sclerosis and other inflammatory neurological diseases. *J Neurol Sci* 1995;129:223–227.

49. Collins T, Read MA, Neish AS, et al. Transcriptional regulation of endothelial cell adhesion molecules: NF-kappa B and cytokine-inducible enhancers. *FASEB J* 1995;9:899–909.

50. Brosnan CF, Cannella B, Battistini L, Raine CS. Cytokine localization in multiple sclerosis lesions: correlation with adhesion molecule expression and reactive nitrogen species. *Neurology* 1995;45(suppl 6):S16–S21.

51. Washington R, Burton J, Todd RF, et al. Expression of immunologically relevant endothelial cell activation antigens on isolated central nervous system microvessels from patients with multiple sclerosis. *Ann Neurol* 1994;35:89–97.

52. Wekerle H, Linington C, Lassmann H, Meyermann R. Cellular immune reactivity within the CNS. *Trends Neurosci* 1986;9:271–277.

53. Hickey WF, Claudio L, Raine CS, Brosnan CF. Migration of hematogenous cells through the blood-brain barrier and the initiation of CNS inflammation. *Brain Pathol* 1991;1:97–105.

54. Dore-Duffy P, Newman W, Balabanov R, et al. Circulating, soluble adhesion proteins in cerebrospinal fluid and serum of patients with multiple sclerosis: correlation with clinical activity. *Ann Neurol* 1995;37:55–62.

55. Hartung HP, Reiners K, Archelos JJ, et al. Circulating adhesion molecules and tumor necrosis factor receptor in

56. Yednock TA, Cannon C, Fritz LC, et al. Prevention of experimental autoimmune encephalomyelitis by antibodies against alpha 4 beta 1 integrin. *Nature* 1992;356:63–66.

57. Cannella B, Cross AH, Raine CS. Anti-adhesion molecule therapy in experimental autoimmune encephalomyelitis. *J Neuroimmunol* 1993;46:43–55.

58. Kostulas VK, Link H, Lefvert AK. Oligoclonal IgG bands in cerebrospinal fluid. Principles for demonstration and interpretation based on findings in 1114 neurological patients. *Arch Neurol* 1987;44:1041–1044.

59. Mattson DH, Roos RP, Arnason BG. Isoelectric focusing of IgG eluted from multiple sclerosis and subacute sclerosing panencephalitis brains. *Nature* 1980;287:335–337.

60. Izquierdo G, Druetta E, Navarro G, et al. Intrathecal secretion of antiviral antibodies in multiple sclerosis in patients in Seville. *Neurologia* 1990;5:151–154.

61. Xiao BG, Linington C, Link H. Antibodies to myelin-oligodendrocyte glycoprotein in cerebrospinal fluid from patients with multiple sclerosis and controls. *J Neuroimmunol* 1991;31:91–96.

62. Warren KG, Catz I. Relative frequency of autoantibodies to myelin basic protein and proteolipid protein in optic neuritis and multiple sclerosis cerebrospinal fluid. *J Neurol Sci* 1994;121:66–73.

63. Linington C, Bradl M, Lassmann H, et al. Augmentation of demyelination in rat acute allergic encephalomyelitis by circulating mouse monoclonal antibodies directed against a myelin/oligodendrocyte glycoprotein. *Am J Pathol* 1988;130:443–454.

64. Genain CP, Nguyen MH, Letvin NL, et al. Antibody facilitation of multiple sclerosis-like lesions in a nonhuman primate. *J Clin Invest* 1995;96:2966–2974.

65. Grundke-Iqbal I, Raine CS, Johnson AB, et al. Experimental allergic encephalomyelitis. Characterization of serum factors causing demyelination and swelling of myelin. *J Neurol Sci* 1981;50:63–79.

66. Scolding NJ, Compston DA. Oligodendrocyte-macrophage interactions in vitro triggered by specific antibodies. *Immunology* 1991;72:127–132.

67. Compston DA, Morgan BP, Campbell AK, et al. Immunocytochemical localization of the terminal complement complex in multiple sclerosis. *Neuropathol Appl Neurobiol* 1989;15:307–316.

68. Scolding NJ, Morgan BP, Houston WA, et al. Vesicular removal by oligodendrocytes of membrane attack complexes formed by activated complement. *Nature* 1989;339:620–622.

69. Weiner HL, Dau PC, Khatri BO, et al. Double-blind study of true vs. sham plasma exchange in patients treated with immunosuppression for acute attacks of multiple sclerosis [see comments]. *Neurology* 1989;39:1143–1149.

70. Moreau T, Coles A, Wing M, et al. Transient increase in symptoms associated with cytokine release in patients with multiple sclerosis. *Brain* 1996;119:225–237.

71. Kitchin LI, Knobler RL, Friedman LS. Crohn's disease in a patient with multiple sclerosis. *J Clin Gastroenterol* 1991;13:331–334.

72. Sadovnick AD, Paty DW, Yannakoulias G. Concurrence of multiple sclerosis and inflammatory bowel disease. *N Engl J Med* 1989;321:762–763.

73. Antel JP, Bania MB, Reder A, Cashman N. Activated suppressor cell dysfunction in progressive multiple sclerosis. *J Immunol* 1986;137:137–141.

74. Antel J, Brown M, Nicholas MK, et al. Activated suppressor cell function in multiple sclerosis–clinical correlations. *J Neuroimmunol* 1988;17:323–330.

75. Challoner PB, Smith KT, Parker JD, et al. Plaque-associated expression of human herpesvirus 6 in multiple sclerosis. *Proc Natl Acad Sci USA* 1995;92:7440–7444.

76. Sanders VJ, Waddell AE, Felisan SL, et al. Herpes simplex virus in postmortem multiple sclerosis brain tissue. *Arch Neurol* 1996;53:125–133.

77. Karpus WJ, Pope JG, Peterson JD, et al. Inhibition of Theiler's virus-mediated demyelination by peripheral immune tolerance induction. *J Immunol* 1995;155:947–957.

78. Njenga MK, Pavelko KD, Baisch J, et al. Theiler's virus persistence and demyelination in major histocompatibility complex class II-deficient mice. *J Virol* 1996;70:1729–1737.

79. Pullen LC, Miller SD, Dal CMC, Kim BS. Class I-deficient resistant mice intracerebrally inoculated with Theiler's virus show an increased T cell response to viral antigens and susceptibility to demyelination. *Eur J Immunol* 1993;23:2287–2293.

80. Rodriguez M, Dunkel AJ, Thiemann RL, et al. Abrogation of resistance to Theiler's virus-induced demyelination in H-2b mice deficient in beta 2-microglobulin. *J Immunol* 1993;151:266–276.

81. Calder V, Owen S, Watson C, et al. MS: a localized immune disease of the central nervous system. *Immunol Today* 1989;10:99–103.

82. Hafler DA, Weiner HL. MS: a CNS and systemic autoimmune disease. *Immunol Today* 1989;10:104–107.

83. Hafler DA, Hemler ME, Christenson L, et al. Investigation of in vivo activated T cells in multiple sclerosis and inflammatory central nervous system diseases. *Clin Immunol Immunopathol* 1985;37:163–171.

84. Zhang J, Vandevyver C, Stinissen P, et al. Activation and clonal expansion of human myelin basic protein-reactive T cells by bacterial superantigens. *J Autoimmun* 1995;8:615–632.

85. Panitch HS. Influence of infection on exacerbations of multiple sclerosis. *Ann Neurol* 1994;36(suppl):S25–S28.

86. Sibley WA, Bamford CR, Clark K. Clinical viral infections and multiple sclerosis. *Lancet* 1985;1:1313–1315.

87. Sharief MK, Hentges R. Association between tumor necrosis factor-alpha and disease progression in patients with multiple sclerosis. *N Engl J Med* 1991;325:467–472.

88. Buhrer C, Berlin C, Thiele HG, Hamann A. Lymphocyte activation and expression of the human leucocyte-endothelial cell adhesion molecule 1 (Leu-8/TQ1 antigen). *Immunology* 1990;71:442–448.

89. Huang K, Beigi M, Daynes RA. Peripheral lymph node-specific and Peyer's patch-specific homing receptors are differentially regulated following lymphocyte activation. *Reg Immunol* 1990;3:103–111.

90. Hamann A, Jablonski-Westrich D, Scholz KU, et al. Regulation of lymphocyte homing. I. Alterations in homing receptor expression and organ-specific high endothelial venule binding of lymphocytes upon activation. *J Immunol* 1988;140:737–743.

91. Cross AH, Cannella B, Brosnan CF, Raine CS. Homing to central nervous system vasculature by antigen-specific lymphocytes. I. Localization of ^{14}C-labeled cells during acute, chronic, and relapsing experimental allergic encephalomyelitis. *Lab Invest* 1990;63:162–170.

92. Raine CS, Cannella B, Duijvestijn AM, Cross AH. Homing to central nervous system vasculature by antigen-specific lymphocytes. II. Lymphocyte/endothelial cell adhesion during the initial stages of autoimmune demyelination. *Lab Invest* 1990;63:476–489.

93. Wucherpfennig KW, Strominger JL. Molecular mimicry in T cell-mediated autoimmunity: viral peptides activate human T cell clones specific for myelin basic protein. *Cell* 1995;80:695–705.

94. Birnbaum G, Kotilinek L, Schlievert P, et al. Heat shock proteins and experimental autoimmune encephalomyelitis (EAE): I. Immunization with a peptide of the myelin protein 2′,3′ cyclic nucleotide 3′ phosphodiesterase that is cross-reactive with a heat shock protein alters the course of EAE. *J Neurosci Res* 1996;44:381–396.

95. Morimoto RI, Tissières A, Georgopoulos C, eds. *Stress proteins in biology and medicine.* Cold Spring Harbor, NY: Cold Spring Harbor Laboratory Press, 1990.

96. Möller G, ed. Heat-shock proteins and the immune system. Copenhagen: Munksgaard, 1991:5–220.

97. Selmaj K, Brosnan CF, Raine CS. Expression of heat shock protein-65 by oligodendrocytes in vivo and in vitro: implications for multiple sclerosis. *Neurology* 1992;42:795–800.

98. Freedman MS, Buu NN, Ruijs TC, et al. Differential expression of heat shock proteins by human glial cells. *J Neuroimmunol* 1992;41:231–238.

99. Allegretta M, Nicklas JA, Sriram S, Albertini RJ. T cells responsive to myelin basic protein in patients with multiple sclerosis. *Science* 1990;247:718–721.

100. Allegretta M, Albertini RJ, Howell MD, et al. Homologies between T cell receptor junctional sequences unique to multiple sclerosis and T cells mediating experimental allergic encephalomyelitis. *J Clin Invest* 1994;94:105–109.

101. Lehmann PV, Sercarz EE, Forsthuber T, et al. Determinant spreading and the dynamics of the autoimmune T-cell repertoire. *Immunol Today* 1993;14:203–208.

102. Lehmann PV, Forsthuber T, Miller A, Sercarz EE. Spreading of T-cell autoimmunity to cryptic determinants of an autoantigen. *Nature* 1992;358:155–157.

103. McRae BL, Vanderlugt CL, Del Canto MC, Miller SD. Functional evidence for epitope spreading in the relapsing pathology of experimental autoimmune encephalomyelitis. *J Exp Med* 1995;182:75–85.

104. Martin R, Utz U, Coligan JE, et al. Diversity in fine specificity and T cell receptor usage of the human CD4+ cytotoxic T cell response specific for the immunodominant myelin basic protein peptide 87-106. *J Immunol* 1992;148:1359–1366.

105. Mustafa M, Vingsbo C, Olsson T, et al. The major histocompatibility complex influences myelin basic protein 63-88-induced T cell cytokine profile and experimental autoimmune encephalomyelitis. *Eur J Immunol* 1993;23:3089–3095.

106. Ebers GC. Genetic factors in multiple sclerosis. *Neurol Clin* 1983;1:645–654.

107. Ebers GC, Bulman DE, Sadovnick AD, et al. A population-based study of multiple sclerosis in twins. *N Engl J Med* 1986;315:1638–1642.

108. Hillert J. Human leukocyte antigen studies in multiple sclerosis. *Ann Neurol* 1994;36(suppl):S15–S17.

109. Hauser SL, Fleischnick E, Weiner HL, et al. Extended major histocompatibility complex haplotypes in patients with multiple sclerosis. *Neurology* 1989;39:275–277.

110. Jain S, Maheshwari MC. Multiple sclerosis: Indian experience in the last thirty years. *Neuroepidemiology* 1985;4:96–107.

111. La Mantia L, Illeni MT, Milanese C, et al. HLA and multiple sclerosis in Italy: a review of the literature. *J Neurol* 1990;237:441–444.

112. al-Din AS, al-Saffar M, Siboo R, Behbehani K. Association between HLA-D region epitopes and multiple sclerosis in Arabs. *Tissue Antigens* 1986;27:196–200.

113. Ebers GC, Kukay K, Bulman DE, et al. A full genome search in multiple sclerosis. *Nat Genet* 1996;13:472–476.

114. Haines JL, Ter-Minassian M, Bazyk A, et al. A complete genomic screen for multiple sclerosis underscores a role for the major histocompatibility complex. The Multiple Sclerosis Genetics Group. *Nat Genet* 1996;13:469–471.

115. Sawcer S, Jones HB, Feakes R, et al. A genome screen in multiple sclerosis reveals susceptibility loci on chromosome 6p21 and 17q22. *Nat Genet* 1996;13:464–468.

116. Kuokkanen S, Sundvall M, Terwilliger JD, et al. A putative vulnerability locus to multiple sclerosis maps to 5p14-p12 in a region syntenic to the murine locus Eae2. *Nat Genet* 1996;13:477–480.

117. Olerup O, Hillert J, Fredrikson S, et al. Primarily chronic progressive and relapsing/remitting multiple sclerosis: two immunogenetically distinct disease entities. *Proc Natl Acad Sci USA* 1989;86:7113–7117.

118. Hillert J, Gronning M, Nyland H, et al. An immunogenetic heterogeneity in multiple sclerosis. *J Neurol Neurosurg Psychiatry* 1992;55:887–890.

119. Beall SS, Concannon P, Charmley P, et al. The germline repertoire of T cell receptor beta-chain genes in patients with chronic progressive multiple sclerosis. *J Neuroimmunol* 1989;21:59–66.

120. Beall SS, Biddison WE, McFarlin DE, et al. Susceptibility for multiple sclerosis is determined, in part, by inheritance of a 175-kb region of the TcR V beta chain locus and HLA class II genes. *J Neuroimmunol* 1993;45:53–60.

121. Seboun E, Robinson MA, Doolittle TH, et al. A susceptibility locus for multiple sclerosis is linked to the T cell receptor beta chain complex. *Cell* 1989;57:1095–1100.

122. Birnbaum G, Van Ness B. T cell receptor gene utilization in the brain, blood, and spinal fluid of patients with multiple sclerosis and other neurologic diseases. *Ann Neurol* 1992;32:24–30.

123. Utz U, Brooks JA, McFarland HF, et al. Heterogeneity of T-cell receptor alpha-chain complementarity-determining region 3 in myelin basic protein-specific T cells increases with severity of multiple sclerosis. *Proc Natl Acad Sci USA* 1994;91:5567–5571.

124. Walter MA, Gibson WT, Ebers GC, Cox DW. Susceptibility to multiple sclerosis is associated with the proximal immunoglobulin heavy chain variable region. *J Clin Invest* 1991;87:1266–1273.

125. Kurtzke JF, Beebe GW, Norman JE Jr. Epidemiology of multiple sclerosis in US veterans: III. Migration and the risk of MS. *Neurology* 1985;35:672–678.

126. Kurtzke JF, Bui-Quoc-Huong. Multiple sclerosis in a migrant population: 2. Half-orientals immigrating in childhood. *Ann Neurol* 1980;8:256–260.

127. Kurtzke JF, Hyllested K. MS epidemiology in Faroe Islands. *Rev Neurol* 1987;57:77–87.

128. Kurtzke JF, Hyllested K. Validity of the epidemics of multiple sclerosis in the Faroe Islands. *Neuroepidemiology* 1988;7:190–227.

129. Kurtzke JF, Gudmundsson KR, Bergmann S. Multiple sclerosis in Iceland: 1. Evidence of a postwar epidemic. *Neurology* 1982;32:143–150.

130. Utz U, Biddison WE, McFarland HF, et al. Skewed T-cell receptor repertoire in genetically identical twins correlates with multiple sclerosis. *Nature* 1993;364:243–247.

131. Gaudet JP, Hashimoto L, Sadovnick AD, Ebers GC. A study of birth order and multiple sclerosis in multiplex families. *Neuroepidemiology* 1995;14:188–192.

132. Ebers GC, Sadovnick AD. The geographic distribution of multiple sclerosis: a review. *Neuroepidemiology* 1993;12:1–5.

133. Ross RT, Nicolle LE, Cheang M. Varicella zoster virus and multiple sclerosis in a Hutterite population. *J Clin Epidemiol* 1995;48:1319–1324.

134. Ebers GC, Sadovnick AD, Risch NJ. A genetic basis for familial aggregation in multiple sclerosis. Canadian Collaborative Study Group. *Nature* 1995;377:150–151.

135. Lafaille JJ, Nagashima K, Katsuki M, Tonegawa S. High incidence of spontaneous autoimmune encephalomyelitis in immunodeficient anti-myelin basic protein T cell receptor transgenic mice. *Cell* 1994;78:399–408.

136. Goverman J, Woods A, Larson L, et al. Transgenic mice that express a myelin basic protein-specific T cell receptor develop spontaneous autoimmunity. *Cell* 1993;72:551–560.

137. Birnbaum G, Kotilinek L, Lehmann PV, Miller SD. Inflammation and environmental infections change the course of chronic, relapsing EAE. *Neurology* 1997;48:A144.

138. Critchfield JM, Racke MK, Zuniga-Pflucker JC, et al. T cell deletion in high antigen dose therapy of autoimmune encephalomyelitis. *Science* 1994;263:1139–1343.

139. Miller A, Lider O, Weiner HL. Antigen-driven bystander suppression after oral administration of antigens. *J Exp Med* 1991;174:791–798.

140. Miller A, al Sabbagh A, Santos LM, et al. Epitopes of myelin basic protein that trigger TGF-beta release after oral tolerization are distinct from encephalitogenic epitopes and mediate epitope-driven bystander suppression. *J Immunol* 1993;151:7307–7315.

141. Weiner HL, Mackin GA, Matsui M, et al. Double-blind pilot trial of oral tolerization with myelin antigens in multiple sclerosis [see comments]. *Science* 1993;259:1321–1324.

142. Acha-Orbea H, Mitchell DJ, Timmermann L, et al. Limited heterogeneity of T cell receptors from lymphocytes mediating autoimmune encephalomyelitis allows specific immune intervention. *Cell* 1988;54:263–273.

143. Urban JL, Kumar V, Kono DH, et al. Restricted use of T cell receptor V genes in murine autoimmune encephalomyelitis raises possibilities for antibody therapy. *Cell* 1988;54:577–592.

144. Owhashi M, Heber KE. Protection from experimental allergic encephalomyelitis conferred by a monoclonal antibody directed against a shared idiotype on rat T cell receptors specific for myelin basic protein. *J Exp Med* 1988;168:2153–2164.

145. Sun D, Hu XZ, Le J, Swanborg RH. Characterization of brain-isolated rat encephalitogenic T cell lines. *Eur J Immunol* 1994;24:1359–1364.

146. Pette M, Fujita K, Wilkinson D, et al. Myelin autoreactivity in multiple sclerosis: recognition of myelin basic protein in the context of HLA-DR2 products by T lymphocytes of multiple-sclerosis patients and healthy donors. *Proc Natl Acad Sci USA* 1990;87:7968–7972.

147. Wucherpfennig KW, Ota K, Endo N, et al. Shared human T cell receptor V beta usage to immunodominant regions of myelin basic protein. *Science* 1990;248:1016–1019.

148. Ben-Nun A, Liblau RS, Cohen L, et al. Restricted T-cell receptor V beta gene usage by myelin basic protein-specific T-cell clones in multiple sclerosis: predominant genes vary in individuals. *Proc Natl Acad Sci USA* 1991;88:2466–2470.

149. Hafler DA, Cohen I, Benjamin DS, Weiner HL. T cell vaccination in multiple sclerosis: a preliminary report. *Clin Immunol Immunopathol* 1992;62:307–313.

150. Medaer R, Stinissen P, Truyen L, et al. Depletion of

myelin-basic-protein autoreactive T cells by T-cell vaccination: pilot trial in multiple sclerosis. *Lancet* 1995;346:807–808.

151. Zhang J, Vandevyver C, Stinissen P, Raus J. In vivo clonotypic regulation of human myelin basic protein-reactive T cells by T cell vaccination. *J Immunol* 1995;155:5868–5877.

152. Vandenbark AA, Chou YK, Whitham R, et al. Treatment of multiple sclerosis with T-cell receptor peptides: results of a double-blind pilot trial. *Nat Med* 1996;2:1109–1115.

153. Chou YK, Morrison WJ, Weinberg AD, et al. Immunity to TCR peptides in multiple sclerosis. II. T cell recognition of V beta 5.2 and V beta 6.1 CDR2 peptides. *J Immunol* 1994;152:2520–2529.

154. Bourdette DN, Whitham RH, Chou YK, et al. Immunity to TCR peptides in multiple sclerosis. I. Successful immunization of patients with synthetic V beta 5.2 and V beta 6.1 CDR2 peptides. *J Immunol* 1994;152:2510–2519.

155. Sakai K, Sinha AA, Mitchell DJ, et al. Involvement of distinct murine T-cell receptors in the autoimmune encephalitogenic response to nested epitopes of myelin basic protein. *Proc Natl Acad Sci USA* 1988;85:8608–8612.

156. Lodge PA, Allegretta M, Steinman L, Sriram S. Myelin basic protein peptide specificity and T-cell receptor gene usage of HPRT mutant T-cell clones in patients with multiple sclerosis. *Ann Neurol* 1994;36:734–740.

Chapter 9
Acute Disseminated Encephalomyelitis

Alex C. Tselis and Robert P. Lisak

Acute disseminated encephalomyelitis (ADEM) is a generally monophasic inflammatory disease of the white matter of the central nervous system (CNS) (1–4). The relation of ADEM to multiple sclerosis (MS), another inflammatory disease of the CNS white matter, is an important issue and is discussed later in the chapter.

It has long been noted that following recovery from a viral infection, a few patients develop an acute or subacute neurologic disease. The original virus probably does not cause this neurologic disease because 1) no virus has been isolated from the brains of fatal cases or from cerebrospinal fluid (CSF) samples of nonfatal cases; 2) the pathology of ADEM in fatal cases is different from that of an acute viral encephalitis; and 3) the same clinical and pathologic disease occurs consequent to other circumstances that do not involve infection, such as vaccination with nonviable organisms.

Postinfectious encephalomyelitis was first reported in 1790. It occurred in a 23-year-old woman who had lower extremity weakness and urinary retention about a week after a measles rash, and who had had a similar syndrome 10 years earlier, after a bout of smallpox (4,5). The prototypical postinfectious encephalomyelitis follows measles. This once was the most common precipitant of ADEM because of the high incidence of measles in the population. No virus could be isolated from, or detected by immunostaining in, the brains of patients with "measles encephalomyelitis" (6), as the measles-associated ADEM was called in the literature. (In the older literature, the nomenclature was confusing, in that a febrile encephalopathy associated with or following a particular viral illness was labeled with that illness, thus, measles encephalomyelitis, varicella encephalomyelitis, rubella encephalomyelitis, and so forth, so that a direct viral infection of the brain and a postinfectious encephalomyelitis were given the same name.)

It soon became apparent that a clinically and pathologically similar illness occasionally followed vaccination with killed or attenuated microorganisms, not necessarily viruses (7). In particular, postvaccination encephalomyelitis frequently followed smallpox (8) and rabies vaccination (9). The post–rabies vaccination encephalomyelitis is also known in the older literature as a *neuroparalytic accident*, a term that broadly encompassed any neurologic complication of rabies vaccination, including acute inflammatory demyelinating polyneuropathy. Indeed, neuroparalytic accidents secondary to immunization with vaccine containing nervous system tissue are, in retrospect, the first instances of experimental allergic encephalomyelitis. The pathology in the cases involving the CNS is indistinguishable from that of other forms of ADEM (10).

Eventually it became clear that ADEM can occur "spontaneously" or can follow a bacterial (11), mycoplasmal (12–14), or viral infection (15); a vaccination (8,16); administration of a medication (18–21) or tetanus antitoxin (22); or other illness (1–4). The disease can also occur after disseminated tuberculosis (23) and possibly neurobrucellosis (24). These types of encephalomyelitis share common clinical and pathologic features (25), and hence are all considered by most as ADEM. In rare instances, there may be concomitant demyelination in both the central and peripheral nervous systems, a combination of ADEM and the Guillain-Barré syndrome (GBS), either simultaneously (26) or in rapid succession (27).

Postinfectious or postvaccination white matter inflammation can be highly focal clinically and even pathologically, and affect only the optic nerve, the spinal cord, or the cerebellum. Such allied syndromes with focal monophasic inflammatory demyelination (optic neuritis, transverse myelitis, and cerebellar ataxia) appear to have triggers similar to those of ADEM. Thus, optic neuritis may follow a vaccination (28), and acute transverse myelitis may follow simultaneous immunization with diphtheria, tetanus, and polio (29) or infection with varicella (30) or *Mycoplasma pneumoniae* (31). Neuromyelitis optica may also follow varicella (32). Bilateral optic neuritis, followed a week later by transverse myelitis, can occur after rubella vaccination (33). Optic neuritis has been associated with Lyme disease, but whether this is due to direct infection by *Borrelia burgdorferi* or is a form of postinfectious white matter inflammation is not clear (34,35). Bilateral optic neuritis has occurred after vaccination with the trivalent measles, mumps, and rubella vaccine (28). Indeed, any vaccination can be followed by dysfunction at any level of the nervous system (36).

Patients also can develop acute hemorrhagic leukoencephalitis (AHLE), a severe form of ADEM (37,38). AHLE is characterized by a more fulminant clinical course, with hemorrhagic necrosis of the white matter and a high fatality rate. The relation of all these conditions to the quintessential inflammatory demyelinating disease of humans, MS, is unclear.

An acute febrile encephalopathy reportedly coincides with or follows systemic infections, viral and possibly also bacterial. The histopathology is not that of an encephalomyelitis. We discuss this in more detail later.

Virus-Induced Demyelination

Occasionally, direct viral infections of the brain and spinal cord can cause demyelination with relative axonal sparing. It is rare for these infections to resemble ADEM. An example may be Epstein-Barr virus (EBV) infection, which is also an associated trigger for ADEM (39,40). In several patients, an acute EBV infection with neurologic manifestations was followed by either a progressive or a relapsing and remitting white matter disease (39). Whether this was a purely demyelinating disease is unknown. Acute infection with human immunodeficiency virus (HIV) is very rarely associated with an ADEM-like syndrome (41–43), with pathologically confirmed demyelination and relative axonal sparing in the lesions, but this is uncommon enough that any causal relation is unclear. Human T-lymphotropic virus (HTLV) type I–associated myelopathy (tropical spastic paraparesis) is documented to have directly demyelinating effects (44–46). It is unknown how these arise, although it is known that HTLV-I infects CD8+ T lymphocytes, which become activated and proliferate. However, these cells are directed against HTLV-I antigens and not myelin. The virus does not infect oligodendrocytes, so that direct viral lysis of myelin-producing cells does not occur. HTLV-I does infect primary cultures of human microglia, activating them and inducing cytokine production, which may be directly toxic to myelin (47). Despite the activation of immune cells in HTLV-I disease, the main clinical outcome of this is a mild immune deficiency, although adult T-cell leukemia/lymphoma and tropical spastic paraparesis are the usual associated diseases, occurring in about 5% of all patients with HTLV-I infections (47). HIV leukoencephalopathy, commonly seen with advanced HIV disease, is characterized by an apparent deficit of myelin (myelin pallor) of unclear nature (48). This has been cited as a possible example of demyelination (49), but further studies showed that the intensity of immunostaining for myelin basic protein (MBP) from affected areas was normal, no lipid-laden macrophages were detected, and neither active demyelination nor demyelinated axons were seen, which suggests that no classic inflammatory demyelination takes place (50). Instead, the pathogenesis appears to have some relationship to alterations in the blood-brain barrier (50), but the nature of this relationship is still not completely clear. These blood-brain barrier alterations are inferred from the presence of serum proteins in the brain parenchyma, localized to neurons and glia, in which they are usually absent. This is different from the alterations in the blood-brain barrier seen with ADEM and MS, in which

there is a more specific inflammatory reaction surrounding small cerebral venules in the deep white matter, with an associated perivenular demyelination in which both cellular and humoral factors have access to the brain parenchyma.

Subacute sclerosing panencephalitis, a chronic progressive measles virus infection of the brain in young persons, is characterized in part by inflammatory demyelination (51). Similarly, progressive rubella encephalitis, a chronic progressive rubella virus disease of the brain, is also characterized by prominent white matter involvement (52). The white matter involvement proceeds beyond demyelination, with axonal fragmentation present as well (53). Neither of these clinically resembles ADEM, however. Progressive multifocal leukoencephalopathy, a papovavirus infection of the brain lytic for oligodendrocytes (and transforming for astrocytes), is seen in patients with advanced immunodeficiency secondary to acquired immunodeficiency syndrome (AIDS), cancer chemotherapy, or immunosuppression after transplantation, and rarely without obvious associations. The characteristic lesions consist of demyelination with little or no accompanying inflammation (54). Demyelination occurs rarely in varicella-zoster virus (VZV) encephalitis in AIDS patients (55,56). Clinically, this is a slowly progressive disease characterized by prominent cognitive difficulties, especially memory loss, and multifocal motor deficits (56). The lesions in AIDS-associated VZV encephalitis cover a broad pathologic spectrum, including a leukoencephalitis in which a vasculopathy gives rise to both necrosis and demyelination, often in the same lesion (55,57). Additionally, demyelination is probably due to direct infection of oligodendrocytes by VZV, since some of the demyelinated areas are ringed with oligodendrocytes containing viral inclusions (56,57). Other cells, including macrophages, endothelial cells, and occasionally neurons, are also infected (57). Finally, it recently was proposed that demyelination can be caused directly by infection of the brain with human herpesvirus-6 (HHV-6) in immunosuppressed transplant recipients and AIDS patients (58). HHV-6 also was recently added to the list of possible etiologic agents in MS (59).

A number of viruses can cause demyelination in animal models (60,61). These include Theiler's virus (an enterovirus) (62), herpesvirus (63), and coronavirus (64,65). Other model viral demyelinating syndromes include those due to Chandipura and vesicular stomatitis viruses (both rhabdoviruses), canine distemper virus, Venezuelan equine encephalomyelitis virus, and Semliki Forest virus (65). Almost all of these are enveloped viruses. A prominent virally induced inflammatory demyelinating disease in nature is the retroviral infection visna, which infects both lungs and brain, in sheep (66).

ADEM can follow a frank viral encephalitis (67), just as it can follow any other viral disease. A patient with biopsy-proved herpes simplex encephalitis who presented with headache, fever, memory loss, and a pleocytosis of 150 was treated with adenine arabinoside, and improved almost back to baseline. After two weeks of therapy, his neurological exam showed only a minimal aphasia, and his CSF pleocytosis had decreased by half. A month later, his condition began to deteriorate, and he did not respond to a second course of adenine arabinoside. A repeat biopsy showed inflammatory demyelination, typical of ADEM. In two patients with rabies, extensive demyelination was found at autopsy, along with the perivenular inflammatory infiltrates typical of ADEM (68,69). The pathogenesis of this finding was unclear, but may well have been due to concurrent rabies encephalitis and ADEM. One of the two patients had received a partial (69) and one had completed (68) a full course of rabies vaccination when the fatal illness began. In one patient, demyelination was seen in the frontal lobes and in the cervical and thoracic regions of the spinal cord as well as the cervical nerve roots (69). In addition, a widespread rabies encephalitis with characteristic viral inclusions (Negri bodies and lyssa bodies) was noted and confirmed by inoculation into suckling mice (69).

With the possible exception of acute EBV infection, which, as noted already, can be a trigger for ADEM and GBS, few viral demyelinating diseases are likely to be confused with ADEM.

Epidemiology

Epidemiologic studies of ADEM are complicated by the fact that this is an uncommon disease. The figures for ADEM vary considerably according to the precipitating disease. ADEM occurs after 1:1000 measles, 1:63 to 1:300,000 vaccinia (given as an inoculation against smallpox) (8), about 1:10,000 varicella, and 1:20,000 rubella cases (15). It has also occurred after mumps and rarely, scarlet fever (15).

The disease has an interesting age dependence: ADEM and the restricted syndromes do not appear to occur in very young children (< about 2 or 3 years old). There are rare apparent exceptions. This rarity of ADEM in young children presumably has to do with the immature state of the myelin. However, an acute toxic encephalopathy can be seen in very young children under circumstances typically associated with ADEM, and is characterized by a rapidly progressive disease with prominent drowsiness and coma, as well as seizures (70). The histopathology is bland, without the white matter perivenular inflammatory infiltrates typical of ADEM. The incidence of this toxic encephalopathy is uncertain (70). We discuss this entity in more detail later.

A very rough estimate of the incidence of ADEM can be obtained from a study of all encephalitis patients admitted to the London Hospital (71) over a 15-year period, between 1963 and 1978. *Encephalitis* was defined as an acute, rapidly progressive illness with diffuse or multifocal inflammatory involvement of the nervous system, with other causes excluded. Three subgroups were defined: 1) one group in which a virus was definitely linked to the encephalitis, 2) one group in which no causal or antecedent virus could be implicated in the encephalitis, and 3) one group in which the viral illness had occurred in the month before the onset of the neurologic illness and was separated from it by a period of normal health. Of 60 patients who fulfilled the criteria for encephalitis, at least one third were thought to have postinfectious encephalomyelitis, by virtue of the fact that they had had an antecedent viral illness that had completely resolved in the month before the onset of the neurologic illness (71). It should be noted that it is possible some cases of postinfectious encephalomyelitis may have been missed, because in some viral exanthems, the associated ADEM can overlap the systemic viral disease (1,4). While there is likely to be some referral bias in this series, and therefore some imprecision in the estimate of the proportion, the above-cited figures provide a rough estimate (probably low) of the proportion of ADEM among all encephalitis patients.

ADEM can occur after immunization with vaccines to prevent measles, diphtheria/tetanus, rubella, and pertussis (7). Given the very large number of vaccinations performed against these diseases, the incidence of ADEM is rare enough to suggest coincidence rather than causality (7). On the other hand, after vaccination with rabies vaccine containing neural antigens, the ADEM incidence is between 1:7000 and 1:50,000 and yet a causal connection is not doubted (72). In a series of 61 patients in Thailand with neurologic complications that occurred after they received Semple-type rabies vaccine, 36 had "major" complications: 12 had encephalitis, 7 had myelitis, 13 had meningitis, and 4 had GBS (72). All were treated with dexamethasone and all recovered completely. The other 25 patients had "minor" complications consisting of headache, backache, fever, and no pleocytosis. It has been estimated in Thailand that between 1 in 400 and 1 in 220 recipients of Semple virus rabies vaccine develop ADEM (72). Other vaccines reported to have ADEM as a sequela include influenza (73–79), hepatitis B (80,81), and Japanese B encephalitis (82,83). The period between influenza vaccination and the onset of the encephalitis could be exceedingly short—only a few hours, in two patients (73–77). Both patients were confused, with one having right-sided weakness and hemisensory loss, and the other having incontinence and marked pleocytosis (73,77). One of the patients (73) had strong local reactions to previous influenza vaccinations. In the other patient (77), skin testing to chicken protein elicited a strong reaction, 35 mm in diameter, within 10 minutes. Hepatitis B vaccination in one patient was followed 21 days later by an illness characterized by headache, backache, flaccid paraplegia, lower extremity areflexia, and urinary retention, which was attributed to transverse myelitis (81). This illness largely resolved in 2 weeks, except for some residual bladder dysfunction. All of these vaccines are of enveloped viruses. We are unaware of any well-documented reports of ADEM following polio vaccination, for example, and the main neurologic complication of this is clinical poliomyelitis resulting from the reversion of an attenuated strain to a virulent strain. The only postvaccination report (29) was of a case of myelitis after multiple vaccination with diphtheria, tetanus, and polio vaccine, which is hardly convincing evidence of poliovirus vaccine—induced myelitis.

ADEM also can occur after administration of a medication (18–21), but such reports are rare enough that a causal link is unlikely. Furthermore, the apparent post-medication ADEM may have been due to the original disease for which the medication was given.

There are additional reasons why we cannot quantify the incidence of ADEM more accurately. For measles, previously a common antecedent, the above-quoted incidence of ADEM may be an underestimate, as patients may have a subclinical form of the disease; indeed, a high proportion of measles patients have minor neurologic and behavioral abnormalities, electroencephalographic (EEG) abnormalities, and CSF pleocytosis (84). Other systemic infections, such as EBV disease (84), chickenpox (86), and mumps, can cause a mild viral encephalitis that can be confused with ADEM clinically, and so its incidence can be overestimated if the illness due to the viral encephalitis is ascribed to ADEM, or underestimated if the illness due to ADEM is ascribed to a viral encephalitis. Indeed, many viral exanthems can be associated with CSF (87) and EEG (88) abnormalities without any obvious brain pathology. Other systemic infections such as legionellosis (89), *B. burgdorferi* infection, and *Mycoplasma* infection can also cause encephalopathies that may erroneously be ascribed to ADEM.

The epidemiology of the clinically and pathologically restricted forms of ADEM mentioned previously, such as optic neuritis, acute cerebellar ataxia, and transverse myelitis, is also not totally understood. These interesting forms of ADEM are discussed in more detail later. Over the years 1951 to 1985, 92 children with a diagnosis of optic neuritis were referred to the Hospital for Sick Children, Great Ormond Street, a major referral center. After exclusion of patients with clear causes of optic neuropathy (leukemia, syphilis, diabetes, hypertension, vitamin deficiency, etc.), there were 39 patients (90). A population-based study of optic neuritis in Olmsted County, Minnesota, was performed using the unique comprehensive Mayo Clinic records-linkage system, and 156 patients who had optic neuritis between 1935 and 1991 were identified (91). Patients were included if 1) there was rapid visual loss with no evidence for any other local or systemic disease, 2) there were clinical signs of optic neuritis, and 3) if the diagnosis was made by a Mayo Clinic ophthalmologist. The incidence rate was found to be 5.5 cases/100,000/yr, based on 156 patients "captured" in the years 1935 to 1991, and the prevalence was 115 per 100,000 (prevalence date, December 1, 1991). The incidence and prevalence were age and sex adjusted to the 1950 US white population. In neither of these studies were there any details about previous infections or other illnesses or vaccinations. In another study of optic neuritis in childhood, 21 patients with optic neuritis (defined as sudden reduction of visual acuity, sudden visual field defects, and an afferent pupillary defect) were seen at the University Children's Hospital in Helsinki from 1970 to 1985 (92). Of these, 5 were diagnosed with other diseases, 9 were diagnosed with optic neuritis associated with MS (either because of previous history or

subsequent events), and 7 were believed to have idiopathic optic neuritis. Of the patients who went on to develop MS, 5 of the 9 had common respiratory infections or vaccinations 3 days to 1 month before the onset of the optic neuritis.

A report from a tertiary medical care center reviewed 40 patients who presented with acute childhood ataxia during a 10-year period (93). All presented to the emergency room and were subsequently admitted. The most common established etiology was postinfectious acute cerebellar ataxia, which was diagnosed in 14 (35%) of the patients. The next most common causes were drug ingestion (32.5%) and GBS (12.5%). Postinfectious cerebellar ataxia (cerebellitis) usually is associated with VZV infections, generally following chickenpox in children (15), but it can follow other viral infections such as EBV mononucleosis (94,95). Its incidence is uncertain, although it is clear that it is high on the list of differential diagnoses for acute cerebellar ataxia in children.

In a population-based study of acute transverse myelitis carried out in Israel, the average annual incidence rate was 1.34/million/yr, based on 62 cases presenting between 1955 and 1975 (96). Patients with other known neurologic disease or injury were excluded. It was found that 23 (37%) of the patients had a preceding infection (96). In a retrospective study, Lipton and Teasdall (97) looked at the records of patients seen at Johns Hopkins Hospital from 1929 to 1967 who had an acute transverse myelopathy as above and for whom follow-up data at 5 years or later or at autopsy could be obtained. Thirty-four such patients were found. Twelve (35%) of these patients had a preceding viral-like illness. Another retrospective study of acute transverse myelitis, using similar criteria, "captured" 32 cases from five neurologic departments in Denmark over a period of 12 years (98). A history of preceding viral infection was obtained in 12 (37.5%) patients.

Clinical Presentation and Outcome

ADEM has a broad clinical spectrum of presentations. It can range from a subclinical episode, detected by the appearance of multifocal white matter abnormalities on brain magnetic resonance images (MRIs) made for other reasons, to a fulminant, rapidly progressive disease with seizures and coma, leading to death. It is likely that ADEM and AHLE have a similar but not identical underlying pathogenesis (99), as both occur under the same circumstances, with ADEM evolving to AHLE in some patients (100). This hypothesis is also supported by work done on the animal models experimental autoimmune encephalomyelitis (EAE) and hyperacute EAE by Levine (101) (see below).

The neurologic symptoms usually begin 1 to 3 weeks after the time of infection, although in exanthems, especially measles, the illness tends to begin sooner, 2 to 7 days after the rash occurs. The onset tends to be abrupt, which may be a point of differentiation (102) from the slightly more gradual onset of a viral encephalitis that ADEM most closely resembles. Rarely, the illness is concurrent with or even precedes the rash. The symptoms consist of headache, fever, nausea, vomiting, confusion, delirium, obtundation, and coma, and evolve over several days. Often superimposed on this global dysfunction are focal abnormalities, including hemiparesis, hemisensory loss, ataxia, visual loss, and paraparesis (15). The latter three may be clinical expressions of a coexistent cerebellar ataxia, optic neuritis, or transverse myelitis, respectively. Seizures, myoclonus, and memory loss have also been reported. Occasionally, there may be dystonia, chorea, athetosis, and rigidity with lesions in the basal ganglia (103). MRIs of the two patients described in that report (103) showed abnormal signal in the putamina and globus pallidus, and extending through the cerebral peduncles to the substantia nigra; interestingly, the lesions were bilaterally symmetric. There is often gradual recovery, which can be surprisingly complete. However, patients with seizures and coma tend to have a less positive outcome (15). The case mortality rate is 10% to 20% (15). It should be clear that the differentiation of ADEM or AHLE from other encephalitides and occasionally from toxic-metabolic encephalopathies can be very difficult.

Of the 62 patients with acute transverse myelitis evaluated by the previously cited Israeli study (96), more than one third had a good recovery, while one third had only a "fair" recovery. The time to maximum improvement was 4 weeks to 3 months. In the study by Lipton and Teasdall (97), most of the patients (85%) had a thoracic sensory level. Half of the patients had CSF pleocytosis at presentation, and one third had an increased CSF protein concentration. Most of the early deaths (5 patients) occurred in the days before respiratory support methods were available, and were due to respiratory failure and pneumonia—all occurred before 1950. Of the patients who survived, roughly two thirds had a good or fair outcome and became ambulatory. Lipton and Teasdall (97) classified the outcomes as follows: 1) *good outcome:* normal gait, normal micturition or minimal urgency, and no or minimally abnormal neurologic signs; 2) *fair outcome:* functional and ambulatory but with an abnormal gait, urinary urgency, and persistent signs of spinal cord dysfunction; and 3) *poor outcome:* chair bound or bedridden, incontinent, and severe sensory deficits. Recovery can take many months, but most of the patients who were able to walk did so within 3 to 6 months. Patients who retained deep tendon reflexes and posterior column function were more likely to recover than were those who did not. Only 3 patients were treated with steroids (doses not reported), and so the efficacy of this therapy could not be evaluated. In the Danish study (98), of the 29 surviving patients who were followed for an average of 12 years, roughly one third each had a good, fair, or poor outcome. Patients with back pain and signs of spinal shock were particularly likely to have a poor outcome. It is interesting to note that only 1 patient (3%) of the 29 in this study eventually developed MS. Another study (104) evaluated 52 patients with acute transverse myelitis at the Massachusetts General Hospital. The investigators noted typically four types of initial symptoms of the disease: 1) bilateral lower

extremity paresthesias, 2) bilateral lower extremity weakness, 3) back pain, and 4) urinary retention, the latter being uncommon. Three distinct tempos of disease were discerned: 1) smoothly progressive over 2 weeks, 2) progressive in a slow or stuttering manner over 10 days to 4 weeks, and 3) explosive in onset. Patients with type 1 or 2 tended to have a fair to good outcome (as classified by Lipton and Teasdall (97)), whereas patients with an explosive onset, especially those with back pain (which may reflect the degree of swelling), had a poor outcome, with only 1 of 11 patients becoming ambulatory again. MS developed in 7 (13%) of the 52 patients, but the mode of onset and tempo could not be used to predict which patients these would be. The degree of pleocytosis and increase in CSF protein concentration were also not predictive of outcome. In a study (105) of incomplete acute transverse myelitis performed prospectively during 1985 to 1987 at the Montreal Neurological Institute, 15 patients with incomplete spinal cord involvement of at least one segment were evaluated and followed. Patients with identifiable causes were excluded, as were patients with complete quadriplegia or paraplegia or spinal shock. In this study, 12 patients (80%) progressed to clinically or laboratory-supported definite MS over an average follow-up time of 38.5 months. Of the patients with periventricular white matter abnormalities at onset, 93% were eventually diagnosed with definite MS. In a study of patients with isolated brainstem or spinal cord demyelinating lesions (106), evaluation included brain MRI as well as CSF examination, at onset. Of the 38 patients with a spinal cord syndrome (almost all of whom had an incomplete transverse myelopathy), 14 (42%) developed MS. The likelihood of progression to MS was strongest in those with disseminated involvement, as determined by MRI or clinical criteria or both (relative risk = 36), and with oligoclonal bands in the CSF (relative risk = 25). There appears to be a greater risk of progression to MS in patients with an incomplete transverse myelitis than in those with a complete transverse myelitis. Thus, an illness characterized by a fever, a depressed level of consciousness, and complete myelitis is unlikely to progress to MS (see below). This is especially likely to be true in patients with only a lesion in the spinal cord and none in the brain, as detected by MRI.

Pathology

The neuropathology of ADEM is that of a perivenular inflammatory myelinopathy. In ADEM, the brain is often grossly swollen, with macroscopic engorgement of veins in the white matter. Microscopically, there is perivascular edema with mononuclear infiltration, mostly with lymphocytes and macrophages (Fig 9-1). Plasma cells and granulocytes are rarely seen. There is proliferation of endothelial cells. The hallmark pathology is that of demyelination, with relative axonal sparing (Fig 9-2). This demyelination occurs around small veins. The pathology is uniform and appears to be independent of the particular inciting agent (107). This appearance is similar to that of EAE in animals (107).

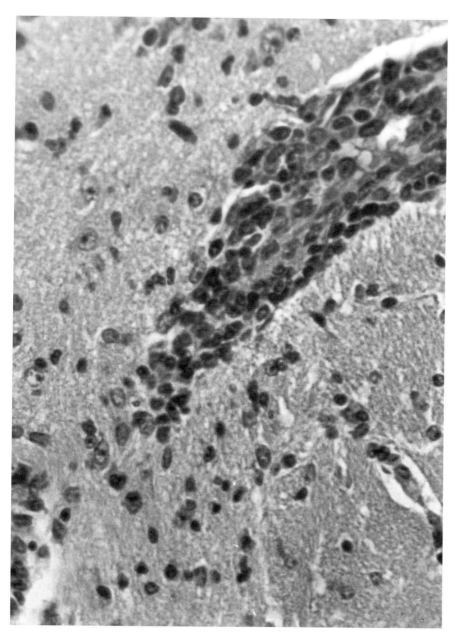

Figure 9-1. Acute disseminated encephalomyelitis. Perivascular edema with mononuclear infiltration, mostly with lymphocytes and macrophages, is seen.

EAE is a disease induced in animals by administration of neural tissue (and certain antigens) with adjuvant, as well as by passive administration of activated sensitized T cells and T-cell lines or clones (101,108). Rabies postvaccinal encephalomyelitis, which used to occur after the inoculation of attenuated (Pasteur and Fermi vaccines) or inactivated (Semple vaccine) rabies virus grown in neural tissue, is an example of EAE in humans (10). The Semple vaccine was replaced by the duck embryo rabies vaccine in the late 1950s, but this was also associated with neuroparalytic accidents, including transverse myelitis, although less commonly than with the earlier vaccines (109). The newer human diploid cell strain vaccine (HDCV), free of neural tissue, is not associated with rabies postvaccinal encephalomyelitis, although one case of a GBS-like syndrome after the administration of HDCV has been reported (110). EAE reportedly occurred in a laboratory worker as a result of a laboratory accident in which a mixture of complete Freund's adjuvant and guinea pig CNS tissue was inoculated via a broken test tube. Twenty-five days later, headache, fever, and a partial lateral rectus palsy developed, and there was a mild pleocytosis with a raised CSF protein concentration. The patient was

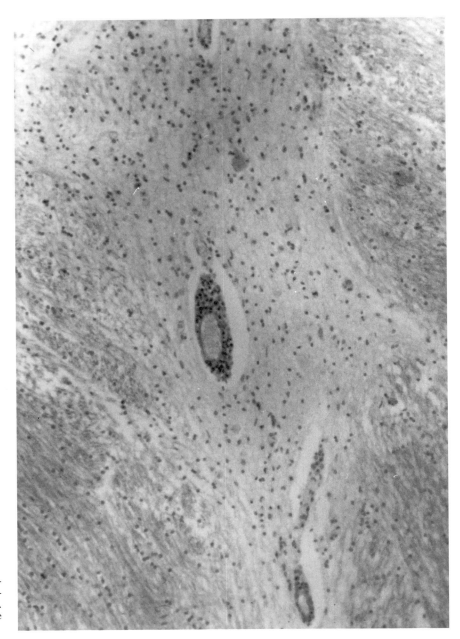

Figure 9-2. Experimental autoimmune encephalomyelitis. Demyelination is seen surrounding a small vein. Intact myelin can be seen at the three corners of the photomicrograph.

treated with corticosteroids and the illness resolved completely. Conversion from protein purified derivative (PPD) negative to PPD positive showed that the amount of Freund's adjuvant was enough to induce a delayed hypersensitivity cell-mediated immune reaction (111).

In AHLE the pathology is a continuation of that seen in ADEM. Macroscopically, the brain is swollen and distended; punctate hemorrhages and ringlike hemorrhagic lesions are seen grossly. Microscopically, there is fibrinoid necrosis and infiltration of the vessels with neutrophils and occasional eosinophils. There is exudation of serum proteins. Red blood cells and granulocytes are distributed around the vessels. Ring hemorrhages associated with venous thrombosis are seen. The pathology does not involve gray matter. The picture is identical to that of hyperacute EAE in animals (101,107) (Fig 9-3). Adams and Kubik (112) and Russell (99) pointed out the continuum between AHLE and ADEM, and Levine (101) demonstrated the continuum between EAE and hyperacute EAE.

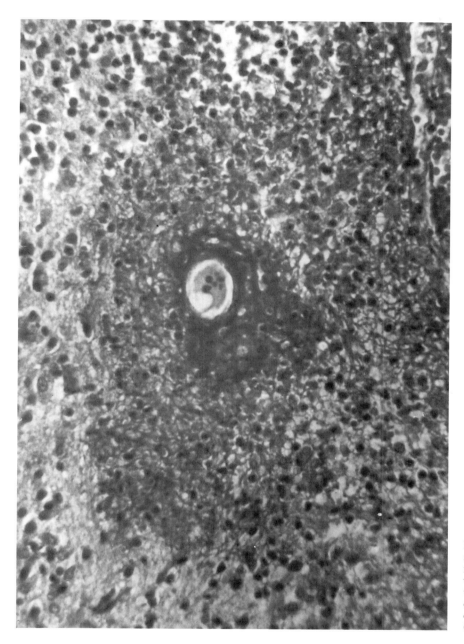

Figure 9-3. Hyperacute experimental autoimmune encephalomyelitis in a rat. A ring hemorrhage associated with venous thrombosis is seen surrounding the venule at the center of the photomicrograph. Red blood cells and granulocytes are distributed around the vessel. (Courtesy of Dr. Seymour Levine.)

Pathogenesis

This is most likely a T cell–mediated autoimmune disease directed against a myelin/oligodendrocyte antigen, probably MBP (113,114). The evidence for this is indirect. First, there is a strong similarity between ADEM and EAE, and between AHLE and hyperacute EAE, which are known to be T cell mediated, since the disease may be transferred to naive recipient animals by lymphocytes but not by serum (115). Second, in vitro studies of blood and CSF lymphocytes from ADEM patients demonstrate increased T-cell reactivity to MBP (113,114). Similar results have been reported for transverse myelopathy (116). However, MBP need not be the only relevant antigen. Proteolipid protein (PLP) and myelin-oligodendrocyte glycoprotein (MOG) would be other possibilities because they also induce EAE. However, no studies have been done to test T-cell reactivity to MBP, PLP, and MOG in the same ADEM patients. It may be pertinent to note that localized models of EAE, corresponding possibly to some of the focal demyelinating syndromes (e.g., optic neuritis and myelitis), have been studied (101). In these, EAE is induced in an animal after mechanical injury to focal areas of the brain. The resulting inflammatory demyelinating lesions localize at the site of the previous mechanical injury (101), and this may be a useful model of the focal forms of EAE.

The reason for the cell-mediated immune reaction directed against myelin is not known. Several possibilities are as follows.

One possible pathogenetic mechanism is that of "molecular mimicry," in which certain peptide, carbohydrate, or lipid epitopes on an infecting virus or other antigen are similar to epitopes on myelin (117,118). Other examples of molecular mimicry of possible pathogenetic significance include the cross-reactivity between *Campylobacter jejuni* and GQ_{1b} ganglioside in the Fisher-Miller variant of GBS (119); *C. jejuni* and GM_1 ganglioside in the acute motor axonal neuropathy variant of GBS (120,121); and some gram-negative bacteria and the α subunit of the acetylcholine receptor (AChR), and herpes simplex virus and the AChR α subunit, in myasthenia gravis (122,123). If cross-reactive T cells are exposed to this antigen, they will expand clonally. Activated cross-reactive T cells can cross the blood-brain barrier. They may then be retained in the CNS, where they could open up the blood-brain barrier and recruit other lymphocytes and macrophages, leading to inflammation and demyelination.

Another possible mechanism is that of viruses or other antigens nonspecifically activating T cells. Such activated T cells can cross the blood-brain barrier. If a nonspecific activated T cell does not find any recognizable epitopes, it will migrate out of the CNS, leaving no real trace of its passage. On the other hand, if the nonspecifically activated T cell happens to be one that recognizes an epitope in myelin, it will expand clonally and trigger the inflammatory reaction, as described already. Some microbial antigens act as "superantigens," which can activate broad classes of CD4+ T cells by binding simultaneously to the major histocompatibility complex (MHC) class II molecule of an antigen-presenting cell and to the V_β region of the T-cell receptor (TCR). Such a superantigen can therefore activate a very large fraction (up to 1 in 50) of the CD4+ T cells in the body. Some of these could be myelin reactive, and will find themselves in the brain, with the consequences discussed above (124).

A third possible pathogenic mechanism is that of inhibition of suppressor T cells. Some viral infections suppress certain types of CD4+ suppressor T cells. If any of these are myelin-specific suppressor cells, the removal of their influence by a virus (or other means) may result in the spontaneous activation of myelin-specific CD4+ T cells, and thence to CNS inflammation and demyelination as described already.

Another less likely possibility includes the direct infection of the oligodendrocytes or astrocytes, leading to an immune reaction. Unlike progressive multifocal leukoencephalopathy or subacute sclerosing panencephalitis, infection of these cells has never been demonstrated in ADEM. Finally, it is possible (though never demonstrated) that endothelial cells are infected, impairing the blood-brain barrier and allowing cells or humoral myelinotoxic factors into the brain, resulting in demyelinating lesions. However, this would not explain how killed microbial products in vaccines could induce ADEM or AHLE, although such vaccines may be compatible with a mechanism requiring systemic cytokine-induced alteration of endothelial cells.

A final possibility is that viral infection of certain cells in the brain induces the expression of MHC class II molecules, which along with viral antigen are necessary for the presentation of viral antigen to helper-inducer T lymphocytes. Some brain cells, such as astrocytes and microglia, can be induced to express MHC class II molecules and act as antigen-presenting cells. It is known that exposure of astrocytes to measles virus or the JHM strain of mouse coronavirus can induce MHC class II molecules. If such glial cells, primed to do so by a previous measles infection, present myelin antigens to T lymphocytes that would otherwise not be stimulated or activated, the stage would be set for an indirect virus-induced demyelination (125).

Some clues to the pathogenesis can be obtained from studies of postmeasles ADEM and post–rabies vaccination encephalomyelitis. In one study of measles patients in Peru (102), the proliferative responses of blood lymphocytes to MBP from patients with postmeasles ADEM were compared with those from patients with uncomplicated measles or with other neurologic diseases, and normal control subjects. The ADEM lymphocytes showed statistically significantly higher reactivity to MBP than did those from the other patient groups. Such T-cell responses were also seen in individual patients with post–rabies vaccination ADEM, postvaricella cerebellar ataxia, and seizures and stupor occurring after rubella (102). In no patient was there intrathecal synthesis of antimeasles antibody. In another study (126), the concentration of soluble CD8 (a measure of immune activation) was measured in CSF samples obtained from patients with postmeasles ADEM and compared with those of control groups with CNS infections and peripheral neuropathy. There was again a statistically significant increase in the levels of soluble CD8 in the CSF from postmeasles ADEM patients compared with those in the other groups. In another study, patients with ADEM after vaccination with Semple rabies vaccine were compared with vaccinated control subjects without neurologic disease and unvaccinated rabies patients (72). In this study, 3 (50%) of the 6 ADEM patients had lymphocytes showing proliferative responses to MBP. No lymphocytes from vaccinated control subjects had such responses. Lymphoproliferation was also seen in 40% (2/5) of unvaccinated rabies patients, however. The results of both of these studies are consistent with ADEM being a cell-mediated immune disease. However, it has not been proved that the cell-mediated immunity in human ADEM is a cause rather than an effect, unlike in EAE. Indeed, there may be a role for humoral immunity to play in ADEM. A study comparing patients who had major neurologic complications (mostly ADEM, and GBS in a few) after vaccination with Semple rabies vaccine with vaccinated control subjects (who did receive Semple rabies vaccine but who did not develop ADEM) found that the levels of serum and CSF antibodies to MBP were higher in the patients (both ADEM and GBS) than the control subjects (127). This is not unprecedented, as in some animal models of EAE, the superimposition of a humoral response on a cell-mediated response enhances the severity and demyelination of the resulting EAE, and some animal species may have involvement of both T- and B-cell responses in EAE (128).

All the viral infections and vaccines that have a proven link to ADEM involve enveloped viruses. The implications of this observation are unclear. However, the literature reports myelitis, along with some brainstem signs, occurring in a patient about 2 or 3 weeks after an episode of acute hepatitis A (a member of the picornaviruses, which are not enveloped) (129). Whether this myelitis occurred as a result of direct infection or postinfectious demyelination was not determinable from the case narrative. It is known that many picornaviruses are neurotropic. However, in many patients with ADEM following nonspecific upper respiratory tract infections or gastroenteritis, a special diagnosis of a virus is never made, and it is possible that adenoviruses and enteroviruses (both are not enveloped) may trigger ADEM. The "classic" triggering viruses, such as measles, cause illnesses that have very characteristic clinical presentations and findings, and are thus easy to diagnose. Since illnesses caused by enteroviruses and adenoviruses are nonspecific, there may be an ascertainment bias in favor of enveloped viruses. However, that said, there is still no well-documented case of a nonenveloped virus triggering ADEM.

Diagnosis

The diagnosis rests on a compatible clinical picture of an acute or subacute febrile neurologic illness, frequently with alterations in mental status, occurring following a nonspecific viral (or other) illness or immunization, along with characteristic findings. Therefore, it is often difficult to diagnose. There is no definitive laboratory test for ADEM or AHLE, short of biopsy. Usually there are no systemic findings in ADEM, while in AHLE there may be an acute-phase reaction, with a significantly increased erythrocyte sedimentation rate (ESR), increased C-reactive protein value, and proteinuria (1). Acute transverse myelitis, optic neuritis, and cerebellar ataxia also have a fairly rapid onset, with characteristic findings on examination, and each has a list of other possible diagnoses to be ruled out. In all cases, a mass lesion needs to be ruled out, because the alternative diagnoses of spinal cord compression and optic nerve compression are neurologic emergencies and demand immediate definitive therapy. Other con-

ditions that generally need to be considered include syphilis, acute viral infections, systemic collagen vascular disease, occasionally CNS vasculitis, and rarely vitamin B_{12} deficiency, all of which can affect both the optic nerve and the spinal cord simultaneously or sequentially. Devic's syndrome can be the presentation of ADEM.

Electroencephalography and Evoked Potentials

There are no specific changes on the EEG. The EEG usually shows nonspecific generalized slowing, often with high voltage, and asymmetry (130), and appears to correlate with disease activity. In a series of patients with acute transverse myelopathy (131), evoked potential testing showed abnormal somatosensory evoked potentials from peroneal but not from median nerve stimulation, as one would expect from disease in the thoracic region of the cord, which is the most commonly involved level. Other modalities, such as visual evoked potentials and brainstem auditory evoked potentials, were normal in patients with acute transverse myelitis (131). At the same center, 72% of MS patients had at least one abnormality in the battery of somatosensory, brainstem auditory, and visual evoked potentials (131). Thus, an evoked potential battery frequently showed at least one abnormality in MS patients while there were few or no abnormalities (other than somatosensory evoked potentials) in patients with acute transverse myelitis (131).

Cerebrospinal Fluid

The CSF findings are often abnormal in ADEM or AHLE but nonspecific. In ADEM, there is often a mild mononuclear pleocytosis, with a mild elevation in protein concentration, but the cell count and protein values are normal in approximately one third of patients (15). In one well-studied group of 18 patients with postmeasles ADEM, 8 (44%) patients had elevated CSF protein levels (although most of these were less than 100 mg/dL) and 13 (72%) had a lymphocytic pleocytosis (although most of these had less than 100 cells/µL) (102). There may be abnormalities of immunoglobulins and increased MBP (a nonspecific indicator of damage to myelin) in a subset of patients, but in a measles ADEM study only 1 of 12 patients had an increased CSF IgG index (102).

In AHLE, there is often a neutrophilic pleocytosis and erythrocytes in the CSF. The protein concentration is usually increased; in 25% of patients it is more than 200 mg/dL, with levels as high as 1000 mg/dL (38). In about 10% of reported patients with AHLE, the CSF is entirely normal (38). It should be noted that an illness of fever, encephalopathy, focal neurologic findings, pleocytosis, and red blood cells in the CSF is also compatible with acute herpes encephalitis.

In a series (97) of 30 patients with acute transverse myelitis, 14 had a normal CSF cell count and protein level. Ten patients had an elevated CSF protein concentration and 15 had pleocytosis. Determinations of CSF IgG concentration and IgG index in 16 patients showed elevations in 6 patients. Oligoclonal bands were found in 1 of 13 CSF samples tested for this abnormality. In another study (104) of 52 patients with transverse myelitis, 18 had pleocytosis of more than 4 cells, with 6 patients having between 200 and 300 white blood cells. All instances of pleocytosis resolved in 3 months. Furthermore, 18 of the patients had an increased CSF protein level (>50 mg/dL), with the highest level being 203 mg/dL. The CSF IgG was more than 12% of the protein in 6 of the 12 patients in which this was tested during the acute illness.

In optic neuritis, pleocytosis is not uncommon, being present in 8 of 21 patients with the isolated disease (90) in the Great Ormond Street study. In that series, only 5 of the 21 patients had an isolated increased CSF protein level, without pleocytosis. In 11 of the 21 patients, the CSF was entirely normal. In another study from Finland of patients with optic neuritis, most were found to have mild pleocytosis at onset, as well as oligoclonal bands and an increased IgG index. However, the numbers from that study were a little difficult to interpret because the series had an admixture of MS patients (92). Of 25 Swedish patients with isolated optic neuritis, 15 (60%) had mononuclear pleocytosis, 6 (24%) had an increased protein level, 6 (24%) had oligoclonal bands, and 4 (16%) had an elevated relative IgG index. The pleocytosis was never very great, with a maximum of 30 cells in one patient, and consisted mostly of lymphocytes. In another series of 48 Finnish patients (133) with optic neuritis, 24 (50%) had a white blood cell count of more than 5 cells/μL. In a recent study (134) of 457 optic neuritis patients, the CSF was examined in 83 patients. A pleocytosis of 6 cells/μL or higher was seen in 30 (36%) of the patients, but the highest count was 27 cells/μL. Oligoclonal bands were seen in 38 (50%) of the 76 patients in whom this was tested. Increased IgG synthesis rates were noted in 10 (43%) of the 23 patients tested, and IgG indexes were elevated in 10 (22%) of the 46 patients in whom this was tested. However, it is difficult to tell what biases might be present, because not all patients in this study had CSF testing.

Neuroimaging

Computed tomography (CT) scans of the brain may show hypodense white matter lesions, occasionally with mass effect, sometimes with enhancement (Fig 9-4). Often, the CT scans appear unremarkable in ADEM, and therefore are not very sensitive. In one series of 11 patients, 4 had normal-appearing brain CT scans, while 7 had abnormalities that included cortical enhancing lesions, lucencies in the deep white matter and basal ganglia, and edema of the brainstem (135). The initial brain CT scan often appeared normal, with abnormalities developing several days after the beginning of the clinical illness. The correlation between the CT abnormalities and clinical findings was limited (135). One pa-

tient with autopsy-confirmed ADEM had a large area of hypodensity in the white matter with no mass effect and no enhancement (136). In three patients with biopsy-proved AHLE, brain CT revealed white matter hypodensities, and enhancement in only one lesion in one patient (137). The results were similar in an autopsied subject: an area of nonenhancing white matter hypodensity, with mass effect, corresponding to the findings of edema with petechial hemorrhages and congested vessels (138). In one patient with a stuttering course of ADEM, the findings on serial brain CT paralleled the clinical state (139). This patient was a 7-year-old girl who developed spastic weakness in the right leg after an upper respiratory tract infection. She was treated with low-dose prednisone. About 6 weeks later, this weakness had resolved and was replaced by right upper extremity weakness. She improved over the next 2 weeks, but then bulbar weakness developed with increased lower extremity tone. Dramatic improvement occurred with prednisone, and symptoms did not recur after the prednisone dose was tapered over the next few months. At the time of each new deficit, brain CT showed enlargement of the old and the emergence of new lesions. The CT abnormalities had completely disappeared by the time of the follow-up examination, when the clinical deficits had completely resolved. In another report of two patients with AHLE, serial brain CT again showed findings that paralleled the patient's state (140).

MRI of the brain is a useful technique and shows multiple prominent white matter lesions, with increased signal on T2-weighted images (Figs 9-5A, 9-6) and proton density–weighted images (Fig 9-5B) and decreased signal on T1-weighted images (Fig 9-7), the latter often enhancing after administration of diethylenetriamine-pentaacetic acid gadolinium (see Fig 9-7) (141–143). The lesions as seen by MRI may vary in size, even in the same patient, and tend to be larger than the pathologic lesions, most likely due to surrounding edema (Fig 9-8). Hyperintense lesions on T2-weighted images (Fig 9-9) and enhancing lesions on T1-weighted images (Fig 9-10) can be quite small and diffuse. In two children with ADEM, both T1- and T2-weighted MRIs of the brain showed multiple white matter abnormalities (144). These tended to resolve with clinical improvement. It should be noted that the MRI appearances of both the brain (145) and the spinal cord (146) can be very similar in ADEM and MS. In acute transverse myelitis, the cord is often enlarged, sometimes with patchy areas of decreased signal on T1-weighted images (Fig 9-11) and increased signal on T2-weighted images (Fig 9-12), as well as diffuse or patchy areas of enhancement (Fig 9-13) (147,148). Cord enlargement can occur in the absence of increased signal on T2-weighted images (149). In one series of seven patients with acute transverse myelopathy (148), the degree of cord enlargement, persistence of increased signal intensity, and poor outcome were correlated. Cord atrophy and persisting increased signal in the cord on late MRIs suggested that further recovery was unlikely (148). The difficulty with this last series, however, is that two of these patients had sys-

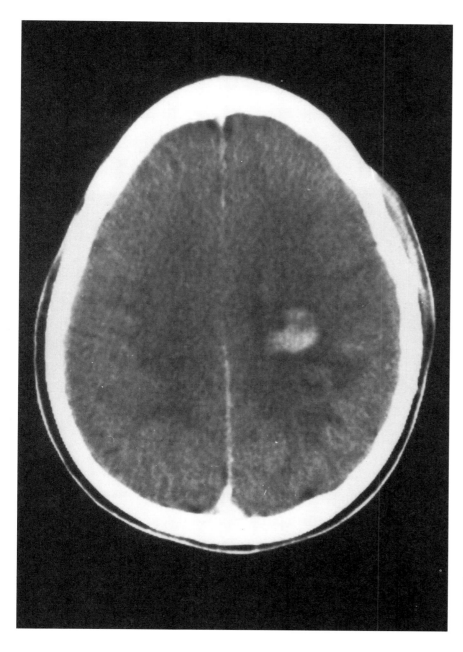

Figure 9-4. Computed tomography (CT) scan of acute disseminated encephalomyelitis showing enhancing lesion in the deep white matter of the left hemisphere.

temic lupus erythematosus, one had sarcoidosis, and one had giant-cell arteritis. Therefore, what the results of that study mean for acute transverse myelitis and ADEM are unclear. The MRI findings of two patients with ADEM (including spinal cord involvement) following *Mycoplasma pneumoniae* infection were reported (150). These showed scattered multifocal lesions of the white matter during a work-up of acute neurologic symptoms that followed *M. pneumoniae*–associated upper respiratory tract illnesses (150). In one of the pa-

tients, who was quadriplegic and ventilator dependent, MRI showed an atrophic cervical region of the cord late in the illness, as well as scattered lesions in the cerebral white matter.

Therapy

There have been no clinical trials of any proposed therapies for this disease, and so there is no proven specific therapy. Symptomatic and supportive therapy is im-

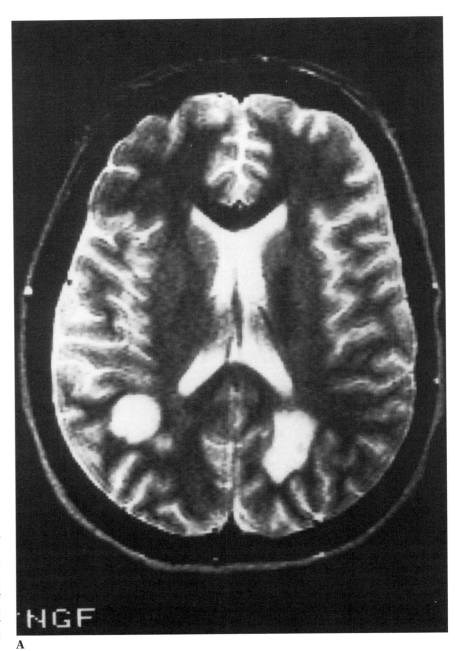

Figure 9-5. (A) T2-weighted MRI of the brain showing bilateral areas of increased intensity in white matter of the occipital lobe on the left and parietal lobe on the right. (B) Proton density–weighted image showing areas of abnormally increased signal in the brainstem (thick arrow), the cerebellar vermis bilaterally (asterisks), and left cerebellar hemisphere (double arrows). **A**

portant, as many patients will recover meaningful function if they survive the acute illness. Clearly, reduction of a malignant fever, maintenance of vital functions (including intubation for respiratory or bulbar compromise) and fluid and electrolyte balance, nutrition, avoidance of decubiti and urinary tract infections, and treatment of seizures are important. Treatment of cerebral edema (by hyperventilation and the use of osmotic agents) is important if there is a threat of herniation of brain matter from one intracranial compartment to

another, especially if vital brainstem centers are involved. Rehabilitation and physical therapy are important in the recovery phase.

Corticosteroids

The rationale for the use of corticosteroids is that they decrease edema, reduce inflammation, and restore the blood-brain barrier (thus reducing the diffusion of plasma proteins and immigration of additional activated

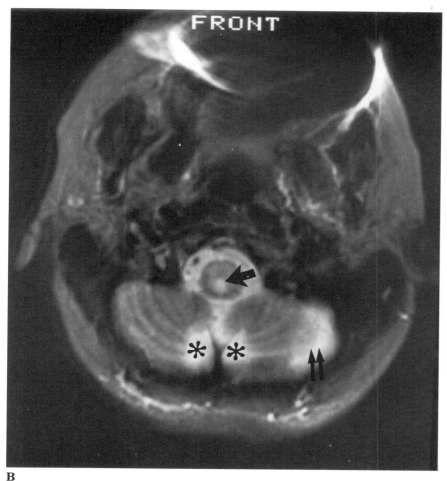

B

Figure 9-5. *Continued*

immune cells into the brain). Many neurologists treat patients with pulse doses of intravenous corticosteroids and then discharge them on a schedule to taper the oral prednisone doses (1). Very good responses have been reported (151), but these remain anecdotal. In a few patients improvement was seen during the administration of corticosteroids, with worsening occurring when the drugs were discontinued and improvement occurring when the drugs were reinstituted, which suggests strongly that corticosteroids do have a genuine effect (130). Patients with AHLE may also respond to corticosteroids (38). However, it is important to be aware that no studies have been done formally to show efficacy.

Plasmapheresis

A few reports on the use of plasmapheresis for ADEM described dramatic recovery in some patients (152–155). However, some of these patients (152) were simultaneously treated with other immunosuppressive therapies, such as corticosteroids and cyclophospha-

mide. In two patients, there appeared to be improvement with plasmapheresis after there was no immediate response to high-dose corticosteroids (156). It is possible that the response ascribed to the plasmapheresis might have been a delayed response to the corticosteroids or spontaneous improvement. Furthermore, a series of six patients who had fulminant MS relapses, confirmed by biopsy, and who were unresponsive to high-dose intravenous methylprednisolone improved dramatically after one or two courses of plasmapheresis (157). Again, the same caveat applies. The rationale for plasmapheresis appears to be that it has efficacy in GBS, an acute or subacute demyelinating disease of the peripheral nervous system, and that a circulating factor may have some role in its pathogenesis (153,158). On the other hand, GBS and ADEM are different diseases. In GBS, humorally mediated mechanisms are likely to be at least as important as cell-mediated ones, whereas ADEM is likely mostly cell mediated. Therefore, one would not expect a treatment targeted at one disease to necessarily work for the other. Given some of the reported improvements, plasmapheresis is reasonable to

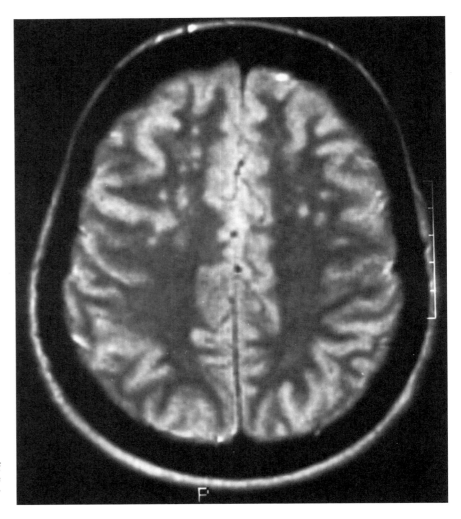

Figure 9-6. Multiple small areas of abnormally increased signal in the white matter of the frontal lobe bilaterally, in a T2-weighted image.

try when more conventional therapy with corticosteroids fails, recognizing that improvement is not proof of efficacy.

Other Modalities

Multiple other treatments have been tried at one time or another. A patient with progressive gait difficulty, fever, somnolence, and anorexia with onset a week after a nonspecific viral syndrome was treated with intravenous immunoglobulin at a dose of 400 mg/kg for 5 days and showed clear clinical improvement with 24 hours. MRI showed the typical white matter lesions (159). There was virtually complete resolution of his clinical deficits 6 days after the intravenous immunoglobulin was started. The MRI abnormalities also resolved 6 months later.

Another patient developed increasing headache and white matter abnormalities on MRI after a bout of viral meningitis. CSF analysis demonstrated pleocytosis and the EEG was abnormal. He had intermittent episodes of delirium and psychosis. The response to dexamethasone (Decadron) was remarkable, and the dose was tapered. Several weeks later, he had a relapse, which responded to methylprednisolone. Further relapses were accompanied by increasing MRI white matter abnormalities, and responded to corticosteroids. One episode consisted of a mass lesion, the biopsy of which revealed demyelination. He was then started on intravenous immunoglobulin, 400 mg/kg every month, and had no further episodes for the next 6 months (160).

A patient with apparent ADEM characterized by progressive spastic paraparesis, ataxia, and dysarthria over 5 months (161) had a mild-to-moderate pleocytosis with increased protein, MBP, and IgG values as well as five oligoclonal bands in the CSF. He was treated with high-dose prednisone, without response. He was then put on polyinosinic-polycytidylic acid-polylysine stabilized with carboxymethylcellulose (poly ICLC) and the prednisone dose was tapered. His improvement was remarkable. Poly ICLC is a potent interferon inducer and probably has immunomodulating effects, but the nature of

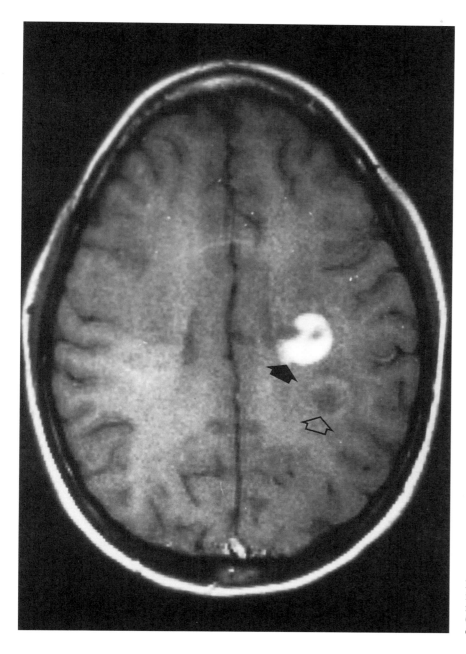

Figure 9-7. T1-weighted image showing an area of enhancement (closed arrow) and an area of decreased intensity (open arrow) in a patient with acute disseminated encephalomyelitis.

these is unclear. Furthermore, the nature of this patient's illness is not completely clear, as the presentation was rather atypical.

In another report (162), three patients with ADEM were treated with copolymer-1, which had previously been shown to prevent or improve EAE, and all three had a complete recovery within 3 weeks, although this would not be unexpected, given the natural history of the disease.

There is no way to fully evaluate these therapeutic modalities short of a controlled clinical trial.

Relationship of Acute Disseminated Encephalomyelitis and Restricted Syndromes to Multiple Sclerosis

The isolated syndromes of acute optic neuritis, transverse myelitis, and acute cerebellar ataxia, which can occur in association with or following a viral illness or vaccination, and in which there is inflammatory white matter involvement, have an uncertain relation to ADEM (1). Some of these syndromes are clearly manifestations of other autoimmune diseases, and some new

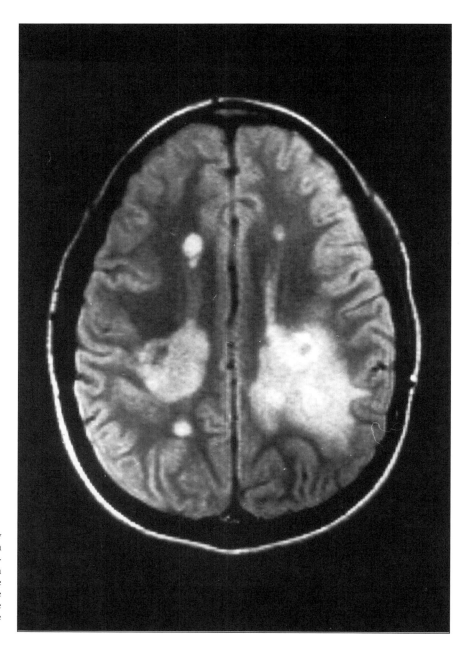

Figure 9-8. The lesions of MRI may vary in size and tend to be larger than the pathologic lesions, most likely because of the surrounding edema as seen in the areas of increased signal on the proton density–weighted image. Note the penetration of the edema along the white matter tracts, especially in the left hemisphere.

associations have been described recently. In two patients, recurrent episodes of acute optic neuritis and transverse myelitis, responsive to corticosteroids, occurred for years. Their illnesses were believed to be consistent with MS, until high antinuclear antibody (ANA) titers developed in both and multiorgan disease in one, years after the onset of the neurologic symptoms (163). However, a coincidence of two diseases was not ruled out and patients with MS may have elevated ANA titers (164,165). Another patient with long-standing ulcerative colitis developed transverse myelitis. Work-up showed a lesion in the cervical region of the spinal cord

and smaller lesions in the brain. She was thought to have MS until dermatomyositis and fibrosing alveolitis developed; the Jo-1 serum antibody titer was positive (166). The occurrence of more than one immunopathologic disorder in an individual patient is always a possibility. Indeed there is abundant evidence for such concordance in the literature (167).

The relation of the various forms of ADEM (including isolated demyelinative syndromes not otherwise linked with systemic autoimmune disease) to MS is unknown. It is clear that some patients with ADEM eventually develop MS, but the proportion is not known

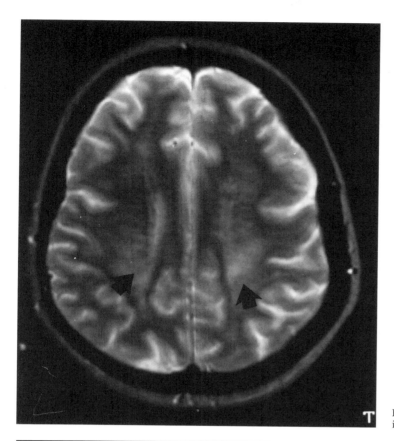

Figure 9-9. Hyperintense lesions on T2-weighted images can be quite small and diffuse (arrows).

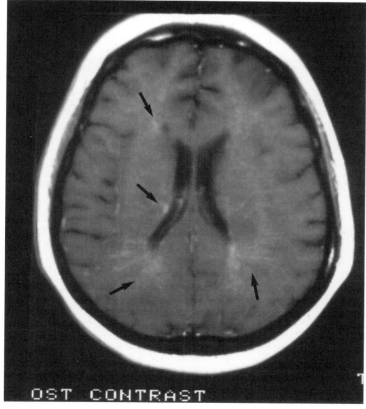

Figure 9-10. Enhancing lesions on T1-weighted images can be quite small and diffuse (arrows).

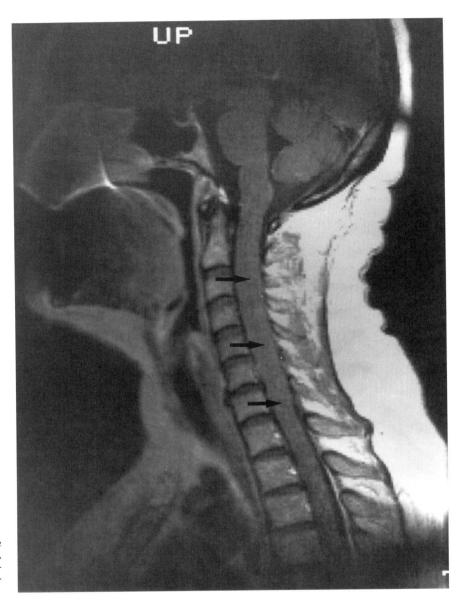

Figure 9-11. In acute transverse myelitis, the cord is often enlarged, sometimes with patchy areas of decreased signal (arrows), as on this T1-weighted image.

exactly. In one study, roughly one fourth of 29 patients with acute disseminated encephalomyelitis went on to develop MS (168). However, this study was done in Denmark, where the prevalence of MS is extremely high, and so it is difficult to generalize this result to other populations. In a series of 27 (of 34) surviving patients with ADEM, acute transverse myelitis, and neuromyelitis optica, MS had not developed by follow-up, over an average of several years, although there were a few recurrences reproducing the original illness (169). The experimental disease induced by inoculating animals with myelin or myelin antigens, EAE, is an excellent model of ADEM. Recurrent or chronic EAE seems to be a reasonable model of MS.

Because optic neuritis is not rare, determining the re-

lation of acute optic neuritis to subsequent MS takes on importance. In the Mayo Clinic study discussed previously (91), the patients with isolated optic neuritis were analyzed using life-table methods to find the risk for progression to MS. Of these patients, 39% had progressed to definite MS by 10 years of follow-up, 49% by 20 years, 54% by 30 years, and 60% by 40 years. Venous sheathing as seen on ophthalmoscopy and recurrent optic neuritis were risk factors for progression. Because CSF examinations were not done, the effect of the presence of oligoclonal bands on the risk of progression to MS could not be examined. Furthermore, brain MRI was not performed, and therefore the relative risk of progression to MS in those with abnormal-appearing MRIs also could not be determined.

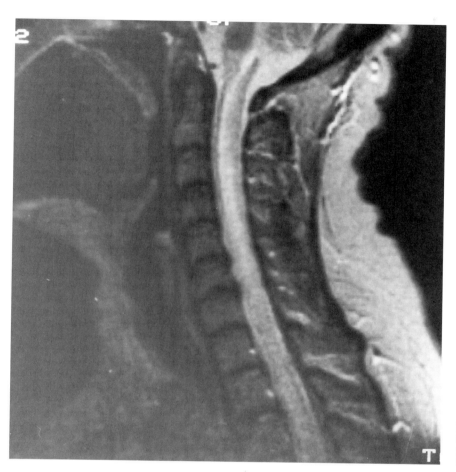

Figure 9-12. In a patient with acute transverse myelitis, T2-weighted MRIs may show patchy and diffuse areas of increased signal.

A recent study examined how three regimens affected visual function of a cohort of patients with acute optic neuritis (170). The regimens were intravenous methylprednisolone followed by tapered doses of oral prednisone, a course of tapered doses of oral prednisone, and placebo designed to resemble the oral prednisone course. Patients were included if they showed signs of optic neuritis but had none of the systemic diseases associated with optic neuritis (such as syphilis or lupus erythematosus), although patients with MS were admitted to the study. The oral prednisone and placebo groups were double blinded, but the intravenous methylprednisolone group was only single blinded. The intravenous methylprednisolone group had the least number of relapses, while the oral prednisone group had the most. In a post hoc analysis (171), after patients with a diagnosis of MS at the time of randomization were excluded, the progression of the different groups to clinically definite MS was examined. The intravenous methylprednisolone group had the lowest rate of progression to MS. The entire cohort was stratified according to the lesion burden seen on cranial MRI, and those with the highest lesion burden had the greatest risk of progression to MS. When the intravenous methyl-

prednisolone group was stratified according to the MRI lesion burden, the subgroup with the highest risk of progression had the most reduction in this risk. In the isolated optic neuritis subgroup, the MRI lesion burden was most predictive of progression to MS, with possibly a separate independent contribution to the risk of progression from the presence of oligoclonal bands (134).

It is possible that the apparent efficacy was only a reflection of the study design. It may reflect the ineffectiveness of the single-blind design (172) in masking who the intravenous methylprednisolone–treated patients were from the study physicians. It is possible that placebo effects, which are known to be strong in MS, were sufficiently different in the intravenous methylprednisolone group to account for some of the effect (172). However, a real effect of the methylprednisolone on the evolution of the disease may also be occurring. A possible mechanism of such a long-term effect is as follows. In EAE, the range of epitopes on the MBP molecule recognized by T cells increases during the course of disease. Initially, only one or a very small number of epitopes is recognized by T cells. As an attack of the disease progresses, more and more epitopes on the MBP molecule are recognized. Also, TCR gene usage to the myelin

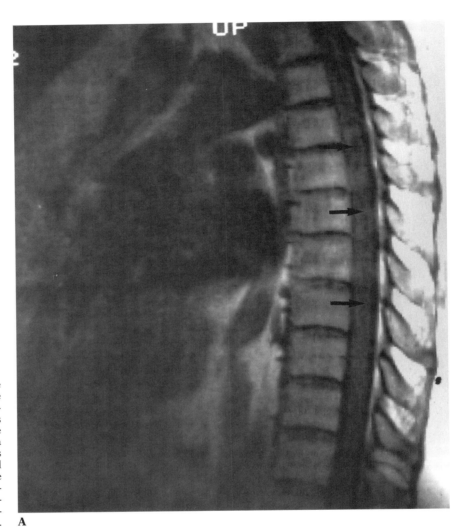

Figure 9-13. Enhancement of the spinal cord in a patient with acute transverse myelitis on T1-weighted images may be diffuse or patchy. (A) This precontrast T1-weighted image of the thoracic region of the spinal cord in a patient with transverse myelitis shows areas of patchy diffuse decreased signal (arrows). (B) This postcontrast image of the same cord shows diffuse enhancement (arrows). Note how the enhancement effaces the patchy abnormalities seen on the noncontrast image. **A**

antigen broadens during the course of the disease, giving an increasing number of distinct TCR molecules reacting to a specific epitope on MBP (and possibly PLP and MOG). There is some evidence that similar dynamics take place in MS (173–177). It is therefore possible that intravenous methylprednisolone had some effect in restricting the progressive broadening of the T-cell response (intra-antigen or interantigen determinant or epitope spreading), and therefore in inhibiting or delaying the subsequent waves of immune reactivity against other myelin antigens and epitopes, which would express clinically as attacks of MS (173,174). In EAE, clonotypic therapy started within the first 3 days can prevent or cure the disease (174). For optic neuritis in humans, all this is speculative, and if the phenomenon of delay of MS is real, other effects of corticosteroids, such as effects on vascular endothelial cell activation (e.g., expression of intercellular adhesion molecules such as ICAM-1 and ICAM-2), need to be evaluated. A trial needs to be carried out to look specif-

ically at the development of MS following treatment with intravenous methylprednisolone for isolated syndromes such as optic neuritis, brainstem events such as internuclear ophthalmoplegia, and myelitis (172).

Another study (178) examined the question of the relation of isolated demyelinative syndromes to the subsequent development of MS. This 5-year follow-up study examined what features (specifically, number of lesions on brain MRI, presence of CSF oligoclonal bands, and HLA haplotype) present at the onset of an isolated optic nerve, brainstem, or spinal cord lesion were predictive of subsequent MS. The predictors, in order from strongest to weakest, were abnormal-appearing brain MRI, the presence of oligoclonal bands in the CSF, and the presence of the HLA-DR2 haplotype. There was a dose-response effect on the risk conferred by an abnormal MRI: Of those with more than four lesions on MRI, 28 (85%) of 33 patients went on to develop clinically definite MS, whereas only 1 (17%) of 6 with a single lesion and only 2 (6%) of 32 with no lesions

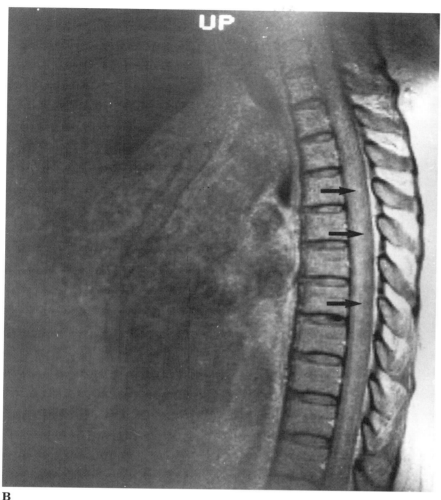

B

Figure 9-13. *Continued*

developed MS during the period of observation. In the three clinical groups, for patients with abnormal-appearing MRIs, those presenting with optic neuritis had the highest risk, and those with isolated spinal cord syndrome, the lowest risk of developing MS. The overall risk ratio (RR) of an abnormal MRI versus a normal MRI was 38. The RR for the presence versus the absence of CSF oligoclonal bands was 5.2 and that for the presence versus the absence of HLA-DR2 was 3.2. While most study results suggest that MRI is the most useful predictor, there have been studies suggesting that oligoclonal bands may be at least as useful (179). The reason for this difference is unclear. The magnetic field strength of the MRI apparatus used in the study by Sandberg-Wollheim et al (179) was 0.3 T, while that used by Morrissey et al (178) was 0.5 T, which may account in part for the discrepancy, since the latter field strength would be somewhat more sensitive and reveal more lesions.

A variant of optic neuritis is bilateral simultaneous optic neuritis. Since 1984, when a study at the Institute of Neurology at Queen Square was conducted, it has been thought that bilateral simultaneous optic neuritis led to MS only rarely in children and uncommonly in adults (180). In that study MS developed in only 2 of 11 adults with simultaneous bilateral optic neuritis, whereas it developed in 8 of 20 with sequential optic neuritis (180). The children were followed for an average of 32 years while the adults were followed for an average of 37 years. A recent follow-up United Kingdom study of bilateral simultaneous optic neuritis analyzed 23 patients (181). The entry criterion was acute (< 14 days from onset to peak) or subacute (14–120 days from onset to peak) visual loss that occurred in both eyes simultaneously, defined as visual loss occurring in the two eyes within 2 weeks of each other. All patients had clinical assessments, brain MRI, HLA typing, and mitochondrial DNA analysis, and 50% had CSF electrophoresis. MS had developed in only 5 patients (22%) by the time of follow-up. MS had not developed in most patients 61% after a mean follow-up of 50 months after the onset of bilateral simultaneous optic neuritis. These latter patients were found to have low rates of risk factors for the subsequent development of MS, such as multiple white matter abnormalities on brain MRI, HLA-DR15/DQw6 haplotype, and the presence of oligoclonal bands. Of interest is that 4 (17%) of the patients with bilateral simultaneous optic neuritis were found to have mitochondrial DNA point mutations indicating Leber's hereditary optic neuropathy. This study concluded that a lower proportion of patients with bilateral simultaneous optic neuritis than with acute unilateral optic neuritis proceed to develop MS. A significant proportion (20% of patients in the United Kingdom study (181)) of patients with bilateral simultaneous optic neuritis have Leber's hereditary optic neuropathy.

As noted already, patients with transverse myelopathy do not seem to develop MS. In the Danish study discussed, of the 29 surviving patients who were followed for an average of 12 years (98), MS developed in only 1 (3%). In the Massachusetts General Hospital study (104), MS developed in 7 (13%) of the 52 patients with acute transverse myelitis. On the other hand, in the Montreal Neurological Institute study (105), 12 (80%) of 15 patients progressed to clinically or laboratory-supported definite MS over an average follow-up of 38.5 months. In the Queen Square study of patients with isolated brainstem or spinal cord demyelinating lesions (106), MS developed in 14 (42%) of 38 patients with transverse myelopathy. The reasons for the discrepancy among these studies are not completely clear, but may have to do with whether the study was prospective or retrospective, with whether the transverse myelitis was complete (with total loss of neurologic function below the affected level) or incomplete, and with differing criteria for MS and follow-up times. Thus, some studies used both clinical and MRI criteria for MS (105,106) whereas others used only clinical criteria (98). Patients with complete transverse myelitis seem to be less likely to progress to MS.

Recurrent and Relapsing Acute Disseminated Encephalomyelitis

Rare recurrent illness has been described for both ADEM (182–184) and AHLE (185). Recurrent acute transverse myelitis has also been reported (185,186). Some points of differentiation between recurrent ADEM and MS, which may resemble each other very closely, include the following. ADEM begins rather abruptly, evolving in an obvious way over several hours or possibly days, whereas an MS exacerbation tends to take longer, although this difference is not absolute. Also, episodes of ADEM tend to be febrile and cause prominent changes in mental status (delirium, confusion, disorientation), whereas MS relapses are afebrile and usually consist of focal neurologic deficits. Finally, recurrences of ADEM usually mimic the first episode. Of course, patients with multiple recurrences of ADEM without delirium or changes in the level of consciousness may be difficult to distinguish from patients with clinically restricted MS.

Acute Disseminated Encephalomyelitis with Mass Lesions

An unusual variant of demyelinating disease, with large demyelinating lesions having mass effect that can be confused with tumors, has been reported (187,188). The diagnosis of tumor was made initially in several such patients, on the basis of imaging and biopsy, and unnecessary therapy with high-dose radiation and chemotherapy agents was given, with rather poor results (188). In about 10% of patients in one study of a total of 31 such patients, the lesions recurred after 9 months to 12 years (187) (Fig 9-14). In 7 of these patients, the lesions were multifocal. Interestingly, 3 patients had systemic malignancies. In 11 patients, the symptoms resolved after treatment with corticosteroids. The disease tends to have a sudden onset, and followed an influenza vaccination in 1 patient. Since there was an abrupt onset, a good response to steroids, and unlikely recurrence, the disease resembled ADEM. It is not clear whether this is a distinct form of demyelinating disease, distinguished by having lesions with a mass effect, or whether it is a form of ADEM. Indeed, mass lesions mimicking neoplasms can also occur with AHLE. In two patients with well-documented AHLE, the entire clinical courses were 6 weeks and 3 months. Instead of an abrupt onset, the patients had a steadily progressive course, with cerebral CT scans showing multiple mass lesions that were diagnosed as tumors (189). The correct diagnosis was made when tissue was obtained at surgery. The disease in some of these patients is reminiscent of an entity known as *myelinoclastic diffuse sclerosis* (the label given to a well-defined subset of patients previously given the vague diagnosis of Schilder's disease) (190,191). The diagnostic criteria for this entity are 1) at least one large, discrete, bilateral, myelin-destroying, axon-sparing ("myelinoclastic") lesion in the centrum semiovale; 2) no other lesions demonstrable in the CNS (by clinical, paraclinical, and imaging methods); 3) normal peripheral nerve, adrenal, and peroxisomal (very-long-chain fatty acids) function; and 4) a histology typical of MS (190). Patients identified to have myelinoclastic diffuse sclerosis have had apparently dramatic responses to corticosteroid therapy and in one patient, to cyclophosphamide (191). A 40-year-old woman showed some response to pulsed methylprednisolone (192).

Acute Toxic Encephalopathy

A small number of reports have described an acute postviral illness that resembles ADEM in some respects but in which only cerebral edema is found at autopsy, with no inflammatory infiltrates (such as are found in ADEM) (191). Some patients, particularly following varicella and influenza B infections (86,193), had concomitant liver failure, and this was recognized as a dis-

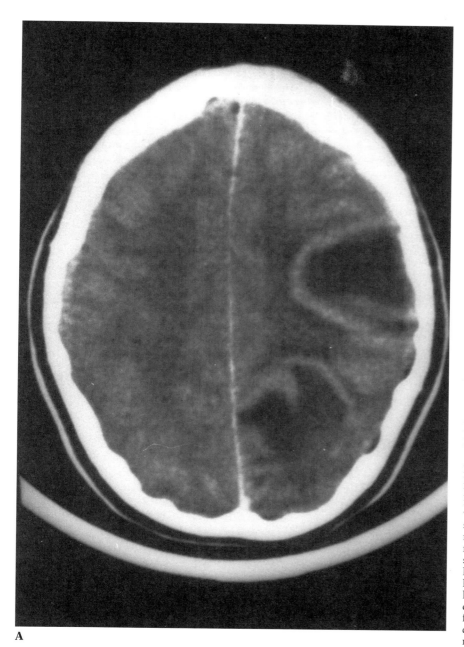

A

Figure 9-14. (A) CT of the brain of a 13-year-old girl with a one-month history of difficulty with speech and clumsiness of the right hand. A biopsy was incorrectly read as a grade III astrocytoma. (B) CT for the same patient, performed after treatment with two courses of chemotherapy using "8 in 1 protocol" (eight drugs—cyclophosphamide, vincristine, cisplatin, methylprednisolone, carmustine, hydroxyurea, procarbazine, and cytarabine—all taken in a 24-hour period) followed two weeks later by radiation therapy for six weeks. The patient had complete resolution of her motor deficits, and returned to school. (C) CT for the same patient, performed four-and-a-half years later after a return of right-handed clumsiness progressing to right hemiparesis. A repeat biopsy showed demyelination. Review of the slides from the previous biopsy also showed demyelination and no evidence of tumor.

tinct postviral syndrome: Reye's syndrome (193,194). Other such syndromes have been seen without liver disease, and seem to occur in children younger than 2 or 3 years (70,195), a population group in which ADEM is rare (70,195,196). However, many of these patients (195) had multiple confounding factors such as prolonged febrile seizures, aspiration pneumonia, and anoxic encephalopathy, and it is unclear whether a truly unique clinicopathologic entity of parainfectious noninflammatory encephalopathy exists, other than Reye's syndrome. Most notorious of these toxic encephalopathies are those purported to occur after pertussis vaccination (197). A review of the studies linking pertussis vaccination to toxic encephalopathies with residual neurologic damage showed that the evidence is at best inconclusive, with such cases being very rare (198). However, there is a slight association of acute encephalopathy with pertussis vaccination, but this is

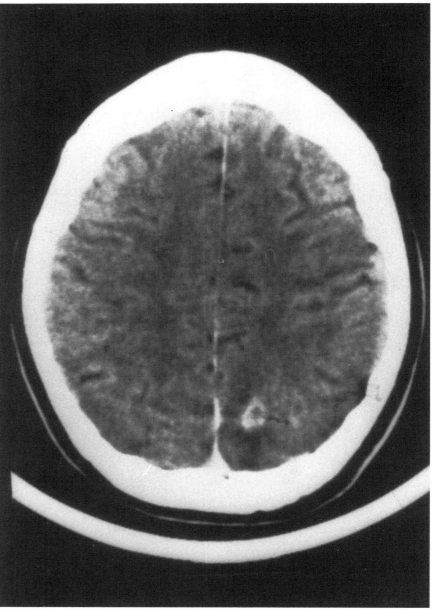

Figure 9-14. *Continued*   **B**

nonspecific: It occurs when febrile seizures occur, developmental delays begin, other diseases are common, or other confounders are present. In some of these patients, pathologic changes are noted in the cerebral microvasculature, and include perivascular edema and lymphocytic infiltrates, fibrinoid necrosis, endothelial proliferation, and neutrophilic and eosinophilic infiltrates in the vascular wall. This vasculopathy was believed to be out of proportion to demyelination, and has been asserted to be an independently existing disease

entity. The pathogenesis of this is unclear, but the direct vascular damage suggests that it is mediated possibly by immune complexes (196,199).

A possible example of such an immune complex–mediated encephalopathy, characterized by a postdiarrheal biphasic illness with fever, rash, seizures, very high ESR (150 mm/hr), positive ANA titer (1:320), and MRI showing more gray than white matter involvement, reportedly occurred in patients who had had *C. jejuni* enteritis (200). A brain biopsy specimen showed

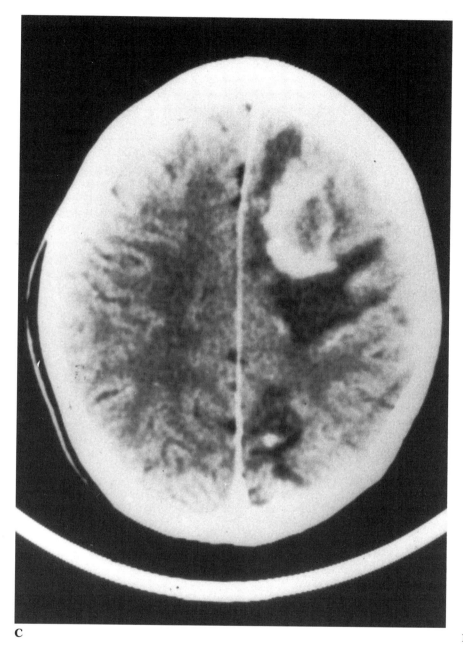

C

Figure 9-14. *Continued*

gliosis and a vasculopathy characterized by scattered lymphocytes and lipid-laden perivascular macrophages. The patient, who had baseline cerebral palsy, responded dramatically to high-dose intravenous methylprednisolone, with resolution of seizures and a return of the ESR and ANA to normal values. Another example is an acute transverse myelopathy that occurred after a febrile upper respiratory tract infection and progressed to a spastic quadriparesis and bilateral optic neuropathy (201). The patient became dependent on a respirator and died 18 months later. Autopsy showed diffuse demyelination in the cerebral hemispheres with occasional perivascular and interstitial mononuclear infiltrates, and necrosis of the cervical and upper thoracic regions of the spinal cord. Scattered areas of vasculitis were seen and deposits of immunoglobulins and complement components were found in blood vessel walls. No viral inclusions were noted and the results of a previous work-up for collagen vascular disease were negative. This appears to be an immune complex–mediated encephalopathy with deposition of immune complexes (and complement) in the cerebral vasculature, leading to inflammatory demyelination.

The clinical picture of acute toxic encephalopathy is by no means unique, and may be seen in any child with prolonged febrile seizures, hypoxia, and metabolic disturbance (195). Furthermore, the pathologic changes are often nonspecific, and many of them are compatible with an agonal state (195). Some of the pathologic changes are variations of normal in the immature brain of a young child. Thus, small vessels in children are often more cellular than those in adults, giving rise to an incorrect impression of endothelial proliferation (195). The existence, therefore, of a separate clinicopathologic entity of acute toxic encephalopathy is still controversial.

Future Directions

Three major issues remain to be resolved: 1) the best therapy for acute disseminated encephalomyelitis, 2) the pathogenesis of the disease, and 3) the relation of a single demyelinative episode to the risk of subsequently developing MS. We have only partial answers. The definitive answers will be difficult to obtain because this is an uncommon disease and in everyday practice is likely underdiagnosed. The first issue, that of the most efficacious therapy, requires a multicenter clinical trial that would need to be sustained for several years. There is a precedent, however, in the multicenter trials for herpes encephalitis, another relatively uncommon disease (202). The pathogenesis of the disease can continue to be explored by investigating the animal model EAE. More direct and clinically relevant clues can be sought by obtaining immune cells from both blood and CSF of patients with the disease and examining the TCR gene usage and state of activation. Finally, the risk of subsequent development of MS after a single demyelinative episode can only be determined by further longitudinal follow-up of such patients.

References

1. Lisak R. Immune-mediated parainfectious encephalomyelitis. In: McKendall R, Stroop W, eds. *Handbook of neurovirology.* New York: Dekker, 1994:173–186.
2. Tselis A, Lisak R. Acute disseminated encephalomyelitis and isolated central nervous system demyelinative syndromes. *Curr Opin Neurol* 1995;8:227–229.
3. Cohen JA, Lisak R. Acute disseminated encephalomyelitis. In: Aarli JA, Behan WMH, Behan PO, eds. *Clinical neuroimmunology.* Oxford: Blackwell Scientific, 1987:192–213.
4. Johnson RT, Griffin DE. Postinfectious encephalomyelitis. In: Kennedy PGE, Johnson RT, eds. *Infections of the nervous system.* New York: Butterworths, 1987: 209–226.
5. Croft PB. Parainfectious and postvaccinal encephalomyelitis. *Postgrad Med J* 1969;45:392–400.
6. Gendelman HE, Wolinsky JS, Johnson RT, et al. Measles encephalomyelitis: lack of evidence of viral invasion of the central nervous system and quantitative study of the nature of demyelination. *Ann Neurol* 1984;15:353–360.
7. Fenichel GM. Neurological complications of immunization. *Ann Neurol* 1982;12:119–128.
8. Spillane JD, Wells CEC. The neurology of Jennerian vaccination. A clinical account of the neurological complications which occurred during the smallpox epidemic in South Wales in 1962. *Brain* 1964;87:1–44.
9. Applebaum E, Greenberg M, Nelson J. Neurological complications following antirabies vaccination. *JAMA* 1953;151:188–191.
10. Shiraki H, Otani S. Clinical and pathological features of rabies post-vaccinal encephalomyelitis in man. Relationship to multiple sclerosis and to experimental "allergic" encephalomyelitis in animals. In: Kies MW, Alvord EC, eds. *Allergic encephalomyelitis.* Springfield, IL: Charles C Thomas, 1959:58–136.
11. Reik L Jr, Smith L, Khan A, Nelson W. Demyelinating encephalopathy in Lyme disease. *Neurology* 1985;35: 267–269.
12. Fernandez CV, Bortolussi R, Gordon K, et al. *Mycoplasma pneumoniae* infection associated with central nervous system complications. *J Child Neurol* 1993;8:27–31.
13. Fisher RS, Clark AW, Wolinsky JS, et al. Postinfectious leukoencephalitis complicating *Mycoplasma pneumoniae* infection. *Arch Neurol* 1983;40:109–113.
14. Decaux G, Szyper M, Ectors M, et al. Central nervous system complications of *Mycoplasma pneumoniae. J Neurol Neurosurg Psychiatry* 1980;43:883–887.
15. Miller HG, Stanton JB, Gibbons JL. Para-infectious encephalomyelitis and related syndromes. A critical review of the neurological complications of certain specific fevers. *Q J Med* 1956;25:427–505.
16. Schlenska GK. Unusual neurological complications following tetanus toxoid administration. *J Neurol* 1977; 215:299–302.
17. Means ED, Barron KD, Van Dyne BJ. Nervous system lesions after sting by yellow jacket. A case report. *Neurology* 1973;23:881–890.
18. Fisher JH, Gilmour JR. Encephalomyelitis following administration of sulphanilamide. *Lancet* 1939;2:301–305.
19. Marsh K. Streptomycin-PAS hypersensitivity treated with ACTH. *Lancet* 1952;2:606–608.
20. Russell DS. Changes in the central nervous system following arsphenamine medication. *J Pathol Bacteriol* 1937;45:357–366.
21. Cohen M, Day CP, Day JL. Acute disseminated encephalomyelitis as a complication of treatment with gold. *BMJ* 1985;290:1170–1180.
22. Williams HW, Chafee FH. Demyelinating encephalomyelitis in a case of tetanus treated with antitoxin. *N Engl J Med* 1961;264:489–491.
23. Kopp N, Groslambert R, Pasquier B, et al. Leucoencephalite aigue hemorrhagique au cours d'une tuberculose. *Rev Neurol (Paris)* 1978;134:313–323.
24. Shakir RA, Al-Din ASN, Araj GF, et al. Clinical categories of neurobrucellosis. *Brain* 1987;110:213–223.
25. Seitelberger F. Autoimmunologic aspects of cerebral diseases. *Pathol Eur* 1967;2:233–256.
26. Kinoshita A, Hayashi M, Miyamoto K, et al. Inflammation demyelination radiculitis in a patient with acute disseminated encephalitis (ADEM). *J Neurol Neurosurg Psychiatry* 1996;60:87–90.
27. Nadkarni N, Lisak RP. Guillain-Barré syndrome (GBS) with bilateral optic neuritis and central white matter disease. *Neurology* 1993;43:842–843.
28. Kazarian EL, Gager WE. Optic neuritis complicating measles, mumps and rubella vaccination. *Am J Ophthalmol* 1978;86:544–547.
29. Whittle E, Roberton NRC. Transverse myelitis after

diphtheria, tetanus, and polio immunisation. *BMJ* 1977; 2:1450.

30. McCarthy JT, Amer J. Postvaricella acute transverse myelitis: a case presentation and review of the literature. *Pediatrics* 1978;62:202–204.

31. Yoshizawa T, Tsukuda A, Maki Y, Kanazawa I. Transverse myelitis associated with *Mycoplasma pneumoniae* infections. *Eur Neurol* 1982;21:48–51.

32. Chusid MJ, Williamson SJ, Murphy JV, Ramey LS. Neuromyelitis optica (Devic disease) following varicella infection. *J Pediatr* 1979;95:737–738.

33. Kline LB, Margulies SL, Oh SJ. Optic neuritis and myelitis following rubella vaccination. *Arch Neurol* 1982;39:443–444.

34. Schechter SL. Lyme disease with associated optic neuropathy. *Am J Med* 1986;81:143–145.

35. Jacobson DM, Marx JJ, Dlesk A. Frequency and clinical significance of Lyme seropositivity in patients with isolated optic neuritis. *Neurology* 1991;41:706–711.

36. Miller HG, Stanton JB. Neurological sequelae of prophylactic inoculation. *Q J Med* 1954;23:1–27.

37. Hurst EW. Acute hemorrhagic leukoencephalitis: a previously undefined entity. *Med J Aust* 1947;2:1.

38. Byers RK. Acute hemorrhagic leukoencephalitis: report of 3 cases and a review of the literature. *Pediatrics* 1975;56:727–735.

39. Bray PF, Culp KW, McFarlin DE, et al. Demyelinating disease after neurologically complicated primary Epstein-Barr virus infection. *Neurology* 1992;42:278–282.

40. Paskavitz JF, Anderson CA, Filley CM, et al. Acute arcuate fiber demyelinating encephalopathy following Epstein-Barr virus infection. *Ann Neurol* 1995;38:127–131.

41. Gray F, Chimelli L, Mohr M, et al. Fulminating multiple sclerosis-like leukoencephalopathy revealing human immunodeficiency virus infection. *Neurology* 1991;41:105–109.

42. Jones HR, Ho DD, Forgacs P, et al. Acute fulminating fatal leukoencephalopathy as the only manifestation of human immunodeficiency virus infection. *Ann Neurol* 1988;23:519–522.

43. von Giesen H-J, Arendt G, Neuen-Jacob E, et al. A pathologically distinct new form of HIV associated encephalopathy. *J Neurol Sci* 1994;121:215–221.

44. Robertson WB, Cruickshank EK. Jamaican (tropical) myeloneuropathy. In: Minckler J, ed. *Pathology of the nervous system.* New York: McGraw-Hill, 1972.

45. Vernant JC, Maurs L, Gessain A, et al. Endemic tropical spastic paraparesis associated with human lymphotropic virus type I: a clinical and seroepidemiological study of 25 cases. *Ann Neurol* 1987;21:123–130.

46. Osame M, Matsumoto M, Usuku K, et al. Chronic progressive myelopathy with elevated antibodies to human lymphotropic virus type I and adult T-cell leukemia-like cells. *Ann Neurol* 1987;21:117–122.

47. McKendall RR. HTLV-I diseases. In: McKendall R, Stroop W, eds, *Handbook of neurovirology.* New York: Dekker, 1994:737–772.

48. Kliehues P, Lang W, Burger PC. Progressive diffuse leukoencephalopathy in patients with acquired immune deficiency syndrome (AIDS). *Acta Neuropathol (Berl)* 1985;68:333–339.

49. Budka H. Human immunodeficiency virus (HIV)-induced disease of the central nervous system: pathology and implications for pathogenesis. *Acta Neuropathol (Berl)* 1989;77:225–236.

50. Power C, Kong PA, Crawford TO, et al. Cerebral white matter changes in acquired immunodeficiency syndrome dementia: alterations of the blood-brain barrier. *Ann Neurol* 1993;34:339–350.

51. Swoveland PT, Johnson KP. Subacute sclerosing panencephalitis and other paramyxovirus infections. In: McKendall RR, ed. *Handbook of clinical neurology.* Vol. 12. *Viral diseases.* Amsterdam: Elsevier Science, 1989: 412–437.

52. Townsend JJ, Baringer JR, Wolinsky JS, et al. Progressive rubella panencephalitis. Late onset after congenital rubella. *N Engl J Med* 1975;292:990–993.

53. Townsend JJ, Wolinsky JS, Baringer JR. The neuropathology of progressive rubella panencephalitis of late onset. *Brain* 1976;99:81–90.

54. Major EO, Amemiya K, Tornatore CS, et al. Pathogenesis and molecular biology of progressive multifocal leukoencephalopathy, the JC virus-induced demyelinating disease of the human brain. *Clin Microbiol Rev* 1992;5:49–73.

55. Ryder JW, Croen K, Kleinschmidt-DeMasters BK, et al. Progressive encephalitis three months after resolution of cutaneous zoster in a patient with AIDS. *Ann Neurol* 1986;19:182–188.

56. Amlie-Lefond C, Kleinschmidt-DeMasters B, Mahalingam R, et al. The vasculopathy of varicella-zoster virus encephalitis. *Ann Neurol* 1995;37:784–790.

57. Gray F, Belec L, Lescs MC, et al. Varicella-zoster virus infection of the central nervous system in the acquired immune deficiency syndrome. *Brain* 1994;117:987–999.

58. Knox KK, Carrigan DR. Active human herpesvirus (HHV-6) infection of the central nervous system in patients with AIDS. *J Acquir Immune Defic Hum Retrovirol* 1995;9:69–73.

59. Challoner PB, Smith KT, Parker JD, et al. Plaque-associated expression of human herpesvirus 6 in multiple sclerosis. *Proc Natl Acad Sci USA* 1995;92:7440–7444.

60. Weller RO. Animal models of demyelinating disease. *Curr Opin Neurol Neurosurg* 1991;4:221–226.

61. Fazakerley JK, Buchmeier MJ. Virus-induced demyelination. In: Martenson RE, ed. *Myelin: biology and chemistry.* Boca Raton, FL: CRC Press, 1992:893–932.

62. Lipton HL. Theiler's virus infection in mice: an unusual biphasic disease process leading to demyelination. *Infect Immun* 1975;11:1147–1155.

63. Kastrukoff LF, Lau AS, Kim SU. Multifocal CNS demyelination following peripheral inoculation with herpes simplex virus type 1. *Ann Neurol* 1987;22:52–59.

64. Lavi E, Weiss SR. Coronaviruses. In: Gilden DH, Lipton HL, eds. *Clinical and molecular aspects of neurotropic virus infection.* Developments in medical virology series. Norwell, MA: Kluwer Academic, 1989:101–139.

65. Dal Canto M, Rabinowitz S. Experimental models of virus-induced demyelination of the central nervous system. *Ann Neurol* 1982;11:109–127.

66. Georgsson G. Neuropathologic aspects of lentiviral infections. *Ann NY Acad Sci* 1994;724:50–67.

67. Koenig H, Rabinowitz SG, Day E, Miller VT. Post-infectious encephalomyelitis after successful treatment of herpes simplex encephalitis with adenine arabinoside. Ultrastructural observations. *N Engl J Med* 1979;300: 1089–1093.

68. Toro G, Vergara I, Roman G. Neuroparalytic accidents of antirabies vaccination with suckling mouse brain vaccine. *Arch Neurol* 1977;34:694–700.

69. Nelson DA, Berry RG. Fatal rabies associated with extensive demyelination. *Arch Neurol* 1993;50:317–322.

70. McNair Scott TF. Postinfectious and vaccinal encephalitis. *Med Clin North Am* 1967;51:701–717.

71. Kennard C, Swash M. Acute viral encephalitis. Its diagnosis and outcome. *Brain* 1981;104:129–148.

72. Hemachudha T, Phanuphak P, Johnson RT, et al. Neurologic complications of Semple-type rabies vaccine: clinical and immunological studies. *Neurology* 1987;37:550–556.

73. Warren WB. Encephalopathy due to influenza vaccine. *Arch Intern Med* 1956;97:803–805.

74. Woods CA, Ellison GW. Encephalopathy following influenza immunization. *J Pediatr* 1964;65:745–748.

75. Rosenberg GA. Meningoencephalitis following an influenza vaccination. *N Engl J Med* 1970;283:1209.

76. Yahr MD, Lobo-Antunes J. Relapsing encephalomyelitis following the use of influenza vaccine. *Arch Neurol* 1972;27:182–183.

77. Gross WL, Ravens KG, Hansen HW. Meningoencephalitis syndrome following influenza vaccination. *J Neurol* 1978;217:219–222.

78. Saito H, Endo M, Takase S, Itahara K. Acute disseminated encephalomyelitis after influenza vaccination. *Arch Neurol* 1980;37:564–566.

79. Cherington C. Locked-in syndrome after "swine flu" vaccination. *Arch Neurol* 1977;34:258.

80. Kaplanski G, Retornaz F, Durand JM, Soubeyrand J. Central nervous system demyelination after vaccination against hepatitis B and HLA haplotype. *J Neurol Neurosurg Psychiatry* 1995;58:758–759.

81. Trevisani F, Gattinari GC, Caraceni P, et al. Transverse myelitis following hepatitis B vaccination. *J Hepatol* 1993;19:317–318.

82. Ohtaki E, Murakami Y, Komori H, et al. Acute disseminated encephalomyelitis after Japanese B encephalitis vaccination. *Pediatr Neurol* 1992;8:137–139.

83. Ohtaki E, Matsuishi T, Hirano Y, Maekawa K. Acute disseminated encephalomyelitis after treatment with Japanese B encephalitis vaccine (Nakayama-Yoken and Beijing strains). *J Neurol Neurosurg Psychiatry* 1995;59:316–317.

84. Hanninen P, Arstila P, Lang H, et al. Involvement of the central nervous system in acute uncomplicated measles virus infection. *J Clin Microbiol* 1980;11:610–613.

85. Gautier-Smith PC. The neurological complications of glandular fever (infectious mononucleosis). *Brain* 1965;88:323–334.

86. Griffith JF, Salam MV, Adams RD. The nervous system diseases associated with varicella. A critical commentary with additional notes on the syndrome of acute encephalopathy and fatty hepatosis. *Acta Neurol Scand* 1970;46:279–300.

87. Gibbs FA, Gibbs EL, Carpenter PR, Spies HW. Electroencephalographic abnormality in "uncomplicated" childhood diseases. *JAMA* 1959;171:1050–1055.

88. Ojala A. On changes in the cerebrospinal fluid during measles. *Ann Med Int Fenn* 1947;36:321–331.

89. Weir AI, Bone I, Kennedy DH. Neurological involvement in legionellosis. *J Neurol Neurosurg Psychiatry* 1982;45:603–608.

90. Kriss A, Francis DA, Cuendet F, et al. Recovery after optic neuritis in childhood. *J Neurol Neurosurg Psychiatry* 1988;51:603–608.

91. Rodriguez M, Siva A, Cross SA, et al. Optic neuritis: a population-based study in Olmsted County, Minnesota. *Neurology* 1995;45:1253–1258.

92. Riikonen R, Donner M, Erkkila H. Optic neuritis in children and its relationship to multiple sclerosis: a clinical study of 21 children. *Dev Med Child Neurol* 1988;30:349–359.

93. Gieron-Korthals MA, Westberry KR, Emmanuel PJ. Acute childhood ataxia: 10-year experience. *J Child Neurol* 1995;9:381–384.

94. Bergen D, Grossman H. Acute cerebellar ataxia of childhood associated with infectious mononucleosis. *J Pediatr* 1975;87:833–834.

95. Cleary TG, Henle W, Pickering LK. Acute cerebellar ataxia associated with Epstein-Barr virus infection. *JAMA* 1980;243:148–149.

96. Berman M, Feldman S, Alter M, et al. Acute transverse myelitis: incidence and etiologic considerations. *Neurology* 1981;31:966–971.

97. Lipton HL, Teasdall RD. Acute transverse myelopathy in adults. A follow-up study. *Arch Neurol* 1973;28:252–257.

98. Christensen PB, Wermuth L, Hinge HH, Bomers K. Clinical course and long-term prognosis of acute transverse myelitis. *Acta Neurol Scand* 1990;81:431–435.

99. Russell DS. The nosological unity of acute haemorrhagic leucoencephalitis and acute disseminated encephalomyelitis. *Brain* 1955;78:369–376.

100. Dangond F, Lacomis D, Schwartz RB, et al. Acute disseminated encephalomyelitis progressing to hemorrhagic encephalitis. *Neurology* 1991;41:1697–1698.

101. Levine S. Hyperacute, neutrophilic and localized forms of experimental allergic encephalomyelitis: a review. *Acta Neuropathol (Berl)* 1974;28:179–189.

102. Johnson RT, Griffin DE, Hirsch RJ, et al. Measles encephalomyelitis—clinical and immunologic studies. *N Engl J Med* 1984;310:137–141.

103. Donovan MK, Lenn NJ. Postinfectious encephalomyelitis with localized basal ganglia involvement. *Pediatr Neurol* 1989;5:311–313.

104. Ropper AH, Poskanzer DC. The prognosis of acute and subacute traumatic myelopathy based on early signs and symptoms. *Ann Neurol* 1978;4:51–59.

105. Ford B, Tampieri D, Francis G. Long-term follow-up of acute transverse myelopathy. *Neurology* 1992;42:250–252.

106. Miller DH, Ormerod IEC, Rudge P, et al. The early risk of multiple sclerosis following isolated acute syndromes of the brainstem and spinal cord. *Ann Neurol* 1989;26:635–639.

107. Hart MN, Earle KM. Haemorrhagic and perivenous encephalitis: a clinical-pathological review of 38 cases. *J Neurol Neurosurg Psychiatry* 1975;38:585–591.

108. Rivers TM, Schwentker FF. Encephalomyelitis accompanied by myelin destruction experimentally produced in monkeys. *J Exp Med* 1935;61:689–702.

109. Label LS, Batts DH. Transverse myelitis caused by duck embryo rabies vaccine. *Arch Neurol* 1982;39:426–430.

110. Bernard KW, Smith PW, Kader FJ, Moran MJ. Neuroparalytic illness and human diploid cell rabies vaccine. *JAMA* 1982;248:3136–3138.

111. Drachman DA, Paterson P, Bornstein MB. Experimental allergic encephalomyelitis in man: a laboratory accident. *Neurology* 1974;24:364.

112. Adams RD, Kubik CS. The morbid anatomy of the demyelinative diseases. *Am J Med* 1952;12:510–546.

113. Lisak RP, Behan PO, Zweiman B, Shetty T. Cell-mediated immunity to myelin basic protein in acute disseminated encephalomyelitis. *Neurology* 1974;24:560–564.

114. Lisak RP, Zweiman B. In vitro cell-mediated immunity of cerebrospinal fluid lymphocytes to myelin basic protein in primary demyelinating diseases. *N Engl J Med* 1977;297:850–853.

115. Paterson PY. Transfer of allergic encephalomyelitis in rats by means of lymph node cells. *J Exp Med* 1960;111:119–136.

116. Abramsky O, Teitelbaum D. The autoimmune features

of acute transverse myelopathy. *Ann Neurol* 1977;2: 36–40.

117. Jahnke U, Fischer EH, Alvord EC Jr. Sequence homology between certain viral proteins and proteins related to encephalomyelitis and neuritis. *Science* 1985;229: 282–284.

118. Fujinami RS, Oldstone MBA. Amino acid homology between the encephalitogenic site of myelin basic protein and virus: mechanism for autoimmunity. *Science* 1985;230:1043–1045.

119. Jacobs BC, Endtz HP, van der Meche FGA, et al. Serun anti-GQ$_{1b}$ IgG antibodies recognize surface epitopes on *Campylobacter jejuni* from patients with Miller-Fisher syndrome. *N Engl J Med* 1995;37:260–264.

120. Oomes PG, Jacobs BC, Hazenberg MPH, et al. Anti-GM1 IgG antibodies and *Campylobacter* bacteria in Guillain-Barré syndrome: evidence of molecular mimicry. *Ann Neurol* 1995;38:170–175.

121. Rees JH, Gregson NA, Hughes RAC. Anti-ganglioside GM1 antibodies in Guillain-Barré syndrome and their relationship to *Campylobacter jejuni* infection. *Ann Neurol* 1995;38:809–816.

122. Stefansson K, Dieperink ME, Richman DP, et al. Sharing of antigenic determinants between the nicotinic acetylcholine receptor and proteins in *Escherichia coli, Proteus vulgaris*, and *Klebsiella pneumoniae*: possible role in the pathogenesis of myasthenia gravis. *N Engl J Med* 1985;312:221–225.

123. Schwimmbeck PL, Dyrberg T, Drachman DB, Oldstone MBA. Molecular mimicry and myasthenia gravis: an autoantigenic site of the acetylcholine receptor α subunit that has biologic activity and reacts immunochemically with herpes simplex virus. *J Clin Invest* 1989;84: 1174–1180.

124. Burns J, Littlefield K, Gill J, Trotter JL. Bacterial toxin superantigens activate human T lymphocytes reactive with myelin antigens. *Ann Neurol* 1992;32:352–357.

125. ter Meulen V. Virus-induced, cell-mediated autoimmunity. In: Notkins AL, Oldstone MBA, eds. *Concepts in viral pathogenesis*. Vol. III. New York: Springer-Verlag, 1989:297–303.

126. Griffin DE, Ward BJ, Jauregui E, et al. Immune activation in measles. *N Engl J Med* 1989;320:1667–1672.

127. Hemachudha T, Griffin DE, Giffels JJ, et al. Myelin basic protein as an encephalitogen in encephalitis and polyneuritis following rabies vaccinations. *N Engl J Med* 1987;316:369–374.

128. Alvord EC Jr, Rose LM, Richards TL. Chronic experimental allergic encephalomyelitis as a model of multiple sclerosis. In: Martenson RE, ed. *Myelin: biology and chemistry*. Boca Raton, FL: CRC Press, 1992:849–891.

129. Tyler KL, Gross RA, Cascino GD. Unusual viral causes of transverse myelitis: hepatitis A virus and cytomegalovirus. *Neurology* 1986;36:855–858.

130. Ziegler DK. Acute disseminated encephalomyelitis. Some therapeutic and diagnostic considerations. *Arch Neurol* 1966;14:476–488.

131. Ropper AH, Miett T, Chiappa KH. Absence of evoked potential abnormalities in acute transverse myelopathy. *Neurology* 1982;32:80–82.

132. Sandberg M, Bynke H. Cerebrospinal fluid in 25 cases of optic neuritis. *Acta Neurol Scand* 1973;49:443–452.

133. Nikoskelainen E, Frey H, Salmi A. Prognosis of optic neuritis with special reference to cerebrospinal fluid immunoglobulins and measles virus antibodies. *Ann Neurol* 1981;9:545–550.

134. Rolak LA, Beck RW, Paty DW, et al. Cerebrospinal fluid

in acute optic neuritis: experience of the optic neuritis treatment trial. *Neurology* 1996;46:368–372.

135. Lukes SA, Norman D. Computed tomography in acute disseminated encephalomyelitis. *Ann Neurol* 1983;13: 567–572.

136. Loizou LA, Cole G. Acute cerebral demyelination: clinical and pathological correlation with computed tomography. *J Neurol Neurosurg Psychiatry* 1982;45:725–728.

137. Valentine AR, Kendall BE, Harding BN. Computed tomography in acute haemorrhagic leukoencephalitis. *Neuroradiology* 1982;22:215–219.

138. Watson RT, Ballinger WE, Quisling RG. Acute hemorrhagic leukoencephalitis: diagnosis by computed tomography. *Ann Neurol* 1984;15:611–612.

139. Walker RWH, Gawler J. Serial cerebral CT abnormalities in relapsing acute disseminated encephalomyelitis. *J Neurol Neurosurg Psychiatry* 1989;52:1100–1102.

140. Sucherowsky O, Sweeney VP, Berry K, Bratty PJA. Acute hemorrhagic leukoencephalopathy. A clinical, pathological and radiological correlation. *Can J Neurol Sci* 1983;10:63–67.

141. Epperson LW, Whittaker J, Kapila A. Cranial MRI in acute disseminated encephalomyelitis. *Neurology* 1988; 38:332–333.

142. Caldemeyer KS, Harris TM, Smith RR, Edwards MK. Gadolinium enhancement in acute disseminated encephalomyelitis. *J Comput Assist Tomogr* 1991;15: 673–675.

143. Atlas SW, Grossman RI, Golberg HI, et al. MR diagnosis of acute disseminated encephalomyelitis. *J Comput Assist Tomogr* 1986;10:798–801.

144. Perdue Z, Bale JF Jr, Dunn VK, Bell WE. Magnetic resonance imaging in childhood disseminated encephalomyelitis. *Pediatr Neurol* 1985;1:370–374.

145. Kesselring J, Miller DH, Robb SA, et al. Acute disseminated encephalomyelitis. MRI findings and the distinction from multiple sclerosis. *Brain* 1990;113:291–302.

146. Sze G. MR imaging of the spinal cord: current status and future advances. *AJR* 1992;159:149–159.

147. Sanders KA, Khandji AG, Mohr JP. Gadolinium-MRI in acute transverse myelopathy. *Neurology* 1990;40: 1614–1616.

148. Holtas S, Basibuyuk N, Fredriksson K. MRI in acute transverse myelopathy. *Neuroradiology* 1993;35:221–226.

149. Merine D, Wang U, Kumar A, et al. CT myelography and MR imaging of acute transverse myelitis. *J Comput Assist Tomogr* 1987;11:606–608.

150. Francis DA, Brown A, Miller DH, et al. MRI appearances of the CNS manifestations of *Mycoplasma pneumoniae*: a report of two cases. *J Neurol* 1988;235:441–443.

151. Pasternak JF, Devivo DC, Prensky AL. Steroid-responsive encephalomyelitis in childhood. *Neurology* 1980;30:481–486.

152. Seales D, Greer M. Acute hemorrhagic leukoencephalitis: a successful recovery. *Arch Neurol* 1991;48: 1086–1088.

153. Stricker RB, Miller RG, Kiprov DD. Role of plasmapheresis in acute disseminated (postinfectious) encephalomyelitis. *J Clin Apheresis* 1992;7:173–179.

154. Newton R. Plasma exchange in acute post-infectious demyelination. *Dev Med Child Neurol* 1981;23:538–543.

155. Cotter FE, Bainbridge D, Newland AC. Neurological deficit associated with *Mycoplasma pneumoniae* reversed by plasma exchange. *BMJ* 1983;286:22.

156. Kanter DS, Horensky D, Sperling RA, et al. Plasmapheresis in fulminant acute disseminated encephalomyelitis. *Neurology* 1995;45:824–827.

157. Rodriguez M, Karnes WE, Bartleson JD, Pineda AA.

Plasmapheresis in acute episodes of fulminant CNS inflammatory demyelination. *Neurology* 1993;43:1100–1104.

158. Guillain-Barré Study Group. Plasmapheresis and acute Guillain-Barré syndrome. *Neurology* 1985;35:1096–1104.

159. Kleiman M, Brunquell P. Acute disseminated encephalomyelitis: response to intravenous immunoglobulin? *J Child Neurol* 1995;10:481–483.

160. Hahn JS, Siegler DJ, Enzmann D. Intravenous gammaglobulin therapy in recurrent acute disseminated encephalomyelitis. *Neurology* 1996;46:1173–1174.

161. Salazar AM, Engel WK, Levy HB. Poly ICLC in the treatment of postinfectious demyelinating encephalomyelitis. *Arch Neurol* 1981;38:382–383.

162. Abramsky O, Teitelbaum D, Arnon R. Effect of a synthetic polypeptide (cop-1) on patients with multiple sclerosis and with acute disseminated encephalomyelitis. *J Neurol Sci* 1977;31:433–438.

163. Kira J, Goto I. Recurrent opticomyelitis associated with anti-DNA antibody. *J Neurol Neurosurg Psychiatry* 1994;57:1124–1125.

164. Dore-Duffy P, Donaldson JO, Rothman BL, Zurier RB. Antinuclear antibodies in multiple sclerosis. *Arch Neurol* 1982;39:504–506.

165. Barned S, Goodman AD, Mattson DH. Frequency of antinuclear antibodies in multiple sclerosis. *Neurology* 1995;45:384–385.

166. Ray DW, Bridger J, Hawnar J, et al. Transverse myelitis as the presentation of Jo-1 antibody syndrome (myositis and fibrosing alveolitis) in long-standing ulcerative colitis. *Br J Rheumatol* 1994;32:1105–1108.

167. Seyfert S, Klapps P, Meisel C, et al. Multiple sclerosis and other autoimmune diseases. *Acta Neurol Scand* 1990;81:37–42.

168. Thygesen P. Prognosis in initial stage of disseminated primary demyelinating disease of the central nervous system. *Arch Psychiatr Neurol* 1949;61:339–351.

169. Miller HG, Evans MJ. Prognosis in acute disseminated encephalomyelitis; with a note on neuromyelitis optica. *Q J Med* 1953;22:347–379.

170. Optic Neuritis Study Group. A randomized, controlled trial of corticosteroids in the treatment of optic neuritis. *N Engl J Med* 1992;326:581–588.

171. Optic Neuritis Study Group. The effect of corticosteroids for acute optic neuritis on the subsequent development of multiple sclerosis. *N Engl J Med* 1993;329:1764–1769.

172. Silberberg DH. Corticosteroids and optic neuritis. *N Engl J Med* 1992;326:1808–1810.

173. Lehmann PV, Sercarz EE, Forsthuber T, et al. Determinant spreading and the dynamics of the autoimmune T-cell repertoire. *Immunol Today* 1993;14:203–208.

174. Lehmann PV, Forsthuber T, Miller A, Sercarz EE. Spreading of T-cell autoimmunity to cryptic determinants of an autoantigen. *Nature* 1992;358:155–157.

175. Mor F, Cohen IR. Shifts in the epitopes of myelin basic protein recognized by Lewis rat T cells before, during and after the induction of experimental allergic encephalomyelitis. *J Clin Invest* 1993;92:2199–2206.

176. Cross AH, Tuohy VK, Raine CS. Development of reactivity to new myelin antigens during chronic relapsing autoimmune demyelination. *Cell Immunol* 1993;146:261–265.

177. Sun D, Le J, Yang S, et al. Major role of antigen-presenting cells in the response of rat encephalitogenic T cells to myelin basic proteins. *J Immunol* 1993;151:111–118.

178. Morrissey SP, Miller DH, Kendall BE, et al. The signifi-

179. Sandberg-Wollheim M, Bynke H, Cronqvist S, et al. A long term prospective study of optic neuritis: evaluation of risk factors. *Ann Neurol* 1990;27:386–393.

180. Parkin PJ, Hierons R, McDonald WI. Bilateral optic neuritis. A long-term follow-up. *Brain* 1984;107:951–964.

181. Morrissey SP, Borruat FX, Miller DH, et al. Bilateral simultaneous optic neuropathy in adults: clinical, imaging, serological, and genetic studies. *J Neurol Neurosurg Psychiatry* 1995;58:70–74.

182. Poser C, Roman G, Emery E. Recurrent disseminated vasculomyelinopathy. *Arch Neurol* 1978;35:166.

183. Alcock N, Hoffman H. Recurrent encephalomyelitis in childhood. *Arch Dis Child* 1962;37:40.

184. Durston JHJ, Milnes JN. Relapsing encephalomyelitis. *Brain* 1970;93:715–730.

185. Lamarche JB, Behan PO, Segarra JM, Feldman RG. Recurrent acute necrotizing hemorrhagic encephalopathy. *Acta Neuropathol (Berl)* 1972;22:79–87.

186. Tippett DS, Fishman PS, Panitch HS. Recurrent transverse myelitis. *Neurology* 1991;41:703–706.

187. Kepes JJ. Large focal tumor-like demyelinating lesions of the brain: intermediate entity between multiple sclerosis and acute disseminated encephalomyelitis? A study of 31 patients. *Ann Neurol* 1993;33:18–27.

188. Peterson K, Rosenblum MK, Powers JM, et al. Effect of brain irradiation on demyelinating lesions. *Neurology* 1993;43:2105–2112.

189. Huang CL, Chu NS, Chen TJ, Shaw CM. Acute hemorrhagic leukoencephalitis with a prolonged clinical course. *J Neurol Neurosurg Psychiatry* 1988;51:870–874.

190. Afifi AK, Bell WE, Menezes AH, Moore SA. Myelinoclastic diffuse sclerosis (Schilder's disease): report of a case and a review of the literature. *J Child Neurol* 1994;9:398–403.

191. Poser CM. Myelinoclastic diffuse sclerosis. In: Koetsier JC, ed. *Handbook of clinical neurology*. Vol. 3. *Demyelinating diseases*. Amsterdam: Elsevier Science, 1985:419–428.

192. Dresser LP, Tourian AY, Anthony DC. A case of myelinoclastic diffuse sclerosis in an adult. *Neurology* 1991;41:316–318.

193. Reye RDK, Morgan G, Baral J. Encephalopathy and fatty infiltration of the viscera. *Lancet* 1963;2:742–752.

194. Davis LE. Influenza virus and Reye's syndrome. In: Gilden DH, Lipton HL, eds. *Clinical and molecular aspects of neurotropic virus infection*. Developments in medical virology series. Norwell, MA: Kluwer Academic, 1989:173–202.

195. Lyon G, Dodge PR, Adams RD. The acute encephalopathies of obscure origin in infants and children. *Brain* 1961;84:680–708.

196. Alvord EC Jr. Pathogenesis of experimental allergic encephalomyelitis: introductory remarks. In: Scheinberg LC, Kies MW, Alvord EC Jr, eds. *Research in demyelinating diseases*. Ann NY Acad Sci Vol. 12. New York: NY Academy of Science, 1965:245–255.

197. Miller DL, Ross EM, Alderslade R, et al. Pertussis immunisation and serious acute neurological illness in children. *BMJ* 1981;282:1595–1599.

198. Wentz KR, Marcuse EK. Diphtheria-tetanus-pertussis vaccine and serious neurological illness: an updated review of the epidemiological evidence. *Pediatrics* 1991;87:287–297.

199. Reik L. Disseminated vasculomyelinopathy: an immune complex disease. *Ann Neurol* 1980;7:291–296.

200. Nasralla CAW, Pay N, Goodpasture HC, et al. Postinfectious encephalopathy in a child following *Campylobacter jejuni* enteritis. *AJNR* 1983;14:444–448.

201. Renkawek K, Majkowska-Wierzbicka J, Krajewski S. Necrotic changes of the spinal cord with immune-complex-mediated vasculitis in a case of allergic encephalomyelitis. *J Neurol* 1985;232:368–373.

202. Schlitt M, Whitley RJ. Viral diseases: herpes simplex encephalitis. In: Porter RJ, Schoenberg BS, eds. *Controlled clinical trials in neurological disease*. Norwell, MA: Kluwer Academic, 1990.

Chapter 10
Paraneoplastic Neurologic Disorders

Jan Verschuuren and Josep Dalmau

Cancer arising outside the nervous system can affect the central and peripheral nervous systems by one of two ways: 1) direct spread or metastases, or 2) indirect mechanisms including vascular disorders, metabolic and nutritional deficits, toxic effects of treatment, and paraneoplastic or "remote effects" of cancer on the nervous system. Therefore, *paraneoplastic disorders of the nervous system* are defined as neurologic disorders pathogenetically related to cancer but not ascribable to nervous system metastases or to any of the other indirect mechanisms just mentioned (1). Paraneoplastic syndromes are the rarest of the neurologic complications in patients with cancer. The exact frequency of these syndromes is unknown, and varies depending on the criteria used to define the paraneoplastic syndrome and the studies done to exclude other nonparaneoplastic neurologic disorders.

Neurologic paraneoplastic disorders may affect any portion of the central or peripheral nervous system (Table 10-1) (1). Frequently, neurologic symptoms develop before the tumor is known to be present and therefore, the correct identification of the disorder permits early detection of the neoplasm. The diagnosis of paraneoplastic neurologic disorders is based mainly on the degree of suspicion by the clinician, which depends on their knowledge of the statistical relationship between the development of characteristic neurologic symptoms and the presence of a specific type of tumor. However, in many instances even when the diagnosis of a paraneoplastic disorder is strongly suspected, the underlying cancer is small and escapes detection despite repetitive thorough clinical and radiologic evaluations.

The discovery that immune-mediated mechanisms, characterized by the presence of antineuronal antibodies, may be involved in some paraneoplastic disorders has provided the opportunity to use these antibodies as diagnostic markers of specific disorders and types of associated tumors (2). This chapter reviews the pathogenesis and clinical approach to the diagnosis and treatment of these disorders, and focuses on specific paraneoplastic neurologic disorders for which immune responses against the tumor, the nervous system, or both, have been demonstrated.

Pathogenesis

The exact pathogenesis of most paraneoplastic neurologic syndromes is unknown. Since these syndromes were initially described, several mechanisms have been proposed (Table 10-2). Although most of these mechanisms have not been demonstrated for the specific disorders that initially suggested them, many of the initial theories have been demonstrated for other disorders. For example, the theory that neurologic symptoms result from toxic substances secreted by the tumor, proposed by Brower in 1919 (3), has not been proved for the disorder that this author reported (paraneoplastic cerebellar degeneration (PCD) associated with ovarian cancer), but has been demonstrated for some other paraneoplastic symptoms (fatigability and cachexia resulting from secretion of tumor necrosis factor) (4). The theory that the tumor competed with the nervous system for essential substrates, proposed by Denny-Brown in 1948 (5), has not been demonstrated for the disorder that he reported (sensory neuronopathy associated with small-cell lung cancer (SCLC)), but is correct for other disorders.

In addition to several pathogenic mechanisms indicated in Table 10-2, current evidence suggests that many paraneoplastic disorders are immune mediated (2). One hypothesis is that the ectopic expression of neuronal antigens by the tumor triggers an immune response against the tumor that affects the nervous system, resulting in the paraneoplastic disorder. An antibody-mediated pathogenesis has been demonstrated for the Lambert-Eaton myasthenic syndrome (LEMS) (6). The IgG of these patients contains antibodies against voltage-gated calcium channels (VGCCs) expressed by the tumor (usually SCLC) (7); these antibodies react with similar epitopes expressed at the presynaptic level of the neuromuscular junction, interfering with the release of acetylcholine and resulting in weakness and fatigue. A similar antibody-mediated mechanism directed against postsynaptic neuromuscular acetylcholine receptors has been demonstrated for myasthenia gravis (8), which is triggered by the presence of thymoma in 10% to 15% of patients. In these antibody-related peripheral nervous system disorders,

Table 10-1.
Paraneoplastic Syndromes of the Nervous System

Paraneoplastic syndromes of the central nervous system
  Paraneoplastic cerebellar degeneration
  Paraneoplastic encephalomyelitis (*) (limbic encephalitis, brainstem encephalitis, myelitis)
  Paraneoplastic opsoclonus-myoclonus
  Cancer-associated retinopathy
  Paraneoplastic stiff-man syndrome
  Paraneoplastic necrotizing myelopathy
  Motor neuron syndromes (amyotrophic lateral sclerosis, subacute motor neuronopathy)
Paraneoplastic syndromes of the peripheral nervous system
  Subacute sensory neuronopathy
  Autonomic neuropathy
  Acute sensorimotor neuropathy
    Polyradiculoneuropathy (Guillain-Barré)
    Brachial neuritis
  Chronic sensorimotor neuropathy
    Sensorimotor neuropathies associated with plasma cell dyscrasias
  Vasculitic neuropathy
  Neuromyotonia
Paraneoplastic syndromes of the neuromuscular junction and muscle
  Lambert-Eaton myasthenic syndrome
  Myasthenia gravis
  Polymyositis-dermatomyositis
  Acute necrotizing myopathy
  Cachectic myopathy
  Carcinomatous neuromyopathy
  Carcinoid myopathy

(*) Can include cerebellar symptoms, autonomic dysfunction, and sensory neuronopathy.

passive transfer of the patients' IgG to animals reproduces the clinical, electrophysiologic, and structural abnormalities of the disorder.

Similar immune-mediated mechanisms have been suggested for antibody-associated paraneoplastic disorders of the central nervous system, such as anti-Hu–associated paraneoplastic encephalomyelitis (PEM) and sensory neuronopathy (PSN) (9,10). Although administration of these antibodies to animals has not reproduced the disease (11–13), the immune origin of these disorders is strongly suggested by several findings, including 1) the presence of high titers of antibodies that react with antigens restricted to the nervous system and tumor (14); 2) intrathecal synthesis of antibodies and deposits of antibodies in neurons and tumor (15–17); 3) the presence of antigen-specific lymphocytes in the nervous system and tumor (18); and 4) absence of similar antibodies in other inflammatory disorders of the central nervous system that are associated with neuronal destruction, or with tumors that do not express the specific antigen (19).

The development of an animal model using IgG from patients with antibody-related paraneoplastic disorders of the central nervous system has been unsuccessful to date and may reflect that the antibodies are not pathogenic (11–13). However, these studies are not conclusive. It is possible that only a small fraction of the antibodies that comprise the polyclonal immune response are pathogenic, and that low but continuous production of a specific antibody is required for neuronal damage. Other factors, such as accessibility of antibodies to the nervous system (persistent intrathecal synthesis of antibodies has not been reproduced in animals), or differences of epitopes between animal species have to be considered as possibly confounding the development of an animal model (12).

Other attempts to develop animal models of antibody-related paraneoplastic disorders of the central nervous system include animal immunization with recombinant paraneoplastic antigens produced in bacteria (11,12). These animals developed high titer of antibodies but no neurologic symptoms; however, pathogenic antibodies directed against conformational epitopes or posttranslational modified forms of the antigen may have been missed in these studies.

In addition to the presence of antineuronal antibodies, the nervous system and the tumor of patients with paraneoplastic disorders of the central nervous system contain inflammatory infiltrates composed of CD4 and CD8 cytotoxic T cells (20,21). In general, B and CD4 cells tend to localize around blood vessels, while CD8 cells have a more widespread interstitial distribution. The tumors of these patients have more inflammatory infiltrates than do the tumors of patients without paraneoplastic disorders (22,23). These findings suggest that a cytotoxic T-cell response may contribute to or be the predominant effector of the neuronal degeneration, and may explain why the tumors of patients with paraneoplastic disorders appear to be more indolent than histologically identical tumors from patients without paraneoplastic symptoms (14). For some disorders, such as anti-Hu–associated PEM, it is typical to find conspicuous inflammatory infiltrates in multiple areas of the nervous system (some of them asymptomatic), with cytotoxic cells surrounding neurons undergoing degeneration (24).

Although all tumors associated with most antibody (anti-Hu, anti-Yo, anti-Ri)-related paraneoplastic disorders of the central nervous system express the antigens that trigger the immune response, tumors from patients who do not develop antineuronal antibodies or paraneoplastic symptoms may also express the same antigens (25,26). It is not known why only a small proportion of tumors expressing these antigens trigger an immune response associated with the paraneoplastic disorder. Factors related to the tumor, such as the coexpression of antigen-presenting molecules (MHC class I and II) (27), and factors related to the patient, such as gender and HLA haplotype (28), may also be involved in the development of the immune response.

Clinical Diagnosis of Paraneoplastic Disorders

It is important to recognize that neurologic disorders that are clinically and pathologically identical to paraneoplastic disorders can occur in the absence of cancer

Table 10-2.
Pathogenesis of Paraneoplastic Neurologic Disorders

Immune-Mediated Disorders	Disorder	Antigens
Antibodies to onco-neuronal antigens, proved with animal model	LEMS	VGCC
	Myasthenia gravis	Acetylcholine receptor
Antibodies to onco-neuronal antigens; no animal model	PEM/PSN	Hu antigens (HuD, HuC, Hel-N1)
	PCD (lung cancer)	Calcium channel
	PCD (breast, ovary)	Yo antigens (CDR34, CDR62)
	Ataxia/opsoclonus	Nova
	Stiff-man syndrome	Amphiphysin
Direct synthesis of IgM or IgG by tumor	Sensorimotor neuropathy (Waldenström)	MAG
	Motor neuronopathy (lymphoma)	GD_1
Competition for substrate	Disorder	Substrate
	Carcinoid myopathy	Tryptophan
	Encephalopathy	Glucose (sarcomas)
	Wernicke encephalopathy	B1 (leukemia)
Viral infection	Disorder	Virus
	Progressive multifocal leukoencephalopathy	JC virus (papovavirus)
	Necrotizing myelopathy	Zoster-varicella virus
	Subacute motor neuronopathy	?
Tumor secretion of toxic substances, cytokines or hormones	Disorder	Hormone-Cytokine
	Cachexia, fatigability	TNF, interleukins-1, -6
	Encephalopathy	SIADH, PTH-like
		ACTH

LEMS = Lambert-Eaton myasthenic syndrome; PEM = paraneoplastic encephalomyelitis; PSN = paraneoplastic sensory neuronopathy; PCD = paraneoplastic cerebrellar degeneration; VGCC = voltage-gated calcium channel; MAG = myelin-associated glycoprotein; TNF = tumor necrosis factor; SIADH = syndrome of inappropriate antidiuretic hormone secretion; PTH = parathyroid hormone; ACTH = adrenocorticotropin.

Table 10-3.
Neurologic Syndromes Suggesting a Paraneoplastic Origin

Syndrome	Tumor
Lambert-Eaton myasthenic syndrome[a]	SCLC
Subacute cerebellar syndrome[b]	Lung, breast, lymphoma, gynecologic
Subacute sensory neuropathy	SCLC
Opsoclonus-myoclonus	
Pediatric population[a]	Neuroblastoma
Adult population	Lung, breast
Subacute autonomic dysfunction (postural hypotension, gastrointestinal, paresis, abnormal pupillary responses)	Lung
Dermatomyositis[b]	Lung, breast, gynecologic, gastrointestinal
Subacute encephalomyelitis	SCLC
Subacute retinopathy	SCLC, melanoma, gynecologic
Subacute limbic encephalopathy	SCLC
Subacute motor neuronopathy and atypical motor neuron disease	SCLC, lymphoma, renal, prostate
Myasthenia gravis	Thymoma

[a]More than 50% of patients with this disorder have the indicated underlying cancer.
[b]In older population (age > 50).
SCLC = small-cell lung cancer.

Table 10-4.
Antineuronal Antibody–Associated Paraneoplastic Disorders

Antibody	Neuronal Reactivity	Neuronal Antigens	Cloned Genes	Tumor	Paraneoplastic Symptoms
Anti-Hu	Nucleus > cytoplasm (all neurons)	35–40 kd	HuD, HuC Hel-N1	SCLC, neuro-blastoma, sarcoma, prostate	PEM, PSN, PCD Autonomic dysfunction
Anti-Yo	Cytoplasm Purkinje cells	34, 62 kd	CDR34, CDR62	Ovary, breast, lung	PCD
Anti-Ri	Nucleus > cytoplasm (CNS neurons)	55, 80	Nova	Breast, gynecologic, lung, bladder	Ataxia, opsoclonus spasms, rigidity
Anti-Tr	Cytoplasm Purkinje cells	?	—	Hodgkin's	PCD
Anti-VGCC	Presynaptic NMJ	P/Q type VGCC 64 kd 37 kd	MysB Synaptotagmin	SCLC	LEMS
Antiretinal	Photoreceptor Ganglion cells	23, 65, 145, 205 kd	Recoverin	SCLC, melanoma, gynecologic	CAR
Antiamphphisin	Presynaptic	128 kd	Amphphisin	Breast, SCLC	Stiff-man, PEM

CNS = central nervous system; VGCC = voltage-gated calcium channel; SCLC = small-cell lung carcinoma; LEMS = Lambert-Eaton myasthenic syndrome; PEM = paraneoplastic encephalomyelitis; PSN = paraneoplastic sensory neuronopathy; PCD = paraneoplastic cerebellar degeneration; CAR = cancer-associated retinopathy.

(29). This, in addition to the fact that the underlying tumor may remain elusive during repetitive examinations for a suspected malignancy, complicates the diagnosis of a paraneoplastic syndrome. The probability that a neurologic disorder is paraneoplastic depends on the type of syndrome; Table 10-3 lists the main neurologic syndromes that suggest paraneoplasia. For some disorders, such as LEMS, the probability of an associated tumor is very high (60%) (30); for others, such as PCD and opsoclonus-myoclonus, while there is a clear statistical association with cancer, this association is increased in some patient populations, such as older patients for PCD and ovarian or breast cancer, and pediatric patients for neuroblastoma and opsoclonus-myoclonus.

The discovery that some paraneoplastic disorders of the central or peripheral nervous system are characteristically associated with antineuronal antibodies (Table 10-4) has had a major impact on the ability to diagnose and manage these disorders. Regardless of whether these antibodies are causal or not, they can 1) be used as markers of the paraneoplastic origin of neurologic symptoms, avoiding unnecessary diagnostic tests, and 2) serve as markers for the presence of specific types of tumors, directing the search for the tumor to a few organs.

Owing to the increasing number of newly described antineuronal antibodies (many with unknown significance at this time), it is important to define these antibodies using rigorous criteria, which must include immunohistochemical and Western blot analysis of cortical neurons or Purkinje cells, or recombinant antigens. The existence of antibodies with different antigen specificities but similar immunohistochemical characteristics, or the coexistence of several antibodies in the same patient, may confuse the diagnosis and lead to unnecessary testing for the presence of a malignancy. In addition, it is important to note that "atypical or not well-defined" antineuronal antibodies may be found in the presence of nonparaneoplastic disorders; thus, identification of "antineuronal antibodies" is not sufficient to diagnose a paraneoplastic disorder. Criteria suggesting that a novel antineuronal antibody can be used as a marker of a paraneoplastic disorder are listed in Table 10-5.

The clinical approach to establish the paraneoplastic origin of a neurologic disorder depends on whether the presence of a cancer is known or not. Because neuro-

Table 10-5.
Criteria Suggesting That a New Antibody Is a Marker for a Paraneoplastic Disorder

Obligatory
   The antibody reacts with the symptomatic area of the nervous system.
   The antibody identifies antigens expressed by the tumor and nervous system.
   The antibody is not detected when a similar neurologic disorder is associated with a tumor that does not express the neuronal antigen.
   The antibody is not present in serum from normal individuals or from patients with nonparaneoplastic neurologic disorders.
   There is intrathecal synthesis of antibody (for paraneoplastic disorders of CNS).
Optional
   In patients with cancer but without paraneoplastic symptoms, either the antibody is not present or its titer does not overlap with the titers detected in patients with paraneoplastic syndromes.
   There are deposits of antibodies in neurons or tumor cells.

logic symptoms usually precede the diagnosis of cancer, most patients are initially seen by a neurologist. The type of syndrome (see Table 10-3), along with the subacute onset and rapid evolution, usually suggest a paraneoplastic etiology (Table 10-6). The detection of paraneoplastic antineuronal antibodies in the serum and cerebrospinal fluid (CSF) establishes the diagnosis, and directs the search for the tumor. If no paraneoplastic antibodies are demonstrated, the evaluation should be directed 1) to examine the CSF, which in the early stages of paraneoplastic disorders of the central nervous system usually contains inflammatory cells and oligoclonal bands, and 2) to demonstrate the presence of a systemic cancer (tumor markers, radiologic studies, etc.).

For patients in whom the presence of cancer is known, efforts should be directed to rule out the possibility that the neurologic symptoms result from metastases or other indirect, nonparaneoplastic mechanisms of neuronal injury (Table 10-7) (1). The detection of paraneoplastic antibodies establishes the paraneoplastic origin of the disorder and avoids extensive evaluations searching for other etiologies. If the tumor is "atypical or unusual" for the type of paraneoplastic antibodies identified, or does not show reactivity with the serum antibodies, the presence of a second neoplasm should be considered (31,32).

Table 10-6.
Approach to the Diagnosis of a Paraneoplastic Disorder in Patients Without Known Cancer

---

Onset and features of neurologic symptoms
  Subacute onset
  Rapid evolution
  Clinical features suggestive of paraneoplastic disorder
CSF studies
  Presence of imflammatory cells
  IgG and IgG index
  Ologoclonal bands
  Antineuronal antibodies
Serum studies
  Cancer markers
  Antineuronal antibodies: CEA, CA-125, BRCA1, PSA
  Immunoelectrophoresis serum and urine (patients with peripheral neuropathy and suspicion of plasma cell dyscrasia)
Neurophysiologic tests
  Nerve conduction studies
  Sensory potentials
  Neuromuscular transmission (repetitive stimulation)
  Electromyography (lower motor neuron dysfunction)
Risk factors of cancer
  Smoking
Work-up for malignancy
  Chest CT
  Mammogram
  Pelvic exam, CT of abdomen/pelvis, ultrasound
  Testis exam, ultrasound
  Lymph node examination
  Stool guaiac
  Bone scan (patients with peripheral neuropathy and suspicion of plasma cell dyscrasia)

CSF = cerebrospinal fluid; CT = computed tomography.

Table 10-7.
Approach to the Diagnosis of a Paraneoplastic Disorder in Patients with Known Cancer

---

Work-up for metastases
  MRI of symptomatic area(s)
  CSF cytology
  Nerve biopsy (patients with leukemia or lymphoma who develop painful, progressive, peripheral neuropathy not related to treatment)
Review of previous treatment(s)
  Radiation therapy
  Chemotherapy
  Immunotherapy and immunologic response modifiers
Review of metabolic and nutritional deficits
  Hypoxia; liver, renal failure
  Deficit B_1 (Wernicke-Korsakoff); B_{12}, folic acid
  Myopathy due to cancer cachexia; carcinoid myopathy
Vascular disorders
  Hypercoagulability
  Hypocoagulability
Opportunistic infections (leukemia, lymphoma, immunosuppression)
  Progressive multifocal leukoencephalopathy (JC virus, papovavirus)
  Acute necrotizing myelopathy (varicella-herpes virus)
  Dementia (herpes)
Coincidental non-cancer-related disorders
  Diabetes, alcohol, uremia
Paraneoplastic or "remote effects" of cancer on the nervous system

---

MRI = magnetic resonance imaging; CSF = cerebrospinal fluid.

Specific Paraneoplastic Syndromes of the Central Nervous System

Paraneoplastic Cerebellar Degeneration

This disorder is characterized by the subacute development of rapidly progressive symptoms of cerebellar dysfunction, which eventually stabilize and leave the patient incapacitated with a pancerebellar syndrome. Initial symptoms typically include dizziness, visual problems (diplopia, blurry vision, or oscillopsia), nausea, vomiting, and dysarthria (1). These symptoms may be considered secondary to a viral process, but in a few days (sometimes hours) the patient develops ataxia of gait and extremities, usually accompanied by dysphagia. The intensity and course of the symptoms, and the association with other neurologic deficits, may vary from patient to patient, but these differences are less noticeable between patients with the same type of tumor, and particularly between patients with the same type of antineuronal antibody in serum and CSF (Table 10-8). Furthermore, the finding of different antineuronal antibodies (33,34), some associated with specific histologic types of tumor, suggests that PCD is a syndrome rather than a disease, and that different pathogenic mechanisms may result in the same symptoms.

The neoplasms most often associated with PCD include cancer of the lung, particularly SCLC, and of the

Table 10-8.
Paraneoplastic Cerebellar Degeneration

Antibody	Antigens	Tumor	Incidence by Sex	Symptoms	Cause of Death/Prognosis
Anti-Hu	HuD, HuC, Hel-N1	SCLC Neuroblastoma	F > M	Pancerebellar, sensory neuropathy, PEM	Paraneoplasia > tumor
Anti-Yo	CDR62, CDR34	Ovary Breast	F >> M	Pancerebellar	Tumor
Anti-Ri	Nova	Breast, gynecologic SCLC	F >> M	Ataxia, opsoclonus, oculomotor dysfunction	Tumor > paraneoplasia; may respond to treatment
Anti-TR	Unknown	Hodgkin's	M > F	Pancerebellar	May respond to treatment
Anti-NMJ	P/Q type VGCC, MysB	SCLC	M = W	Pancerebellar, LEMS	Unknown

SCLC = small-cell lung carcinoma; PEM = paraneoplastic encephalomyelitis; LEMS = Lambert-Eaton myasthenic syndrome; VGCC = voltage-gated calcium channel.

ovary, and breast and lymphoma (35). Classic postmortem studies demonstrate nearly total or total loss of Purkinje cells with relative preservation of other cerebellar neurons, and Bergmann astrogliosis. Inflammatory infiltrates, if present, usually involve the deep cerebellar nuclei. Demyelinating changes may be present in the cerebellum and dorsal spinocerebellar and posterior columns of the spinal cord (36).

The diagnosis of PCD should be suspected in any patient older than 50 years who shows subacute symptoms of cerebellar dysfunction. The diagnostic approach depends on whether the patient is known to have cancer or not (see Tables 10-6 and 10-7). In the early stages of symptoms, examination of the CSF usually demonstrates pleocytosis, increased protein concentrations, increased IgG index, and oligoclonal bands. The detection of a well-characterized paraneoplastic antibody establishes the diagnosis and directs the search for the neoplasm (see Table 10-8). Other tests, such as magnetic resonance imaging (MRI) of the head, do not usually demonstrate changes in the acute phase of the disease; atrophy of the cerebellum may be seen several months after the development of neurologic symptoms (1).

The response to treatment may be different for these disorders. While the cerebellar dysfunction associated with anti-Hu or anti-Yo antibodies does not usually improve with any treatment (31,37,38), the cerebellar symptoms of patients with anti-Tr antibodies and Hodgkin's disease (39) may improve spontaneously or with treatment of the tumor.

Anti-Yo–Associated Paraneoplastic Cerebellar Degeneration

This disorder is the best-characterized PCD (37,38). Typically, patients are postmenopausal women with no history of cancer (two thirds of patients), or with a recent diagnosis of cancer of the breast or the ovary (one third of patients) who develop dizziness, nausea, double or blurry vision, slurred speech, and motor incoordination.

Within a few weeks the disorder evolves toward a pancerebellar deficit, with dysarthria, dysphagia, and downbeat nystagmus. Most of the patients are unable to read, watch television, feed themselves, or walk without assistance. In some patients the clinical syndrome develops acutely (overnight), mimicking a stroke. Symptoms progress for a few weeks until stabilization; depending on the course of the tumor, these patients may remain wheelchair bound for years. Autopsy studies demonstrate total or near-total loss of Purkinje cells (Fig 10-1) (23,38).

The anti-Yo antibodies react with 34- and 62-kd protein antigens expressed in the cytoplasm of Purkinje cells and tumor (Fig 10-2) (40). The genes encoding both antigens (CDR34 and CDR62) have been cloned and are located on chromosome X and 16, respectively (1,41–43). The function of these proteins is unknown, but CDR62 contains leucine-zipper and zing-finger motifs, suggesting a role in the regulation of gene expression (42).

In these patients, detection of anti-Yo antibodies in the serum or CSF confirms the paraneoplastic origin of the disorder and should prompt the search for a breast or gynecologic cancer, mainly ovarian (38). In some patients, the presence of axillary adenopathies without a known primary tumor is suggestive of breast cancer. All paraneoplastic tumors express Yo antigens, but these proteins are also expressed in 20% of ovarian cancers from patients without anti-Yo antibodies and without PCD (26). Among 90 patients with anti-Yo–associated PCD whose serum was studied at Memorial Sloan-Kettering Cancer Center, the few exceptions to the previous findings include one woman with adenocarcinoma of the lung, one man with mediastinal adenopathy highly suggestive of a primary lung tumor (32), and one man with adenocarcinoma of the salivary gland (44). The tumors of these three patients expressed Yo antigens, indicating that no other occult neoplasms were involved in the disorder.

Low titers of anti-Yo antibodies can be detected in 1% of patients with ovarian cancer, without neurologic

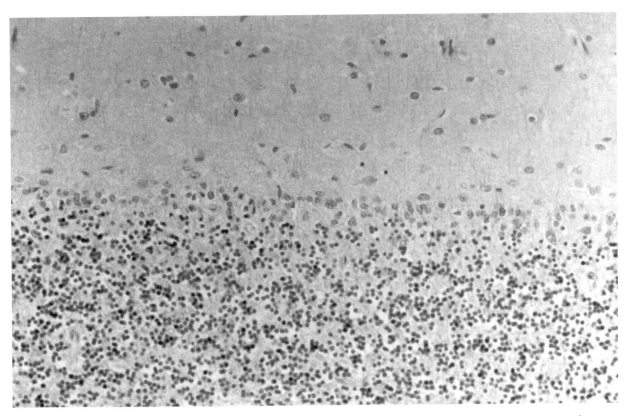

Figure 10-1. Section of cerebellum from a patient with anti-Yo–associated paraneoplastic cerebellar degeneration, demonstrating absence of Purkinje cells and Bergmann gliosis.

symptoms (26). High titers of antibodies are always associated with PCD. Owing to the strong correlation between detection of this antibody and the presence of breast or gynecologic tumors, anti-Yo–positive patients should undergo mammography and computed tomography (CT) of the pelvis and abdomen. If the tumor is not found, repeat mammography and pelvic examination under anesthesia with dilation and curettage are recommended. If the results of these tests and tests for other cancer markers (CA-125, CA 15-3, BRCA1) are negative, a chest CT should be obtained. Removal of the ovaries and uterus should be considered for postmenopausal women whose test results remain negative (38,45).

Treatment of the tumor, plasmapheresis, and administration of intravenous immunoglobulin (IVIg) do not usually affect the course of this paraneoplastic disorder (38,46,47). There is one report of two patients who improved with cyclophosphamide treatment (48).

Paraneoplastic Cerebellar Dysfunction Associated with Hodgkin's Disease

This disorder predominates in men, and the patients are usually younger than patients with PCD associated with other tumors. Neurologic symptoms usually de-

velop after the diagnosis of the lymphoma, or when the tumor is in remission. Paraneoplastic cerebellar symptoms may be the first sign of tumor recurrence. Neurologic deficits are usually less severe than those for the cerebellar dysfunction associated with anti-Yo or anti-Hu antibodies (39). The first anti–Purkinje cell antibody identified was from the serum of a patient with Hodgkin's disease and PCD. This antibody, identified by Trotter et al (49), reacts diffusely with the cytoplasm of Purkinje cells. The exact incidence of this antibody in the serum and CSF of patients with this disorder is unknown. Using immunohistochemical studies, Hammack et al (39) identified similar antibodies in 6 of 22 patients with PCD and Hodgkin's disease. The results of Western blot analysis with homogenate of cerebellum or Purkinje cells are usually negative, and the exact nature of the antigen(s) remains unknown. An important limitation to identifying this antibody is that treatment of the lymphoma results in a rapid and marked decrease of antibody titers. Another limitation is that the antigen appears to degrade rapidly and is difficult to identify in human cerebellum obtained at autopsy (Graus F, et al, unpublished data). The paraneoplastic cerebellar dysfunction in patients with Hodgkin's disease may improve spontaneously, after treatment of the

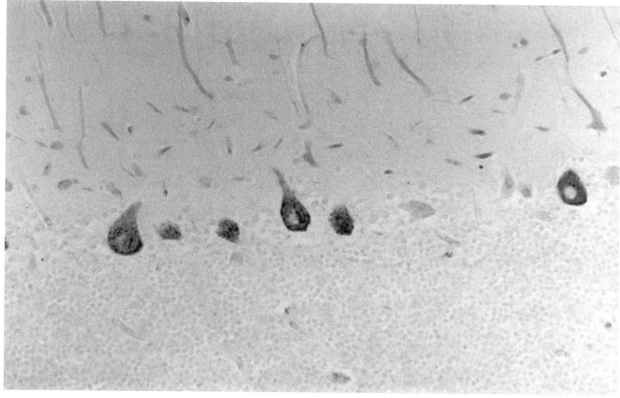

Figure 10-2. Reactivity of anti-Yo antibodies with a section of cerebellum obtained at autopsy of a neurologically normal individual. Note the predominant granular reactivity of the anti-Yo antibodies with the cytoplasm of Purkinje cells. (Section mildly counterstained with hematoxylin.)

tumor, or after symptomatic treatment with clonazepam (39).

Paraneoplastic Cerebellar Degeneration and Opsoclonus, Associated with Anti-Ri Antibodies

In some women with subacute cerebellar dysfunction, the predominant symptoms are gait difficulty, truncal ataxia, and opsoclonus. These patients may harbor in their serum and CSF an antineuronal antibody, called *anti-Ri* (50,51). This antibody reacts with 55- and 80-kd proteins expressed in the nuclei of most neurons of the central nervous system (Fig 10-3) as well as in the associated tumor, usually a breast cancer. The tumor is usually identified after the neurologic symptoms develop. Other associated cancers include gynecologic tumors, carcinoma of the lung, and carcinoma of the bladder (50,52). In some patients, no tumor is identified (50,53,54). A gene encoding an Ri antigen, called *Nova*, has recently been cloned (55).

Different from other PCDs in which symptoms are pancerebellar, in patients with anti-Ri antibodies the motor incoordination predominantly affects the trunk and gait, and oscillopsia (opsoclonus) is present in 75%

of patients. The opsoclonus may improve spontaneously or with medications (clonazepam, triazolam, prednisone), leaving the patient with ocular flutter or dysmetria (50). Other symptoms include vertigo, nausea, dysphagia, ocular paresis, axial rigidity, muscle spasms, and confusion (50,52–54). All reported patients have been women; one of our patients is a man with carcinoma of the bladder. Clinical responses (usually partial) to treatment have been noted with clonazepam, triazolam, thiamine, steroids, cyclophosphamide, and treatment of the tumor (50,52–54). A patient who developed episodes of muscle spasms, axial rigidity, and hyperventilation improved with baclofen (53).

Paraneoplastic Cerebellar Degeneration Without Antineuronal Antibodies or Antibodies of Unknown Clinical Significance

Paraneoplastic cerebellar dysfunction can occur without identifiable antineuronal antibodies, which makes the diagnosis more difficult. The diagnostic approach depends on whether or not a tumor is known to be present (see Tables 10-6 and 10-7). The neoplasms more commonly involved are SCLC and non-Hodgkin's lym-

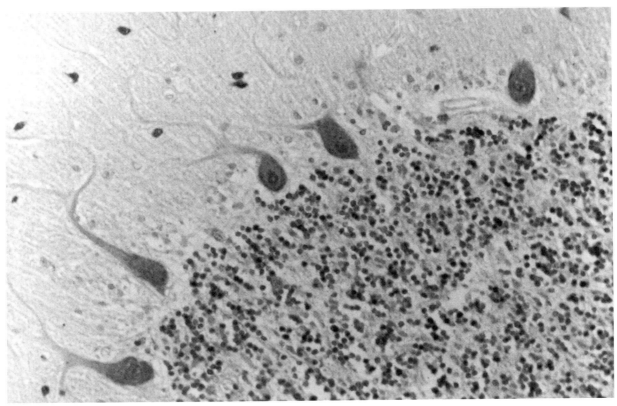

Figure 10-3.   Reactivity of anti-Ri antibodies with a section of cerebellum obtained at autopsy of a neurologically normal individual. Note that the anti-Ri antibodies react predominantly with the nuclei of all neurons (Purkinje cells and neurons of the granular and molecular layers). (Section mildly counterstained with hematoxylin.)

phoma (1,35). Patients with SCLC and pure or predominantly cerebellar dysfunction may not harbor anti–Hu antibodies; differentiation between anti-Hu-positive and –negative patients has significant clinical and prognostic implications (see Paraneoplastic Encephalomyelitis).

Results of one study suggested that antibodies to a variety of non–N-methyl-D-aspartate (NMDA) glutamate receptors are present in the serum of patients with paraneoplastic disorders, and that these antibodies through excitotoxic mechanisms may contribute to the neuronal degeneration (56). Using serum from patients with anti-Yo–, anti-Hu–, and anti-Ri–associated paraneoplastic disorders, other authors were not able to identify anti–glutamate receptor antibodies (57). In addition, the presence of several antineuronal antibodies against uncharacterized antigens has been documented in anecdotal or isolated case reports (58–60). The significance of these antibodies as clinical markers of paraneoplastic disorders, as well as the prognostic implications and the specific association to certain types of tumors, remain unknown.

The development of cerebellar dysfunction in association with LEMS and anti-VGCC antibodies suggests that antibodies to calcium channels may be involved in the pathogenesis of some PCDs (61,62). The most common tumor is SCLC; one patient with LEMS and paraneoplastic cerebellar dysfunction had lymphoma (62). The detection of different types of calcium channel antibodies in patients with SCLC without paraneoplastic neurologic symptoms, as well as in patients with non-neoplastic disorders and normal individuals (63), makes it difficult to use these antibodies as markers of paraneoplastic central nervous system disorders.

Paraneoplastic Encephalomyelitis

Patients with this disorder develop symptoms of multifocal involvement of the nervous system, which can include dementia (limbic encephalopathy), brainstem encephalopathy, cerebellar dysfunction, myelopathy (lower motor neuron), sensory deficits due to dorsal root ganglia (DRG) involvement, and autonomic dysfunction. The distribution of symptoms as well as the pathologic findings along the neuraxis are variable, giving rise to several syndromes that can occur alone or in association. The areas with prominent pathologic abnormalities are almost always symptomatic, but pathologic findings are usually far more extensive than the distribution of clinical symptoms (31,64). The main pathologic abnormalities include interstitial and perivascular inflammatory infiltrates, neuronal degeneration, lymphocytic neuronophagic nodules (microglial nodules), and gliosis (24,31,64).

In 80% of patients the associated tumor is SCLC, but the disorder has been documented in the setting of almost any type of neoplasm (64). Most patients with PEM and SCLC harbor high titers of anti-Hu antibodies in their serum and CSF (14,31). Anti-Hu antibodies react with a family of RNA-binding proteins (HuD, Hel-N1, HuC) expressed in the nuclei, and to a lesser degree the cytoplasm of all neurons of the central and peripheral nervous systems, and tumor cells (Fig 10-4) (18,65–67). Because paraneoplastic symptoms usually develop before a tumor is known to be present, detection of anti-Hu antibodies is highly indicative of the presence of SCLC. In a few pediatric patients with brainstem dysfunction, detection of anti-Hu antibodies suggests the presence of neuroblastoma (27,68). Low titers of anti-Hu antibodies (usually orders of a magnitude lower than the titers in paraneoplastic patients) are present in 17% of patients with SCLC without paraneoplastic symptoms (14).

The distribution of symptoms in a series of patients with anti-Hu–associated PEM/PSN is shown in Figure 10-5.

Limbic encephalopathy includes the presence of personality changes, irritability, depression, agitation, anxiety, sleep disturbances, hallucinations, memory deficits (predominantly short-term memory), and dementia (69). Partial complex seizures and general seizures may be the presentation of the disorder. More than two thirds of patients with paraneoplastic limbic encephalopathy develop symptoms of involvement of other areas of the nervous system, indicating that the disorder is a fragment of PEM (31). In this situation, when SCLC is the associated tumor, the anti-Hu antibody is almost always present in the serum and CSF. This antibody, however, may be absent in patients with SCLC and "pure" limbic encephalopathy, and is almost always absent when tumors other than SCLC are involved (70).

Symptoms of *cerebellar dysfunction* (see Paraneoplastic Cerebellar Degeneration) may be the presentation of PEM and PSN (31). Patients with SCLC who develop symptoms of pure or predominant cerebellar dysfunction may not harbor anti-Hu antibodies. The detection of anti-Hu antibodies usually predicts that other areas of the nervous system will become involved (sensory

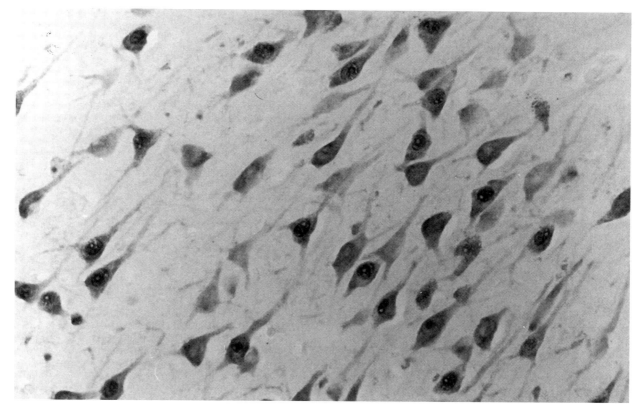

Figure 10-4.   Reactivity of anti-Hu antibodies with a section of cerebral cortex (hippocampus) obtained at autopsy of a neurologically normal individual. Note that the anti-Hu antibodies react predominantly with the nuclei of all neurons.

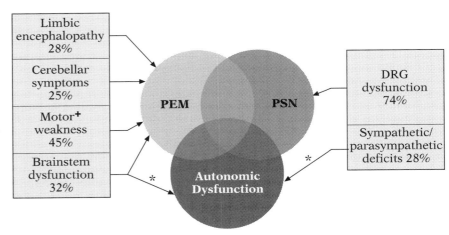

Figure 10-5. Distribution of neurologic symptoms in a series of 71 patients with anti-Hu–associated paraneoplastic neurologic symptoms. +Twenty percent of patients with motor weakness had signs of lower motor neuron dysfunction. *The exact contribution of the brainstem dysfunction or peripheral sympathetic and parasympathetic neuronal involvement to the autonomic symptoms of these patients is unknown. PEM = paraneoplastic encephalomyelitis; PSN = paraneoplastic sensory neuronopathy; DRG = dorsal root ganglion.

neuronopathy, brainstem dysfunction). Whereas anti-Hu–negative patients usually die of tumor progression, most anti-Hu–positive patients die as a result of the neurologic disease (71).

Autopsies of patients with PEM usually demonstrate inflammatory changes involving the *brainstem*, particularly the medulla (24,31,64). In a study of 71 patients with anti-Hu–associated PEM/PSN, symptoms of brainstem encephalopathy were identified in 32% of the patients (31). Symptoms may include diplopia, hearing loss, dysphagia, dysarthria, gaze abnormalities, trigeminal-distribution sensory deficits, and rarely oscillopsia (opsoclonus).

Motor weakness, muscle atrophy, and fasciculations are prominent in 20% of patients with diffuse PEM. Although some of these symptoms result from inflammatory involvement of motor nerve roots, the pathologic studies of these patients usually demonstrate involvement of the *spinal cord (myelitis)*, including inflammatory infiltrates and neuronal degeneration. In one of our patients the autopsy demonstrated loss of most of the neurons of the anterior horn of the spinal cord (31). If spinal cord involvement is the leading and predominant dysfunction, the diagnosis of subacute motor neuron dysfunction (or atypical amyotrophic lateral sclerosis (ALS)) may be entertained until other areas of the nervous system become involved.

Autonomic dysfunction, resulting from central and peripheral nervous system involvement, affects about 30% of patients with diffuse anti-Hu–associated PEM. Symptoms include orthostatic hypotension, gastrointestinal paresis and pseudo-obstruction, impotence, dry mouth, bladder dysfunction, abnormal pupillary responses, and sweating disturbances (31,72,73). Involvement of autonomic nerves (sympathetic ganglia, myenteric plexus) has been demonstrated in some patients with this disorder.

SCLC is the neoplasm most commonly associated with paraneoplastic autonomic dysfunction; carcinoma of the pancreas (74) and carcinoid tumor (75) of the

lung have also been reported. In some patients an acute pandysautonomia is the predominant or isolated manifestation of the paraneoplastic disorder. The autonomic dysfunction, including hypothermia, hypoventilation, sleep apnea, and cardiac arrhythmias, may be the cause of sudden death of these patients (75). Pathologic studies can demonstrate widespread central and peripheral involvement of the autonomic nervous system, which make the clinicopathologic correlations very difficult to assess. Involvement of sympathetic and parasympathetic nerves, reticular formation of the medulla oblongata, or locus ceruleus may explain the variety of symptoms (75).

About 75% of patients with anti-Hu–associated PEM develop an asymmetric neuropathy, often with painful dysesthesias, that involves all modalities of sensation and results from DRG inflammation and neuronal degeneration (see Paraneoplastic Sensory Neuronopathy) (31).

Analysis of CSF obtained during the early stages of PEM with or without dorsal root ganglionitis usually demonstrates pleocytosis, increased protein concentrations, and intrathecal synthesis of IgG; oligoclonal bands are frequently detected. Intrathecal synthesis of anti-Hu antibodies is demonstrated in most patients with SCLC, and in a few with other tumors (prostate cancer, neuroblastoma, chondromyxosarcoma) (31). In patients with anti-Hu–associated paraneoplastic symptoms, tumors other than SCLC are extremely rare, and when detected they express the Hu antigens. If no tumor is detected, periodic (every 6 months) clinical follow-up and CT of the chest are recommended. If the anti-Hu antibody titer is negative, the search for a neoplasm should have a wider spectrum, including other (non-SCLC) lung tumors and breast cancer.

Except for the detection of anti-Hu antibodies, there are no other markers of PEM/PSN, or specific diagnostic tests. MRIs of the head or spinal cord usually appear normal, but in some patients with limbic encephalitis, T2-weighted images show abnormalities and

T1-weighted images of the medial aspect of the temporal lobes show small areas of contrast enhancement (76). In patients with dorsal root ganglionitis, the electrophysiologic studies typically demonstrate an absence or severe reduction of the sensory potentials, with relative preservation of motor conduction velocities and compound muscle action potentials (77); signs of motor denervation are usually absent unless there is a concomitant myelitis with anterior horn involvement, or anterior root nerve inflammation (78).

The prognosis for patients with anti-Hu–associated encephalomyelitis is poor. Treatment of the tumor and immunosuppression do not modify the course of the paraneoplastic symptoms, which usually result in death. For the patients with anti-Hu–associated sensory neuronopathy who do not develop other symptoms of central nervous system dysfunction (about 25% of all patients with anti-Hu–associated paraneoplastic disorders), treatment of the tumor or immunosuppression may stabilize the disorder or, more rarely, result in some improvement (79).

Paraneoplastic Opsoclonus-Myoclonus

The syndrome opsoclonus-myoclonus consists of spontaneous, arrhythmic, large-amplitude conjugate saccades occurring in all directions of gaze, which are associated with myoclonus of the head, trunk, or extremities (80). The pathogenesis of opsoclonus remains unclear, but it has been suggested that it results from disruption of the tonic inhibitory control of saccadic neurons by the "omnipause neurons" in the pontine reticular formation. However, autopsy studies of two patients with SCLC and paraneoplastic opsoclonus failed to demonstrate damage of these neurons (81). Opsoclonus-myoclonus may also occur as a result of viral, toxic, metabolic, and vascular disorders (82). Paraneoplastic opsoclonus-myoclonus has been described in three clinical settings: 1) pediatric patients with neuroblastoma; 2) adult patients with anti-Ri antibodies, usually female with breast cancer (see Paraneoplastic Cerebellar Degeneration); and 3) adult patients with other tumors, or without anti-Ri antibodies (these patients usually have SCLC).

For all these subgroups of patients with paraneoplastic opsoclonus-myoclonus, the pathologic basis of the disorder remains unknown. Pathologic findings vary from mild to severe inflammatory infiltrates, involving the brainstem, cerebellum, and leptomeninges; there may be also a variable loss of Purkinje cells (83). The development of opsoclonus in subgroups of patients characterized by the presence of different types of tumors, sometimes associated with well-characterized antineuronal antibodies (such anti-Ri), and divergent pathologic findings suggests that paraneoplastic opsoclonus may result from involvement of several structures in the central nervous system.

In children, the clinical features of paraneoplastic opsoclonus-myoclonus are similar to those of the syndrome unrelated to the presence of a tumor (viral cause). Symptoms develop acutely, and include irritability, vomiting, hypotonia, ataxia, and opsoclonus-myoclonus (82). In most pediatric patients, these symptoms lead to the discovery of the neuroblastoma. However, the disorder may develop after tumor diagnosis, during tumor remission, or at tumor recurrence. The exact incidence of the paraneoplastic disorder associated with neuroblastoma is unknown, but 2% to 3% of patients with neuroblastoma develop opsoclonus-myoclonus. Treatment with steroids or adrenocorticotropin (ACTH), or treatment of the tumor, results in improvement of the opsoclonus-myoclonus and ataxia in one half to two thirds of patients. Symptoms may relapse with steroid withdrawal or during intercurrent febrile illnesses. Despite an initial response to steroids and treatment of the tumor, a substantial number of patients (25%–50%) are left with permanent neurologic deficits, including tremor, ataxia, and cognitive dysfunction (84–86).

It has been suggested that the presence of opsoclonus-myoclonus predicts indolent tumor behavior, independently of the patient's age, and stage of disease (87). Compared with the tumor of patients without paraneoplastic symptoms, which usually have multiple copies of the N-*myc* oncogene, the tumors of patients with opsoclonus-myoclonus show evidence for maturation to ganglioneuromas, and most, but not all, contain a single copy of N-*myc* (88,89).

Antibodies directed against neurofilaments and other neuronal antigens have been identified in serum from patients with neuroblastoma and opsoclonus-myoclonus (90). The incidence of these antibodies and their clinical significance as markers of this paraneoplastic disorder remain unknown.

In adult patients, there is a syndrome characterized by ataxia, ocular movement disorders (usually opsoclonus), and myoclonus that develops in association with anti-Ri antibodies (see Paraneoplastic Cerebellar Degeneration). Although the role of these antibodies in the pathogenesis of the disorder is unclear, the identification of the antibody is usually indicative of the paraneoplastic nature of the disorder, and the presence of an underlying tumor (usually breast or gynecologic tumor) (50).

In adults, paraneoplastic opsoclonus can develop in association with other tumors, SCLC being the most common (83,91). In these patients, the disorder may vary from opsoclonus and mild truncal ataxia to a more severe clinical syndrome characterized by opsoclonus, myoclonus, ataxia, and encephalopathy that leads to stupor and death. No antineuronal antibodies have been identified in most of these patients (91,92). Treatment with steroids, clonazepam, or plasma exchange with a protein A column may result in improvement in some patients.

A few patients with brainstem encephalopathy associated with anti-Hu antibodies may develop opsoclonus (93). One of these patients had improvement of opsoclonus with IVIg (Fadul C, et al, unpublished observations).

Paraneoplastic Retinopathy

Patients with this disorder develop subacute visual loss due to degeneration of the photoreceptor or ganglion cells of the retina (94,95). Symptoms usually precede the diagnosis of the tumor, which usually is SCLC, but other associated tumors include melanoma (96,97), gynecologic cancers (98–100), and breast cancer (101). Symptoms develop abruptly, involving one eye first, and become bilateral over days or weeks; they include photosensitivity, light-induced glare, color vision deficits, and intermittent visual obscuration, and progress to gradual loss of vision. Ophthalmologic examination demonstrates peripheral and ringlike scotomata, impaired visual acuity and color vision, and narrowing of the retinal arteries (102). Inflammatory cells in the vitreous can be identified with slit-lamp examination. The visual evoked responses may be normal, but electroretinography demonstrates reduced or flat photopic and scotopic responses, indicating involvement of the photoreceptor. The pathologic abnormalities include loss of photoreceptors or less frequently, involvement of ganglion cells. The inner retinal layers, optic nerves, and visual tracts are usually preserved (94,99). The presence of antibodies reacting with several retinal proteins (see Table 10-4) suggests an immune-mediated mechanism of retinal injury (95). A 23-kd photoreceptor calcium-binding protein of the calmodulin family, called *recoverin*, is identified by some of these antibodies (103,104). The role of these antibodies in the pathogenesis of the disorder is unknown, as recoverin affinity-purified antibodies do not react with SCLC proteins (104), and other antiretinal antibodies with other antigen reactivities have been identified (105–107). Treatment of cancer-associated retinopathy with steroids or plasmapheresis may result in symptom stabilization, but no improvement of symptoms.

Paraneoplastic Muscle Rigidity and Stiffness (Including Neuromyotonia and Stiff-Man Syndrome)

Paraneoplastic muscle rigidity and stiffness can result from several disorders of the central and peripheral nervous systems including neuromyotonia (108), encephalomyelitis (109), and stiff-man syndrome (110). The small number of patients reported, as well as the lack of rigorous electrophysiologic studies in some cases and antineuronal antibody studies in others, make it difficult to compare and identify physiopathologic mechanisms shared by these disorders.

Neuromyotonia is characterized by continuous muscle fiber activity, associated with progressive aching, stiffness, muscle cramps, myokymia, and hyperhidrosis, and can be encountered as a paraneoplastic disorder. Neuromyotonia is thought to be secondary to abnormal activity generated in the peripheral nerves, resulting in continuous muscle fiber activity. The neurologic examination may demonstrate an associated sensorimotor neuropathy, and electrophysiologic studies show bursts of high-frequency, atypical, motor unit discharges that persist after a voluntary muscle contraction has stopped. These motor discharges may continue during sleep, general anesthesia, and proximal nerve block, but disappear upon blockade of the neuromuscular junction (108). The tumors more commonly involved include SCLC (111,112) and thymoma (113). The autoimmune basis of this disorder is suggested by the demonstration of antibodies that interfere with the function of K^+ channels in patients with nonparaneoplastic neuromyotonia (114,115). Passive transfer of IgG from patients with nonparaneoplastic neuromyotonia to mice resulted in increased resistance to *d*-tubocurarine at the neuromuscular junction. For patients with paraneoplastic neuromyotonia, it is tempting to suggest that the abnormal expression of K^+ channels by some tumors triggers the production of antibodies, which results in the same neurophysiologic abnormality identified in nonparaneoplastic patients.

Paraneoplastic rigidity and "spinal myoclonus" may result from widespread dysfunction of the central nervous system, characterized by perivascular inflammatory infiltrates and neuronal degeneration mainly involving the cervical portion of the spinal cord (109,116). This disorder, called *progressive encephalomyelitis with rigidity*, is associated with SCLC (109). Patients with this disorder have not been examined for the presence of antineuronal antibodies. A woman with breast cancer and typical anti-Ri–associated opsoclonus-myoclonus and ataxia developed rigidity and muscle spasms, resulting in hip fracture (53) (see previous sections on anti-Ri and opsoclonus-myoclonus syndrome).

Stiff-man syndrome is characterized by progressive muscle stiffness, aching, muscle spasms, and rigidity. Muscle spasms are triggered by different stimuli and can lead to limb deformities and fractures. Electrophysiologic studies demonstrate continuous discharge of motor unit potentials. The tumors more commonly involved include SCLC (117), thymoma, and breast cancer (110). An autoimmune basis of the disorder was initially suggested by the identification of antibodies against glutamic acid decarboxylase (GAD) in patients who had nonparaneoplastic stiff-man syndrome (118). More recently, a subset of patients with paraneoplastic stiff-man syndrome and breast cancer were found to harbor antibodies that react with a 128-kd neuronal synaptic protein (amphiphysin) (110,119,120). Antibodies against 125- to 130-kd proteins were also identified in one patient with carcinoma of the colon and one with Hodgkin's disease (121). In patients with breast cancer, paraneoplastic stiff-man, and antiamphiphysin antibodies, treatment of the tumor and steroids may result in neurologic improvement (110).

Specific Paraneoplastic Syndromes of the Peripheral Nervous System

Paraneoplastic Sensory Neuronopathy

PSN resulting from DRG dysfunction is a usual component of PEM (31,64). About three fourths of patients with PEM have symptoms of PSN. The typical onset of

PSN includes pain and paresthesias asymmetrically involving one limb, which can lead to the misdiagnosis of radiculopathy or multineuropathy (31,77). Usually, symptoms progress rapidly (weeks) to involve other extremities and sometimes the face and trunk. Other cranial nerves may be affected, resulting in loss of taste and sensorineural deafness. Eventually, there is severe involvement of all modalities of sensation, which interferes with walking and movement of the extremities. Deep tendon reflexes are asymmetrically decreased or abolished. In more than 80% of patients with PSN, the associated tumor is SCLC (1,31,64). Sensory symptoms usually precede the diagnosis of the tumor. In patients with no known cancer, PSN should be suspected when sensory symptoms develop asymmetrically or involve the trunk and cranial nerves. Electrophysiologic studies demonstrate decreased or abolished somatosensory evoked potentials and action potentials of sensory nerves (77). Motor conduction is normal; signs of motor denervation are absent unless there is a concomitant myelitis with anterior horn involvement (78).

The pathologic hallmark of PSN is the degeneration of DRG neurons, associated with inflammatory infiltrates (mainly of T cells) surrounding neurons (Fig 10-6), and proliferation of the capsular cells (Nageotte nodules) (5,31,64). Inflammatory infiltrates are usually not restricted to DRG, and may be found in other areas of the neuraxis (encephalomyelitis) including the anterior and posterior nerve roots.

As occurs with other components of PEM, the detection of the anti-Hu antibody in the serum or CSF should direct the search for a SCLC (31). If no tumor is detected, periodic (every 6 months) clinical follow-up and CT of the chest are recommended. If the anti-Hu antibody titer is negative, the search for a neoplasm should have a wider spectrum, including other (non-SCLC) lung tumors and breast cancer.

An asymmetric sensory neuropathy may be the only presenting symptom of Sjögren's syndrome (122,123). The disorder cannot be differentiated clinically from PSN, but usually in Sjögren's syndrome patients the sensory neuropathy evolves less rapidly. Other symptoms of Sjögren's syndrome, such as xerostomia and xerophthalmia, may be absent for years (123); the diagnosis may be suspected by the detection of Ro antibodies (not always present), and confirmed by salivary gland biopsy. Pathology studies demonstrate inflammatory infiltrates and neuronal degeneration in DRG. The anti-Hu antibody is absent in patients with sensory neuropathy and Sjögren's syndrome (122,124).

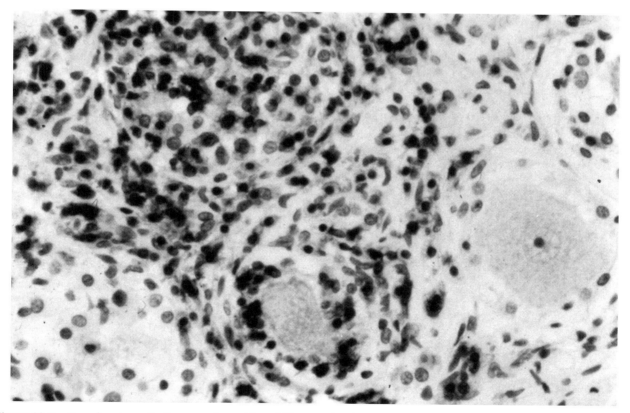

Figure 10-6.   Dorsal root ganglia from a patient with anti-Hu–associated paraneoplastic sensory neuronopathy. Note the presence of inflammatory infiltrates surrounding degenerating neurons. In the top left of the figure, there is a nodule of Nageotte. Most of the lymphocytes reacted with the T-cell marker UCHL-1.

Patients with SCLC and anti-Hu–associated PSN may develop Sjögren's syndrome as a concurrent disorder (31,124).

PSN should be distinguished from toxic neuropathies, including taxol (125–128) and *cis*-platinum neuropathy (129). The neuropathy caused by *cis*-platinum predominantly affects large fibers (proprioception and vibratory sensation), in contrast to PSN which usually affects all modalities of sensation. The properties that render the DRG selectively liable to immune and toxic attacks are poorly understood, but a contributing factor might be the incomplete blood-brain barrier at this site (130).

In patients with anti-Hu–associated PEM, the prognosis is poor, with the neurologic dysfunction being a frequent cause of death (31). If the symptoms remain limited to PSN, the prognosis is somewhat better. In a few patients, PSN may be mildly debilitating and have a more indolent course (79).

Paraneoplastic Motor Neuron Dysfunction

Of patients with cancer, those with motor neuron disorders have been divided into three groups (131,132): 1) patients with cancer and typical motor neuron disease; 2) patients with motor neuron disease as a component of paraneoplastic encephalomyelitis; and 3) patients with subacute motor neuronopathy, usually associated with lymphoma.

Motor Neuron Disease

A pathogenic association between cancer and motor neuron disease remains controversial. Although epidemiologic studies indicate that the incidence of motor neuron disorders is not increased in patients with cancer (133,134), there are well-documented patients whose motor neuron symptoms improved after treatment of the tumor, suggesting a causal relationship between the cancer and the motor neuron dysfunction. The neoplasms most commonly involved include carcinoma of the lung and kidney, and lymphoma (131,132).

Patients with lymphoma may develop a motor neuron syndrome (ALS or lower motor neuron dysfunction) associated with paraproteinemia, and increased protein concentrations and oligoclonal bands in the CSF. Electrophysiologic studies show denervation with normal conduction velocities. Two patients (one with chronic lymphocytic leukemia and the other with Hodgkin's disease) demonstrated multifocal conduction blocks on nerve conduction studies; no antibodies against GM_1 or myelin-associated glycoprotein (MAG) were identified. The postmortem study of two patients (Hodgkin's disease and follicular mixed large-cell–lymphoma) showed severe loss of motor neurons in the spinal cord, brainstem, and motor cortex, and bilateral degeneration of corticospinal tracts (135).

These findings suggest that patients with motor neuron symptoms associated with paraproteinemia, or increased protein concentrations or oligoclonal bands in

the CSF should undergo bone marrow biopsy to rule out a lymphoproliferative disorder (135,136).

Motor Neuron Dysfunction as a Component of Paraneoplastic Encephalomyelitis

Another situation in which a motor neuron syndrome can be considered paraneoplastic is when a marker of paraneoplasia, such as the anti-Hu antibody, is identified. A paraneoplastic motor neuron syndrome, which in rare instances resembles ALS, may form part of PEM (see Paraneoplastic Encephalomyelitis). These patients usually develop symptoms involving other areas of the nervous system, but in some patients the presentation of the disorder can be a subacute, rapidly evolving, motor neuron dysfunction including weakness, muscle atrophy, fasciculations, and loss or more rarely, increased reflexes and extensor plantar responses (31,137).

In patients with motor neuron disease and SCLC, other antibodies reacting with several areas of the nervous system have been described (138,139). The exact nature of the associated neuronal antigens is unknown.

Subacute Motor Neuronopathy

This disorder develops subacutely, over days or weeks, usually in patients with Hodgkin's lymphoma. Symptoms include proximal muscle weakness that predominates in the lower extremities; reflexes are decreased or abolished. Initially, symptoms may be asymmetric; fasciculations are rare, and bulbar muscles are usually spared (136). Pain and symptoms of upper motor neuron dysfunction are absent. Sensory symptoms, if any, are mild and transitory. The CSF is normal or may have mildly increased protein concentrations. This disorder usually has a benign course, independent of the activity of the neoplasm. Neurologic stabilization or spontaneous improvement is common (140,141).

Electrophysiologic studies show denervation with normal or mild slowness of motor nerve velocities. Pathologic studies demonstrate neuronal degeneration predominantly involving the anterior horn of the spinal cord, and patchy areas of segmental demyelination involving spinal nerve roots and brachial and lumbar plexuses. Inflammatory infiltrates are mild or absent.

There is some evidence that this disorder may be caused by an opportunistic viral infection of the anterior horn neurons (141,142): 1) The pathologic abnormalities resemble those of burnt-out poliomyelitis; 2) viral-like particles were found in the anterior horn of the spinal cord of one patient (141); and 3) two retroviruses, the murine leukemia virus and the human T-cell lymphotropic virus type I, can cause lymphoma and myelopathy (143). In these viral disorders it is unclear whether the virus is both neurotropic and oncogenic, or whether it induces an autoimmune response that affects the motor neurons.

Paraneoplastic motor neuronopathy should be differentiated from a lower motor neuron syndrome secondary to radiation therapy (144,145). In these patients, motor weakness predominates in the distal muscles of the lower extremities. Symptoms may stabilize, but usually do not improve. Symptoms of lower motor neuron involvement, with severe atrophy involving paraspinal muscles, flexors and extensors of the neck, and muscles of the shoulder may develop in patients with Hodgkin's lymphoma, years after mantle irradiation was completed.

Sensorimotor Neuropathies Associated with Plasma Cell Dyscrasias

Approximately 10% of patients with peripheral neuropathy of unknown origin have monoclonal gammopathy (M protein). Plasma cell dyscrasias associated with peripheral neuropathy include monoclonal gammopathy of uncertain significance (MGUS), multiple myeloma, Waldenström's macroglobulinemia, cryoglobulinemia, monoclonal gammopathy with solid tumors, monoclonal gammopathy with benign lymph node hyperplasia, gamma heavy-chain disease, and POEMS syndrome.

The main two mechanisms by which M proteins can result in neurologic dysfunction include 1) deposition of amyloid in peripheral nerves, and 2) binding of antibodies to glycoconjugates, such as MAG, GM_1, and GD_{1b}, or chondroitin sulfate C. Antibodies to glycoconjugates are mainly found in patients with IgM monoclonal gammopathy (146).

Patients with *osteolytic multiple myeloma* may develop peripheral neuropathy as a result of 1) compression of nerve roots secondary to involvement of the spine by the disease; 2) amyloid neuropathy, including symptoms of carpal tunnel compression, autonomic dysfunction (postural hypotension, sphincter dysfunction, impotence, and anhydrosis), and lancinating and burning dysesthesias; and 3) paraneoplastic dysfunction. This paraneoplastic neuropathy resembles the chronic axonal sensorimotor neuropathy seen in patients with carcinoma. The incidence is probably less than 5%. Treatment of the osteolytic myeloma with chemotherapy does not result in neurologic improvement (147).

About 2% of patients with myeloma develop *osteosclerotic myeloma*, which is characterized by a high incidence (50%) of peripheral neuropathy (148). Sensory deficits and paresthesias usually precede the diagnosis of myeloma, but eventually the motor deficits predominate. In contrast with amyloid neuropathy, pain and autonomic deficits are absent. Almost all patients have elevated protein concentrations in the CSF, with normal glucose values and cell counts. The results of nerve conduction studies are consistent with demyelinating sensorimotor neuropathy. Examination of a sural nerve biopsy specimen may reveal small foci of perivascular mononuclear cells in the epineurium, and decreased density of myelinated fibers. The serum level of M protein is relatively low (0.5–1.7 g/dL), rarely more than 3 g/dL. The paraprotein is composed of λ-light chains with IgG or IgA heavy chains. In contrast, the serum level of M protein in patients with osteolytic myeloma is higher and usually composed of κ-light chains. Also, patients with osteosclerotic myeloma are younger than those with osteolytic myeloma, have less involvement of

the bone marrow, and often have sparing of the renal function. Radiologic studies typically show sclerotic lesions in the spine, pelvic bones, and ribs. Skull and the distal aspect of long bones are usually spared. Resection or tumoricidal radiation therapy of solitary lesions results in improvement of the neuropathy (148,149).

Frequently patients with osteosclerotic myeloma develop symptoms included in the *POEMS* syndrome: *p*olyneuropathy, *o*rganomegaly (hepatosplenomegaly, lymphadenopathy), *e*ndocrinopathy (gynecomastia, impotence, testicular atrophy, low serum testosterone and thyroxine levels, high serum estrogen level, hyperglycemia), *M* protein, and *s*kin changes (hirsutism, thickening of the skin, hyperpigmentation, hyperhidrosis). Less frequently, some of these symptoms are also associated with plasma cell dyscrasias other than osteosclerotic myeloma (150).

Patients with *Waldenström's macroglobulinemia* may develop a demyelinating sensorimotor neuropathy with marked slowing of nerve conduction velocities. Sensory symptoms are prominent, as occur with the neuropathy of patients with IgM MGUS. At least one third of patients with MGUS eventually develop multiple myeloma, macroglobulinemia, amyloidosis, or a malignant lymphoproliferative disorder (151,152). About 50% of patients with IgM monoclonal proteins and peripheral neuropathy harbor IgM antibodies against MAG (147), which may be implicated in the pathogenesis of the neuropathy. The IgM paraprotein may react with MAG (anti-MAG), but in some cases the IgM paraprotein may lack anti-MAG reactivity. A minority of patients have predominant axonal degeneration. Reduction of IgM levels can improve the neuropathy.

Brachial Neuritis

Although rare, brachial neuritis similar to that observed in patients without cancer develops with increased frequency in patients with Hodgkin's disease (153,154). Pain usually precedes the development of paresthesias and motor weakness. The nerve biopsy of one patient demonstrated a decreased density of myelinated fibers with single or small groups of T cells between nerve bundles, suggesting a cytotoxic T cell–mediated immune mechanism. Treatment with prednisone can be effective.

This rare disorder should be differentiated from other frequent causes of brachial plexopathy in patients with cancer, including tumor infiltration, traumatic injury during surgery or anesthesia, and radiation injury of the plexus (1).

Acute Polyradiculoneuropathy

Acute paraneoplastic polyradiculoneuropathy can develop in association with Hodgkin's disease (155,156) and non-Hodgkin's lymphoma (152). Clinical and pathologic features resemble those of the Guillain-Barré syndrome. Pathologic studies demonstrate perivascular lymphocytic infiltration in peripheral nerve trunks, or lymphocytes penetrating Schwann cells. It has been postulated that a selective depression of cell-mediated immunity, together with an increased occurrence of viral infections, may explain the increased incidence of acute polyradiculoneuropathies in patients with Hodgkin's disease.

Patients with Hodgkin's disease (157) and other histologic tumor types (158) may develop a sensory neuropathy, which is probably a variant of chronic inflammatory demyelinating neuropathy, or a sensory variant of Guillain-Barré syndrome (159,160). Symptoms may resemble a subacute sensory neuronopathy but usually improve. The anti-Hu antibody is not detected in serum and CSF.

In patients with leukemia or lymphoma, diffuse neoplastic infiltration of the peripheral nerves may also mimic acute neuritis. Lymphomatous infiltration of the peripheral nerves has been observed in the presence of B- and and T-cell lymphomas, angiotropic lymphomas, and leukemias. The diagnosis can be made by nerve biopsy or demonstration of malignant cells in the CSF, but the absence of malignant cells does not completely rule out this complication (161,162).

Vasculitic Neuropathy

In some patients with cancer, paraneoplastic vasculitis may be confined to nerve and muscle. The tumors more commonly involved include SCLC, adenocarcinoma of the lung, prostate, and endometrium, and Hodgkin's and non-Hodgkin's lymphoma (163–165). Symptoms of mononeuritis multiplex, or painful, asymmetric sensorimotor polyneuropathy, precede the diagnosis of the tumor in about half of the patients. As a result of the muscle vasculitis, some patients may develop proximal muscle weakness. The diagnosis is suggested by the presence of elevated protein concentrations in the CSF, and confirmed by biopsy of nerve and muscle. In the nerve biopsy specimen there is infiltration of small epineural vessels by mononuclear cells. This disorder may respond to steroids.

Peripheral nerve vasculitis can develop in association with PEM and SCLC (166). It is not known whether these patients harbor anti-Hu antibodies, but at least in one patient with SCLC and vasculitic neuropathy, high titers of anti-Hu antibodies were identified (167).

Polymyositis-Dermatomyositis

The association of these disorders with cancer remains controversial, but older patients with polymyositis and particularly dermatomyositis have an increased incidence of cancer (168,169). About 15% of patients with dermatomyositis develop cancer, which is usually diagnosed by the time the neurologic symptoms develop. This risk appears to be higher for women than men (170). Cancers of the breast, lung, ovary, and stomach are the most commonly associated tumors, but Hodgkin's disease has also been reported (1).

Clinical symptoms are similar in patients with and those without cancer, and the course of the disease is independent from the tumor. Patients with dermatomyositis may present with a reddish or purplish skin rash that often precedes the proximal muscle weakness. The flexor muscles of the neck and pharyngeal and respiratory muscles may also be involved. Dysphagia occurs in at least one third of the patients (171). Respiratory muscle weakness may lead to ventilatory failure and contribute to death. Other symptoms include arthralgias and muscle contractures, myocardial inflammation leading to congestive heart failure, and interstitial lung disease. The serum creatine kinase level is usually, but not always, elevated. Electrophysiologic studies demonstrate signs of myopathy (169).

The muscle biopsy specimen shows varying degrees of mononuclear inflammatory infiltrates, which in some patients can be virtually absent. Lymphocytes are mainly found in the interstitial and perivascular areas, with B cells and CD4+ T cells predominating (172). A characteristic finding of dermatomyositis is the presence of perifascicular muscle fiber atrophy involving type I and type II fibers, believed to result from endofascicular hypoperfusion (173).

An immune-mediated intramuscular angiopathy appears to be involved in the pathogenesis of dermatomyositis. Deposits of IgG and IgM, as well as deposits of complement (including C3, C9, and membrane attack complex), are identified in muscle blood vessels (172). In patients with polymyositis, however, the endomysial inflammatory infiltrates are mainly composed of CD8+ T cells and macrophages; B cells are less prominent and have a perivascular distribution (169,172).

In as many as 20% of patients with dermatomyositis or polymyositis, other autoantibodies against several nuclear or cytoplasmic antigens have been found. An antibody against histidyl-transfer RNA synthetase, called *anti-Jo-1*, is identified in 80% of patients with associated interstitial lung disease (173).

Dermatomyositis and polymyositis usually respond to corticosteroids, which should be considered as the first therapeutic choice. It is recommended to start with a high dose, and taper to an alternate-day schedule once symptoms start improving (169,173). High-dose IVIg has proved to be effective for dermatomyositis (174).

A severe, rapidly evolving *acute necrotizing myopathy* has been observed in patients with cancer of the lung, bladder, breast, and gastrointestinal tract (175,176). Symptoms include painful proximal muscle weakness, which also involves pharyngeal and respiratory muscles, resulting in death in a few weeks. The serum creatine kinase level is elevated, and the electrophysiologic findings are consistent with myopathy. Muscle biopsy demonstrates necrosis with minimal or absent inflammation. Thick "pipestem" capillaries with deposits of complement membrane attack complex were identified in the muscle biopsy specimen of one patient, suggesting that the disorder may result from an immune-mediated microangiopathy (177).

Carcinoid Myopathy

In patients with carcinoid, a progressive myopathy may develop many years after the diagnosis of the tumor (178–180). Symptoms include proximal muscle weakness, and cramps and tenderness in the shoulder muscles. Pathologic studies show atrophy of type II fibers, with minimal or absent inflammation. It has been suggested that the myopathy is related to the increased level of circulating serotonin secreted by the tumor. Serotonin antagonists, such as cyproheptadine, might be effective in treating this myopathy (178,181).

Treatment of Paraneoplastic Neurologic Disorders

Most paraneoplastic disorders evolve independently of the course of the tumor (1). Although the paraneoplastic disorder is usually the first sign of the tumor, it may develop after the tumor is diagnosed or treated, or even when the tumor is in remission. With a few exceptions (usually disorders of the peripheral nervous system), most paraneoplastic syndromes do not improve with treatment of the tumor. Furthermore, treatment of antibody-related paraneoplastic disorders of the central nervous system with immunosuppression or immunomodulation is usually unsatisfactory (Table 10-9).

There are isolated anecdotal reports of central nervous system disorders of probable paraneoplastic ori-

gin that improved dramatically after treatment of the tumor (182–185). Antineuronal antibodies confirming the paraneoplastic nature of the disorder were not studied or identified in most of these patients, and therefore, other mechanisms of neuronal damage cannot be completely ruled out. In a large series of patients with antibody-associated paraneoplastic disorders of the central nervous system, no significant neurologic improvement was seen after treatment of the tumor, or after treatment of the paraneoplastic disorder with plasmapheresis or IVIg (46,47).

Removal or treatment of the tumor (source of antigen) can be very effective for paraneoplastic disorders of the peripheral nervous system, particularly those involving the neuromuscular junction, such as LEMS (usually associated with SCLC) (186) and myasthenia gravis (associated with thymoma) (8). Treatment of osteosclerotic myeloma can result in dramatic improvement of the sensorimotor neuropathy associated with this disorder (148,149), although most paraneoplastic peripheral neuropathies do not usually improve with treatment of the tumor. It is important to recognize that some peripheral neuropathies, such as brachial neuritis, acute polyradiculoneuritis (Guillain-Barré syn-

Table 10-9.
Paraneoplastic Disorders: Response to Therapy

Paraneoplastic disorders that usually respond to treatment
  Dermatomyositis (steroids, IVIg, immunosuppression)
  Lambert-Eaton myasthenic syndrome (tumor, plasmapheresis, IVIg)
  Myasthenia gravis (tumor, plasmapheresis, IVIg, immunosuppression)
  Carcinoid myopathy (tumor, cyproheptadine)
  Opsoclonus-myoclonus (pediatrics) (steroids, ACTH, tumor)
  Peripheral neuropathy and osteosclerotic myeloma (tumor resection)
Paraneoplastic disorders that may respond to treatment
  Paraneoplastic vasculitis of nerve and muscle (steroids)
  Opsoclonus-myoclonus (adult population) (steroids, tumor, protein A column, clonazepam, diazepam, baclofen)
  Paraneoplastic cerebellar degeneration and Hodgkin's disease (tumor)
  Opsoclonus/ataxia and anti-R antibodies (steroids, cyclophosphamide)
  Acute polyradiculopathy (Guillain-Barré) associated with Hodgkin's lymphoma (tumor, plasmapheresis, IVIg)
Paraneoplastic disorders that usually do not respond to treatment
  Paraneoplastic cerebellar degeneration associated with:
    Anti-Hu antibodies (SCLC)
    Anti-Yo antibodies (cancer of ovary, breast)
    SCLC without anti-Hu antibodies
  Paraneoplastic sensory neuronopathy and encephalomyelitis associated with anti-Hu antibodies (may include):
    Limbic encephalopathy (steroids)
    Brainstem encephalopathy
    Cerebellar degeneration
    Myelopathy
    Autonomic dysfunction (central or peripheral)
  Cancer-associated retinopathy
Paraneoplastic disorders that may improve spontaneously
  Acute motor neuronopathy and lymphoma
  Paraneoplastic cerebellar disorder associated with Hodgkin's
  Acute polyradiculopathy associated with Hodgkin's
  Limbic encephalopathy
  Opsoclonus-myoclonus (pediatric and adult population)

IVIg = intravenous immunoglobulin; ACTH = adrenocorticotropin; SCLC = small-cell lung carcinoma.

drome), and acute sensory neuropathies (probably sensory variants of Guillain-Barré syndrome) associated with Hodgkin's disease may improve spontaneously.

In addition to treating the tumor, there have been several endeavors to treat the immune response known, or suspected, to be involved in the paraneoplastic disorder. Table 10-9 summarizes the response of these disorders to treatment, including plasma exchange, IVIg, and immunosuppressant drugs. In general, the antibody-mediated disorders of the neuromuscular junction and peripheral nervous system are the disorders that give more satisfactory results. Plasma exchange is effective for LEMS and myasthenia gravis (8,187); these disorders along with dermatomyositis may also respond to IVIg (174,188). Steroids may result in dramatic improvement of paraneoplastic vasculitis of peripheral nerve and muscle.

Although there are reports of patients with paraneoplastic disorders of the central nervous system who may have benefited from immunosuppression (54,91,189–191), large series of patients with anti-Hu– or anti-Yo–related syndromes did not show significant improvement after plasmapheresis or IVIg, with or without concomitant treatment of the tumor (46,47).

The design and evaluation of treatments of paraneoplastic syndromes have important limitations (Table 10-10), including the following: 1) These diseases are very uncommon; thus, no isolated medical center is likely to accrue enough patients to conduct a prospective clinical trial. 2) The diagnosis is difficult, particularly for those disorders not associated with markers (such as paraneoplastic antineuronal antibodies), or for which no specific tests (such as repetitive stimulation for LEMS) are available. It might be that some patients who had improvement of a neurologic disorder after treatment of the tumor had central nervous system micrometastases that escaped conventional radiologic techniques. 3) Most paraneoplastic syndromes of the central nervous system are associated with subacute and severe neuronal destruction. For example, patients who die from anti-Hu–, anti-Yo–, or anti-Ri–associated paraneoplastic disorders usually have a severe loss of neurons or Purkinje cells that explains the lack of improvement of symptoms, even when treatments are initiated very early (23,31,38,192). Therefore, one can only evaluate treatment if it is given very early in the course of the disease, when neurons are not irreversibly damaged. 4) Because the disease tends to stabilize sponta-

Table 10-10.
General Problems in Designing Therapy for Paraneoplastic Disorders

Paraneoplastic syndromes are rare
Difficulty to confirm the diagnosis
Subacute neuronal destruction
Spontaneous stabilization of symptoms
Spontaneous remission of symptoms
Pathogenesis not well understood
Lack of animal models

Table 10-11.
Immunologic Treatment of Paraneoplastic Syndromes

Remove source of antigen (treat the tumor)
 Surgery
 Radiation therapy
 Chemotherapy
Suppress B-cell response/remove antineuronal antibodies
 Plasmapheresis
 Protein A immunoadsorption
 Intravenous immunoglobulin
 Immunosuppressive drugs
 Radiation of lymph nodes, central nervous system
Suppress cytotoxic T cells (CD8)
 Irradiation, steroids, cyclosporine, FK 506
Increase the function of suppressor T cells
 Interferon beta
Suppress the function of helper T cells
 Anti-CD4 antibodies
Interfere with autoreactive T-cell activation
 Compete for antigen binding with "designed" peptides
 Anti-MHC monoclonal antibodies to inhibit MHC
  recognition
 Anti-TCR
 Anti-CD4
Induce tolerance
 Oral administration of paraneoplastic antigen
Suppress inflammation
 Steroids
 Nonsteroidal anti-inflammatory drugs

MHC = major histocompatibility complex proteins; TCR = T-cell receptor.

neously, any treatment that appears to result in arrest or stabilization of symptoms does not indicate that the therapy has been effective. 5) Some disorders (opsoclonus, myoclonus, acute sensory neuropathy associated with Hodgkin's) may improve dramatically without treatment. Therefore, any other treatment given concurrently may seem to be effective.

All investigators of paraneoplastic disorders and the physicians who take care of these patients should recognize these problems and caveats in designing and evaluating treatments for these disorders. Until the pathogenesis of paraneoplastic disorders is better understood, the management of these patients should be based on the prompt detection and treatment of the tumor. For the disorders in which no clear responses to any therapy have been identified, the efforts should be directed to early diagnosis of the syndrome and, probably, aggressive immunotherapy (Table 10-11), which may include plasma exchange, IVIg, high-dose steroids, and immunosuppressants such as cyclophosphamide and cyclosporine.

References

1. Posner JB. *Neurologic complications of cancer*. Philadelphia: FA Davis, 1995.
2. Posner JB, Furneaux HM. Paraneoplastic syndromes. In: Waksman BH, ed. *Immunologic mechanisms in neu-*

rologic and psychiatric disease. New York: Raven, 1990:187–219.

3. Brouwer B. Beitrag zur Kenntnis der chronischen diffusen Kleinhirnerkrankungen. *Mendels Neurol Zentralbl* 1919;38:674–682.

4. Lowry SF, Moldawer LL. Tumor necrosis factor and other cytokines in the pathogenesis of cancer cachexia. *Princ Pract Oncol Updates* 1990;4:1–12.

5. Denny-Brown D. Primary sensory neuropathy with muscular changes associated with carcinoma. *J Neurol Neurosurg Psychiatry* 1948;11:73–87.

6. Lang B, Newsom-Davis J, Wray D, et al. Autoimmune aetiology for myasthenic (Eaton-Lambert) syndrome. *Lancet* 1981;2:224–226.

7. Chester KA, Lang B, Gill J, et al. Lambert-Eaton syndrome antibodies: reaction with membranes from a small cell lung cancer xenograft. *J Immunol* 1988;18:97–104.

8. Drachman DB. Myasthenia gravis. *N Engl J Med* 1994; 330:1797–1810.

9. Graus F, Cordon-Cardo C, Posner JB. Neuronal antinuclear antibody in sensory neuronopathy from lung cancer. *Neurology* 1985;35:538–543.

10. Graus F, Elkon KB, Cordon-Cardo C, Posner JB. Sensory neuronopathy and small cell lung cancer: antineuronal antibody that also reacts with the tumor. *Am J Med* 1986;80:45–52.

11. Tanaka K, Tanaka M, Onodera O, et al. Passive transfer and active immunization with the recombinant leucine-zipper (Yo) protein as an attempt to establish an animal model of paraneoplastic cerebellar degeneration. *J Neurol Sci* 1994;127:153–158.

12. Sillevis Smitt PAE, Manley GT, Posner JB. Immunization with the paraneoplastic encephalomyelitis antigen HuD does not cause neurologic disease in mice. *Neurology* 1995;45:1873–1878.

13. Graus F, Illa I, Agusti M, et al. Effect of intraventricular injection of anti-Purkinje cell antibody (anti-Yo) in a guinea pig model. *J Neurol Sci* 1991;106:82–87.

14. Dalmau J, Furneaux HM, Gralla RJ, et al. Detection of the anti-Hu antibody in the serum of patients with small cell lung cancer—a quantitative Western blot analysis. *Ann Neurol* 1990;27:544–552.

15. Furneaux HM, Reich L, Posner JB. Autoantibody synthesis in the central nervous system of patients with paraneoplastic syndromes. *Neurology* 1990;40:1085–1091.

16. Graus F, Segurado OG, Tolosa E. Selective concentration of anti-Purkinje cell antibody in the CSF of two patients with paraneoplastic cerebellar degeneration. *Acta Neurol Scand* 1988;78:210–213.

17. Brashear HR, Caccamo DV, Heck A, Keeney PM. Localisation of antibody in the CNS of a patient with paraneoplastic encephalomyelitis. *Neurology* 1991;41:1583–1587.

18. Szabo A, Dalmau J, Manley G, et al. HuD, a paraneoplastic encephalomyelitis antigen, contains RNA-binding domains and is homologous to Elav and Sex-lethal. *Cell* 1991;67:325–333.

19. Anderson NE, Rosenblum MK, Graus F, et al. Autoantibodies in paraneoplastic syndromes associated with small-cell lung cancer. *Neurology* 1988;38:1391–1398.

20. Graus F, Ribalta T, Campo E, et al. Immunohistochemical analysis of the immune reaction in the nervous system in paraneoplastic encephalomyelitis. *Neurology* 1990;40:219–222.

21. Jean WC, Dalmau J, Ho A, Posner JB. Analysis of the IgG subclass distribution and inflammatory infiltrates in patients with anti-Hu associated paraneoplastic encephalomyelitis. *Neurology* 1994;44:140–147.

22. Hetzel DJ, Stanhope R, O'Neill BP, Lennon VA. Gynecologic cancer in patients with subacute cerebellar degeneration predicted by anti-Purkinje cell antibodies and limited in metastatic volume. *Mayo Clin Proc* 1990;65: 1558–1563.

23. Verschuuren J, Chuang L, Rosenblum MK, et al. Inflammatory infiltrates and complete absence of Purkinje cells in anti-Yo associated paraneoplastic cerebellar degeneration. *Acta Neuropathol (Berl)* 1996;91:519–525.

24. Dalmau J, Furneaux HM, Rosenblum MK, et al. Detection of the anti-Hu antibody in specific regions of the nervous system and tumor from patients with paraneoplastic encephalomyelitis/sensory neuronopathy. *Neurology* 1991;41:1757–1764.

25. Dalmau J, Furneaux HM, Cordon-Cardo C, Posner JB. The expression of the Hu (paraneoplastic encephalomyelitis/sensory neuronopathy) antigen in human normal and tumor tissues. *Am J Pathol* 1992;141:881–886.

26. Liu S, Mezrich J, Berk J, et al. Expression of Purkinje-cell antigens in ovarian tumor, and presence of anti-Purkinje cell antibodies in the serum of patients without paraneoplastic cerebellar degeneration. *Neurology* 1995; 45(suppl 4):A228–A229. Abstract.

27. Dalmau J, Graus F, Cheung N-K V, et al. Major histocompatibility (MHC) proteins, anti-Hu antibodies and paraneoplastic encephalomyelitis in neuroblastoma and small cell lung cancer. *Cancer* 1995;75:99–109.

28. Tanaka M, Tanaka K, Tsuji S. HLA antigens in paraneoplastic cerebellar degeneration associated with anti-Yo antibody. *Neurodegeneration* 1994;3:341–342.

29. Torvik A, Slettebo M. Encephalomyelitis with polyneuropathy. *Acta Neurol Scand* 1980;61:287–297.

30. O'Neill JH, Murray NM, Newsom-Davis J. The Lambert-Eaton myasthenic syndrome. A review of 50 cases. *Brain* 1988;111:577–596.

31. Dalmau J, Graus F, Rosenblum MK, et al. Anti-Hu-associated paraneoplastic encephalomyelitis/sensory neuronopathy. A clinical study of 71 patients. *Medicine* 1992;71:59–72.

32. Krakawer J, Balmaceda CM, Posner JB, Dalmau J. Anti-Yo associated paraneoplastic cerebellar degeneration in a man with adenocarcinoma of unknown origin. *Neurology* 1996;46:1486–1487.

33. Greenlee JE, Brashear HR. Antibodies to cerebellar Purkinje cells in patients with paraneoplastic cerebellar degeneration and ovarian carcinoma. *Ann Neurol* 1983;14:609–613.

34. Jaeckle KA, Graus F, Houghton A, et al. Autoimmune response of patients with paraneoplastic cerebellar degeneration to a Purkinje cell cytoplasmic protein antigen. *Ann Neurol* 1985;18:592–600.

35. Henson RA, Urich H. Cortical cerebellar degeneration. In: Henson RA, Urich H, eds. *Cancer and the nervous system.* Oxford, UK: Blackwell Scientific, 1982:346–367.

36. Brain WR, Daniel PM, Greenfield JG. Subacute cortical cerebellar degeneration and its relation to carcinoma. *J Neurol Neurosurg Psychiatry* 1951;14:59–75.

37. Anderson NE, Rosenblum MK, Posner JB. Paraneoplastic cerebellar degeneration: clinical-immunological correlations. *Ann Neurol* 1988;24:559–567.

38. Peterson K, Rosenblum MK, Kotanides H, Posner JB. Paraneoplastic cerebellar degeneration. I. A clinical analysis of 55 anti-Yo antibody-positive patients. *Neurology* 1992;42:1931–1937.

39. Hammack JE, Kotanides H, Rosenblum MK, Posner JB. Paraneoplastic cerebellar degeneration. II. Clinical and

immunologic findings in 21 patients with Hodgkin's disease. *Neurology* 1992;42:1938–1943.

40. Furneaux HM, Rosenblum MK, Dalmau J, et al. Selective expression of Purkinje-cell antigens in tumor tissue from patients with paraneoplastic cerebellar degeneration. *N Engl J Med* 1990;322:1844–1851.

41. Dropcho EJ, Chen Y-T, Posner JB, Old LJ. Cloning of a brain protein identified by autoantibodies from a patient with paraneoplastic cerebellar degeneration. *Proc Natl Acad Sci USA* 1987;84:4552–4556.

42. Fathallah-Shaykh H, Wolf S, Wong E, et al. Cloning of a leucine zipper protein recognized by the sera of patients with antibody-associated paraneoplastic cerebellar degeneration. *Proc Natl Acad Sci USA* 1991;88:3451–3454.

43. Sakai K, Mitchell DJ, Tsukamoto T, Steinman L. Isolation of a complementary DNA clone encoding an autoantigen recognized by an anti-neuronal cell antibody from a patient with paraneoplastic cerebellar degeneration. *Ann Neurol* 1990;28:692–698.

44. Felician O, Renard JL, Vega F, et al. Paraneoplastic cerebellar degeneration with anti-Yo antibody in a man. *Neurology* 1995;45:1226–1227.

45. Lennon VA. Anti-Purkinje cell cytoplasmic and neuronal nuclear antibodies aid diagnosis of paraneoplastic autoimmune neurological disorders. *J Neurol Neurosurg Psychiatry* 1989;52:1438–1439.

46. Graus F, Vega F, Delattre J-Y, et al. Plasmapheresis and antineoplastic treatment in CNS paraneoplastic syndromes with antineuronal autoantibodies. *Neurology* 1992;42:536–540.

47. Uchuya M, Graus F, Vega F, et al. Intravenous immunoglobulin therapy in paraneoplastic neurologic syndromes with antineuronal autoantibodies. *J Neurol Neurosurg Psychiatry* 1996;60:388–392.

48. Stark E, Wurster U, Patzold U, et al. Immunological and clinical response to immunosuppressive treatment in paraneoplastic cerebellar degeneration. *Arch Neurol* 1995;52:814–818.

49. Trotter JL, Hendin BA, Osterland CK. Cerebellar degeneration with Hodgkin's disease: an immunological study. *Arch Neurol* 1976;33:660–661.

50. Luque FA, Furneaux HM, Ferziger R, et al. Anti-Ri: an antibody associated with paraneoplastic opsoclonus and breast cancer. *Ann Neurol* 1991;29:241–251.

51. Budde-Steffen C, Anderson NE, Graus F, et al. An anti-neuronal autoantibody in paraneoplastic opsoclonus. *Ann Neurol* 1988;23:528–531.

52. Escudero D, Barnadas A, Codina M, et al. Anti-Ri associated paraneoplastic neurologic disorder without opsoclonus in a patient with breast cancer. *Neurology* 1993;43:1605–1606.

53. Casado JL, Gil-Peralta A, Graus F, et al. Anti-Ri antibodies associated with opsoclonus and progressive encephalo-myelitis with rigidity. *Neurology* 1994;44: 1521–1522.

54. Dropcho EJ, Kline LB, Riser J. Antineuronal (anti-Ri) autoantibodies in a patient with steroid-responsive opsoclonus myoclonus. *Neurology* 1993;43:207–211.

55. Buckanovich RJ, Posner JB, Darnell RB. Nova, the paraneoplastic Ri antigen, is homologous to an RNA-binding protein and is specifically expressed in the developing motor system. *Neuron* 1993;11:657–672.

56. Gahring LC, Twyman RE, Greenlee JE, Rogers SW. Autoantibodies to neuronal glutamate receptors in patients with paraneoplastic neurodegenerative syndrome enhance receptor activation. *Mol Med* 1995;1:245–253.

57. Degenhardt A, Hoard R, Duvoisin RM, et al. Glutamate receptor antibodies and paraneoplastic neurologic disorders. *Neurology* 1996;46:A410. Abstract.

58. Tanaka K, Yamazaki M, Sato S, et al. Antibodies to brain proteins in paraneoplastic cerebellar degeneration. *Neurology* 1986;36:1169–1172.

59. Anderson NE, Budde-Steffen C, Wiley RG, et al. A variant of the anti-Purkinje cell antibody in a patient with paraneoplastic cerebellar degeneration. *Neurology* 1988; 38:1018–1026.

60. Tsukamoto T, Yamamoto H, Iwasaki Y, et al. Antineural autoantibodies in patients with paraneoplastic cerebellar degeneration. *Arch Neurol* 1989;46:1225–1229.

61. Clouston PD, Saper CB, Arbizu T, et al. Paraneoplastic cerebellar degeneration. III. Cerebellar degeneration, cancer, and the Lambert-Eaton myasthenic syndrome. *Neurology* 1992;42:1944–1950.

62. Goldstein JM, Waxman SG, Vollmer TL, et al. Subacute cerebellar degeneration and Lambert-Eaton myasthenic syndrome associated with antibodies to voltage-gated calcium channels: differential effect of immunosuppressive therapy on central and peripheral defects. *J Neurol Neurosurg Psychiatry* 1994;57:1138–1139.

63. Lennon VA, Kryzer TJ, Griesmann GE, et al. Calcium-channel antibodies in the Lambert-Eaton syndrome and other paraneoplastic syndromes. *N Engl J Med* 1995; 332:1467–1474.

64. Henson RA, Urich H. Encephalomyelitis with carcinoma. In: Henson RA, Urich H, eds. *Cancer and the nervous system.* Oxford, UK: Blackwell Scientific, 1982:314–345.

65. Levine TD, Gao F, King PH, et al. Hel-N1: an autoimmune RNA-binding protein with specificity for 3'uridylate-rich untranslated regions of growth factor mRNAs. *Mol Cell Biol* 1993;13:3494–3504.

66. Dropcho EJ, King PH. Autoantibodies against the Hel-N1 RNA-binding protein among patients with lung carcinoma: an association with type I anti-neuronal nuclear antibodies. *Ann Neurol* 1994;36:200–205.

67. Manley GT, Sillevis Smitt P, Dalmau J, Posner JB. Hu antigens: reactivity with Hu antibodies, tumor expression, and major immunogenic sites. *Ann Neurol* 1995;38:102–110.

68. Fisher PG, Wechsler DS, Singer HS. Anti-Hu antibody in a neuroblastoma associated paraneoplastic syndrome. *Pediatr Neurol* 1994;10:309–312.

69. Corsellis JAN, Goldberg GJ, Norton AR. "Limbic encephalitis" and its association with carcinoma. *Brain* 1968;91:481–496.

70. Alamowitch S, Graus F, Benyahia B, et al. Limbic encephalitis and small-cell lung cancer: clinical and immunological features. *Neurology* 1995;45:319–320. Abstract.

71. Mason WP, Graus F, Valldeoriola F, et al. Paraneoplastic cerebellar degeneration (PCD) in small cell lung cancer (SCLC): impact of anti-Hu antibody (HuAb) on clinical presentation and survival. *Neurology* (in press).

72. Lennon VA, Sas DF, Busk MF, et al. Enteric neuronal autoantibodies in pseudoobstruction with small cell lung carcinoma. *Gastroenterology* 1991;100:137–142.

73. Condom E, Vidal A, Rota R, et al. Paraneoplastic intestinal pseudo-obstruction associated with high titres of Hu autoantibodies. *Virchows Arch A Pathol Anat* 1993;423:507–511.

74. Thomas JP, Shields R. Associated autonomic dysfunction and carcinoma of the pancreas. *BMJ* 1970;4:32.

75. Veilleux M, Bernier JP, Lamarche JB. Paraneoplastic encephalomyelitis and subacute dysautonomia due to an occult atypical carcinoid tumor of the lung. *Can J Neurol Sci* 1990;17:324–328.

76. Dirr LY, Elster AD, Donofrio PD, Smith M. Evolution of brain MRI abnormalities in limbic encephalitis. *Neurology* 1990;40:1304–1306.

77. Chalk CH, Windebank AJ, Kimmel DW, McManis PG. The distinctive clinical features of paraneoplastic sensory neuronopathy. *Can J Neurol Sci* 1992;19:346–351.

78. Graus F, Elkon KB, Lloberes P. Neuronal antinuclear antibody (anti-Hu) in paraneoplastic encephalomyelitis simulating acute polyneuritis. *Acta Neurol Scand* 1987; 75:249–252.

79. Graus F, Bonaventura I, Uchuya M, et al. Indolent anti-Hu associated paraneoplastic sensory neuropathy. *Neurology* 1994;44:2258–2261.

80. Dropcho E, Payne R. Paraneoplastic opsoclonus-myoclonus: association with medullary thyroid carcinoma and review of the literature. *Arch Neurol* 1986;43: 410–415.

81. Ridley A, Kennard C, Scholtz CL, et al. Omnipause neurons in two cases of opsoclonus associated with oat cell carcinoma of the lung. *Brain* 1987;110:1699–1709.

82. Dyken P, Kolar O. Dancing eyes, dancing feet: infantile polymyoclonia. *Brain* 1968;91:305–320.

83. Anderson NE, Budde-Steffen C, Rosenblum MK, et al. Opsoclonus, myoclonus, ataxia, and encephalopathy in adults with cancer: a distinct paraneoplastic syndrome. *Medicine* 1988;67:100–109.

84. Lott I, Kinsbourne M. Myoclonic encephalopathy of infants. *Adv Neurol* 1986;43:127–136.

85. Boltshauser E, Deonna T, Hirt HR. Myoclonic encephalopathy of infants, or "dancing eyes syndrome." *Helv Paediat Acta* 1979;34:119–133.

86. Marshall PC, Brett EM, Wilson J. Myoclonic encephalopathy of childhood (the dancing eye syndrome): a long-term follow-up study. *Neurology* 1978;28:348.

87. Altman AJ, Baehner RL. Favorable prognosis for survival in children with coincident opso-myoclonus and neuroblastoma. *Cancer* 1976;37:846–852.

88. Cohn SL, Salwen H, Herst CV, et al. Single copies of the N-myc oncogene in neuroblastomas from children presenting with the syndrome of opsoclonus-myoclonus. *Cancer* 1988;62:723–726.

89. Hiyama E, Yokoyama T, Ichikawa T, et al. Poor outcome in patients with advanced stage neuroblastoma and coincident opsomyoclonus syndrome. *Cancer* 1994;74: 1821–1826.

90. Connolly AM, Pestronk A, Noetzel MJ, et al. Autoantibodies in childhood opsoclonus-myoclonus syndrome. *Ann Neurol* 1995;38:505.

91. Cher LM, Hochberg FH, Teruya J, et al. Therapy for paraneoplastic neurologic syndromes in six patients with protein A column immunoadsorption. *Cancer* 1995;75:1678–1683.

92. Graus F, Cordon-Cardo C, Cho ES, Posner JB. Opsoclonus and oat cell carcinoma of the lung: lack of evidence for anti-CNS antibodies. *Lancet* 1984;1:1479.

93. Hersh B, Dalmau J, Dangond F, et al. Paraneoplastic opsoclonus-myoclonus associated with anti-Hu antibody. *Neurology* 1994;44:1754–1755.

94. Buchanan TAS, Gardiner TA, Archer DB. An ultrastructural study of retinal photoreceptor degeneration associated with bronchial carcinoma. *Am J Ophthalmol* 1984;97:277–287.

95. Thirkill CE, Fitzgerald P, Sergott RC, et al. Cancer-associated retinopathy (CAR syndrome) with antibodies reacting with retinal, optic nerve, and cancer cells. *N Engl J Med* 1989;321:1589–1594.

96. Berson EL, Lessell S. Paraneoplastic night blindness with malignant melanoma. *Am J Ophthalmol* 1988;106: 307–311.

97. Milam AH, Saari JC, Jacobson SG, et al. Autoantibodies against retinal bipolar cells in cutaneous melanoma-associated retinopathy. *Invest Ophthalmol Vis Sci* 1993; 34:91–100.

98. Campo E, Brunier MN, Merino MJ. Small cell carcinoma of the endometrium with associated ocular paraneoplastic syndrome. *Cancer* 1992;69:2283–2288.

99. Sawyer RA, Selhorst JB, Zimmerman LE, Hoyt WF. Blindness caused by photoreceptor degeneration as a remote effect of cancer. *Am J Ophthalmol* 1976;81: 606–613.

100. Keltner JL, Roth AM, Chang RS. Photoreceptor degeneration. *Arch Ophthalmol* 1983;101:564–569.

101. Klingele TG, Burde RM, Rappazzo JL, et al. Paraneoplastic retinopathy. *J Clin Neuroophthalmol* 1984;4: 239–245.

102. Jacobson DM, Thirkill CE, Tipping SJ. A clinical triad to diagnose paraneoplastic retinopathy. *Ann Neurol* 1990;28:162–167.

103. Polans AS, Buczylko J, Crabb J, Palczewski K. A photoreceptor calcium binding protein is recognized by autoantibodies obtained from patients with cancer-associated retinopathy. *J Cell Biol* 1991;112:981–989.

104. Adamus G, Guy J, Schmied JL, et al. Role of anti-recoverin autoantibodies in cancer-associated retinopathy. *Invest Ophthalmol Vis Sci* 1993;34:2626–2633.

105. Rizzo JF, Gittinger JW. Selective immunohistochemical staining in the paraneoplastic retinopathy syndrome. *Ophthalmology* 1992;99:1286–1295.

106. Grunwald GB, Kornguth SE, Towfighi J, et al. Autoimmune basis for visual paraneoplastic syndrome in patients with small cell lung carcinoma. *Cancer* 1987;60: 780–786.

107. Kornguth SE, Klein R, Appen R, Choate J. Occurrence of anti-retinal ganglion cell antibodies in patients with small cell carcinoma of the lung. *Cancer* 1982;50: 1289–1293.

108. Newsom-Davis J, Mills KR. Immunological associations of acquired neuromyotonia (Isaacs' syndrome). *Brain* 1993;116:453–469.

109. Whitely AM, Swash M, Urich H. Progressive encephalomyelitis with rigidity. *Brain* 1976;99:27–42.

110. Folli F, Solimena M, Cofiell R, et al. Autoantibodies to a 128-kd synaptic protein in three women with the stiff-man syndrome and breast cancer. *N Engl J Med* 1993;328:546–551.

111. Waerness E. Neuromyotonia and bronchial carcinoma. *Electromyogr Clin Neurophysiol* 1974;14:527–535.

112. Walsh JC. Neuromyotonia: an unusual presentation of intrathoracic malignancy. *J Neurol Neurosurg Psychiatry* 1976;39:1086–1091.

113. Garcia-Merino A, Cabello A, Mora JS, Liaño H. Continuous muscle fiber activity, peripheral neuropathy, and thymoma. *Ann Neurol* 1991;29:215–218.

114. Sinha S, Newsom-Davis J, Mills K, et al. Autoimmune etiology for acquired neuromyotonia (Isaacs' syndrome). *Lancet* 1991;338:75–77.

115. Shillito P, Molenaar PC, Vincent A, et al. Acquired neuromyotonia: evidence for autoantibodies directed against K+ channels of peripheral nerves. *Ann Neurol* 1995;38:714–722.

116. Roobol TH, Kazzaz BA, Vecht CHJ. Segmental rigidity and spinal myoclonus as a paraneoplastic syndrome. *J Neurol Neurosurg Psychiatry* 1987;50:628–631.

117. Bateman DE, Weller RO, Kennedy P. Stiffman syndrome: a rare paraneoplastic disorder? *J Neurol Neurosurg Psychiatry* 1990;53:695–696.

118. Solimena M, Folli F, Aparisi R, et al. Autoantibodies to GABA-ergic neurons and pancreatic beta cells in stiffman syndrome. *N Engl J Med* 1990;322:1555–1560.

119. De Camilli P, Thomas A, Cofiell R, et al. The synaptic vesicle-associated protein amphiphysin is the 128-kD autoantigen of stiff-man syndrome with breast cancer. *J Exp Med* 1993;178:2219–2223.

120. David C, Solimena M, De Camilli P. Autoimmunity in stiff-man syndrome with breast cancer is targeted to the C-terminal region of human amphiphysin, a protein similar to the yeast proteins, Rvs167 and Rvs161. *FEBS Lett* 1994;351:73–79.

121. Grimaldi LM, Martino G, Braghi S, et al. Heterogeneity of autoantibodies in stiff-man syndrome. *Ann Neurol* 1993;34:57–64.

122. Graus F, Pou A, Kanterewizc E, Anderson NE. Sensory neuronopathy and Sjögren's syndrome: clinical and immunologic study of two patients. *Neurology* 1988;38:1637–1639.

123. Font J, Valls J, Cervera R, et al. Pure sensory neuropathy in patients with primary Sjögren's syndrome: clinical, immunological, and electromyographic findings. *Ann Rheumat Dis* 1990;49:775–778.

124. Sillevis-Smitt P, Manley G, Moll JWB, et al. Pitfalls in the diagnosis of auto-antibodies that are associated with paraneoplastic neurological disease. *Neurology* (in press).

125. Lipton RB, Apfel SC, Dutcher JP. Taxol produces a predominantly sensory neuropathy. *Neurology* 1989;39:368–373.

126. Philips WEJ, Mills JHL, Charbonneau SM, et al. Subacute toxicity of pyridoxine hydrochloride in the beagle dog. *Toxicol Appl Pharmacol* 1978;44:323–333.

127. Spencer PS, Schaumburg HH. Pathobiology of neurotoxic axonal degeneration. In: Waxman SG, ed. *Physiology and pathobiology of axons*. New York: Raven, 1978:265–282.

128. Schaumburg HH, Kaplan J, Windebank A, et al. Sensory neuropathy from pyridoxin abuse. *N Engl J Med* 1983;309:445–448.

129. Roelofs RI, Hrushesky W, Robin J, Rosenberg L. Peripheral sensory neuropathy and cisplatin chemotherapy. *Neurology* 1984;34:934–938.

130. Jacobs JM, MacFarlane RM, Cavanagh JB. Vascular leakage in the dorsal root ganglia of the rat, studied with horseradish peroxidase. *J Neurol Sci* 1976;29:95–107.

131. Rosenfed MR, Dalmau J. Paraneoplastic syndromes and progressive motor dysfunction. *Semin Neurol* 1993;13:291–298.

132. Rosenfeld MR, Posner JB. Paraneoplastic motor neuron disease. *Adv Neurol* 1991;56:445–459.

133. Jokelainen M. The epidemiology of amyotrofic lateral sclerosis in Finland: a study based on the death certificates of 421 patients. *J Neurol Sci* 1976;29:55–63.

134. Bharucha NE, Schoenberg BS, Raven RH, et al. Geographic distribution of motor neuron disease and correlation with possible etiologic factors. *Neurology* 1983;33:911–915.

135. Younger DS, Rowland LP, Latov N, et al. Lymphoma, motor neuron diseases, and amyotrophic lateral sclerosis. *Ann Neurol* 1991;29:78–86.

136. Rowland LP, Schneck SA. Neuromuscular disorders associated with malignant neoplastic disease. *J Chronic Dis* 1963;16:777–795.

137. Forsyth PA, Dalmau J, Graus F, Posner JB. Paraneoplastic motor neuron disease (MND). *Ann Neurol* 1993;34:277.

138. Dhib-Jalbut S, Liwnicz BH. Immunocytochemical binding of serum IgG from a patient with oat cell tumor and paraneoplastic motor neuron disease to normal human cerebral cortex and molecular layer of the cerebellum. *Acta Neuropathol (Berl)* 1986;69:96–102.

139. Wong MCW, Salanga VD, Chou S, et al. Immune associated paraneoplastic motor neuron disease and limbic encephalopathy. *Muscle Nerve* 1987;10:661–662.

140. Schold SC, Cho ES, Somasundaram M, Posner JB. Subacute motor neuronopathy: a remote effect of lymphoma. *Ann Neurol* 1979;5:271–287.

141. Walton JN, Tomlinson BE, Pearce GW. Subacute poliomyelitis and Hodgkin's disease. *J Neurol Sci* 1968;6:435–445.

142. Andrews Jm, Gardner MB. Lower motor neuron degeneration associated with type C RNA virus infection in mice; neuropathological features. *J Neuropathol Exp Neurol* 1974;33:2288–2297.

143. Vernant JC, Maurs L, Gesain A, et al. Endemic tropical spastic paraparesis associated with human T-lymphotropic virus type I: a clinical and seroepidemiologic study of 25 cases. *Ann Neurol* 1987;21:123–131.

144. Sadowsky CH, Sachs E Jr, Ochoa J. Postradiation motor neuron syndrome. *Arch Neurol* 1976;33:786–787.

145. Kristensen O, Melgard B, Schiodt AV. Radiation myelopathy of the lumbosacral spinal cord. *Acta Neurol Scand* 1977;56:217–222.

146. Nobile-Orazio E, Manfredini E, Carpo M, et al. Frequency and clinical correlates of anti-neural IgM antibodies in neuropathy associated with IgM monoclonal gammopathy. *Ann Neurol* 1994;36:416–424.

147. Kelly JJ. Peripheral neuropathies associated with monoclonal proteins. A clinical review. *Muscle Nerve* 1985;8:138–150.

148. Kelly JJ, Kyle RA, Miles JM, Dyck PJ. Osteosclerotic myeloma and peripheral neuropathy. *Neurology* 1983;33:202–210.

149. Philips ED, El-Mahdi AM, Humprey RL. The effect of the radiation treatment on the polyneuropathy of multiple myeloma. *J Can Assoc Radiol* 1972;23:103–106.

150. Miralles GD, O'Fallon JR, Talley NJ. Plasma cell dyscrasia with polyneuropathy. *N Engl J Med* 1992;327:1919–1923.

151. Kyle RA. Multiple myeloma: review of 869 cases. *Mayo Clinic Proc* 1975;50:29–40.

152. Vallat JM, De Mascarel HA, Bordessoule D, et al. Non-Hodgkin malignant lymphomas and peripheral neuropathies—13 cases. *Brain* 1995;118:1233–1245.

153. Lachance DH, O'Neill BP, Harper CM, et al. Paraneoplastic brachial plexopathy in a patient with Hodgkin's disease. *Mayo Clin Proc* 1991;66:97–101.

154. Pezzimenti JF, Bruckner HW, De Conti RC. Paralytic brachial neuritis in Hodgkin's disease. *Cancer* 1973;31:626–629.

155. Lisak RP, Mitchell M, Zweiman B, et al. Guillain-Barré syndrome and Hodgkin's disease: three cases with immunological studies. *Ann Neurol* 1977;1:72–78.

156. Hussein KK, Shaw MT, Oleinick SR. Autoimmune thrombocytopenia and peripheral neuropathy heralding Hodgkin's disease. *South Med J* 1975;68:1414–1416.

157. Plante-Bordeneuve V, Baudrimont M, Gorin NC, Gherardi RK. Subacute sensory neuropathy associated with Hodgkin's disease. *J Neurol Sci* 1994;121:155–158.

158. Croft PB, Urich H, Wilkinson M. Peripheral neuropathy of sensorimotor type associated with malignant disease. *Brain* 1967;90:31–36.

159. Oh SJ, Joy JL, Kuruoglu R. "Chronic sensory demyelinating neuropathy": chronic inflammatory demyelinating polyneuropathy presenting as a pure sensory neuropathy. *J Neurol Neurosurg Psychiatry* 1992;55:677–680.

160. Dawson DM, Samuels MA, Morris J. Sensory form of acute polyneuritis. *Neurology* 1988;38:1728–1731.

161. Krendel DA, Stahl RL, Chan WC. Lymphomatous polyneuropathy. Biopsy of clinically involved nerve and successful treatment. *Arch Neurol* 1991;48:330–332.

162. Kuroda Y, Nakata H, Kakigi R, et al. Human neurolymphomatosis by adult T-cell leukemia. *Neurology* 1989;39:144–146.

163. Oh SJ, Slaughter R, Harrell L. Paraneoplastic vasculitic neuropathy: a treatable neuropathy. *Muscle Nerve* 1991;14:152–156.

164. Vincent D, Dubas F, Hauw JJ, et al. Nerve and muscle microvasculitis in peripheral neuropathy: a remote effect of cancer? *J Neurol Neurosurg Psychiatry* 1986;49:1007–1010.

165. Matsumuro K, Izumo S, Umehara F, et al. Paraneoplastic vasculitic neuropathy: immunohistochemical studies on a biopsed nerve and post-mortem examination. *J Intern Med* 1994;236:225–230.

166. Johnson PC, Rolak LA, Hamilton RH, Laguna JF. Paraneoplastic vasculitis of nerve: a remote effect of cancer. *Ann Neurol* 1979;5:437–444.

167. Younger DS, Dalmau J, Inghirami G, et al. Anti-Hu-associated peripheral nerve and muscle microvasculitis. *Neurology* 1994;44:181–183.

168. Richardson JB, Callen JP. Dermatomyositis and malignancy. *Med Clin North Am* 1989;73:1211–1220.

169. Dalakas MC. Polymyositis, dermatomyositis and inclusion-body myositis. *N Engl J Med* 1991;325:1487–1498.

170. Sigurgeirsson B, Lindelöf B, Edhag O, Allander E. Risk of cancer in patients with dermatomyositis or polymyositis. *N Engl J Med* 1992;326:363–367.

171. Horowitz M, McNeill JD, Maddern GJ, et al. Abnormalities of gastric and esophageal emptying in polymyositis and dermatomyositis. *Gastroenterology* 1986;90:434–439.

172. Engel AG, Hohlfeld R, Banker BQ. The polymyositis and dermatomyositis syndromes. In: Engel AG, Franzini-Armstrong C, eds. *Myology.* New York: McGraw-Hill, 1994:1335–1383.

173. Dalakas MC. Immunopathogenesis of inflammatory myopathies. *Ann Neurol* 1995;37:S74–S86.

174. Dalakas MC, Illa I, Dambrosia JM, et al. A controlled trial of high-dose intravenous immune globulin infusions as treatment for dermatomyositis. *N Engl J Med* 1993;329:1993–2000.

175. Brownell B, Hughes JT. Degeneration of muscle in association with carcinoma of the bronchus. *J Neurol Neurosurg Psychiatry* 1975;38:363–370.

176. Vosskamper M, Korf B, Franke F, Schachenmayer W. Paraneoplastic necrotizing myopathy: a rare disorder to be differentiated from polymyositis. *J Neurol* 1989;236:489–492.

177. Emslie AM, Engel AG. Necrotizing myopathy with pipestem capillaries, microvascular deposits of the complement membrane attack complex (MAC) and minimal cellular infiltration. *Neurology* 1991;41:936–939.

178. Swash M, Fox KP, Davidson AR. Carcinoid myopathy. Serotonin-induced muscle weakness in man? *Arch Neurol* 1975;32:572–574.

179. Berry EM, Maunder C, Wilson M. Carcinoid myopathy and treatment with cyproheptadine (Periactin). *Gut* 1974;15:34–38.

180. Lederman RJ, Bukowski RM, Nickerson P. Carcinoid myopathy. *Cleve Clin J Med* 1987;54:299–303.

181. Moertel CG, Kvols LK, Rubin J. A study of cyproheptadine in the treatment of metastatic carcinoid tumor and the malignant carcinoid syndrome. *Cancer* 1991;67:33–36.

182. Paone JF, Jeyasingham K. Remission of cerebellar dysfunction after pneumonectomy for bronchogenic carcinoma. *N Engl J Med* 1980;302:156.

183. Kearsley JH, Johnson P, Halmagyi M. Paraneoplastic cerebellar disease. Remission with excision of the primary tumor. *Arch Neurol* 1985;42:1208–1210.

184. Burton GV, Bullard DE, Walther PJ, et al. Paraneoplastic limbic encephalopathy with testicular carcinoma. A reversible neurologic syndrome. *Cancer* 1988;62:2248–2251.

185. Carr I. The Ophelia syndrome: memory loss in Hodgkin's disease. *Lancet* 1982;1:844–845.

186. Chalk CH, Murray NMF, Newsom-Davis J, et al. Response of the Lambert-Eaton myasthenic syndrome to treatment of associated small-cell lung carcinoma. *Neurology* 1990;40:1552–1556.

187. Newsom-Davis J, Murray NMF. Plasma exchange and immunosuppressive drug treatment in the Lambert-Eaton myasthenic syndrome. *Neurology* 1984;34:480–485.

188. Bird SJ. Clinical and electrophysiologic improvement in Lambert-Eaton syndrome with intravenous immunoglobulin therapy. *Neurology* 1992;42:1422–1423.

189. Cocconi G, Ceci G, Juvarra G. Successful treatment of subacute cerebellar degeneration in ovarian carcinoma with plasmapheresis. A case report. *Cancer* 1985;56:2318–2320.

190. Verschuuren J, Twijnstra A, De Baets M, et al. Hu-antigen and anti-Hu antibodies in a patient with myxoid chondrosarcoma. *Neurology* 1994;44:1551–1552.

191. Counsell CE, McLeod M, Grant R. Reversal of subacute paraneoplastic cerebellar syndrome with intravenous immunoglobulin. *Neurology* 1994;44:1184–2011.

192. Hormigo A, Dalmau J, Rosenblum M, et al. Immunological and pathological study of anti-Ri associated encephalopathy. *Ann Neurol* 1994;36:896–902.

Chapter 11

Involvement of Inflammation and Complement in Alzheimer's Disease

Douglas G. Walker, Edith G. McGeer, and Patrick L. McGeer

The involvement of the immune system in neurodegenerative disorders, in particular, multiple sclerosis (MS), Alzheimer's disease (AD), Parkinson's disease (PD), and amyotrophic lateral sclerosis (ALS), has been intensively studied in the last 8 to 10 years. There is increasing evidence that inflammatory-associated changes are playing a significant role in contributing to the progression of these neurodegenerative disorders. The long-held concept that the brain is immunologically privileged is no longer realistic. Now what has to be considered is the extent of the *difference* between inflammatory- and immune-associated changes in the brain, compared to the rest of the body.

This chapter reviews the findings concerning the nature and extent of inflammatory and immune reactions in human neurodegenerative diseases, with particular emphasis on AD. These findings are related to relevant in vitro experimental data. There is also considerable literature on inflammatory-associated changes in MS. This area is dealt with in detail in other sections of this book and here the literature is only discussed in relation to AD.

Clinical and Pathologic Features of Alzheimer's Disease

The possible involvement of inflammatory-associated changes in AD has gained credibility in recent years. How these changes might fit into accepted understanding of the pathogenesis of AD needs to be considered. AD is a degenerative disorder whose pathology is believed to originate in the cerebral cortex, with the hippocampus being particularly vulnerable, and then to spread to select subcortical regions, particularly the basal forebrain, as the disease progresses (1). Clinically, it is characterized by memory loss leading to progressive dementia. AD can present as a range of clinical symptoms including a progressive decline in memory function, initially as a poor recall of recent information while earlier memories remain intact. As the disease progresses, all memory function becomes affected. Also seen is a decline in language function, initially as a loss of fluency but leading to aphasia, and visuospatial impairment. Behavioral changes are also frequently observed and include delusions, depression, agitation,

and wandering. The progressive mental decline invariably leads to the patient showing symptoms described as dementia (2). Most patients with late-stage AD are unable to look after themselves and reside in nursing homes or similar institutions. With the increased life span of both men and women in the latter part of the twentieth century, the increased numbers of AD patients put an enormous cost on public and private health care systems. An estimate of the direct annual cost of looking after an AD patient was $47,000 in 1991, for a total of $20.6 billion in the United States of America (3).

Pathologic Features

It is clear that dementia is the consequence of synaptic loss; however, the cause of this is not clear. Initially observed by Alzheimer (4), and confirmed by numerous others, was the presence of insoluble structures in the brains of patients affected by AD that are not normally seen in the brains of nonaffected individuals. These structures are classified primarily as β amyloid (Aβ)–containing extracellular plaques and intraneuronal neurofibrillary tangles (NFTs). The subclassification of these structures is extensive; however, all have the characteristic of persistence in vivo, and insolubility when analyzed chemically. Aβ is a peptide of 39 to 43 amino acids and is the major constituent of the extracellular plaques. Glenner and Wong (5) isolated and sequenced vascular amyloid and Masters et al (6) did the same for plaque amyloid. Screening of complementary DNA libraries showed that the Aβ peptide was derived from a larger protein that was designated as the amyloid precursor protein (APP) (7–9). Subsequent studies demonstrated that several variants of APP arise, due to alternative transcription and differential glycosylation (10–12). Since then, much research has been carried out on characterization of these proteins, to understand the function of APP, how APP is processed to the Aβ peptide and becomes deposited in plaques, and how this is related to AD pathology (for detailed reviews, see other publications (13–15)). Since the initial finding that the carboxyl 100–amino acid segment and also synthetic Aβ peptide can be directly toxic to cultured neurons (16,17), it had been assumed that the presence of extracellular amyloid was the direct cause of the AD pathology (18). This conclusion has been difficult to confirm, as direct proof of toxicity of Aβ peptide in vivo has not been shown conclusively (19). AD has proven to be a difficult disease on which to ascertain the cause. In 15% to 20% of patients there is clear evidence of a genetic cause for inherited AD. In rare patients, it has been shown that specific mutations in the APP gene invariably lead to clinical AD (20–22); however, mutations at a neighboring position can lead to hereditary cerebral hemorrhage with amyloidosis (HCHWA) (23). In addition, those affected by Down syndrome, who acquire an extra copy of the APP gene, also invariably develop AD pathology. These findings were interpreted as evidence of an amyloid cause for AD. However, there is now evidence that possession of the apolipoprotein E4 (apoE) allele, which is present on chromosome 19, represents a significant risk factor in developing late-onset AD (24–26). ApoE is a cholesterol transport protein that can be produced by astrocytes in the human brain (27). It exists as three different forms in the human population, arising from polymorphism at two amino acids. While the possession of an apoE4 allele is a significant risk factor to developing AD, the possession of the apoE2 allele is believed to be a significant protection factor from AD (28). The most common allele in the human population is apoE3. The mechanism of apoE4 involvement in AD is unclear. The protein is deposited on amyloid plaques in AD brains (29), and forms a sodium dodecyl sulfate (SDS)-resistant interaction with Aβ in vitro (30). Purified apoE4 forms a much tighter association with Aβ peptide than does apoE3 (31). However, the significance of apoE interactions with Aβ has been questioned, and some research has focused on the interaction of apoE with microtubules, including the microtubule-associated proteins MAP2c and tau (32,33). While neurons do not appear to produce apoE, they have receptors for the protein, and can be immunoreactive for apoE (34). Based on in vitro experiments apoE4 has a weaker interaction with tau than does apoE3, and phosphorylation of tau at serine 262 abolishes apoE3 binding and in so doing also reduces tau binding to microtubules (35). The significance of these observations needs to be proven in vivo.

Two distinct genes for early-onset familial AD, present on chromosomes 1 and 14, have been identified (36,37). These genes share a significant degree of homology, and appear to encode for classic type membrane-associated proteins, designated presenilins. Antibodies to presenilin proteins appear to detect subpopulations of neurons with intracellular NFTs in AD brains (38). Although the mechanism is unclear, the possession of either presenilin mutation leads to increased production of β amyloids 1 through 42 (39).

The mechanisms of NFT formation are still not clearly understood. There is a differential tendency of different populations of neurons to develop tangles. In AD, the NFTs are composed mainly of bundles of helically twisted filaments called *paired helical filaments*. The fibrils have diameters of 10 to 22 nm consisting mainly of the microtubule-associated protein tau, but also contain ubiquitin (40). The tau protein present in NFTs is abnormally phosphorylated, particularly at serine 199 and serine 202 (40). The abnormal phosphorylation of tau is believed to be responsible for the instability of neuronal microtubules. At present, it is not known if the defect that leads to abnormal tau phosphorylation is due to excess activity of protein kinases or a defect in protein phosphatase activity (39). The abnormal phosphorylation of tau appears to represent an early event preceding the development of neurofibrillary pathology (40).

Nongenetic (Sporadic) Causes

There has still not been clear evidence as to the nongenetic cause (or causes) for AD. As AD occurs in 80% to 85% of individuals with no clear history of inherited dementia, other causes have been actively pursued over the years. These include environmental aluminum, viruses, head trauma, and substandard education (42–45). Possession of the apoE4 allele appears to be a contributing risk factor, even in sporadic AD (24). A number of studies demonstrated a positive association of AD with head trauma (e.g., the study by Rasmusson et al (45)). It has been suggested that head trauma may lead to an increased production of APP, which can be induced in response to injurious stimuli such as brain trauma. The increased APP production could then lead to increased deposition of Aβ peptide. This has been demonstrated in brains from patients diagnosed with dementia pugilistica (46). It should be added that other studies do not support the positive correlation of AD with head trauma (e.g., study by Mendez et al (47)). In spite of what now appears to be evidence for several different causes to the disease, the postmortem pathologic features are similar, namely, the presence of extracellular Aβ plaques, NFTs, and dystrophic neurites, along with significant neuronal loss.

One prominent additional feature observed in brain tissue from AD patients is the presence of large numbers of activated microglia and reactive astrocytes. It seems evident that this reactive gliosis is a secondary event in the disease, but there is abundant experimental data that it may play a significant role in the progression of the disease. In addition, it now appears that therapy directed at the inflammation occurring in AD may be effective in slowing the progression of the disease (48–50).

Inflammation and Alzheimer's Disease

Over the years, different individuals have identified microglia as the brain resident representatives of the mononuclear phagocytic system, and as having immune effector properties. Initial observations were made on the basis of a silver staining technique developed by del Rio Hortega (51). Penfield (52) confirmed the concept of a population of brain resident phagocytes. In 1927, Bolsoi (53) observed the clustering of these types of cells around senile plaques. The rapid advances in characterizing the role of microglia in the brain and the possible contribution to neurodegenerative processes have occurred since the development of monoclonal antibody probes and modern sensitive immunocytochemical methodology. Initial identification of reactive microglia in AD tissue employed antibodies to the class II major histocompatibility complex (MHC) protein HLA-DR. It was known that this protein was more readily detectable on the surface of macrophages after inflammatory stimulus. McGeer et al (54) showed that the HLA-DR protein is more abundantly expressed on microglia that are closely associated with areas of degenerative pathology, in tissue from AD patients. Staining for HLA-DR is not as readily detectable in tissue from neurologically normal patients (Fig 11-1A, B). It is particularly prominent on microglia that are in close association with Aβ-containing senile plaques (Fig 11-1C). Luber-Narod and Rogers (55) made similar observations on the expression of HLA-DR, and also showed the induction of the other MHC class II antigens, HLA-DP and HLA-DQ. In addition, the induction of HLA-DR–positive microglia has been observed in association with the pathology of other degenerative disorders, including PD, acquired immunodeficiency syndrome (AIDS) dementia, Parkinson's dementia complex of Guam, and ALS (56). The expression of the HLA-DR glycoprotein remains one of the best markers for microglial activation in tissue. Its role in immune responses is to present processed antigens to CD4+ T cells and its expression on cells is increased by treatment with the cytokine interferon (IFN)-γ (57). Similarly, expression of MHC class I antigens (HLA-A, -B, -C) has been detected on reactive microglia in AD-affected tissue (58). These were not as numerous as microglia expressing HLA-DR. It is possible to demonstrate cells that coexpress both proteins. The function of MHC class I antigens is to present processed peptides to CD8+ T cells. The demonstration of these proteins on microglia indicates that they are immunocompetent antigen-presenting cells. However, the function of these proteins is not clearly understood in diseases like AD. CD4+ (helper-inducer) and CD8 (cytotoxic-suppressor) T cells have been detected in AD tissue, but they are very sparse in comparison to the number of class II immunoreactive cells (59). This has led to the hypothesis that the immune system changes in AD are of a chronic inflammatory nature, in comparison to MS where there is evidence for an antigen-driven autoimmune response (60). This distinction was confirmed by the demonstration of the presence of B7, a costimu-

latory molecule required for antigen presentation to T cells, on microglia in active MS lesions, but not in AD or normal brains (61). The expression of HLA-DR was not readily detectable in the gray matter of neurologically normal tissue, but became abundantly expressed where neurodegeneration was evident. How-

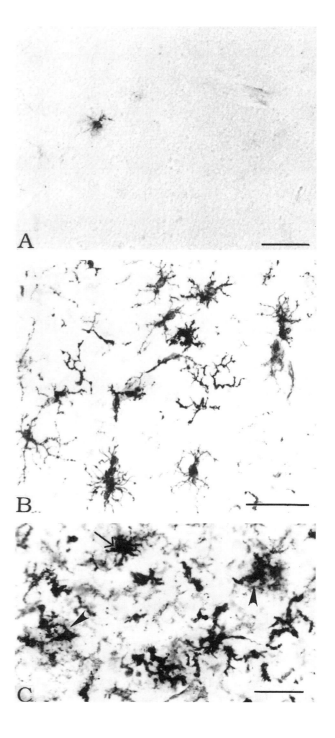

Figure 11-1. (A) Photomicrograph of a section from the entorhinal cortex from a neurologically normal patient, stained for MHC class II antigen. Bar = 50 mm. (B) Photomicrograph of a section from the entorhinal cortex from an Alzheimer's disease patient, stained for MHC class II antigen. The intense staining is of cells with profiles of activated microglia. (C) Photomicrograph of a section from the entorhinal cortex from an Alzheimer's disease patient, doubly stained for MHC class II antigen (darker staining) and with an antibody specific for β amyloid peptide (lighter staining). The dark staining is of microglial clusters (arrow) arranged on top of extracellular β amyloid–containing plaques (arrowheads).

ever, some investigators (62,63) reported that HLA-DR expression can be detected on microglia in normal tissue, especially in white matter, and proposed that microglia constitutively express this protein. The ability to detect HLA-DR immunoreactivity in normal and pathologically affected tissue highly depends on the particular monoclonal antibodies being used, and also on tissue fixation conditions (64). Regular fixation conditions employed for routine pathology (long fixation time in 10% formalin, along with paraffin embedding) normally denature this antigen, though some monoclonal antibodies to HLA-DR that have been developed recognize epitopes that are less sensitive to fixation denaturation (65). With these new antibodies, examination for activated microglia may be a useful test in routine neuropathology.

Characterization of Antigens Expressed on Microglia

Since the time of the initial studies using HLA-DR as the marker for reactive microglia, a number of studies have characterized the expression of other immune system antigens on microglia in AD-affected brain tissue. The antigens for both microglia and astrocytes are summarized in Table 11-1 (54,55,58,66–85) which has to be considered incomplete as additional markers are consistently being identified. The macrophage antigens CD11a, CD11b, CD11c (members of the β_2 integrin family), leukocyte common antigen (LCA), and the Fcγ receptor (FcγR) class of immunoglobulin receptors are readily detectable on resting microglia, though their expression is also greatly increased in reactive microglia in AD-affected tissue (66–70). LCA is a cell surface receptor that has phosphotyrosine phosphatase activity (68,69). Its expression is restricted to cells of hematopoietic origin (except erythrocytes). One study (66) showed that there is an increase in the number and intensity of staining of LCA-positive microglia in AD cortex compared to control samples. A further study identified that the majority of microglia were immunoreactive for the CD45RB isoform, while a subset of reactive microglia in AD tissue stained for the CD45RO isoform (68). Owing to alternative patterns of messenger RNA (mRNA) splicing and protein glycosylation, six to eight different isoforms of CD45 have been identified.

Table 11-1.
CD Surface Antigens, MHC Antigens, and Some Other Inflammatory-Associated Antigens Detected on Glial Cells in Degenerative Diseases

Antigen Designation	Function	Expression in AD (ref)
MHC class I	Antigen presentation to CD8+ cells	Increased (58)
MHC class II	Antigen presentation to CD4+ cells	Increased (54,55)
CD11a (LFA-1)	Intercellular adhesion molecule (IACM)-1 and ICAM-2 receptor	Increased (66,67)
CD11b (CR3)	C3bi receptor	Increased (66,67)
CD11c (p150)	C3bi receptor	Increased (66,67)
CD18 (β_2 integrin)	Subunit of CD11 complex	As for CD11a, b, c
CD25 (Tac)	Interleukin-2 receptor	Increased (54)
CDw32 (FcγRII)	IgG Fc fragment receptor	Increased (66,70)
CD44 (Pgp-1)	Hyaluronate receptor	Increased (71)
CD45 (LCA)	Receptor with phosphotyrosine phosphatase activity	Increased CD45RO (68,69)
CD49 (VLA)	Cell adhesion molecule	No change (72)
CD51 (αv integrin)	Vitronectin receptor	Increased (73)
CD54 (ICAM-1)	Ligand for leukocyte function–associated antigen (LFA)-1	Increased (74)
CD64 (FcγRI)	IgG Fc fragment receptor	Increased (70)
CD68 (macrosialin)	Unknown	Not changed
Interleukin-1α	Inflammatory cytokine	Increased (75)
Interleukin-1β	Inflammatory cytokine	Increased (76)
Interleukin-6	Inflammatory cytokine	Increased (76)
Tumor necrosis factor (TNF)-α	Inflammatory cytokine	Increased (76)
Granulocyte-macrophage colony-stimulating factor (GM-SF)	Macrophage growth factor	Increased (77)
Macrophage colony-stimulating factor receptor (MCSF-R) (c-fms)	CSF-1 receptor	Increased (78)
α₂-Macroglobulin receptor	Binds α₂-macroglobulin	Increased (79)
Interferon-α	Inflammatory cytokine	Increased (68)
Lactotransferrin	Iron transport protein	Increased (80)
Ferritin	Iron transport protein	Increased (81)
Plasminogen activator inhibitor	Serpin protease inhibitor	Increased (82)
Acidic fibroblast growth factor (aFGF)	Growth factor	Increased (astrocytes) (83)
Phosphotyrosine	Product of tyrosine kinases	Increased (84)
Gelatinase A	Protease	Increased (85)

The β_2 integrin complement receptors, also called the *leukocyte integrins*, consist of CD11a (LFA-1), CD11b (complement receptor 3, Mac 1), and CD11c (complement receptor 4, p150,95). Functionally they consist of a unique α integrin chain and a common β integrin (CD18) chain that are noncovalently associated (66,67). Although designated as complement receptors, they also can bind to a number of extracellular matrix proteins. For example, CD11c can bind to fibrinogen. The FcγR family consists of FcγRI (CD64), FcγRII (CDw32), and FcγRIII (CD16) (66,70). The receptors share structural similarity and approximately 50% homology in the C2 immunoglobulin superfamily domain. FcγRI is a high-affinity receptor, while FcγRII and FcγRIII are low-affinity receptors. The presence of the complement and immunoglobulin receptors on microglia/macrophages is associated with their role in phagocytosis of complement and immunoglobulin opsonized tissue debris. Ligand binding to the FcγRs can cause the microglia to become activated, as shown by increased NADPH oxidase activity (86). As discussed later, there is evidence for activation of the complement system in AD-affected tissue; however, the role of immunoglobulin in the process has not been demonstrated. The upregulation of the FcγRs on brain resident microglia may be as a result of cytokine induction, particularly by interleukin (IL)-1, IL-6, or tumor necrosis factor (TNF)-α, whose expression is increased in microglia in AD tissue (75,76). Treatment of cultured rat brain microglia with IL-1, TNF-α, IFN-γ, or lipopolysaccharide (LPS) increased Fc receptor expression (87). Immunocytochemical staining of AD tissue sections has not consistently demonstrated the presence of immunoglobulins colocalized with AD pathologic structures (88), even though the activated microglia associated with these structures highly express the Fc receptors. It has been suggested that immunoglobulin immunoreactivity in the tissue parenchyma of the brain may be a postmortem artifact (88).

Microglia can also be immunostained for IL-1α and -1β, IL-6, and TNF-α in AD brains (75,76). These cytokines have the potential to coordinate the majority of inflammatory changes found in AD brain tissue. They can induce a number of genes in astrocytes and neurons, including increasing the expression of the APP, complement, and acute-phase response genes (89–91). Staining for these cytokines is more intense on microglia in the vicinity of senile plaques (75,76). The intensity of staining appears to be related to the state of activation. Cytokine staining is also detectable in normal brains from patients who died from infectious processes (76). Owing to the secreted nature of these proteins, brains with a short postmortem delay, along with a short fixation time, are needed to demonstrate cell-associated immunoreactivity. Another marker for activated microglia is phosphotyrosine. Tyrosine kinases are rapidly induced in macrophages as a result of most forms of activation, and protein tyrosine phosphorylation appears to be a crucial signaling pathway for many inflammatory-associated events (92). Subsets of microglia as well as tangles in AD brains stain for phosphotyrosine (93). These changes tend to be short-lived owing to the action of phosphatases, and staining could identify populations of microglia that are highly active.

Characterization of Complement Proteins

A number of studies demonstrated the presence of activated complement proteins colocalized on senile amyloid plaques and vascular amyloid. This was demonstrated in tissue sections from AD patients by staining with antibodies to C1q, C3b, C3c, C3d, and C4d (94–97). The different stages of the classic complement pathway, along with the places where the various complement inhibitory molecules act, are shown in Figure 11-2. The positive staining with antibodies to C1q and the C4 cleaved fragment C4d indicated that the classic pathway of the complement system is activated in AD tissue. Staining for protein markers of the alternative pathway was negative (94). In addition, antibodies to C1q, C3d, and C4d stained dystrophic neurites and some NFTs. Furthermore, with sensitive immunohistochemical techniques, the C5b-9 neoantigen was detected on dystrophic neurites and NFTs in AD tissue (94). This is evidence of formation of the membrane attack complex, the membrane-penetrating, cell lysis–inducing complex of the complement system. The assembly of the terminal components of the complement system (C5-C9) into the membrane attack complex requires a lipid membrane for anchoring. Examples of immunohistochemical staining for complement components in AD brain tissue are shown in Figure 11-3. An additional pathogenic structure was demonstrated by complement immunohistochemistry. Complement-activated

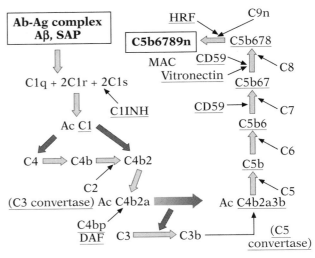

Figure 11-2. Diagram demonstrating the different stages of the classic complement pathway, and the stage of intervention of crucial complement inhibitory molecules. Ab-Ag = antibody-antigen; Aβ = β-amyloid; SAP = serum amyloid P; MAC = membrane attack complex; Ac = activated; DAF = decay accelerating factor; HRF = homologous restriction factor.

oligodendroglia can be seen in a number of degenerative neurologic conditions, and also are detectable in normal aged brains, though less abundant in numbers (98). Owing to the potential pathologic consequences to normal cells of unregulated complement activation (known as *bystander lysis*), a number of regulatory proteins exist to inhibit different stages of the complement pathway. The stages of intervention of these proteins in

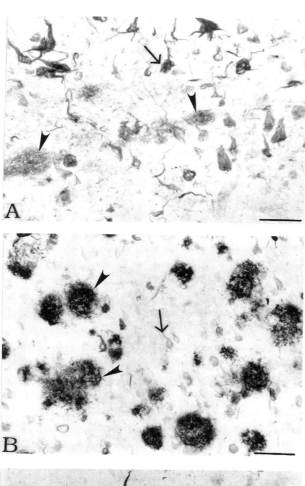

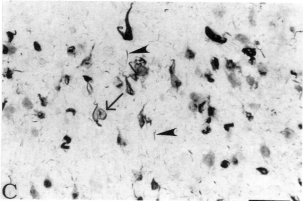

the pathway are shown in Figure 11-2. C1 inhibitor, also known as *C1 esterase inhibitor*, a serine protease inhibitor, functions by binding and inactivating activated C1r and C1s, thus preventing the complement pathway from proceeding to the second stage. The protein can be detected in pyramidal neurons in normal and AD brains, and also on some senile plaques in AD (99) (Fig 11-4A). Neuropil threads and dystrophic neurites are also immunoreactive. In addition to C1, C1 inhibitor is active against kallikrein, plasmin, and coagulation factors XIa and XIIa. The distribution of clusterin (100), vitronectin (68,73), and CD59 (protectin) (101) in AD brains has also been studied. These proteins are active in inhibiting the assembly of the membrane attack complex. There is evidence of increased expression of these complement regulatory proteins in AD tissue. Staining for vitronectin and CD59 is shown in Figure 11-4. Staining for CD59 is prominent in tangles and dystrophic neurites (see Fig 11-4C), structures that also are immunoreactive for the membrane attack complex antigen C5b-9. This could be indicative of increased expression in response to complement activation. Similar patterns of staining are observed using antibodies to vitronectin (see Fig 11-4B) and clusterin (100). In comparison to CD59, vitronectin and clusterin are secreted proteins and can also be detected localized on amyloid plaques (see Fig 11-4B). This may represent nonspecific adherence to these structures, or else these proteins could have functions in addition to inhibiting the formation of the membrane attack complex. Clusterin (also referred to as *apoJ*) is a lipid transport protein, and its expression is upregulated in cells undergoing programmed cell death (apoptosis) (102). Microglia stain prominently for the vitronectin receptor (68,73). These cells were observed colocalized on vitronectin immunoreactive plaques in AD brains (73). In this case, vitronectin may be acting as an opsonizing agent rather than in a complement inhibitory role. Vitronectin is a multifunctional plasma and extracellular matrix glycoprotein involved in cell attachment, coagulation, phagocytosis, and the protection of bystander cells from complement and T cell–mediated lysis (103). The vitronectin

Figure 11-3. (A) Photomicrograph of a section from the entorhinal cortex from an Alzheimer's disease patient, stained for the complement protein C1q. Staining is present on structures with the appearance of neurofibrillary tangle–containing neurons (arrow) and extracellular amyloid plaques (arrowheads). (B) Photomicrograph of a section from the entorhinal cortex from an Alzheimer's disease patient, stained for the complement protein subfragment C4d. Staining is present on structures with the appearance of neurofibrillary tangle–containing neurons (arrow) and extracellular amyloid plaques (arrowheads). Note the more intense staining of extracellular amyloid plaques compared to A. (C) Photomicrograph of a section from the entorhinal cortex from an Alzheimer's disease patient, stained for the complement protein C5b-9, a neoantigen formed as a result of assembly of the membrane attack complex. Staining is present on structures with the appearance of neurofibrillary tangle–containing neurons (arrow) and dystrophic neurites (arrowheads), but absent from extracellular amyloid plaques.

receptor, consisting of the αv integrin chain (CD51) and the β_3 integrin chain (CD61), can also bind to von Willebrand's factor, fibrinogen, and thrombospondin (104).

The complement proteins are present in the circulation in relatively high concentrations. The cells of the liver have the capacity to synthesize all these proteins. Initially it was assumed that the complement proteins that were detected in AD brain tissue were derived from the peripheral circulation and were entering the brain because of defects in the blood-brain barrier. However,

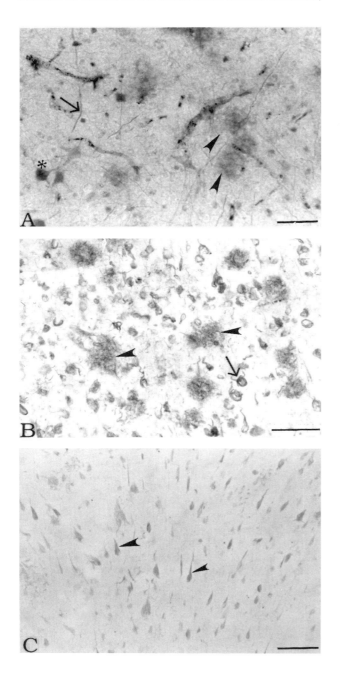

two studies clearly demonstrated the capacity of the brain to produce the proteins of the complement pathway (105,106). These studies demonstrated the presence of mRNA for the complement proteins in RNA extracted from brain tissue from both AD and control subjects. There appears to be increased expression of complement genes (especially C1qB, C3, and C4) in brain tissue affected by AD degenerative processes (105,106). Additional studies (107,108) demonstrated increased complement gene expression in brain tissue from animals that had been given different types of artificial lesions. Interestingly, in one set of studies, different classes of neurons were positive for complement C1qB and C4 mRNA as shown by the in situ hybridization technique (106,107). C1q immunoreactive neurons have been detected in AD brains (109). Also, some neuroblastoma cell lines can express C3, C4, and C9 mRNA (110). It is well established that macrophages can express the proteins of the complement system (111), and it would be expected that brain microglia share this property. Human microglia derived from postmortem brains can express the C1qB, C3, and C4 genes, and also the C1 inhibitor gene (99,111). In addition, astrocytes from human and rat brains can express a number of complement genes, in particular C3 (112). The significance of complement production by neurons remains a matter for investigation. There is clearly increased localized complement production at the site of pathology in damaged brains and this may have a role in contributing to the inflammatory changes in the tissue. Increased complement gene expression can occur in macrophages and astrocytes in response to cytokine activation (113,114).

Interaction of Microglia and Inflammatory-Associated Proteins with Aβ Plaques

Studies on the role of activated microglia in AD have attempted to answer the question, At what point in the degenerative process do microglia become involved? Namely, when do they become activated, and what is the consequence of this? Due to the persistence of the amyloid plaques, it has been suggested that microglia in their vicinity remain in a state of constant activation, as they remain "frustrated" in their attempts to remove

Figure 11-4. (A) Photomicrograph of a section from the occipital cortex from an Alzheimer's disease patient, stained for complement C1 inhibitor. Staining is present on structures with the appearance of neuropil threads (arrow), and extracellular amyloid plaques (arrowheads). Pyramidal neurons immunoreactive for C1 inhibitor can also be observed (asterisk). (B) Photomicrograph of a section from the entorhinal cortex from an Alzheimer's disease patient, stained for vitronectin. Staining is present on structures with the appearance of neurofibrillary tangle–containing neurons (arrow) and extracellular amyloid plaques (arrowheads). (C) Photomicrograph of a section from the entorhinal cortex from an Alzheimer's disease patient, stained for the complement inhibitor CD59 (protectin). Staining is present on structures with the appearance of neurofibrillary tangle–containing neurons (arrowheads).

this material. The interaction of microglia with NFTs has not been investigated to the same extent although they also appear resistant to degradation and removal. Reactive (HLA-DR immunopositive) microglia colocalize in clusters on nearly all mature amyloid plaques, whereas they are associated with only half of the diffuse amyloid plaques (115,116). The initial deposition of Aβ immunoreactive structures is believed to be as diffuse amyloid plaques. These are seen in various number in different regions of the elderly brain, including regions that do not usually show AD-type pathology, for example, the cerebellar cortex (115). These deposits do not generally have associated HLA-DR immunoreactive microglia. However, diffuse amyloid plaques, including those in the cerebellum, are immunoreactive for the complement proteins C1q, C3d, and C4d (115,116). The presence of serum amyloid P (SAP) on diffuse cerebellar plaques has also been observed (115). SAP is an acute-phase reactant that is associated with all forms of amyloid plaques in amyloidoses of different origins (117). Binding of SAP to amyloid appears to make the amyloid resistant to proteolytic digestion (118). SAP immunoreactivity in AD brains invariably colocalizes with markers for complement activation, for example, C4d (119). Immunoreactivity for α_1-antichymotrypsin was observed on 60% of cerebellar diffuse plaques (115). The presence of these acute phase–associated proteins on mature senile plaques has been well documented. A large number of different proteins have been demonstrated to colocalize on Aβ plaques in AD brains. A partial list is presented in Table 11-2 (31,67,73,74,94–96,99,100,115,120–140). Many of these proteins are the products of activated glial cells. From the inflammatory point of view, the most prominent proteins are believed to be those of the complement pathway. As stated, immunohistochemical studies demonstrated that complement activation is an early event

following the appearance of amyloid deposits in brain tissue (115,118). Other prominent Aβ deposited proteins, which are believed to be astrocytic in origin, are α_1-antichymotrypsin (120), apoE (27), apoJ (clusterin) (100), and heparan and chondroitin sulfate proteoglycans (121). The origin of SAP in the brain has not been determined. It has not been possible to obtain evidence that this protein is expressed by brain resident cells. Analysis of mRNA extracted from human brains (AD and control subjects) by polymerase chain reaction techniques failed to detect SAP mRNA (141). At present, only liver cells are known to synthesize this protein. The interactions of these proteins with Aβ have been well characterized in vitro, each one forming stable complexes with Aβ. In vitro studies showed that SAP binding to Aβ is calcium dependent (142). α_1-Antichymotrypsin, apoE, and SAP promote Aβ fibril formation, which may make it neurotoxic and resistant to proteolytic digestion (143–145). However, the significance of the interaction of these proteins with Aβ remains unclear. Soluble Aβ, which can be secreted by a number of different cell types, is complexed with apoJ in vivo. ApoJ has been identified bound to soluble Aβ isolated from plasma and cerebrospinal fluid, while apoE is also found bound to Aβ isolated from cerebrospinal fluid, but at much lower concentrations (146). There is evidence that binding of apoJ to Aβ inhibits its ability to form fibrils (147). However, these forms of Aβ remain toxic to neurons (148). The findings that binding of apoE, α_1-antichymotrypsin, and C1q to Aβ promotes fibril formation have given rise to the hypothesis that these proteins may act as "pathologic chaperones" (143,149). A change in the balance in the concentrations of these different proteins may be one of the events that transforms the benign diffuse amyloid to the consolidated form that is associated with neuritic plaques, and that can be stained by thioflavine S or Congo red.

Table 11-2.
Extracellular Molecules Reported in Aβ-Containing Plaques

Complement proteins	Coagulation factors	Growth factors
C1q (94–96, 109)	Tissue plasminogen activator (130)	bFGF (137)
C3d, C3c (94–96)	Thrombin (131)	TGF-β1 (138)
C4d (94–96)	Hageman factor (132)	Midkine (139)
C7, C9 (94)	Acute-phase reactants	Interleukin-6 (140)
Proteases	Heat shock proteins (133)	Complement inhibitors
α_1-Trypsin (122)	Serum amyloid P (115)	C1 inhibitor (99)
Cathepsin B, D (123)	Proteoglycans	C4-binding protein (115)
Protease inhibitors	HSPG (121)	Vitronectin (73)
α_1-Antichymotrypsin (120)	CSPG (121)	Clusterin (100)
α_1-Antitrypsin (124)	DSPG (134)	Others
α_2-Macroglobulin (125)	Receptors	Apolipoprotein E (31)
Tissue inhibitor of	EGFR (135)	Collagen (67)
metalloproteinase (126)	α_2-Macroglobulin receptor (136)	Laminin (67)
Cystatin A (127)		ICAM-1 (74)
Other enzymes		Lactotransferrin (80)
AChE (128)		
BuChE (129)		

AChE = acetylcholinesterase; BuChE = butyrylcholinesterase; HSPG = heparan sulfate proteoglycan; CSPG = chondroitin sulfate proteoglycan; EGFR = epidermal growth factor receptor; bFGF = basic fibroblast growth factor; TGF = transforming growth factor; ICAM = intercellular adhesion molecule.

There still remains to be determined the events that transform the amyloid plaque to a form that causes it to be a target for activated microglia. It has been observed that reactive microglia, using the expression of the class II MHC antigen HLA-DR as the index for activation, do not colocalize with diffuse amyloid plaques in AD, even though inflammatory-inducing complement proteins have been deposited on them. However, Griffin et al (75) used immunoreactivity for the cytokine IL-1α as the index for microglial activation. These authors observed that 78% of diffuse nonneuritic plaques in AD brains contained IL-1α–positive microglia. Diffuse neuritic plaques had the greatest number of associated IL-1α–positive microglia, whereas there were fewer in association with dense-core neuritic plaques. These results indicate that the initial appearance of Aβ may be sufficient to activate brain resident microglia, even though it may not induce the expression of HLA-DR. The stimulus for HLA-DR induction in AD brain remains to be defined. It is well documented that HLA-DR can be induced on cultured microglia by IFN-γ, but not by IL-1α or -1β or TNF-α (57). In a disease such as MS, where there are large numbers of T cells, there is a clear source for IFN-γ. As referred to earlier, there are only scarce T cells detected in AD brains, and we have not been able to detect IFN-γ mRNA in RNA samples from AD brains. Evidence exists for a neuronal form of IFN-γ. This protein has been isolated from small neurons of the peripheral sensory ganglia of rats, has a molecular size of 54 to 66 kd, and is capable of inducing MHC class I and II antigens on macrophages (150). Recent evidence indicates that this protein also exists in the brain. Its existence may account for the rapid induction of class II antigens on microglia under neurotoxic conditions. IL-3, which can be made by cultured rat microglia and astrocytes, can also increase the expression of MHC class II antigens on microglia in vitro (151,152).

A number of tissue culture studies that used microglia and macrophages from humans and rats showed that synthetic Aβ peptides have inflammatory-inducing properties by activating microglia/macrophages to produce IL-1 (153), basic fibroblast growth factor (153), nitric oxide (154), and reactive oxygen intermediates (155) and that the peptide has chemotactic properties for microglia/macrophages (156). In addition, one study (157) showed that Aβ increases the synthesis of complement C3 protein by rat microglia, though this may have been an indirect consequence of an initial induction of IL-1β.

The aforementioned study by Griffin et al (75) demonstrated the possible role for microglia in the generation of neuritic plaques. A number of researchers have reported the colocalization of reactive microglia with amyloid plaques, particularly mature senile plaques. These studies are commonly interpreted as indicating that the microglia are attempting phagocytosis and removal of the Aβ plaque. However, a series of studies by Wisniewski et al (158,159) demonstrated evidence that microglia may play a role in the production of fibrillar Aβ. By electron microscopic study of Aβ plaques, they observed that the amyloid fibrils are associated with al-

tered cisternae of the endoplasmic reticulum and deep infoldings of cell membranes of cells with the characteristics of microglia (158). They also observed continuity between the amyloid fibrils present in the periphery of amyloid plaques, and those present in the cytoplasmic channels of microglial cells. In comparison, when partially purified amyloid cores from AD brains were added to cultures of microglia isolated from adult dog brains, the immunoreactive Aβ remained associated with intracellular phagosomes (159). The amyloid was detected in phagosomes, apparently undigested, 20 days after its addition to the cultures. These authors proposed that there may be a neuronal origin for the diffuse amyloid deposit, and a microglial origin for the fibrillar form of Aβ.

Complement Activation by Aβ Peptide

Complement activation not only can lead to the generation of cytolytic complexes (membrane attack complex), but also can generate potent inflammatory-inducing subfragments during the formation of this complex (C3a, C5a). Aβ peptide directly activates the classic complement pathway by binding to C1q in the absence of specific immunoglobulins (88). Similar in vitro assays revealed that the Aβ needs to be partially aggregated for efficient complement activation to occur, as monomeric Aβ cannot bind C1q (160). Synthetic Aβ (1–42), which has a tendency to aggregate rapidly in aqueous solution, is more efficient at complement activation than Aβ 1 through 40 (161). Binding of C1q to Aβ peptide occurs between residues 4 and 11 of Aβ, and residue 7 appears to be critical. C1q binding to Aβ is abolished if residue 7 (aspartic acid) is substituted with isoaspartic acid (162). The true situation in vivo may not be quite so straightforward, as SAP, which has been detected on all Aβ plaques, can also activate the classic complement pathway by an antibody-independent mechanism. Similar to Aβ, complement activation by SAP requires that it be in an aggregated state (163).

Evidence for Neurotoxicity by Activated Microglia or Astrocytes

A number of studies have shown the potential for activated microglia to produce substances that are potentially neurotoxic (154,162,164–166). These substances include complement components, reactive oxygen intermediates, reactive nitric oxide, cytokines, glutamate, and a stable N-methyl-D-aspartate (NMDA) receptor–binding excitotoxic product (or products). It needs to be suggested at this stage that the inflammatory events occurring in AD-affected brains are more complicated than simply a result of microglial activation. A number of studies have utilized experimental insults to rat brains that cause neuronal cell death (e.g., see work by Akiyama et al (167) and Jorgensen et al (168)). A common feature of these studies has been the rapid activation of microglia (usually demonstrated by increased class I and/or class II immunoreactivity on microglia), which gradually resolves to control levels with time.

This demonstrates that once the cell debris is removed, the microglia resume their resting properties, and do not appear to cause additional neuronal cell death. A difference between these experimental studies and the events occurring in AD may be that a specific interaction between microglia and astrocytes, both of which become associated with the senile plaques and NFTs, is established and could gradually amplify the localized inflammation. This could be explained by the fact that IL-1β, which is secreted by activated microglia, may be responsible for the proliferation of astrocytes in vivo. Astrocytes have IL-1 receptors (169). In comparison, the major growth factors for microglia are colony-stimulating factor (CSF)-1 and granulocyte-macrophage CSF (GM-CSF). Both CSFs are produced by astrocytes. CSF-1 is detectable in unstimulated human astrocyte cultures and is upregulated by IL-1, whereas GM-CSF is only detectable in astrocyte cultures after IL-1β treatment (170). Receptors for IL-1 are detectable on microglia (171). In addition, the astrocytes in senile plaques in AD brain sections can be immunostained for GM-CSF, as can those in active lesions of MS (78). Increased expression of macrophage CSF receptor (MCSF-R) is detected on microglia in AD brains (79). The production of microglial growth factors by astrocytes may be detrimental to the brain that has undergone sufficient degeneration to induce microglial activation. The contribution of apoE and α₁-antichymotrypsin to the degenerative process is unclear. Both products have been localized to astrocytes in the human AD brain. Because they can induce the formation of Aβ fibrils, the binding of these proteins to Aβ plaques could contribute to the pathologic process. Recent studies showed that the synthesis of both apoE and α₁-antichymotrypsin by astrocytes is increased by treatment with IL-1 (Walker DG, et al, unpublished results, 1993) (172). This could be added evidence for the detrimental consequences of plaque-associated microglia-astrocyte interactions.

There is limited evidence for a direct toxic effect by astrocyte-produced products, though a role for astrocyte-produced nitric oxide needs to be considered. A number of studies showed that nitric oxide production can be induced in rodent brain–derived microglia. One inducing agent for this is the Aβ peptide (154). Interestingly, the induction of nitric oxide by human microglia (or macrophages) has not been possible using the same stimuli. In our laboratory, the production of nitric oxide or the induction of the inducible nitric oxide synthase gene has not been convincingly demonstrated in human postmortem brain–derived microglia (109). Similar results were shown using human fetal brain microglia (173). However, one recent study (174) did not agree with these observations, and claimed ready induction of nitric oxide and inducible nitric oxide synthase mRNA in human fetal microglia. There are similar controversies in the published literature as to whether nitric oxide can be produced by human blood macrophages. In comparison, production of nitric oxide by human astrocytes has been readily demonstrated. In human astrocytes, this can be induced by treatment of cells with a combination of IL-1β and IFN-γ or

TNF-α (173,175). The significance of astrocyte nitric oxide production is indicated by the staining of astrocytes for NADPH-diaphorase (a histochemical marker for nitric oxide synthase activity) in the vicinity of MS plaques. In comparison, microglia were not reactive though they did stain for IL-1β and TNF-α (176). Similar studies using AD tissue have not been done at this time. Studies using mixed cultures of rodent brain–derived cells demonstrated that induction of nitric oxide by microglia can lead to neurotoxicity (154,165). The toxicity of nitric oxide appears to be mediated by peroxynitrite, which is formed by the interaction of nitric oxide with superoxide anion.

Reactive Oxygen Intermediates

It has been shown that reactive oxygen intermediates, which can be generated by activated microglia in large amounts as a result of NADPH oxidase activation, could potentially play a role in causing toxicity in the brain, particularly in brain ischemia (e.g., see article by Banati et al (177)). The concepts of oxidative stress, reactive oxygen intermediates, and tissue damage in AD are well accepted; however, at present there is little direct evidence that microglia-generated reactive oxygen intermediates contribute to AD pathology. It is believed that free radical generation, as a by-product of mitochondrial respiration or other chemical reactions that can occur in any cell type, becomes a significant factor in aging owing to a decline in activity of various antioxidant enzymes, including catalase, superoxide dismutase, and glutathione peroxidase, or owing to increased free radical generation as a result of head injury, aluminum toxicity, or exposure to organic solvents, among other factors (178). There is evidence that reactive oxygen intermediates contribute to the toxicity caused by Aβ peptide on neurons in vitro. It has been suggested that the Aβ peptide can generate free radicals by chemical decay in a manner that will cause membrane damage (179,180). In related experiments, the toxicity of Aβ peptide to cultured neurons can be attenuated by treatment with the lipoxygenase inhibitor nordihydroguaiaretic acid (181). Although this agent has anti-inflammatory activity, in these experiments there was no evidence that microglia were involved in the Aβ toxicity. Similarly, vitamin E, a free radical scavenger, and diphenylene iodonium, an inhibitor of NADPH oxidase, can reduce Aβ toxicity to neuron cultures (182). Markers for oxidative stress can be seen in AD brains. Immunohistochemical examination of AD brains for superoxide dismutase, an antioxidant enzyme, showed increased immunoreactivity in tangles, senile plaques, and reactive glial cells (183).

NMDA Receptor–Mediated Toxins

In a series of studies, Giulian et al (166,184,185) identified a microglial neurotoxin that mediates its effect through the neuronal NMDA receptor. This toxin appears to have a molecular size of less than 500 daltons and is resistant to protease action (indicating that it is not a peptide) and to freezing and boiling (indicating that it is not a reactive oxygen or nitrite intermediate). Its neurotoxic action was blocked by the NMDA receptor antagonist AP5 and the NMDA receptor ion channel blocker MK-801, but not by non-NMDA receptor antagonists or calcium L-channel blockers. This toxin (or closely related toxins) is secreted by activated rat microglia, produced in rat brains following ischemic and traumatic injury, produced by mononuclear phagocytes infected with the human immunodeficiency virus, and produced by human and rat microglia that are cocultured with amyloid isolated from AD brains and with synthetic Aβ peptides (166,184, 185). The first study on AD (166) showed that the presence of amyloid purified from senile plaques induces the production of this toxin by microglia, whereas extracts of brains that do not contain plaques are not able to induce toxin production. A compound with the same properties was extracted and partially purified from AD brain, but not from normal or ALS brains. The highest levels of toxin activity were extracted from AD brain regions that are more severely affected by AD degeneration, and the lowest levels were from the cerebellum and white matter, regions not normally affected by AD.

The most recent study showed in more detail that synthetic human Aβ could induce the production of this toxin by microglia (185). Using Aβ peptides of different sizes, it was shown that microglial toxin induction required two separate sequences present in the human Aβ peptide. Binding of the peptide to microglia was mediated by residues 12—16, while toxin induction required the residues at the carboxy terminus of Aβ (residues 29–40/42) (185). Rodent Aβ (1–40), which only differs from the human sequence at residues 5, 10, and 13, was not effective in inducing the production of this microglial toxin (185).

Therapy Aimed at Inflammatory Changes

At this point in time the only pharmaceutical agent licensed for the treatment of AD is tacrine, an acetylcholinesterase inhibitor. Although a number of clinical trials for tacrine have been performed, its effectiveness appears to be limited. The potential effectiveness for anti-inflammatory therapy in AD was first examined by reviewing the incidence of AD in rheumatoid arthritis patients who have a long history of taking anti-inflammatory drugs, particularly nonsteroidal anti-inflammatory drugs (NSAIDs) for controlling that condition (186). Since 1988, a number of studies have generally shown that the incidence of AD is significantly lower in rheumatoid arthritis patients (e.g., see articles by Jenkinson et al (187) and Li et al (188)). Similarly, studies in AD patients showed a significant protective effect from onset and course of the disease by use of NSAIDs (189–191). One study elegantly confirmed this by comparing the onset of AD in groups of twins. The one consistent factor in delaying or preventing the onset of AD

in one of the twins was the use of NSAIDs or steroids (192). To date, only one double-blind, placebo-controlled trial of anti-inflammatory treatment has been carried out on AD patients; it tested the cyclooxygenase inhibitor indomethacin. The results showed that over a 6-month period there appeared to be a significant protection in the rate of cognitive decline in the patients receiving indomethacin. Although the study only had 14 patients in each group, and was carried out for a relatively short time, it has provided the impetus to many others to look at this avenue as a way of treating AD (193).

Epidemiologic studies showing a reduced incidence of dementia in leprosy patients indicated another class of drugs that might be effective in delaying or preventing AD. The incidence of dementia in a group of leprosy patients over 65 years old was 2.9% in those continuously treated with dapsone or closely related drugs for many years. The incidence rose to 6.25% in those untreated for at least 5 years (194). Examination of the brains from a group of leprosy patients indicated that they had reduced numbers of senile amyloid plaques. Dapsone has anti-inflammatory properties, possibly by inhibiting the synthesis of prostaglandins and leukotrienes (195).

Conclusions

As a result of immunocytochemical studies on brains of AD patients, along with experimental data from various models, the basis for considering some of the pathologic changes in AD as part of a chronic inflammatory condition has become established. In addition, retrospective clinical studies, and one controlled drug trial, showed that anti-inflammatory treatment offers real promise as a means for slowing the progression of this disease. The time course of events for the involvement of microglia and inflammatory-associated molecules remains undetermined. A theoretical sequence of these events is presented in Figure 11-5.

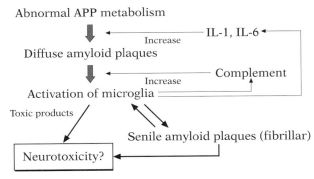

Figure 11-5. Hypothetical scheme outlining the involvement of neuroinflammatory mechanisms with Alzheimer's disease pathology. APP = amyloid precursor protein; IL = interleukin.

Acknowledgments

The authors are indebted to the Alzheimer Society of British Columbia for constant support over the years. Additional support was provided by the Jack Brown and Family AD Research Fund and the British Columbia Health Research Foundation.

References

1. Braak H, Braak E. Pathology of Alzheimer's disease. In: Calne DB, ed. *Neurodegenerative diseases*. Philadelphia: WB Saunders, 1994:585–613.
2. Corey-Bloom J, Galasko D, Thal LJ. Clinical features and natural history of Alzheimer's disease. In: Calne DB, ed. *Neurodegenerative diseases*. Philadelphia: WB Saunders, 1994:631–645.
3. Ernst RL, Hay JW. The US economic and social costs of Alzheimer's disease revisited. *Am J Public Health* 1994; 84:1261–1264.
4. Alzheimer A. Uber eine eigenartige Erkrankung der Hirnrinde. *Centralbl Nervenheilk Psychiatr (Leipzig)* 1907;30:177–179.
5. Glenner GG, Wong CW. Alzheimer's disease: initial report of the purification and characterization of a novel cerebrovascular amyloid protein. *Biochem Biophys Res Commun* 1984;120:885–890.
6. Masters CL, Multhaup G, Simms G, et al. Neuronal origin of a cerebral amyloid: neurofibrillary tangles of Alzheimer's disease contain the same protein as the amyloid of plaque cores and blood vessels. *EMBO J* 1985;4:2757–2763.
7. Tanzi RE, Gusella JF, Watkins PC, et al. Amyloid beta protein gene: cDNA, mRNA distribution, and genetic linkage near the Alzheimer locus. *Science* 1987;235: 880–884.
8. Kang J, Lemaire HG, Unterbeck A, et al. The precursor of Alzheimer's disease amyloid A4 protein resembles a cell-surface receptor. *Nature* 1987;325:733–736.
9. Goldgaber D, Lerman MI, McBride OW, et al. Characterization and chromosomal localization of a cDNA encoding brain amyloid of Alzheimer's disease. *Science* 1987;235:877–880.
10. Tanzi RE, McClatchey AI, Lamperti ED, et al. Protease inhibitor domain encoded by an amyloid protein precursor mRNA associated with Alzheimer's disease. *Nature* 1988;331:528–530.
11. Kitaguchi N, Takahashi Y, Tokushima Y, et al. Novel precursor of Alzheimer's disease amyloid protein shows protease inhibitory activity. *Nature* 1988;331:530–532.
12. Neve RL, Finch EA, Dawes LR. Expression of the Alzheimer amyloid precursor gene transcripts in the human brain. *Neuron* 1988;1:669–677.
13. Selkoe DJ. Alzheimer's disease: a central role for amyloid. *J Neuropathol Exp Neurol* 1994;53:438–447.
14. Selkoe DJ. Amyloid beta-protein and the genetics of Alzheimer's disease. *J Biol Chem* 1996;271:18295–18298.
15. Cordell B. β-Amyloid formation as a potential therapeutic target for Alzheimer's disease. *Annu Rev Pharmacol Toxicol* 1994;34:69–89.
16. Yankner BA, Dawes LR, Fisher S, et al. Neurotoxicity of a fragment of the amyloid precursor associated with Alzheimer's disease. *Science* 1989;245:417–420.
17. Yankner BA, Duffy LK, Kirschner DA. Neurotrophic and neurotoxic effects of amyloid beta protein: reversal by tachykinin neuropeptides. *Science* 1990;250:279–282.
18. Yankner BA. Amyloid and Alzheimer's disease—cause or effect? *Neurobiol Aging* 1989;10:470–471.
19. Stephenson DT, Clemens JA. In vivo effects of beta-amyloid implants in rodents: lack of potentiation of damage associated with transient global forebrain ischemia. *Brain Res* 1992;586:235–246.
20. Chartier HM, Crawford F, Houlden H, et al. Early-onset Alzheimer's disease caused by mutations at codon 717 of the beta-amyloid precursor protein gene. *Nature* 1991; 353:844–846.
21. Mullan M, Tsuji S, Miki T, et al. Clinical comparison of Alzheimer's disease in pedigrees with the codon 717 Val→Ile mutation in the amyloid precursor protein gene. *Neurobiol Aging* 1993;14:407–419.
22. Lannfelt L, Johnston J, Bogdanovich N, Cowburn R. Amyloid precursor protein gene mutation at codon 670/671 in familial Alzheimer's disease in Sweden. *Biochem Soc Trans* 1994;22:176–179.
23. Levy E, Carman MD, Fernandez MI, et al. Mutation of the Alzheimer's disease amyloid gene in hereditary cerebral hemorrhage, Dutch type. *Science* 1990;248: 1124–1126.
24. Saunders AM, Schmader K, Breitner JC, et al. Apolipoprotein E epsilon 4 allele distributions in late-onset Alzheimer's disease and in other amyloid-forming diseases. *Lancet* 1993;342:710–711.
25. Saunders AM, Strittmatter WJ, Schmechel D, et al. Association of apolipoprotein E allele epsilon 4 with late-onset familial and sporadic Alzheimer's disease. *Neurology* 1993;43:1467–1472.
26. Corder EH, Saunders AM, Strittmatter WJ, et al. Gene dose of apolipoprotein E type 4 allele and the risk of Alzheimer's disease in late onset families. *Science* 1993; 261:921–923.
27. Diedrich JF, Minnigan H, Carp RI, et al. Neuropathological changes in scrapie and Alzheimer's disease are associated with increased expression of apolipoprotein E and cathepsin D in astrocytes. *J Virol* 1991;65: 4759–4768.
28. Oyama F, Shimada H, Oyama R, Ihara Y. Apolipoprotein E genotype, Alzheimer's pathologies and related gene expression in the aged population. *Brain Res Mol Brain Res* 1995;29:92–98.
29. Namba Y, Tomonaga M, Kawasaki H, et al. Apolipoprotein E immunoreactivity in cerebral amyloid deposits and neurofibrillary tangles in Alzheimer's disease and kuru plaque amyloid in Creutzfeldt-Jakob disease. *Brain Res* 1991;541:163–166.
30. Strittmatter WJ, Saunders AM, Schmechel D, et al. Apolipoprotein E: high-avidity binding to beta-amyloid and increased frequency of type 4 allele in late-onset familial Alzheimer disease. *Proc Natl Acad Sci USA* 1993;90:1977–1981.
31. Strittmatter WJ, Weisgraber KH, Huang DY, et al. Binding of human apolipoprotein E to synthetic amyloid beta peptide: isoform-specific effects and implications for late-onset Alzheimer disease. *Proc Natl Acad Sci USA* 1993;90:8098–8102.
32. Huang DY, Goedert M, Jakes R, et al. Isoform-specific interactions of apolipoprotein E with the microtubule-associated protein MAP2c: implications for Alzheimer's disease. *Neurosci Lett* 1994;182:55–58.
33. Strittmatter WJ, Saunders AM, Goedert M, et al. Isoform-specific interactions of apolipoprotein E with microtubule-associated protein tau: implications for Alzheimer disease. *Proc Natl Acad Sci USA* 1994; 91:11183–11186.

34. Han SH, Einstein G, Weisgraber KH, et al. Apolipoprotein E is localized to the cytoplasm of human cortical neurons: a light and electron microscopic study. *J Neuropathol Exp Neurol* 1994;53:535–544.

35. Huang DY, Weisgraber KH, Goedert M, et al. ApoE3 binding to tau tandem repeat 1 is abolished by tau serine(262) phosphorylation. *Neurosci Lett* 1995;192:209–212.

36. Levylahad E, Wasco W, Poorkaj P, et al. Candidate gene for the chromosome 1 familial Alzheimer's disease locus. *Science* 1995;269:973–977.

37. Sherrington R, Rogaev EI, Liang Y, et al. Cloning of a gene bearing missense mutations in early-onset familial Alzheimer's disease. *Nature* 1995;375:754–760.

38. Murphy GM Jr, Forno LS, Ellis WG, et al. Antibodies to presenilin proteins detect neurofibrillary tangles in Alzheimer's disease. *Am J Pathol* 1996;149:1839–1846.

39. Scheuner D, Eckman C, Jensen M, et al. Secreted amyloid beta-protein similar to that in senile plaques of Alzheimer's disease is increased in vivo by the presenilin 1 and 2 APP mutations linked to familial Alzheimer's disease. *Nature Med* 1996;2:864–870.

40. Iqbal K, Grundke-Iqbal I. Neurofibrillary tangles. In: Calne DB, ed. *Neurodegenerative diseases*. Philadelphia: WB Saunders, 1994:71–81.

41. Gong CX, Shaikh S, Wang JZ, et al. Phosphatase activity toward abnormally phosphorylated tau: decrease in Alzheimer disease brain. *J Neurochem* 1995;65:732–738.

42. Martyn CN, Barker DJ, Osmond C, et al. Geographical relation between Alzheimer's disease and aluminum in drinking water. *Lancet* 1989;1:59–62.

43. Pogo BG, Casals J, Elizan TS. A study of viral genomes and antigens in brains of patients with Alzheimer's disease. *Brain* 1987;110:907–915.

44. Stern Y, Alexander GE, Prohovnik I, Mayeux R. Inverse relationship between education and parietotemporal perfusion deficit in Alzheimer's disease. *Ann Neurol* 1992;32:371–375.

45. Rasmusson DX, Brandt J, Martin DB, Folstein MF. Head injury as a risk factor in Alzheimer's disease. *Brain Injury* 1995;9:213–219.

46. Gentleman SM, Graham DI, Roberts GW. Molecular pathology of head trauma: altered beta APP metabolism and the aetiology of Alzheimer's disease. *Prog Brain Res* 1993;96:237–246.

47. Mendez MF, Underwood KL, Zander BA, et al. Risk factors in Alzheimer's disease: a clinicopathologic study. *Neurology* 1992;42:770–775.

48. McGeer PL, Rogers J. Anti-inflammatory agents as a therapeutic approach to Alzheimer's disease. *Neurology* 1992;42:447–449.

49. McGeer PL, McGeer EG. The inflammatory response system of the brain: implications for therapy of Alzheimer's disease and other neurodegenerative diseases. *Brain Res Rev* 1995;21:195–218.

50. Rich JB, Rasmusson DX, Folstein MF, et al. Nonsteroidal anti-inflammatory drugs in Alzheimer's disease. *Neurology* 1995;45:51–55.

51. del Rio Hortega P. El "tercer elemento" de centros nervisos: poder fagocitario y movilidad de la microglia. *Biol Soc Exp Biol Ano* 1919;9:154–166.

52. Penfield W. Microglia and the process of phagocytosis in gliomas. *Am J Pathol* 1925;1:77–89.

53. Bolsoi D. Placche senile e microglia. *Riv Patol Nerv Mental* 1927;32:65–68.

54. McGeer PL, Itagaki S, Tago S, McGeer EG. Reactive microglia in patients with senile dementia of the Alzheimer's type are positive for the histocompatibility glycoprotein HLA-DR. *Neurosci Lett* 1987;79:1285–1291.

55. Rogers J, Luber NJ, Styren SD, Civin WH. Expression of immune system-associated antigens by cells of the human central nervous system: relationship to the pathology of Alzheimer's disease. *Neurobiol Aging* 1988;9:339–349.

56. McGeer PL, Itagaki S, McGeer EG. Expression of the histocompatibility glycoprotein HLA-DR in neurological disease. *Acta Neuropathol (Berl)* 1988;76:550–557.

57. Loughlin AJ, Woodroofe MN, Cuzner ML. Modulation of interferon-β induced major histocompatibility complex class II and Fc receptor expression on isolated microglia by transforming growth factor-β1, interleukin-4, noradrenaline and glucocorticoids. *Immunology* 1993;79:125–130.

58. Tooyama I, Kimura H, Akiyama H, McGeer PL. Reactive microglia express class I and class II major histocompatibility complex antigens in Alzheimer's disease. *Brain Res* 1990;523:273–280.

59. Itagaki S, McGeer PL, Akiyama H. Presence of T-cytotoxic suppressor and leucocyte common antigen cells in Alzheimer's disease brain tissue. *Neurosci Lett* 1988;91:59–64.

60. Vannoort JM, Vansechel AC, Bajramovic JJ, et al. The small heat-shock protein alpha-b-crystallin as candidate autoantigen in multiple sclerosis. *Nature* 1995;375:798–801.

61. Desimone R, Giampaolo A, Giometto B, et al. The costimulatory molecule B7 is expressed on human microglia in culture and in multiple sclerosis acute lesions. *J Neuropathol Exp Neurol* 1995;54:175–187.

62. Gehrmann J, Banati RB, Kreutzberg GW. Microglia in the immune surveillance of the brain: human microglia constitutively express HLA-DR molecules. *J Neuroimmunol* 1993;48:189–198.

63. Perlmutter LS, Scott SA, Barron E, Chui HC. MHC class II-positive microglia in human brain: association with Alzheimer lesions. *J Neurosci Res* 1992;33:549–558.

64. Mattiace LA, Davies P, Dickson DW. Detection of HLA-DR on microglia in the human brain is a function of both clinical and technical factors. *Am J Pathol* 1990;136:1101–1114.

65. Colloby PS, West KP, Fletcher A. Is poor prognosis really related to HLA-DR expression by melanoma cells. *Histopathology* 1992;20:411–416.

66. Akiyama H, McGeer PL. Brain microglia constitutively express beta-2 integrins. *J Neuroimmunol* 1990;30:81–93.

67. Eikelenboom P, Zhan SS, Kamphorst W, et al. Cellular and substrate adhesion molecules (integrins) and their ligands in cerebral amyloid plaques in Alzheimer's disease. *Virchows Arch* 1994;424:421–427.

68. Akiyama H, Ikeda K, Katoh M, et al. Expression of MRP14, 27E10, interferon-alpha and leukocyte common antigen by reactive microglia in postmortem human brain tissue. *J Neuroimmunol* 1994;50:195–201.

69. Masliah E, Mallory M, Hansen L, et al. Immunoreactivity of CD45, a protein phosphotyrosine phosphatase, in disease. *Acta Neuropathol (Berl)* 1991;83:12–20.

70. Peress NS, Fleit HB, Perillo E, et al. Identification of Fc gamma RI, II and III on normal human brain ramified microglia and on microglia in senile plaques in Alzheimer's disease. *J Neuroimmunol* 1993;48:71–79.

71. Akiyama H, Tooyama I, Kawamata T, et al. Morphological diversities of CD44 positive astrocytes in the cortex of normal subjects and patients with Alzheimer's disease. *Brain Res* 1993;632:249–259.

72. McGeer PL, Zhu SG, Dedhar S. Immunostaining of human brain capillaries by antibodies to very late antigens. *J Neuroimmunol* 1990;26:213–218.

73. Akiyama H, Kawamata T, Dedhar S, McGeer PL. Immunohistochemical localization of vitronectin, its receptor and beta-3 integrin in Alzheimer brain tissue. *J Neuroimmunol* 1991;32:19–28.

74. Akiyama H, Kawamata T, Yamada T, et al. Expression of intercellular adhesion molecule (ICAM)-1 by a subset of astrocytes in Alzheimer disease and some other degenerative neurological disorders. *Acta Neuropathol (Berl)* 1993;85:628–634.

75. Griffin WS, Sheng JG, Roberts GW, Mrak RE. Interleukin-1 expression in different plaque types in Alzheimer's disease: significance in plaque evolution. *J Neuropathol Exp Neurol* 1995;54:276–281.

76. Dickson DW, Lee SC, Mattiace LA, et al. Microglia and cytokines in neurological disease, with special reference to AIDS and Alzheimer's disease. *Glia* 1993;7:75–83.

77. Lee SC, Liu W, Brosnan CF, Dickson DW. GM-CSF promotes proliferation of human fetal and adult microglia in primary cultures. *Glia* 1994;12:309–318.

78. Akiyama H, Nishimura T, Kondo H, et al. Expression of the receptor for macrophage colony stimulating factor by brain microglia and its upregulation in brains of patients with Alzheimer's disease and amyotrophic lateral sclerosis. *Brain Res* 1994;639:171–174.

79. Tooyama I, Kawamata T, Akiyama H, et al. Immunohistochemical study of alpha 2 macroglobulin receptor in Alzheimer and control postmortem human brain. *Mol Chem Neuropathol* 1993;18:153–160.

80. Kawamata T, Tooyama I, Yamada T, et al. Lactotransferrin immunocytochemistry in Alzheimer and normal human brain. *Am J Pathol* 1993;142:1574–1585.

81. Connor JR, Menzies SL, St. Martin MS, Mufson EJ. A histochemical study of iron, transferrin, and ferritin in Alzheimer's diseased brains. *J Neurosci Res* 1992;31:75–83.

82. Akiyama H, Ikeda K, Kondo H, et al. Microglia express the type 2 plasminogen activator inhibitor in the brain of control subjects and patients with Alzheimer's disease. *Neurosci Lett* 1993;164:233–235.

83. Yasuhara O, Tooyama I, Akiyama H, et al. Reactive astrocytes express acidic fibroblast growth factor in Alzheimer's disease brain. *Dementia* 1991;2:64–70.

84. Wood JG, Zinsmeister P. Tyrosine phosphorylation systems in Alzheimer's disease. *Neurosci Lett* 1992;121:12–16.

85. Yamada T, Miyazaki K, Koshikawa N, et al. Selective localization of gelatinase A, an enzyme degrading beta-amyloid protein, in white matter microglia and in Schwann cells. *Acta Neuropathol (Berl)* 1995;89:199–203.

86. Ulvestad E, Williams K, Matre R, et al. Fc receptors for IgG on cultured human microglia mediate cytotoxicity and phagocytosis of antibody-coated targets. *J Neuropathol Exp Neurol* 1994;53:27–36.

87. Loughlin AJ, Woodroofe MN, Cuzner ML. Regulation of Fc receptor and major histocompatibility complex antigen expression on isolated rat microglia by tumour necrosis factor, interleukin-1 and lipopolysaccharide: effects on interferon-gamma induced activation. *Immunology* 1992;75:170–175.

88. Rogers J, Cooper NR, Webster S, et al. Complement activation by beta-amyloid in Alzheimer disease. *Proc Natl Acad Sci USA* 1992;89:10016–10020.

89. Donnelly RJ, Friedhoff AJ, Beer B, et al. Interleukin-1 stimulates the beta-amyloid precursor protein promoter. *Cell Mol Neurobiol* 1990;10:485–495.

90. Barnum SR, Jones JL, Benveniste EN. Interleukin-1 and tumor necrosis factor-mediated regulation of C3 gene expression in human astroglioma cells. *Glia* 1993;7:225–236.

91. Das S, Potter H. Expression of the Alzheimer amyloid-promoting factor antichymotrypsin is induced in human astrocytes by IL-1. *Neuron* 1995;14:447–456.

92. Green SP, Philips WA. Activation of the macrophage respiratory burst by phorbol myristate acetate: evidence for both tyrosine-kinase-dependent and independent pathways. *Biochim Biophys Acta* 1994;1222:241–248.

93. Wood JG, Zinsmeister P. Tyrosine phosphorylation systems in Alzheimer's disease pathology. *Neurosci Lett* 1991;121:12–16.

94. McGeer PL, Akiyama H, Itagaki S, McGeer EG. Activation of the classical complement pathway in brain tissue of Alzheimer patients. *Neurosci Lett* 1989;107:341–346.

95. Eikelenboom P, Stam FC. An immunohistochemical study on cerebral vascular and senile plaque amyloid in Alzheimer's dementia. *Virchows Arch B Cell Pathol Mol Pathol* 1984;47:17–25.

96. Eikelenboom P, Hack CE, Rozemuller JM, Stam FC. Complement activation in amyloid plaques in Alzheimer's dementia. *Virchows Arch B Cell Pathol Mol Pathol* 1989;56:259–262.

97. Ishii T, Haga S. Immuno-electron-microscopic localization of complements in amyloid fibrils of senile plaques. *Acta Neuropathol (Berl)* 1984;63:296–300.

98. Yamada T, Akiyama H, McGeer PL. Complement-activated oligodendroglia: a new pathogenic entity identified by immunostaining with antibodies to human complement proteins C3d and C4d. *Neurosci Lett* 1990;112:161–166.

99. Walker DG, Yasuhara O, Patston PA, et al. Complement C1 inhibitor is produced by brain tissue and is cleaved in Alzheimer disease. *Brain Res* 1995;675:75–82.

100. McGeer PL, Kawamata T, Walker DG. Distribution of clusterin in Alzheimer brain tissue. *Brain Res* 1992;579:337–341.

101. McGeer PL, Walker DG, Akiyama H, et al. Detection of the membrane inhibitor of reactive lysis (CD59) in diseased neurons of Alzheimer brain. *Brain Res* 1991;544:315–319.

102. Wong P, Taillefer D, Lakins J, et al. Molecular characterization of human TRPM-2/clusterin, a gene associated with sperm maturation, apoptosis and neurodegeneration. *Eur J Biochem* 1994;221:917–925.

103. Preissner KT. The role of vitronectin as multifunctional regulator in the hemostatic and immune systems. *Blut* 1989;59:419–431. Review.

104. Kieffer N, Fitzgerald LA, Wolf D, et al. Adhesive properties of the beta 3 integrins: comparison of GP IIb-IIIa and the vitronectin receptor individually expressed in human melanoma cells. *J Cell Biol* 1991;113:451–461.

105. Walker DG, McGeer PL. Complement gene expression in human brain: comparison between normal and Alzheimer disease cases. *Brain Res Mol Brain Res* 1992;14:109–116.

106. Johnson SA, Lampert EM, Pasinetti GM, et al. Complement mRNA in the mammalian brain: responses to Alzheimer's disease and experimental brain lesioning. *Neurobiol Aging* 1992;13:641–648.

107. Pasinetti GM, Johnson SA, Rozovsky I, et al. Complement C1qB and C4 mRNAs responses to lesioning in rat brain. *Exp Neurol* 1992;118:117–125.

108. Liu L, Tornqvist E, Mattsson P, et al. Complement and clusterin in the spinal cord dorsal horn and nucleus fol-

lowing sciatic nerve injury in the adult rat. *Neuroscience* 1995;68:167–179.

109. Afagh A, Cummings BJ, Cribbs DH, et al. Localization and cell association of C1q in Alzheimer's brain. *Exp Neurol* 1996;138:22–32.

110. Walker DG, McGeer PL. Complement gene expression in neuroblastoma and astrocytoma cell lines of human origin. *Neurosci Lett* 1993;157:99–102.

111. Walker DG, Kim SU, Mcgeer PL. Complement and cytokine gene expression in cultured microglia derived from postmortem human brains. *J Neurosci Res* 1995;40:478–493.

112. Gasque P, Fontaine M, Morgan BP. Complement expression in human brain—biosynthesis of terminal pathway components and regulators in human glial cells and cell lines. *J Immunol* 1995;154:4726–4733.

113. Lappin DF, Birnie GD, Whaley K. Interferon-mediated transcriptional and post-transcriptional modulation of complement gene expression in human monocytes. *Eur J Biochem* 1990;194:177–184.

114. Barnum SR, Jones JL, Benveniste EN. Interleukin-1 and tumor necrosis factor-mediated regulation of C3 gene expression in human astroglioma cells. *Glia* 1993; 7:225–236.

115. Kalaria RN, Perry G. Amyloid P component and other acute-phase proteins associated with cerebellar A beta-deposits in Alzheimer's disease. *Brain Res* 1993;631: 151–155.

116. Lue L-F, Rogers J. Full complement activation fails in diffuse plaques of the Alzheimer's disease cerebellum. *Dementia* 1992;3:308–313.

117. Pepys MB, Rademacher TW, Amatayakul CS, et al. Human serum amyloid P component is an invariant constituent of amyloid deposits and has a uniquely homogeneous glycostructure. *Proc Natl Acad Sci USA* 1994; 91:5602–5606.

118. Tennent GA, Lovat LB, Pepys MB. Serum amyloid P component prevents proteolysis of the amyloid fibrils of Alzheimer disease and systemic amyloidosis. *Proc Natl Acad Sci USA* 1995;92:4299–4303.

119. Akiyama H, Yamada T, Kawamata T, McGeer PL. Association of amyloid P component with complement proteins in neurologically diseased brain tissue. *Brain Res* 1991;548:349–352.

120. Abraham CR, Selkoe DJ, Potter H. Immunochemical identification of the serine protease inhibitor alpha 1-antichymotrypsin in the brain amyloid deposits of Alzheimer's disease. *Cell* 1988;52:487–501.

121. Snow AD, Mar H, Nochlin D, et al. Early accumulation of heparan sulfate in neurons and in the beta-amyloid protein-containing lesions of Alzheimer's disease and Down's syndrome. *Am J Pathol* 1990;137:1253–1270.

122. Smith MA, Kalaria RN, Perry G. α1-Trypsin immunoreactivity in Alzheimer disease. *Biochem Biophys Res Commun* 1993;193:579–584.

123. Nakamura Y, Takeda M, Suzuki H, et al. Abnormal distribution of cathepsins in the brain of patients Alzheimer's disease. *Neurosci Lett* 1991;30:195–198.

124. Gollin PA, Kalaria RN, Eikelenboom P, et al. Alpha 1-antitrypsin and alpha 1-antichymotrypsin are in the lesions of Alzheimer's disease. *Neuroreport* 1992;3: 201–203.

125. Van Gool D, De Strooper B, Van Leuven F, et al. Alpha 2-macroglobulin expression in neuritic-type plaques in patients with Alzheimer's disease. *Neurobiol Aging* 1993; 14:233–237.

126. Peress N, Perillo E, Zucker S. Localization of tissue inhibitor of matrix metalloproteinases in Alzheimer's disease and normal brain. *J Neuropathol Exp Neurol* 1995;54:16–22.

127. Bernstein HG, Rinne R, Kirschke H, et al. Cystatin A-like immunoreactivity is widely distributed in human brain and accumulates in neuritic plaques of Alzheimer disease subjects. *Brain Res Bull* 1994;33:477–481.

128. Tago H, McGeer PL, McGeer EG. Acetylcholinesterase fibers and the development of senile plaques. *Brain Res* 1987;406:363–369.

129. Moran MA, Mufson EJ, Gomez RP. Colocalization of cholinesterases with beta amyloid protein in aged and Alzheimer's brains. *Acta Neuropathol (Berl)* 1993;85: 362–369.

130. Rebeck GW, Harr SD, Strickland DK, Hyman BT. Multiple, diverse senile plaque-associated proteins are ligands of an apolipoprotein E receptor, the α2-macroglobulin receptor/low density-lipoprotein receptor-related protein. *Ann Neurol* 1995;37:211–217.

131. Akiyama H, Ikeda K, Kondo H, McGeer PL. Thrombin accumulation in brains of patients with Alzheimer's disease. *Neurosci Lett* 1992;146:152–154.

132. Yasuhara O, Walker DG, McGeer PL. Hageman factor and its binding sites are present in senile plaques of Alzheimer's disease. *Brain Res* 1994;654:234–240.

133. Shinohara H, Inaguma Y, Goto S, et al. Alpha B crystallin and HSP28 are enhanced in the cerebral cortex of patients with Alzheimer's disease. *J Neurol Sci* 1993; 119:203–208.

134. Snow AD, Mar H, Nochlin D, et al. Peripheral distribution of dermatan sulfate proteoglycans (decorin) in amyloid-containing plaques and their presence in neurofibrillary tangles of Alzheimer's disease. *J Histochem Cytochem* 1992;40:105–113.

135. Birecree E, King LE Jr, Nanney LB. Epidermal growth factor and its receptor in the developing human system. *Brain Res Dev Brain Res* 1991;60:145–154.

136. Tooyama I, Kawamata T, Akiyama H, et al. Immunohistochemical study of alpha 2 macroglobulin receptor in Alzheimer and control postmortem human brain. *Mol Chem Neuropathol* 1993;18:153–160.

137. Cummings BJ, Su JH, Cotman CW. Neuritic involvement within bFGF immunopositive plaques of Alzheimer's disease. *Exp Neurol* 1993;124:315–325.

138. van der Wal EA, Gomez-Pinilla F, Cotman CW. Transforming growth factor-beta 1 is in plaques in Alzheimer and Down pathologies. *Neuroreport* 1993;4:69–72.

139. Yasuhara O, Muramatsu H, Kim SU, et al. Midkine, a novel neurotrophic factor, is present in senile plaques of Alzheimer disease. *Biochem Biophys Res Commun* 1993;192:246–251.

140. Huell M, Strauss S, Volk B, et al. Interleukin-6 is present in early stages of plaque formation and is restricted to the brains of Alzheimer's disease patients. *Acta Neuropathol (Berl)* 1995;89:544–551.

141. Kalaria RN, Golde TE, Cohen ML, Younkin SG. Serum amyloid P in Alzheimer's disease. Implications for dysfunction of the blood-brain barrier. *Ann NY Acad Sci* 1991;640:145–148.

142. Hamazaki H. Ca^{2+}-dependent binding of human serum amyloid P component to Alzheimer's β-amyloid. *J Biol Chem* 1995;270:10392–10394.

143. Ma J, Yee A, Brewer HJ, et al. Amyloid-associated proteins alpha 1-antichymotrypsin and apolipoprotein E promote assembly of Alzheimer beta-protein into filaments. *Nature* 1994;372:92–94.

144. Wisniewski T, Castano EM, Golabek A, et al. Acceleration of Alzheimer's fibril formation by apolipoprotein E in vitro. *Am J Pathol* 1994;145:1030–1035.

145. Hamazaki H. Amyloid P component promotes aggregation of Alzheimer's β-amyloid peptide. *Biochem Biophys Res Commun* 1995;211:349–353.

146. Golabek A, Marques MA, Lalowski M, Wisniewski T. Amyloid beta binding proteins in vitro and in normal human cerebrospinal fluid. *Neurosci Lett* 1995;191:79–82.

147. Oda T, Pasinetti GM, Osterburg HH, et al. Purification and characterization of brain clusterin. *Biochem Biophys Res Commun* 1994;204:1131–1136.

148. Oda T, Wals P, Osterburg HH, et al. Clusterin (apoJ) alters the aggregation of amyloid beta-peptide (A beta 1–42) and forms slowly sedimenting A beta complexes that cause oxidative stress. *Exp Neurol* 1995;136:22–31.

149. Webster S, O'Barr S, Rogers J. Enhanced aggregation and beta structure of amyloid beta peptide after coincubation with C1q. *J Neurosci Res* 1994;39:448–456.

150. Olsson T, Kelic S, Edlund C, et al. Neuronal interferon-gamma immunoreactive molecule: bioactivities and purification. *Eur J Immunol* 1994;24:308–314.

151. Gebicke-Haerter PJ, Appel K, Taylor GD, et al. Rat microglial interleukin-3. *J Neuroimmunol* 1994;50:203–214.

152. Imamura K, Suzumura A, Sawada M, et al. Induction of MHC class II antigen expression on murine microglia by interleukin-3. *J Neuroimmunol* 1994;55:119–125.

153. Araujo DM, Cotman CW. Beta-amyloid stimulates glial cells in vitro to produce growth factors that accumulate in senile plaques in Alzheimer's disease. *Brain Res* 1992;569:141–145.

154. Meda L, Cassatella MA, Szendrei GI, et al. Activation of microglial cells by beta-amyloid protein and interferon-gamma. *Nature* 1995;374:647–650.

155. Klegeris A, Walker DG, and McGeer PL. Activation of macrophages by Alzheimer beta amyloid peptide. *Biochem Biophys Res Commun* 1994;199:984–991.

156. Davis JB, McMurray HF, Schubert D. The amyloid beta-protein of Alzheimer's disease is chemotactic for mononuclear phagocytes. *Biochem Biophys Res Commun* 1992;189:1096–1100.

157. Haga S, Ikeda K, Sato M, Ishii T. Synthetic Alzheimer amyloid beta/A4 peptides enhance production of complement C3 component by cultured microglial cells. *Brain Res* 1993;601:88–94.

158. Wisniewski HM, Wegiel J, Wang KC, et al. Ultrastructural studies of the cells forming amyloid fibers in classical plaques. *Can J Neurol Sci* 1989;16:535–542.

159. Frackowiak J, Wisniewski HM, Wegiel J, et al. Ultrastructure of the microglia that phagocytose amyloid and the microglia that produce beta-amyloid fibrils. *Acta Neuropathol (Berl)* 1992;84:225–233.

160. Snyder SW, Wang GT, Barrett L, et al. Complement C1q does not bind monomeric beta-amyloid. *Exp Neurol* 1994;128:136–142.

161. Jiang H, Burdick D, Glabe CG, et al. Beta-amyloid activates complement by binding to a specific region of the collagen-like domain of the C1q A chain. *J Immunol* 1994;152:5050–5059.

162. Valazquez P, Cribbs DH, Poulos TL, Tenner AJ. Aspartate residue 7 in amyloid beta-protein is critical for classical complement pathway activation—Implications for Alzheimers disease pathogenesis. *Nature Med* 1997;3:77–79.

163. Ying SC, Gewurz AT, Jiang H, Gewurz H. Human serum amyloid P component oligomers bind and activate the classical complement pathway via residues 14–26 and 76–92 of the A chain collagen-like region of C1q. *J Immunol* 1993;150:169–176.

164. Banati RB, Gehrmann J, Schubert P, Kreutzberg GW. Cytotoxicity of microglia. *Glia* 1993;7:111–118. Review.

165. Boje KM, Arora PK. Microglial-produced nitric oxide and reactive nitrogen oxides mediate neuronal cell death. *Brain Res* 1992;587:250–256.

166. Giulian D, Haverkamp LJ, Li J, et al. Senile plaques stimulate microglia to release a neurotoxin found in Alzheimer brain. *Neurochem Int* 1995;27:119–137.

167. Akiyama H, Itagaki S, McGeer PL. Major histocompatibility complex antigen expression on rat microglia following epidural kainic acid lesions. *J Neurosci Res* 1988;20:147–157.

168. Jorgensen MB, Finsen BR, Jensen MB, et al. Microglial and astroglial reactions to ischemic and kainic acid-induced lesions of the adult rat hippocampus. *Exp Neurol* 1993;120:70–88.

169. da Cunha A, Jefferson JJ, Tyor WR, et al. Control of astrocytosis by interleukin-1 and transforming growth factor-beta 1 in human brain. *Brain Res* 1993;631:39–45.

170. Lee SC, Liu W, Roth P, et al. Macrophage colony-stimulating factor in human fetal astrocytes and microglia. Differential regulation by cytokines and lipopolysaccharide, and modulation of class II MHC on microglia. *J Immunol* 1993;150:594–604.

171. Ban EM, Sarlieve LL, Haour FG. Interleukin-1 binding sites on astrocytes. *Neuroscience* 1993;52:725–733.

172. Das S, Potter H. Expression of the Alzheimer amyloid-promoting factor antichymotrypsin is induced in human astrocytes by IL-1. *Neuron* 1995;14:447–456.

173. Liu J, Zhao ML, Brosnan CF, Lee SC. Expression of type II nitric oxide synthase in primary human astrocytes and microglia: role of IL-1 beta and IL-1 receptor antagonist. *J Immunol* 1996;157:3569–3576.

174. Colasanti M, Dipucchio T, Persichini T, et al. Inhibition of inducible nitric oxide synthase mRNA expression by basic fibroblast growth factor in human microglial cells. *Neurosci Lett* 1995;195:45–48.

175. Hu S, Sheng WS, Peterson PK, Chao CC. Differential regulation by cytokines of human astrocyte nitric oxide production. *Glia* 1995;15:491–494.

176. Brosnan CF, Battistini L, Raine CS, et al. Reactive nitrogen intermediates in human neuropathology—an overview. *Dev Neurosci* 1994;16:152–161.

177. Banati RB, Schubert P, Rothe G, et al. Modulation of intracellular formation of reactive oxygen intermediates in peritoneal macrophages and microglia/brain macrophages by propentofylline. *J Cereb Blood Flow Metab* 1994;14:145–149.

178. Friedlich AL, Butcher LL. Involvement of free oxygen radicals in β amyloidosis: an hypothesis. *Neurobiol Aging* 1994;15:443–455.

179. Hensley K, Carney JM, Mattson MP, et al. A model for β-amyloid aggregation and neurotoxicity based on free radical generation by the peptide: relevance to Alzheimer disease. *Proc Natl Acad Sci USA* 1994;91:3270–3274.

180. Butterfield DA, Hensley K, Harris M, et al. β-Amyloid peptide free radical fragments initiate synaptosomal lipoperoxidation in a sequence-specific fashion: implications to Alzheimer's disease. *Biochem Biophys Res Commun* 1994;200:710–715.

181. Goodman Y, Steiner MR, Steiner SM, Mattson MP. Nordihydroguaiaretic acid protects hippocampal neurons against amyloid β-peptide toxicity, and attenuates free radical and calcium accumulation. *Brain Res* 1994;654:171–176.

182. Behl C, Davis JB, Lesley R, Schubert D. Hydrogen per-

oxide mediates amyloid β protein toxicity. *Cell* 1994; 77:817–827.

183. Pappolla MA, Omar RA, Kim KS, Robakis NK. Immunohistochemical evidence of antioxidant stress in Alzheimer's disease. *Am J Pathol* 1992;140:621–628.

184. Giulian D, Vaca K, Noonan CA. Secretion of neurotoxins by mononuclear phagocytes infected with HIV-1. *Science* 1990;250:1593–1596.

185. Giulian D, Haverkamp LJ, Yu JH, et al. Specific domains of beta-amyloid from Alzheimer plaque elicit neuron killing in human microglia. *J Neurosci* 1996;16:6021–6037.

186. McGeer PL, McGeer E, Rogers J, Sibley J. Anti-inflammatory drugs and Alzheimer disease. *Lancet* 1990;335:1037.

187. Jenkinson ML, Bliss MR, Brain AT, Scott DL. Rheumatoid arthritis and senile dementia of the Alzheimer's type. *Br J Rheumatol* 1988;28:86–88.

188. Li G, Shen YC, Li YT, et al. A case-control study of Alzheimer's disease in China. *Neurology* 1992;42:1481–1488.

189. Breitner JCS, Welsh KA, Helms MJ, et al. Delayed onset of Alzheimer's disease with nonsteroidal anti-inflamma-

tory and histamine H2 blocking drugs. *Neurobiol Aging* 1995;16:523–530.

190. Andersen K, Launer LJ, Ott A, et al. Do nonsteroidal anti-inflammatory drugs decrease the risk for Alzheimer's disease? The Rotterdam Study. *Neurology* 1995; 45:1441–1445.

191. McGeer PL, Schulzer M, McGeer EG. Arthritis and anti-inflammatory agents as possible protective factors for Alzheimer's disease: a review of 17 epidemiologic studies. *Neurology* 1996;47:425–432.

192. Breitner JC, Gau BA, Welsh KA, et al. Inverse association of anti-inflammatory treatments and Alzheimer's disease: initial results of a co-twin control study. *Neurology* 1994;44:227–232.

193. Rogers J, Kirby LC, Hempelman SR, et al. Clinical trial of indomethacin in Alzheimer's disease. *Neurology* 1993;43:1609–1611.

194. McGeer PL, Harada N, Kimura H, et al. Prevalence of dementia amongst elderly Japanese with leprosy: apparent effect of chronic drug therapy. *Dementia* 1992;3:146–149.

195. Bonney RJ, Humes JL. Physiological and pharmacological regulation of prostaglandin and leukotriene production by macrophages. *J Leukoc Biol* 1984;35:1–10.

Chapter 12

HIV-1 Infection and Its Related Neurologic Diseases

Leslie P. Weiner, Rodrigo Rodriguez, and David Hinton

In 1981, Masur et al (1) described *Pneumocystis carinii* pneumonia in homosexual males. These immunoincompetent patients had depressed T-cell counts and defects in cellular immunity. A series of observations and reports of a rare skin cancer, Kaposi's sarcoma, and a variety of opportunistic infections in male homosexuals, intravenous drug users, and hemophiliacs suggested that a transmissible agent may be responsible for this acquired immunodeficiency syndrome (AIDS). In 1983, Barre-Sinoussi et al (2) at the Pasteur Institute isolated a retrovirus from the lymph node of such an immune-impaired patient. This virus was subsequently named *human immunodeficiency virus* or *HIV-1*. Gallo et al (3) also reported the isolation of a retrovirus from patients with AIDS. Montagnier et al (4) clarified the issue, showing that the AIDS agent was a human retrovirus similar to human T-cell leukemia virus (HTLV), but distinct in growing to high concentration in CD4+ T lymphocytes and also killing these cells, in contrast to HTLV.

AIDS has evolved as a major public health problem and a worldwide distribution has been recognized. In North and South America and in western Europe, AIDS is most prominent in male homosexuals, intravenous drug users, and female prostitutes, many of whom are drug abusers or have had contact with bisexual men. In Africa, males and females are equally affected and most infections are via heterosexual contacts. The patterns in Asia are changing, but appear to be primarily heterosexual contacts with prostitutes and drug users.

The US prevalence of AIDS has been reported to be up to 130 per 100,000 persons in endemic areas. AIDS is now reported to be the most common cause of death in males in the 25- to 40-year age group (5). In 1991 it was estimated that 2 million people were infected with HIV-1 and, most disturbing, 206,392 AIDS cases and 133,232 AIDS-related deaths were reported in the United States alone (6).

Neurologic disease associated with HIV-1 infection is common and the clinical syndromes diverse. It is believed that more than 50% of HIV seropositive patients will develop symptomatic neurologic disease during the course of their illness (7). In most instances, the neurologic problems occur when severe immunosuppression

is present; however, between 10% and 20% of HIV-infected patients present with neurologic problems prior to other clinical evidence of immunoincompetence (7,8). The clinical syndromes are believed to be the result of either a direct effect of HIV through lytic, toxic, or immunopathologic mechanisms (Table 12-1), or the results of severe immunosuppression (Table 12-2). In 1994, Bacellar et al (9) reported the temporal trends of HIV-1–related neurologic disease and examined toxoplasmosis, cryptococcal meningitis, primary central nervous system (CNS) lymphoma, progressive multifocal leukoencephalopathy (PML), HIV dementia, and sensory neuropathy. Between 1985 and 1992 there appeared to be an upward trend in all conditions except dementia. The incidence of sensory neuropathy seemed to increase and that of HIV dementia declined slightly. Antiretroviral agents were not protective and, in fact, sensory neuropathy was more likely to develop in men receiving antiviral treatment.

The neurologic manifestations of HIV-1 infection are common and at autopsy 80% of brains and 100% of peripheral nerves are abnormal (10–13). Most of the neurologic disease occurs late, and hence as patients live longer, more neurologic problems are likely to occur.

HIV-1 infection is a growing epidemic, most likely affecting far more people than currently reported. The Center for Disease Control and Prevention (CDC) has included HIV-1–related neurologic illness as a separate subcategory.

Biology of HIV

Virology

HIV is a lentivirus and constitutes a separate genus of the retroviral family. Lentiviruses infect a diverse group of animals, including horses (equine infectious anemia virus), sheep (visna), goats (caprine arthritis/encephalitis virus), and a wide variety of nonhuman primates (simian immunodeficiency virus). Bovine and feline immunodeficiency viruses have also been found. HIV-2 is distinct from HIV-1 and is prevalent in western Africa (14).

Lentiviruses contain an RNA genome with an RNA-

Table 12-1.
Central Nervous System Manifestations of HIV Infection

Encephalitis
Meningitis
Dementia
   Leukoencephalopathy
   Cortical atrophy
Vasculitis
Vacuolar myelopathy

dependent DNA polymerase (reverse transcriptase (RT)) (15). There is a prolonged incubation period and an infection of the cells of the immune system that persist in the natural host. HIV, as other lentiviruses, are nontransforming retroviruses and produce a cytopathic effect on immune cells. The effect on T cells can be lytic and the effect on macrophages can result in the formation of syncytia, the so-called multinucleated giant cells (MGCs).

The virus has a large, icosahedral structure with envelope spikes and a lipid bilayer. The cone-shaped core is composed of the Gag protein (p24). Within this capsid or nucleoid are two identical RNA strands with RT and the nucleocapsid proteins. The inner portion of the viral membrane is surrounded by another protein, p17, that provides the matrix for viral structure. Thus, the

Table 12-2.
Opportunistic Infections and Tumors Associated with HIV-Induced Immunoincompetence

Central nervous system
  Viral
    Cytomegalovirus, herpes simplex virus (HSV)-1, HSV-2, varicella-zoster virus, papovaviruses, and adenovirus-2 infections
  Fungal
    Cryptococcosis, candidiasis, aspergillosis, coccidioidosis, mucormycosis, rhizopus infection, acremoniosis, histoplasmosis, and zygomycosis
  Bacterial
    Listeriosis, *Treponema pallidum* infection, *Mycobacterium hominis* tuberculosis, *Mycobacterium avian-intracellulare* infection, and *Bartonella henselae* infection
  Parasitic
    Toxoplasmosis, acanthamebiasis, nocardiosis, *Trypanosoma cruzi* infection, and strongyloidiasis
  Neoplasms
    Lymphoma and metastatic Kaposi's sarcoma
Peripheral nervous system
  Viral
    Cytomegalovirus infection
  Bacterial
    Staphylococcus aureus and mycobacterium infections
  Parasitic
    Toxoplasmosis

Sources: Adapted from Britton CB. HIV infection. *Neurol Clin* 1993;11:605–624; and Levy RM, Berger JR. HIV and HTLV infections of the nervous system. In: Tyler KL, Martin JB, eds. *Infectious diseases of the central nervous system.* Philadelphia: FA Davis, 1993:47–75.

core proteins are coded for by the *gag* gene that produces the nucleocapsid proteins, p24, matrix protein, and nucleic acid–binding protein. The core also contains the proteins coded by the *pol* gene, namely RT, endonuclease (integrase), and protease (16,17). Detection of p24 is considered the most reliable indicator of HIV-1 infection. Antiviral agents such as zidovudine (AZT) interfere with RT and the new protease inhibitors work on proteases involved in the formation of Gag and Pol proteins.

The envelope spikes consist of knobs with a transmembrane element. The envelope spike is composed of glycoprotein (gp) 120 and the transmembrane component is gp41. The *env* gene encodes the envelope gp160, which is cleaved. The gp120 attaches the virus to the cell utilizing CD4 as a viral receptor. The gp41 fuses with the cell membrane and allows the virus to enter the cell (16,17).

Thus, there are three genes coding for structural proteins, *gag*, *pol*, and *env*. However, there are a number of regulatory genes that code for proteins essential for viral replication. These include *tat* (transactivation), *rev* (viral messenger RNA (mRNA) expression), *nef* (negative factor for replication), *vif* (increases infectivity), *vpr* (transcription activator), *vpx* (transcription activator), and *vpu* (virus release) (16,17).

Life Cycle

HIV-1 as a free virus can be found in most body fluids. The highest concentrations of virus are in blood plasma and cerebrospinal fluid (CSF). Ten percent to 30% of seminal and vaginal fluid specimens have virus or virus-infected cells. Surprisingly, the quantity of virus in the fluids is low when compared to that in blood (15). The major forms of transmission remain intimate sexual contact and contamination of blood. The transmission from mother to child appears to occur in as many as 25% to 30% of children born to HIV-positive mothers (18).

HIV-1 infects CD4+ lymphocytes and macrophages (19–21). The gp120 binds with high affinity to CD4+ on the surface of the T cell. In cells derived from neural sources, galactocerebroside C may be an alternative receptor for HIV-1 (22). HIV-1 enters the cell by fusion of gp41 with the cell membrane. At entry, the virion becomes an active nucleoprotein complex. The RT transcribes genomic RNA into unintegrated double-stranded DNA. Activation of the cell is required and enables viral DNA (provirus) to integrate into the cell's chromosomal DNA. HIV-1 DNA can be unintegrated as well, contributing to the cytopathology. With integration, the provirus will express viral genes with the aid of cellular factors. The initial viral genes expressed have regulatory functions. The most critical is *tat*. It is essential for replication and initiates RNA transcription by stimulating the production of full-length RNA transcripts that are expressed as regulatory proteins. Rev, another of these proteins, effects the transport of unspliced and singly spliced mRNA from the nucleus to the cytoplasm. These mRNAs encode the structural and enzymatic proteins needed for assembly of the virus mRNA core and envelope proteins at the cell membrane. The mature virion buds from the cell surface (16,17,21).

Immunology

The most important event in the establishment of HIV infection is the localization of the virus in lymphoid tissues. Even though no clinical manifestations may be evident for many years, this latent phase is characterized by active disease in lymphoid tissues. The persistence of virus causes chronic stimulation of the immune response and eventual destruction of lymphoid tissue, resulting in progressive immunoincompetence (23). Thus, the primary infection is often accompanied by nonspecific mononucleosis-like symptoms. The period of latency is an asymptomatic phase with a median duration of 10 years and is followed, with rare exceptions, with clinical AIDS. The clinical manifestations of AIDS involve specific syndromes directly related to the virus and complications of immunosuppression such as neoplasms and opportunistic infections.

There is a discrepancy between continued HIV replication and progression of disease accompanied by a progressive loss of CD4+ T lymphocytes. Both HIV-specific antibodies and specific cytotoxic T lymphocytes (CTLs) can be detected very early during the course of infection. There is no general agreement regarding the primary mechanisms of HIV disease. Pantaleo and Fauci (23) reviewed the early immune response and suggested that the same events seen during a normal immune response against pathogens paradoxically favor HIV infection. The basis for this is activation of T cells, B cells, and macrophages. HIV replication depends on the activation of target cells and the production of such cytokines as tumor necrosis factor (TNF)-α, interleukin (IL)-10, and IL-6.

HIV dissemination from the first lymphoid infection probably occurs prior to the HIV-specific immune response (23–25). However, both CTL–mediated immune (CMI) and humoral responses are detected very early in the course of the primary HIV infection; in fact, CTLs appear prior to neutralizing antibody (26). The neutralizing antibody appears at a time when the transition from the acute to the chronic or latent phase has already occurred (27). Downregulation of the plasma viremia and viral replication in blood and lymph node mononuclear cells are seen during the transition from the acute to the chronic phase.

The role of antibodies is still not completely understood. Most infected individuals have antibodies that neutralize HIV. Early in the course of infection, subjects may have antibodies that neutralize viruses isolated from their own bodies, but later will not have neutralizing effects against that same strain; in fact, antibodies may actually enhance infectivity of that particular strain (28). Levy (29) reviewed this and showed that the same monoclonal antibody can neutralize or enhance activity, depending on the HIV strain used (29). The mechanism for enhancement is not clear and it cannot always be attributed to the CD4 molecule. The envelope region responsible for enhanced infectivity is located within gp120 for the Fc-mediated response and gp41 for protein complement–mediated activity (30). Changes in the V3 loop of gp120 seem to be critical in determining whether a virus is neutralized or enhanced. The V3 loop of gp120 plays a critical role in viral infectivity and tropism, and contains the major neutralizing determinant. Antibodies to the V3 loop inhibit entry, even after binding of gp120 to CD4, as well as syncytial formation, suggesting a role of V3 loop in membrane fusion events (31).

The HIV-specific primary immune response probably plays a critical role in determining clinical outcome. The two major associations between disease and immune response have focused on the major histocompatibility complex (MHC) as just described as well as the restricted T-cell receptor (TCR) variable-gene repertoire. In their recent review of HLA associations, Westby et al (32) indicated that HLA-A2 and -DR13 are linked to resistance and A1/B8/DR3 is associated with increased susceptibility and rapid disease progression. When A1/B8 is split from DR3, increased rate of progression segregates with A1/B8. Other MHC class I alleles linked to rapid progression include HLA-A24 and -B35 and class II alleles include HLA-DR2 and -DR5 (32,33). MHC class II DR5 and DR6 correlate with slow progression and are believed to be due to mimicry between the gp120 V3 loop and the DR sequences (34). The underlying mechanisms are unclear but an appealing theory of associations relates to HIV structural and sequence motifs similar to HLA that may elicit a response resulting in a depletion of CD4+ cells.

Pantaleo et al (23,35) analyzed TCR repertoire during primary infection. Their studies showed an expansion of the CD8+ T-cell subset with a predominant Vβ usage driven by HIV. These restricted expansions are oligoclonal. Although the number of patients studied is small, certain patterns seem to correlate with clinical outcome. Vβ expansions appear to differ qualitatively and quantitatively from patient to patient. Antigen levels themselves, secondary to the viral load, do not explain the diversity of the response. More likely, the diversity corresponds to the evolution of the responding TCR repertoire.

Additional research has focused on the possibility of an HIV-encoded superantigen. Superantigens stimulate a broad range of T cells binding to the (chain of MHC class II and interacting with TCR Vβ families. Westby et al (32) reviewed evidence supporting the superantigen in maintaining a T-cell reservoir, but whether the superantigen is encoded by HIV is not known (32).

There have been several explanations to account for the existence and persistence of B-cell function and CD8+ T-cell activation in spite of a lack of significant CD4+ T-cell function. The first is evidence of programmed cell death or apoptosis (36). Amersen et al (37) reviewed the evidence for apoptosis, including the following: In vitro studies of HIV-1–infected lymphocytes demonstrate that dysfunction is prevented by an inhibition of protein synthesis; the cytolytic effects of HIV-1 in infected CD4 cells appear to be related to the induction of programmed cell death; cross-linking of gp120 or anti-CD4 antibodies to CD4 can produce apoptosis in uninfected human CD4+ T cells; severe combined immunodeficient (SCID)-mice infected with HIV-1, when reconstituted with human T cells (thus becoming SCID-human mice), show rapid loss of CD4+ T cells in vivo by apoptosis; and experimental models of AIDS in primate and feline AIDS demonstrate in vitro programmed death of peripheral T cells. Evidence also exists of abnormal amounts of apoptotic cells in the lymph nodes of HIV-1–infected patients (38).

Cytokines have also been implicated in the pathogenesis of HIV-1. IL-10, a cytokine present in CD4+ Th2 cells, inhibits HIV-1 in macrophages but not in T cells. However, CD8+ T cells have increased levels of IL-10 mRNA, suggesting that they may be one of the sources of IL-10 in HIV-infected patients. IL-12, a proinflammatory cytokine, is reduced in macrophages infected with HIV-1, independent of enhanced IL-10 production. IL-12 enhances CMI responses such as natural killer (NK) cell activity, the production of IL-2 and interferon (IFN)-γ, and the proliferation of T cells in HIV-positive patients (39). However, IL-12 can enhance HIV replication in prestimulated peripheral blood mononuclear cells. Thus, IL-10 and IL-12 are important in viral latency and tropism.

Neurologic Syndromes: AIDS Dementia Complex

A consensus report in 1991 proposed terminology based on neuropathology (40). The report concluded that HIV encephalitis, HIV leukoencephalopathy, and diffuse poliodystrophy appear to be the pathologic substrates of the AIDS dementia complex (ADC). Synonyms for ADC include HIV encephalopathy, HIV dementia, HIV-associated dementia complex, and HIV-1–associated cognitive/motor complex. In 1987, the Centers for Disease Control (CDC) added HIV encephalopathy as an AIDS-defining illness.

Clinical-Pathologic Findings

HIV-1 enters the brain almost immediately after the initial onset of infection. At first it may be clinically silent, but within 4 to 6 weeks an infectious mononucleosis-like systemic illness, an acute meningitis, or meningoencephalitis occur. Such patients have headache, stiff neck, altered mental state, and occasionally, seizures. In most patients the acute illness resolves, although in rare instances a persistent illness continues with chronic headaches and CSF lymphocytosis (41). Following the acute infection, most patients with HIV-1 enter an asymptomatic phase. Eventually dementia develops in 20% to 30% of adults. In 3%, dementia is the AIDS-defining illness (42).

The cognitive and motor deficits manifested in patients with ADC are listed in Table 12-3. The onset of symptoms is usually insidious and difficult to discern from depression. A mild illness with only fatigue, malaise, headaches, and slowness of thinking can oc-

Table 12-3.
Clinical Manifestations of AIDS Dementia Complex

Cognitive
  Psychomotor slowing to retardation
  Forgetfulness to severe memory impairment
  Concentration difficulty
Behavioral
  Apathy and withdrawal
  Mutism
  Insight loss
  Hallucinations
  Mood changes
  Psychosis
Motor
  Spastic weakness
  Ataxia
  Myoclonus
  Seizures
  Handwriting difficulty
  Leg weakness

cur. The severe signs and symptoms of ADC include a progressive memory loss, concentration problems, difficulty reading, and general apathy. Language problems and depression are common. The motor deficits include incoordination, gait disturbances, tremors, and parkinsonian rigidity and bradykinesia. Seizures, sleep disturbances, and a variety of corticospinal and frontal release signs can also be present. Eventually, the patient may be completely immobile and incontinent (43–46).

Snider et al (43) originally described myelin pallor. Figure 12-1 shows the myelin pallor with diffuse damage to the white matter including myelin loss as well as MGCs in both the brain and the spinal cord. The MGCs are of the macrophage/microglia lineage and contain HIV-1 antigens (47–49). Figure 12-2 shows a microglial nodule containing macrophages, astrocytes, and MGCs. The MGCs are of macrophage origin and contain HIV p24 antigen. In addition to the MGCs and white matter pallor, the major findings are marked astrocytosis and basophilic mineralization with calcium deposition in the putamen and globus pallidum (50,51). Less common is the finding of a perivascular infiltration with vasculitis (40). A vacuolar myelopathy in the lateral and dorsal columns is also found and is characterized by a spongiform change with MGC and macrophage infiltrates (52). Macrophages and MGCs contain HIV-1, as demonstrated by in situ hybridization (53,54).

The brains of ADC patients invariably have significant neuronal loss and cortical atrophy despite the lack of evidence of HIV-1 invasion of neurons. In fact, the only brain cells that consistently contain HIV-1 are those of macrophage/microglial lineage. Astrocytes, endothelial cells, and oligodendrocytes rarely contain virus, with the exception of pediatric patients, in whom astrocytes have been found to contain evidence of HIV-1 infection (55,56).

Neuronal loss can be found in the cerebellum, inferior olivary nucleus, substantia nigra, and putamen, but rarely in the hippocampus. The major neuronal loss oc-

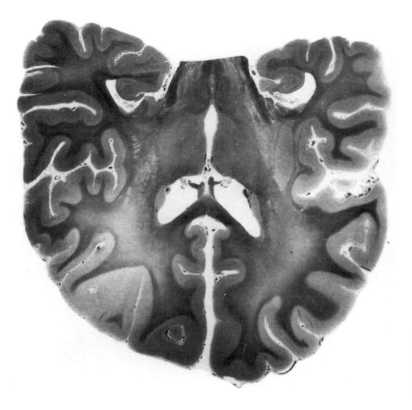

Figure 12-1. White matter palor. The diffuse white matter palor pathologically includes myelin loss, reactive astrogliosis, and macrophages. (Reproduced by permission from *Brain Pathology* 1993;1: (cover photograph). International Society of Neuropathology.)

curs in the fronto-orbital region and the superior frontal gyrus. Neuronal loss is not uniform, even in a susceptible population (57). Synaptophysin staining indicates a loss of synapses associated with dendritic damage (58).

The relationship between the clinical syndrome of ADC and the neuropathology has remained problematic. In some studies only half of the patients with ADC have MGCs (44,45,54) and in fact many patients had no pathologic findings. Patients can be found with severe encephalitis and no documentation of dementia (59,60).

HIV can be demonstrated in the brains of most patients with ADC. Using p24 as an indicator, Brew et al (60) found the infection to be more limited than one would expect from the degree of clinical dysfunction. Thus, the major studies of Navia et al (44,45), Glass et al (54), and Brew et al (60) found a discordance between HIV infection in the brain and the presence of ADC. In a recent study of brains from patients infected with HIV-1, Johnson et al (61) found no significant differences between demented and nondemented patients in the quantity of HIV DNA measured by quantitative polymerase chain reaction. This suggested qualitative differences in the virus rather than the virus load, and supports previous work suggesting strain differences and tropism for infection of the brain (62).

The diagnosis of HIV-associated cognitive/motor complex depends on ruling out opportunistic infection and lymphoma. Magnetic resonance imaging (MRI) may show either cortical atrophy (Fig 12-3) or white matter changes (Fig 12-4). Many studies have focused on CSF findings and have attempted correlations with ADC and prediction of progression. Table 12-4 catalogues the CSF findings (63–79). HIV-1 is inconsistently found in the CSF at the time of seroconversion. The IgG1 subclass seems to predominate. The CSF of ADC patients has higher anti-pol and anti-env gp120 IgG3 antibodies than does corresponding serum (79). Increased IgG synthesis, oligoclonal bands, IgM, and IgG1-G4 antibodies are also found in ADC patients (65). Immune markers such as cytokines (TNF receptor, TNF-α, IL-6) as well as β$_2$-microglobulin, neopterin, prostaglandins, and fibronectin can be found in ADC patients. Cytotoxic CD8+ cells found in the CSF may be the source of some of the cytokines (75).

The study by Tyor et al (80) of cytokine expression in the brain was one of the more comprehensive; however, there appeared to be no correlation between levels of cytokines and the presence or absence of central nervous system (CNS) disease. The investigators found upregulation of MHC class II on macrophage/microglia cells. Endothelial cells were positive for IL-1 and IFN-γ and less frequently for the TNF-α cytokines known to upregulate TNF receptors. Figure 12-5 shows the upregulation of TNF receptor p55 in cells appearing to be macrophages and TNF-α in cells with astrocyte and macrophage mor-

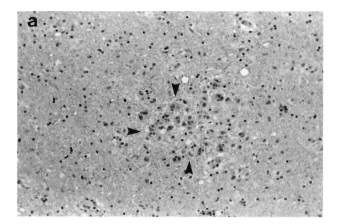

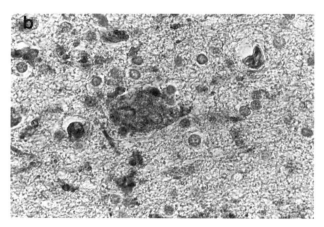

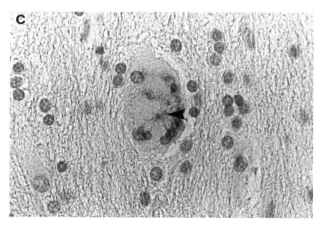

Figure 12-2. HIV encephalopathy. (A) Hematoxylin and eosin–stained section of the white matter shows a microglial nodule (arrowheads) containing macrophages, astrocytes, and multinucleated giant cells (× 35). (B) Immunoperoxidase staining with HAM-56 reveals a multinucleated giant cell with strong cytoplasmic positivity, indicating macrophage origin (× 350). (C) Immunoperoxidase staining for HIV p24 reveals strong linear positivity (arrowhead) within a multinucleated giant cell (× 350).

phology. Thus, both CSF and brain studies show that HIV-1 infection is associated with activation of the cytokine cascade. There is a discrepancy between the CSF findings and brain findings in some patients.

The presence of quinolinic acid and kynurenines, neuroactive metabolites, in the CSF is diagnostic, reflecting the neurodegenerative changes in ADC (72).

Pathogenesis

HIV-1 is localized to blood-derived macrophages and microglia within the perivascular areas and brain parenchymal tissue. Most importantly, neurons, oligodendrocytes, astrocytes, and endothelial cells are rarely infected if at all. The predilection for white matter, deep gray matter, and brainstem does not explain the extensive cortical neuronal dropout. Finally, the viral load does not always correlate with either clinical ADC or neuropathologic findings.

Nottet and Gendelman (81) recently reviewed the neuroimmune mechanisms involved in ADC. The entry of HIV-1 into the brain is an initial event that must overcome the blood-brain barrier (BBB). A number of theories have been suggested: infection of the endothelial cells that form the BBB; entry by means of infected macrophages, the so-called Trojan horse theory; and finally, the induction by HIV-1–infected macrophages of adhesion molecules on microvascular endothelial cells. HIV-1–infected monocytes induce expression of E-selectin on vascular endothelial cells in the brain (82). Activation of infected cells even further induces the production of E-selectin and vascular cell adhesion molecule (VCAM)-1 on endothelial cells. This suggests that E-selectin may play a role in the penetration of the CNS by HIV-1–infected macrophages. Adhesion molecules are probably not the only factor. HIV-infected monocytes secrete leukotrienes that increase the permeability of the BBB (83,84). There appears to be a role for astrocytes in regulating activated macrophages (84). Transforming growth factor (TGF)-β is also found in HIV-infected brains and is a chemoattractant for macrophages (85).

After entry into the CNS, HIV-1 is replicated in macrophages/microglia, suggesting that these cells are key to the neuronal loss. The neurotoxicity may be due to the interaction of virus with a variety of host factors (86). A monocyte-secreted, low-molecular-weight, heat-stable, proteinase-resistant molecule has been shown to kill neurons via the N-methyl-D-aspartate (NMDA) receptor (87). HIV gp120 also is toxic to neurons (88). One mechanism of gp120 neurotoxicity is its antagonism to vasoactive intestinal peptide (VIP) function (89). The gp120 also can elevate intracellular Ca^{2+} levels (90). In another example of viral-host interaction, HIV Tat protein has been shown to be involved in neuronal damage (91).

Activated infected brain macrophages produce a number of potential neurotoxins including eicosanoids, platelet-activating factor, TNF-α, quinolinate, and nitric oxide (NO) (84,86). NO appears to be an important element of gp120 toxicity. The toxicity requires external glutamate and calcium and is blocked by glutamate re-

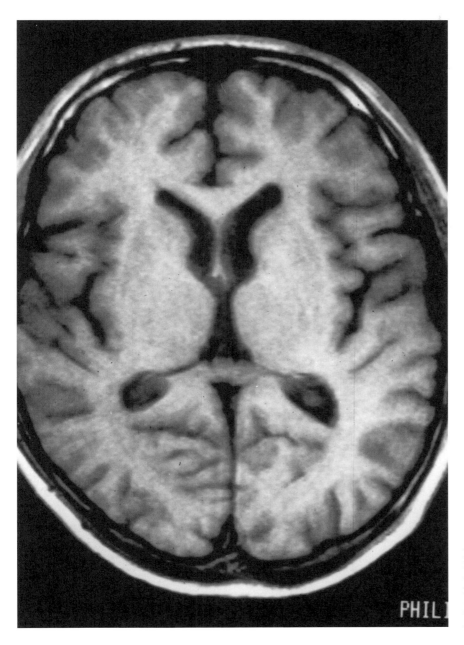

Figure 12-3. MRI of a 25-year-old HIV-1–positive patient with advanced dementia shows marked frontal atrophy and palidystrophy. (Courtesy of Chi S. Zee, MD, of the University of Southern California School of Medicine, Los Angeles.)

ceptor antagonists. The NO mechanism is critical in gp120 neurotoxicity, as inhibitors of NO synthase block the toxicity, as does superoxide dismutase (92).

Cytokines are also critical in the concept of neurotoxicity of HIV-1–infected macrophages. TNF-α and IL-1β stimulate astrocytosis and upregulate NO. IFN-γ can induce quinolate, an NMDA agonist. NO induced by cytokines may react with superoxide anion to yield a neurotoxic substance (93).

Thus, there appear to be direct effects of HIV-1 on neural cells in the form of viral proteins such as gp120 and Tat, and indirect effects mitigated by cytokines and other macrophage-associated molecules that cause BBB penetration, toxicity, and astrocyte proliferation. Autoimmunity has also been suggested to play a role in the pathogenesis of ADC via cross-reactivity between viral proteins and host proteins. Finally, NMDA receptor and calcium influx may be the common pathway for neuronal loss, whether the mechanism is a direct viral or an indirect macrophage-associated toxicity.

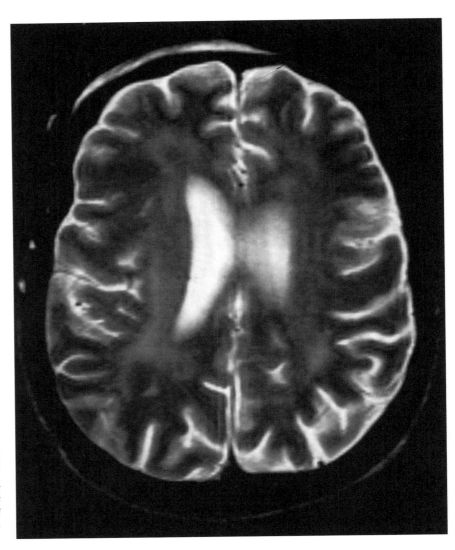

Figure 12-4. MRI of a 31-year-old patient with AIDS dementia complex and leukoencephalopathy shows diffuse white matter changes. Postmortem examination confirmed the diagnosis of AIDS dementia complex. (Courtesy of Chi S. Zee, MD, of the University of Southern California School of Medicine, Los Angeles.)

Therapeutic Inventions

It is important to recognize that the incidence of ADC is significantly lower in patients receiving zidovudine (AZT) versus those who never receive the drug (94,95). The percentage of patients with ADC decreased when treated with AZT from 1987 to 1990, comparing to the time period of 1982 to 1987, when they were not treated. When treatment was terminated, the incidence of ADC increased. In 1991 and 1992 the incidence decreased, coinciding with the use of dideoxyinosine (ddI). Combinations of AZT with ddI are effective. AZT and zalcitabine (ddC) are associated with a high frequency of peripheral neuropathy (96). Clinical improvement with AZT is associated with decreased quinolinate and β-macroglobulin levels in the CSF (97). Treatments designed to protect neurons from excitotoxic injury including Ca^{2+} channel blockers and NMDA receptor antagonists may well have a role in inhibiting ADC (98,99). The role of RT inhibitors and protease inhibitors in the treatment of ADC has not been determined (100).

Alteration of the immune response also shows promise for the treatment of HIV-1. The presence of HIV-1–specific cytotoxic lymphocytes in the CSF suggests that with either proper stimulation or removal of inhibiting factors, the host has the means to destroy cells containing virus by CMI (75). Perhaps the most promising immunotherapies relate to the use of proinflammatory cytokines such as IL-12. Peripheral blood mononuclear cells are usually unresponsive in HIV-positive patients as measured by T-cell proliferation, IL-2 production, and failure to respond to IFN-γ. These functions are restored by IL-12 in vitro and show promise in augmenting the diminished immune response in HIV-1 infection (101). More recently, Cocchi et al (102)

Table 12-4.
Cerebrospinal Fluid Findings in AIDS Dementia Complex

Study	Comment	Reference No.
General findings		
Viral		
Viral population	± Dementia	64
p24	Dementia	64, 65
gp120	Nerotoxic activity	66
Biochemical-immune markers		
β₂-Microglobulin	Dementia	67
Prostaglandins	Dementia	68
Ferritin	Neurologic disease	69
Fibronectin	Increase in dementia, PML	70, 71
Neopterin	± Dementia	72
Quinolinic acid	Increase in dementia	72
Neuroactive kynurenines	± Dementia	72
Immunologic findings		
Immune cells—cytokines		
T-cell antigens	sCD25 increase	73
(sCD25, sCD27)	sCD27 decrease	73
TNF soluble receptors	Increase in dementia	74
Interleukin-6	Slight increase in dementia	75
Cytotoxic lymphocytes (CD8+)	Dementia	76
TNF-α	± Dementia	77
Immunoglobulins		
IgM, IgG1-G4	Dementia	78
IgG synthesis	Dementia	65, 79
Oligoclonal bands	± Dementia	65, 78, 79

± = positive or negative for; PML = progressive multifocal leukoencephalopathy; TNF = tumor necrosis factor.

demonstrated HIV-1 suppression from soluble substances secreted by CD8+ CTLs. These suppressive factors are the chemokines RANTES (regulated on activation normal T cell expressed and secreted), macrophage inflammatory protein (MIP)-1α, and MIP-1β (102). Chemokines exert proinflammatory effects and function as chemoattractants for T cells and mononuclear cells. It is possible these substances have a direct antiviral effect rather than have an effect through their action as chemoattractants.

Neuromuscular Manifestations of HIV Infection

The neuromuscular manifestations are in the form of both peripheral nerve pathology and muscle disease (Table 12-5).

Peripheral Neuropathies

Diverse involvement of the peripheral nervous system is the rule and up to approximately 10% of asymptomatic HIV patients will have nerve conduction findings con-

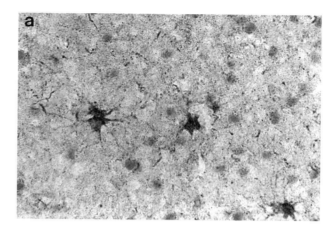

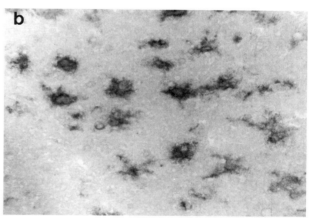

Figure 12-5. Cytokines in HIV encephalopathy. (a) Immunoperoxidase staining for tumor necrosis factor (TNF)-α shows strong positivity in scattered cells with the morphology of reactive astrocytes and macrophages (× 350). (b) Immunoperoxidase staining for TNF receptor (p55) reveals strong positivity in many macrophages (× 350). Normal brain does not stain for TNF-α and shows only focal weak staining for TNF receptor.

sistent with a distal symmetric polyneuropathy (DSPN) (103). Generally, most patients with peripheral nerve disease have CD4/CD8 cell ratios lower than 0.8 (104,105). The major clinical categories of peripheral nerve involvement in HIV-1 infection can be separated into DSPN, acute and chronic inflammatory demyelinating polyneuropathy (CIDP), mononeuritis multiplex, and polyradiculopathy (104).

Clinical-Pathologic Manifestations

Histologic studies often demonstrate multiple peripheral nerve processes including axonal degeneration, demyelination, and mononuclear cell inflammation. Moreover, de la Monte et al (10), in their histologic re-

Table 12-5.
Peripheral Nervous System Manifestations of HIV Infection

Polyneuropathy
  Acute inflammatory demyelinating polyradiculoneuropathy
  Chronic inflammatory demyelinating polyradiculoneurop-
    athy
  Distal sensory axonal neuropathy
  Mononeuritis multiplex
  Vasculitic neuropathy
  Autonomic neuropathy
  Ganglioradiculoneuritis
  Neuropathy associated with lymphoma
Muscle
  Polymyositis
  Necrotizing myopathy
  Nemaline myopathy
  Mitochondrial myopathy
  Wasting in advanced AIDS
  Necrotizing vasculitis
  Zidovudine (AZT)-associated toxic myopathy

---

view of sural and popliteal nerve specimens and brachial and lumbar plexi from 21 asymptomatic and symptomatic patients, showed histologic evidence of demyelination in nearly 80%, axonal degeneration in 36%, and mononuclear cell inflammation in 37%. MGCs seen in the CNS were not found in the peripheral nervous system. Both CIDP and DSPN appear to involve the same degree of demyelination and axonal degeneration.

In DSPN, weakness begins in the distal aspect of the lower extremities and progresses to the knees before affecting the upper extremities. The sensory component of DSPN is the major element and is most disturbing, particularly in the late stage of AIDS. It affects up to 30% of all patients (43). Often, sensory polyneuropathy is the most frequent reason for neurologic consultation. The initial complaints are of burning dysesthesias at the soles of the feet, severe enough to functionally disable the patient. However, patients may also describe their feet as "frostbitten" (106). HIV-infected patients receiving ddC and ddI treatment may have sensory symptoms as a complication (96). Griffin et al (104) performed more detailed histologic examination of sural nerve specimens and found that the predominant feature in sensory polyneuropathy is wallerian degeneration of myelinated fibers. Interestingly, however, retrograde axonal degeneration, or "dying" back is also present in HIV sensory neuropathy (106,107). Rance et al (108) demonstrated loss of myelin in the fasciculus gracilis correlating with sensory neuropathy.

Typical electrophysiologic findings for DSPN have included evidence of active degeneration as indicated by fibrillation potentials and positive waves and decreased recruitment consistent with a loss of functioning motor units. Primary loss of axons is further supported, as compound muscle action potential and sensory nerve action potential studies show severely decreased amplitudes in the setting of at most, mildly decreased conduction velocities (105).

Pathogenesis

The cause of the loss of axons and the secondary demyelination is not understood. Implication for a T cell–mediated mechanism as a result of coinfection by cytomegalovirus has not been confirmed. The majority of T cells are CD8+ lymphocytes, but the primary infiltrating cell is the macrophage. Macrophage infiltration is also found in dorsal root ganglia and gracile tracts. Macrophage activation is indicated by the expression of MHC class II and cytokines IL-1, TNF-α, IL-6, and IFN-γ (107,109). Neither immunoglobulin nor complement have been demonstrated in peripheral nerves of AIDS patients (10,107).

In contrast to DSPN, both acute inflammatory demyelinating peripheral neuropathy and CIDP present at an early stage of infection and may well represent an autoimmune process. This process often is found in an asymptomatic patient with normal CD4 counts. Studies of peripheral nerves show very little evidence of HIV-1 infection of the nerve itself, suggesting the involvement of factors other than direct infection (110).

HIV-1–infected patients even without evidence of peripheral nerve disease show inflammatory changes in both sensory and sympathetic ganglia. The ganglia contain infiltrates of activated macrophages and T lymphocytes. In seven patients gp41 and p24 were found in ganglionic macrophages in both sensory and sympathetic ganglia (111).

HIV-1–Associated Muscle Disorders

The two major forms of myopathy seen with HIV-1 infection include polymyositis and toxic myopathy associated with AZT. Table 12–5 lists other rare myopathic processes. The wasting-cachectic syndrome is quite common in patients with far-advanced AIDS.

Polymyositis

Clinical-Pathologic Manifestations
Polymyositis can present during any stage of HIV infection. The patient may have muscle pain and progressive proximal weakness. Polymyositis often occurs during the phase of illness in which there is an increase in HIV antibody, and often at the same stage of disease associated with CIDP or idiopathic thrombocytopenic purpura. Creatine kinase levels are often elevated and the electromyogram is myopathic.

Muscle biopsy findings vary from inflammatory myopathy to noninflammatory muscle fiber necrosis with nemaline bodies and mitochondrial changes (112).

Pathogenesis
Chad et al (113) observed gp41 antigen in infiltrating macrophages in inflammatory polymyositis (113). There has not been any evidence of HIV-1 infection to the muscle fibers themselves. The mechanism of the muscle damage in HIV-infected patients is not clear, although an autoimmune mechanism has been suggested.

Treatment

The treatment of polymyositis may include pulse intravenous methylprednisolone, plasmapheresis, and intravenous immunoglobulin. The latter seems to be best tolerated (114). A controlled trial has not been carried out

Zidovudine-Associated Toxic Myopathy

AZT-associated toxic myopathy appears to be more common than the other myopathic processes associated with HIV. This myopathy is a mitochondrial myopathy with atrophic ragged-red fibers, marked myofibrillar changes, and inflammation (115,116). AZT-associated toxic myopathy most frequently occurs in symptomatic AIDS patients who clinically show proximal weakness with marked muscle pain. Creative kinase levels are elevated and the electromyogram is myopathic.

Pathogenesis

The pathogenetic mechanism for toxic myopathy is not clear. A toxic effect directly on mitochondria has been postulated. Gherardi et al (117) demonstrated IL-1 reactivity in vessels and inflammatory cells including macrophages from patients with HIV-1 myopathy associated with AZT. IL-1 expression is much stronger in AZT-treated patients with this form of myopathy than in patients with other mitochondrial myopathies. IL-1 message was also found in muscle cells from HIV-1–infected patients with AZT-associated myopathy, suggesting IL-1 induction in the muscle and an important role in muscle damage (117).

Opportunistic Infections and Neoplasms

In almost all patients with HIV-1–associated neurologic disease, the differential involves distinguishing the direct effects of the virus versus the complications of the patient's immune incompetence. It has been estimated that close to 90% of patients dying of AIDS have significant nervous system involvement (11). In most instances, a wide variety of opportunistic infections including those caused by bacteria, mycobacteria, fungi, protozoa, viruses, and other parasites have been reported. Table 12–2 lists the known infections associated with the defective cellular immune response in HIV-1–infected patients (118,119).

Toxoplasmosis

The most common opportunistic infection seen in the CNS in AIDS patients is caused by the protozoan *Toxoplasma gondii*. Toxoplasmosis is a common infection in cats. In humans it usually presents as multiple necrotic lesions of the brain. It is likely that in the HIV-1–infected patient toxoplasmosis results from activation of a latent infection. The incidence is thought to be between 2% and 13% in HIV-positive patients (119). The clinical presentation includes seizures, increased intracranial pressure, facial palsy, focal neurologic signs, and dif-

fuse encephalopathy with confusion, weakness, and lethargy. Computed tomography (CT) is usually diagnostic in that the finding of multiple ring enhancing lesions, particularly in the basal ganglia, is likely to indicate toxoplasmosis in about 90% to 95% of HIV-1–positive patients with CD4 counts of 200 cells/μL or less. The problem of diagnosis arises in the setting of a single lesion, which must be differentiated from lymphoma. CSF findings are varied and often nondiagnostic and because most HIV-1–infected patients have antibody to *T. gondii*, it is not particularly helpful for establishing the diagnosis. Most patients respond to antibiotic therapy within days or weeks, confirming the diagnosis.

Cryptococcosis

The most common CNS fungal infection is cryptococcal meningitis, although the CNS can be involved secondary to disseminated candidal infection. Cryptococcal infections will develop in about 5% of all AIDS patients. There is usually a fever, headache, confusion, and stiff neck. The onset is most often abrupt. CSF analysis is diagnostic, showing pleocytosis, elevated protein concentrations, and at times reduced glucose levels. India ink staining is usually positive but the presence of cryptococcal antigen in the CSF is definitive. Cryptococcal meningitis often results in either normal- or low-pressure hydrocephalus that can be treated by repeated spinal taps. However, dilated ventricles with increased pressure and clinical and radiographic evidence of progressive hydrocephalus must be treated with intraventricular shunt and not by spinal taps.

Cryptococcal meningitis is associated with CD4 counts below 200 cells/μL and the spinal fluid may have but a few cells in more advanced stages. In those instances, the yeast invades the brain parenchyma to form cryptococcomas, microinfarcts, and diffuse cerebral swelling. MRI and CT frequently do not reflect the extensive tissue necrosis seen with this disease.

The treatment is amphotericin and modern drugs such as fluconazole and 5-flucytosine, particularly in patients with more advanced stages of disease. Maintenance antifungal therapy is always essential (120).

Herpesvirus Infections

The most common viral infections of the nervous system in HIV-1–positive patients are herpesvirus infections. In AIDS patients, cytomegalovirus, herpes simplex virus (HSV)-1 and -2, and varicella-zoster virus (VZV) can produce a wide variety of clinical neurologic syndromes (42). These include meningitis, encephalitis, myelitis, radiculoneuritis, and retinitis.

Cytomegalovirus can be detected in the brains of AIDS patients and usually can be demonstrated in the CSF by polymerase chain reaction. Pathologically, microglial nodules are not uncommon. The treatment of cytomegalovirus retinitis is generally ineffective and CNS infection with cytomegalovirus, HSV-1, HSV-2, and VZV in late AIDS usually suggests a poor prognosis. The

CSF may show a mild pleocytosis with slightly elevated protein levels and normal glucose concentrations.

HSV-2 is more commonly the cause of encephalitis in AIDS patients than is HSV-1. The disease is less acute, the encephalitis less hemorrhagic, and the lesions are usually not restricted to the frontotemporal lobes. Electroencephalography usually does not reveal the repetitive discharges seen with HSV-1 encephalitis in nonimmunocompromised patients. Five percent to 10% of HIV-1–infected patients have clinical VZV infection. For the most part, this is dermal. Postherpetic neuralgia is common although a small number of patients develop a myeloradiculitis with severe spinal cord sensory and motor findings. Invasion of the brain is rare but brainstem encephalitis can occur after trigeminal or cervical VZV involvement. Ophthalmic VZV infection can be followed with granulomatous angiitis and thrombotic occlusion of the ipsilateral middle cerebral and carotid arteries (121). Therapy with antiherpes agents can alter the clinical course although the treatments for postherpetic neuroglias are less effective.

Progressive Multifocal Leukoencephalopathy

Progressive multifocal leukoencephalopathy (PML) is caused by the human papovavirus JC virus (JCV). It is usually associated with an immunocompromised state such as in patients with lymphomas, transplant recipients, and patients with an iatrogenic clinical condition (122). PML is a rare disorder in the general population, but JCV is a common human infectious agent. Evidence suggests that JCV infection often remains latent and becomes activated with immune suppression. As many as 60% of people worldwide have antibody to JCV after the age of 10. PML patients have IgG antibody, suggesting that JCV is not a primary infection in immunodeficiency states (123). PML has become an important complication of AIDS. The autopsy incidence of PML in AIDS is reported to be 3% to 5% (124,125).

In AIDS patients the course of PML is quite fulminant and death may occur within 2 months of clinical presentation. Clinical signs and symptoms include visual defects, focal motor weakness, cerebellar ataxia, and mental deficits including memory loss, confusion, and dementia (126). Pathologic examination shows focal areas of white matter degeneration that is visible on gross inspection of the sliced brain. Microscopically these areas are foci of demyelination with relative sparing of axons, oligodendroglial loss, and astrogliosis. Oligodendroglial cells have inclusions containing JCV antigen and viral particles and astroglia have enlarged, irregularly lobulated hyperchromatic nuclei with JCV mRNA but only on a rare occasion virions (127).

MRI is diagnostic, showing nonenhancing lesions of the white matter in HIV-1–positive patient with focal signs and normal CSF. Polymerase chain reaction of the CSF demonstrating JCV makes diagnostic brain biopsy unnecessary for the diagnosis of PML (128).

Thus far, the treatment of PML has been unsuccessful in most HIV-1–infected patients; PML is the terminal illness.

Conclusions

There has been a significant body of information accumulated on HIV-1 infection in a very short time. Therapies have prolonged and improved the quality of life for many AIDS patients. New treatments for opportunistic infections and neoplasms such as lymphoma have improved. Central and peripheral nervous system effects have continued to be a problem, particularly in patients with more advanced AIDS. The incidence of ADC has declined but sensory neuropathies have become very frequent and opportunistic CNS and PNS infections continue to produce major difficulties and often are the cause of death. It is likely that with newer and less toxic therapies, the incidence of neurologic manifestations of AIDS will decline.

References

1. Masur H, Michelis MA, Greene JB. An outbreak of community acquired *Pneumocytis carnii* pneumonia: initial manifestations of immune dysfunction. *N Engl J Med* 1981;305:1431–1438.
2. Barre-Sinoussi F, Nugeyre M, Daugnet C. Isolation of a T-lymphotrophic retrovirus from a patient at risk for acquired immune deficiency syndrome. *Science* 1983;220:868–871.
3. Gallo RC, et al. Isolation of human T-cell leukemia virus in acquired immune deficiency syndrome (AIDS). *Science* 1983;220:865–867.
4. Montagnier L, et al. A new human T-lymphotrophic retrovirus: characterization and possible role in lymphadenopathy and acquired immune deficiency syndromes. In: Gallo RC, Essex ME, Gross L, eds. *Human T cell leukemia/lymphoma virus*. Cold Spring Harbor, NY: Cold Spring Harbor Laboratory, 1984:363–379.
5. Centers for Disease Control and Prevention. *HIV/AIDS surveillance report*. Vol. 5. Atlanta, GA: Centers for Disease Control and Prevention, 1993:3–19.
6. Surveillance Branch, Division of HIV-AIDS, National Center for Infectious Diseases, CDC. The second 100,000 cases of the acquired immunodeficiency syndrome—United States, June 1981-December 1991. *MMWR* 1991;41(2):28–29.
7. Berger JR, Kaderman R. HIV encephalopathy: clinical and diagnostic considerations. In: Major EO, Levey JA, eds., Technical Advances in AIDS in the Human Nervous System. New York: Plenum, 1995:3–26.
8. Bredesen DE, Messing R. Neurological syndromes heralding the acquired immune deficiency syndrome. *Ann Neurol* 1983;14:141. Abstract.
9. Bacellar H, et al. Temporal trends in incidence of HIV-1 related neurologic diseases: multicenter AIDS cohort study, 1985–1992. *Neurology* 1994;44:1982–1900.
10. de la Monte SM, et al. Peripheral neuropathy in the acquired immunodeficiency syndrome. *Ann Neurol* 1988;23:485–492.
11. Levy RM, Bredesen DE, Rosenblum ML. Neurological manifestations of the acquired immune deficiency syndrome (AIDS): experience at UCSF and review of the literature. *J Neurosurg* 1985;62:475–495.
12. Petito CK. Review of central nervous system pathology in human immunodefiency virus infection. *Ann Neurol* 1988;23(suppl):S54–S57.
13. Marshall DW, Brey RW, Cahill WT, et al. Immunologic abnormalities of cerebrospinal fluid (CSF) in asymp-

tomatic (AS) human immunodeficiency virus (HIV) infected individuals. *Neurology* 1988;38:167.

14. De-The G, et al. Human retroviruses HTLV-1, HIV-1 and HIV-2 and neurological diseases in some equatorial areas of Africa. *J Acquir Immune Defic Syndr* 1989; 2:550–556.

15. Levy J. Pathogenesis of human immunodeficiency virus infection. *Microbiol Rev* 1993;57:183–289.

16. Greene WC. The molecular biology of human immunodeficiency virus type 1 infection. *N Engl J Med* 1991;324:308–317.

17. Haseltine WA. Molecular biology of human immunodeficiency virus type 1. *FASEB J* 1991;5:2349–2360.

18. Gwinn M, et al. Prevalence of HIV infection in child bearing women in the United States. Surveillance using newborn blood samples. *JAMA* 1991;265:1704–1708.

19. Dalgleish AG, Beverly PCL, Claoham PR. The CD4 antigen is an essential component of the receptor for AIDS retrovirus. *Nature* 1984;312:763–767.

20. Ho DD, Rota TR, Hirsch MS. Infection of monocyte/macrophages by HTLV-III. *J Clin Invest* 1986;77: 1712–1715.

21. Schnittmann SM, Fauci AS. Human immunodeficiency virus and acquired immunodeficiency syndrome: an update. *Adv Intern Med* 1994;39:305–355.

22. Harouse JM, et al. Inhibition of entry of HIV-1 in neural cell lines of antibodies against galactosyl ceramide. *Science* 1991;253:320–323.

23. Pantaleo G, Fauci AS. New concepts in the immunopathogenesis of HIV infection. *Annu Rev Immunol* 1995;13:487–512.

24. Pantaleo G, Graziosi C, Fauci, AS. The immunopathogenesis of human immunodeficiency virus infection. *N Engl J Med* 1993;328:327–335.

25. Pantaleo G, et al. HIV infection is active and progressive in lymphoid tissue during the clinically latent stage of disease. *Nature* 1993;362:355–358.

26. Safarit JT, et al. Characterization of human immunodeficiency virus type 1 specific cytotoxic T lymphocyte clones isolated during acute seroconversion: recognition of autologous virus sequences within a conserved immunodominant epitope. *J Exp Med* 1994;179: 463–472.

27. Koup RA, et al. Temporal association of cellular immune responses with the initial control of viremia in primary human immunodeficiency virus type 1 syndrome. *J Virol* 1994;68:4650–4655.

28. Homsy J, Meyer M, Levy JA. Serum enhancement of human immunodeficiency virus (HIV) correlates with disease in HIV-1 infected individuals. *J Virol* 1990;64: 1437–1440.

29. Levy JA. Features of human immunodeficiency virus infection and disease. *Pediatr Res* 1993;33:S63–S70.

30. Robinson EW Jr, et al. Two immunodominant domains of gp41 bind antibodies which enhance human immunodeficiency virus type 1 infection in vitro. *J Virol* 1991; 65:4169–4176.

31. Ghiara JB, et al. Crystal structure of the principal neutralization site of HIV-1. *Science* 1994;264:82–85.

32. Westby M, Manca F, Dalgeish AG. The role of host immune responses in determining the outcome by HIV infection. *Immunol Today* 1996;17:120–126.

33. Jeanne H, Sztajzel R, Carpentier N, et al. HLA antigens are risk factors for development of AIDS. *AIDS* 1989; 1:28–32.

34. Itescu S, Rose S, Dwyer E, Winchester R. Certain HLA-DR5 and -DR6 major histocompatibility complex class II alleles are associated with a CD8 lymphocytic host response to immunodeficiency virus type 1 characterized by low lymphocyte viral strain heterogeneity and slow disease progression. *Proc Natl Acad Sci USA* 1994;91: 11472–11476.

35. Pantaleo G, et al. Major expansion of CD8+ T cells with a predominant Vβ usage during the primary immune response of HIV. *Nature* 1994;370:463–467.

36. Groux H, et al. Activation-induced death by apoptosis in CD4+ T cells from HIV-infected asymptomatic individuals. *J Exp Med* 1992;175:331–340.

37. Amersen JC, Estaquier J, Idziorek T. From AIDS to parasitic infection: pathogen-mediated subversion of programmed cell death as a mechanism for immune dysfunction. *Immunol Rev* 1994;142:9–52.

38. Pantaleo G, Fauci AS. HIV-1 infection in lymphoid organs: a model of disease development. *J NIH Res* 1993;5:68–72.

39. Haraguchi S, Good RA, Day NK. Immunosuppressive retroviral peptides: cAMP and cytokine patterns. *Immunol Today* 1995;16:595–603.

40. Budka H. Human immunodeficiency virus (HIV-l)-induced disease of the central nervous system: pathology and implications for pathogenesis. *Acta Neuropathol (Berl)* 1989;77:225–236.

41. Hollander H, Stringari S. Human immunodeficiency virus-associated meningitis. Clinical course and correlations. *Am J Med* 1987;83:813–816.

42. McArthur JC, et al. Dementia in AIDS patients: incidence and risk factors. *Neurology* 1993;43:2245–2252.

43. Snider WD, et al. Neurologic complications of acquired immune deficiency syndrome: analysis of 50 patients. *Ann Neurol* 1983;14:403–418.

44. Navia BA, Jordan BD, Price RW. The AIDS dementia complex: I. Clinical features. *Ann Neurol* 1986;19: 517–524.

45. Navia BA, Cho ES, Petito CK, Price RW. The AIDS dementia complex: II. Neuropathology. *Ann Neurol* 1986; 19:525–535.

46. Janssen RS, et al. Nomenclature and research case definitions for neurological manifestation of human immunodeficiency virus type-1 (HIV-1) infection. Report of a Working Group of the American Academy of Neurology AIDS Task Force. *Neurology* 1991;41:778–785.

47. Koenig S, et al. Detection of AIDS virus in macrophages in brain tissue from AIDS patients with encephalopathy. *Science* 1986;233:1089–1093.

48. Epstein LG, et al. HTLV-III/LAV-like retrovirus particles in the brains of patients with AIDS encephalopathy. *AIDS Res* 1985;1:447–454.

49. Dickson DW. Multinucleated giant cells in acquired immunodeficiency syndrome. Origin from endogenous microglia? *Arch Pathol Lab Med* 1986;110:967–968.

50. Rhodes RH. Histopathologic features in the central nervous system of 400 acquired immunodeficiency syndrome cases: implications of rates of occurrence. *Hum Pathol* 1993;24:1189–1198.

51. Sharer LR. Pathology of HIV-l infection of the central nervous system. A review. *J Neuropathol Exp Neurol* 1992;51:3–11.

52. Petito CK, et al. Vacuolar myelopathy pathologically resembling subacute combined degeneration in patients with the immunodeficiency syndrome. *N Engl J Med* 1985;132:874–879.

53. Petito CK, Cho E-S, Lemann W, et al. Neuropathology of acquired immunodeficiency syndrome (AIDS): an autopsy review. *J Neuropathol Exp Neurol* 1986;45: 635–646.

54. Glass JD, Wesselingh SL, Selnes OA, McArthur JC. Clin-

ical-neuropathologic correlation in HIV-associated dementia. *Neurology* 1993;43:2230–2237.

55. Saito Y, et al. Overexpression of nef as a marker for restricted HIV-1 infection of astrocytes in postmortem pediatric central nervous tissues. *Neurology* 1994;44: 471–481.

56. Tornatore C, Chandra R, Berger JR, Major EO. HIV-1 infection of subcortical astrocytes in the pediatric central nervous system. *Neurology* 1994;44:481–487.

57. Wiley CA, et al. Neocortical damage during HIV infection. *Ann Neurol* 1991;29:651–657.

58. Masliah E, Ge N, Achim CL, et al. Selective neuronal vulnerability in HIV encephalitis. *J Neuropathol Exp Neurol* 1992;51:585–593.

59. Wiley CA, Achim C. Human immunodeficiency virus encephalitis is the pathological correlate of dementia in the acquired immunodeficency syndrome. *Ann Neurol* 1994;36:673–676.

60. Brew BJ, et al. AIDS dementia complex and HIV-1 brain infection: clinical-virological correlations. *Ann Neurol* 1995;38:563–570.

61. Johnson RT, Glass JD, McArthur JC, Chesebro BW. Quantitation of human immunodeficiency virus in brains of demented and non-demented patients with acquired immunodeficiency syndrome. *Ann Neurol* 1996; 39:392–395.

62. Power C, et al. Distinct HIV-1 env sequences are associated with neurotropism and neurovirulence. *Curr Top Microbiol Immunol* 1995;202:89–104.

63. Steuler H, Stroch-Hagenlocher B, Wildemann B. Distinct population of human immunodeficiency virus type 1 in blood and cerebrospinal fluid. *AIDS Res Hum Retroviruses* 1992;8:53–59.

64. Royal W, Selnes OA, Concha M, et al. Cerebrospinal fluid human immunodeficiency virus type 1 (HIV-1) p24 antigen levels in HIV-1 related dementia. *Ann Neurol* 1994;36:32–39.

65. Singer EJ, Syndulko K, Fahy-Chandon BN, et al. Cerebrospinal fluid p24 antigen levels and intrathecal immunoglobulin G synthesis are associated with cognitive disease severity in HIV-1. *AIDS* 1994;8:197–204.

66. Buzy J, Brenneman DE, Pert CB, et al. Potent gp120-like neurotoxic activity in the cerebrospinal fluid of HIV-infected individuals is blocked by peptide T. *Brain Res* 1992;598:10–18.

67. McArthur JC, et al. The diagnostic utility in cerebrospinal fluid β2-microglobulin in HIV-1 dementia. *Neurology* 1992;42:1707–1712.

68. Griffen DE, Wesselingh SL, McArthur JC. Elevated central nervous system prostaglandins in human immunodeficiency virus-associated dementia. *Ann Neurol* 1994; 35:592–597.

69. Perrella O, Finelli L, Munno I, et al. Cerebrospinal fluid ferritin in human immunodeficiency virus infection: a marker of neurologic involvement? *J Infect Dis* 1993; 168:1079–1080.

70. Wiley CA, Achim CL, Schrier RD, et al. Relationship of cerebrospinal fluid immune activation associated factors to HIV encephalitis. *AIDS* 1992;6:1299–1307.

71. Torre D, Zeroli C, Ferrario G, et al. Cerebrospinal fluid concentration of fibronectin in patients with HIV-1 infection and central nervous system disorders. *J Clin Pathol* 1993;46:1039–1041.

72. Heyes MP, et al. Interrelationships between quinolinic acid, neuroactive kynurenines, neopterin and β2 microglobulin in cerebrospinal fluid and serum of HIV-1 infected patients. *J Neuroimmunol* 1992;40:71–80.

73. Portegies P, et al. Low levels of specific T cell activation marker CD27 accompanied by elevated levels of markers for non-specific immune activation in the cerebrospinal fluid of patients with AIDS dementia complex. *J Neuroimmunol* 1993;48:241–248.

74. Torre D, et al. Cerebrospinal fluid levels of IL-6 in patients with acute infections of the central nervous system. *Scand J Infect Dis* 1992;24:787–791.

75. Jassoy C, Johnson RP, Navia BA, et al. Detection of vigorous HIV-1-specific cytotoxic T lymphocyte response of cerebrospinal fluid from infected persons with AIDS dementia complex. *Immunology* 1992;149:3113–3119.

76. Mastroianni CM, et al. Tumor necrosis factor (TNF-α) and neurologic disorders in HIV infection. *J Neurol Neurosurg Psychiatry* 1992;55:219–221.

77. Shasken EG, Thompson RM, Price RW. Undetectable tumor necrosis factor-alpha in spinal fluid from HIV-1 infected patients. *Ann Neurol* 1992;31:687–688.

78. Elovaara I, et al. CSF follow-up in HIV-1 infection: intrathecal production of HIV-specific and unspecific IgG, and beta-2 microglobulin increase with duration of HIV-1 infection. *Acta Neurol Scand* 1993;83:388–396.

79. Elovarra I, Albert PS, Ranki A, et al. HIV-1 specificity of cerebrospinal fluid and serum IgG, IgM, and IgG1-G4 antibodies in relation to clinical disease. *J Neurol Sci* 1993;117:111–119.

80. Tyor WR, et al. Cytokine expression in the brain during the acquired immunodeficiency syndrome. *Ann Neurol* 1992;31:349–360.

81. Nottet HSLM, Gendelman HE. Unraveling the neuroimmune mechanisms for the HIV-1 associated cognitive/motor complex. *Immunol Today* 1995;16:441–448.

82. Nottet HSLM, et al. Mechanisms for the transendothelial migration of HIV-1 infected monocytes into the brain. *J Immunol* 1996;156:1284–1295.

83. Genis P, et al. Cytokines and arachidonic metabolites produced during human immunodeficiency virus (HIV)-infected macrophage-astroglia interactions: implications for the neuropathogenesis of HIV disease. *J Exp Med* 1992;176:1703–1718.

84. Nottet HSLM, et al. A regulatory role for astrocytes in HIV-1 encephalitis: an over-expression of eicosanoids, platelet-activating factor and tumor necrosis factor-α by activated HIV-1 infected monocytes is attenuated by primary human astrocytes. *J Immunol* 1995;154: 3567–3581.

85. Wahl SM, et al. Macrophage and astrocyte-derived transforming growth factor β as a mediator of central nervous system dysfunction in acquired immune deficiency syndrome. *J Exp Med* 1991;173:981–991.

86. Achim CL, Heyes MP, Wiley CA. Quantitation of human immunodeficiency virus, immune activation factors, and quinolinic acid in AIDS brains. *J Clin Invest* 1993; 91:2769–2775.

87. Giulian D, Wendt E, Vaca K, Noonan CA. Secretion of neurotoxins in mononuclear phagocytes infected with HIV-1. *Science* 1990;250:1593–1596.

88. Giulian D, Wendt E, Vaca K, Noonan CA. The envelope glycoprotein of human immunodeficiency virus type-1 stimulates release of neurotoxins from monocytes. *Proc Natl Acad Sci USA* 1993;90:2769–2773.

89. Brenneman D, Buzy J, Ruff M. Peptide T sequences prevent neuronal cell death produced by the protein gp120 of the human immunodeficiency virus. *Drug Dev Res* 1988;15:361–369.

90. Dreyer EB, et al. HIV-1 coat protein neurotoxicity prevented by calcium channel antagonists. *Science* 1990; 248:364–367.

91. Sabatier JM, et al. Evidence for neurotoxic activity of tat

from human immunodeficiency virus type 1. *J Virol* 1991;65:961–967.

92. Dawson VL, et al. Human immunodeficiency virus type 1 coat protein neurotoxicity mediated by nitric oxide in primary cortical cultures. *Proc Natl Acad Sci USA* 1993;90:3256–3259.

93. Lipton SA, et al. A redox-based mechanism for the neuroprotective and neurodestructive effects of nitric oxide and related nitric oxide and related nitroso-compounds. *Nature* 1993;364:626.

94. Gray F, Belec L, Keohane C, et al. Zidovudine therapy and HIV encephalitis: a 10-year neuropathological survey. *AIDS* 1994;8:489–493.

95. Gray F, et al. Neuropathological evidence that zidovudine reduces incidence of HIV infection of the brain. *Lancet* 1991;337:852–853.

96. Brew BJ, et al. Cerebrospinal fluid β_2 microglobulin in patients with AIDS dementia complex: an expanded series including response to zidovudine treatment. *AIDS* 1992;6:461–465.

97. Berger AR, et al. 2'3'-Dideoxycytidine (ddc) toxic neuropathy: a study of 52 patients. *Neurology* 1993;43:358.

98. Lipton SA. Models of neuronal injury in AIDS: another role for the NMDA receptor? *Trends Neurosci* 1992;15:75–79.

99. Lipton SA. HIV displays its coat of arms. *Nature* 1994;367:113–114.

100. Vella S. Rationale and experience with reverse transcriptase inhibitors and protease inhibitors. *J Acquir Immune Defic Syndr Hum Retrovirol* 1995;10:S58–S61.

101. Clerici M, et al. Restoration of HIV-specific cell-mediated immune responses by interleukin-12 in vitro. *Science* 1993;262:1721–1724.

102. Cocchi F, et al. Identification of RANTES, MIP-1(and MIP-1(as the major HIV-suppressive factors produced by CD8+ T cells. *Science* 1995;270:1811–1813.

103. Chavanet PY, et al. Altered peripheral nerve conduction in HIV-patients. *Cancer Detect Prev* 1988;12:249–255.

104. Griffin JW, et al. Peripheral nerve disorders HIV infection: similarities and contrast with CNS disorders. In: Price RW, Perry SW III, eds., *HIV, AIDS and the Brain*. New York: Raven, 1994:159–182.

105. Miller RG, Gareth JP, Pfieffl W, et al. The spectrum of peripheral neuropathy associated with ARC and AIDS. *Muscle Nerve* 1988;11:857–863.

106. Cornblath DR, McArthur JC. Predominately sensory neuropathy in patients with AIDS and AIDS-related complex. *Neurology* 1988;38:794–796.

107. Harrison MHG, McArtheur JC. *AIDS and neurology.* Edinburgh: Churchill Livingstone, 1995:87–108.

108. Rance NE, et al. Gracile tract degeneration in patients with sensory neuropathy and AIDS. *Neurology* 1988;38:265–271.

109. Cornblath DR, et al. Quantitative analysis of endoneurial T-cells in human sural nerve biopsies. *J Neuroimmunol* 1990;26:113–118.

110. Ho DD, et al. Isolation of HTLV-III from cerebrospinal fluid and neural tissue of patients with neurological syndromes related to acquired immunodeficiency syndrome. *N Engl J Med* 1995;313:1493–1497.

111. Esiri M, Morris C, Millard P. Sensory and sympathetic ganglia in HIV-1 infection: immunocytochemical demonstration of HIV-1 viral antigens, increased MHC class II antigen expression and mild reactive inflammation. *J Neurol Sci* 1994;114:178–187.

112. Simpson DM, Wolfe DE. Neuromuscular complications of HIV infection and its treatment. *AIDS* 1991;5:917–926.

113. Chad DA, et al. Human immunodeficiency virus (HIV)-associated myopathy: immunocytochemical identification of an HIV antigen (gp41) in muscle macrophages. *Ann Neurol* 1990;28:579–582.

114. Viard J-P, Vittecoq D, Lacroix C, Bach J-F. Response of HIV-1 associated polymyositis to intravenous immunoglobulin. *Am J Med* 1992;92:580–581. Letter.

115. Dalakas MC, Illa I, Pezeshkpour GH, et al. Mitochondrial myopathy caused by long-term zidovudine therapy. *N Engl J Med* 1990;322:1098–1105.

116. Grau JM, et al. Human immunodeficiency virus type 1 infection and myopathy: clinical relevance of zidovudine myopathy. *Ann Neurol* 1993;34:206–211.

117. Gherardi RK, Florea-Strat A, Fromont G, et al. Cytokine expression in the muscle of HIV-infected patients: evidence for interleukin-1α accumulation in mitochondria of AZT fibers. *Ann Neurol* 1994;36:752–758.

118. Britton CB. HIV infection. *Neurol Clin* 1993;11:605–624.

119. Levy RM, Berger JR. HIV and HTLV infections of the nervous system. In: Tyler KL, Martin JB, eds. *Infectious diseases of the central nervous system*. Philadelphia: FA Davis, 1993:47–75.

120. Larsen RA, Leal MA, Chan LS. Fluconazole compared with amphotericin B plus flucytosine for cryptococcal meningitis in AIDS. A randomized trial. *Ann Intern Med* 1990;113:183–197.

121. Eidelberg D, et al. Thrombotic cerebral vasculopathy associated with herpes zoster. *Ann Neurol* 1986;19:7–14.

122. Weiner LP. Chronic and slow infections of the central nervous system. In: Tyler KL, Martin JB, eds. *Infectious diseases of the central nervous system*. Philadelphia: FA Davis, 1993:131–154.

123. Padgett BL, Walker DL. Virologic and serologic studies of progressive multifocal leukoencephalopathy . In: Sever JL, Madden DL, eds. *Polyomaviruses and human neurological diseases*. New York: Liss, 1983:107–118.

124. Berger E, Kaszovitz B, Donovan Post JM, Dickinson G. Progressive multifocal leukoencephalopathy associated with human immunodeficiency virus infection. *Ann Intern Med* 1987;107:78–87.

125. Navia BA, Jordan BD, Price RW. Central nervous system complications of immunosuppression. In: Parsillo JE, Masier H, eds. *The critically ill immunosuppressed patient*. Rockville, MD: Aspen, 1987:119–142.

126. Brooks BR, Walker DL. Progressive multifocal leukoencephalopathy. *Neurol Clin* 1984;2:299–313.

127. Aksamit AJ, Mourrain P, Sever JL. Progressive multifocal leukoencephalopathy: investigation of three cases using in situ hybridization with JC virus biotinylated DNA probe. *Ann Neurol* 1985;18:490–494.

128. Telenti A, Akasmit AJ, Smith TF. Detection of JC virus DNA by polymerase chain reaction in patients with progressive multifocal leukoencephalopathy. *J Infect Dis* 1990;162:858–861.

Chapter 13

Infectious Immune Disorders: HTLV-I

Steven Jacobson, Michael Levin, Ursula Utz, and Paul Drew

The purpose of this chapter is to review the current information on the human T-cell lymphotropic virus type I (HTLV-I) and a number of human disorders that have been definitively associated with HTLV-I infection. HTLV-I is a member of the retrovirus family, which is a group of RNA viruses that replicate through a DNA intermediate and are defined by common morphology, genetic organization, and mode of replication (1–4). Similar to the human immunodeficiency virus (HIV), HTLV-I is transmitted vertically (mother to child), through sexual contact, and parenterally through blood transfusion or intravenous drug use. Epidemiologically, HTLV-I infection is defined by seroreactivity, determined either by an HTLV-I enzyme-linked immunosorbent assay (ELISA) or more specifically by Western blot analysis. Interestingly, the HTLV-I Western blot patterns can vary markedly among different geographic populations (5). HTLV-I is endemic in many regions throughout the world, most notably in the southern region of Japan (Kyushu, Shikoku, Okinawa), the Caribbean (Jamaica, Trinidad, Martinique, Barbados, Haiti), and the equatorial regions of Africa (Ivory Coast, Nigeria, Zaire, Kenya, Tanzania) and South America (Colombia, Brazil) (1,6,7). The seroprevalence rate in some of these endemic areas can be extraordinarily high, for example, exceeding 30% in Kagoshima, Japan. In the general population of the United States, the seroprevalence of HTLV-I is approximately 0.025% but can be as high as 2.1% in southeastern regions (8). It is important, however, to appreciate that unlike HIV, the majority of individuals infected with HTLV-I remain clinically asymptomatic throughout their lives.

Two human diseases are causally associated with HTLV-I infection: a malignant T-cell leukemia/lymphoma termed *adult T-cell leukemia* (ATL) (9–11) and a chronic progressive neurologic disease termed *HTLV-I–associated myelopathy/tropical spastic paraparesis* (HAM/TSP) (2,6,7). Indeed, HTLV-I was the first human retrovirus to be identified and was originally isolated from a patient with ATL (10). Why one group of HTLV-I seropositive individuals develop neurologic symptoms, another a neoplastic condition, and the majority remain asymptomatic carriers is unknown. One goal of this review is to discuss possible mechanisms whereby infection with the same viral agent can lead to dramat-

ically different clinical outcomes. The focus of this review is on the relationship of HTLV-I with the progressive neurologic disorder HAM/TSP, as considerable information on the molecular virology, pathology, and immunology of this disease is known.

HTLV-I Genomic Structure

HTLV-I transcription is principally determined by *cis*-acting, long terminal repeat (LTR) sequences present in the 5' and 3' termini of the HTLV-I genome (Fig 13-1). As with other retroviruses, open reading frames (ORFs) that encode Gag, Pol, and Env proteins are required for replication and are present in the 5' portion of the HTLV-I genome. In addition, human retroviruses including HTLV-I possess ORFs between Env and the 3' LTR. This region (pX) of HTLV-I contains four ORFs. The complexity of the proteins produced from these ORFs is increased owing to alternative splicing of viral messenger RNA (mRNA) from the pX region (reviewed elsewhere (12–15)). The viral regulatory proteins Tax and Rex are encoded in the pX region (see Fig 13-1). Tax functions as an activator of HTLV-I transcription (16,17) and Rex regulates expression of the virus via a posttranscriptional mechanism. Tax and Rex are encoded by the same spliced polycistronic mRNA. The phosphoprotein p21$^{Rex III}$ (14), and p12, p13, and p30^{TOF} proteins (18) are also encoded in the pX region.

HTLV-I Tax

HTLV-I Tax is a 42-kd nuclear phosphoprotein encoded in the pX region of the HTLV-I genome (12,17,19) and is of fundamental importance for viral replication (20), its effect on a number of cellular genes, and its immunogenicity. The immune response to this protein is thought to play a key role in the pathogenesis of HTLV-I–associated disease and is discussed in detail later. Tax activates the transcription of viral genes through Tax-responsive elements (TREs) located in the U3 region of the viral LTR (12,16,17). HTLV-I Tax transactivates the expression of a variety of cellular genes, listed in Table 13-1. The gene encoding the DNA-repair enzyme, β-polymerase, is the sole gene reported to be repressed

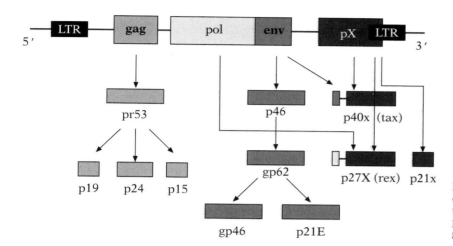

Figure 13-1. Schematic representation of the HTLV-I proviral genome and some of the immunologically relevant HTLV-I gene products encoded by the *gag, env,* and *pX* genes. LTR = long terminal repeat.

by HTLV-1 Tax (21). Tax is believed to regulate the expression of cellular genes by affecting the binding of cellular transcription factors to the promoter elements of the genes. Tax-mediated transactivation of genes encoding lymphokines, lymphokine receptors, growth factors, cellular oncogenes, and important gene regulatory molecules appears to play an important role in HTLV-I–mediated cell proliferation. Tax may induce T-cell activation and proliferation via an autoregulatory pathway involving increased interleukin (IL)-2 and IL-2 receptor α production (22). Tax can also be secreted from HTLV-I–infected cells and can induce the proliferation of cells

exposed to soluble Tax protein (23), suggesting that HTLV-I, via Tax, can also mediate the proliferation of uninfected cells in vivo. Activation of gene transcription also appears important in Tax-mediated immortalization of T cells, transformation of fibroblasts, and tumor formation in transgenic mice (19). Tax repression of the DNA repair enzyme β-polymerase (21) also likely functions in HTLV-I–mediated pathogenesis.

Regulation of Gene Expression by HTLV-I Tax

HTLV-I Tax mediates viral transcription through TREs (TRE-1 and TRE-2) located in the U3 region of the HTLV-1 LTR (16,17). Tax does not bind directly to these viral regulatory elements, but instead affects viral transcription indirectly, by inducing binding of cellular transcription factors to the TREs (24,25). The TRE-1 element of the HTLV-I LTR is characterized by 21-bp repeats. The cyclic adenosine monophosphate (cAMP)–responsive element binding protein (CREB)/activating transcription factor (ATF) proteins, a family of leucine zipper–containing transcription factors, are capable of binding to TRE-1 (26,27). At least partial specificity of these interactions is suggested by the fact that not all CREB/ATF pathway proteins bind Tax, and Tax mutants incapable of transactivating the HTLV-I LTR are unable to interact with CREB proteins (27). Recently, the protein domains involved in Tax-CREB interactions were identified. These studies demonstrated that the amino terminus of Tax (28) interacts with the basic region of basic leucine zipper (bZIP) proteins (29). However, both the basic and leucine zipper regions of CREB-1 physically interact with Tax (28). Interaction between Tax and bZIP proteins including CREB may promote protein dimerization and transcription factor binding to the cAMP-responsive element (CRE), and modify DNA binding site selection (19,29).

CREB proteins are activated to bind DNA following

Table 13-1.
Cellular Genes Transactivated by HTLV-I Tax

Upregulated
  Interleukin (IL)-2
  IL-2 receptor-α chain (tac)
  IL-3
  IL-6
  Tumor necrosis factor (TNF)-α
  TNF-β
  Transforming growth factor-β1
  Nuclear factor β proteins
  Immunoglobulin light chain
  Proenkephalin
  Major histocompatibility complex class I
  Nerve growth factor
  Granulocyte-macrophage colony-stimulating factor
    (GM-CSF)
  Parathyroid hormone–related protein
  Vimentin
  c-*fos*, c-*myc*, c-*sis*, fra-1
  A20 zinc finger protein
  Krox 20 and Krox 24
  Globin
Downregulated
  β-Polymerase

protein kinase A–mediated phosphorylation in response to cAMP (30). Tax is capable of binding unphosphorylated CREB and inducing CREB binding to the CRE. Thus, Tax may substitute for phosphorylation during CREB activation and DNA binding. CREB-binding protein (CBP) binds both phosphorylated CREB and the basal transcription factor TFIIB. CBP is believed to serve as a coactivator molecule by linking CREB, which is associated with the upstream enhancer CRE, to the basal transcription machinery. Tax physically interacts with basal transcription proteins, and HTLV-I LTR activation requires holo-TFIID and TFIIA. Thus, Tax may substitute for CBP in HTLV-I LTR activation and bypass the requirement of CREB phosphorylation in transcriptional activation (12,19,24).

The mechanisms that regulate HTLV-I LTR transactivation through TRE-2 are less clear. However, binding sites for a variety of transcription factors are present in the TRE-2 region and can activate the HTLV-I LTR (reviewed elsewhere (31)).

HTLV-I–Associated Diseases

Adult T-Cell Leukemia/Lymphoma

In 1980, the first human retrovirus was discovered; it was isolated from a patient with ATL (10). ATL is a lymphoproliferative malignancy of mature CD4+ T cells characterized by non-Hodgkin's lymphoma with leukemia (1,32). Histologically, there is a characteristic flower shape, a pleomorphic appearance of convoluted nuclei in the leukemic cells. Clinically, this disorder can be associated with hypercalcemia, hepatomegaly, splenomegaly, enlarged lymph nodes, or cutaneous involvement. ATL is classified into four subtypes: acute, chronic, smoldering, and lymphoma (32), with the acute form representing prototypic ATL. Acute ATL is a rapidly aggressive disease with a mean survival time of less than 9 months from the date of diagnosis. Chronic ATL is associated with increased white blood cell counts and skin disease whereas smoldering ATL involves few ATL-like cells in the peripheral blood although skin lesions may be present. Importantly, both chronic and smoldering ATL often progress to prototypic ATL after a long duration (32). HTLV-I monoclonally integrates into malignant CD4+ T-cells, although the site of integration varies among patients (11,33). Recently, the virus was found in these cells in a latent or defective state (34). Long-term CD4+ T-cell lines from ATL patients have been propagated in vitro and shown to be "transformed" in that they no longer require exogenous growth factors (35). This property of transformation has been attributed to HTLV-I. HTLV-I has the property to immortalize normal T cells in vitro (12). Possible mechanisms for this HTLV-I–induced lymphocyte transformation include transactivation of cellular IL-2 and IL-2 receptor genes by the HTLV-I regulatory protein Tax (see Fig 13-1), activation of cellular oncogenes such as c-*fos*, downregulation of DNA repair enzymes such as β-polymerase (see Table 13-1), and chromosomal aberrations (12,36–39).

HTLV-I–Associated Myelopathy/Tropical Spastic Paraparesis

In 1985 and 1986, studies from the Caribbean and Japan, respectively, described high HTLV-I seroprevalence rates in patients with a chronic progressive neurologic disease termed *HAM/TSP* (6,7). In HAM/TSP patients, unlike patients with ATL, HTLV-I proviral DNA randomly integrates into peripheral blood lymphocytes (PBLs) (40). The incubation period from the time of infection to the onset of disease is in the order of years to decades (41) but can be as short as 18 weeks, as reported in an individual who received a transfusion with HTLV-I–contaminated blood (42). The age at onset is usually between 35 and 45 years but can be as early as 12 years (1). HAM/TSP is three times more prevalent in females than males. Clinically, HAM/TSP is characterized by spasticity and hyperreflexia of the lower extremities, urinary bladder disturbance, lower-extremity muscle weakness, and sensory disturbances (43,44). Patients may have a mild pleocytosis with increased protein levels and oligoclonal bands (45–47). Magnetic resonance imaging (MRI)–detected abnormalities include atrophy of the spinal cord. Lesions in the white matter of the brain are found in approximately 50% of patients and are similar to those observed in patients with multiple sclerosis (MS) (48,49). Because of the clinical similarity of HAM/TSP with the primary progressive form of MS (Table 13-2), a search for an association of HTLV-I with MS was undertaken. While there have been conflicting reports on the involvement of HTLV-I in this disorder (50–57), based on both serologic and polymerase chain reaction (PCR) techniques, it is generally believed today that prototypic HTLV-I/II is not involved in the pathogenesis of MS. However, this does not rule out the possibility that a closely related human retrovirus may be associated with some clinical forms of MS. Since the clinical profiles of HAM/TSP and primary progressive MS are so similar (see Table 13-2), an understanding of the pathogenesis of HTLV-I–associated neurologic disease could lead to insights into the pathogenesis of MS, a disease in which viruses (and potentially retroviruses) have long been suspected to play a role (58).

HTLV-I–Associated Arthropathy

It is clear that both a leukemic and a neurologic disorder are associated with HTLV-I infection, and more recently, a number of other diseases have also been linked to HTLV-I. A chronic inflammatory arthropathy (termed *HTLV-I–associated arthropathy*) has been proposed to be related to HTLV-I infection (59,60). Clinical and pathologic characteristics of this disorder were different from those of other rheumatic diseases and HTLV-I proviral DNA was detected in T cells and non-T cells in the synovium of affected patients (60–62).

HTLV-I–Associated Uveitis

HTLV-I–associated uveitis is another clinical disorder in which seroepidemiologic, ophthalmologic, and virologic data indicate HTLV-I involvement. In some areas

Table 13-2.
HTLV-I–Associated Myelopathy/Tropical Spastic Paraparesis (HAM/TSP): Similarities with Multiple Sclerosis (MS)

	HAM/TSP	MS
Clinical	Chronic progressive myelopathy	Resembles primary progressive "spinal" form of MS
Oligoclonal bands	Yes, to HTLV-I antigens	Yes, to unknown antigens
Magnetic resonance imaging	Atrophy of spinal cord; occasionally mimics CNS demyelination in brain similar to that of MS	Demyelinating lesions of CNS white matter
Disease for life	Yes	Yes
Response to steroids	Typically not effective	Typically not effective
Etiologic agent	HTLV-I	Unknown, viruses considered
Demyelination	Yes, predominantly of corticospinal tracts, mild in posterior columns	Yes, diffuse involvement of spinal cord white matter, corticospinal and posterior columns severely affected
Inflammation	Yes, present at all levels of CNS; predominates in spinal cord at levels of severe demyelination	Yes, moderate in CNS lesions
Lymphocytes in lesions	Yes, CD4 and CD8 early in disease, CD8 persist in late disease	Yes, combination of CD4 and CD8
Immune response	Yes, spontaneous lymphoproliferation; high HTLV-I–specific antibody and CTLs	Yes, activated T cells in CSF and blood
HLA association	Yes, Japanese-associated alleles	Yes, DR2 in white patients

CNS = central nervous system; CTLs = cytotoxic T lymphocytes; CSF = cerebrospinal fluid.

of Japan, 20% of all uveitis cases are associated with HTLV-I (63,64), with the infiltrating cells in the anterior chamber containing HTLV-I DNA sequences.

HTLV-I–Associated Polymyositis

An HTLV-I–associated polymyositis with clinical similarities to sporadic polymyositis has also been reported (65,66). Epidemiologic studies indicate a significantly higher seroprevalence rate of HTLV-I in histologically proved polymyositis than in the general population in the Caribbean and Japan (67). Histologically, inflammatory cells are seen in muscle biopsy specimens, with HTLV-I–specific DNA sequences detected within the bulk of the muscle biopsy homogenate (65,68). The muscle fiber itself does not harbor HTLV-I but the endomysial macrophage does (65).

Other Disorders Suggested To Be Associated with HTLV-I Infection

HTLV-I has also been suggested to be associated with a T-cell alveolitis (69,70), Behçet's syndrome (71), infective dermatitis (72), and Sjögren's syndrome (62,70,71). Typically the disease descriptions involve HTLV-I seropositivity in patients with the corresponding clinical manifestations. In any of these HTLV-I disease associations, it is difficult to determine whether HTLV-I is directly related to disease pathogenesis or whether these disorders are coincidental in these patients, as many of them come from HTLV-I endemic areas. A more complete understanding of the pathophysiology of these diseases will allow us to better define the role of HTLV-I in them. Since considerably more informa-

tion is available on the neurologic disease HAM/TSP, the involvement of HTLV-I in this disorder serves as a framework to define the role that a human retrovirus can play in human disease.

Pathology of HTLV-I–Associated Myelopathy/Tropical Spastic Paraparesis

The neuropathology of central nervous system (CNS) autopsy specimens from patients with HAM/TSP has been carefully studied, and provides a model for the study of retrovirus-associated, immune-mediated damage to CNS tissues. The neuropathology of HAM/TSP patients is characterized by extensive damage and immune cell inflammation of the spinal cord, predominantly but not exclusively at the thoracic level (73–76) (Table 13-3). Specifically, the spinal cord is atrophic and the leptomeninges and blood vessels are thickened and fibrotic (74,77). There is symmetric, widespread loss of myelin (74,78) and axonal dystrophy (79) of the lateral columns, particularly of the corticospinal tracts of the spinal cord. Damage is most severe in the thoracic and lumbar regions; however, corticospinal damage has been clearly observed in the cervical region of the spinal cord (77,80–82) and the brainstem (80,82), and may be consistent with wallerian degeneration (74). Damage to the anterior and posterior columns is more variable and less extensive compared to corticospinal tract damage (74,79). Gliosis may also be present in the white matter of the spinal cord (79,82,83). All of these findings are consistent with a patient's clinical presentation, in which corticospinal signs such as paraparesis, spasticity, hyperreflexia, and Babinski signs predominate,

Table 13-3.
Pathologic Changes Found in the Central Nervous System (CNS) of HAM/TSP Patients

	Stage of Disease	
CNS Lesion	*Early*	*Late*
Inflammatory response		
Lymphocytic infiltration of spinal cord leptomeninges, blood vessels, and parenchyma	Extensive	Moderate
% CD8+ T cells	Equal to CD4+	Predominates
% CD4+ T cells	Equal to CD8+	Minimal
% B cells/plasma cells	Moderate	Minimal
% Foamy macrophages	Moderate	Minimal
Inflammatory cytokines (IL-2, TNF-α)	ND	Present
Neuropathologic damage		
Spinal cord atrophy	Moderate	Extensive
Leptomeningeal and blood vessel thickening	Present	Extensive
Lateral column degeneration (demyelination and axonal damage)	Moderate	Extensive
HTLV-I		
Viral particles	Present (EM)	ND
DNA sequences	Present (PCR)	Present (PCR)
RNA expression	ND	Present (ISH)
Colocalization with resident CNS cells	ND	Astrocyte

IL = interleukin; TNF = tumor necrosis factor; EM = electron microscopy; PCR = polymerase chain reaction; ISH = in situ hybridization; ND = not determined

compared to neurologic signs referable to other parts of the CNS (4).

In addition to parenchymal damage, there is an extensive immune response in the spinal cord of HAM/TSP patients (84). The leptomeninges and blood vessels are infiltrated with lymphocytes that may also penetrate the surrounding parenchyma. The phenotype of the infiltrating immune cells depends on the length of time the patient had neurologic disease prior to autopsy. In all patients, infiltrating cells contain CD8+ lymphocytes (85), and CD8+ cells in active lesions stain for TIA-1 (a marker for cytotoxic T lymphocytes) (86). Early in the course of the disease, there are greater numbers of inflammatory cells consisting of both CD8+ and CD4+ T cells, as well as B lymphocytes (77,78,85). In addition, foamy macrophages are present in damaged areas of spinal cord parenchyma (77,78). In chronic HAM/TSP specimens, inflammatory cells persist but are less frequent, and almost exclusively are of the CD8+ T-cell phenotype (74,79,85). In these specimens, CD4+ cells are rare and B lymphocytes and foamy macrophages are typically absent (74,79,82). Recently, we analyzed a spinal cord biopsy specimen from a patient with disease for longer than 10 years. The specimen showed inflammation of the leptomeninges and parenchyma. Analysis of the mononuclear infiltrate showed CD3+, CD45R0+ cells (activated T cells) that were almost entirely CD8+ (unpublished observation, 1995). One study evaluated inflammatory cytokines and major histocompatibility molecules (MHC) in autopsy specimens of a patient with HAM/TSP for more than 20 years (79). In this study, CD8+ cells predominated in areas of class I MHC molecule (β-microglobulin and HLA-ABC) expression and there were minimal numbers of CD4+ cells and class II MHC molecule (HLA-DRα) ex-

pression (which was attributed to activation rather than CD4 interaction) (79). Also, IL-1β and tumor necrosis factor (TNF)-α were detected by immunohistochemistry in the glial cells of these spinal cord sections (79).

Many studies have attempted to localize HTLV-I in the CNS of HAM/TSP patients. With electron microscopy, HTLV-I–like viral particles were found in the spinal cord of a HAM/TSP patient (87). Also, HTLV-I *gag* DNA sequences were localized to the thoracic region of the spinal cord (88). HTLV-I *pX* and *env* (89) DNA sequences were localized to the spinal cord but did not correlate with areas of lymphocyte infiltration (89,90). These studies give the impression that the virus in the CNS may not be localized to infiltrating immune cells, such as CD4+ cells, where the virus is localized to peripheral blood (91,92), but may be present in resident CNS cells. In fact, HTLV-I *pX* and *gag* RNAs were localized to degenerating lateral columns of the thoracic region of the cord in areas where lymphocyte infiltration was minimal (92). Further evidence that HTLV-I may infect resident CNS cells was provided by a recent study demonstrating HTLV-I *tax* RNA in the astrocytes of HAM/TSP patients (93).

Immune Response to HTLV-I

The neuropathology of HAM/TSP provided some of the earliest evidence that immune-mediated mechanisms play a major role in the pathogenesis of this disease. Indeed, a number of humoral and cellular immune parameters are abnormal in HAM/TSP patients compared to normal HTLV-I seronegative control subjects or more relevantly, compared to HTLV-I seropositive asymptomatic carriers. The sera and cerebrospinal fluid (CSF) of HAM/TSP patients have high antibody titers to

HTLV-I, which are diagnostic for this disorder (6,7). Patients may have hypergammaglobulinemia, oligoclonal bands in the CSF, and elevated levels of lymphokines such as IL-6 and soluble IL-2 in the serum and CSF (4,94,95). In addition, abnormal cellular immune responses include decreased natural killer cell activity and natural killer subsets as well as decreased antibody-dependent cellular cytotoxicity (ADCC) (96,97). In the peripheral blood and CSF of HAM/TSP patients, activated T lymphocytes are present (95,98,99), as demonstrated by an increase in the number of large CD3+ cells that express markers of T-cell activation such as HLA-DR and IL-2 receptor molecules (95,98). T-cell activation can also be demonstrated by the capacity of the PBLs of HAM/TSP patients to spontaneously proliferate in vitro in the absence of exogenously added antigen (95,98,99). This spontaneous lymphoproliferation has also been documented for PBLs of asymptomatic HTLV-I seropositive individuals (100) and individuals infected with HTLV-II, although the magnitude of the response is higher in HAM/TSP patients (101). While the exact mechanism for this spontaneous lymphoproliferation is not known, it is thought to be a consequence of T-cell transactivation that is driven by the HTLV-I–encoded Tax protein (22,102) (see Fig 13-1), or perhaps due to a physiologic response of viral antigen immune recognition and subsequent activation and expansion of regulatory immune cells.

It has been reported that the PBLs of HAM/TSP patients have up to 50 times more HTLV-I proviral DNA compared to the PBLs of asymptomatic carriers, which may be related to many of the immunologic responses discussed already (103,104). The amount of this HTLV-I proviral load as measured by PCR can range from 2 to 20 copies per 100 PBLs from HAM/TSP patients, compared to 0.04 to 8.00 copies per 100 PBLs in asymptomatic carriers (105). However, these figures may overrepresent the amount of HTLV-I in the PBLs if the virus integrates at more than 1 copy per cell. This was suggested by a study using in situ PCR technology, which demonstrated that as little as 1 in 10,000 HAM/TSP patients' PBLs contain HTLV-I in situ (106) and is comparable to what is seen in the PBLs of asymptomatic carriers. Even if these immune responses are driven by the high viral load in HAM/TSP patients, the hope is to define an HTLV-I–specific immune response that is unique to or over-represented in this disorder and determine the role that these particular responses play in disease pathogenesis. By defining such antigen-specific, functional cellular host responses to HTLV-I, we hope to better understand the underlying mechanisms involved in the neuro-pathology of HTLV-I–associated neurologic disease.

HTLV-I–Specific Cytotoxic T-Cell Responses

This review focuses on HTLV-I–specific, CD8+, HLA class I–restricted cytotoxic T lymphocytes (CTLs) that have been demonstrated in the peripheral blood and CSF of HAM/TSP patients (107–115). Characteristics of these CD8+ CTLs are emphasized and evidence is presented for the role that these CTLs may play in the pathogenesis of HTLV-I–associated neurologic disease.

CTLs play an important role in the normal, immunologically mediated recovery from infectious disease, by recognizing and subsequently eliminating foreign antigens (116–119). Through their antigen-specific T-cell receptor (TCR), CTLs recognize foreign proteins as short peptide fragments in association with human histocompatibility molecules (HLA). Two subsets of CTLs have been identified. CD8+ CTLs recognize foreign antigens, typically as short 9–amino acid peptide fragments, in the context of HLA class I molecules, and CD4+ CTLs recognize somewhat longer peptides in association with HLA class II molecules. Both populations are beneficial in eliminating infected cells and in recovery from viral infection (117). However, virus-specific CTLs can also be immunopathologic and cause disease, particularly if they destroy essential cellular structures (118,119). When defining a virus-specific CTL response, it is important to determine whether these responses are beneficial or detrimental. This will dictate a strategy for potential clinical therapies that can either augment a CTL response, to help eliminate virus-infected cells, or inhibit the CTL response to reduce the associated immunopathology.

HTLV-I–specific, CD8+, HLA class I–restricted CTLs have been demonstrated directly (without the need for in vitro expansion) from fresh mononuclear cells isolated from either the peripheral blood or CSF of HAM/TSP patients (107–115). Surprisingly, lysis was predominantly restricted to a product of the HTLV-I tax gene, although other HTLV-I antigens, most notably the envelope region of HTLV-I, were also recognized (108–111). Moreover, the frequency of these HTLV-I tax–specific CTLs in the peripheral blood was exceptionally high, ranging from 1 in 75 to 1 in 320 circulating CD8+ cells (109,110). Lower frequencies of HTLV-I env– and gag–specific CTLs were also demonstrated for some patients (110). This extraordinarily high frequency of HTLV-I–specific CD8+ CTLs explains why it is possible to directly detect these responses from PBLs of HAM/TSP patients.

Activated T cells in the CSF of HAM/TSP patients (95,110) are also cytotoxic and lyse HTLV-I expressing targets in an HLA class I–restricted manner. HTLV-I Tax was the predominant HTLV-I protein recognized by CSF CTLs. In addition, precursor frequency analysis of HTLV-I–specific CTLs from CSF lymphocytes also showed an increased frequency (as high as 1 in 60 CD8+ cells) in this compartment (110). Given the predominance of CD8+ T cells in the CSF of HAM/TSP patients, this would suggest that the absolute numbers of CD8+, HTLV-I–specific CTLs in the CSF may be even greater than the numbers in the peripheral blood.

In contrast to the high frequency of CD8+ HTLV-I–specific CTLs from HAM/TSP patients, HTLV-I seropositive, asymptomatic individuals have no or significantly lower CTL responses (108,110,111). Precursor frequency analysis also confirmed these observations:

The number of HTLV-I–specific CD8+ CTLs was 40- to 100-fold lower in asymptomatic carriers than HAM/TSP patients (110). In addition, HTLV-I–specific CTLs from circulating peripheral blood were not detected from two ATL patients. Collectively, these results suggest that the presence of circulating HTLV-I–specific CD8+ CTLs is a major immunologic feature of patients with HAM/TSP, reflective of the exceptionally high frequency of these CTLs in the peripheral blood, and therefore may contribute to the pathogenesis of this disorder. Support for the role of HTLV-I–specific CD8+ CTLs in disease pathogenesis may be extended to other disorders associated with HTLV-I (1,59–72). HTLV-I–specific CD8+ CTLs have also been demonstrated in some HTLV-I seropositive patients with arthritis, uveitis, Sjögren's syndrome (107), and a chronic muscle disorder (113).

HTLV-I Tax Peptide Specificity of HTLV-I–Specific Cytotoxic T Lymphocytes

As all HAM/TSP patients demonstrate high levels of CD8+ HTLV-I–specific CTLs directed toward the Tax protein of HTLV-I (107–115), a more precise characterization of the Tax epitopes recognized by these CTLs has been undertaken. Mapping of the predominant CTL epitopes is important because such an analysis could lead to tailored immunotherapeutic strategies that could specifically affect CTL function and potentially alter disease progression. This would be similar to the successful approaches that have been pioneered in the treatment and prevention of T cell–mediated experimental allergic encephalomyelitis (EAE) (120–122).

As discussed previously, CD8+ HLA class I–restricted CTLs recognize short peptide fragments (usually 9 amino acids) endogenously processed within virus-infected cells and conformationally bound to an HLA class I molecule (123–125). Different HLA class I molecules bind different peptides and unique binding motifs have been identified for a number of HLA class I alleles (126). HTLV-I–specific CTLs that recognize HTLV-I Tax protein are specific for the 9–amino acid peptide LLFGYPVYV (tax11–19), in association with the HLA-A2 allele (110–113). This peptide conforms to a known HLA-A2 binding motif of leucine or isoleucine in the second position and valine or leucine in the ninth position (126,127). Figure 13-2 depicts the binding of HTLV-I tax11–19 to an HLA-A2 molecule in which the HLA contact residues are shown. The tax11–19 peptide has an extraordinarily high affinity for the HLA-A2 molecule and can sensitize an HLA-A2 target for lysis by HTLV tax11–19–specific CTLs at a concentration as low as 10^{-16} M (0.1 femtomoles). Biochemical binding studies demonstrated that the HTLV-I tax11–19 peptide has one of the highest affinities known for any peptide-HLA complex with a half-life of 6400 minutes in association with HLA-A2 (128). Precursor frequency analysis of HTLV-I tax11–19–specific CTLs from the peripheral blood of HLA-A2–positive HAM/TSP patients (at a level of 1 in 300 CD8+ cells) is also consistent with the immunodominance of this peptide (110).

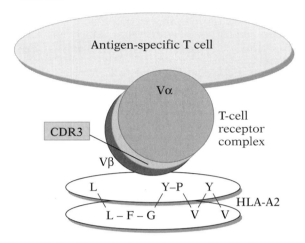

Figure 13-2. Through its antigen-specific T-cell receptor (TCR) consisting of a heterodimer of one α and one β chain, an HTLV-I tax11–19 peptide–specific T cell recognizes a 9–amino acid peptide bound to an HLA-A2 molecule. Amino acids in the first (L= leucine), fifth (Y = tyrosine), sixth (P = proline), and eighth (Y = tyrosine) positions of HTLV-I tax11–19 are thought to make contact with the TCR while amino acids in the second (L = leucine), third (F = phenylalanine), fourth (G = glycine), seventh (V = valine), and ninth (V = valine) positions are bound in a pocket of the HLA-A2 molecule. Highly variable complementary determining regions (CDR3) have been defined within the TCR and are thought to bind directly to the antigenic peptide-HLA complex.

T-Cell Receptor Usage in HTLV-I–Associated Myelopathy/Tropical Spastic Paraparesis

T cells recognize foreign antigens by a trimolecular interaction involving an MHC-bound antigenic peptide with an antigen-specific TCR consisting of a heterodimer of one α and one β chain (129–131). To recognize the enormous spectrum of peptide-MHC combinations, TCR heterogeneity is generated by the somatic rearrangement of noncontiguous V, D, and J genes (129–131). Highly variable complementary determining regions (CDR3) have been defined within the TCR and are thought to bind directly to the antigenic peptide-MHC complex (129–131). The salient features of this trimolecular interaction are depicted in Figure 13-2 with specific reference to HTLV-I–specific CTL recognition of HTLV-I tax11–19 in association with HLA-A2. With the molecular resolution of the crystal structure of the HTLV-I tax11–19–HLA-A2 complex (126), it is possible to suggest potential HTLV-I tax11–19 amino acid contact points with the TCR (see Fig 13-2). Proline appeared to be the most prominently exposed amino acid with two tyrosine residues and one phenylalanine accessible for TCR contact (126).

As discussed previously, the vast majority of virus-specific CTLs from HLA-A2–positive HAM/TSP patients recognize HTLV-I tax11–19. It is important to define whether these CTLs are dominated by a single, limited, or heterogeneous set of TCRs. In this way, therapeutic strategies could be devised to target a specific set of TCRs of potentially immunopathogenic T cells. Such therapies have been successfully used in murine models of neurologic disease, such as EAE (122,132–134) and have recently been evaluated in trials of patients with MS (135,136).

A recent study investigating HLA-A2–restricted, tax11–19–specific CTLs demonstrated an expansion of oligoclonal CD8+ CTLs in all HAM/TSP patients examined (137). The virus-specific TCRs were analyzed by PCR using two sets of TCR Vα- and Vβ family–specific primers and the CDR3 regions were determined (137). A comparison of 11 unique TCR α-chain sequences revealed heterogeneity of the CDR3 regions, and varying Vα and Jα gene usage. However, at least one T-cell clone from each patient utilized Vα2 rearranged with Jα24. Six unique TCRs with this combination were identified. Their sequences were identical except for one amino acid within the CDR3 region. The two preceding hydrophobic amino acids were composed of combinations of alanine, valine, and leucine.

The 11 TCR β-chain sequences were preferentially (8/11) rearranged with Jβ2.1 and 2.7, two Jβ genes with strong homologies. Half of the TCR α-chain sequences contained proline followed by glycine in their CDR3. The proline/glycine motif was found in combination with Vβ12.3, Vβ16, and Vβ17. The CDR3 lengths (139) ranged from 6 to 11 amino acids for TCR β chains and 6 to 12 amino acids for TCR β chains. No correlation was found between the CDR3 lengths of pairing α and β chains. TCR α chains with a CDR3 11 amino acids long were observed to pair with β chains with a CDR3 6 to 12 amino acids long (137). Therefore, the length of the CDR3 of one chain seems not to restrict the length of the chain partner.

Interestingly, one of the HLA-A2–restricted, tax11–19–specific CTL clones was traceable in one patient over a period of 3 years. The persistence of individual T-cell clones has been observed for myelin basic protein–specific T cells in MS patients (139,140). The fact that HLA-A2–restricted, HTLV-I tax11–19–specific CTLs are oligoclonally expanded in HAM/TSP patients is indicative of an in vivo activation and expansion of virus-specific CTLs, and corresponds well with the documented high precursor frequencies for HTLV-I–specific T cells in HAM/TSP patients (109,110). A dramatic expansion of a limited number of CD4+ as well as CD8+ T cells following viral infection had been demonstrated in the past, most recently in patients newly infected with influenza (141).

While there may be oligoclonal expansion of specific HTLV-I tax11–19–specific CTLs in some patients, the recognition of this peptide can be facilitated by diverse TCR αβ combinations with no apparent homologies. Highly heterogeneous CDR3 regions despite identical restriction and epitope specificity has also been reported

for class II–restricted TCRs specific for tetanus toxin 830–843 (142). This TCR diversity argues for a concerted action of both TCR chains and an involvement of all CDR regions. The primary TCR contact residues may vary within a given peptide-TCR combination. While there may be an overrepresentation of certain Vβ chains as reported for responses to other immunodominant viral epitopes, such as the HLA-A2–restricted influenza A matrix peptide M1$_{57-68}$ (143,144), an H-2K^b–restricted antigenic peptide from vesicular stomatitis virus (145), and an HLA-B8–restricted peptide from Epstein-Barr virus nuclear antigen 3 (146), this was not observed for HTLV-I tax11–19.

Restricted TCR Vβ-region usage has also been reported for a number of autoimmune diseases (147–149). One of the best-studied autoreactive T-cell responses is the one to myelin basic protein in MS (147,150–154). MS is a demyelinating disease with striking clinical similarities to HAM/TSP (see Table 13-2), and both diseases have been postulated to involve an autoimmune mechanism. Consequently, TCR genes expressed by T cells that infiltrate the spinal cord or CNS of HAM/TSP and MS patients have been studied and compared to TCRs expressed by myelin basic protein–specific T cells (155,156). Hara et al (155) and Oksenberg et al (156) postulated CDR3 region homologies between these TCRs. A comparison of oligoclonally expanded HTLV-I tax11–19–specific TCRs (137) and TCRs expressed by infiltrating T cells (155) from HAM/TSP patients did not reveal sequence homologies. However, HTLV-I–specific T cells recognizing epitopes other than HTLV-I tax11–19 and restricted by other HLA class I molecules might be present in the CNS. Therefore, the question of whether T cells that infiltrate the spinal cords of HAM/TSP patients represent virus-specific CTLs or autoreactive T cells recognizing myelin antigens is still not answered. The information obtained from the analysis of TCR usage by HTLV-I Tax–specific CTLs from HAM/TSP patients and the potential use of immunotherapeutic strategies to eliminate these cells could be extended to other CNS diseases of retroviral origin. Such therapies have been initially developed for use in EAE and more recently have been extended to patients with MS (120–122,132–136).

Immunopathogenic Model of HTLV-I–Associated Diseases

A number of models of HAM/TSP pathogenesis have been proposed (4,84,94), incorporate many of the virologic and immunologic features described, and are based on HTLV-I–induced immune-mediated responses that recognize either specific viral antigen(s) or cross-reactive self-peptides in the affected organ. The model detailed in this review reflects two major experimental observations: 1) inflammatory T cells in affected HAM/TSP spinal cord areas (74–76) that have a predominant CD8+ T-cell phenotype which increases in number as the disease progresses (92,105) and 2) the extraordinarily high frequency of CD8+ HTLV-I Tax–specific CTLs demonstrated in the peripheral blood and CSF of

HAM/TSP patients (107–113). In addition, the fact that virus-specific CTL responses are lower or absent in HTLV-I seropositive asymptomatic carriers supports further the hypothesis that immunopathogenic cytotoxic T cells may be directly involved in the pathogenesis of HAM/TSP. It is intriguing to ask whether the CD8+ inflammatory T cells present in HAM/TSP lesions are the same HTLV-I–specific CTLs detected in the periphery and CSF. If so, what could be the target for these CTLs in the CNS of HAM/TSP patients?

Because it is virtually impossible to obtain functionally active T cells from autopsy specimens, other approaches must be considered to determine whether inflammatory CD8+ T cells in HAM/TSP lesions are HTLV-I–specific CTLs. HAM/TSP patients are known to have a pleocytosis (45) and lymphocytes that have migrated into the CSF are readily accessible. Therefore, cells migrating into the CSF may reflect events in the CNS. As discussed already, experimental observations made with these CSF cells provide insight about the immunologic events in the CNS of affected patients and reveal CD8+ HTLV-I peptide–specific CTLs comparable, if not increased, to the CTL responses detected in peripheral blood. Alternatively, if a unique set of TCR genes were used by these CTLs, then it might be possible to probe HAM/TSP autopsy material for the in situ expression of defined TCR α and β chains. Results indicate, however, that while there may be oligoclonal expansion of specific HTLV-I tax11–19 peptide–specific CTLs in some HLA-A2 patients, the recognition of this peptide can be facilitated by diverse TCR αβ combinations with no apparent homologies (137,157). Potentially, a unique set of TCR chains may be used by HTLV-I Tax–specific CTLs in HAM/TSP patients early in the course of the disease (157) but CNS material from these individuals will be difficult to obtain.

To date, the most direct demonstration of HTLV-I–specific CTLs in the CNS of HAM/TSP patients is based on a biopsy specimen from a patient with HAM/TSP of long disease who had a large MRI enhancing lesion in the spinal cord (158). Inflammatory T cells were present in this spinal cord specimen and were almost entirely CD8+. This material was cultured in vitro without antigenic stimulation, in an attempt to expand these cells. CD8+ T-cell lines were generated and demonstrated to be cytotoxic, HTLV-I specific, and HLA class I restricted (158). This patient was not HLA-A2 positive. The HTLV-I peptide specificity of these CD8+ HTLV-I–specific CTL lines derived from the spinal cord specimen was not determined. Although these results are based on CTL lines derived after short-term culture, they argue strongly for the presence of functionally active HTLV-I–specific CTLs in the pathogenesis of HTLV-I–associated neurologic disease.

If CD8+ T cells in HAM/TSP CNS material are cytotoxic, what is the target for these cells? It has been difficult to demonstrate HTLV-I antigens in HAM/TSP CNS material by immunocytochemical techniques (74). This is not surprising as the PBLs of these patients known to be infected with HTLV-I do not express HTLV-I antigens (159). HTLV-I DNA sequences in the CNS of HAM/TSP patients have been determined by solution-phase PCR (92,105), although with this technique, it is not possible to determine which cell in the CNS contains these HTLV-I DNA sequences. Recent reports of studies using in situ hybridization techniques showed that HTLV-I is present in spinal cord material obtained at autopsy of HAM/TSP patients (93,160). In one, HTLV-I DNA was localized to inflammatory CD4+ cells, by a novel in situ hybridization PCR technique (155). In contrast, by more conventional in situ hybridization procedures, HTLV-I RNA was not found in inflammatory infiltrates but rather in cells that appeared to be astrocytes (93,160).

A number of possibilities can be envisioned by which cytotoxic inflammatory CD8+ cells in HAM/TSP CNS lesions are associated with HTLV-I neuropathology. Infiltrating HTLV-I–infected CD4+ cells early in the course of the disease (92) could result in HTLV-I infection of resident glial cells, which could induce the elements necessary for recognition by inflammatory cytotoxic CD8+ cells, including viral antigen in association with the appropriate HLA molecule. These CTLs could cause CNS damage by direct lysis or through the release of inflammatory cytokines such as TNF-α, which induces demyelination in experimental models. Alternatively, HTLV-I infection of cells far from CNS lesion sites, either within other regions of the CNS or even in the peripheral blood, may result in the release of HTLV-I proteins or immunodominant peptides which can be processed by cells in affected CNS areas that become targets for HTLV-I–specific CTLs.

This model of HAM/TSP immunopathogenesis may also be applied to other HTLV-I–associated disorders that may be immunopathologically mediated (59–72). This theory would suggest that HTLV-I immunoreactive T cells are present in the affected organs and the expression of HTLV-I at these sites may be targets for these pathogenic infiltrates. In support of this hypothesis, both HTLV-I DNA sequences and inflammatory T cells are found in the synovial fluid or aqueous humor of patients with HTLV-I–associated arthropathy or HTLV-I–associated uveitis (61). The critical component of this theory is the inappropriate expression of HTLV-I in at least one organ system. Immune recognition of HTLV-I in the CNS may lead to HAM/TSP; in the synovium it may lead to arthritis; in muscle, to polymyositis; and so on. Importantly, these theories give a rationale for immunotherapeutic strategies in attempts to clinically intervene in this disease.

References

1. McFarlin DE, Blattner WA. Non-AIDS retroviral infections in humans. *Annu Rev Med* 1991;42:97–105.
2. Bucher B, Poupard JA, Vernat JC, DeFreitas EC. Tropical neuropathies and retroviruses: a review. *Rev Infect Dis* 1990;12:890–899.
3. Wong Staal F, Gallo RC. Human T lymphotropic retroviruses. *Nature* 1985; 317:395–403.
4. Hollsberg P, Hafler DA. Pathogenesis of diseases induced by human lymphotropic virus type I infection. *N Engl J Med* 1993;328:1173–1182.

5. Gessain A, Mathieux R. HTLV-I indeterminate Western blot patterns observed in sera from tropical regions: the situation revisited *J Acquir Immune Defic Syndr Hum Retrovirol* 1995;9:316–319.

6. Gessain A, Vernant JC, Maurs L, et al. Antibodies to human T-lymphotropic virus I in patients with tropical spastic paraparesis. *Lancet* 1985;2:407–410.

7. Osame M, Usuku K, Izumo S, et al. HTLV-I associated myelopathy: a new clinical entity. *Lancet* 1986;1:1031–1032.

8. Kabbaz RF, Darrow WW, Hartley TM, et al. Seroprevalence and risk factors for HTLV-I/II infection among female prostitutes in the United States. *JAMA* 1990;263:60–64.

9. Uchiyama T, Yodoi J, Sagawa K, et al. Adult T cell leukemia: clinical and hematologic features of 16 cases. *Blood* 1977;50:481–492.

10. Poeisz BJ, Ruscetti FW, Gazdar AF, et al. Detection and isolation of type C retrovirus particles from fresh and cultured lymphocytes of a patient with cutaneous T cell lymphoma. *Proc Natl Acad Sci USA* 1980;77:7415–7419.

11. Yoshida M, Seiki M, Yamaguchi K, Takasuki K. Monoclonal integration of human T cell leukemia provirus in all primary tumors of adult T cell leukemia suggests a causative role of human T cell leukemia virus in the disease. *Proc Natl Acad Sci USA* 1984;81:2534–2537.

12. Franchini G. Molecular mechanisms of human T cell leukemia/lymphotropic virus type I infection. *Blood* 1995;86:3619–3639.

13. Seiki M, Hikikoshi A, Taniguchi T, Yoshida M. Expression of the pX gene of HTLV-I: general splicing mechanism in the HTLV family. *Science* 1985;228:1532–1534.

14. Berneman ZN, Gartenhaus RB, Reitz MS, et al. Expression of alternatively spliced human T-lymphotropic virus type I (HTLV-I) pX mRNA in infected cell lines and in primary uncultured cells from patients with adult T cell leukemia/lymphoma and healthy carriers. *Proc Natl Acad Sci USA* 1992;89:3005–3009.

15. Koralnick IJ, Gessain A, Klotman ME, et al. Protein isoforms encoded by the pX region of human T-leukemia/lymphotropic virus type I. *Proc Natl Acad Sci USA* 1992;89:8813–8817.

16. Sodroski JC, Rosen WC, Haseltine WA. Transactivating transcriptional activation of the long terminal repeat of human T-lymphotropic viruses in infected cells. *Science* 1984;226:177–179.

17. Felber BK, Paskalis H, Wong-Staal F, Pavlakis GN. The pX protein of HTLV-I is a transcriptional activator of its long terminal repeat. *Science* 1985;229:675–679.

18. Koralnick IJ, Fullen J, Franchini G. The p12, p13, and p30 proteins encoded by human T-leukemia/lymphotropic virus type I open reading frames I and II are localized in three different cellular compartments. *J Virol* 1993;67:2360–2366.

19. Yoshida M. Host HTLV-I type I interaction at the molecular level. *AIDS Res Hum Retroviruses* 1994;10:1193–1197.

20. Chen ISY, Slamon DJ, Rosenblatt JD, et al. The pX gene is essential for HTLV replication. *Science* 1985;229:54–58.

21. Jeang KT, Widen SG, Semmens OJ, Wilson SH. HTLV-I transactivator protein Tax is a trans-repressor of the human β-polymerase. *Science* 1990;247:1082–1084.

22. Siekevitz M, Feinberg M, Holbrook N, et al. Activation of interleukin 2 and interleukin 2 receptor (tac) promoter expression by the transactivator (tat) gene product of human T cell leukemia virus type I. *Proc Natl Acad Sci USA* 1987;84:5389–5393.

23. Marriott SJ, Lindholm PF, Reid RL, Brady JN. Soluble HTLV-I TaxI protein stimulates proliferation of human peripheral blood lymphocytes. *New Biol* 1991;3:678–686.

24. Gitlin SD, Dittmer J, Reid RL, Brady JN. The molecular biology of human T cell leukemia viruses. In: Cullen BR, ed. *Frontiers in molecular biology.* Oxford, UK: Oxford, 1993:159–192.

25. Marriott SJ, Lindholm PF, Brown KM, et al. A 36-kilodalton cellular transcription factor mediates an indirect interaction of human T cell leukemia/lymphoma virus type I Tax with a responsive element in the viral long terminal repeat. *Mol Cell Biol* 1990;10:4192–4201.

26. Jeang KT, Boros I, Brady M, et al. Characterization of cellular factors that interact with the human T-lymphotropic virus type I p40 responsive 21 base pair sequence. *J Virol* 1988;62:4499–4509.

27. Suzuki T, Fujisawa J, Toita M, Yoshida M. The trans activator tax of human T-lymphotropic virus type I (HTLV-I) interacts with cAMP responsive element (CRE) binding and CRE modulator proteins that bind to the 21 base pair enhancer of HTLV-I. *Proc Natl Acad Sci USA* 1993;90:610–614.

28. Yin MJ, Paulssen EJ, Seeler JS, Gaynor RB. Protein domains involved in both in vivo and in vitro interactions between human T-cell leukemia virus type I tax and CREB. *J Virol* 1995;69:3420–3432.

29. Baranger AM, Palmer CR, Hamm MK, et al. Mechanism of DNA-binding enhancement by the human T-cell leukaemia virus transactivator Tax. *Nature* 1995;376:606–608.

30. Gonzales GA, Montminy MR. Cyclic AMP stimulates somatostatin gene transcription by phosphorylation of CREB at serine. *Cell* 1989;59:675–680.

31. Gitlin SD, Dittmer J, Shin RC, Brady JN. Transcriptional activation of the human T-lymphotropic virus type I long terminal repeat by functional interaction of Tax1 and Ets1. *J Virol* 1993;67:7307–7316.

32. Yamaguchi K, Kiyokawa T, Futami G, et al. Pathogenesis of adult T cell leukemia from clinical pathologic features. In: Blattner WA, ed. *Human retrovirology: HTLV.* New York: Raven, 1990:163–171.

33. Wong-Staal F, Hahn B, Manzari V, et al. A survey of human leukemias for sequences of a human retrovirus. *Nature* 1983;302:626–628.

34. Franchini G, Wong-Staal, F, Gallo RC. Molecular studies on human T cell leukemia virus and adult T cell leukemia. *J Invest Dermatol* 1984;83:S63–S66.

35. Miyoshi I, Kubonishi I, Yoshimoto S, et al. Type C virus particles in a cord T cell line derived by co-cultivating normal human cord leukocytes and human leukemic T cells. *Nature* 1981;294:770–771.

36. Yoshida M. Expression of the HTLV-I genome and its association with a unique T cell malignancy. *Biochem Biophys Acta* 1987;970:145–161.

37. Smith MR, Greene WC. Identification of HTLV-I transactivator mutants exhibiting novel transcriptional phenotypes. *Genes Dev* 1990;4:1875–1885.

38. Fujii M, Sassone-Corsi P, Verma IM. c-fos Promoter transactivation by the tax protein of human T cell leukemia virus type 1. *Proc Natl Acad Sci USA* 1988;85:8526–8530.

39. Jeang KT, Widen SG, Semmes OJ, Wilson SH. HTLV-I transactivator protein tax is a transrepressor of the human β-polymerase gene. *Science* 1990;247:1082–1084.

40. Greenberg SJ, Jacobson, S, Waldmann TA, McFarlin DE. Molecular analysis of HTLV-I proviral integration and T cell receptor rearrangement indicates that T cells

in tropical spastic paraparesis are polyclonal. *J Infect Dis* 1989;159:741–744.

41. Osame K, Izumo S, Igata A, et al. Blood transfusion and HTLV-I associated myelopathy. *Lancet* 1986;104–105.

42. Gout O, Baulac M, Gessain A, et al. Rapid development of myelopathy after HTLV-I infection acquired by transfusion during cardiac transplantation. *N Engl J Med* 1990;322:383–388.

43. Osame M, McArthur JC. Neurologic manifestations of infection with human T cell lymphotropic virus type I. In: Asbury AK, McKhann GM, McDonald WI, eds. *Diseases of the nervous system: clinical neurobiology.* Philadelphia: WB Saunders, 1990:1331–1339.

44. Virus diseases: human T cell lymphotropic virus type I, HTLV-I. In: *Weekly epidemiological record.* Geneva: World Health Organization, 1989:382–383.

45. Jacobson S, Gupta A, Mattson D, et al. Immunological studies in tropical spastic paraparesis. *Ann Neurol* 1990;27:149–156.

46. Ceroni M, Piccardo P, Rodgers-Johnson P, et al. Intrathecal synthesis of IgG antibodies to HTLV-I supports an etiological role for HTLV-I in tropical spastic paraparesis. *Ann Neurol* 1988;23(suppl):S188–S191.

47. Link H, Cruz M, Gessain A, et al. Chronic progressive myelopathy associated with HTLV-I: oligoclonal IgG and anti-HTLV-I IgG antibodies in the cerebrospinal fluid and serum. *Neurology* 1989;39:1566–1572.

48. Mattson DH, McFarlin DE, Mora C, Zaninovic V. Central nervous system lesions detected by magnetic resonance imaging (MRI) of tropical spastic paraplegia. *Lancet* 1987;2:49.

49. Cruickshank JK, Rudge P, Dalgleish AG, et al. Tropical spastic paraparesis and human T cell lymphotropic virus type I in the United Kingdom. *Brain* 1990;112:1057–1090.

50. Koprowski H, DeFrietas EC, Harper ME, et al. Multiple sclerosis and human T cell lymphotropic retroviruses. *Nature* 1985;318:154–160.

51. Ohta M, Ohta K, Fumiyo M, et al. Sera from patients with multiple sclerosis react with human T cell lymphotropic virus-I gag proteins but not env proteins—Western blotting analysis. *J Immunol* 1986;137:3440–3443.

52. Rice GPA, Armstrong HA, Bulman DE, et al. Absence of antibodies to HTLV-I and III in sera from Canadian patients with multiple sclerosis and chronic myelopathy. *Ann Neurol* 1986;20:533–534.

53. Hauser S, Aubert C, Burks JS, et al. Analysis of human T lymphotropic virus sequences in multiple sclerosis tissue. *Nature* 1986;322:176–177.

54. Reddy EP, Sandberg-Wollheim M, Mettus RV, et al. Amplification and molecular cloning of HTLV-I sequences from DNA of multiple sclerosis patients. *Science* 1989;243:529–533.

55. Greenberg SJ, Ehrlich GD, Abbott MA, et al. Detection of sequences homologous to human retroviral DNA in multiple sclerosis by gene amplification. *Proc Natl Acad Sci USA* 1989;86:2878–2882.

56. Bangham CRM, Nightingale S, Cruickshank JK, Daenke S. PCR analysis of DNA from multiple sclerosis patients for the presence of HTLV-I. *Science* 1989;246:821.

57. Richardson JH, Endo N, Rudge P, et al. PCR analysis of DNA from multiple sclerosis patients for the presence of HTLV-I. *Science* 1989;246:821–823.

58. Johnson RT. The virology of demyelinating diseases. *Ann Neurol* 1994;36(suppl):54–60.

59. Nishioka K, Maruyama I, Sato K, et al. Chronic inflammatory arthropathy associated with HTLV-I. *Lancet* 1989;1:441.

60. Sato K, Maruyama I, Maruyama Y, et al. Arthritis in patients infected with human lymphotropic virus type I: clinical and immunopathologic features. *Arthritis Rheum* 1991;34:714–721.

61. Kitajima I, Yamamoto K, Sato K, et al. Detection of human T cell lymphotropic virus type I proviral DNA and its gene expression in synovial cells in chronic inflammatory arthropathy. *J Clin Invest* 1991;88:1315–1322.

62. Nishioka K, Nakajima T, Hasanuma T, Sato K. Rheumatic manifestation of human leukemia virus infection. *Rheum Dis Clin North Am* 1993;2:489–503.

63. Mochizuki M, Watanabe T, Yamaguchi K, et al. HTLV-I uveitis: a distinct clinical entity caused by HTLV-I. *Jpn J Cancer Res* 1992;5:29–42.

64. Watanabe T, Ono A, Mochizuki M, et al. Analysis of the infiltrating cells of HTLV-I uveitis. *AIDS Res Hum Retroviruses* 1994;10:444. Abstract.

65. Leon-Monzon M, Illa I, Dalakas C. Polymyositis in patients infected with human T cell lymphotropic virus type I: the role of the virus in the cause of the disease. *Ann Neurol* 1994;36:643–649.

66. Morgan OS, Rodgers-Johnson P, Mora C, Char G. HTLV-I and polymyositis in Jamaica. *Lancet* 1989;2:1184–1187.

67. Higuchi I, Montemayor ES, Izumo S, et al. Immunohistochemical characteristics of polymyositis in patients with HTLV-I associated myelopathy and carriers. *Muscle Nerve* 1993;16:472–476.

68. Ijichi T, Higuchi I, Fukunaga H, et al. Lymphocyte subsets in muscle biopsies of human T cell lymphotropic virus type I carriers with polymyositis. *Intern Med* 1992;31:973–977.

69. Sugimoto M, Nakashima H, Watanabe S, et al. T lymphocyte alveolitis in HTLV-I associated myelopathy. *Lancet* 1987;2:1220.

70. Vernat JC, Buisson G, Magdelaine J, et al. T lymphocyte alveolitis, tropical spastic paraparesis and Sjögren's syndrome. *Lancet* 1988;1:177.

71. Kanazama H, Ijichi I, Eiraku N, et al. Behçet's syndrome and Sjögren syndrome in a patient with HTLV-I associated myelopathy. *J Neurol Sci* 1993;119:121–122.

72. LeGrande K, Hanchard B, Fletcher V, et al. Infective dermatitis of Jamaican children: a marker for HTLV-I infection. *Lancet* 1990;336:1345–1347.

73. Piccardo P, Ceroni M, Rodgers-Johnson P, et al. Pathological and immunological observations on tropical spastic paraparesis in patients from Jamaica. *Ann Neurol* 1988;23(suppl):S156–S160.

74. Moore GRW, Traugott U, Scheinberg LC, Raine CS. Tropical spastic paraparesis: a model of virus-induced cytotoxic T-cell mediated demyelination? *Ann Neurol* 1989;26:523–530.

75. Iwasaki I. Pathology of chronic myelopathy associated with HTLV-I infection (HAM/TSP). *J Neurol Sci* 1990;96:103–123.

76. Yoshioka A, Hirose G, Ueda Y, et al. Neuropathological studies of the spinal cord in early stage HTLV-I–associated myelopathy (HAM). *J Neurol Neurosurg Psychiatry* 1993;56:1004–1007.

77. Akizuki S. The first autopsy case of HAM. In: Iwasaki Y, ed. *Neuropathology of HAM/TSP in Japan. Proceedings of the first workshop on neuropathology of retrovirus infections.* Sendai, Japan: Tohoku University School of Medicine, 1989:1–6.

78. Izumo S, Higuchi I, Ijichi T, et al. Neuropathological

study in two autopsy cases of HTLV-I associated myelopathy (HAM). In: Iwasaki Y, ed. *Neuropathology of HAM/TSP in Japan. Proceedings of the first workshop on neuropathology of retrovirus infections.* Sendai, Japan: Tohuku University School of Medicine, 1989:7–17.

79. Wu E, Dickson DW, Jacobson S, Raine CS. Neuroaxonal dystrophy in HTLV-I associated myelopathy/tropical spastic paraparesis: neuropathologic and neuroimmunologic correlations. *Acta Neuropathol (Berl)* 1993;86: 224–235.

80. Akizuki S. An autopsy case of HAM with prolonged steroid therapy. In: Iwasaki Y, ed. *Neuropathology of HAM/TSP in Japan. Proceedings of the first workshop on neuropathology of retrovirus infections.* Sendai, Japan: Tohuku University School of Medicine, 1989:25–32.

81. Kobayashi I, Ota K, Yamamoto K, et al. Clinical and pathological observations in HTLV-I associated myelopathy. In: Iwasaki Y, ed. *Neuropathology of HAM/TSP in Japan. Proceedings of the first workshop on neuropathology of retrovirus infections.* Sendai, Japan: Tohuku University School of Medicine, 1989:33–46.

82. Hara M, Sano J, Watanabe R, Honda M. An autopsy case of HAM with a history of blood transfusions. In: Iwasaki Y, ed. *Neuropathology of HAM/TSP in Japan. Proceedings of the first workshop on neuropathology of retrovirus infections.* Sendai, Japan: Tohuku University School of Medicine, 1989:75–82.

83. Kishikawa M, Kurihara K, Kitai K, Kondo T. An autopsy case of HTLV-I associated myelopathy (HAM) caused by blood transfusions for uterine adenocarcinoma. In: Iwasaki Y, ed. *Neuropathology of HAM/TSP in Japan. Proceedings of the first workshop on neuropathology of retrovirus infections.* Sendai, Japan: Tohuku University School of Medicine, 1989:18–24.

84. Jacobson S. HTLV-I myelopathy: an immunopathologically mediated chronic progressive disease of the central nervous system. *Curr Opin Neurol* 1995;8:179–183.

85. Umehara F, Izumo S, Nakaga M, et al. Immunocytochemical analysis of the cellular infiltrates in the spinal cord lesions in HTLV-I associated myelopathy. *J Neuropathol Exp Neurol* 1993;52:424–430.

86. Umehara F, Nakamura A, Izumo S, et al. Apoptosis of T lymphocytes in the spinal cord lesions of HTLV-I associated myelopathy: a possible mechanism to control viral infection in the central nervous system. *J Neuropathol Exp Neurol* 1994;53:617–624.

87. Liberski PP, Rodgers-Johnson P, Char G, et al. HTLV-I-like viral particles in spinal cord cells in Jamaican tropical spastic paraparesis. *Ann Neurol* 1988;23(suppl): S185–S187.

88. Bhigjee AI, Wiley CA, Wachsman W, et al. HTLV-I associated myelopathy: clinicopathologic correlation with localization of provirus to the spinal cord. *Neurology* 1991;41:1990–1992.

89. Kira J, Itohama Y, Koyanagi Y, et al. Presence of HTLV-I proviral DNA in central nervous system of patients with HTLV-I-associated myelopathy. *Ann Neurol* 1992;31:39–45.

90. Ohara Y, Iwasaki Y, Izumo S, et al. Search for human T-cell leukemia virus type I (HTLV-I) proviral sequences by polymerase chain reaction in the central nervous system of HTLV-I-associated myelopathy. *Arch Virol* 1992;124: 31–43.

91. Richardson JH, Edwards AJ, Cruickshank JK, et al. In vivo cellular tropism of human T-cell leukemia virus type I. *J Virol* 1990;64:5682–5687.

92. Kubota R, Umehara F, Izumo S, et al. HTLV-I proviral

93. Lehky TJ, Fox CH, Koenig S, et al. Detection of human T lymphotropic virus type I (HTLV-I) tax RNA in the central nervous system of HTLV-I associated myelopathy/tropical spastic paraparesis by in situ hybridization. *Ann Neurol* 1995;37:246–254.

94. Jacobson S. Immune response to retroviruses in the central nervous system: role in the neuropathology of HTLV-I associated neurologic disease. *Semin Neurosci* 1992;4:285–290.

95. Jacobson S, Gupta A, Mattson D, et al. Immunologic studies in tropical spastic paraparesis (TSP). *Ann Neurol* 1990;27:149–156.

96. Morimoto C, Matsuyama T, Oshige C, et al. Functional and phenotypic studies of Japanese adult T cell leukemia cells. *J Clin Invest* 1985;75:836–843.

97. Kitajima I, Osame M, Izumo S, Igata A. Immunological studies of HTLV-I associated myelopathy. *Autoimmunity* 1988;1:125–131.

98. Jacobson S, Zaninovic V, Mora C, et al. Immunological findings in neurological diseases: activated lymphocytes in tropical spastic paraparesis. *Ann Neurol* 1988;23: 196–200.

99. Itoyama Y, Minato S, Kira J, et al. Spontaneous proliferation of peripheral blood lymphocytes increased in patients with HTLV-I associated myelopathy. *Neurology* 1988;38:1302–1307.

100. Kramer A, Jacobson S, Reuben JF, et al. Spontaneous lymphocyte proliferation is elevated in asymptomatic HTLV-I positive Jamaicans. *Lancet* 1989;(2)8668: 923–924.

101. Wiktor SZ, Jacobson S, Reuben JS, et al. Spontaneous lymphocyte proliferation in HTLV-II infected intravenous drug users. *Lancet* 1991;337:327–328.

102. Inoue J, Seiki M, Taniguichi T, et al. Induction of interleukin 2 receptor gene expression by p40x encoded by human T cell lymphotropic virus type I. *EMBO J* 1986;5:2883–2888.

103. Gessain A, Saal F, Gout O, et al. High human T cell lymphotropic virus type I proviral DNA load with polyclonal integration in peripheral blood mononuclear cells from French West Indian patients with tropical spastic paraparesis. *Int J Cancer* 1989;43:327–333.

104. Kira J, Koyanagi Y, Yamada T, et al. Increased HTLV-I proviral DNA in HTLV-I associated myelopathy: a quantitative polymerase chain reaction study. *Ann Neurol* 1991;29:194–201.

105. Kubota R, Fujiyoshi T, Izumo S, et al. Fluctuation of HTLV-I proviral DNA in peripheral blood mononuclear cells of HTLV-I associated myelopathy. *J Neuroimmunol* 1993;42:147–154.

106. Levin MC, Fox RJ, Lehky T, et al. Polymerase chain reaction/in situ hybridization detection of HTLV-I tax proviral DNA in peripheral blood lymphocytes of patients with HTLV-I associated neurologic disease. *J Virol* 1996;70:924–933.

107. Kannagi M, Matsushita S, Shida H, Harada S. Cytotoxic T cell response and expression of the target antigen in HTLV-I infection. *Leukemia* 1994;8(suppl 1):S54–S59.

108. Jacobson S, Shida H, McFarlin DE, et al. Circulating CD8+ cytotoxic lymphocytes specific for HTLV-I in patients with HTLV-I associated neurological disease. *Nature* 1990;348:245–248.

109. Jacobson S, McFarlin D, Robinson S, et al. Demonstration of HTLV-I specific cytotoxic T lymphocytes in the

cerebrospinal fluid of patients with HTLV-I associated neurologic disease. *Ann Neurol* 1992;32:651–657.

110. Elovaara I, Koenig S, Brewah A, Jacobson S. High HTLV-I specific precursor cytotoxic T lymphocyte frequencies in patients with HTLV-I associated neurological disease. *J Exp Med* 1993;177:1567–1573.

111. Koenig S, Woods R, Brewah AH, et al. Characterization of major histocompatibility complex-(MHC) class I restricted cytotoxic T cell (CTL) responses to Tax in HTLV-I infected patients with neurological disease. *J Immunol* 1993;156:3874–3883.

112. Kannagi M, Harada S, Maruyama I, et al. Predominant recognition of human T cell leukemia virus type I (HTLV-I) pX gene products by human CD8+ cytotoxic T cells directed against HTLV-I infected cells. *Int Immunol* 1991;3:761–767.

113. Parker CE, Daenke S, Nightingale S, Bangham CR. Activated, HTLV-I specific cytotoxic T lymphocytes are found in healthy seropositives as well as patients with tropical spastic paraparesis. *Virology* 1992;188:628–636.

114. Shida H, Tochikura T, Sato T, et al. Effect of recombinant vaccinia viruses that express HTLV-I envelope gene on HTLV-I infection. *EMBO J* 1987;6:3379–3384.

115. Daenke S, Kermode AG, Hall SE, et al. High cytotoxic effector frequencies occur in healthy HTLV-I carriers and patients with tropical spastic paraparesis. *J Acquir Immune Defic Syndr Hum Retrovirol* 1995;10:243. Abstract.

116. Battisto JR, Plate J, Shearer G, eds. Cytotoxic T cells: biology and relevance to disease. *Ann NY Acad Sci* 1988; 532:1–489.

117. Askonas BA, Taylor PM, Esquivel F. Cytotoxic T cells in influenza virus infection. *Ann NY Acad Sci* 1988;532:230–237.

118. Sun D, Meyerman R, Wekerle H. Cytotoxic T cells in autoimmune disease of the central nervous system. *Ann NY Acad Sci* 1988;532:221–229.

119. Leist TP, Cobbold SP, Waldmann H, et al. Functional analysis of T lymphocytes subsets in antiviral host defense. *J Immunol* 1987;138:2278–2281.

120. Wraith DC, Smilek DE, Mitchell JD, et al. Antigen recognition in autoimmune encephalomyelitis and the potential for peptide mediated immunotherapy. *Cell* 1989;59:247–255.

121. Sakai K, Zamvil SS, Mitchell DJ, et al. Prevention of experimental encephalomyelitis with peptides that block interaction of T cells with major histocompatibility complex proteins. *Proc Natl Acad Sci USA* 1989;86:9470–9474.

122. Howell MD, Winters ST, Olee T, et al. Vaccination against experimental allergic encephalomyelitis with T cell receptor peptides. *Science* 1989;246:668–670.

123. Zinkernagel RM, Doherty PC. Restriction of in vitro cell mediated cytotoxicity in lymphocytic choriomeningitis within a syngeneic or semiallogeneic system. *Nature* 1974;248:701–702.

124. Townsend ARM, Rothbard J, Gotch FM, et al. The epitopes of influenza nucleoprotein recognized by cytotoxic T lymphocytes can be defined by short synthetic peptides. *Cell* 1986;44:959–968.

125. Townsend ARM, Bodmer H. Antigen recognition by class I restricted T lymphocytes. *Annu Rev Immunol* 1989;7:601–624.

126. Madden DR, Garboczi DN, Wiley DC. The antigenic identity of peptide-MHC complexes: a comparison of the conformations of five viral peptides presented by HLA A2. *Cell* 1993;75:693–708.

127. Utz U, Koenig S, Coligan JE, Biddison WE. Presentation of 3 different viral peptides, HTLV-I tax, HCMV gB, and influenza virus M1 is determined by common structural features of the HLA A2.1 molecule. *J Immunol* 1992; 149:214–221.

128. Parker KC, DiBrino M, Hull L, Coligan JE. The beta 2-microglobulin dissociation rate is an accurate measure of the stability of MHC class I heterotrimers and depends on which peptide is bound. *J Immunol* 1992;149:1896–1904.

129. Davis MM, Bjorkman PJ. T cell antigen receptor genes and T cell recognition. *Nature* 1988;344:395–402.

130. Chothia C, Boswell DR, Lesk AM. The outline structure of the T cell αβ receptor. *EMBO J* 1988;7:3745–3755.

131. Marrack P, Kappler J. The T cell receptor. *Science* 1987;238:1073–1079.

132. Vandenbark AA, Hashim G, Offner H. Immunization with a synthetic T cell receptor V region peptide protects against experimental allergic encephalomyelitis. *Nature* 1989;341:541–544.

133. Offner H, Hasim G, Vandenbark AA. T cell receptor therapy triggers autoregulation of experimental allergic encephalomyelitis. *Science* 1990;251:430–432.

134. Vandenbark AA, Chou YK, Bourdette DN, et al. T cell receptor peptide therapy for autoimmune disease. *J Autoimmunol* 1992;5:83–92.

135. Chou YK, Morrison WJ, Weinberg AD, et al. Immunity to TCR peptides in multiple sclerosis. II. T cell recognition of V beta 5.2 and V beta 6.1 CDR2 peptides. *J Immunol* 1994;152:2520–2529.

136. Bourdette DN, Whitham RH, Chou YK, et al. Immunity to TCR peptides in multiple sclerosis. I. Successful immunization of patients with synthetic V beta 5.2 and V beta 6.1 CDR2 peptides. *J Immunol* 1994;152:2510–2519.

137. Utz U, Banks D, Jacobson S, Biddison WE. Analysis of the T cell receptor repertoire of HTLV-I Tax-specific CD8+ CTL from patients with HTLV-I associated disease: evidence for oligoclonal expansion. *J Virol* 1995;70:843–851.

138. Rock EP, Sibbald PE, Davis MM, Chien YH. CDR3 length in antigen-specific immune receptors. *J Exp Med* 1994;179:323–328.

139. Salvetti M, Ristori G, D'Amato M, et al. Predominant and stable T cell responses to regions of myelin basic protein can be detected in individual patients with multiple sclerosis. *Eur J Immunol* 1993;23:1232–1239.

140. Wucherpfennig K, Zhang MJ, Witek C, et al. Clonal expansion and persistence of human T cells specific for an immunodominant myelin basic protein peptide. *J Immunol* 1994;152:5581–5592.

141. Masuko K, Kato T, Ikeda Y, et al. Dynamic changes of accumulated T cell clonotypes during antigenic stimulation in vivo and in vitro. *Int Immunol* 1994;6:1959–1966.

142. Boitel B, Blank U, Mege D, et al. Strong similarities in antigen fine specificity among DRB1*1302-restricted tetanus toxin tt830–843-specific TCRs in spite of highly heterogeneous CDR3. *J Immunol* 1995;154:3245–3255.

143. Lehner PJ, Wang ECY, Moss PAH, et al. Human HLA-A0201-restricted cytotoxic T lymphocyte recognition of influenza A is dominant by T cells bearing the Vβ17 gene segment. *J Exp Med* 1995;181:79–91.

144. Moss PA, Moots RJ, Rosenberg WM, et al. Extensive conservation of alpha and beta chains of the human T-cell antigen receptor recognizing HLA-A2 and influenza A matrix peptide. *Proc Natl Acad Sci USA* 1991;88:8987–8990.

145. Imarai M, Goyarts EC, van Bleek GM, Nathenson SG.

Diversity of T cell receptors specific for the VSV antigenic peptide (N52–59) bound by the H-2K^b class I molecule. *Cell Immunol* 1995;160:33–42.

146. Argaet VP, Schmidt CW, Burrows SR, et al. Dominant selection of an invariant T cell antigen receptor in response to persistent infection by Epstein-Barr virus. *J Exp Med* 1994;180:2335–2340.

147. Ben-Nun A, Liblau RS, Cohen L, et al. Restricted T-cell receptor V beta gene usage by myelin basic protein-specific T-cell clones in multiple sclerosis: predominant genes vary in individuals. *Proc Natl Acad Sci USA* 1991; 88:2466–2470.

148. Kotzin BL, Karuturi S, Chou YK, et al. Preferential T-cell receptor β-chain variable gene use in myelin basic protein-reactive T-cell clones from patients with multiple sclerosis. *Proc Natl Acad Sci USA* 1991;88:161–165.

149. Zamvil SS, Mitchell DJ, Lee NE, et al. Predominant expression of a T cell receptor V beta gene subfamily in autoimmune encephalomyelitis. *J Exp Med* 1988;167: 1586–1596. (Published erratum appears in *J Exp Med* 1988;168:455.)

150. Utz U, McFarland HF. The role of T cells in multiple sclerosis: implications for therapies targeting the T cell receptor. *J Neuropathol Exp Neurol* 1994;53:351–358.

151. Martin R, Utz U, Coligan JE, et al. Diversity in fine specificity and T cell receptor usage of the human CD4+ cytotoxic T cell response specific for the immunodominant myelin basic protein peptide 87–106. *J Immunol* 1992;148:1359–1366.

152. Oksenberg JR, Stuart S, Begovich AB, et al. Limited heterogeneity of rearranged T-cell receptor V alpha transcripts in brains of multiple sclerosis patients. *Nature* 1990;345:344–346. (Published erratum appears in *Nature* 1991;353:94.)

153. Rotteveel FT, Kokkelink I, van Walbeek HK, et al. Analysis of T cell receptor-gene rearrangement in T cells from the cerebrospinal fluid of patients with multiple sclerosis. *J Neuroimmunol* 1987;5:243–249.

154. Wucherpfennig KW, Ota K, Endo N, et al. Shared human T cell receptor V beta usage to immunodominant regions of myelin basic protein. *Science* 1994;248: 1016–1019.

155. Hara H, Mortia M, Iwaki T, et al. Detection of human T lymphotropic virus type I (HTLV-I) proviral DNA and analysis of T cells receptor Vβ CDR3 sequences in spinal cord lesions of HTLV-I associated myelopathy/tropical spastic paraparesis. *J Exp Med* 1984;180:831–839.

156. Oksenberg JR, Panzara MA, Begovich AB, et al. Selection for T-cell receptor V beta-D beta-J beta gene rearrangements with specificity for a myelin basic protein peptide in brain lesions of multiple sclerosis. *Nature* 1993;362:68–70.

157. Elovaara I, Utz U, Smith S, Jacobson S. Limited T cell receptor usage by HTLV-I specific HLA class I restricted cytotoxic T lymphocytes from patients with HTLV-I associated neurologic disease. *J Neuroimmunol* 1995; 63:47–53.

158. Levin MC, Lehky TJ, Flerlage N, et al. Immunopathogenesis of HTLV-I–associated chronic progressive neurologic disease: in vivo evidence based on a spinal cord biopsy from a patient with HTLV-I–associated myelopathy/tropical spastic paraparesis (HAM/TSP). *New Engl J Med* 1997; 336:839–845.

159. Jacobson S, Raine C, Mingioli E, McFarlin DE. Isolation of an HTLV-I-like retrovirus from patients with tropical spastic paraparesis (TSP) by activation with antibodies to the CD3 complex. *Nature* 1988;331:540–543.

160. Kuroda Y, Matsui M, Kikuchi M, et al. In situ demonstration of the HTLV-I genome in the spinal cord of a patient with HTLV-I associated myelopathy. *Neurology* 1994;44:2295–2299.

Chapter 14
Lyme Disease

John J. Halperin

The past two decades has witnessed an explosion of information about Lyme borreliosis (also known as Lyme disease), the multisystem infectious disease caused by the tick-borne spirochete *Borrelia burgdorferi*. However, despite the application of extremely powerful research techniques, and even the development of animal models, the pathophysiology of this disorder, particularly with regard to nervous system manifestations, remains obscure. In attempting to understand the underlying disease mechanisms, there has been a nearly irresistible, though not necessarily valid, temptation to compare Lyme disease to the other extensively studied neurospirochetosis, neurosyphilis. Both are caused by a slowly reproducing spirochete, capable of causing a chronic infection with relapsing symptoms. Both elicit persistent but not necessarily effective immune responses. In both, the immune reaction may play a role in end-organ damage. In both, appropriate antimicrobial therapy appears to arrest disease progression.

Likewise, in both infections the diagnosis is challenging, in large part because of the difficulty of culturing the organism from infected patients. In both, this is probably due to the rather small number of organisms present during the later stages of disease. However, unlike *Treponema pallidum*, it is technically possible to culture *B. burgdorferi* from patients, though the sensitivity of culture is quite low, with cultures being positive in only about 10% of patients with Lyme meningitis (1). Even with polymerase chain reaction (PCR) techniques, organisms can be detected in the cerebrospinal fluid (CSF) of only a subset of presumably infected individuals (2–4); even then, the number of organisms appears to be quite small. This striking dissociation between the severity of signs and symptoms, and the apparently small bacterial load has led to the suggestion that a number of immunologic processes might be responsible for disease amplification. Although this is plausible, the data at this point are far from conclusive.

History

The disorder commonly referred to in North America as Lyme disease, and first characterized by Steere et al at Yale (5), has actually been well known by other names for many years in Europe. In the United States, attention was first focused on what appeared to be an epidemic of juvenile rheumatoid arthritis in Lyme, Connecticut. Epidemiologic studies demonstrated an association between the development of arthritis and both bites of hard-shelled *Ixodes* ticks and a characteristic rash; subsequently a variety of other non-rheumatologic difficulties was also linked to this disorder (5,6). Shortly thereafter, the causative tick-borne spirochete, *B. burgdorferi*, was identified (7–9). The characteristic skin lesion, an erythematous, typically painless, slowly expanding, classically round to ovoid macular rash, often at the site of the tick bite, had been labeled *erythema chronicum migrans* (now usually referred to just as *erythema migrans*) by a Scandinavian physician, Afzelius, in 1910 (10). In 1922 the French physicians Garin and Bujadoux (11) first recognized the association of meningitis and a painful radiculoneuritis with the same tick bites. In 1941 Bannwarth (12) expanded on this observation in a series of papers that also recognized this disorder as associated with rheumatologic symptoms. Although the responsible microorganism was identified in European patients in 1984 (13), a year after its identification in American patients with Lyme disease, European physicians recognized as early as the 1950s that this disorder responded well to penicillin and other antimicrobial agents.

Detailed microbiologic studies rapidly demonstrated that the organisms responsible for European Garin-Bujadoux-Bannwarth syndrome, and North American Lyme disease, were similar, if not identical. The clinical signs and symptoms are extremely similar in both populations of patients, although there has been a persistent impression that North American patients are more likely to have prominent rheumatologic symptoms, whereas in European patients neurologic phenomena predominate. Because the European disease was first described as neurologic, and the American form as rheumatologic, ascertainment bias may well play a role in this apparent difference. However, recent work applying molecular biologic techniques in the study of *B. burgdorferi* suggests that there may be true biologic differences in the microorganisms present on the two sides of the Atlantic (14). The broad group of responsible spirochetes is now known as *B. burgdorferi sensu lato;* the North American group, as *B. burgdorferi sensu stricto;* and in Europe, at least three groups of *Borrelia* have been identified—*B. burgdorferi sensu stricto, B. afzelii,* and *B. garinii.*

Diagnosis

Microbiologic diagnosis is generally difficult, because of at least three factors. First, the organism is technically difficult to grow in culture, although with the development of specialized media, culture can now be successful for 70% or more of skin biopsy specimens of the acute lesion (15). Second, once the acute phase of the illness has passed, the bacterial load is probably quite small, particularly in the nervous system. Third, this organism has high affinity for tissue (with specific affinity demonstrated for endothelial cells, fibroblasts, and oligodendroglia, for example), and probably only briefly resides in body fluids such as the blood and CSF.

Because of the limitations of direct microbiologic methods, diagnosis has generally relied on immunologic techniques. Serologic testing, though frequently maligned, has generally provided the mainstay of diagnosis. Initially, efforts were marred by a complete lack of standardization of methodology, with different laboratories using different strains of *Borrelia,* different techniques for antigen preparation, different fractions of bacterial antigens, different technologies (immunofluorescence, standard enzyme-linked immunosorbent assay (ELISA), capture ELISA), different criteria for positivity, and different methods of reporting results. Not surprisingly, comparative studies demonstrated a striking lack of concordance of results from different laboratories on the same samples (16–18).

Superimposed on this has been a striking misuse of the data provided. Although the usual method of applying serodiagnosis in virtually all other infections has been the demonstration of an evolving antibody titer, in Lyme borreliosis the usual practice has been to use a single titer measurement. Because there is antigenic cross-reactivity among the antigens of *B. burgdorferi* and those of many other spirochetes, including those responsible for much periodontal disease, this has been particularly problematic. In addition, seropositivity clearly cannot differentiate between prior exposure and acute infection. Moreover, the concepts of positive and negative predictive values have been much neglected (19). As Lyme disease is a highly locally endemic disease, there are many areas of the world (including much of the United States) where the local prevalence is vanishingly small. Since "Lyme seropositivity" is generally defined statistically to compensate for the high background rate of cross-reactivity, 1% to 5% of all samples studied (depending on the statistical criteria used) will necessarily be considered positive, assuming values are normally distributed (which may not necessarily be valid either). If the true local prevalence is substantially below this 1% to 5%, the number of positive results due to cross-reactivity will vastly exceed the number of true positives, making the test results uninterpretable. Therefore, it is only reasonable to interpret a serologic test result as indicative of exposure to this microorganism if it comes from a patient with a reasonable a priori basis for making the diagnosis in the first place.

In the past several years, considerable effort has been devoted to improving the technical aspects of the assays, and most laboratories now have improved technical concordance significantly, although disparities still occur. As a result of a recent consensus meeting, it is now standard practice to confirm positive serologic test results with a Western blot (Table 14-1) (20,21), just as with human immunodeficiency virus (HIV) infection. Hopefully with further refinement of methodology, at least the technical differences among laboratories can be largely eliminated.

One unusual observation has led to particular insecurity in interpreting serologic results. Several centers have described small subpopulations of patients who appear to have typical Lyme disease, but never demonstrate an appropriate antibody response (22,23). Most of these patients have had demonstrable T-cell responses to *B. burgdorferi,* measurement of which is subject to even more dramatic interlaboratory variability than antibody testing. Since most of these patients have received low doses of antimicrobial therapy early in the course of *B. burgdorferi* infection, the hypothesis has been that the antibiotics decrease the antigen load very early, abrogating the development of an appropriate antibody response but leaving enough viable organisms in protected sites (joints, nervous system) to permit persistent infection. Unfortunately, this rather rare observation has tremendously amplified the uncertainty in the interpretation of serologic test results, and has led to a widespread superstition that a negative Lyme serologic test result is of absolutely no import. In fact, the preponderance of data indicate that in a patient significantly at risk for Lyme disease, the negative predictive value of such a test is extremely high.

Clinical Phenomena

Lyme disease, virtually without exception, begins with the bite of a hard-shelled *Ixodes* tick. Although one re-

Table 14-1.
Western Blot Criteria*

IgG (5/10)	IgM (2/3)
18	23
23	39
28	41
30	
39	
41	
45	
60	
66	
93	

*The data are in kilodaltons. Western blots are considered positive if 5 or more of the indicated bands are present on an IgG blot, or 2 or more of the indicated bands are present on an IgM blot (20,21).

port of possible transfusion-associated Lyme disease has been published (24), spirochetemia seems to be such an insignificant phenomenon in this disease that this would seem likely to be an extremely rare event. Similarly, although *B. burgdorferi* has been isolated from other blood-feeding insects, the unique relationship between *Ixodes* ticks and their hosts—with the tick remaining attached for several days and ingesting blood, which then triggers spirochete proliferation within the tick, and then the tick injecting spirochetes along with other salivary contents into the host 24 to 48 hours into the feeding—makes it seem very unlikely that other vectors would transmit this infection. Following inoculation, spirochetes proliferate locally and migrate centrifugally, resulting in an erythematous macular rash at the site of the bite in at least two thirds of patients. Because this rash is typically asymptomatic, and can occur in areas that are difficult to see, it frequently goes unnoticed despite the fact that it can expand to a foot or more in diameter and persist for several weeks. In a subset of patients, spirochetes disseminate rapidly and patients may develop a multifocal rash. Spirochete dissemination is typically accompanied by a febrile illness, with malaise, myalgias, headache, and so on, commonly referred to as flulike (although respiratory and gastrointestinal symptoms do not typically occur). Bacteria disseminate rapidly; there is good evidence that the central nervous system (CNS) may be seeded early in the course of infection (3,25,26), although not necessarily frequently (27) or with prominent symptomatology. Whether this early seeding necessarily leads to development of persistent CNS infection has not been established. Once the acute dissemination of bacteria ends, the illness can become quiescent. Subsequently, more focal signs of disseminated infection may become apparent. Some patients develop otherwise unexplained heart block—something that is generally transient, although a temporary pacemaker may be necessary. Joint involvement may be prominent; this typically involves large joints (elbows, hips, knees), affecting one joint at a time for a period of days to weeks, then subsiding, only to recur later affecting a different joint (i.e., a relapsing large-joint oligoarthritis). Signs of true arthritis (swelling, erythema) are typically apparent.

Nervous system involvement can be particularly prominent. Although a tremendous range of pheno-

Table 14-2.
Peripheral Nerve Disorders in Lyme Disease

Disorder	Cause
Cranial neuropathy	Mononeuropathy multiplex
Radiculopathy	(the mechanism for all
Diffuse peripheral neuropathy	peripheral nerve dis-
Mononeuropathy multiplex	orders in Lyme disease)
Brachial plexopathy	
Lumbosacral plexopathy	
Motor neuronopathy	
"Guillain-Barré like"	

Table 14-3.
CNS Disorders in Lyme Disease

Disorder	Cause
Meningitis	Infection
Encephalomyelitis	?Infection
	?Immune
Encephalopathy	?Encephalomyelitis
	?Neuroimmunomodulators

mena has been attributed to this infection, most can be included within one of the following four groups (Tables 14-2, 14-3): 1) lymphocytic meningitis; 2) peripheral neuropathy, usually a form of mononeuropathy multiplex; 3) encephalomyelitis, a focal inflammation within the CNS of unclear pathophysiology; and 4) encephalopathy, a reversible change in mental status that in some instances may be due to CNS infection and in others may be a remote effect of systemic infection.

Meningitis

Meningitis typically occurs as a monophasic illness early in infection and is almost certainly attributable to bacterial infection within the subarachnoid space. *B. burgdorferi* can be cultured from CSF in about 10% of patients. The low sensitivity of culture is probably in part due to the technical difficulties inherent in culturing this spirochete, but is also probably related to a rather low bacterial load, as suggested by semiquantitative PCR studies. This illness clinically resembles most other "aseptic" meningitides, with a lymphocytic pleocytosis, modest elevation of protein in the CSF, usually normal glucose level in the CSF, and clinical findings of headache, photophobia, and mild meningismus, typically without clinical evidence of altered CNS function.

Peripheral Neuropathy

A tremendous range of peripheral nervous system (PNS) disorders has been described. Garin and Bujadoux described what has come to be recognized as a characteristic disorder involving prominent radicular signs and symptoms (often in the dermatome involved by the tick bite), typically accompanied by a CSF pleocytosis. The classic triad described in North America (6,28) emphasized cranial neuropathies, particularly unilateral or bilateral seventh cranial nerve palsies, in addition to the meningitis and radiculoneuritis described in Europe. Other studies described other cranial neuropathies, plexopathies, typical mononeuropathy multiplex, a Guillain-Barré–like syndrome (i.e., an acute to subacute symmetric severe disseminated polyneuropathy; interestingly most such patients have not shown compelling evidence of demyelination, and most have had a CSF pleocytosis), as well as more indolent and diffuse polyneuropathies. Detailed neurophysiologic and pathologic studies (29–31) suggested that all these forms are attributable to a mononeuropathy multiplex, varying merely in severity and distribution (32,33).

Encephalomyelitis

Rare patients (probably approximately 0.1% of untreated infected individuals) develop focal inflammation in the CNS (34,35). Myelopathic presentations are particularly common but brainstem, cerebellar, and cerebral involvement also occurs. Foci of inflammation are generally demonstrable on magnetic resonance images (MRIs). CSF analysis typically reveals evidence of chronic inflammation with a mild CSF lymphocytic pleocytosis or elevated protein levels. In most patients there is evidence of intrathecal production of immunoglobulins; an elevated IgG index is seen frequently and oligoclonal bands have been demonstrated in many patients, particularly in European studies. Intrathecal production of anti–B. burgdorferi antibodies has been demonstrated with variable frequency. In European series, it is reported to occur in essentially all described cases (36–38) (although most European authorities consider demonstration of intrathecal production of specific antibody an essential requirement to make this diagnosis, rendering this argument somewhat circular). In North American series, intrathecal antibody production is reported to occur in more than 90% of patients with acute disease (39), but in a variable proportion of those with chronic disorders (39,40).

Encephalopathy

A significant number of patients with clear evidence of nonneurologic Lyme disease manifest objectively demonstrable cognitive difficulties (41,42). Findings on brain MRIs and CSF analysis are variable, but often normal (43); the etiology of this disorder remains controversial. Notably significant numbers of these patients have completely normal CSF, including no evidence of intrathecal production of specific antibody, but have clear evidence of rheumatologic or other extraneurologic involvement. In these patients the encephalopathy clears in parallel with the other (nonneurologic) evidence of disease.

Pathophysiology

Since all forms of neurologic impairment typically improve following antimicrobial therapy (except for residua attributable to remaining structural damage), ongoing infection with B. burgdorferi must be responsible for each. However, microbiologic evidence of nervous system infection is scanty in all forms but meningitis, and even in patients with meningitis, the bacterial load is clearly low. The dissociation between apparent bacterial load and disease severity has led to a great deal of conjecture regarding the mechanisms by which disease amplification can occur. Similarly, the wide variability in clinical manifestations among different infected individuals has led to speculation that host factors must also play a role in the illness's pathophysiology. The most obvious focal point for all this conjecture has been the host's immune response.

Numerous studies have demonstrated significant immune activation in this disease. Both serum and CSF antibody responses are persistent, if somewhat unusual. In addition to the normally anticipated early IgM response with a subsequent IgG response, IgM production often persists in both CSF and serum compartments long after the IgG response matures (36,44,45). Patients develop antibody responses to different epitopes in sequential fashion, with responses to the 41-kd (flagellar) and 39-kd antigens occurring early, and responses to outer surface proteins C (23 kd), A (31 kd), and B (34 kd) evolving over time (20), suggesting perhaps that the spirochete only slowly exposes its different antigens to the host. In patients with CNS infection, specific anti–B. burgdorferi antibody is produced locally within the neuraxis, with clonal proliferation of targeted B cells demonstrable in the CSF (46). Oligoclonal bands are not uncommon, particularly in patients with inflammatory disease of some duration, and there is often sufficient overall immune stimulation such that more global markers of intrathecal immunoglobulin production, such as the IgG index, are elevated. A more recent study suggested similar clonal proliferation of specific T cells in this disease as well (47). Apparent intrathecal production of specific antibody often persists long after the causative bacteria have been eradicated, with some studies indicating persistent intrathecal antibody production as long as a decade or more after presumed clinical cure with antimicrobial therapy (48).

While animal models would be helpful in furthering our understanding of the pathogenesis of this disorder, unfortunately it has been very difficult to create valid models with nervous system involvement. Rodent models of rheumatologic involvement have been developed, but other than an occasional very transient meningitis, these animals do not develop significant neurologic involvement. Recent work in primates succeeded in developing models of meningitis and peripheral neuropathy; to date none of the animals has been reported to develop parenchymal CNS involvement (49,50). Therefore, even in primates, the applicability of data derived from animal models cannot be assumed.

Immunopathogenesis

Several mechanisms have been proposed to explain potential immune amplification of disease. These hypotheses can be grouped into the following five categories:

1. *B. burgdorferi* adheres to cells within the peripheral or central nervous system, precipitating a local immune response targeting the bacteria but incidentally damaging the nervous system.
2. *B. burgdorferi* or its constituent proteins are bound by antibodies, with a resultant immune complex disease.
3. *B. burgdorferi* shares epitopes with nervous system antigens, and the immune response designed to

fend off the bacterial infection results in an autoimmune-type disease.

4. *B. burgdorferi* infection causes a vasculitis within the nervous system with secondary damage to the nervous system.

5. *B. burgdorferi* infection stimulates high levels of lymphokine production, which in turn has significant modulatory effects on the nervous system.

Each of these models has potential strengths and weaknesses. There is now considerable evidence that *B. burgdorferi* penetrates the CNS early in infection, although this appears to be a relatively infrequent occurrence (27). The spirochete can adhere to oligodendroglia, with specific binding to galactocerebroside (51,52). Activation of an immune response in these circumstances could easily lead either to "innocent bystander" damage to adjacent brain or nerve tissue, or alternatively to an adjuvant-like effect stimulating an immune response against nearby glial epitopes, particularly if these were not normally exposed, but became exposed as part of the glial-bacterial interaction.

Either of these hypotheses could explain a persistent immune-mediated attack on CNS white matter, which would be consistent with the clinical observations. In the rare patients who do develop parenchymal CNS disease, MRI abnormalities are primarily, but not exclusively, seen in the white matter. Clinical manifestations tend to be "white matter" abnormalities, that is, spasticity, ataxia, and sensory symptoms (with some patients misdiagnosed as having multiple sclerosis), whereas seizures and major cognitive abnormalities (more typically considered signs of "gray matter" involvement) are comparatively uncommon. Either of these hypotheses could also explain the observation of anti–myelin basic protein antibodies in the CSF of some patients (53,54), as well as the more recent demonstration of antiganglioside antibodies (55).

While it has been exceptionally difficult to demonstrate spirochetes in biopsy specimens of affected nerve or brain, arguing against an innocent bystander mechanism, the arguments against the adjuvant immunization hypothesis (with an ensuing autoimmune-type process) seem even more compelling. First, it is notable that neither a peripheral neuropathy nor an encephalomyelitis develop in the very animal models in which these cross-reactivities have been demonstrated. Second, it has been well documented that anti-*Borrelia* antibody production persists within the CNS for years or even decades following successful treatment of the underlying infection, yet the observed encephalomyelitis appears to cease with successful antimicrobial response, as demonstrable both clinically and by PCR analysis of CSF. This dissociation between the persistence of the immune response and the elimination of the causative organism, with resolution of disease in parallel with elimination of the organism, argues strongly for an essential role for persistent spirochetes in persistent disease. In contrast, there is now good evidence that Lyme arthritis can be caused by just such an innocent bystander mechanism. When inbred hamsters

were given *B. burgdorferi*–specific T lymphocytes, obtained from animals immunized with a whole-cell *B. burgdorferi* vaccine, and then infected with *B. burgdorferi*, a severe destructive arthritis developed. Thus in this model, the combination of active infection and a primed immune response appears essential to cause one of the most dramatic clinical phenomena seen in Lyme disease (47).

Although PNS disease has been, in many ways, more accessible to analysis, here too it has been difficult to prove a pathogenesis. Initially thought to be an extremely confusing mixture of many types of pathologic processes, it is likely that most peripheral nerve manifestations are in fact manifestations of a mononeuropathy multiplex (32,33). Interestingly, laboratory studies demonstrated several potential interactions between *B. burgdorferi* and peripheral nerve. On the one hand, Garcia Monco et al (51) demonstrated that *B. burgdorferi* binds specifically to peripheral nerve Schwann cells. On the other, Sigal and Tatum (56) demonstrated that IgM antibodies from patients with nervous system Lyme disease bind to human peripheral nerve axons. Additional work demonstrated that a monoclonal antibody directed at a domain of the 41-kd flagellar protein interacts specifically with human axonal proteins and the neuritic processes of neuroblastoma cells (57). The significance of both sets of observations must be viewed in the context of the clinical phenomena observed. Since Lyme disease is only rarely associated with peripheral nerve demyelination, the implications of the interaction between *B. burgdorferi* and Schwann cells are not at all clear. Although the interaction with axons is more pertinent in view of the typical neurophysiologic observations indicative of axonal damage, it is at best curious that anti–41-kd activity is one of the earliest, most commonly observed and most persistent specific immunoreactivities seen in patients with Lyme disease, yet by no means every patient with this immunoreactivity develops peripheral neuropathy. Similarly, this observation leaves unanswered the question of why disease abates with the elimination of the responsible organisms. If in fact infection triggers the production of antiaxonal antibodies, which in turn damage axons, disease should progress as long as antibody production persists. Finally, most patients with Lyme disease–related neuropathies in fact have a mononeuropathy multiplex, a class of neuropathies usually occurring on a vasculopathic basis. Thus neither interactions with Schwann cells nor those with axons would specifically explain the observed process.

Several other lines of evidence suggest that a vasculitis may underlie the nervous system damage seen in this disease. Several cerebral arteriographic studies demonstrated large-artery vasculitis in patients with positive results on Lyme serologic studies (58–60). Curiously, none of these patients had demonstrable intrathecal antibody production. Although it might be argued that these large arteries could be involved by infection limited to the intra-arterial side of the blood-brain barrier, this would then beg the question of how this process relates to true CNS involvement, in which intrathecal antibody production is usually present, which in turn is considered compelling evidence of intra-CNS infection. On the other hand, false-positive serologic results are particularly common in patients with significant immune stimulation (e.g., subacute bacterial endocarditis (61) or vasculitis), rendering the significance of these observations unclear.

In contrast, in the PNS, neurophysiologic studies generally indicate a mononeuropathy multiplex, and biopsy specimens of peripheral nerve typically contain perivascular inflammatory infiltrates (29–31). Yet none of these studies has ever demonstrated a true vasculitis, with vessel wall necrosis. Consequently, the observed pathologic changes may be more a reflection of a reactive immune response with migration of lymphocytes out of vessels (perhaps attacking spirochetes adherent to endothelial or glial cells) rather than a true vasculitis.

Other studies suggest an immune-complex basis for this disease. One laboratory repeatedly demonstrated immune complexes in the CSF of patients with presumed CNS Lyme disease (62–64). Interestingly, immune complexes were initially thought to be responsible for rheumatologic disorders in Lyme disease, a hypothesis that fell out of favor when it became increasingly difficult to demonstrate immune complexes in the serum or tissue of affected patients. In patients with neurologic disease, either peripheral or central, no laboratory has been able to demonstrate deposition of antibodies or antigens in biopsy specimens of involved tissue. Patients do not have other manifestations of immune-complex disease; in particular, significant renal involvement is extremely uncommon. Finally, it is surprising that immune complexes and free antigens are detectable in such a high proportion of patients, when PCR techniques have been so much less sensitive. Since PCR can detect DNA from as few as one to five organisms, while ELISA techniques can only detect antigens with several orders of magnitude less sensitivity, it is paradoxical that free antigens and immune complexes should be demonstrable with such frequency.

Finally, it has been proposed that some nervous system processes, particularly some of the cognitive difficulties, occur on the basis of production of lymphokines or other potential neuroimmunomodulators (65). That some lymphokines, as well as other molecules such as the kynurenines, 1) are produced in response to infection, 2) can cross the blood-brain barrier, and 3) can modulate neuronal function provides an appealing hypothetical mechanism to explain altered neurologic function in patients who do not have other evidence (intrathecal antibody production, microbiologic evidence of infection by PCR or culture) of CNS infection.

Several studies indicate that *B. burgdorferi* infection induces production of interleukin (IL)-1 (66,67). As with other CNS infections, elevated levels of IL-6 have been demonstrated in the CSF of patients with active Lyme meningitis (67,68). Perhaps of greatest interest has been evidence indicating elevations in tumor necrosis factor (TNF)-α concentrations. It has been suggested that TNF-α may play a role in arthritis (69). Evidence

of a role for this molecule in neurologic disease is more indirect. In a series of studies, Heyes et al (70–72) demonstrated elevated concentrations of quinolinic acid in the serum and CSF of patients with infections. This *N*-methyl-D-aspartate (NMDA) agonist is produced normally both within and outside the CNS, with its production regulated by both interferon-γ and TNF-α. In patients with Lyme disease, the most significant elevations of quinolinic acid concentration in the CSF were noted in patients with active CNS infection. However, in patients with systemic infection but with no evidence of direct CNS involvement, both CSF and serum concentrations were elevated, with the CSF concentration rising in parallel to that in serum, suggesting diffusion either of the molecule itself or of its regulating cytokines across the blood-brain barrier. Because many of these molecules, in addition to quinolinic acid itself, have direct neuromodulatory activity, such a phenomenon could potentially explain altered CNS function (e.g., encephalopathy) in patients with systemic evidence of Lyme disease, but without anything to suggest direct CNS infection.

Finally, the question remains as to why there is such variability in host response to this infection. Although recent evidence suggests that this is in part attributable to species differences among different strains of *B. burgdorferi*, this cannot explain all the differences. Presumably some of the variability must relate to differences in the host response to infection, something that could be influenced by previous immunologic experience, coinfections, or immunologic predisposition as reflected in HLA haplotype. Results from several studies indicate that persistent Lyme arthritis, with recurrent attacks despite antimicrobial therapy, relates to HLA haplotype, with patients with HLA-DR4 being particularly at risk (73). Studies in patients with persistent CNS inflammation are far less compelling, with associations suggested with DQw1 (39,74).

Treatment

While it is true that occasional treatment failures occur, currently recommended regimens (Table 14-4) are successful in eradicating infection in the vast majority of patients, even those with late disseminated disease.

Table 14-4.
Treatment Recommendations

Drug	Dose	Duration
Early disease		
Doxycycline	100 mg 2–3 times/day	14–28 days
Amoxicillin	500 mg 4 times/day	14–28 days
Late disease		
Ceftriaxone	2 g/day	14–28 days
Cefotaxime	2 g 3 times/day	14–28 days
Penicillin	20–24 million U/day	14–28 days

Note: Tetracyclines such as doxycycline should not be used in pregnant women or in children up to age 8. Ceftriaxone should probably not be used during the third trimester of pregnancy.

If arthritis has resulted in joint destruction, or encephalomyelitis has resulted in areas of gliosis in the brain or spinal cord, obviously recovery may be incomplete. However, barring such phenomena, this is an antibiotic-responsive disease. In vitro the organism is quite sensitive to a variety of antimicrobial agents (tetracyclines, cephalosporins, erythromycin and its new congeners). In vivo, treatment with tetracyclines or cephalosporins is successful in most patients.

Following initial inoculation of the spirochete, organisms disseminate rapidly. The nervous system in particular is subject to early invasion (25). It is presumed that the need for antibiotics to penetrate the blood-brain barrier explains the apparent superiority of some agents over others. In early disease (rash, acute febrile illness), both amoxicillin and doxycycline are effective in more than 90% of patients (75). Although numerous other oral agents have been tried, none has improved on this success rate, and all are considerably more expensive.

In patients with severe CNS disease, or those who do not respond to oral regimens, parenteral treatment with high-dose penicillin or a third-generation cephalosporin is necessary. Ceftriaxone appears to be superior to penicillin (76). Presumably this is related to several factors. First, in vitro the organism is more sensitive to ceftriaxone than to penicillin. Second, in the absence of significant blood-brain barrier disruption, ceftriaxone enters the CNS far more readily than does penicillin. Finally, ceftriaxone's long elimination half-life results in prolonged exposure of the organism to sustained, high levels of antibiotic, an important consideration for slowly reproducing organisms such as spirochetes. Results of other studies indicate that cefotaxime is as effective as ceftriaxone, even though it has a shorter half-life (77), and the results of at least one study indicate that oral doxycycline may be as effective as high-dose penicillin, at least in Lyme meningitis (78).

The optimum duration of treatment remains controversial. Early studies indicated that even for late disease, treatment for 14 days was as effective as a more prolonged course (76). Since symptoms typically do not resolve completely immediately with treatment, there has been a tendency to extend therapy. More importantly, some patients develop late neurologic sequelae after receiving parental antimicrobial agents for 14 days. As a result, most centers now use 21- to 28-day courses of therapy, although there are few systematic data to support this. In rare instances of severe parenchymal CNS damage, patients have been treated for as long as 6 weeks. However, courses longer than this are generally considered to be without scientific basis.

Vaccination

In comparison to many other infectious diseases, Lyme disease is a relatively easily treated and uncommon disorder (approximately 13,000 cases reported in the United States in 1994 (79)). However in endemic areas it is quite frequent (seroprevalence rates as high as 10% or more in some areas (80,81)), and is the cause of tremendous anxiety in the at-risk population. Because of this, there has been great interest in the development of a vaccine. This poses a problem of considerable theoretical interest. Three issues in particular must be considered. First is the historic precedent: Development of effective vaccines for other major spirochetoses, particularly syphilis, has been extraordinarily difficult. Second is the observation that in Lyme disease, natural infection is not necessarily protective against reinfection. Finally, until it is clear what the role of the host immune response is in the pathogenesis of the more complex manifestations of this disease (e.g., arthritis, encephalomyelitis, neuropathy), there is the inherent risk that immunization could in fact induce some of the most significant morbidity that it is intended to prevent. In at least one animal model of Lyme disease, severe arthritis is readily created by first immunizing animals with a whole-cell vaccine, then transferring their reactive T cells to other animals, and then infecting these passively immunized animals (47).

Results of studies to date have been mixed. Vaccination has generally been attempted with selected antigens, most commonly either 41-kd flagellin or outer surface protein A, B, or C (Osp A, B, or C). Although somewhat variable in their sequences, the outer surface proteins are relatively *B. burgdorferi* specific. Flagellar antigens tend to be far more cross-reactive with flagellae of other bacterial species (82). In rodent models these selective vaccines have been safe, and have protected against the immunizing strain, and in some studies against multiple strains (83). However, recent work demonstrated a great deal of antigenic variability among wild strains, as well as rapid antigenic evolution in hosts after infection (much like in the relapsing fevers) such that as soon as the host develops an effective response to one set of epitopes, a substrain of *Borrelia* emerges with different immunodominant markers (84). Finally, although no significant neurologic abnormalities have developed in immunized rodents, it must be remembered that these species do not develop significant neurologic disease in natural infection. Preliminary reports of immunization in primate hosts and in humans appear to indicate that serious neurologic complications do not occur (85), but to date the numbers are small and in natural infection these are relatively rare occurrences. A great deal more data will be necessary before it becomes clear that a vaccine is both safe and effective.

Conclusions

In the past two decades a great deal has been learned about infection with *B. burgdorferi*. The manifestations occurring in any given individual are heavily influenced both by the infecting strain and by the host immune response. Meningitis, probably the most common CNS manifestation, appears to be the result of simple invasion of the CNS by bacteria. All other manifestations—encephalomyelitis, peripheral neuropathy, and encephalopathy—appear to involve a much more complex interplay of the bacteria, its adherence to host cells, and the host immune response. A better understanding of these interactions should facilitate the development of better therapeutic strategies for patients with this disease. It is hoped that the lessons learned will provide more general insights into bacteria-host interactions, improving our understanding of other complex infectious diseases as well.

References

1. Karlsson M, Hovind HK, Svenungsson B, Stiernstedt G. Cultivation and characterization of spirochetes from cerebrospinal fluid of patients with Lyme borreliosis. *J Clin Microbiol* 1990;28:473–479.
2. Rosa PA, Schwan TG. A specific and sensitive assay for the Lyme disease spirochete *Borrelia burgdorferi* using the polymerase chain reaction. *J Infect Dis* 1989;160:1018–1029.
3. Keller TL, Halperin JJ, Whitman M. PCR detection of *Borrelia burgdorferi* DNA in cerebrospinal fluid of Lyme neuroborreliosis patients. *Neurology* 1992;42:32–42.
4. Luft BJ, Steinman CR, Neimark HC, et al. Invasion of the central nervous system by *Borrelia burgdorferi* in acute disseminated infection. *JAMA* 1992;267:1364–1367. (Published erratum appears in *JAMA* 1992;268:872.)
5. Steere AC, Malawista SE, Hardin JA, et al. Erythema chronicum migrans and Lyme arthritis. The enlarging clinical spectrum. *Ann Intern Med* 1977;86:685–698.
6. Reik L, Steere AC, Bartenhagen NH, et al. Neurologic abnormalities of Lyme disease. *Medicine* 1979;58:281–294.
7. Burgdorfer W, Barbour AG, Hayes SF, et al. Lyme disease: a tick borne spirochetosis? *Science* 1982;216:1317–1319.
8. Benach JL, Bosler EM, Hanrahan JP, et al. Spirochetes isolated from the blood of two patients with Lyme disease. *N Engl J Med* 1983;308:740–742.
9. Steere AC, Grodzicki RL, Kornblatt AN, et al. The spirochetal etiology of Lyme disease. *N Engl J Med* 1983;308:733–740.
10. Afzelius A. Verhandlugen der dermatorischen Gesellshaft zu Stockholm. *Arch Derm Syphiligr* 1910;101:404.
11. Garin, Bujadoux. Paralysie par les tiques. *J Med Lyon* 1922;71:765–767.
12. Bannwarth A. Chronische lymphocytare meningitis, entzundliche polyneuritis und "rheumatismus." *Arch Psychiatr Nervenkr* 1941;113:284–376.
13. Asbrink E, Hederstedt B, Hovmark A. The spirochetal etiology of acrodermatitis chronica atrophicans Herxheimer. *Acta Derm Venereol* 1984;64:506–512.
14. Baranton G, Postic D, Saint GI, et al. Delineation of *Borrelia burgdorferi sensu stricto, Borrelia garinii* sp. *nov.*, and group VS461 associated with Lyme borreliosis. *Int J Syst Bacteriol* 1992;42:378–383.
15. Berger BW, Johnson RC, Kodner C, Coleman L. Cultivation of *Borrelia burgdorferi* from erythema migrans lesions and perilesional skin. *J Clin Microbiol* 1992;30:359–361.
16. Schwartz BS, Goldstein MD, Ribeiro JM, et al. Antibody testing in Lyme disease. A comparison of results in four laboratories [see comments]. *JAMA* 1989;262:3431–3434.
17. Greene RT, Hirsch DA, Rottman PL, Gerig TM. Interlaboratory comparison of titers of antibody to *Borrelia burgdorferi* and evaluation of a commercial assay using canine sera. *J Clin Microbiol* 1991;29:16–20.
18. Schmitz JL, Powell CS, Folds JD. Comparison of seven commercial kits for detection of antibodies to *Borrelia*

19. *burgdorferi*. *Eur J Clin Microbiol Infect Dis* 1993;12:419–424.
19. Golightly MG. Laboratory considerations in the diagnosis and management of Lyme borreliosis. *Am J Clin Pathol* 1993;99:168–174.
20. Dressler F, Whalen JA, Reinhardt BN, Steere AC. Western blotting in the serodiagnosis of Lyme disease. *J Infect Dis* 1993;167:392–400.
21. Recommendations for Test Performance and Interpretation from the Second National Conference on Serologic Diagnosis of Lyme Disease. *MMWR* 1995;44:590–591.
22. Dattwyler RJ, Volkman DJ, Luft BJ, et al. Seronegative Lyme disease. Dissociation of specific T- and B-lymphocyte responses to *Borrelia burgdorferi*. *N Engl J Med* 1988;319:1441–1446.
23. Steere AC. Seronegative Lyme disease. *JAMA* 1993;270.
24. Aoki SK, Holland PV. Lyme disease—another transfusion risk? *Transfusion* 1989;29:646–655.
25. Garcia Monco JC, Villar BF, Alen JC, Benach JL. *Borrelia burgdorferi* in the central nervous system: experimental and clinical evidence for early invasion. *J Infect Dis* 1990;161:1187–1193.
26. Logigian EL, Steere AC. Invasion of the central nervous system by *Borrelia burgdorferi* in acute disseminated infection. *JAMA* 1992;267:1364–1367.
27. Kuiper H, de Jongh BM, van Dam AP, et al. Evaluation of central nervous system involvement in Lyme borreliosis patients with a solitary erythema migrans lesion. *Eur J Clin Microbiol Infect Dis* 1994;13:379–387.
28. Steere AC, Pachner AR, Malawista SE. Neurologic abnormalities of Lyme disease: successful treatment with high-dose intravenous penicillin. *Ann Intern Med* 1983;99:767–772.
29. Vallat JM, Hugon J, Lubeau M, et al. Tick bite meningoradiculoneuritis. *Neurology* 1987;37:749–753.
30. Camponovo F, Meier C. Neuropathy of vasculitic origin in a case of Garin-Bujadoux-Bannwarth syndrome with positive *Borrelia* antibody response. *J Neurol* 1986;233:69–72.
31. Halperin JJ, Little BW, Coyle PK, Dattwyler RJ. Lyme disease—a treatable cause of peripheral neuropathy. *Neurology* 1987;37:1700–1706.
32. Halperin JJ, Luft BJ, Volkman DJ, Dattwyler RJ. Lyme neuroborreliosis—peripheral nervous system manifestations. *Brain* 1990;113:1207–1221.
33. Logigian EL, Steere AC. Clinical and electrophysiologic findings in chronic neuropathy of Lyme disease. *Neurology* 1992;42:303–311.
34. Ackermann R, Gollmer E, Rehse KB. [Progressive *Borrelia* encephalomyelitis. Chronic manifestation of erythema chronicum migrans disease of the nervous system]. *Dtsch Med Wochenschr* 1985;110:1039–1042.
35. Halperin JJ, Luft BJ, Anand AK, et al. Lyme neuroborreliosis: central nervous system manifestations. *Neurology* 1989;39:753–759.
36. Stiernstedt GT, Granstrom M, Hederstedt B, Skoldenberg B. Diagnosis of spirochetal meningitis by enzyme linked immunosorbent assay and indirect immunofluorescence assay in serum and cerebrospinal fluid. *J Clin Microbiol* 1985;21:819–825.
37. Wilske B, Schierz G, Preac-Mursic V, et al. Intrathecal production of specific antibodies against *Borrelia burgdorferi* in patients with lymphocytic meningoradiculitis. *J Infect Dis* 1986;153:304–314.
38. Hansen K, Lebech AM. Lyme neuroborreliosis: a new sensitive diagnostic assay for intrathecal synthesis of *Borrelia burgdorferi*-specific immunoglobulin G, A, and M. *Ann Neurol* 1991;30:197–205.

39. Halperin JJ, Volkman DJ, Wu P. Central nervous system abnormalities in Lyme neuroborreliosis. *Neurology* 1991;41:1571–1582.
40. Steere AC, Berardi VP, Weeks KE, et al. Evaluation of the intrathecal antibody response to *Borrelia burgdorferi* as a diagnostic test for Lyme neuroborreliosis. *J Infect Dis* 1990;161:1203–1209.
41. Halperin JJ, Pass HL, Anand AK, et al. Nervous system abnormalities in Lyme disease. *Ann NY Acad Sci* 1988;539:24–34.
42. Logigian EL, Kaplan RF, Steere AC. Chronic neurologic manifestations of Lyme disease. *N Engl J Med* 1990;323:1438–1444.
43. Halperin JJ, Krupp LB, Golightly MG, Volkman DJ. Lyme borreliosis-associated encephalopathy. *Neurology* 1990;40:1340–1343.
44. Henriksson A, Link H. Prolonged IgM response within the central nervous system in lymphocytic meningoradiculitis (Bannwarth's syndrome). *N Engl J Med* 1985;313:1231. Letter.
45. Henriksson A, Link H, Cruz M, Stiernstedt G. Immunoglobulin abnormalities in cerebrospinal fluid and blood over the course of lymphocytic meningoradiculitis (Bannwarth's syndrome). *Ann Neurol* 1986;20:337–345.
46. Link H, Baig S, Olsson T, Zachau A. Antibody-producing cells in CSF and peripheral blood. *Ann NY Acad Sci* 1988;540:277–281.
47. Lim LC, England DM, DuChateau BK, et al. *Borrelia burgdorferi* specific T-lymphocytes induce severe destructive Lyme arthritis. *Infect Immun* 1995;63:1400–1408.
48. Hammers-Berggren S, Hansen K, Lebech AM, Karlsson M. *Borrelia burgdorferi*-specific intrathecal antibody production in neuroborreliosis: a follow-up study. *Neurology* 1993;43:169–175.
49. Philipp MT, Aydintug MK, Bohm RJ, et al. Early and early disseminated phases of Lyme disease in the rhesus monkey: a model for infection in humans. *Infect Immun* 1993;61:3047–3059.
50. Pachner AR, Delaney E, O'Neill T, Major E. Inoculation of nonhuman primates with the N40 strain of *Borrelia burgdorferi* leads to a model of neuroborreliosis faithful to the human disease. *Neurology* 1995;45:165–172.
51. Garcia Monco JC, Fernandez VB, Rogers RC, et al. *Borrelia burgdorferi* and other related spirochetes bind to galactocerebroside. *Neurology* 1992;42:1341–1348.
52. Garcia Monco JC, Fernandez-Villar B, Benach JL. Adherence of the Lyme disease spirochete to glial cells and cells of glial origin. *J Infect Dis* 1989;160:497–506.
53. Garcia Monco JC, Coleman JL, Benach JL. Antibodies to myelin basic protein in Lyme disease. *J Infect Dis* 1988;158:667–668. Letter.
54. Baig S, Olsson T, Hojeberg B, Link H. Cells secreting antibodies to myelin basic protein in cerebrospinal fluid of patients with Lyme neuroborreliosis. *Neurology* 1991;41:581–586.
55. Garcia Monco JC, Wheeler CM, Benach JL, et al. Reactivity of neuroborreliosis patients (Lyme disease) to cardiolipin and gangliosides. *J Neurol Sci* 1993;117:206–214.
56. Sigal LH, Tatum AH. Lyme disease patients' serum contains IgM antibodies to *Borrelia burgdorferi* that cross-react with neuronal antigens. *Neurology* 1988;38:1439–1442.
57. Sigal LH. Cross-reactivity between *Borrelia burgdorferi* flagellin and a human axonal 64,000 molecular weight protein. *J Infect Dis* 1993;167:1372–1378.
58. May EF, Jabbari B. Stroke in neuroborreliosis. *Stroke* 1990;21:1232–1235.
59. Uldry PA, Regli F, Bogousslavsky J. Cerebral angiopathy and recurrent strokes following *Borrelia burgdorferi* infection. *J Neurol Neurosurg Psychiatry* 1987;50:1703–1704.
60. Veenedaal-Hilbers JA, Perquin WVM, Hoogland PH, Doornbos L. Basal meningovasculitis and occlusion of the basilar artery in two cases of *Borrelia burgdorferi* infection. *Neurology* 1988;38:1317–1319.
61. Kaell AT, Volkman DJ, Gorevic PD, Dattwyler RJ. Positive Lyme serology in subacute bacterial endocarditis. A study of four patients. *JAMA* 1990;264:2916–2918.
62. Coyle PK, Schutzer SE, Belman AL, et al. Cerebrospinal fluid immune complexes in patients exposed to *Borrelia burgdorferi*: detection of *Borrelia*-specific and -nonspecific complexes. *Ann Neurol* 1990;28:739–744.
63. Coyle PK, Deng Z, Schutzer SE, et al. Detection of *Borrelia burgdorferi* antigens in cerebrospinal fluid. *Neurology* 1993;43:1093–1097.
64. Schutzer SE, Coyle PK, Belman AL, et al. Sequestration of antibody to *Borrelia burgdorferi* in immune complexes in seronegative Lyme disease. *Lancet* 1990;335:312–315.
65. Halperin JJ, Heyes MP. Neuroactive kynurenines in Lyme borreliosis. *Neurology* 1992;42:43–50.
66. Habicht GS, Beck G, Benach JL. The role of interleukin-1 in the pathogenesis of Lyme disease. *Ann NY Acad Sci* 1988;539:80–86.
67. Habicht GS, Katona LI, Benach JL. Cytokines and the pathogenesis of neuroborreliosis: *Borrelia burgdorferi* induces glioma cells to secrete interleukin-6. *J Infect Dis* 1991;164:568–574.
68. Weller M, Stevens A, Sommer N, et al. Cerebrospinal fluid interleukins, immunoglobulins, and fibronectin in neuroborreliosis. *Arch Neurol* 1991;48:837–841.
69. Pfister HW, Wilske B, Weber K. Lyme borreliosis: basic science and clinical aspects. *Lancet* 1994;343:1013–1016.
70. Heyes MP, Rubinow D, Lane C, Markey SP. Cerebrospinal fluid quinolinic acid concentrations are increased in acquired immune deficiency syndrome. *Ann Neurol* 1989;26:275–277.
71. Heyes MP, Brew BJ, Price RW, Markey SP. Cerebrospinal fluid quinolinic acid and kynurenic acid in HIV-1 infection. In: Guidotti A, ed. *Neurotoxicity of excitatory amino acids*. New York: Raven, 1990:217–221.
72. Heyes MP, Lackner A. Increased cerebrospinal fluid quinolinic acid, kynurenic acid, and L-kynurenine in acute septicemia. *J Neurochem* 1990;55:338–341.
73. Steere AC, Dwyer E, Winchester R. Association of chronic lyme arthritis with HLA-DR4 and HLA-DR2 alleles. *N Engl J Med* 1990;323:219–223.
74. Wokke JH, van DPA, Brand A, et al. Association of HLA-DR2 antigen with serum IgG antibodies against *Borrelia burgdorferi* in Bannwarth's syndrome. *J Neurol* 1988;235:415–417.
75. Dattwyler RJ, Volkman DJ, Conaty SM, et al. Amoxycillin plus probenecid versus doxycycline for treatment of erythema migrans borreliosis. *Lancet* 1990;336:1404–1406.
76. Dattwyler RJ, Halperin JJ, Volkman DJ, Luft BJ. Treatment of late Lyme disease. *Lancet* 1988;1:1191–1193.
77. Pfister HW, Preac Mursic V, Wilske B, et al. Randomized comparison of ceftriaxone and cefotaxime in Lyme neuroborreliosis. *J Infect Dis* 1991;163:311–318.
78. Karlsson M, Manners-Berggren S, Lindquist L, et al. Comparison of intravenous penicillin G and oral doxycycline for treatment of Lyme neuroborreliosis. *Neurology* 1994;44:1203–1207.
79. Lyme Disease—United States, 1994. *MMWR* 1995;44:459–462.

80. Hanrahan JP, Benach JL, Coleman JL, et al. Incidence and cumulative frequency of endemic Lyme disease in a community. *J Infect Dis* 1984;150:489–496.

81. Steere AC, et al. Longitudinal assessment of the clinical and epidemiologic features of Lyme disease in a defined population. *J Infect Dis* 1986;154:295–300.

82. Luft BJ, Dunn JJ, Dattwyler RJ, et al. Cross reactive antigenic domains of the flagellin protein of *Borrelia burgdorferi*. *Res Microbiol* 1993;144:251–257.

83. Fikrig E, Telford SR, Wallich R, et al. Vaccination against Lyme disease caused by diverse *Borrelia burgdorferi*. *J Exp Med* 1995;181:215–221.

84. Fikrig E, Tao H, Kantor FS, et al. Evasion of protective immunity by *Borrelia burgdorferi* by truncation of outer surface protein B. *Proc Natl Acad Sci USA* 1993;90:4092–4096.

85. Keller D, Koster FT, Marks DH, et al. Safety and immunogenicity of a recombinant outer surface protein A Lyme vaccine. *JAMA* 1994;271:1764–1768.

Chapter 15

Central Nervous System Tumors and the Immune System

Pierre-Yves Dietrich, Paul R. Walker, Philippe Saas, and Nicolas de Tribolet

Whether the immune system plays a role in the control of cancer development, growth, and dissemination has been a subject of great controversy for the past few decades. Many previous issues have now been settled and it is clear that immune cells, in a complex network of intercellular interactions and cytokine-mediated signals, in some circumstances can contribute to protect the host against cancer. Tumor immunology is now an exciting research field, with significant advances made every year, and the fine manipulation of the immune system is a new promising strategy to treat cancer. This development is based mainly on the dramatic advances in our understanding of basic immunology at a molecular level (e.g., antigen presentation and recognition, tumor antigens, costimulatory signals, three-dimensional structure of several surface molecules), as well as the strides made in unraveling the complex cellular interactions involved in tumor immunology.

Several clinical and experimental observations demonstrate the existence of an antitumor response. The incidence of some cancer types is increased in immunosuppressed individuals. Lymphocytes infiltrate the majority of tumors, and some of the former have the ability to lyse autologous tumor cells in vitro. More convincingly, cytolytic T cells have been derived from a spontaneously regressing melanoma (1). In addition, administration of interleukin (IL)-2 to melanoma and renal cell carcinoma patients induces partial or complete responses at a low but reproducible rate (2). Perhaps the most demonstrative arguments in favor of an immune response against human cancer can be drawn from a series of clinical features observed in bone marrow transplant recipients. First, allogeneic bone marrow grafts confer a better prognosis in chronic and acute leukemia patients than do syngeneic or autologous grafts, because minor (or major) histocompatibility disparities lead to an antitumor effect provided by the transplant itself (graft versus leukemia effect). Second, T lymphocytes clearly mediate this graft versus leukemia effect, since T-cell depletion in transplants increases the rate of relapse (3). Third, chronic myeloid leukemia patients who relapse after allogeneic bone marrow grafting may be rescued with a single administration of donor lymphocytes (adoptive immunotherapy) (4). More recently, donor lymphocytes have also been used successfully to treat posttransplantation Epstein-Barr virus (EBV)–related lymphomas (5).

With respect to tumors arising within the central nervous system (CNS), crucial questions are whether and how such an antitumor response develops against a tumor within the CNS, a long-believed immune-privileged site (6). In this chapter, we summarize the current understanding and some of the hypotheses in this field, and briefly discuss the most promising treatment strategies currently being developed. We focus on astrocytic tumors, which form the majority of CNS malignancies and are certainly the most lethal. Indeed, despite aggressive multimodality therapy, the prognosis of patients with malignant astrocytomas remains poor. For glioblastoma, the median survival time after surgery and adjuvant radiotherapy is less than 1 year, with only a few patients still alive 2 years after diagnosis (7–9).

The initiation of an immune response against glioma is undoubtedly a critical step. This may involve interactions not only between T lymphocytes and tumor cells, but also possibly professional antigen-presenting cells (APCs), with both specific and nonspecific intercellular contacts (Fig 15-1). The subsequent development of effector mechanisms and the regulation of the response require further cellular cooperation and both positive and negative signals. For didactic reasons, this review concentrates on the cell surface molecules involved in specific immune interactions and discusses how an effective or an abortive immune response may develop. We are aware that this focus may underestimate the complexity of these biologic processes. Therefore, other aspects are integrated in a more realistic network in a later section of this chapter. It must be emphasized that an antitumor immune response is not a static process. There may be stages of intense immune activity and other periods of apparent immunologic anergy.

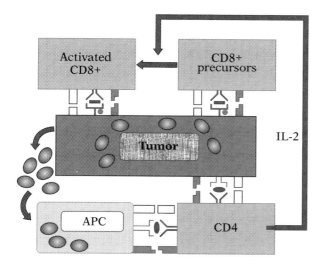

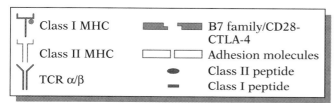

Figure 15-1. Hypothetical and schematic view of antigen presentation by glioma cells to T lymphocytes. Activation of both helper (CD4+ T cells) and cytolytic (CD8+ T cells) pathways is probably needed to elicit an effective antitumor response. A specific contact may be created by the interaction between the MHC class I–peptide complexes on tumor cells surface and the T-cell receptor (TCR) of CD8+ T cells. Interaction between MHC class II peptides and CD4+ T cells, with subsequent production of cytokines (e.g., interleukin (IL)-2) activating resting CD8+ T lymphocytes, may also be necessary. This step may be provided by professional antigen-presenting cells (APC) or glioma cells themselves. Nonspecific intercellular contacts by costimulatory and adhesion molecules are also crucial.

Thus, apparently conflicting data from in vitro and in vivo studies may in fact be reconcilable when the dynamics of the immune response are considered.

Antigen-Specific Interaction Between Glioma Cells and Immune Cells

As schematically shown in Figure 15-1, there are three principal components to an antigen-specific immune interaction: major histocompatibility complex (MHC) molecules, antigenic peptides, and T-cell receptors (TCRs). During the last few years, major advances in basic immunology have led to a better understanding of this pivotal biologic process. We will discuss this in the context of antitumor immune responses.

How Tumor Antigens Can Be Presented to and Recognized by T Cells

Antigen Presentation and the Major Histocompatibility Complex

Self and foreign antigenic proteins are continuously presented to T cells with the help of class I and II MHC molecules. Since T cells recognize small peptides rather than naive protein, antigens follow an intracellular pathway in which proteolytic cleavage can occur (*antigen processing*) (10). At the end of this complex process, class I molecules present peptides to CD8 T lymphocytes that are 8 to 10 amino acids in length and generally originate from endogenously expressed proteins (11). Class II molecules present peptides to CD4+ T cells (14–22 residues) that usually derive from exogenous protein (12).

The different steps for processing and assembly of antigens with MHC class I molecules are well defined, even if several unresolved questions remain (Fig 15-2). Briefly, endogenous proteins are first degraded into small peptides by the proteasome: a 2000-kd cytosolic structure comprising about 1% of protein in mammalian cells. They contain two major components, the 20S proteasome exhibiting proteolytic function and a 19S particle containing several adenosinetriphosphatases (ATPases). They are able to unfold the proteins and engulf them into a degradative tunnel (13). Whereas the majority of peptides degraded in proteasomes are rapidly hydrolyzed to amino acids by cytosolic exopeptidases, a minority of them, having an appropriate size, are transported into the endoplasmic reticulum by peptide transporters associated with antigen processing (TAP molecules). The peptide transporter is a heterodimeric protein formed of two homologous polypeptides encoded by the *TAP1* and *TAP2* genes located in the MHC class II region (14). Mutant cell lines not expressing this transporter and knock-out mice lacking the *TAP1* or *TAP2* gene do not present antigen to CD8+ T cells and show strongly reduced expression of surface class I MHC molecules. The reason for this is that the stable assembly of MHC class I molecules relies on peptide: "Empty" class I heterodimers either do not exit from the endoplasmic reticulum or traffic inefficiently through the Golgi compartment. Moreover, the low number of class I molecules that nevertheless reach the cell surface are unstable because of the lack of peptide in their peptide groove. In humans, a genetic defect in TAP was recently described; it resulted in an inherited immune deficiency (15). Thus, in addition to various cytokines (such as interferon (IFN)-γ), TAP molecules play a key role in the regulation of MHC class I molecule expression. This point may be relevant in understanding the possible mechanisms by which tumor cells escape from immune surveillance, by downregulation of class I molecule expression (see below).

The processing of proteins resulting in the assembly of class II MHC molecules with peptides and their expression at the cell surface is very complex and still in-

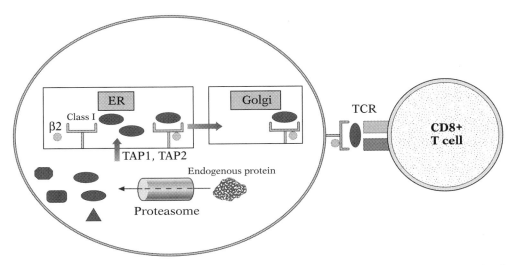

Figure 15-2. Antigen processing and presentation. The intracellular pathway of antigenic proteins presented by class I molecules (see text). ER = endoplasmic reticulum; TAP = peptide transporter; TCR = T-cell receptor.

completely understood (16), even if major advances have been achieved recently (17). Briefly, exogenous antigens undergo endocytosis in cells and proteolysis in successive intracellular compartments (endosomes, lysosomes). At some stage, the peptides must interact with the α and β chains of class II molecules that assemble in the endoplasmic reticulum and then travel to the cell surface in vesicles. The intracellular location where vesicles containing MHC molecules fuse with vesicles containing peptides probably varies depending on the cell type and the antigen presented (18). Then, MHC class II molecules loaded with peptides are transported to the cell surface in a way that is not clearly established. The understanding of MHC class II gene regulation has progressed following the elucidation of the molecular basis of a rare inherited disease, the bare lymphocyte syndrome, one of the two forms of MHC class II deficiency. The defect of MHC class II expression in this syndrome is due to mutations in the genes encoding the transcription factors involved in the regulation of MHC class II gene expression (19–22). One of these genes, *CIITA*, appears to be of particular interest and its expression is regulated by IFN-γ (21). Whether these regulatory mechanisms are defective or silent in tumor cells, and how they might be used as tools to improve the antigen presentation by the tumor cells themselves provide exciting and ongoing areas of research (23).

Which cells have the capacity to present antigens? Most nucleated cells of the body, if one excludes the CNS and the reproductive tissues, usually express class I molecules (at various levels) and can present peptides to CD8 T cells, at least under certain conditions. In contrast, antigen presentation to CD4 T cells is limited to those few cell types that express class II molecules (24). Monocytes, macrophages, B lymphocytes, and dendritic

cells are particularly implicated in this APC function. Dendritic cells are particularly potent APCs, especially for initiating primary immune responses. They take their origin from bone marrow progenitors (25,26) and are found in nearly all tissues of the body (Langerhans' cells in the skin, interdigitating dendritic cells in the thymus and lymph nodes, interstitial dendritic cells in the heart, kidney, gut, or lung). They are characterized by a dendritic morphology, the presence of intracytoplasmic Birbeck granules, the expression of CD1a and high levels of MHC class II molecules, and the expression of accessory molecules (e.g., B7, CD58 or LFA-3, CD54 or ICAM-1) implicated in giving a second signal to T cells (see below) (27,28). Even if their role in eliciting an effective antitumor immune response has not been directly demonstrated, the therapeutic effects achieved in animal models with dendritic cells pulsed with tumor peptides (29) strongly suggest their involvement in this process.

Antigen Recognition by T Cells

Two molecules are involved in antigen recognition, antibodies and the TCR. In the 1980s tumor immunologists focused on antibodies that were used as hooks for tumor antigen "fishing." In the 1990s, it is increasingly recognized that T cells are the critical mediators of the immune response against tumors. More than 80% of peripheral blood lymphocytes are T lymphocytes expressing either α/β TCRs (95% of T cells) or γ/δ TCRs (2%–5% only) at their surface (30). Mature α/β T lymphocytes recognize antigenic peptides presented by MHC molecules through their heterodimeric α/β TCR, whereas the noncovalently linked CD3 molecular complex is involved in intracellular signal transduction (31) (Fig 15-3). CD3 functions as well as the alterations in

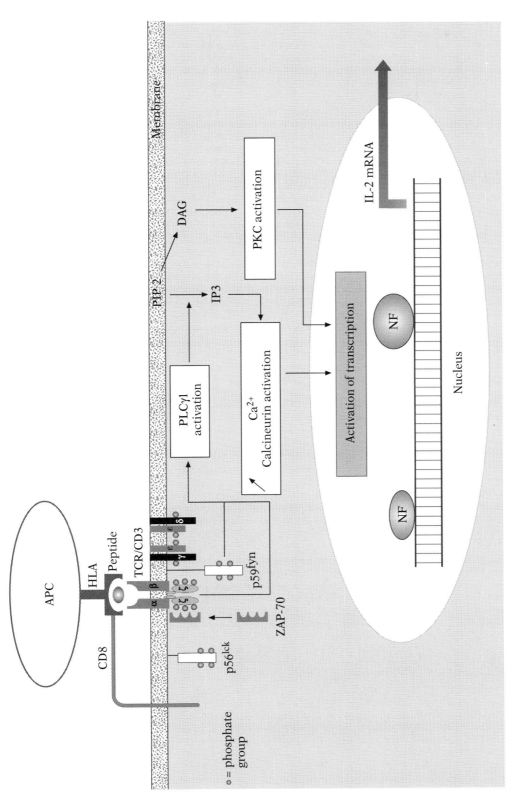

Figure 15-3. Simplified illustration of the intracellular steps leading to T-cell activation. After the HLA-peptide complex and T-cell receptor (TCR) have interacted, the first biochemical events consist of a series of tyrosine phosphorylations on several protein tyrosine kinases (PTK). Such enzymes possess the ability to add a phosphate group on tyrosine residues. Belonging to the Src family, p56^lck is a membrane PTK that interacts with the cytoplasmic domain of CD4 or CD8 α chain. The phosphorylation of p56^lck tyrosine residues favors the bringing together of p56^lck and CD3 ζ chains, with subsequent phosphorylation of tyrosine located in specific domains termed *ARAM* (antigen recognition activation motif) or *TAM* (tyrosine-based activation motif) in ζ chains (and probably also in the other chains of CD3). Another member of the Src family, p59^fyn, is directly associated with the ζ chain and works in a similar manner. Phosphorylation of ζ chains induces the recruitment of cytoplasmic ZAP-70, which is a 70-kd PTK belonging to the Syk family not constitutively localized at the membrane. This tyrosine phosphorylation cascade results in the activation of the phospholipase Cγ1 (PLCγ1), which in turn induces the hydrolysis of phosphatidylinositol 4,5-diphosphate (PIP2) into phosphatidylinositol 2,4,5-triphosphate (IP3) and diacylglycerol (DAG). DAG activates protein kinase C (PKC), which enhances specific nuclear transcription factors (NF). On the other hand, IP3 increases the free intracytoplasmic calcium level with subsequent activation of calcineurin. Calcineurin, a serine phosphatase whose enzymatic function is inhibited by cyclosporine, acts in transferring the cytoplasmic subunit of the transcription factor NF-AT in close contact to its nuclear subunit (not shown on the figure), leading to the transcription of the interleukin (IL)-2 gene. Note that IL-2 transcription can be enhanced by other factors, such as Oct-1, AP-1 (which is a dimeric protein composed of *fos* and *jun* products), and NFκB. Interestingly, NFκB is also implicated in the regulation of the IL-2 receptor α chain (see text). Finally, activation of T cells probably also requires other complex signal cascades under the CD28 molecule and IL-2 receptor α chain (277,278).

signaling pathways observed in cancer patients are discussed in a subsequent paragraph.

Each TCR α and β chain includes a variable and a constant region. Variable regions determine the antigen specificity. The repertoire of TCR specificities that an individual must create to face the huge diversity of antigenic determinants is immense. Complex molecular mechanisms contribute to the shaping of this diversification (32–34). During T-cell differentiation, unique variable-region genes are created by recombination of variable (V), diversity (D), and joining (J) segments for the β locus, and of V and J segments for the α locus. The random joining of these segments generates what is referred to as *combinatorial diversity* (Fig 15-4). In humans, 63 Vβ and more than 65 Vα gene segments have been molecularly characterized and are classified into 25 and 32 subfamilies, respectively, based on nucleotide sequence similarity in their coding region (35,36). There are also 13 Jβ and 61 Jα gene segments (37). In addition to the combinatorial diversity, TCR diversity is greatly increased by nibbling of V, D, or J segments as well as by the addition of untemplated N-region nucleotides between these gene segments during the recombination process (*junctional diversity*) (38). Corresponding to the hypervariable regions of immunoglobulin molecules, N regions (also termed *CDR3*) are essential for binding to the antigenic peptide presented by a MHC molecule. Expression of unique rearranged TCR gene products thus determines the specificity of a given T cell (34,39). Finally, the random combination of the α and β chains encoded by these genes further increases the diversity of the TCR repertoire.

Given the crucial role of T cells in antigen recognition, major efforts have been made to characterize the function of tumor-infiltrating lymphocytes (TILs). After in vitro culture in the presence of high concentrations of IL-2, TILs isolated from various tumors often acquire nonspecific lytic properties, such that not only autologous tumor cells, but also allogeneic tumor cell lines and natural killer (NK) or lymphokine-activated killer (LAK) target cell lines (K562, Daudi) are lysed. The biologic interest of such a nonspecific cytolysis is probably faint. In contrast, the in vitro generation of cytotoxic T lymphocyte (CTL) lines or CTL clones exhibiting a MHC-restricted cytotoxicity against only autologous tumor cell lines is proof that tumor-specific antigenic peptides exist. Such CTL clones have been derived mainly, but not exclusively, from melanoma (40,41) and have been used as biologic reagents to identify tumor-specific antigens, such as MAGE (see below). However, it is now obvious that many TILs exhibit profound functional defects induced by diverse mechanisms (see below).

The molecular analysis of TCRs in TILs is another powerful way to define whether a T-cell immune response has occurred in vivo against tumor (42). Indeed, identification of recurrent TCR transcripts (same rearrangement and same N region) in large T-cell populations suggests antigen-driven expansion of the corresponding T-cell clones. Several polymerase chain reaction (PCR)–based methods have been developed in the last years, allowing the detection of T-cell clonal expansions occurring in vivo (43–49). With such methods, major T-cell clonal expansions have been observed in various tumor types, such as melanoma, renal cell carcinoma, head and neck cancer, and chronic lymphatic leukemia (1,50–54). This molecular approach is not informative per se concerning the significance of de-

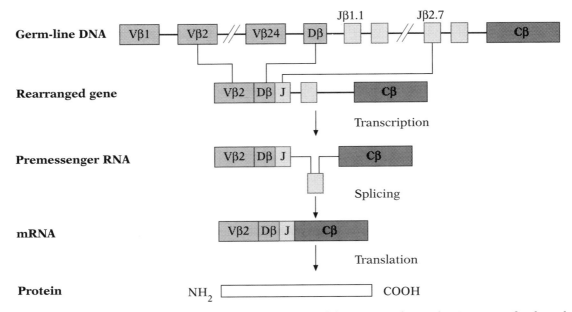

Figure 15-4. Gene rearrangement generating β-chain *combinatorial diversity*. Similar mechanisms occur for the α chain.

tected clonal expansions, but when coupled with subsequent analyses of function and specificity, it is a powerful tool. Indeed, the recent demonstration in a patient with melanoma (1) and one with renal cell carcinoma (54) that T-cell clonal expansions detected by TCR molecular analysis were actually cytolytic against autologous tumor cells in a MHC-restricted fashion highlights the interest of this approach.

Tumor Antigens

The existence on tumor cell surfaces of antigens that can be recognized by immune cells is the sine qua non condition for the generation of a specific immune response against tumor. In more than four decades, a high number of tumor-specific transplantation antigens (TSTAs) have been identified in experimental tumors. TSTAs are defined as antigens expressed on tumor cells that can be recognized and rejected in graft experiments using syngeneic mice (55,56). However, TSTAs have been considered artifacts for a long time, since their existence appeared to be restricted to experimental tumors. Such tumors are artificially induced by oncogenic viruses (e.g., polyoma, SV40) (57), ultraviolet irradiation (58), or chemical carcinogens (e.g., methylcholanthrene) (59,60). In contrast, spontaneous tumors appeared nonimmunogenic, unable to elicit an immune response in transplantation experiments.

This generally accepted notion acted as a strong brake in tumor antigen research until 1991 when Boon et al (61) identified the first gene encoding a human *tumor-specific antigen* recognized by CTLs, *MAGE-1* (melanoma antigen) (Fig 15-5). This gene is unrelated to known genes and is silent in normal tissues with the exception of the testis and placenta. The encoded antigenic peptide is a nonamer presented by the HLA-A1 molecule (62). In fact, *MAGE-1* belongs to a gene family of several members, of which *MAGE-3* also has been characterized extensively (63,64). Besides melanomas, a significant proportion of breast tumors, non-small-cell lung tumors, and head and neck carcinomas, as well as glioma cell lines express *MAGE-1* or *MAGE-3* (65,66). More recently, other tumor-specific gene families have been identified, namely, the *BAGE, GAGE,* and *RAGE* genes (67).

Tumor-specific antigens are not the unique candidates able to elicit CTL responses in melanoma. Indeed, a series of *differentiation antigenic peptides* have been identified during the last few years. These peptides are derived from tyrosinase, Melan-A (also called MART-1), gp100, and gp75 (68–71) proteins. Melanoma differentiation antigens are defined by their expression in tumor cells and also in the normal cell counterpart (i.e., melanocytes). In contrast to specific tumor antigens, they are not expressed in other tumor types. Interestingly, it was recently demonstrated that certain peptides derived from such antigens are very common immunogenic epitopes shared by a high proportion of HLA-A2 melanomas, and are thus interesting candidates for immunotherapy (70). In addition, a peptide derived from tyrosinase is also presented by a class II molecule (HLA-DR4), implicating CD4+ helper T-cell involvement in at least some antitumor responses (72).

A further area of interest has been peptides encoded by mutated human proto-oncogenes or by chimeric genes resulting from chromosomal translocations. Such peptides (e.g., fusion protein Bcr-Abl in chronic myeloid leukemia) may be able to elicit T-cell immunity (73,74). Indeed proteins structurally altered during tumoral transformation appear to be the best candidates for inducing a specific immune response. In vitro responses to mutated *ras* oncogene were demonstrated in murine and human systems (75–77). In addition, immunization of mice with vaccinia virus expressing mutant Ras protein allows the generation of CTLs that lyse target cells infected with vaccinia virus carrying the mutated but not the normal *ras* gene (78). Similarly, a tumor antigen may also be the product of a tumor suppressor gene, and specific cytotoxic T-cell clones have been generated in vitro against mutated p53 protein (79–81). Furthermore, in a murine model, in vivo immunization with a mutated p53 peptide induces specific CTL clones that can lyse H-2–matched tumor cells expressing the mutated p53 gene (82).

How Specific Tumor Cell Recognition May Induce Effective or Abortive T-Cell Responses in Glioma

Antigen Presentation

Which cells in the CNS have the intrinsic ability to present antigens to immune cells is the first issue to address regarding how an immune response can occur in an "immunologically privileged site" (6). A prerequisite is the appropriate expression of MHC class I or class II

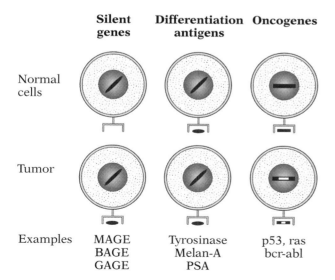

Figure 15-5. Schematic representation of tumor antigens into three major categories.

molecules on the cell surface. In theory, tumor cells themselves or APCs localized in the tumor microenvironment can be involved in tumor-antigen presentation to immune cells.

Microglial cells are probably the most promising candidates. They comprise 5% to 15% of the total cellular composition of brain tissue, they are distributed throughout the CNS (83), and they belong to the dendritic cell lineage, possessing many of their characteristics (84), discussed earlier. Recently, their hematopoietic origin was demonstrated directly in transplantation studies in animals, in which the grafting of a new bone marrow induced a new microglia population of donor origin in the host (85). Other APC candidates may be endothelial cells and capillary pericytes, on which class II molecule and adhesion molecule expression is inducible by IFN-γ, tumor necrosis factor (TNF)-α, and IL-1 (6,86,87). The perivascular location of pericytes and endothelial cells is particularly appropriate for APC function and the communication between CNS cells and immune cells. Indeed, the recent demonstration of lymphatic connections between the brain and draining deep cervical lymph nodes is consistent with such a function (88). Using such a route, microglial cells and other endovascular and perivascular cells could migrate to cervical lymph nodes to elicit an immune response, in a similar manner as Langerhans' cells or dendritic cells, which migrate to regional lymph nodes and the spleen from skin, cardiac, or renal transplants (89–92).

Tumor cells of astrocytic lineage might also participate in antigen presentation. Conflicting data emerge from the extensive literature concerning the expression of MHC class I and II molecules by normal astrocytes and their putative ability to present antigens. These controversies may be due to the facts that most of the studies were performed on in vitro cultured astrocytes and that the CNS probably has to be considered an inducible rather than a constitutive site for the expression of MHC molecules (93–96). For example, the variable expression of MHC class I and II molecules on the surface of in vitro cultured astrocytes is constantly enhanced after incubation with IFN-γ. Some murine as well as human IFN-γ–treated astrocytes may present foreign antigens to class I– and class II–restricted human CTLs (96), but seem unable to stimulate T-cell proliferation and thus to trigger a complete T-cell activation program (95). Can glioma cells themselves present antigens to T cells? Some human glioblastoma cell lines are able to activate T cells in an antigen-specific MHC class II–dependent manner (96). Even if some normal or tumoral glial cells possess the intracellular machinery to present antigens, these in vitro data and their biologic relevance should be considered with some caution. Therefore, analysis of in vivo expression of MHC molecules may be more informative (97). Interestingly, class II expression by glioma cells was often associated with expression of intercellular adhesion molecule (ICAM)-1, suggesting the potential ability of some glioma cells to elicit a CD4+ T-cell response in vivo (98).

The regulation of MHC class I and class II expression is thus a critical component that will influence tumor cell–immune cell interactions. Indeed, the loss of MHC class I molecule expression in cancer cells may lead to immune escape (99–105). In virally infected cells, for example, virus proteins (e.g., E3 glycoprotein of adenovirus, H301 of cytomegalovirus) may bind to class I heavy chain or (β$_2$-microglobulin, inducing the retention of class I MHC in the endoplasmic reticulum (106–109). Downregulation of MHC class I molecules can also be related to transcriptional inhibition of heavy-chain or β$_2$-microglobulin gene expression (110, 111). However, normal levels of heavy-chain and β$_2$-microglobulin RNAs are observed in some cancers devoid of class I MHC surface molecules. This situation is frequently related to the absence of TAP1/2 expression, leading to aberrant class I assembly and trafficking as previously discussed. Interestingly, this mechanism has been most convincingly documented in a virus-associated cancer, human cervical carcinoma (112). Indeed, the results of two independent studies (113,114) suggest that this could be a common mechanism used by viruses to escape from T-cell killing. It was demonstrated that an immediate early protein of herpes simplex virus binds to TAP and thus inhibits peptide transport across the endoplasmic reticulum membrane.

T Lymphocytes

T-Cell Function in Glioma Patients

A high proportion of high-grade astrocytomas are infiltrated by lymphocytes that are mostly CD8 T cells, whereas B cells, NK cells, and CD4 T cells are much more scattered (115,116). The intensity of this infiltration is variable and predominant at the tumor periphery and around vessels. T-lymphocyte infiltration is not clearly related to a good prognosis in glioma patients (117,118), although exceptions to this conclusion have been reported (119). This apparent paradox may be the consequence of the series of defects in immune functions that have been identified in glioma patients. These defects include an abnormal delayed hypersensitivity to antigens, such as *Mycobacterium tuberculosis* or *Candida albicans;* a low count of circulating T cells; a depressed proliferative response to mitogens, such as phytohemagglutinin, concanavalin A, and phorbol ester; a decreased antibody response to tetanus toxoid, influenza virus, or other antigens, probably related to a failure of CD4 T cells to function as helper cells for immunoglobulin secretion; and deficient antibody-mediated and T-cell cytotoxicity in vitro (120–127). The lytic functions of TILs appear particularly suppressed (124,128) (see below). Even if it is possible to expand high numbers of TILs with nonspecific cytolytic activities (128,129), only rare CTL clones with MHC-restricted cytotoxicity have been reported (130), and their characterization was incomplete. The biologic significance of such CTL clones must be considered carefully. Indeed, CTL clones are usually obtained after repeated in vitro stimulation of T cells by autologous and allogeneic tumor cells in the presence of IL-2 and APCs. Although such an in vitro approach is very useful in melanoma research, where in vitro derived CTL clones are used as reagents to identify the antigens recognized, several artifacts may minimize the real biologic relevance of CTLs when no antigen is subsequently identified. Indeed, a tumor cell line represents a selection of a few tumor cells among the highly heterogeneous cellular population of a given tumor. In addition, it undergoes multiple genetic alterations during in vitro passages. It is also clear that the growth rate of T cells is not uniform: Some lymphocytes either do not grow or expand slowly, whereas other cells have significant growth advantage, inducing an important skewing of the TCR repertoire after culture as compared with the in situ TCR repertoire (131).

Intense research is currently ongoing to characterize the molecular events underlying the global T-cell unresponsiveness observed in glioma patients. We now discuss the abnormalities in IL-2 receptor expression and in intracellular signal transduction mechanisms, the alteration of peptides presented by MHC molecules, and finally the immunosuppressive agents secreted by glioma cells themselves.

Interleukin-2 Receptor Abnormalities. Ex vivo, glioma TILs lose their ability to proliferate in culture after a few weeks, when IL-2 receptor (IL-2R) expression declines progressively in spite of the addition of IL-2 in the culture medium (129). Moreover, the in vitro production of IL-2 by lectin-stimulated T cells obtained from glioma patients is less than that obtained from cells of normal individuals, and the addition of recombinant IL-2 does not restore their impaired proliferative abilities (127). Such data suggest defective IL-2R expression by T cells. IL-2 exerts its biologic effects through specific binding to its receptor. The IL-2R is a complex structure with low, intermediate, or high affinity for its ligand, depending on its composition. IL-2Rs composed of either α chain or βγ chains have low or intermediate affinity, respectively, and require high IL-2 concentrations to be saturated. Activated T cells and a small subset of NK cells express the α, β, and γ chains of the IL-2R, forming a high-affinity trimer requiring very low concentrations of IL-2 for an activation signal. It has been demonstrated that T cells obtained from glioma patients express reduced levels of the α chain (p55) after mitogenic stimulation, and therefore fail to assemble normal levels of the high-affinity IL-2R (132). The molecular basis of the failure of p55 expression remains to be determined. Indeed, these T cells express normal levels of p55 messenger RNA (mRNA) as well as adequately glycosylated p55 protein. In the absence of transcription, translation, or posttranslation abnormalities, several hypotheses may be evoked to explain the inability of glioma T cells to express high-affinity IL-2Rs. These may include, for example, an unstable p55 mRNA or an insufficient rate of its synthesis, an intracellular sequestration, or degradation of the normal p55 protein. The failure of many glioma T cells to express adequate α-chain levels is a crucial defect, since T-cell proliferation in response to physiologic concentrations of IL-2 is clearly related

to the expression of the high-affinity heterotrimeric αβγ IL2-R. However, it is noteworthy that the data concerning α-chain defects were obtained at a time when the γ chain was not yet identified. The γ chain is a common subunit to IL-2, IL-4, IL-7, IL-9, and IL-15 receptors, and is able to regulate the commitment of T cells to either clonal expansion or anergy (133). The analysis of the γ chain on glioma T cells may improve our understanding of the role of IL-2R abnormalities in T-cell functional defects. Furthermore, it will be informative to better define the causes of these IL2-R abnormalities. A first step in this direction was achieved with the demonstration that transforming growth factor (TGF)-β can downregulate the IL-2R α chain (134).

Abnormalities in T-Cell Signal Transduction. The recognition of the MHC-peptide complex by TCRs induces a cascade of intracellular events transducing the information to the cell nucleus (135–139) (see Fig 15-3). Any blockade in this complex pathway may explain why T cells do not efficiently respond to an adequate signal delivered by antigen. Several abnormalities in T-cell signaling of cancer patients were described recently.

A first possible alteration is the lack of CD3 ζ chain and p56lck PTK in T lymphocytes infiltrating tumors (140,141). One or two missing CD3 ζ chains are replaced by one or two γ chains of the receptor for IgE. This abnormality induces a decreased ability to mobilize intracellular calcium in response to activation signals and, in parallel, a marked decrease of the antitumor effects mediated by such T cells (142,143). Both CD4 and CD8 T cells are affected. First described in mice bearing colon carcinoma (MCA-38) or renal cell carcinoma (Renca), this abnormality was also demonstrated in human pathology. Western blot and immunohistology revealed a marked decrease in TCR ζ chain and p56lck expression in the TILs of 10 of 11 patients with renal cell carcinoma (144) and in all 14 patients with colorectal cancers analyzed (145). TILs are more severely affected than peripheral blood lymphocytes (PBLs), suggesting that a factor within the tumor microenvironment may induce this defect. The recent observation that macrophages at certain activation stages are able to induce the loss of ζ chain strengthens this thesis (146). On the other hand, the systemic alteration of the T cells, albeit less pronounced, may reflect the metastatic progression of the malignancy. Whether CD3 ζ chains are absent in T lymphocytes of high-grade astrocytomas remains to be determined. Moreover, the secretion of numerous immunosuppressive agents by glioma cells (as will be discussed) may potentially further impede T-cell signaling, although this has yet to be examined.

Another interesting alteration in downstream signaling events was recently identified. The kB enhancer-binding proteins is a family of related proteins including NF-κB1 (p50), RelA (p65), and c-Rel. They are mainly involved in the regulation of many cellular gene products associated with T-cell activation including IFN-γ, IL-2, and IL-2R α chain. In resting T cells, p65 is associated with its inhibitor in cytoplasm, whereas p50 is located in the nucleus. Activation of T lymphocytes results in the release of p65 from its inactive complex with its inhibitor (termed *IκBa*), allowing the translocation of p65 into the nucleus and its binding to the nuclear p50 to form an active heterodimeric transcription factor (p50/p65). In TILs isolated from animal and human renal cell carcinomas, p65 does not translocate into the nucleus and there is no induction of a normal NF-κB complex (p50/p65) after in vitro stimulation (147,148), resulting in the repression of several gene promoter activities including IL-2 and IL-2R α chain (149). Whether such a molecular event occurs in T lymphocytes infiltrating glioma has not been investigated. In particular, whether the NF-κB1 failure to translocate to the nucleus contributes to the IL2-R α-chain expression defect is still unknown. A further important issue is to determine whether NF-κB abnormalities are only consecutive to defects in upstream signaling environments. Indeed, the release of NF-kB1 from its inhibitor needs the phosphorylation of the latter, a step that is mediated by activated PKC. Cells packing CD3 ζ chains, p56^{lck}, and p59^{fyn} (see above) are unable to activate PKC. Thus, the lack of such early events in T-cell signaling may hinder the phosphorylation of IκBa and the consecutive binding of p50 with p65 into the nucleus.

However, a serious "caveat" has been reported concerning the significance of the alterations of proteins involved in signal transduction (150). Indeed, except when tumors constituted more than 20% of the mice body weight (i.e., unrepresentative of the human situation), only subtle abnormalities were observed in four different models using chemically or ultraviolet light–induced tumors. Moreover, the severe tumor-specific immunodeficiency occurring during their growth was not related to these alterations.

Alteration of Antigenic Peptides. An additional mechanism that may lead to signaling impairment involves slight alterations of the peptide presented by the MHC molecule. Indeed, minor modifications in amino acid sequence may either affect the interaction between the peptide and MHC molecule (e.g., amino acids at positions 2 and 9 are particularly implicated in the interaction with HLA-A2 class I molecules) or suppress the recognition by TCR (151,152). Moreover, it was recently reported that subtle amino acid substitutions can yield analogue peptides (mutated peptides) that can still interact with the TCR but are unable to deliver a full stimulatory signal. T cells stimulated in vitro by such peptides become anergic to subsequent stimulation with the nonmutated peptide. In vitro models show that anergy is consistently correlated with a unique pattern of TCR ζ-chain phosphorylation and a subsequent lack of association with ZAP-70 (153–159). It was recently suggested that hepatitis B virus and human immunodeficiency virus (HIV) type 1 may exploit such mechanisms to evade protective immune responses critical for their clearance (160,161). The contribution of this phenomenon to the escape of cancer from immune surveillance is still hypothetical. Nevertheless, it is an attractive concept that immune control of tumor growth can occur when T cells recognize tumor epitopes, and that cancer progression is at least partly related to subtle residue changes in one or several tumor peptides. Recent data support this hypothesis. The substitution of an arginine by a glycine at position 3 of a 9–amino acid peptide derived from human papillomavirus (HPV16) was detected in 30% of invasive cervical cancers associated with the HLA-B7 haplotype (a genotype associated with a significant poor prognosis) (162).

Immunosuppressive Factors. During recent years, cumulative data suggest that soluble factors produced within the local glioma environment may hinder an adequate immune response. Indeed, the addition of culture supernatants obtained from glioblastoma cell lines, fresh glioma, or glioma cyst fluid inhibits several lymphocyte functions (see above). Moreover, T lymphocytes from normal individuals exhibit similar immunologic abnormalities when cultured in the presence of glioma supernatant (163). Such results imply the existence of soluble suppressor factors derived from gliomas. The role of several candidate immunosuppressive molecules was investigated in recent studies.

Immunosuppressive Factors: Transforming Growth Factor-β. TGF-β was temporarily called *glioblastoma cell–derived T-cell suppressor factor* (G-Tsf), because it was first identified in 1984 in the supernatant of a human glioblastoma cell line exhibiting suppression of T-cell growth activity (164). It was later renamed *TGF-β2* after purification and cloning, due to sequence homology with the previously described TGF-β1. TGF-β is secreted as a precursor molecule that must be cleaved by proteases such as plasmin and cathepsin to become biologically active (165). In glioma research, two main issues determine which TGF-β isoforms are produced by glioma cells and the qualitative differences observed in normal and tumoral astrocytes. Murine astrocytes in culture express all three TGF-β isoform mRNAs but secrete TGF-β2 in its inactive *latent* form. In contrast, glioblastoma cell lines, also able to synthesize all three TGF-β isoform transcripts, secrete mainly the TGF-β2 isoform in its *active cleaved* form (166,167). Indeed, an elegant well-controlled study using protease inhibitors demonstrated that TGF-β2–mediated T-cell suppression (see below) requires the action of proteases produced by glioma cells (168).

Many immune effects can be mediated by the TGF-β2 active isoform produced by glioma cells. TGF-β2 inhibits NK- and LAK-cell activity, B-cell proliferation and differentiation, as well as the secretion or function of numerous cytokines (IFN-γ, TNF-α, TNF-β, IL-1, IL-2, IL-3, IL-6, and granulocyte-macrophage colony-stimulating factor (GM-CSF)). TGF-β2 induces a strong inhibition of T-cell growth, an effect mediated through the TGF-β receptors on the membrane of T cells (169,170). Furthermore, TGF-β2 can downregulate MHC class II molecules on glioma cells in vitro (171), thus decreasing their potential abilities to act as APCs (96). Finally, TGF-β produced by some skin macrophages inhibits immune responses against defined antigens by decreasing IL-2R α-chain expression (134). The biologic relevance of these in vitro data has been extended by in vivo observations. TGF-β2 immunostaining, observed in the majority of glioma, appears to be inversely correlated with the presence of IL-2R–positive lymphocytes (169,172). More recently, antisense TGF-β2 phosphorothioate oligonucleotides were used to inhibit TGF-β2 secretion by glioblastoma cell lines, thus reversing certain immunosuppressive effects of TGF-β2 in vitro (173). Such properties suggest that TGF-β2 may play a role in glioma escape from immune surveillance. The new avenues opened by this concept in the treatment strategy of glioma are discussed later.

Immunosuppressive Factors: Interleukin-10. IL-10 is a newly identified cytokine with a broad spectrum of biologic activities, including immunosuppressive effects. Located on chromosome 1q, the human IL-10 gene was cloned based on its homology to the mouse gene. Interestingly, both genes exhibit strong DNA sequence homology with an open reading frame termed *BCRF1* in the EBV genome. *BCRF1* could provide a selective advantage to the virus by inhibiting cell-mediated antiviral immune responses (174). T-cell secretion of IL-10 appears to be limited to one of the helper T-cell subsets defined on the basis of cytokine secretion profiles. Th1 cells produce IL-2, IFN-γ, and TNF-α, and strongly activate cell-mediated responses, whereas Th2 cells produce IL-4, IL-5, IL-6, IL-10, and IL-13 and stimulate B cells to generate an antibody response. IFN-γ inhibits the proliferation of Th2 clones, while IL-4 and IL-10 inhibit that of Th1 clones, providing a partial explanation of the common mutual exclusion of these two types of immune responses in vivo (175). Mainly but not exclusively produced by T cells, IL-10 displays numerous biologic activities through binding to its widely expressed receptor, which was recently cloned (176). It inhibits the antigen-dependent and mitogen-dependent proliferation of T cells; inhibits the production of IFN-γ, IL-1, IL-6, IL-8, IL-12, granulocyte colony-stimulating factor (G-CSF), and GM-CSF in activated monocytes as well as their phagocytosis abilities and their nitric oxide production; and downregulates MHC class II molecule expression and the APC abilities of macrophages (174).

Whether IL-10 contributes to the escape of glioma from immune surveillance is still not clear. IL-10 mRNA was observed in a high proportion of glioblastomas (177,178), but with reverse transcriptase (RT)-PCR only. Since IL-10 can also be observed after amplification in normal brain tissue and lymphocytes infiltrating glioma, the biologic significance of these data should be considered with some caution. More recently, it was reported that glioma cell line supernatant can abrogate the release of IFN-γ by lymphocytes and inhibit MHC class II expression by monocytes. The first inhibitory effect was reversed by anti–IL-10 monoclonal antibody (suggesting the major contribution of IL-10 in this effect), while the second one appeared to be only partly due to IL-10 (179). Unfortunately, the direct demonstration of IL-10 in glioma supernatants was not described in this work. Further studies are warranted to

better define the precise role of IL-10 in the immune suppression observed in glioma.

Other Immunosuppressive Factors. The secretion of prostaglandin E_2 (PGE_2) by glioblastoma in vitro was in fact the first observation of the production of a potential immunosuppressive agent by these cells (180). PGE_2 is also produced in vivo (181). The immunosuppressive effects of PGE_2 are now better defined. PGE_2 profoundly suppresses the production of IL-2 and IFN-γ by Th1 cells, while it enhances the antibody-mediated immune responses (182). Thus, together with IL-10 and TGF-β, PGE_2 may contribute to the defect in cellular immunity observed in gliomas.

The more recent description of the production of an IL-1 receptor antagonist by glioma is intriguing (183). Indeed, IL-1α and IL-1β are produced by a significant proportion of high-grade astrocytomas (184). Moreover 10 of 11 glioblastomas tested expressed IL-1 receptor (185). The production of IL-1 by glioma might play a role in initiating a cascade of events, such as the secondary release of other cytokines (IL-6, IL-8, macrophage chemoattractant protein (MCP)-1) and the upregulation of adhesion molecules such as ICAM-1 or vascular cell adhesion molecule (VCAM) on tumor and endothelial cells. Such effects might therefore promote attraction and extravasation of circulating lymphocytes and macrophages. Whether IL-1 is involved in tumor growth by an autocrine or a paracrine manner, whether IL-1 actually initiates an immune response in vivo, and finally whether such effects are inhibited by an IL-1 receptor antagonist also produced by glioma cells remain to be determined.

T-Cell Receptor Molecular Analysis

As mentioned in an earlier section (Antigen Recognition by T Cells), the molecular characterization of the receptor involved in antigen recognition (i.e., the TCR) is a powerful approach to detect the presence of antigen-driven T-cell populations in a variety of tumors (186). In TILs of most malignant astrocytomas studied, Nitta et al (187) found a limited usage of TCR Vα and Vβ gene segments, with a preferential expression of Vα7 and Vβ13 genes in TILs from the majority of gliomas studied. The sequencing of TCR Vα7 and Vβ13 amplified transcripts showed recurrent sequences reflecting T-cell clonal expansions (188). More surprisingly, and for the first time in tumor immunology to our knowledge, identical clones were expanded in several distinct patients sharing the same HLA haplotype. These data suggest that T cells clonally expanded in vivo may be driven by a common antigen shared by several gliomas. However, a strange result is the report of this same recurrent TCR sequence in a patient expressing a different HLA haplotype. In a series of caucasian patients, we also found a constantly high expression of Vβ13 transcripts within gliomas. However, other Vβ gene segment subfamilies can also be overrepresented. Furthermore, the recurrent and highly prominent Vβ13 sequence described by Ebato et al (188) was not detected in nine glioblastoma and aplastic astrocytoma patients

(Dietrich P-Y, et al, unpublished results, 1997), despite two patients expressing the HLA-B24 allele assumed to be the restriction element. Finally, using a new high-resolution RT-PCR method based on the determination of TCR β-chain CDR3 transcript length, we also observed the presence of several oligoclonal expansions, thus suggesting that an immune response may develop within the CNS against still putative glioma antigens. These conflicting results underline the absolute necessity to combine TCR molecular analysis with phenotypic and functional studies, in order to define the activation state and the biologic significance of in vivo expanded T-cell populations, and hopefully to characterize the glioma antigen recognized by such cells.

Tumor Antigens in Glioma

No glioma-specific antigen able to elicit an immune response has been identified to date. *MAGE* family genes are expressed in some of glioblastoma cell lines, but never in uncultured tumors (66). This discrepancy could be due to a variation in DNA methylation level, since this mechanism regulates *MAGE* expression. Results of recent studies suggest but do not demonstrate that specific glioma antigens exist. The screening of astrocytoma complementary DNA (cDNA) expression libraries by autologous serum led to the discovery that IgG molecules react with the expression product of the *TEGT* gene, a gene developmentally regulated in the testis. These antibodies were detected in 2 of 13 glioma patients but never in the serum of healthy control subjects or other cancer patients (189). As discussed by the authors, this antibody response may reflect a CD4+ helper T-cell involvement in the antiglioma immune response.

Similarly, no differentiation antigen has been characterized in astrocytic tumors. The therapeutic usefulness of such antigens in glioma patients would probably be limited, because of the potential autoimmunity and the severe toxicity against normal brain structure generated by their use. Nevertheless, T-cell activation occurs only after a certain threshold of MHC-specific peptide complexes is available for TCR engagement (190). Therefore, it could be assumed that the level of expression of such antigens may be different in normal cells than in tumor cells, leading to a specific recognition of tumor cells by effectors and an acceptable therapeutic window (191). In the case of melanoma, some melanocyte-specific antigens are also expressed in certain cells of the retina, inner ear, and brain. However, whereas melanoma patients occasionally develop vitiligo (either spontaneously or after treatment), they never develop abnormalities of the visual system, vestibula, or CNS.

As discussed previously (see Tumor Antigens), the frequent p53 alterations observed in astrocytic tumors could provide new antigenic peptides that may trigger an immune response. Another quite common molecular event observed with glioma is the amplification and the mutation of the epidermal growth factor (EGF) receptor gene (192). Whether these alterations can serve

as targets for the immune system in the case of glioma is still unknown. Even if a mutated EGF receptor can be targeted by monoclonal antibodies for use in diagnosis, its ability to elicit an immune response in man has not been established (193). A tumor antigen is a much more useful tool for immunization strategies if there is some evidence for at least some immunogenicity that could be potentially enhanced.

There has been little effort to date to specifically search for glioma antigens. However, the phenotypical, functional, and molecular studies of T cells infiltrating gliomas strongly suggest that an antitumor immune response against gliomas can in some circumstances take place in the CNS, even if it is ultimately unable to control tumor growth. The identification of glioma antigens would represent a major advance in understanding the interaction between glioma cells and the immune system, and would facilitate the design of new treatment strategies for glioma patients.

Nonspecific Interactions Between Glioma Cells and Immune Cells

In addition to the specific signal delivered by the MHC-peptide complex to T cells, other nonspecific contacts exist between tumor cells, professional APCs, and lymphocytes. Several types of surface molecules are involved in this critical phenomenon. Their respective roles are complex and still poorly understood. Here we summarize the contribution of adhesion molecules and costimulatory molecules (Fig 15-6).

Adhesion Molecules

The central role of adhesion molecules in mediating cell–extracellular matrix and specific cell-cell interactions has been elucidated in recent years. Adhesion molecules are transmembrane receptors that comprise the integrins, cadherins, selectins, CD44, and immunoglobulin superfamilies (194). A detailed description of all adhesion molecules potentially implicated in cell-cell and cell–extracellular matrix interactions in glioma is beyond the scope of this chapter (for an excellent review, see (195)). We focus on a few examples showing the biologic significance of such molecules. During an immune response against glioma, adhesion molecules play an important role in two types of interactions: first between glioma cells and T lymphocytes, and second between CNS endothelial cells and immune cells.

The Role of Adhesion Molecules in Contact Between Glioma Cells and Immune Cells

A first critical interaction occurs between ICAM-1 and lymphocyte function–associated antigen (LFA)-1. ICAM-1 is a member of the immunoglobulin superfamily, whose other members include TCR, platelet-derived growth factor receptor, MHC molecules, neural cellular adhesion molecule (NCAM), and carcinoembryonic antigen (CEA). ICAM-1 is weakly expressed or absent

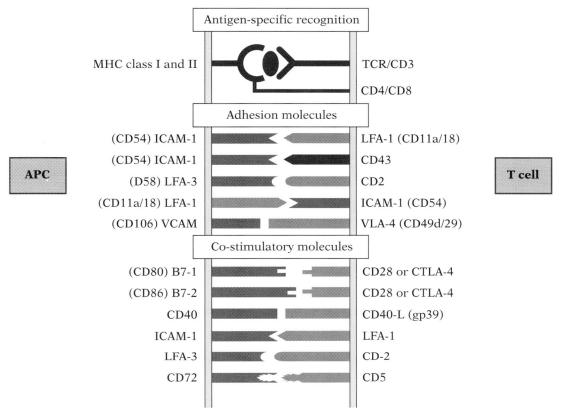

Figure 15-6. Interactions between antigen-presenting cells (APC) and T cells. As illustrated by the nonexhaustive list of molecules shown in this figure, three types of interactions appear to be required to induce a T-cell response. First, intercellular contact is mediated by *adhesion molecules* and their respective ligands. Some of them are lineage restricted (CD2 is exclusively expressed on T cells), while others may be expressed on both cell types involved in the interaction (ICAM-1 and LFA-1 are expressed on both T cells and APCs). Second, the antigen-specific signal is delivered by the interaction between the MHC-peptide complex and the T-cell receptor (TCR). A third type of interaction is required to induce an effective response consisting of cytokine production, cellular proliferation, and effector function. This is provided by costimulatory molecules, such as B7-CD28. Certain adhesion molecules, such as ICAM-1 and LFA-1, also are able to deliver costimulatory signals. ICAM = intercellular adhesion molecule; VCAM = vascular cell adhesion molecule; LFA = leukocyte function–associated antigen; VLA = very late activation antigen.

from low-grade astrocytomas and absent from normal brain, but is strongly expressed by glioma cells in vivo (196). The natural ligand of ICAM-1 is LFA-1, a member of the integrin family present on the surface of lymphocytes infiltrating gliomas. The interaction between ICAM-1 and LFA-1 seems a necessary cell-cell contact for efficient binding between glioma cells and immune cells and for efficient killing mediated by LAK cells and T cells. Indeed, monoclonal antibodies against ICAM-1 and LFA-1 are able to inhibit the binding of TILs or LAK cells to human glioblastoma cells (195). Another finding suggesting the importance of this interaction is that soluble ICAM-1 shed from melanoma cell surface abrogates the non-MHC-restricted as well as the MHC-restricted cytotoxicity mediated by NK cells and T-cell clones, respectively (197,198). The clinical relevance of an ICAM-1–LFA-1 interaction is further substantiated by the observation that mutation of the β2 subunit of

LFA-1 is correlated with fatal recurrent infections in children resulting from a lack of effective lymphocyte adherence (199).

Other adhesion molecules expressed by glioblastoma cells include LFA-3 and CD44 (200). LFA-3 is one of the ligands for the lymphocyte CD2 molecule. CD44 is a broadly distributed cell surface glycoprotein implicated in lymphocyte homing, T-cell activation (201), and adhesion to hyaluronate, a major component of extracellular matrix (202). In fact, several CD44 isoforms are generated by mRNA differential splicing and by cell type–specific glycosylation. Overexpression of certain isoforms has been associated with metastasis in a range of human tumors (203). CD44 is strongly expressed in glioblastomas and weakly expressed in other CNS tumors and normal brain. More importantly, glioblastomas express splice variants that are not detected in meningiomas, for example (204). Such findings could partly explain the differences in invasive behavior of these tumors. On the other hand, the role of CD44 in attracting and activating T cells in high-grade astrocytomas remains hypothetical, even if CD44 could be implicated in the adhesion between T cells and endothelial cells.

The Role of Adhesion Molecules for the Recruitment of Immune Cells into the CNS

A second key question to address is how adhesion molecules are involved in the recruitment of immune cells from the periphery and their retention within the CNS. While this has yet to be systematically investigated, recent advances in the understanding of leukocyte migration will undoubtedly be instructive (for an excellent review, see (205)). In particular, leukocyte arrest by endothelial cells schematically requires three sequential steps. First, L-selectin (CD62) expressed at the surface of many circulating lymphocytes (although downregulated or shed after T-cell activation) recognizes carbohydrate ligands (namely, glyCAM-1, CD34) on the surface or in the proximity of endothelial cells. Second, T cells and monocytes produce chemokines (e.g., MCP-1, macrophage inflammatory protein (MIP)-1α and -1β, and RANTES (regulated on activation, normal T cell expressed and secreted)), which are 70- to 80-residue polypeptides. Chemokines act by linking membrane receptors coupled to G proteins on endothelial cells. This interaction leads to the third step, the upregulation of various integrin molecules (e.g., LFA-1, vary late activation antigen (VLA)-4) and their subsequent binding with several members of the immunoglobulin family (e.g., ICAM-1, ICAM-3, VCAM).

CNS endothelial cells appear to express all the necessary adhesion molecules to ensure the attraction and arrest of immune cells, even if this has not been assessed functionally in vivo. Three major adhesion molecules are present at the surface of endothelial cells: ICAM-1, VCAM-1, and endothelial-leukocyte adhesion molecule (ELAM)-1. ELAM-1 may partly contribute to the monocyte infiltration observed in glioma. The role of ICAM-1 and VCAM-1 is particularly significant, since their respective ligands, LFA-1 and VLA-4, are expressed by T cells and monocytes infiltrating glioma. Furthermore, MCP-1 is often highly expressed in astrocytic tumors and their cyst fluid, as well as in the cerebrospinal fluid of glioma patients (206). Moreover, it should be noted that MCP-1 is not solely a monocyte chemoattractant, but also a major lymphocyte chemoattractant (205). Together, these observations suggest that the development of glioma induces a series of events that may lead to the migration of mononuclear cells into the CNS and to their adhesion to endothelial cells. It has yet to be established whether lymphocyte homing into the CNS is dependent on expression of particular surface molecules, analogous to the carbohydrate cutaneous lymphocyte-associated antigen (CLA) implicated in skin tropism.

While the mechanisms governing leukocyte traffic through the body have been partly elucidated, much re-

mains to be learned about the cell migration across the endothelium and the regulation of their localization inside specific anatomic compartments. Finally, it is noteworthy that adhesion molecule expression is inducible and may be transient. For example, TNF-α, IL-1β, and IFN-γ enhance ICAM-1 expression, whereas other cytokines also secreted in the environment of gliomas do not (172) (for an excellent review, see (207)). Therefore, as cytokines are also regulated in a very complex network, the studies analyzing the expression of such molecules do not necessarily reflect the subtle dynamics of the in vivo situation.

Costimulatory Molecules

Recent attention has focused on a subgroup of surface molecules called *costimulatory molecules*. Schematically, antigen-specific T-cell clonal activation and expansion require two signals (Fig 15-7). The first signal, which confers the antigen specificity, is delivered by the interaction between the MHC-peptide complex and the TCR. The second signal, which is nonspecific, enables lymphokine secretion, T-cell clonal expansion, and enhancement of effector functions. The absence of a second signal results in the specific unresponsiveness of T cells, a state termed *anergy*. Cumulative data suggest that B7-CD28 interactions play a pivotal role in determining immune reactivity versus anergy (208,209). Two members of the B7 family (B7-1 and B7-2) have been cloned so far (210–212). Both are located on chromosome 3q, and are members of the immunoglobulin superfamily with two immunoglobulin-like domains. Their expression on B cells and professional APCs is enhanced by IFN-γ. B7-1 and B7-2 have probably complementary costimulatory functions, as suggested by the differences of their expression after B-cell activation. Activation of B cells, which do not express either B7-1 or B7-2 in the resting state, induces the expression of B7-2 within 24 hours, whereas B7-1 appears later (213).

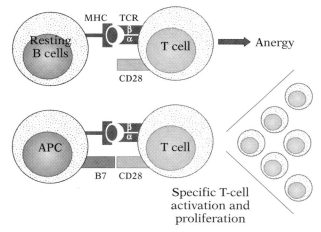

Figure 15-7. B7-mediated costimulatory signal. APC = antigen-presenting cell; TCR = T-cell receptor.

There are two counterreceptors on T cells. A member of the immunoglobulin superfamily, CD28 is a homodimeric glycoprotein, the expression of which is restricted to T cells and plasma cells. A molecule highly homologous to CD28 has been cloned and called *CTLA-4* (214). Interestingly, CTLA-4 binds both B7-1 and B7-2 with higher affinities than does CD28. Furthermore, recent results suggest that the costimulation system is more complex than initially thought. Indeed, it is likely that CD28 mediates stimulatory effects, whereas CTLA-4 may be a negative regulator of T-cell responses. In accordance with this assumption, impressive antitumor responses recently were documented in several animal models when CTLA-4 function was blocked by antibodies (215).

Glioma cells do not constitutively express B7-1 and B7-2 molecules, as demonstrated by Northern blot analysis and immunocytochemistry (216). Moreover, B7 expression is not inducible by IFN-γ. In vivo, glioblastoma cells are also B7 negative. Interestingly, macrophages infiltrating glioma are B7-1/B7-2 negative, whereas those at the tumor boundary remain positive. Therefore, it is unlikely that glioblastoma cells or infiltrating monocytes have the capacities to trigger a CD4 helper T-cell response. Indeed, an anergic state could be induced. Thus, gene therapy designed to simultaneously improve the MHC class II and B7 molecules expression may be a powerful approach.

Future Immunotherapy of Glioma

There is an increasing body of evidence that tumor cells can in theory communicate with immune cells, with or without the help of professional APCs. Such interactions are potentially controlled not only by receptors and ligands pairing during cell-cell contact but also by a plethora of cytokines. The complexity of this surveillance system implies that the equilibrium can be disrupted by a wide series of events. In the last few years, numerous mechanisms explaining how tumor cells escape from the immune system have been identified. Taken together, these advances (which represent only the beginning of a long story) allow us to envisage the development of new therapy strategies, based on selective boosting of the immune system. One must remember that the infiltrative behavior of gliomas is a major impediment to the success of classic cytotoxic approaches (e.g., chemotherapy, irradiation, suicide genes or other gene therapy with prodrug-activating system). Thus, the specific targeting of tumor cells by the immune system is perhaps the only means to achieve their complete elimination. Several approaches can be envisaged. Well-defined tumor antigens could be used as immunogens, as for melanoma patients. Several types of immunization are now in clinical development, such as peptides alone or with adjuvant, recombinant protein, and dendritic cells pulsed with specific peptides. The absence of well-characterized glioma antigens with immunogenic properties to date is a serious obstacle to this approach. On the other hand, gene therapy approaches designed to induce or enhance a specific immune response against gliomas is currently the most promising strategy, because it circumvents the need to identify tumor antigens.

Vaccines with Genetically Modified Tumor Cells

Perhaps because gliomas arise within the CNS, few studies have examined the potential of transfected glioma cells to be used as vaccines. Therefore, we first summarize results obtained in tumors other than gliomas.

Tumors Other Than Gliomas

The development or the progression of a cancer may be related to a large number of defects in immune surveillance. In the last few years, a new concept of therapy has been progressively emerging from the major advances supporting this thesis. Tumor cells can be genetically modified, in order to artificially build ideal interactions between tumor cells and immune cells. The goals of gene transfections into tumor cells are to repair one or several defects in this complex system, and therefore to restore a strong and specific immune response against cancer cells. For example, IFN-γ increases the expression of MHC class I and II molecules, B7 delivers the obligatory costimulatory signal, GM-CSF improves APC abilities, and IL-2 induces a global immune activation (Fig 15-8). It was hypothesized that transfected tumor cells can be used as immunogens after irradiation. Such cells may be optimally immunogenic to induce a systemic response. With this ambitious objective, a large number of different genes have been transfected into tumor cells in various animal models. These in vivo assays are helpful tools to examine a series of critical issues for understanding the biology of cytokine-induced antitumor activity.

First, they allow a fine analysis of the *localized* action of a given cytokine in vivo, therefore recapitulating the physiologic paracrine and autocrine delivery of cytokines much better than the systemic administration of cytokines.

Second, the tumorigenicity of transfected tumor cell lines injected into syngeneic animals can be compared to that of the parental (nontransfected) tumor cell line. Studies of series of different animal models using various tumor cell lines showed that tumor cells transfected with several genes including IL-2, IFN-γ, IL-4, IL-1, IL-3, IL-6, IL-7, TNF-α, IL-12, GM-CSF, and B7 (217–243) were generally vigorously rejected by the host immune response, whereas corresponding parental cell lines grew. To better define the host effector mechanisms taking place in vivo, two types of experiments were undertaken. A given transfected tumor was successively tested in immunocompetent mice and in a panel of genetically immunodeficient mouse strains, such as nude mice (T cell deficient), bg/bg mice (NK cell deficient), or severe combined immunodeficient (SCID) mice (B and T cell deficient). In addition, experiments in immunocompetent hosts were per-

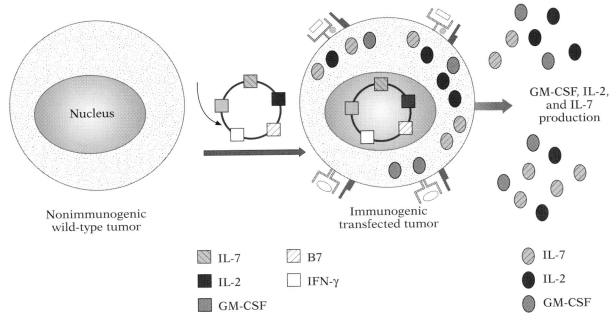

Figure 15-8. Gene transfer into tumor cells. Wild-type human tumors are poorly immunogenic. They can be genetically modified to express a high level of MHC molecules and costimulatory molecules, or to produce adequate amounts of cytokines. IL = interleukin; GM-CSF = granulocyte-macrophage colony-stimulating factor; IFN = interferon.

formed after selective depletion of different cell subsets, such as CD8 T cells, CD4 T cells, NK cells, monocytes, and eosinophils. Thus it was established that tumor cells producing IL-2 or IFN-γ were rejected mainly by CD8 T cells (218,221), while the rejection of those producing IL-4 was mainly mediated by eosinophils (226). In marked contrast to what was observed with the cytokines listed above, the transfection of TGF-β promoted the growth of highly immunogenic tumors that were rejected in their parental state (244,245). This is a very interesting observation in light of the critical role of TGF-β in glioma immunity.

Third, of particular significance to cancer vaccination strategies, is the ability of transfected tumor cells to protect the host against simultaneous or subsequent challenge with parental (or wild-type) tumor. Again, the majority of engineered tumor cells producing IL-2, IFN-γ, IL-4, IL-6, IL-7, TNF-α, IL-12, and GM-CSF or expressing B7 possess such immunostimulatory properties (217,219,221,223,228,229,231,232,234,236). However, in many models, transfected tumor cells were injected only simultaneously with parental tumors, and not a few days or weeks before.

Fourth, to further define the interests of this new treatment approach in a human setting, it is crucial to investigate in animal models whether transfected tumor cells lead to the regression of pre-established parental tumors. Few studies have examined this critical issue carefully. With this objective, tumors transfected with IL-2, GM-CSF, IFN-γ, IL-6, or B7 appear to be effective in some models, albeit only against small tumor burdens (220,223,229,236,243). These data suggest

that the T cells primed locally at the site of injection of transfected tumor cells are able to recirculate and to provide systemic immunity to parental tumor cells.

Finally, few studies reported that the immune response induced by transfected tumors is tumor specific (219,221,242,246). Similarly, the duration of the protection (or the memory) has not been investigated except in rare cases (221). Both these critical elements should be examined in further studies.

Malignant Glioma

The Paradox of Interleukin-2

When IL-2 was administered by intravenous infusion, high serum concentrations of IL-2 were obtained, leading to an overall immune stimulation and severe adverse events. In contrast, the IL-2 concentration at the tumor site was low and probably unable to stimulate T cells. In order to circumvent this difficulty, IL-2 was injected directly to the site of an existing tumor, resulting in low systemic concentrations and high intratumor concentrations. These pioneering studies performed more than 10 years ago showed that lymphocytes, macrophages, neutrophils, and eosinophils migrate into the tumor after local injections of IL-2, leading to its rejection (247,248). Based on these data, the next step was to genetically engineer tumor cells to produce IL-2 and to test their potential to be used as vaccines in animal models (217–220). In most in vivo assays, IL-2–producing tumor cells induced a strong T cell–mediated immune response able to protect against subsequent challenge with wild-type tumor. It is noteworthy that numerous human gene therapy programs using IL-2–transduced tumor cells are ongoing.

In glioma, IL-2 transfection has been less studied, and mostly to better understand how "suicide" gene therapy induces tumor regression. Because suicide gene therapy is not a topic in this review, we only briefly summarize it here. In a rat brain tumor model (9L gliosarcoma), the in vivo retrovirus-mediated transduction of tumor cells with the herpes simplex thymidine kinase (*Hstk*) gene renders these glioma cells sensitive to ganciclovir therapy (249). However, immunodeficient mice are less responsive to this therapy than are immunocompetent animals, suggesting that tumor eradication induced by this genetic modification is partly related to the immune system. Moreover, at least in animal models, complete regression has been achieved despite a low efficiency of gene transfer into brain tumor cells. This hypothesis was examined in another study (250). Surprisingly, the in vivo transfection of the tumor with the IL-2 gene failed to induce an immune response sufficient to influence tumor regression in the brain. This unexpected result may be due to the decreased expression of high-affinity IL-2Rs on glioma lymphocytes (132). An alternative explanation may be considered before drawing definitive conclusions. The IL-2–transduced clones chosen for this study produced high levels of IL-2. In light of recent data, such a choice might explain the poor responses observed in this study. Indeed, in a model of melanoma cells genetically engineered to produce IL-2, the most successful immunizations were achieved with vaccines producing intermediate IL-2 levels, whereas vaccines producing low or high levels of IL-2 were ineffective in protecting against parental tumor challenge (251). The reason for this is not clear. These recent data highlight the importance of the amount of cytokine produced by tumor cells in vaccine protocols.

Interleukin-7

Human IL-7 is a 152–amino acid glycoprotein exhibiting several immunostimulatory properties. Among them, IL-7 induces CD4 and CD8 T-cell proliferation, enhances the cytotoxicity of CTLs and LAK cells, and induces perforin mRNA in the CD8 subset. The immunoregulatory effects of cells engineered to produce IL-7 were analyzed in a murine glioma (ependymoblastoma) model (252), where tumor cells were transfected with an expression vector containing murine IL-7 cDNA. In proportion to the level of IL-7 production, IL-7–transfected glioma cells were vigorously rejected by a CD8 T cell–mediated immune response taking place in C57BL/6 mice. Moreover, the antitumor effect observed was tumor specific, as there was no protection against syngeneic tumors (melanoma B-16 and fibrosarcoma YM-12). These in vivo data show that IL-7 should be investigated further (230). Furthermore, some immunologic effects mediated by IL-7 render this cytokine particularly attractive in the setting of malignant glioma. Indeed, IL-7 increases IL-2R α-chain expression in CD4 cells (253), and inhibits TGF-β1

mRNA expression and its production by murine macrophages (254).

Insulin Growth Factor-I Antisense

Insulin growth factors (IGFs)-I and -II are polypeptides crucially involved in normal growth and development during fetal, neonatal, and pubertal stages. Interacting with a common IGF-I receptor, they are growth factors for a variety of cells including fibroblasts, epithelial cells, smooth muscle cells, osteoclasts, and bone marrow stem cells. Their vital role in development has been highlighted by the observation that IGF-I or IGF-I receptor knock-out mice have profound fetal growth retardation (255). Cumulative data support the view that IGF-I and IGF-II are involved in the normal growth and differentiation of the CNS. IGFs are expressed in the developing brain of rodents and humans (256) and in fetal astrocytes in culture. IGF receptors have been identified in normal human and rat brain tissue. IGF-I stimulates the in vitro growth of fetal brain cells (257), increases the expression of cytoskeletal proteins, and promotes the proliferation and differentiation of normal rat oligodendroglia cells. IGF-II is expressed in abundance in the human adult brain (258). It is now evident that IGF-I may function as a growth factor in a variety of tumors (259). Neuroblastoma, for example, produces IGF-I and IGF-II peptides that promote the growth of these cells in an autocrine manner.

Originally obtained from a *N*-nitrosomethylurea–induced tumor, rat C6 glioma cells express glial fibrillary acidic protein (GFAP), produce IGF-I and IGF-I receptor, and are therefore an appropriate animal model to study the IGF-I–mediated effects on tumor behavior. Indeed, Trojan et al (246) observed that C6 glioma cells lose tumorigenicity when transfected with an episome-based vector encoding antisense IGF-I cDNA, with a mononuclear cell infiltrate of mainly CD8 T cells at the site of tumor cell injection. Furthermore, the subcutaneous injection of IGF-I antisense–transfected C6 cells prevented the development of tumors induced by non-transfected (parental) C6 cells, and pre-established parental glioblastomas regressed after treatment with transfected cells at sites distal to the parental tumor. Finally, cell mixing experiments using different tumor types suggested the antitumor immune response was C6 glioma–specific. Overall, these data suggest that the inhibition of IGF-I expression restores an adequate and specific immune response. However, how long such an antitumor immune response persists (the duration of immunologic memory), and the consequences of CD8 T-cell depletion were not investigated in this study.

The role of IGF-I in rat C6 glioma growth was further examined using an antisense RNA to IGF-I *receptor*, to inhibit the effects of both IGF-I and -II (260). Results similar to those of Trojan et al were obtained. However, given the crucial properties of IGF-I in cell proliferation, it would be surprising that the dramatic effects mediated by an inhibition of IGF-I expression are only consecutive to immunologic mechanisms. Indeed, IGF-I is now considered a survival factor that can inhibit, for example, the apoptosis mediated by c-*myc* (261). A direct effect on cellular transformation and tumor growth was suggested in a model of human melanoma in nude mice, using the same antisense to IGF-I receptor (262). Unfortunately these studies did not provide any data concerning the putative immunologic changes induced by the inhibition of IGF-I.

Only rare reports have explored the immunologic properties of IGF-I; they indicate immunostimulating properties, such as inducing the repopulation of atrophied thymus in diabetic rats (263) or stimulating lymphopoeisis (264). These observations conflict with the dramatic immune effects apparently induced by the blocking of IGF-I expression of rat glioblastoma cells using antisense IGF-I RNA (246,265).

Whatever the mechanisms involved, this approach appears to offer new possibilities for therapy. If antisense treatment specifically inhibits the production of IGF-I, the obligatory condition for the application of this approach would be the production of IGF-I by human glioma. This has yet to be fully assessed in vivo. Alternatively, it cannot be excluded that the impressive results observed in this model were due to nonspecific and unexpected effects of antisense, such as the modulation of surface molecules involved in T-cell activation. Before this strategy is applied to human therapy, further studies are warranted to better define the real effects of IGF-I on in vivo glioma growth, and in parallel, on tumor immunogenicity.

Transforming Growth Factor-β2 Antisense

The critical role of TGF-β2 in glioma T-cell immunosuppression has been summarized already (see T-Cell Function in Glioma Patients). In vitro, the inhibition of TGF-β2 production by glioma cells using antisense technology restores the proliferative and cytolytic functions of autologous lymphocytes (173). No in vivo data have been published until very recently, when a report confirmed the therapeutic potential of this approach (266). Using a TGF-β2 antisense plasmid vector to inhibit TGF-β2 expression of rat 9L gliosarcoma, the authors demonstrated that transfected cells, when inoculated subcutaneously, are highly immunogenic and eradicate established wild-type tumor. Unfortunately, as in most studies using fast-growing experimentally induced tumors, the pre-establishment of the wild-type tumor was only performed a short time (5 days) before the immunization. However, the data convincingly demonstrated that a partial memory response (at 12 weeks) was induced. Finally, lymphocytes isolated ex vivo from the lymph nodes of animals immunized with TGF-β2 antisense–modified tumor cells exhibited significant higher cytotoxicity properties, compared with animals immunized with wild-type or IL-2 gene–modified tumor cells, although the specificity of the lysis was not thoroughly investigated.

Transfection of Oncogenes with Subsequent Immunologic Effects

Surprising data concerning the s-myc gene were recently reported. The s-myc gene belongs to the MYC family, the proteins of which play a pivotal role in cellular proliferation, transformation, and apoptosis. The s-Myc protein inhibits the progression of the glioma cell cycle toward the S phase and induces the apoptosis of tumor cells (267). In in vivo models (rat 9L and C6 gliomas), the coinjection of the s-myc gene linked to a viral promoter with the glioma cell lines prevented the formation of both subcutaneous and brain tumors. Moreover, the inhibitory effect was clearly restricted to the glioma tested, strongly supporting the view that a specific immune response was taking place (268). Such results are reminiscent to those observed with antisense anti–IGF-I. Indeed, the inhibition of a survival factor (i.e., IGF-I) appears to have similar immunostimulant properties as the expression of an apoptotic factor (i.e., s-myc) to mediate a strong antitumor effect. In both cases, further studies are needed to explore the immune mechanisms underlying such effects, and therefore to build an adequate related strategy for treatment in humans.

Other Immune-Based Gene Therapy Approaches

Intratumoral Delivery of Cytokines

Gene therapy may also be designed to administer cytokines within the target tumor, at a place where an immune response should develop. For this purpose, most studies in gliomas have been performed with IL-4. Mainly produced by CD4 T cells, IL-4 exhibits pleiotropic functions, including activation of B cells, enhancement of IgE production in activated B lymphocytes, increase of T-cell proliferation and cytotoxicity, and enhancement of eosinophil proliferation and differentiation. IL-4 may also exert in vitro direct antiproliferative effects against diverse tumor cell lines originating from lung cancer, gastric cancer, renal cell carcinoma, multiple myeloma, and so on (269,270). Its potent antitumor effect in vivo against a wide variety of murine tumor types has been demonstrated in cytokine transfected–tumor assays. In most of these models, the antitumoral effect of IL-4–transfected tumor was maintained in nude mice, suggesting the IL-4 action is T cell independent (269). The ability of IL-4 to mediate an antitumor response against human gliomas was studied in a nude mice model where a human glioma cell line (U87) was mixed with a transfected IL-4–producing plasmocytoma cell line (LT-1) (271). Subcutaneous injection induced a strong recruitment of eosinophils with subsequent growth inhibition. More interestingly, the intracerebral injection by stereotactic surgery of U87 plus IL-4–producing cells resulted in a prolongation of survival, when compared to U87 and IL-4–negative mock cell lines. However, even if this effect was accompanied by a dramatic eosinophil infiltrate, a direct antiproliferative effect mediated by IL-4 cannot be totally excluded because no eosinophil depletion was performed in this study. This interesting approach is not a vaccination strategy, but a tool to obtain a local and long-lasting delivery of IL-4, leading to an in vivo antitumor effect within the CNS. The non-T-cell–dependent nature of this antitumor effect could be an advantage in glioma patients showing several T-cell abnormalities, although whether this benefit will be counteracted by poor memory T-cell induction remains to be clarified.

Transfection of Tumor Suppressor Genes with Subsequent Immunologic Effects

Cytokine expression is under the control of several gene products, for example, oncogenes and tumor suppressor genes. The transfection of wild-type tumor suppressor genes into gliomas as a therapy may be accompanied by significant modification of glioma immunogenicity. For example, the wild-type *p53* represses the expression of genes having a TATA-box promoter sequence (272). Therefore, wild-type *p53* diminishes the transcription of many cytokines, such as TGF-β2, as the TATA box is found in its promoter region (273). In contrast, the mutant p53 protein upregulates the secretion of TGF-β2, and also that of vascular endothelial growth factor (VEGF), which is a crucial angiogenic factor in glioma. It is likely that *p53* and other genes involved in glioma pathogenesis exert numerous other forms of control of cytokine or surface molecule expression. Since *p53* alteration is an early event in glioma pathogenesis, gene therapy of gliomas using wild-type *p53* transfection is intensively explored. This single gene modification might induce a series of favorable events (immunoenhancement and antiangiogenesis) that may synergize to produce a therapeutic effect.

Antibodies Against Fas Receptor

Recently, a new exciting way to treat malignant gliomas emerged from the discovery that these tumors often express Fas/APO-1, whereas normal cells in the CNS do not (274). Fas/APO-1 (CD95) is a transmembrane glycoprotein belonging to the nerve growth factor/TNF receptor superfamily: like TNF receptor 1, it can transduce an apopoptic signal through its cytoplasmic domain. Apoptosis is triggered by the binding of Fas with its natural ligand (FasL) or by cross-linking with anti-Fas antibodies (275). A high proportion of human glioma cell lines are sensitive to Fas/APO-1 antibody–mediated apoptosis in vitro. Others are resistant, either because they do not express Fas protein in an adequate level or because Fas protein is not membrane associated. However, these resistant cell lines have been rendered highly sensitive to Fas/APO-1 antibody–mediated apoptosis by stable transfection of a human Fas cDNA (276). These results open new promising avenues to treat gliomas with Fas antibodies combined with a gene therapy approach designed to increase Fas expression at the surface of target tumor cells.

Conclusions

In the last few years, remarkable insights into the molecular interactions occurring between tumor cells and immune cells have fostered the current excitement in the development of new strategies for treating malignant astrocytomas. There is currently a large body of accumulated data demonstrating that manipulation of the immune system may be an appropriate approach to treat gliomas, albeit their location inside the CNS. However, there are many questions for basic and clinical research to answer before this ambitious objective can be achieved. In the next few years, major efforts will be devoted to identify putative glioma antigens. The ideal finding would be the discovery of a tumor-specific antigenic protein expressed exclusively at the surface of glioma cells, or the identification of an oncogene or tumor suppressor gene product differentially expressed by normal and tumor astrocytes. In any case, the characterization of still hypothetical glioma antigens would provide new avenues in the biologic treatment approaches currently investigated. One of the most promising approaches is the use of genetically modified glioma cells as immunogens. Results of current studies suggest that T cells primed in the periphery may recirculate and reach the CNS to exert their function, at least in certain circumstances. In further studies, the precise mechanisms underlying the migration and the properties of these cells must be characterized better. The interest and perhaps the synergism of different genes transfected into glioma cells will be compared, to determine the best candidates for human therapy (IL-2, IFN-γ, B7, GM-CSF, antisense anti–TGF-β). In addition, other biologic treatment strategies have been elaborated in the last few years. For example, glioma cells may be rendered sensitive to ganciclovir therapy with the transfection of the *Hstk* gene (249). They may also be transfected by the wild-type *p53* gene with subsequent loss of malignant phenotype, and inhibition of neoangiogenesis (279). Finally, the selective expression of Fas/APO-1 by tumoral astrocytes suggests that the induction of glioma cell apoptosis using Fas targeting may be a new promising treatment strategy in glioma.

In conclusion, there is no doubt that further basic and clinical research will improve the understanding of glioma immunobiology, and hopefully, generate more effective treatments against glioma, and therefore ameliorate the current disastrous prognosis of patients suffering from this cancer.

Additional Findings

After the original construction of this chapter, we hypothesised that cell contact–mediated events might also play a role in glioma-induced immunosuppression, and we focused on FasL. FasL, a 40-kd type II membrane protein belonging to the TNF family, is implicated in several biological functions through its interaction with Fas, a member of the TNF receptor (TNFR)/nerve growth factor receptor (NGFR) family. FasL not only is used as a cytotoxic effector mechanism by T cells to induce apoptosis in Fas expressing targets, but is also implicated in clonal downsizing of these cells once they have eliminated antigen (280). More recently, FasL was shown to be expressed by nonlymphoid tissues. Investigators have proposed that expression of FasL by cells of the anterior chamber of the eye and Sertoli cells of the testis maintains a state of immune privilege in their respective organs by eliminating infiltrating Fas+ leukocytes (281,282).

We demonstrated the in vivo expression of FasL by human glioma, and the efficient killing of Fas-bearing cells by glioma lines (human and rodent) in vitro and by human tumor cells ex vivo (283). Furthermore, CD4+ and CD8+ T-cell lines derived from tumor-infiltrating lymphocytes were killed in vitro by autologous glioma cells (284). FasL expression is not restricted to glioma and has been reported in large granular lymphocytic leukemia of T cell or NK origin (285), in colon carcinoma (286), in melanoma (287), and in hepatocellular carcinoma (288). These results show that FasL expression by different tumors including glioma may potentially impede an appropriate immune response. However, whether the expression of FasL inhibits specific T-cell responses and plays a significant role in vivo is still to be explored.

In addition, since glioma potentially express both Fas and FasL, the Fas/FasL interaction may regulate tumor growth by autocrine suicide or "fratricide". This has to be considered in therapeutic strategies designed to exploit the Fas death pathway to directly reduce tumor growth. To minimize the deleterious effects on potentially useful antitumor immune responses, it will be necessary to understand how the components of the Fas pathway are regulated not only in normal immune homeostasis, but also in pathologic situations.

References

1. Mackensen A, Carcelain G, Viel S, et al. Direct evidence to support the immunosurveillance concept in a human regressive melanoma. *J Clin Invest* 1994;93:1397–1402.
2. Jones M, Philip T, Palmer P, et al. The impact of interleukin-2 alone on survival in renal cancer: a multivariate analysis. *Cancer Biother* 1993;8:275–288.
3. Horowitz MM, Gale RP, Sondel PM, et al. Graft-versus-leukemia reactions after bone marrow transplantation. *Blood* 1990;75:555–562.
4. Helg C, Roux E, Beris P, et al. Adoptive immunotherapy for recurrent CML after BMT. *Bone Marrow Transplant* 1993;12:125–129.
5. Papadopoulos EB, Ladanyi M, Emanuel D, et al. Infusions of donor leukocytes to treat Epstein-Barr virus-associated lymphoproliferative disorders after allogeneic bone marrow transplantation. *N Engl J Med* 1994;330:1185–1191.
6. Fabry Z, Raine CS, Hart MN. Nervous tissue as an immune compartment: the dialect of the immune response in the CNS. *Immunol Today* 1994;15:218–224.
7. Fine HA, Dear KGB, Loeffler JS, et al. Meta-analysis of radiation therapy with and without adjuvant chemotherapy for malignant gliomas in adults. *Cancer* 1993;71:2585–2597.
8. Chang CH, Horton J, Schoenfeld D, et al. Comparison of postoperative radiotherapy and combined postoperative radiotherapy and chemotherapy in the multidisciplinary management of malignant gliomas. A joint Radiation Therapy Oncology Group and Eastern Cooperative Oncology Group study. *Cancer* 1983;52:997–1007.
9. Lesser GJ, Grossman S. The chemotherapy of high-grade astrocytomas. *Semin Oncol* 1994;21:220–235.
10. Goldberg AL, Rock KL. Proteolysis, proteasomes and antigen presentation. *Nature* 1992;357:375–379.
11. Monaco JJ. A molecular model of MHC class-I-restricted antigen processing. *Immunol Today* 1992;13:173–178.
12. Rudensky AY, Preston-Hurlburt P, Hong SC, et al. Sequence analysis of peptides bound to MHC class II molecules. *Nature* 1991;353:622–627.
13. Goldberg AL. Functions of the proteasome: the lysis at the end of the tunnel. *Science* 1995;268:522–523.
14. Suh WK, Cohen-Doyle MF, Fruh K, et al. Interaction of MHC class I molecules with the transporter associated with antigen processing. *Science* 1994;264:1322–1325.
15. De la Salle H, Hanau D, Fricker D, et al. Homozygous human TAP peptide transporter mutation in HLA class I deficiency. *Science* 1994;265:237–241.
16. Neefjes JJ, Ploegh HL. Intracellular transport of MHC class II molecules. *Immunol Today* 1992;13:179–184.
17. Kropshofer H, Vogt AB, Stern LJ, Hämmerling GJ. Self-release of CLIP in peptide loading of HLA-DR molecules. *Science* 1995;270:1357–1359.
18. Wade WF, Davoust J, Salamero J, et al. Structural compartmentalization of MHC class II signaling function. *Immunol Today* 1993;14:539–546.
19. Mach B. MHC class II regulation: lessons from a disease. *N Engl J Med* 1995;332:120–122.
20. Steimle V, Otten LA, Zufferey M, Mach B. Complementation cloning of an MHC class II transactivator mutated in hereditary MHC class II deficiency (or bare lymphocyte syndrome). *Cell* 1993;75:135–146.
21. Steimle V, Siegrist CA, Mottet A, et al. Regulation of MHC class II expression by interferon-gamma mediated by the transactivator gene CIITA. *Science* 1994;265:106–109.
22. Reith W, Siegrist CA, Durand B, et al. Function of major histocompatibility complex class II promoters requires cooperative binding between factors RFX and NF-Y. *Proc Natl Acad Sci USA* 1994;91:554–558.
23. Siegrist CA, Martinez-Soria E, Kern I, Mach B. A novel antigen-processing-defective phenotype in major histocompatibility complex class II-positive CIITA transfectants is corrected by interferon-gamma. *J Exp Med* 1995;182:1793–1799.
24. Caux C, Liu YJ, Banchereau J. Recent advances in the study of dendritic cells and follicular dendritic cells. *Immunol Today* 1995;16:2–4.
25. Romani N, Gruner S, Brang D, et al. Proliferating dendritic cell progenitors in human blood. *J Exp Med* 1994;180:83–93.
26. Galy A, Travis M, Cen D, Chen B. Human T, B, natural killer, and dendritic cells arise from a common bone marrow progenitor cell subset. *Immunity* 1995;3:459–473.
27. Lenz A, Heine M, Schuler G, Romani N. Human and murine dermis contain dendritic cells: isolation by means of a novel method and phenotypical and functional characterization. *J Clin Invest* 1993;92:2587–2596.
28. Kosco-Vilbois MH, Gray D, Scheidegger D, Julius M. Follicular dendritic cells help resting B cells to become effective antigen-presenting cells: induction of B7/BB1 and upregulation of major histocompatibility complex class II molecules. *J Exp Med* 1993;178:2055–2066.
29. Zitvogel L, Mayordomo JI, Tjandrawan T, et al. Therapy of murine tumors with tumor peptide-pulsed dendritic cells: dependence on T cells, B7 costimulation, and T

helper cell 1-associated cytokines. *J Exp Med* 1996;183: 87–97.

30. Meuer SC, Fitzgerald KA, Hussey RE, et al. Clonotypic structures involved in antigen-specific human T cell function. *J Exp Med* 1983;157:705–719.

31. Chien YH, Davis MM. How αβ T-cell receptors see peptide/MHC complexes. *Immunol Today* 1993;14:597–601.

32. Lieber MR. The mechanism of V(D)J recombination: a balance of diversity, specificity, and stability. *Cell* 1992;70:873–876.

33. Lefranc MP. Organization of the human T-cell receptor genes. *Eur Cytokine Netw* 1990;1:121–130.

34. Chothia C, Boswell DR, Lesk AM. The outline structure of the T-cell alpha/beta receptor. *EMBO J* 1988;7:3745–3755.

35. Ferradini L, Roman-Roman S, Azocar J, et al. Analysis of T-cell receptor alpha/beta variability in lymphocytes infiltrating a melanoma metastasis. *Cancer Res* 1992;52: 4649–4654.

36. Roman-Roman S, Ferradini L, Azocar J, et al. Studies on the human T cell receptor alpha/beta variable region genes. I. Identification of 7 additional Valpha subfamilies and 14 Jalpha gene segments. *Eur J Immunol* 1991;21:927–933.

37. Wei S, Charmley P, Robinson MA, Concannon P. The extent of the human germline T cell receptor V beta gene segment repertoire. *Immunogenetics* 1994;40:27–36.

38. Davis MM, Bjorkman PJ. T-cell antigen receptor genes and T-cell recognition. *Nature* 1988;334:395–402.

39. Matis LA. The molecular basis of T cell specificity. *Annu Rev Immunol* 1990;8:65–82.

40. Belldegrun A, Muul LM, Rosenberg SA. Interleukin 2 expanded tumor-infiltrating lymphocytes in human renal cell cancer: isolation, characterization, and antitumor activity. *Cancer Res* 1988;48:206–214.

41. Topalian SL, Muul LM, Solomon D, Rosenberg SA. Expansion of human tumor infiltrating lymphocytes for use in immunotherapy trials. *J Immunol Methods* 1987;102:127–141.

42. Houghton AN. Cancer antigens: immune recognition of self and altered peptides. *J Exp Med* 1994;180:1–4.

43. Cochet M, Pannetier C, Regnault A, et al. Molecular detection and in vivo analysis of the specific T cell response to a protein antigen. *Eur J Immunol* 1992;22:2639–2647.

44. Pannetier C, Cochet M, Darche S, et al. The sizes of the CDR3 hypervariable regions of the murine T-cell receptor β chains vary as a function of the recombined germ-line segments. *Proc Natl Acad Sci USA* 1993;90:4319–4323.

45. Genevee C, Diu A, Nierat J, et al. An experimentally validated panel of sub-family-specific oligonucleotide primers (Vα1-w29/Vβ1-w24) for the study of human T cell receptor variable V gene segment usage by polymerase chain reaction. *Eur J Immunol* 1992;22: 1261–1269.

46. Pannetier C, Even J, Kourilsky P. T cell repertoire diversity and clonal expansions in normal and clinical samples. *Immunol Today* 1995;16:176–180.

47. Even J, Lim A, Puisieux I, et al. T-cell repertoire in healthy and diseased human tissues analysed by T-cell receptor β-chain CDR3 size determination: evidence for oligoclonal expansions in tumours and inflammatory diseases. *Res Immunol* 1995;146:65–80.

48. Dietrich PY, Caignard A, Diu A, et al. Analysis of T cell receptor variability in transplanted patients with human cutaneous acute graft versus host disease. *Blood* 1992;80:2419–2424.

49. Dietrich PY, Caignard A, Lim A, et al. In vivo T-cell clon-

al amplification in human acute graft versus host disease. *Blood* 1994;84:2815–2820.

50. Ferradini L, Mackensen A, Genevee C, et al. Analysis of T cell receptor variability in tumor-infiltrating lymphocytes from a human regressive melanoma. Evidence for in situ T cell clonal expansion. *J Clin Invest* 1993;91:1183–1190.

51. Mackensen A, Ferradini L, Carcelain G, et al. Evidence for in situ amplification of cytotoxic T-lymphocytes with antitumor activity in a human regressive melanoma. *Cancer Res* 1993;53:3569–3573.

52. Caignard A, Dietrich PY, Morand V, et al. Evidence for T-cell clonal expansion in patients with squamous cell carcinoma of the head and neck. *Cancer Res* 1994;54:1292–1297.

53. Farace F, Kremer F, Dietrich PY, et al. T-cell repertoire in patients with B-chronic lymphocytic leukemia: evidence for in vivo T cell clonal expansions. *J Immunol* 1994;153:4281–4290.

54. Caignard A, Guillard M, Gaudin C, et al. In situ demonstration of renal-cell-carcinoma–specific T-cell clones. *Int J Cancer* 1996;66:564–570.

55. Klein G, Sjogren HO, Klein E, Hellstrom KE. Demonstration of resistance against methylcholanthrene-induced sarcomas in the primary autochthonous host. *Cancer Res* 1960;20:1561–1572.

56. Basombrio MA. Search for common antigenicities among twenty-five sarcomas induced by methylcholanthrene. *Cancer Res* 1970;30:2458–2462.

57. Khera KS, Ashkenasi A, Rapp F, Melnick JL. Immunity in hamsters to cells transformed in vitro and in vivo by SV40. Tests for antigenic relationship among the papovaviruses. *J Immunol* 1963;91:604–613.

58. Kripke ML. Antigenicity of murine skin tumors induced by ultraviolet light. *J Natl Cancer Inst* 1974;53:1333–1336.

59. Prehn RT, Main JM. Immunity to methylcholanthrene-induced sarcomas. *J Natl Cancer Inst* 1957;18:769–777.

60. Baldwin RW. Immunity to methylcholanthrene-induced tumors in inbred rats following atrophy and regression of the implanted tumours. *Br J Cancer* 1955;9:652–657.

61. Van der Bruggen P, Traversari C, Van der Eynde B, et al. A gene encoding an antigen recognized by cytolytic T lymphocytes on a human melanoma. *Science* 1991; 254:1643–1647.

62. Traversari C, Van der Bruggen P, Luescher IF, et al. A nonapeptide encoded by human gene MAGE-1 is recognized on HLA-A1 by CTL directed against tumor antigen MZ2-E. *J Exp Med* 1992;176:1453–1457.

63. Gaugler B, Van den Eynde B, Van der Bruggen P, et al. Human gene MAGE-3 codes for an antigen recognized on a melanoma by autologous cytolytic T lymphocytes. *J Exp Med* 1994;179:921–930.

64. Van der Bruggen P, Bastin J, Gajewski T, et al. A peptide encoded by human gene MAGE-3 and presented by HLA-A2 induces cytolytic T lymphocytes that recognize tumor cells expressing MAGE-3. *Eur J Immunol* 1994;24:3038–3043.

65. Boon T. Toward a genetic analysis of tumor rejection antigens. *Adv Cancer Res* 1992;58:177–210.

66. Boon T, Cerottini JC, Van den Eynde B, et al. Tumor antigens recognized by T lymphocytes. *Annu Rev Immunol* 1994;12:337–365.

67. Boon T, Van der Bruggen P. Human tumor antigens recognized by T lymphocytes. *J Exp Med* 1996;183:725–729.

68. Brichard V, Van Pel A, Wölfel T, et al. The tyrosinase gene codes for an antigen recognized by autologous cytolytic

T lymphocytes on HLA-A2 melanomas. *J Exp Med* 1993;178:489–495.

69. Coulie PG, Brichard V, Van Pel A, et al. A new gene coding for a differentiation antigen recognized by autologous cytolytic T lymphocytes on HLA-A2 melanomas. *J Exp Med* 1994;180:35–42.

70. Kawakami Y, Eliyahu S, Sakaguchi K, et al. Identification of the immunodominant peptides of the MART-1 human melanoma antigen recognized by the majority of HLA-A2-restricted tumor infiltrating lymphocytes. *J Exp Med* 1994;180:347–352.

71. Bakker ABH, Schreurs MWJ, de Boer AJ, et al. Melanocyte lineage-specific antigen gp100 is recognized by melanoma-derived tumor-infiltrating lymphocytes. *J Exp Med* 1994;179:1005–1009.

72. Topalian SL, Rivoltini L, Mancini M, et al. Human CD4+ T cells specifically recognize a shared melanoma-associated antigen encoded by the tyrosinase gene. *Proc Natl Acad Sci USA* 1994;91:9461–9465.

73. Chen W, Peace DJ, Rovira DK, et al. T cell immunity to the joining region of p210 bcr-abl protein. *Proc Natl Acad Sci USA* 1992;89:1468–1472.

74. Gambacorti-Passerini C, Grignani F, Arienti F, et al. Human CD4 lymphocytes specifically recognize a peptide representing the fusion region of the hybrid protein pml/RARa present in acute promyelocytic leukemia cells. *Blood* 1993;81:1369–1375.

75. Jung S, Schluesener HJ. Human T lymphocytes recognize a peptide of single point-mutated, oncogenic ras proteins. *J Exp Med* 1991;173:273–276.

76. Gedde-Dahl TI, Fossum B, Eriksen JA, et al. T cell clones specific for p21 ras-derived peptides: characterization of their fine specificity and HLA restriction. *Eur J Immunol* 1993;23:754–760.

77. Fossum B, Gedde-Dahl T, Hansen T, et al. Overlapping epitopes encompassing a point mutation (12 gly-arg) in p21 ras can be recognized by HLA-DR, -DP, and -DQ restricted T cells. *Eur J Immunol* 1993;23:2687–2691.

78. Skipper J, Stauss HJ. Identification of two cytotoxic T lymphocyte-recogized epitopes in the Ras protein. *J Exp Med* 1993;177:1493–1498.

79. Houbiers JGA, Nijman HW, van der Burg SH, et al. In-vitro induction of human cytotoxic T lymphocyte responses against peptides of mutant and wild type p53. *Eur J Immunol* 1993;23:2072–2077.

80. Stuber G, Leder GH, Storkus WJ, et al. Identification of wild type and mutant p53 peptides binding to HLA-A2 assessed by a peptide loading-deficient cell line assay and a novel major histocompatibility complex class I peptide binding assay. *Eur J Immunol* 1994;24:765–768.

81. Yanuck M, Carbone DP, Pendleton CD, et al. A mutant p53 tumor suppressor protein is a target for peptide-induced CD8+ cytotoxic T-cells. *Cancer Res* 1993;53:3257–3261.

82. Noguchi Y, Chen YT, Old LJ. A mouse mutant p53 product recognized by CD4+ and CD8+ T cells. *Proc Natl Acad Sci USA* 1994;91:3171–3175.

83. Davis EJ, Foster TD, Thomas WE. Cellular forms and functions of brain microglia. *Brain Res Bull* 1994;34:73–78.

84. Wucherpfennig KW. Autoimmunity in the central nervous system: mechanisms of antigen presentation and recognition. *Clin Immunol Immunopathol* 1994;72:293–306.

85. Krivit W, Sung JH, Shapiro EG, Lockman L. Microglia: the effector cell for reconstitution of the central nervous system following bone marrow transplantation for lysosomal and peroxisomal storage diseases. *Cell Transplant* 1995;4:385–392.

86. Fabry Z, Waldschmidt MM, Hendrickson D, et al. Adhesion molecules on murine brain microvascular endothelial cells: expression and regulation of ICAM-1 and Lgp 55. *J Neuroimmunol* 1992;36:1–11.

87. Pardridge WM, Yang J, Buciak J, Tourtellotte WW. Human brain microvascular DR-antigen. *J Neurosci Res* 1989;23:337–341.

88. Cserr HF, Knopf PM. Cervical lymphatics, the blood-brain barrier and the immunoreactivity of the brain: a new view. *Immunol Today* 1992;13:507–512.

89. Larsen CP, Steinmann RM, Witmer-Plack M, et al. Migration and maturation of Langerhans cells in skin transplants and explants. *J Exp Med* 1990;172:1483–1493.

90. Austyn JM, Larsen CP. Migration patterns of dendritic leukocytes: implications for transplantation. *Transplantation* 1990;49:1–7.

91. Barker CF, Billingham RE. The role of regional lymphatics in the skin homograft response. *Transplantation* 1967;5:962–966.

92. Macatonia SE, Knight SC, Edwards AJ, et al. Localization of antigen on lymph node dendritic cells after exposure to the contact sensitizer fluorescein isothiocyanate. *J Exp Med* 1987;166:1654–1667.

93. Yamada M, Kakimoto K, Shinbori T, et al. Accessory function of human glioma cells for the induction of CD3-mediated T cell proliferation: a potential role of glial cells in T cell activation in the central nervous system. *J Neuroimmunol* 1992;38:263–273.

94. Kim SU, Moretto G, Shin DH. Expression of Ia antigens on the surface of human oligodendrocytes and astrocytes in culture. *J Neuroimmunol* 1985;10:141–149.

95. Weber F, Meinl E, Aloisi F, et al. Human astrocytes are only partially competent antigen presenting cells: possible implications for lesion development in multiple sclerosis. *Brain* 1994;117:59–69.

96. Däubener W, Zennati SS, Wernet P, et al. Human glioblastoma cell line 86HG39 activates T cells in an antigen specific major histocompatibility complex class II-dependent manner. *J Neuroimmunol* 1992;41:21–28.

97. Lampson LA, Hickey WF. Monoclonal antibody analysis of MHC expression in human brain biopsies: tissue ranging from histologically normal to that showing different levels of glial tumor involvement. *J Immunol* 1986;136:4054–4062.

98. Kuppner MC, van Meir E, Hamou MF, de Tribolet N. Cytokine regulation of intercellular adhesion molecule-1 (ICAM-1) expression on human glioblastoma cells. *Clin Exp Immunol* 1990;81:142–148.

99. Bodmer WF, Browning MJ, Krausa P, et al. Tumor escape from immune response by variation in HLA expression and other mechanisms. *Ann NY Acad Sci* 1993;690:42–49.

100. Maudsley DJ, Pound JD. Modulation of MHC antigen expression by viruses and oncogenes. *Immunol Today* 1991;12:429–431.

101. D'Urso CM, Wang Z, Cao Y, et al. Lack of HLA class I expression by cultured melanoma cells FO-1 due to a defect in $\beta 2m$ gene expression. *J Clin Invest* 1991;87:284–292.

102. Connor ME, Stern PL. Loss of MHC class-I expression in cervical carcinomas. *Int J Cancer* 1990;46:1029–1034.

103. Cromme FV, Meijer CJ, Snijders PJ, et al. Analysis of MHC class I and II expression in relation to presence of HPV genotypes in premalignant and malignant cervical lesions. *Br J Cancer* 1993;67:1372–1380.

104. Restifo NP, Esquivel F, Kawakami Y, et al. Identification of human cancers deficient in antigen processing. *J Exp Med* 1993;177:265–272.

105. Ruiz-Cabello F, Klein E, Garrido F. MHC antigens on human tumors. *Immunol Lett* 1991;29:181–189.

106. Andersson ML, Paabo S, Nilsson T, Peterson PA. Impaired intracellular transport of class I MHC antigens as a possible means for adenoviruses to evade immune surveillance. *Cell* 1985;43:215–222.

107. Paabo S, Sverinsson L, Andersson M, et al. Adenovirus proteins and MHC expression. *Adv Cancer Res* 1989;52:151–163.

108. Browne H, Smith G, Beck S, Minson T. A complex between the MHC class I homologue encoded by human cytomegalovirus and β2-microglobulin. *Nature* 1990;347:770–772.

109. Del Val M, Hengel H, Häcker H, et al. Cytomegalovirus prevents antigen presentation by blocking the transport of peptide-loaded major histocompatibility complex class I molecules into the medial-Golgi compartment. *J Exp Med* 1992;176:729–738.

110. Lassam N, Jay G. Suppression of MHC class I RNA in highly oncogenic cells occurs at the level of transcriptional initiation. *J Immunol* 1989;143:3792–3797.

111. Doyle A, Martin WJ, Funa K, et al. Markedly decreased expression of class I histocompatibility antigens, proteins, and mRNA in human small-cell lung cancer. *J Exp Med* 1985;161:1135–1151.

112. Cromme FV, Airey J, Heemels MT, et al. Loss of transporter protein, encoded by the TAP-1 gene, is highly correlated with loss of HLA expression in cervical carcinomas. *J Exp Med* 1994;179:335–340.

113. Hill A, Jugovic P, York I, et al. Herpes simplex virus turns off the TAP to evade host immunity. *Nature* 1995;375:411–415.

114. Früh K, Ahn K, Djaballah H, et al. A viral inhibitor of peptide transporters for antigen presentation. *Nature* 1995;375:415–418.

115. Paine JT, Hajime H, Yamasaki J, Miyatake S. Immunohistochemical analysis of infiltrating lymphocytes in central nervous system tumors. *Neurosurgery* 1986;18:766–772.

116. Kuppner MC, Hamou MF, de Tribolet N. Immunohistological and functional analyses of lymphoid infiltrates in human glioblastomas. *Cancer Res* 1988;48:6926–6932.

117. Rossi ML, Hughes JT, Esiri MM, et al. Immunohistological study of mononuclear cell infiltrate in malignant glioma. *Acta Neuropathol (Berl)* 1987;74:269–277.

118. Stavrou D, Anzil AP, Weidenbach W. Immunofluorescence study of lymphocytic infiltration in gliomas. Identification of T lymphocytes. *J Neurol Sci* 1977;33:275–282.

119. Brooks WH, Markesbery WR, Gupta GD, et al. Relationship of lymphocyte invasion and survival of brain tumor patients. *Ann Neurol* 1978;4:219–224.

120. Mahaley MS, Brooks WH, Roszman TL, et al. Immunobiology of primary intracranial tumors. Part I. Studies of the cellular and humoral general immune competence of brain-tumor patients. *J Neurosurg* 1977;46:467–476.

121. Brooks WH, Roszman TL, Mahaley MS, Woosley RE. Immunobiology of primary intracranial tumors. II. Analysis of lymphocyte subpopulations in patients with primary brain tumors. *Clin Exp Immunol* 1977;29:61–66.

122. Brooks WH, Roszman TL, Rogers AS. Impairment of rosette-forming T lymphocytes in patients with primary intracranial tumors. *Cancer* 1976;37:1869–1873.

123. Young HF, Sakalas R, Kaplan AM. Inhibition of cell mediated immunity in patients with brain tumors. *Surg Neurol* 1976;5:19–23.

124. Roszman TL, Brooks WH, Elliot LH. Immunobiology of primary intracranial tumors. VI. Suppressor cell function and lectin-binding lymphocyte subpopulations in patients with cerebral tumors. *Cancer* 1982;50:1273–1279.

125. Wood GW, Morantz RA. In vitro reversal of depressed T-lymphocyte function in the peripheral blood of brain tumor patients. *J Natl Cancer Inst* 1982;68:27–33.

126. Miescher S, Whiteside TL, Carrel S, Von Fliedner V. Functional properties of tumor infiltrating and blood lymphocytes in patients with solid tumors: effects of tumor cells and their supernatants on proliferative responses of lymphocytes. *J Immunol* 1986;136:1899–1907.

127. Elliot LH, Brooks WH, Roszman TL. Activation of immunoregulatory lymphocytes obtained from patients with malignant gliomas. *J Neurosurg* 1987;67:231–236.

128. Miescher S, Whiteside TL, de Tribolet N, Von Fliedner V. In situ characterization, clonogenic potential, and antitumor cytolytic activity of T lymphocytes infiltrating human brain cancers. *J Neurosurg* 1988;68:438–448.

129. Sawamura Y, Hosokawa M, Kuppner MC, et al. Antitumor activity and surface phenotypes of human glioma-infiltrating lymphocytes after in vitro expansion in the presence of interleukin-2. *Cancer Res* 1989;49:1843–1849.

130. Miyatake S, Kikuchi H, Iwasaki K, et al. Specific cytotoxic activity of T lymphocyte clones derived from a patient with gliosarcoma. *J Neurosurg* 1988;69:751–759.

131. Dietrich PY, Walker PR, Schnuriger V, et al. T cell receptor analysis reveals significant repertoire selection during in vitro lymphocyte culture. *Int Immunol* 1997 (August), in press.

132. Elliott L, Brooks W, Rozman T. Inability of mitogen-activated lymphocytes obtained from patients with malignant primary intracranial tumors to express high affinity interleukin-2 receptors. *J Clin Invest* 1990;86:80–86.

133. Boussiotis VA, Barber DL, Nakarai T, et al. Prevention of T cell anergy by signaling through the γ chain of the IL-2 receptor. *Science* 1994;266:1039–1042.

134. Stevens SR, Shibaki A, Meunier L, Cooper KD. Suppressor T cell-activating macrophages in ultraviolet-irradiated human skin induce a novel, TGF-β dependent form of T cell activation characterized by deficient IL-2r alpha expression. *J Immunol* 1995;155:5601–5607.

135. Straus DB, Weiss A. Genetic evidence for the involvement of the lck tyrosine kinase in signal transduction through the T cell antigen receptor. *Cell* 1992;70:585–593.

136. Appleby MW, Gross JA, Cooke MP, et al. Defective T cell receptor signaling in mice lacking the thymic isoform of p59^{fyn}. *Cell* 1992;70:751–763.

137. Weiss A, Littman DR. Signal transduction by lymphocyte antigen receptors. *Cell* 1994;76:263–274.

138. Chan AC, Iwashima M, Turck CW, Weiss A. ZAP-70: a 70 kd protein-tyrosine kinase that associates with the TCR ζ chain. *Cell* 1992;71:649–662.

139. Iwashima M, Irving BA, Van Oers NSC, et al. Sequential interactions of the TCR with two distinct cytoplasmic tyrosine kinases. *Science* 1994;263:1136–1139.

140. Mizoguchi H, O'Shea JJ, Longo DL, et al. Alterations in signal transduction molecules in T lymphocytes from tumor-bearing mice. *Science* 1992;258:1795–1797.

141. Travis J. Do tumor-altered T cells depress immune responses? *Cancer Res* 1992;258:1732–1733.

142. Shores EW, Huang K, Tran T, et al. Role of TCR ζ chain in T cell development and selection. *Science* 1994;266: 1047–1050.

143. Loeffler CM, Smyth MJ, Longo DL, et al. Immunoregulation in cancer-bearing hosts: down-regulation of gene expression and cytotoxic function in CD8+ T cells. *J Immunol* 1992;149:949–956.

144. Finke JH, Zea AH, Stanley J, et al. Loss of T-cell receptor ζ chain and p56^{lck} in T-cells infiltrating human renal cell carcinoma. *Cancer Res* 1993;53:5613–5616.

145. Nakagomi H, Petersson M, Magnusson I, et al. Decreased expression of the signal-transducing zeta chains in tumor-infiltrating T cells and NK cells of patients with colorectal carcinoma. *Cancer Res* 1993;53:5610–5612.

146. Aoe T, Okamoto Y, Saito T. Activated macrophages induce structural abnormalities of the T cell receptor-CD3 complex. *J Exp Med* 1995;181:1881–1886.

147. Ghosh P, Sica A, Young HA, et al. Alterations in NFKB/Rel family proteins in splenic T-cells from tumor-bearing mice and reversal following therapy. *Cancer Res* 1994;54:2969–2972.

148. Li X, Liu J, Park JK, et al. T cells from renal cell carcinoma patients exhibit an abnormal pattern of KB-specific DNA-binding activity: a preliminary report. *Cancer Res* 1994;54:5424–5429.

149. Kang SM, Tran AC, Grilli M, Leonardo MJ. NF-κB subunit regulation in nontransformed CD4+ T lymphocytes. *Science* 1992;256:1452–1456.

150. Levey DL, Srivastava PK. T cells from late tumor-bearing mice express normal levels of p56^{lck}, p59^{fyn}, ZAP-70, and CD3ζ despite suppressed cytolytic activity. *J Exp Med* 1995;182:1029–1036.

151. Weiss A, Koretzky G, Schatzman R, Kadlecek T. Functional activation of the T-cell antigen receptor induces tyrosine phosphorylation of phospholipase C-γ1. *Proc Natl Acad Sci USA* 1991;88:5484–5488.

152. Nolan GP, Ghosh S, Liou HC, et al. DNA binding and IkB inhibition of the cloned p65 subunit of NF-κB, a rel-related peptide. *Cell* 1991;64:961–969.

153. Evavold BD, Sloan-Lancaster J, Allen PM. Tickling the TCR: selective T-cell functions stimulated by altered peptide ligands. *Immunol Today* 1993;14:602–609.

154. Sloan-Lancaster J, Evavold BD, Allen PM. Induction of T-cell anergy by altered T-cell-receptor ligand on live antigen-presenting cells. *Nature* 1993;363:156–159.

155. Sloan-Lancaster J, Shaw AS, Rothbard JB, Allen PM. Partial T cell signaling: altered phospho-ζ and lack of Zap70 recruitment in APL-induced T cell anergy. *Cell* 1994;79:913–922.

156. Hogquist KA, Jameson SC, Heath WR, et al. T cell receptor antagonist peptides induce positive selection. *Cell* 1994;76:17–27.

157. Marx J. The T cell receptor begins to reveal its many facets. *Science* 1995;267:459–460.

158. Madrenas J, Wange RL, Wang JL, et al. ζ Phosphorylation without ZAP-70 activation induced by TCR antagonists or partial agonists. *Science* 1995;267:515–518.

159. Isakov N, Wange RL, Burgess WH, et al. ZAP-70 binding specificity to T cell receptor tyrosine-based activation motifs: the tandem SH2 domains of ZAP-70 bind distinct tyrosine-based activation motifs with varying affinity. *J Exp Med* 1995;181:375–380.

160. Klenerman P, Rowland-Jones S, McAdam S, et al. Cytotoxic T-cell activity antagonized by naturally occuring HIV-1 gag variants. *Nature* 1994;369:403–407.

161. Bertoletti A, Sette A, Chisari FV, et al. Natural variants of cytotoxic epitopes are T-cell receptor antagonists for antiviral cytotoxic T-cells. *Nature* 1994;369:407–410.

162. Ellis JRM, Keating PJ, Baird J, et al. The association of an HPV16 oncogene variant with HLA-B7 has implications for vaccine design in cervical cancer. *Nat Med* 1995;1:464–470.

163. Elliott LH, Brooks WH, Roszman TL. Suppression of high affinity IL-2 receptors on mitogen activated lymphocytes by glioma-derived suppressor factor. *J Neurooncol* 1992;14:1–7.

164. Fontana A, Hengartner H, de Tribolet N, Weber E. Glioblastoma cells release interleukin-1 and factors inhibiting interleukin-2-mediated effects. *J Immunol* 1984;132:1837–1844.

165. Border WA, Noble NA. Transforming growth factor β in tissue fibrosis. *N Engl J Med* 1994;331:1286–1292.

166. Couldwell WT, Yong VW, Dore-Duffy P, et al. Production of soluble autocrine inhibitory factors by human glioma cell lines. *J Neurol Sci* 1992;110:178–185.

167. Bodmer S, Strommer K, Frei K, et al. Immunosuppression and transforming growth factor β in glioblastoma. Preferential production of transforming growth factor-beta 2. *J Immunol* 1989;143:3222–3229.

168. Huber D, Philipp J, Fontana A. Protease inhibitors interfere with the transforming growth factor-β-dependent but not the transforming growth factor-β-independent pathway of tumor cell-mediated immunosuppression. *J Immunol* 1992;148:277–284.

169. Maxwell M, Galanopoulos T, Neville-Golden J, Antoniades HN. Effect of the expression of transforming growth factor-β2 in primary human glioblastomas on immunosuppression and loss of immune surveillance. *J Neurosurg* 1992;76:799–804.

170. Kehrl JH, Wakefield LM, Roberts AB, et al. Production of transforming growth factor β by human T lymphocytes and its potential role in the regulation of T cell growth. *J Exp Med* 1986;163:1037–1050.

171. Zuber P, Kuppner MC, de Tribolet N. Transforming growth factor-β2 down-regulates HLA-DR antigen expression on human malignant glioma cells. *Eur J Immunol* 1988;18:1623–1626.

172. Schneider J, Hofman FM, Apuzzo ML, Hinton DR. Cytokines and immunoregulatory molecules in malignant glial neoplams. *J Neurosurg* 1992;77:265–273.

173. Jachimczak P, Bogdahn U, Schneider J, et al. The effect of TGF-β2-specific phosphorothioate-anti-sense oligodeoxynucleotides in reversing immunosuppression in malignant glioma. *J Neurosurg* 1993;78:944–951.

174. Mosmann TR. Properties and functions of interleukin-10. *Adv Immunol* 1994;56:1–26.

175. Romagnani S. Human TH1 and TH2 subsets: "eppur si muove." *Eur Cytokine Netw* 1994;5:7–12.

176. Liu Y, Wei SH, Ho AS, et al. Expression cloning and characterization of a human IL-10 receptor. *J Immunol* 1994;152:1821–1829.

177. Nitta T, Hishii M, Sato K, Okumura K. Selective expression of interleukin-10 gene within glioblastoma multiforme. *Brain Res* 1994;649:122–128.

178. Merlo A, Juretic A, Zuber M, et al. Cytokine gene expression in primary brain tumours, metastases and meningiomas suggests specific transcription patterns. *Eur J Cancer* 1993;29A:2118–2125.

179. Hishii M, Nitta T, Ishida H, et al. Human glioma-derived interleukin-10 inhibits antitumor immune responses in vitro. *Neurosurgery* 1995;37:1160–1167.

180. Fontana A, Kristensen F, Dubs R, et al. Production of prostaglandin and interleukin-1 like factor by culture astrocytes in C6 glioma cells. *J Immunol* 1982;129: 2413–2419.

181. Sawamura Y, Diserens AC, de Tribolet N. In vitro

prostaglandin E2 production by glioblastoma cells and its effect on interleukin-2 activation of oncolytic lymphocytes. *J Neurooncol* 1990;9:125–130.

182. Phipps RP, Stein SH, Roper RL. A new view of prostaglandin E regulation of the immune response. *Immunol Today* 1991;12:349–352.

183. Tada M, Diserens AC, Desbaillet I, et al. Production of interleukin-1 receptor antagonist by human glioblastoma cells in vitro and in vivo. *J Neuroimmunol* 1994;50:187–194.

184. Gauthier T, Hamou MF, Monod L, et al. Expression and release of interleukin-1 by human glioblastoma cells in vitro and in vivo. *Acta Neurochir (Wien)* 1993;121:199–205.

185. Tada M, Diserens AC, Desbaillet I, de Tribolet N. Analysis of cytokine receptor messenger RNA expression in human glioblastoma cells and normal astrocytes by reverse-transcription polymerase chain reaction. *J Neurosurg* 1994;80:1063–1073.

186. McHeyzer-Williams MG, Altman JD, Davis MM. Tracking antigen-specific helper T cell responses. *Curr Opin Immunol* 1996;8:278–284.

187. Ebato M, Nitta T, Yagita H, et al. Skewed distribution of TCR Va 7-bearing T cells within tumor infiltrating lymphocytes of HLA-A24(9) positive patients with malignant glioma. *Immunol Lett* 1994;39:53–64.

188. Ebato M, Nitta T, Yagita H, et al. Shared amino acid sequences in the NDβN and Nα regions of the T cell receptors of tumor-infiltrating lymphocytes within malignant glioma. *Eur J Immunol* 1994;24:2987–2992.

189. Sahin U, Türeci Ö, Schmitt H, et al. Human neoplasms elicit multiple specific immune responses in the autologous host. *Proc Natl Acad Sci USA* 1995;92:11810–11813.

190. Harding CV, Unanue ER. Quantitation of antigen-presenting cell MHC class II/peptide complexes necessary for T-cell stimulation. *Nature* 1990;346:574–576.

191. Pardoll DM. Tumour antigens: a new look for the 1990s. *Nature* 1994;369:357–358.

192. Libermann TA, Nusbaum HR, Razon N, et al. Amplification, enhanced expression and possible rearrangement of EGF receptor gene in primary human brain tumors of glial origin. *Nature* 1985;313:144–147.

193. Wong AJ, Zoltick PW, Moscatello DK. The molecular biology and molecular genetics of astrocytic neoplams. *Semin Oncol* 1994;21:139–148.

194. Pignatelli M, Vessey CJ. Adhesion molecules: novel molecular tools in tumor pathology. *Hum Pathol* 1994;25:849–856.

195. Couldwell WT, de Tribolet N, Antel JP, et al. Adhesion molecules and malignant gliomas: implications for tumorigenesis. *J Neurosurg* 1992;76:782–791.

196. Kuppner MC, Hamou MF, de Tribolet N. Activation and adhesion molecule expression on lymphoid infiltrates in human glioblastomas. *J Neuroimmunol* 1990;29:229–238.

197. Becker JC, Dummer R, Hartmann AA, et al. Shedding of ICAM-1 from human melanoma cell lines induced by IFN-gamma and tumor necrosis factor-alpha. Functional consequences on cell-mediated cytotoxicity. *J Immunol* 1991;147:4398–4401.

198. Becker JC, Termeer C, Schmidt RE, Brocker EB. Soluble intercellular adhesion molecule-1 inhibits MHC-restricted specific T cell/tumor interaction. *J Immunol* 1993;151:7224–7232.

199. Springer TA. Adhesion receptors of the immune system. *Nature* 1990;346:425–434.

200. Kuppner MC, Van Meir E, Gauthier T, et al. Differential expression of the CD44 molecule in human brain tumours. *Int J Cancer* 1992;50:572–577.

201. Huet S, Groux H, Caillou B, et al. CD44 contributes to T cell activation. *J Immunol* 1989;143:798–803.

202. Bartolazzi A, Peach R, Aruffo A, Stamenkovic I. Interaction between CD44 and hyaluronate is directly implicated in the regulation of tumor development. *J Exp Med* 1994;180:53–66.

203. Matsumara Y, Tarin D. Significance of CD44 gene products for cancer diagnosis and disease evaluation. *Lancet* 1992;340:1053–1058.

204. Li H, Hamou MF, de Tribolet N, et al. Variant CD44 adhesion molecules are expressed in human brain metastases but not in glioblastomas. *Cancer Res* 1993;53:5345–5349.

205. Springer TA. Traffic signals for lymphocyte recirculation and leukocyte emigration: the multistep paradigm. *Cell* 1994;76:301–314.

206. Desbaillets I, Tada M, de Tribolet N, et al. Human astrocytomas and glioblastomas express MCP-1 in vivo and in vitro. *Int J Cancer* 1994;58:240–247.

207. Van Meir E. Cytokines and tumors of the central nervous system. *Glia* 1995;15:264–288.

208. Guinan EC, Gribben JG, Boussiotis VA, et al. Pivotal role of the B7:CD28 pathway in transplantation tolerance and tumor immunity. *Blood* 1994;84:3261–3282.

209. June CH, Bluestone JA, Nadler LM, Thompson CB. The B7 and CD28 receptor families. *Immunol Today* 1994;15:321–325.

210. Hathcock KS, Laszlo G, Dickler HB, et al. Identification of an alternative CTLA-4 ligand costimulatory for T cell activation. *Science* 1993;262:905–911.

211. Azuma M, Ito D, Yagita H, et al. B70 antigen is a second ligand for CTLA-4 and CD28. *Nature* 1993;366:76–79.

212. Freeman GJ, Gribben JG, Boussiotis VA, et al. Cloning of B7-2: a CTLA-4 counter-receptor that costimulates human T cell proliferation. *Science* 1993;262:844–845.

213. Boussiotis VA, Freeman GJ, Gribben JG, et al. Activated human B lymphocytes express three CTLA-4 counter-receptors that costimulate T-cell activation. *Proc Natl Acad Sci USA* 1993;90:11059–11063.

214. Wu Y, Guo Y, Liu Y. A major costimulatory molecule on antigen-presenting cells, CTLA4 ligand A, is distinct from B7. *J Exp Med* 1993;178:1789–1793.

215. Leach DR, Krummel MF, Allison JP. Enhancement of antitumor immunity by CTLA-4 blockade. *Science* 1996;271:1734–1736.

216. Tada M, Diserens AC, Hamou MF, et al. Suppressed expression of T-cell costimulatory molecules B7 and B70 in human glioblastomas in vivo. In: Nagai M, ed. *Brain tumor research and therapy*. Tokyo: Springer, 1996:327–337.

217. Bannerji R, Arroyo CD, Cordon-Cardo C, Gilboa E. The role of IL-2 secreted from genetically modified tumor cells in the establishment of antitumor immunity. *J Immunol* 1994;152:2324–2332.

218. Fearon ER, Pardoll DM, Itaya T, et al. Interleukin-2 production by tumor cells bypasses T helper function in the generation of an antitumor response. *Cell* 1990;60:397–403.

219. Gansbacher B, Zier K, Daniels B, et al. Interleukin-2 gene transfer into tumor cells abrogates tumorigenicity and induces protective immunity. *J Exp Med* 1990;172:1217–1224.

220. Connor J, Bannerji R, Saito S, et al. Regression of bladder tumors in mice treated with interleukin-2 gene modified tumor cells. *J Exp Med* 1993;177:1127–1134.

221. Gansbacher B, Bannerji R, Daniels B, et al. Retroviral

vector-mediated γ-interferon gene transfer into tumor cells generates potent and long lasting antitumor immunity. *Cancer Res* 1990;50:7820–7825.

222. Watanabe Y, Kuribayashi K, Miyatake S, et al. Exogenous expression of mouse interferon γ cDNA in mouse neuroblastoma C1300 cells results in reduced tumorigenicity by augmented anti-tumor immunity. *Proc Natl Acad Sci USA* 1989;86:9456–9460.

223. Porgador A, Bannerji R, Watanabe Y, et al. Antimetastatic vaccination of tumor-bearing mice with two types of IFN-γ gene inserted tumor cells. *J Immunol* 1993;150:1458–1470.

224. Golumbek PT, Lazenby AJ, Levitsky HI, et al. Treatment of established renal cancer by tumor cells engineered to secrete interleukin-4. *Science* 1991;254:713–716.

225. Tepper RI, Pattengale PK, Leder P. Murine interleukin-4 displays potent antitumor activity in vivo. *Cell* 1989;57:503–512.

226. Tepper RI, Coffmann RL, Leder P. An eosinophil-dependent mechanism for the antitumor effect of IL-4. *Science* 1992;257:548–551.

227. Tepper RI, Mule JJ. Experimental and clinical studies of cytokine gene-modified tumor cells. *Hum Gene Ther* 1994;5:153–164.

228. Mullen CA, Coale M, Levy AT, et al. Fibrosarcoma cells transduced with the IL-6 gene exhibit reduced tumorigenicity, increased immunogenicity and decreased metastatic potential. *Cancer Res* 1992;52:6020–6024.

229. Porgador A, Tzehoval E, Katz A, et al. Interleukin-6 gene transfection into Lewis lung carcinoma tumor cells suppresses the malignant phenotype and confers immunotherapeutic competence against parental metastatic cells. *Cancer Res* 1992;52:3679–3686.

230. Hock H, Dorsch M, Diamanstein T, Blankenstein T. Interleukin-7 induces CD4+ T cell-dependent tumor rejection. *J Exp Med* 1991;174:1291–1298.

231. McBride WH, Thacker JD, Comora S, et al. Genetic modification of a murine fibrosarcoma to produce interleukin-7 stimulates host cell infiltration and tumor immunity. *Cancer Res* 1992;52:3931–3937.

232. Asher AL, Mule JJ, Kasid A, et al. Murine tumor cells transduced with the gene for tumor necrosis factor-α. *J Immunol* 1991;146:3227–3234.

233. Blankenstein T, Qin Z, Uberla K, et al. Tumor suppression after tumor cell-targeted tumor necrosis-α gene transfer. *J Exp Med* 1991;173:1047–1052.

234. Tahara H, Zeh HJ, Storkus WJ, et al. Fibroblasts genetically engineered to secrete interleukin 12 can suppress tumor growth and induce antitumor immunity to a murine melanoma in vivo. *Cancer Res* 1994;54:182–189.

235. Colombo MP, Ferrari G, Stoppacciaro A, et al. Granulocyte-colony stimulating factor gene suppresses tumorigenicity of a murine adenocarcinoma in vivo. *J Exp Med* 1991;173:889–897.

236. Dranoff G, Jaffee E, Lazenby A, et al. Vaccination with irradiated tumor cells engineered to secrete murine granulocyte-macrophage colony-stimulating factor stimulates potent, specific, and long-lasting anti-tumor immunity. *Proc Natl Acad Sci USA* 1993;90:3539–3543.

237. Baskar S, Ostrand-Rosenberg S, Nabavi N, et al. Constitutive expression of B7 restores immunogenicity of tumor cells expressing truncated MHC class II molecules. *Proc Natl Acad Sci USA* 1993;90:5687–5690.

238. Chen L, Ashe S, Brady W, et al. Costimulation of antitumor immunity by the B7 counterreceptor for the T lymphocyte molecules CD28 and CTLA4. *Cell* 1992;71:1093–1102.

239. Townsend S, Allison J. Tumor rejection after direct cos-timulation of CD8+ T cells by B7-transfected melanoma cells. *Science* 1993;259:368–370.

240. Chen L, McGowan P, Ashe S, et al. Tumor immunogenicity determines the effect of B7 costimulation on T cell-mediated tumor immunity. *J Exp Med* 1994;179:523–532.

241. Amato I. A stimulating new approach to cancer treatment. *Science* 1993;259:310–311.

242. Chen L, Linsley PS, Hellström KE. Costimuation of T cells for tumor immunity. *Immunol Today* 1993;14:483–486.

243. Matulonis UA, Dosio C, Lamont C, et al. Role of B7-1 in mediating an immune response to myeloid leukemia cells. *Blood* 1995;85:2507–2515.

244. Chang HL, Gillett N, Figari I, et al. Increased transforming growth factor β expression inhibits cell proliferation in vitro, yet increases tumorigenicity and tumor growth of Meth A sarcoma cells. *Cancer Res* 1993;53:4391–4398.

245. Torre-Amione G, Beauchamp RD, Koeppen H, et al. A highly immunogenic tumor transfected with a murine transforming growth factor β1 cDNA escapes immune surveillance. *Proc Natl Acad Sci USA* 1990;87:1486–1490.

246. Trojan J, Johnson TR, Rudin SD, et al. Treatment and prevention of rat glioblastoma by immunogenic C6 cells expressing antisense insulin-like growth factor I RNA. *Science* 1993;259:94–96.

247. Forni G, Giovarelli M, Santoni A. Lymphokine-activated tumor inhibition in vivo. I. The local administration of interleukin-2 triggers nonreactive lymphocytes from tumor bearing mice to inhibit tumor growth in vivo. *J Immunol* 1985;134:1305–1312.

248. Forni G, Fujiwara H, Martino F, et al. Helper strategy in tumor immunology: expansion of helper lymphocytes and utilization of helper lymphokines for experimental and clinical immunotherapy. *Cancer Metastasis Rev* 1988;7:289–309.

249. Culver KW, Ram Z, Wallbridge S, et al. In vivo gene transfer with retroviral vector-producer cells for treatment of experimental brain tumors. *Science* 1992;256:1550–1552.

250. Ram Z, Walbridge S, Heiss JD, et al. In vivo transfer of the human interleukin-2 gene: negative tumoricidal results in experimental brain tumors. *J Neurosurg* 1994;80:535–540.

251. Schmidt W, Schweighoffer T, Herbst E, et al. Cancer vaccines: the interleukin 2 dosage effect. *Proc Natl Acad Sci USA* 1995;92:4711–4714.

252. Aoki T, Tashiro K, Miyatake SI, et al. Expression of murine interleukin 7 in a murine glioma cell line results in reduced tumorigenicity in vivo. *Proc Natl Acad Sci USA* 1992;89:3850–3854.

253. Armitage RJ, Namen AE, Sassenfeld HM, Grabstein KH. Regulation of human T cell proliferated by IL-7. *J Immunol* 1990;144:938–941.

254. Dubinett SM, Huang M, Dhanani S, et al. Down-regulation of macrophage transforming growth factor-beta messenger RNA expression by IL-7. *J Immunol* 1993;151:6670–6680.

255. Liu JP, Baker J, Perkins AS, et al. Mice carrying null mutations of the genes encoding insulin-like growth factor I (IGF-I) and type 1 IGF receptor. *Cell* 1993;75:59–72.

256. Chernausek SD. Insulin-like growth factor-I (IGF-I) production by astroglial cells: regulation and importance for epidermal growth factor-induced cell replication. *J Neurosci Res* 1993;34:189–197.

257. Lenoir D, Honegger P. Insulin-like growth factor I (IGF

I) stimulates DNA synthesis in fetal rat brain culture. *Brain Res* 1983;283:205–213.

258. Sandberg AC, Engberg C, Lake M, et al. The expression of insulin-like growth factor I and insulin-like growth factor II genes in the human fetal and adult brain and in gliomas. *Neurosci Lett* 1988;93:114–119.

259. LeRoith D, Baserga R, Helman L, Roberts CT. Insulin-like growth factors and cancer. *Ann Intern Med* 1995;122:54–59.

260. Resnicoff M, Sell C, Rubini M, et al. Rat glioblastoma cells expressing an antisense RNA to the insulin-like growth factor-1 (IGF-1) receptor are nontumorigenic and induce regression of wild-type tumors. *Cancer Res* 1994;54:2218–2222.

261. Harrington EA, Bennett MR, Fanidi A, Evan G. c-myc Induced apoptosis fibroblasts is inhibited by specific cytokines. *EMBO J* 1994;13:3286–3295.

262. Resnicoff M, Coppola D, Sell C, et al. Growth inhibition of human melanoma cells in nude mice by antisense strategies to the type 1 insulin-like growth factor receptor. *Cancer Res* 1994;54:4848–4850.

263. Binz K, Joller P, Froesh P, et al. Repopulation of the atrophied thymus in diabetic rats by insulin-like growth factor I. *Proc Natl Acad Sci USA* 1990;87:3690–3694.

264. Clark R, Strasser J, McCabe S, et al. Insulin-like growth factor-1 stimulation of lymphopoiesis. *J Clin Invest* 1993;92:540–548.

265. Trojan J, Blossey BK, Jonson TR, et al. Loss of tumorigenicity of rat glioblastoma directed by episome-based antisense cDNA transcription of insulin-like growth factor 1. *Proc Natl. Acad Sci USA* 1992;89:4874–4878.

266. Fakhrai H, Dorigo O, Shawler DL, et al. Eradication of established intracranial rat gliomas by transforming growth factor β antisense gene therapy. *Proc Natl Acad Sci USA* 1996;93:2909–2914.

267. Asai A, Miyagi Y, Sugiyama A, et al. The s-Myc protein having the ability to induce apoptosis is selectively expressed in rat embryo chondrocytes. *Oncogene* 1994;9:2345–2352.

268. Asai A, Miyagi Y, Hashimoto H, et al. Modulation of tumor immunogenicity of rat glioma cells by s-Myc expression: eradication of rat gliomas in vivo. *Cell Growth Differ* 1994;5:1153–1158.

269. Tepper RI. The anti-tumour and pro-inflammatory actions of IL-4. *Res Immunol* 1993;144:633–637.

270. Romagnani S. Regulatory role of IL-4 and other cytokines in the function and the development of human T-cell clones. *Res Immunol* 1993;144:625–628.

271. Yu JS, Wei MX, Chiocca EA, et al. Treatment of glioma by engineered interleukin 4-secreting cells. *Cancer Res* 1993;53:3125–3128.

272. Mack DH, Vartilar J, Pipas JM, et al. Specific repression of TATA-mediated but not initiator-mediated transcription by wild-type p53. *Nature* 1993;363:281–283.

273. McCartney-Francis NL, Wahl SM. Transforming growth factor-β: a matter of life and death. *J Leukoc Biol* 1994;55:401–409.

274. Weller M, Frei K, Groscurth P, et al. Anti-Fas/APO-1 antibody-mediated apoptosis of cultured human glioma cells. *J Clin Invest* 1994;94:954–964.

275. Lynch DH, Ramsdell F, Alderson MR. Fas and FasL in the homeostatic regulation of immune responses. *Immunol Today* 1995;16:569–574.

276. Weller M, Malipiero U, Rensing-Ehl A, et al. Fas/APO-1 gene transfer for human malignant glioma. *Cancer Res* 1995;55:2936–2944.

277. Ward SG, June CH, Olive D. PI 3-kinase: a pivotal pathway in T-cell activation? *Immunol Today* 1996;17:187–197.

278. Zier K, Gansbacher B, Salvadori S. Preventing abnormalities in signal transduction of T cells in cancer: the promise of cytokine gene therapy. *Immunol Today* 1996;17:39–45.

279. Van Meir EG, Polverini PJ, Chazin VR, et al. Release of an inhibitor of angiogenesis upon induction of wild type p53 expression in glioblastoma cells. *Nat Genet* 1994;8:171–176.

280. Lynch DH, Ramsdell F, Alderson MR. Fas and FasL in the homeostatic regulation of immune responses. *Immunol Today* 1995;16:569–574.

281. Griffith TS, Brunner T, Fletcher SM, et al. Fas ligand-induced apoptosis as a mechanism of immune privilege. *Science* 1995;270:1189–1192.

282. Bellgrau D, Gold D, Selawry H, et al. A role for CD95 ligand in preventing graft rejection. *Nature* 1995;377:630–632.

283. Saas P, Walker PR, Hahne M, et al. Fas Ligand expression by astrocytoma in vivo: maintaining immune privilege in the brain? *J Clin Invest* 1997;99:1173–1178.

284. Walker PR, Saas P, Dietrich P-Y. The role of Fas ligand (CD95L) in immune escape: the tumor cell strikes back. *J Immunol* 1997 (May), in press.

285. Tanaka M, Suda T, Haze K, et al. Fas ligand in human serum. *Nat Med* 1996;2:317–322.

286. O'Connell J, O'Sullivan GC, Collins JK, Shanahan F. The Fas counterattack: Fas-mediated T cell killing by colon cancer cells expressing Fas ligand. *J Exp Med* 1996;184:1075–1082.

287. Hahne M, Rimoldi D, Schröter M, et al. Melanoma cell expression of Fas(Apo-1/CD95) ligand: Implications for tumor immune escape. *Science* 1996;274:1363–1366.

288. Strand S, Hofmann WJ, Hug H, et al. Lymphocyte apoptosis induced by CD95 (Apo-1/Fas) ligand-expressing tumor cells—a mechanism of immune evasion? *Nat Med* 1996;2:1361–1366.

Chapter 16

Neurologic Manifestations of CNS Vasculitides

Patricia M. Moore

Background

The vasculitides are a group of diseases and disorders sharing the central feature of inflammation of the blood vessel wall with attendant tissue ischemia. Because involvement of the blood vessel is intrinsic to inflammation of any type, vasculitis may be a manifestation of diverse diseases. When inflammation targets the vasculature and tissue injury results from ischemia, the disease itself is called a *vasculitis*. Many varieties of vasculitis exist. Some are named on the basis of distinctive clinical features; others are recognized on the basis of a known etiology. Classification of the primary and secondary vasculitides still depends on clinical and histologic characteristics, although recent advances in the understanding of the immunopathogenic mechanisms offer additional diagnostic tools.

Clinically, preferential involvement of certain organs renders many of the diseases characteristic. Histologically, the type and size of vessel, the character of the inflammatory infiltrate, and the presence of necrosis, aneurysm formation, and cicatrization in the vessel wall contribute distinct information. Recent studies of adhesion molecules, cytokines and their receptors, and neuropeptides add to the histopathologic repertoire. Factors that contribute to the tissue ischemia include physical disruption of the vessel wall from the cellular infiltrate, hemorrhage from altered wall competence, increased coagulation from changes in the normally anticoagulant endothelial cell surface, and increased vasomotor reactivity from released neuropeptides.

Early studies of vasculitis focused on the histologic features. In the past century, papers detailed clinical features of patients with sundry disorders. More recently, identification of a prominent cellular infiltration in the vessel wall enabled numerous authors to distinguish among diseases and name them (1–4). Corticosteroids and later immunosuppressant medications ushered a third era of interest in vasculitis (5–7). Current studies are re-examining the initial interpretations and the natural history of the disease, as well as inaugurating debate about the risks and benefits of aggressive therapy in individual diseases. Recent symposia on the criteria for diagnosis of vasculitis have both clarified certain issues and stimulated debate over others (8–11).

Immunopathogenic Mechanisms in the Development of Inflammation

Multiple processes can stimulate inflammation in and around the vessel wall. These include leukocyte-endothelial interactions, immune complex–induced inflammation and autoantibody-associated vascular inflammation. In the idiopathic vasculitides, physicians can often identify immediate processes that result in vascular damage but remain unaware of the inciting events (12,13) (Table 16-1). Recent understanding of the cell-mediated interactions between T cells and endothelial cells exemplifies this. Both cells can "activate" each other and participate in the normal physiologic processes of immune surveillance and clearing the body of microbial pathogens. Pertinent yet unanswered questions include the following: Which cell is the initial stimulus in vasculitis? Why do processes that are normally subject to tight regulatory control persist? Why do leukocytes that normally traverse the vessel wall remain in the vessel wall? Why does the endothelium, which normally facilitates development of inflammation without self-injury, become a target for injury in vasculitis? Future therapies depend on the answers to these questions.

Leukocyte-Endothelial Interactions

Inflammation begins with leukocyte adhesion to endothelial cells and subsequent recruitment of additional leukocytes to the region. The location of the vasculitis, type of inflammatory infiltrate, and persistence of vascular inflammation are determined by adhesion molecules, cytokines, leukotrienes, and activated complement components. Subsequent steps of inflammation, penetration in the vessel wall, and release of injurious products vary with particular immunopathogenic mechanisms.

The vascular endothelium, a highly specialized, metabolically active monolayer of cells, contributes to functional specialization of different organs, maintains thromboresistance and vascular tone, directs lymphocyte circulation, and regulates inflammation and immune interactions. Dynamic interactions between endothelial cells, leukocytes, and platelets contribute to numerous physiologically important mechanisms (14).

Table 16-1.
Vasculitides Affecting the Nervous System

	Participating Immunopathogenic Mechanisms		
Vasculitis	Immune Complex	Auto-antibody	Cell Mediated
Polyarteritis nodosa	+	—	+
Churg-Strauss angiitis	—	—	+
Hypersensitivity vasculitis	+ +	—	—
Wegener's granulomatosis	—	+	+
Lymphomatoid granulo-matosis	—	—	+
Temporal arteritis	—	—	+
Takayasu's arteritis	—	—	—
Isolated angiitis of the CNS	—	—	+
Vasculitis secondary to:			
Infection	+ +	—	+ +
Toxins	—	—	+ +
Neoplasia	+ +	+	+

+ = present, possibly involved in pathogenesis; + + = prominent, likely involved in pathogenesis; — = not present or conflicting results.

Endothelial cells communicate with cells of the immune system and tissue parenchyma by expression of a variety of cell surface molecules (such as adhesion molecules and homing receptors) and secretion of biologically active substances such as cytokines. The constitutive and inducible expression of these molecules in endothelial cells varies with the size of the vessel, the organ, and the genetic makeup of the host. In the development of inflammation, a pivotal step involves leukocyte recruitment and attachment in the presence of blood flow. Leukocyte attachment to the endothelium and infiltration of tissue are mediated by a multiple receptor-ligand system belonging to three families of related proteins: the selectins, the integrins, and the immunoglobulin superfamily. The spatial and temporal development of selectins, chemoattractants, adhesion molecules, and integrins results in the recruitment of leukocytes to a specific tissue site (15–18).

The initial attachment of leukocytes to endothelial cells, which must occur in flowing blood, results from the sequential binding of selectins to carbohydrate moieties on the leukocyte cell surface. Endothelial P-selectin expressed at high densities or leukocyte L-selectin can mediate the initial capture of leukocytes (19–21). Subsequently, E-selectin confers a loose binding, which enables the leukocyte to roll along the endothelial cell surface. This reduction in the shear forces (associated with flow rates) enables leukocyte integrins and ligands to exert their effects. At this stage another set of molecules, the chemokines, exerts a prominent effect on the recruitment of specific cells from the circulation. Chemokines, a group of small secreted proteins such as monocyte chemoattractant protein (MCP)-1, interleukin (IL)-8, and platelet-activating factor (PAF) recruit additional specific cells to the site. Chemokines

lead to transendothelial migration via chemotaxis (migration along a gradient in solution) and haptotaxis (migration along a gradient bound to extracellular matrices or cell membranes) (22,23) (Fig 16-1).

Integrins predominate in the next step of the developing inflammation. Although they have some effect on rolling, integrins largely mediate the adhesion (arrest) stage. PAF, a biologically active phospholipid, is coexpressed with P-selectin at the time of endothelial cell activation and appears to signal activation of integrins on the leukocyte surface. Leukocyte β_1 and β_2 integrins binding to their ligands such as vascular cell adhesion molecule (VCAM) and intercellular adhesion molecule (ICAM) (members of the immunoglobulin superfamily of adhesion molecules) mediate firmer adhesion of the leukocyte to the endothelium. ICAM-1 is at least one ligand for the CD18 family of leukocyte integrins. There exists some constitutive expression on several nonhematopoietic cells. Proinflammatory cytokines such as IL-1, IL-8, tumor necrosis factor (TNF), MCP-1, PAF, leukotriene B_4, and C5a upregulate expression of these receptor ligand molecules on endothelial cells and leukocytes. After firm adhesion, leukocytes then traverse the vessel wall. This last step, diapedesis of the leukocytes between endothelial cells, involves homotypic adhesion of platelet–endothelial cell adhesion molecule (PECAM-1, CD31) expressed on both leukocytes and endothelium.

Tissue injury depends on the ultimate location of fully activated leukocytes. In neutrophil-mediated tissue injury, neutrophils, following a chemoattractant gradient, completely traverse the wall and enter the tissue parenchyma. In this scenario, the final stages of ac-

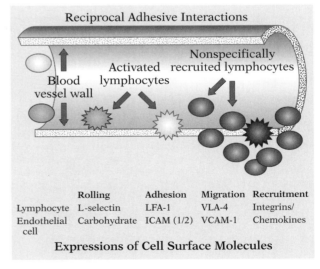

	Rolling	Adhesion	Migration	Recruitment
Lymphocyte	L-selectin	LFA-1	VLA-4	Integrins/
Endothelial cell	Carbohydrate	ICAM (1/2)	VCAM-1	Chemokines

Expressions of Cell Surface Molecules

Figure 16–1.   The sequential expression of molecules on the cell surface of lymphocytes and endothelial cells mediates the rolling, adhesion, and migration of lymphocytes to and through the blood vessel wall. The cell surface molecules shown (LFA-1, ICAM (1/2)) are examples; the exact specificity varies with cell type and tissue source (see text).

tivation, degranulation, and generation of toxic oxygen metabolites occur in the tissue with minimal changes in the vessel wall. However, if neutrophils are fully activated within the vessel wall (as they are in many cases of vasculitis), then the release of lytic granules (including collagenases, proteases, and elastases) and toxic radicals (including hydroxyl radicals and hydrogen peroxide) injures the vessel wall itself (24–27). The most severe injuries cause mural necrosis, leading to hemorrhage and thrombosis.

T lymphocyte–mediated infiltration of the vessels appears often but the final sequences are well defined. T cell–mediated vascular inflammation may be antigen specific or antigen nonspecific (15,28–30). Antigen-specific adhesion of T lymphocytes to endothelial cells (such as seen in transplantation rejection and graft-versus-host disease) requires the binding of T-cell antigen receptors (TCRs) and major histocompatibility complex (MHC) molecule receptors (CD4 and CD8) on T lymphocytes to antigen in the antigen-presenting groove of MHC molecules on endothelial cells. The presence of lymphocytes in an inflammatory lesion, however, does not identify an antigen-specific process. Cytokine-initiated and -amplified activation of either lymphocytes or endothelial cells provides a mechanism for cellular attachment in the absence of antigen. The families of adhesion molecules such as selectin, integrins, and immunuglobulin cellular adhesion molecules (IgCAMs), as described above, promote lymphocyte-endothelial binding in the absence of a specific antigen. Another characteristic of lymphocytes that distinguishes them from neutrophils is their egress from the tissue and re-entry into the circulation (31). These recirculating lymphocytes impart a pivotal feature of immunologic memory. Memory lymphocytes respond more quickly to stimuli and are often more refractory to deletion.

Other cells participate in the cell-mediated vasculitides. Important cells, particularly in the progression of inflammation from acute to chronic, are the mononuclear cells, which when activated become macrophages (32,33). These cells also release cytokines that recruit more monocytes, macrophages, and lymphocytes to the site of injury. Notably, they also possess regulatory functions and may crucially downregulate the inflammatory responses.

Platelets contribute to vascular damage by mechanisms in addition to their role in coagulation. Their cell surface receptors include class I MHC, P-selectin, IgG receptors, low-affinity IgE receptors, and receptors for von Willebrand's factor and fibrinogen (34). A wide variety of substances activate platelets. These include epinephrine, adenosine diphosphate, collagen, serotonin, membrane attack complex of complement, vasopressin, PAF, and immune complexes. Platelets then release a variety of proinflammatory mediators that generate complement activation and augment neutrophil-mediated injury.

The eosinophil, characteristically present in lesions of patients with Churg-Strauss angiitis, may also participate in the pathogenesis of vascular injury (35,36).

Autoantibody-Mediated Mechanisms

Until recently, investigators thought autoantibodies played a minor role in the pathogenesis of vasculitis (37). Several specific situations now illustrate real or potential immunopathogenic mechanisms. In Goodpasture's syndrome, a vasculitis of the pulmonary alveolar capillaries and renal glomeruli, autoantibodies to type IV collagen in the capillary basement membrane bind to their target and activate complement and leukocytes. The subsequent inflammation results in vascular injury. In vitro studies of Kawasaki disease, an acute viral vasculitis of children, revealed that antiendothelial antibodies bind to neoantigens induced by IL-1 and TNF on cultured endothelial cells and lyse their targets (38). The in vivo role is not as clear.

One of the most widely investigated autoantibodies was described in 1985 (39). Anti–neutrophil cytoplasmic antibodies (ANCAs) are a group of antibodies reactive with the neutrophils (40,41). ANCAs have two histologic patterns, c-ANCA and p-ANCA, which correlate with two different autoantigens, PC3 and myeloperoxidase, respectively. c-ANCAs are strongly associated with Wegener's granulomatosis and microscopic polyarteritis (42). Their role in the pathogenesis of disease is not certain but proposed mechanisms do account for many features of disease. Binding of ANCAs to neutrophils or monocytes in vitro stimulates the cells to undergo a respiratory burst. After this burst, the cell generates toxic oxygen metabolites and secretes proinflammatory mediators such as leukotriene B_4, IL-8, and MCP-1 that recruit more neutrophils and monocytes to the area. Neutrophils degranulate, releasing lytic enzymes that also injure the vascular endothelium. ANCA-associated vasculitides are characterized histologically by a neutrophil-rich inflammatory infiltrate.

Immune Complex–Mediated Mechanisms

Immune complexes (antigen-antibody complexes) are a normal part of the immune response and usually are cleared from the body without causing vascular inflammation. Immune complexes localized in vessel walls, either by deposition from the circulation or by in situ formation, may be pathogenic (43–45). Conditions conducive to pathogenicity are certain biophysical properties of the complexes or particularly receptive features of a vessel wall (increased vascular permeability secondary to platelets, complement activation, or presence of mast cells). Complexes near equivalence to antibodies and antigens are more likely to precipitate; those with a negative charge are more likely to interact with vessel walls.

Immune complexes can then initiate a series of events that recruit an inflammatory response. The Fc portion of the IgG and IgM antibody molecules in the complexes engages Fc receptors on neutrophils and monocytes, both attaching these cells to the site of immune complex localization and inducing degranulation and release of proinflammatory molecules. Immune complexes also activate complement components that induce a variety of inflammatory events. C2a and C3a increase vascular permeability and neutrophil degranulation. C5a attracts neutrophils and monocytes to the region (46–50). The membrane attack complex, C5b-9, injures matrix materials and cells in the vessel wall. The results of these events include necrosis of the vessel wall, an exudative inflammatory response, and usually healing with prominent scarring.

The types of antigens identified in immune complexes include both heterologous antigens (sulfonamides, mouse monoclonal antibodies, microbial antigens) and autoantigens (nuclear antigens and rheumatoid factor). Antigens in in situ complex formation are less completely studied but DNA complexes are found in the kidney. Immune complex–mediated vasculitides are characterized histologically by mixed neutrophil and mononuclear cell infiltrates, with prominent necrosis and evidence of immunoglobulin, complement, and fibrin deposition.

Features of the Central Nervous System Vasculature

Biochemical and immunologic features of endothelial cells and smooth muscle cells vary regionally. Arteries with smooth muscle cells in the vessel wall possess characteristics distinct from microvasculature and the venous system. Endothelial cells of the central nervous system (CNS) are physically and biochemically conspicuously distinctive. Their tight junctions between cells, paucity of micropinocytic vessels, and high levels of γ-glutamyltranspeptidase are three examples of their distinctive characteristics. Several other properties of cerebral endothelial cells result in differences in inflammation of the cerebral blood vessels compared with the systemic blood vessels. Although cerebral endothelial cells are capable of expressing MHC class I molecules (restriction elements for antigen presentation to the TCR of CD8+ T cells) and MHC class II (restriction elements for CD4+ helper T cells), they appear to do this less often than does the endothelium of the systemic vasculature (51–55). A low constitutive expression of adhesion molecules also contributes to the lower proclivity of cerebral vessels for vasculitis. For example, ICAM-1 appears to be expressed constituently only at low levels on brain endothelium in vivo in contrast to other tissue endothelium. Molecules regulating inflammation such as transforming growth factor (TGF)-β, which downregulates the adhesion of leukocytes, may play a more prominent role in the CNS than the systemic vasculature.

CNS endothelium readily presents adhesion molecules but may leave antigen presentation to parenchymal brain cells (56–58). Lymphocyte traffic through the CNS is normally limited. The level of lymphocyte adhesion to brain endothelium is less than 5% compared with 15% to 20% in other organs (59,60). Activated lymphocytes do traverse the cerebral endothelium and enter the CNS. This may have survival advantages because inflammation within the cerebral vessel wall disrupts the tight endothelial junctions and integrity of the blood-brain barrier. Supporting evidence for the relative resistance of CNS blood vessels to inflammation is found in the systemic vasculitides where CNS vasculitis occurs less frequently than does vasculitis of the visceral vessels. Many of the central neurologic complications in polyarteritis nodosa (PAN), for example, appear later in the course of disease and might result from hypertensive or chronic vaso-occlusive changes rather then segmental inflammation of the vessel wall. Another disease supporting this assertion that inflammation of the CNS vasculature is tightly regulated is systemic lupus erythematosus. Degenerative or vaso-occlusive vasculopathy is present in the CNS but inflammatory vascular disease rarely occurs, despite the presence and deposition of circulating immunoglobulins that cause inflammation elsewhere.

Processes That Exacerbate or Modify Tissue Injury Associated with Inflammation

Coagulation

Several events intimately connected with but temporally dispersed from the initial events contribute to the clinical features of vasculitis. Of these, coagulation is the best studied. Resting endothelium provides a non-thrombogenic, anticoagulant surface. Additional endothelial antiplatelet and fibrinolytic properties contribute to the maintenance of thromboresistance. During inflammation, the balance changes and the endothelial surface exerts a net procoagulant effect (61–64). IL-1 and TNF-α activation of the endothelium stimulates the intrinsic and extrinsic coagulation pathways and also reduces its fibrinolytic activity. Further, tissue factor, the principal procoagulant of human brain, resides in specific regions of the nervous system and is increased during inflammation. Acute-phase reactants, including IL-6, also induce fibrinogen. This confluence of procoagulant effects may in part serve a physiologic function. Reduction of blood flow through the inflamed vasculature would reduce the cascade that recruits additional cells to the area. Nonetheless, excessive coagulation would perpetuate tissue damage from ischemia.

Vascular Tone

Similarly, maintenance of vascular tone is carefully regulated under normal circumstances. Intrinsic modulation of vascular tone depends in part on elaboration of both vasorelaxants and vasoconstrictors (65). Endothelins, which are powerful vasoconstrictors, and nitric oxide, which is a potent vasodilator, are part of a balanced system that regulates blood flow in the brain and other organs (65–68). Endothelins can provoke a long-lasting vasoconstriction in cerebral vessels of all sizes including those in the microcirculation (69). Under physiologic conditions, endothelins do not penetrate the blood-brain barrier or influence permeability. However, endothelins are produced by brain endothelial cells, smooth muscle cells, astrocytes, and neurons. Potential sources within the brain for this vasoconstrictor are numerous. Nitric oxide, a free radical with high lipid solubility and an extremely short half-life of only a few seconds, is also produced widely within the brain by endothelial cells, astrocytes, and neurons. In inflammation, cytokine (particularly IL-1)-associated release of endothelin induces an overriding vasoconstriction (70). The functional effect, to reduce flow through the injured vessels, is likely an appropriate physiologic response. Persistent endothelin release also stimulates vascular smooth muscle proliferation. Thus, excessive or persistent vasoconstriction may add to ischemic tissue injury (71–73).

PAF is produced and released from platelets, leukocytes, endothelial cells, and neurons as well as numerous other cells. Its secretion is often accompanied by the secretion of prostacyclin and other vasoactive lipid mediators. PAF is a prominent stimulator of inflammation, of the production of reactive oxygen intermediates, and of coagulation. The effects of PAF are numerous but include hemodynamic effects (profound hypotension and perfusion changes) and induction of neuronal differentiation in vitro. Cerebrovascular effects include disruption of the blood-brain barrier, edema formation, and vasospasm.

Regulation of Vascular Inflammation

Vascular inflammation is normally transient. Mechanisms of persistent vasculitis include not only the obvious cause, persistence of antigenic stimulation, but also other abnormalities that are less well defined. Better understanding of regulatory mechanisms in vasculitis could provide more effective, less toxic therapies. Current clinical studies of IL-8 and granulocyte-macrophage colony-stimulating factor (GM-CSF), which induce rapid shedding of L-selectin from leukocytes, and TGF-β, which in many tissues downregulates the expression of adhesion molecules, may prove useful.

Clinical Features of Idiopathic Vasculitides

Polyarteritis Nodosa

PAN, a systemic necrotizing vasculitis, affects medium-sized muscular arteries throughout the body with the notable exceptions of the spleen and lungs. The varying severity and often restricted disease are notable (74–78). Systemic symptoms of fever, malaise, and weight loss often herald the disease. Over half the patients have either arthralgias or an erythematous, purpuric, or vasculitic rash. Some extent of renal involvement occurs in more than 70% of patients, although an abnormal urinary sediment is more frequent than uremia. Hypertension develops in at least half the patients.

Histologically, there is a segmental, transmural vascular inflammation with a mixture of lymphomononuclear cells and variable numbers of neutrophils and eosinophils (79). Fibrinoid necrosis is typical but not diagnostic. Infiltration is followed by intimal proliferation and thrombosis. A temporal spectrum of vascular changes appears in vessels throughout the body. Strikingly, active necrotizing lesions and proliferative fibrotic healing lesions coexist in close proximity. The lesions have a predilection for vessel bifurcations.

Neurologically, both central and peripheral nervous system abnormalities occur, but the frequency, tempo, and histology vary (80). Peripheral neuropathies occur in 50% to 60% of patients and are often the presenting manifestation of disease. Most frequent are classic mononeuritis multiplex and polyneuropathies, either pattern occurring in over half the patients with neuropathy (80–83). An ascending sensorimotor quadriparesis occurs, resulting from infarction of watershed blood vessels supplying nerves in the mid-arm and mid-thigh (84). The clinical presentation is that of an extensive mononeuropathy multiplex. Cutaneous neuropathies, frequently evident at careful sensory examination, may not be symptomatic. More troublesome diagnostically are the plexopathies and radiculopathies. These are relatively infrequent and usually attributed to vasculitis only in patients with other known manifestations of disease. Sural nerve biopsies of carefully selected patients reveal histologic evidence of vascular inflammation in the vasonervorum, and active axonal degeneration with asymmetric involvement appears between or within fascicles. The cellular infiltrate consists mainly of macrophages and T lymphocytes, particularly the CD4+ subset. Infiltrating cells exhibit immunologic activation of markers such as IL-2 receptor, transferrin receptor, and MHC class II antigen expression (85,86).

CNS abnormalities develop in 40% of patients, and include encephalopathy, focal and multifocal lesions of the brain and spinal cord, subarachnoid hemorrhage, seizures, strokes, and cranial neuropathies (87–89). These usually occur later in the course of disease than the peripheral neuropathies. Hypertension sometimes accompanies or follows the encephalopathy and the additional marginal ischemia may further compromise neurologic function. Visual symptoms are numerous; blurred vision and visual loss may result from inflammation of the choroidal, retinal, or brain parenchymal arteries (90–92). Vasculitis of the optic nerve, chiasm, and tract and the occipital cortex occurs. Diplopia results from inflammation of the arteries supplying cranial nerve III, IV, or VI (93–95).

Laboratory evidence of systemic inflammation is reflected nonspecifically as anemia, leukocytosis, thrombocytosis, C reactive proteins, and elevated sedimentation rate. Antinuclear antibodies (ANAs) may be present in 20% of patients but are characteristically of low titer and a nonspecific pattern. Although its role in the pathogenesis of PAN is not clear, about 20% to 30% of patients have a hepatitis B antigenemia. ANCAs, particularly to myeloperoxidase, are associated with microscopic polyarteritis, possibly aiding diagnosis. Abnormalities in the urine sediment are common, even if the blood urea nitrogen (BUN) and creatinine values are normal. Creatinine clearance is the best measure of renal function and may indicate otherwise inapparent renal disease. Angiography is a useful diagnostic test and often suggests the diagnosis in patients when biopsy has been unrewarding. Notable and prominent radiographic changes in about 65% of patients are aneurysms, particularly in the hepatic and renal vasculature. Segmental narrowings of vessels, variations in caliber, and pruning of the vascular tree all occur.

Although the criteria are evolving, the diagnosis of PAN remains largely dependent on the classic methods of angiography and biopsy. The triad that alerts a physician to a diagnosis of PAN is systemic inflammation, angiographic evidence of enteric vascular diseases, and histologic evidence of vasculitis, often in a peripheral nerve.

Churg-Strauss Angiitis

In 1951, Churg and Strauss described distinctive features found at autopsy of 13 patients who died after an illness characterized by fever, asthma, eosinophilia, and systemic disorder (96). Churg-Strauss angiitis appears as a vasculitis of small to medium-sized vessels with clinically distinctive features. The disease is often heralded by rhinitis and then increasingly severe asthma (97–99). This prodrome may precede the development of eosinophilia and systemic vasculitis by 2 to 20 years. Clinical and hematologic features distinguish it from PAN. Early features may include anemia, weight loss, heart failure, recurrent pneumonia, and bloody diarrhea. Pulmonary involvement is typical in Churg-Strauss angiitis and rare in PAN. Similarly, the eosinophilia that is characteristic in Churg-Strauss angiitis is not a feature of PAN (77,100). Cutaneous manifestations include palpable purpura, erythema, and subcutaneous nodules. Peripheral nerves and kidneys are typically involved in 65% and 60% of patients, respectively.

Histologically, medium-sized and small vessels are affected. Debate continues over the necessity for strict histologic criteria (necrotizing vasculitis, tissue infiltration by eosinophils, and extravascular granuloma) to establish a diagnosis. Study of the potential mechanisms for vascular and tissue injury center on the eosinophil (35,36). The two diagnostically essential lesions are angiitis and extravascular necrotizing granulomas usually with eosinophilic infiltrates (99). In any single biopsy specimen, however, the changes may appear very similar to those of PAN.

Neurologic abnormalities are similar to those in PAN, but encephalopathies occurring early in the course of the disease are more frequent, probably reflecting the small size of the vessels involved (101). CNS abnormalities include memory loss, confusion, seizures, subarachnoid hemorrhage, and chorea (102–104). Visual abnormalities are a prominent part of the disease (105,106). In the absence of histologic evidence of vasculitis in the brain, however, the frequency of cerebrovascular inflammatory disease remains conjectural. Peripheral neuropathies predominate (50%–75% of patients) over CNS changes (25%). Peripheral neurop-

athies classically present as mononeuropathy multiplex but polyneuropathies also occur (107,108). Histologically, vasculitis in the peripheral nerve blood vessel may have the typical features of eosinophils and granulomas but as often appears similar to PAN.

Laboratory features reflect general systemic inflammation. Although the sedimentation rate is elevated, and ANAs may be present in low titer, no autoantibodies are diagnostic of the disease. ANCA titers are not a reliable parameter. Thus, the clinical features again provide important information for diagnosis. Characteristically, the triad of asthma, eosinophilia, and vasculitis in two extrapulmonary organs defines the disease.

Hypersensitivity Vasculitis

Hypersensitivity vasculitis (HSV), the most frequently encountered of all the vasculitides, is a heterogeneous group of clinical syndromes characterized by an inflammation of small vessels, typically venules (109–111). The predominant target organ is the skin; this feature unifies these diseases. In many instances, the vessel inflammation can be identified as a response to a precipitating antigen such as a drug, foreign protein, or microbe (112–115). Endogenous antigens, such as tumor antigens or serum proteins, can also serve as the sensitizing antigen.

Clinically, lesions appear as purpura or urticaria. Histologically, the presence of fragmentation and phagocytosis of nuclear debris (leukocytoclasia) is a typical pathologic feature. Damage to the vessel wall appears to result from deposition of immune complexes with activation of the complement cascade. Although the ensuing infiltrate is usually neutrophilic, a distinct lymphocytic subset may exist. Henoch-Schönlein purpura (HSP), a disorder featuring palpable purpura and colicky abdominal pain in children, often exhibits evidence of IgA in the walls of the arterioles and glomeruli (116). Isolated cutaneous lesions may occur in cryoglobulinemia, connective tissue diseases, and malignancies. Histologic and clinical features are typically monophasic. ANCA autoantibodies are not present and ANAs present only in low titers. One third of the patients have elevated IgA as demonstrated by serum immunoelectrophoresis.

Involvement of the nervous system varies. In serum sickness, encephalopathies, seizures, and brachial plexopathies occur although the incidence is unknown (117,118). In other HSVs, subarachnoid hemorrhage or seizures are occasionally reported (119). In most patients with cutaneous venulitis, the nervous system is not affected.

To the neurologist and internist, the prominent clinical dilemma in the diagnosis and therapy of HSV is whether the vasculitis will remain restricted to the skin or is the presenting manifestation of systemic vasculitis such as PAN, Churg-Strauss angiitis, or Wegener's granulomatosis. For this reason, evaluation of patients with HSV includes analyses of renal function, immunoglobulins, and autoantibodies that may suggest alternative diseases. In all of these, the main goals are to identify any inciting causes, remove the cause, and observe the patients. Evidence of systemic disease (renal, cardiac, gastrointestinal, neurologic) warrants glucocorticoid or immunosuppressive therapy.

Wegener's Granulomatosis

Wegener's granulomatosis is characterized by a necrotizing, granulomatous vasculitis of the upper and lower respiratory tract, glomerulonephritis, and small-vessel vasculitis. Prominent cranial neuropathies reflect erosion from contiguous extension of the sinus granulomas. Hearing loss, proptosis, ophthalmoplegias, and facial and trigeminal neuropathies are prominent. The small-vessel vasculitis affects the CNS parenchyma as well as the peripheral nervous system (120–125).

Presenting features of disease may be respiratory, renal, or neurologic and are usually accompanied by features of systemic inflammation, including malaise, fever, and weight loss. Chest radiography is useful diagnostically as is head magnetic resonance imaging (MRI). In active disease the sedimentation rate is invariably elevated. Autoantibodies to c-ANCAs are present sufficiently often that they may be used as markers of disease, although their role in pathogenesis is still debated (126).

Isolated Angiitis of the Central Nervous System

Idiopathic, recurrent vasculitis is an uncommon disease of the CNS characterized by inflammation of small and medium-sized vessels (127–133). Historically, the disease was called *granulomatous angiitis* on the basis of granulomas found at postmortem examination. Histologic examinations antemortem reveal that granulomas are a variable and often absent feature. The current term is *isolated angiitis of the CNS (IAC)*. Some authors use the term *primary angiitis of the CNS* but this includes a variety of disorders and histologic confirmation is often lacking. IAC has been recognized with increasing frequency in the past decade, possibly because current treatment methods are so effective.

Symptoms and signs are restricted to the nervous system and typically include headaches, encephalopathies, strokes, cranial neuropathies, and myelopathies. Headache is prominent in at least half the patients. The clinical situations that should suggest the diagnosis are new onset of headaches and encephalopathy, particularly in association with multifocal signs. Notably, symptoms and laboratory evidence of systemic inflammation are absent. In addition, because an occasional self-limited vasculopathy occurs, evidence of recurrent or persistent disease should be confirmed in individual patients prior to immunosuppression.

The findings on neurodiagnostic studies, including computed tomography (CT) and MRI, are often non-specifically abnormal (134). Cerebrospinal fluid analysis reveals abnormalities in only half the patients, and even then the abnormalities may be a mild pleocytosis or protein elevation. Angiography is the most sensitive diagnostic study, although an occasional patient with only small-vessel disease may have a normal-appearing angiogram. Of greater concern to accurate diagnosis is the fact that the angiographic features are not specific for vasculitis; similar abnormalities can occur in non-inflammatory vasculopathies as well as vasculitis secondary to infections, drugs, and neoplasia. Angiography often shows single or multiple areas of beading along the course of a vessel, abrupt vessel terminations, hazy vessel margins, and neovascularization (135–137). Classically, appropriate clinical features, absence of evidence of systemic inflammation, and angiographic and histologic data are important. Rigorous evaluations are necessary to exclude the numerous secondary causes of CNS vascular inflammation and alternative causes of vasculopathy.

Isolated Peripheral Nervous System Vasculitis

Vasculitis restricted to the peripheral nervous system occurs and in some series comprises one third of all patients with vasculitic neuropathy (138–141). A major difficulty in establishing this as a distinct clinical diagnosis is that vasculitis of the peripheral nerve is often the presenting feature of systemic vasculitis. Since the distribution and histology of isolated vasculitis of the peripheral nervous system are identical to those of PAN, it is difficult to determine whether patients, if untreated, would go on to develop systemic disease. Until more information on the etiology or pathogenic mechanisms of the peripheral nervous system vasculature is available, careful and repeated studies of these patients including funduscopic examination, fresh urinalysis for occult blood and protein, measurement of creatinine clearance rates, and evaluation for evidence of systemic inflammation are prudent.

Temporal Arteritis

Temporal arteritis is a systemic panarteritis although symptoms below the neck are distinctly unusual. Clinical features typically appear in people over the age of 50. New-onset headache and jaw claudication are frequent early symptoms. Visual abnormalities including visual loss and ophthalmoplegias occur tragically, often from infarction of branches of the extracranial circulation. Histologically, there is also evidence of vascular inflammation in the posterior circulation, and this appears to explain the symptoms and signs referable to the posterior fossa. Encephalopathies develop in patients with temporal arteritis but the histologic associations in this older population are not yet clear. There is a distinctive overlap of temporal arteritis with the systemic inflammatory disease polymyalgia rheumatica. Temporal artery biopsy is important because the two diseases require different dosages of corticosteroids for effective therapy.

Other Vasculitides

There are several reports and series of patients with neurologic abnormalities not readily classifiable in the disease groups described above (142). There is a small-vessel vasculitis restricted to the CNS, skin, and muscle (143). Retinocochlear encephalopathy, another disorder of small vessels, is more likely a microvasculopathy than a vasculitis (144). The syndrome consists of a subacute encephalopathy (often with early psychiatric features), sensorineural hearing loss, and retinal arteriolar occlusions. This hearing loss in association with vascular disease must be distinguished from Cogan's syndrome (nonsyphilitic interstitial keratitis and vestibuloauditory symptoms). Some patients with Cogan's syndrome have a vasculitic component that is predominantly an aortitis (145,146).

Clinical Features of the Secondary Vasculitides

Vasculitis of the nervous system secondary to a known cause or underlying process is both frequent and clinically important. The numbers of patients with CNS vasculitis from secondary causes far exceed the numbers of those with a primary, idiopathic vasculitis. A high index of suspicion enables a clinician to promptly institute therapy for a vasculitis that may be secondary to infection, neoplasia, or a toxin.

Infectious organisms that elicit a prominent vascular inflammation are numerous and include bacteria, fungi, viruses and protozoa. Mechanisms of infection-mediated inflammation include toxic disruption of the endothelium, infection of the endothelial cells, and immune complex–mediated inflammation. The prolific inflammation induced by bacteria includes conspicuous accumulation of cells in the vessel wall with associated thrombosis and hemorrhage (147–149). This accounts for the frequent strokes that are part of acute bacterial meningitis and responsible for much of the neurologic sequelae. Other infectious agents frequently causing a vasculitis but more difficult to detect are fungi. Aspergilli, cryptococci, *Coccidioides immitis*, *Histoplasma capsulatum*, and fungi causing mucormycoses, in particular, infiltrate cerebral vessels (150–158). Neuroborelliosis also results in vasculitis (159,160). The clinical features range from subtle changes in cognition to fatal hemorrhagic infarctions. Other common infections such as tuberculosis (161,162) and syphilis (163) can cause a vasculitis. Strokes associated with viral infection usually demonstrate more pleomorphic features. Histologically, inflammation and necrosis of the cerebral blood vessel wall certainly appear as a result of infections with herpes simplex virus, herpes zoster virus, cytomegalovirus, *Toxoplasma gondii*, human immunodeficiency virus, and varicella virus (164–169). However, viruses such as herpes zoster may also cause vaso-occlusive disease without inflammatory changes.

Toxins are another distinct cause of vasculitis (154,170–173). The cutaneous disorder HSV is associated with a wide variety of inciting agents but CNS complications are few. However, CNS vasculitis can occur after use of illicit drugs, notably those with a prominent sympathomimetic effect, such as amphetamines. Cocaine and crack cocaine do cause stroke and have occasionally been associated with a vasculitis.

Neoplasias exert several effects on the blood vessel. Encasement of the vessel by tumor itself is far more common than inflammation of a vessel remote from the neoplasm (174–178). The mechanism of the paraneoplastic vasculitis is not understood but current studies suggest that overexpression of certain cytokines may play a role. Hodgkin's disease, however, is associated with a vasculitis that resolves with the treatment of the underlying disease. Other lymphomas, including lymphomatoid granulomatosis and angioendotheliosis, are vasocentric and may present with central or peripheral nervous system abnormalities, illustrating the importance of histology in accurate diagnosis and therapy.

Connective tissue diseases are systemic inflammatory diseases in which a component of the disease is often a vasculitis. However, with the possible exception of Sjögren's disease, vasculitis of the CNS rarely occurs (179–182). In systemic lupus erythematosus, neurologic abnormalities are frequent but histologic evidence of vasculitis is rare. The pathogeneses of the neurologic abnormalities are undefined but multiple contributions from autoantibodies reactive with neuronal tissue, ischemia from coagulopathies, and behavioral changes from activation of the hypothalamic-pituitary-adrenal axis all appear likely. The CNS abnormalities in systemic lupus erythematosus are clearly multifactorial. Vascular disease occurs from emboli, coagulopathies, and a degenerative process in the vessel wall. The cause of the vasculopathy is not clear. Despite the absence of inflammation in the vessel wall, an immune-mediated process is the likely basis. Studies of the coronary vascular system in autoimmune mice of varying genetic backgrounds provide clues. The histologic result of circulating immune complex deposition depended on the titer and chronicity of the circulating complexes as well as the genetic features of the host. Predisposed animals with low levels of immune complexes developed a degenerative process without a cellular infiltrate.

A vasculitic neuropathy can occur in association with rheumatoid arthritis, although a compressive neuropathy is more frequently encountered (183–186). Similarly in the nonspecific systemic inflammatory diseases such as associated with cryoglobulins, a mononeuropathy multiplex, polyneuropathy, or autonomic neuropathy may occur associated with vascular inflammation. In the peripheral nervous system, lupus vasculitis accounts for only 1% of patients presenting to a neurologist with a vasculitic neuropathy.

Sjögren's disease is a systemic disorder manifested by sicca complex and a variety of extraglandular features. Both central and peripheral nervous system abnormalities occur, although the histology is not convincingly vasculitic. In one series of nerve biopsies, however, 8 of 11 patients had findings consistent or highly suggestive of vasculitis; other patients had a perivascular inflammatory response. An alternative, distinctive neuropathy in Sjögren's disease is not vasculitis but a dorsal root ganglionitis. These patients present with a sensory neuropathy and ataxia usually associated with autonomic insufficiency (187,188).

Diagnostic Consideration and Neuroradiographic Studies

Clinical neurologic abnormalities merit neurodiagnostic studies but these are of variable utility in detecting underlying vascular inflammation. Cerebrospinal fluid analysis is neither sensitive nor specific for vasculitis but may identify underlying causes of vascular inflammation such as infections or tumors. Electroencephalography is also neither specific nor sensitive for vasculitis but occasionally provides a supportive clue in the small-vessel vasculitides affecting the brain. MRI often detects vascular disease but the signals result from fluid changes in ischemic tissue (134,189,190). Thus, the result of vascular inflammation rather than the inflammation itself is identified (Table 16-2). Nonetheless, the presence of multifocal abnormalities often suggests vascular disease and the need for further studies. Magnetic resonance angiography (MRA) promises to provide more information about vascular abnormalities prior to infarction but current studies do not have sufficient resolution to exclude many cases of CNS vasculitis.

Cerebral angiography remains the gold standard for detecting intracranial vasculopathies. There are, however, limitations (135,137,191–193). It is an invasive, expensive procedure. Its utility also varies with the underlying vasculitis. Although angiographic findings are abnormal in 75% to 90% of patients with primary CNS vasculitis, vascular inflammation may occur in vessels beyond the resolution of angiography, as demonstrated in several biopsy-proved cases of IAC. The utility of cerebral angiography in systemic vasculitis remains undetermined. Abnormal findings are seldom found in PAN or Wegener's granulomatosis, although it has been useful in lymphomatoid granulomatosis. Angiography of other regions of the body is often useful and occasionally the critical diagnostic study in systemic vasculitis. Aortic arch arteriography is central to a diagnosis of Takayasu's arteritis. PAN may be revealed by renal or mesenteric angiography performed for the evaluation of persistent visceral pain or hemorrhage.

Cortical/leptomeningeal biopsy is an important part of the diagnosis of the intracranial vasculitides because no other study distinguishes between inflammatory and noninflammatory causes of angiographically demonstrable vascular irregularities. Further, in those patients with vascular inflammation, biopsy may provide the only information on an underlying cause requiring alternative therapy such as infection. A major limitation of biopsy is the false-negative rate, which remains at 20% to 40%. Because biopsy samples vessels of a different size than those recognized by angiography or MRI, these latter studies do not yet provide a useful guide for biopsy site.

Diagnosis of vasculitis in individual patients often evolves over time as the pattern and extent of clinical facets appear. For this reason, a clinician must periodically re-evaluate the diagnosis. A repeated, careful history with direct questions about renal, gastrointestinal, cardiac, pulmonary, and CNS function is essential. Further studies, including urinalysis, determination of creatinine clearance rate, and measurement of BUN, are useful.

Therapy

In current nosology, clinical and pathologic features divide the vasculitides into groups. Perhaps the single most important division to the clinician is that of primary (or idiopathic) and secondary vasculitis. Prompt identification of the secondary vasculitides results in better therapy. Clinical and pathologic features distin-

Table 16-2.
Clinical Features of Disease in Neurovasculitis

Vasculitis	E	Sz	S	Myel	CN	PN	SAH	Myo
Polyarteritis nodosa	++	+	++	+	++	+++	++	+
Churg-Strauss angiitis	+++	+	+	+	+	++	+	+
Hypersensitivity vasculitis	−	+	−	−	−	−	+	−
Wegener's granulomatosis	++	+	++	+	+++	++	++	+
Lymphomatoid granulomatosis	++	+	+	+	++	++	−	−
Temporal arteritis	+	−	−	−	++	+	−	−
Takayasu's arteritis	+	−	++	−	−	+	+	−
Behçet's disease	++	+	+	−	+	−	++	−
Isolated angiitis of the CNS	+++	++	++	+	+	−	+	−
Vctd	++	++	+	+	++	++	+	−
Secondary vasculitis	+++	+++	+++	++	+	++	+	−

The relative frequency of occurrence of groups of neurologic abnormalities is listed above. +++ indicates feature is a prominent component of disease; ++, frequent occurrence; +, feature is occasionally present; −, unusual or not present.
E = encephalopathy; Sz = seizures; S = stroke; Myel = myelopathy; CN = cranial neuropathy; PN = peripheral neuropathy; SAH = subarachnoid hemorrhage; Myo = myopathies; Vctd = vasculitis associated with connective tissue diseases.

guish among the primary vasculitides. Early in any of the diseases, the diagnosis may be enigmatic. As the diseases progress, the diagnosis is clearer. Several reviews on therapy in vasculitis are available (194–198).

Treatment of vasculitis ranges from the simple measures of removing the cause of the chronic inflammation, to the corticosteroid/cyclophosphamide immunosuppressive mainstays of some diseases, to experimental measures in refractory vasculitis. As information on the mechanisms of vascular inflammation increases, more specific, less toxic therapies can be developed. Treatment of patients with vasculitis requires expertise with a spectrum of vasculitides and autoimmune diseases so that there will be an appreciation for the potential of overlap syndromes or evolution of a specific diagnosis over time. Experience in the use of immunosuppressant medications is also important because of the wide range of potential and actual side effects. Side effects occur with any of these agents and the physician should be thoroughly acquainted with all potential side effects before initiating treatment. Most patients do well on the standard regimens. More difficult are those patients who only partially respond to treatment. The physician must determine whether the clinical effects are from persistent inflammation or other causes. Excluding infection should remain a high priority. Ischemia may result not only from the inflammation but also from chronic changes in the vessel wall accompanied by thrombosis or hemorrhage.

Corticosteroids remain a mainstay in the therapy of vasculitis, and in some types of vasculitis, corticosteroids alone are effective. Corticosteroids affect the immune system at numerous sites (199). Intracellularly, steroids bind to a cytoplasmic receptor protein and enter the cell where they alter the rate of ribosomal and messenger RNA synthesis. Among the effects are inhibition of synthesis of IL-1, IL-2, IL-6, and GM-CSF; decreased production of proinflammatory mediators such as eicosamide; and diminished lipocortin action (200).

The efficacy of glucocorticoids, usually prednisone or methylprednisolone, varies among the vasculitic syndromes. Undoubtedly it is the single most effective treatment in temporal arteritis. In some HSVs and in microangiopathic renal vasculitis, prednisone therapy alone may suffice. In other disorders, either the high dosage is unsustainable because of the considerable side effects or it is effective only as adjunct therapy. It is ineffective in well-established Wegener's granulomatosis. Patients with PAN may develop new neurologic side effects while their disease is apparently quiescent during prednisone treatment. In these disorders, experience with the underlying disease will enable the physician to determine when to use another agent such as cyclophosphamide.

The side effects of corticosteroids are numerous and frequent. In addition to the well-described side effects of acute and chronic corticosteroid therapy, there are specific effects that impact vascular diseases, particularly a potential to augment vasoconstriction and platelet aggregation. This may complicate the treatment of vasculitic syndromes (201,202). More recent studies of the effects of chronically elevated corticosteroids on glucocorticoid receptors in the hippocampus and associated changes in cognition underly the need for careful use of these medications (203). There is currently increased use of immunosuppressive agents for their steroid-sparing effects.

Cyclophosphamide, an alkylating nitrogen mustard, cross-links DNA, thus interfering with cell division and diminishing clonal expansion of B and T lymphocytes. Immunologic effects include suppression of immunoglobulin production, diminished antigen-induced proliferation of helper and effector T cells, and reduced cytotoxicity of macrophages. Early evaluations of cyclophosphamide suggested that acute high doses principally suppress humoral immunity while chronic doses affect cell-mediated immune mechanisms. More recently, influences of cyclophosphamide on endothelial cells are also being explored.

Cyclophosphamide was effectively added to therapeutic immunosuppressive regimens of systemic necrotizing vasculitis in 1979, dramatically reducing the mortality of Wegener's granulomatosis. Its efficacy as treatment of IAC and PAN is well established. It is also a useful adjunct either to reduce the dosage and side effects of prednisone or for treatment when corticosteroid therapy is ineffective. It is most often prescribed either in a daily oral dose or as an intermittent intravenous bolus. Oral cyclophosphamide is usually prescribed at a dose of 1 to 2 mg/kg/day. Hydration is important to prevent hemorrhagic cystitis and potentially reduce the incidence of bladder malignancies. Monitoring the white blood cell count for a limiting factor of neutropenia of more than 1500 cells minimizes the likelihood of infection.

More recently, bolus intravenous cyclophosphamide has been tried with the aim of reducing the total dosage and side effects. Different protocols of pulse cyclophosphamide administration have been employed. Pulse cyclophosphamide has been effective in lupus nephritis (204) and systemic vasculitis (205), but despite initial improvement, in Wegener's granulomatosis there may be a higher relapse rate than with standard cyclophosphamide therapy (206).

Cyclosporine is a cyclic endecapeptide extracted from the fungus *Tolypocladium inflatum Gams*. Cyclosporine's immune effects are selective; it inhibits the production of IL-2 by T lymphocytes (207). It has dramatically impacted the treatment of organ transplantation; the efficacy of cyclosporine in various autoimmune diseases is under investigation. The side effects of nephrotoxicity and hypertension limit its widespread use in human vasculitis, although further studies are needed to investigate a possible therapeutic benefit.

Azathioprine, a purine analogue, inhibits protein and antibody synthesis in vitro. Both immunoglobulin production and cell-mediated effector function are diminished by azathioprine. Azathioprine's role in the therapy of systemic vasculitides is restricted to those patients who cannot tolerate cyclophosphamide. It appears to be less effective than cyclophosphamide in inducing remission but may be used later in the course in place of cyclophosphamide to sustain a remission.

Pheresis (plasma exchange and leukopheresis), the selective removal of plasma or cellular components from the blood, is demonstrably effective in controlled studies of Goodpasture's syndrome, certain hyperviscosity states, thrombotic thrombocytopenic purpura, Guillain-Barré syndrome, and myasthenia gravis. Its efficacy in connective tissue and vasculitic diseases is unsubstantiated (208). Pheresis has been used in PAN, particularly that associated with hepatitis B viremia (209), and in a series of patients with rapidly progressive renal disease, pheresis with immunosuppression appeared to be more effective than immunosuppression alone (210,211). In the absence of controlled studies it is difficult to determine whether pheresis improves the morbidity and mortality over the standard treatment of prednisone and cyclophosphamide.

Intravenous immunoglobulin (IGIV), initially used about 10 years ago for the treatment of primary immunodeficiency disease, effectively supplies anti-infectious agent antibodies by passive immunization. It was incidentally noted at the time to improve thrombocytopenia. Although the exact mechanism of this effect remains unknown, several possible explanations include 1) an effect on the Fc receptor of phagocytic cells and B lymphocytes, reducing their effector functions; 2) production of anti-idiotypic antibodies; and 3) prevention of activated complement components from reaching their targets (212). IVIG is demonstrably effective therapy of Kawasaki syndrome (a childhood vasculitis associated with high cytokine levels and coronary arteritis). Some recent studies showed that IVIG may be effective in some patients with systemic vasculitis, particularly those with refractory vasculitis (213,214). The occasional reversible impairment of renal function requires further study (213).

The *nonsteroidal anti-inflammatory medications (NSAIDs)* have anti-inflammatory, analgesic, antipyretic, and platelet inhibitory actions. Those currently available come from a variety of chemical classes that affect their distribution in the body and to some extent their therapeutic performance. The similarities among them are large, and as a group, they are potentially useful adjuncts in autoimmune disease. A major mechanism of action of NSAIDs is the inhibition of cyclooxygenase activity and therefore the synthesis of prostaglandins (215). Although not yet studied systematically, this effect may reduce some of the chronic changes in vasculitis.

Antiprostaglandin medications may also be effective. In the diseased blood vessel, endothelium-dependent smooth muscle relaxation is impaired. Both vasoconstriction and secondary platelet aggregation accelerate. An endothelial peptide, endothelin, is a smooth muscle contractor; increased levels of endothelin are present in some diseases. In several patients prostaglandin E_1 infusion resulted in anti-inflammatory and antivasospastic effects (216). The size of the vessel involved appears to be a restricting factor in the efficacy of anti–prostaglandin E_1 therapy. There would be limited

effects in peripheral neuropathy due to vasonervorum infarction and other small vessels too small to contain muscle cells. Side effects are unusual but noteworthy. The vasodilatory effect could result in hypotension (potentially serious in patients with ischemic bowel) and steal syndromes.

In certain of the vasculitides, there is evidence of a coagulopathy, and so *antiplatelet agents and anticoagulation* have been tried. Active Takayasu's disease is associated with hyperfibrinogenemia and hypofibrinolytic activity. Studies in patients with Kawasaki disease reveal thrombocytosis, diminished fibrinolytic activity, and increased platelet-derived β-thromboglobulin. Less data exist for other vasculitides, but thrombosis is a common clinical and histologic feature. A potentially simple solution with minimal side effects would be to continue low-dose aspirin during immunosuppressive therapy. This, however, has not been rigorously studied. Anticoagulation with heparin or warfarin therapy has both theoretical and practical limitations. First, parts of the coagulation in the vessels may be a physiologic effect to protect the vessel and tissue. In addition, many of the vasculitides demonstrate histologic evidence of perivascular hemorrhage. The risk of intracranial hemorrhage with these medications is potentially high.

Immunotherapy is directed at interrupting the inflammatory or proliferative cascade at key points. The goal is to downregulate the process to the point of disease remission. There is clear scientific rationale but prominent clinical limitations in the application of these focused therapies.

Monoclonal antibodies directed against surface markers on lymphocytes are potentially useful as selective therapeutic agents in a variety of immunologically mediated diseases (217). Antibodies directed at crucial components of the early phase of the immune response include anti–class II MHC antibodies, anti–IL receptor antibodies, and anti-CD4 antibodies. Such monoclonal antibodies successfully induced a short-term remission in one patient with systemic vasculitis refractory to conventional immunosuppression (218). Monoclonal antibodies to the IL-2 receptor might also modify recurrent inflammation. Generation of interferon-γ, and NK-cell function are all highly dependent on IL-2 synthesis and IL-2 receptor–driven endocytosis. Early studies of anti–IL-2Ra (expressed only on the surface of activated T cells) showed a benefit in the therapy of human T-cell leukemia with minimal immunosuppressive side effects. Studies in inflammatory diseases have not yet been reported. Antibodies to cell adhesion molecules such as ICAM reduce histologic evidence of inflammation in experimental studies; results in human studies are pending.

Cytokines, or their inhibitors, in pharmacologic dosages could downregulate inflammatory and proliferative pathways. Interferon-α is therapeutically effective in hemangiomatosis and, at least anecdotally, in Behçet's disease refractory to conventional immunosuppression (219). The effects of interferon-α include inhibition of locomotion of capillary endothelium in vitro and angiogenesis in mice and may prove useful in minimizing chronic vessel changes in patients with vasculitis. The clinical effects of TGF-β are untested but a prominent and severe immunosuppression is anticipated.

Conclusions

Studies of the vasculitides illustrate recent advances and convergence of information in the biology of inflammation, clinical diagnostic studies, and newer therapies. Over the next decade, we anticipate that more focused, less toxic treatments will result from our studies of immunopathogenesis today.

References

1. Kernohan JW, Woltman HW. Periarteritis nodosa; a clinicopathologic study with special reference to the nervous system. *Arch Neurol Psychiatry* 1938;39:655–686.
2. Zeek PM, Smith CC, Weeter JC. Studies on periarteritis nodosa. III. The differentiation between the vascular lesions of periarteritis nodosa and of hypersensitivity. *Am J Pathol* 1948;24:889–917.
3. Zeek PM. Periarteritis nodosa: a critical review. *Am J Clin Pathol* 1952;22:777–790.
4. Zeek PM. Periarteritis nodosa and other forms of necrotizing angiitis. *N Engl J Med* 1953;248:764–772.
5. Baggenstoss AH, Shick RM, Polley HF. The effect of cortisone on the lesions of periarteritis nodosa. *Am J Pathol* 1951;27:537–551.
6. Fauci AS, Doppmann JL, Wolff SM. Cyclophosphamide-induced remissions in advanced polyarteritis nodosa. *Am J Med* 1978;64:890–894.
7. Fauci AS, Haynes BF, Katz P. The spectrum of vasculitis. Clinical, pathologic, immunologic, and therapeutic considerations. *Ann Intern Med* 1978;89:660–676.
8. Hunder GG, Arend WP, Bloch DA, et al. The American College of Rheumatology 1990 criteria for the classification of vasculitis. Introduction. *Arthritis Rheum* 1990;33:1065–1067.
9. Jennette JC, Falk RJ, Andrassy K, et al. Nomenclature of systemic vasculitides. Proposal of an international consensus conference. *Arthritis Rheum* 1994;37:187–192.
10. Bloch DA, Michel BA, Hunder GG, et al. The American College of Rheumatology 1990 criteria for the classification of vasculitis. Patients and methods. *Arthritis Rheum* 1990;33:1068–1073.
11. Fries JF, Hunder GG, Bloch DA, et al. The American College of Rheumatology 1990 criteria for the classification of vasculitis. Summary. *Arthritis Rheum* 1990;33:1135–1136.
12. Hasler F. Vasculitis: immunologic aspects. *Eur Neurol* 1984;23:389–393.
13. Savage COS, Ng YC. The aetiology and pathogenesis of major systemic vasculitides. *Postgrad Med J* 1986;62:627–636.
14. Savage COS, Cooke SP. The role of the endothelium in systemic vasculitis. *J Autoimmun* 1993;6:237–249.
15. Springer TA. Traffic signals for lymphocyte recirculation and leukocyte emigration: the multistep paradigm. *Cell* 1994;76:301–314.
16. Luscinskas FW, Brock AF, Arnaout MA, Gimbrone MA Jr. Endothelial-leukocyte adhesion molecule-1 dependent and leukocyte (CD11/CD18)-dependent mechanisms contribute to polymorphonuclear leukocyte adhesion to cytokine-activated human vascular endothelium. *J Immunol* 1989;142:2257–2263.
17. Argenbright LW, Barton RW. Interactions of leukocyte integrins with intercellular adhesion molecule 1 in the production of inflammatory vascular injury in vivo. *J Clin Invest* 1992;89:259–272.
18. Osborn L. Leukocyte adhesion to endothelium in inflammation. *Cell* 1990;62:3–6.
19. Lawrence MB, Springer TA. Leukocytes roll on a selectin at physiological flow rates: distinction from and prerequisite for adhesion through integrins. *Cell* 1991;65:859–873.
20. Picker LJ, Warnock RA, Burns AR, et al. The neurophil selectin LECAM-1 presents carbohydrate ligands to the vascular selectins ELAM-1 and GMP-140. *Cell* 1991;66:921–933.
21. Okada Y, Copeland BR, Mori E, et al. P-selectin and intercellular adhesion molecular-1 expression after focal brain ischemia and reperfusion. *Stroke* 1994;25:202–211.
22. Matsushima KV, Oppenheim JJ. Interleukin-8 and MCAF. Novel inflammatory cytokines induced by TNF and IL-1. *Cytokine* 1989;1:2–10.
23. Rollins BJ, Yoshimera T, Leonard EJ, Pober JS. Cytokine-activated human endothelial cells synthesize and secrete a monocyte chemoattractant, MCP-1/JE. *Am J Pathol* 1990;136:1229–1241.
24. Sacks T, Moldow C, Craddock P, et al. Oxygen radicals mediate endothelial cell damage by complement-stimulated granulocytes. An in vitro model of immune vascular damage. *J Clin Invest* 1978;61:1161–1167.
25. Blann AD, Scott DGI. Activated, cytotoxic lymphocytes in systemic vasculitis. *Rheumatol Int* 1991;11:69–72.
26. das Neves FC, Suassuna J, Leonelli M. Cell activation and the role of cell-mediated immunity in vasculitis. *Contrib Nephrol* 1991;94:13–21.
27. Rothlein R, Kishimoto TK, Mainolfi E. Cross-linking of ICAM-1 induces co-signaling of an oxidative burst from mononuclear leukocytes. *J Immunol* 1994;152:2488–2495.
28. Stevens SK, Weissman IL, Butcher EC. Differences in the migration of B and T lymphocytes: organ-selective localization in vivo and the role of lymphocyte-endothelial cell recognition. *J Immunol* 1982;128:844–851.
29. Pober JS, Gimbrone MA Jr, Collins T, et al. Interactions of T lymphocytes with human vascular endothelial cells: role of endothelial cell surface antigens. *Immunobiology* 1984;168:483–494.
30. Dustin ML, Springer TA. Lymphocyte function-associated antigen-1 (LFA-1) interaction with intercellular adhesion molecule-1 (ICAM-1) is one of at least three mechanisms for lymphocyte adhesion to cultured endothelial cells. *J Cell Biol* 1988;107:321–331.
31. Cox JH, Ford WL. The migration of lymphocytes across specialized vascular endothelium. IV. Prednisolone acts at several points on the recirculation pathways of lymphocytes. *Cell Immunol* 1982;66:407–422.
32. Snyder DS, Beller DI, Unanue ER. Prostaglandins modulate macrophage Ia expression. *Nature* 1982;299:163–165.
33. Merrill JE, Chen ISY. HIV-1, macrophages, glial cells, and cytokines in AIDS nervous system disease. *FASEB J* 1991;5:2391–2397.
34. Johnson RJ. Platelets in inflammatory glomerular injury. *Semin Nephrol* 1991;11:276–284.
35. Tai PC, Holt ME, Denny P, et al. Deposition of eosinophil cationic protein in granulomas in allergic granulomatosis and vasculitis: the Churg-Strauss syndrome. *BMJ* 1984;289:400–402.

36. Nagata M, Segdwick J, Bates M, et al. Eosinophil adhesion to vascular cell adhesion molecule-1 activates superoxide anion generation. *J Immunol* 1995;155: 2194–2202.

37. Kallenberg CGM. Autoantibodies in vasculitis: current perspectives. *Clin Exp Rheumatol* 1993;11:355–360.

38. Leung DYM, Geha RS, Newburger JW, et al. Two monokines, interleukin 1 and tumor necrosis factor, render cultured vascular endothelial cells susceptible to lysis by antibodies circulating during Kawasaki syndrome. *J Exp Med* 1986;164:1958–1972.

39. van der Woude FJ, Rasmussen N, Lobatto S, et al. Autoantibodies against neutrophils and monocytes: tool for diagnosis and marker of disease activity in Wegener's granulomatosis. *Lancet* 1985;1:425–429.

40. Gross WL, Schmitt WH, Csernok E. ANCA and associated diseases: immunodiagnostic and pathogenetic aspects. *Clin Exp Immunol* 1993;91:1–12.

41. Falk RJ, Jennette JC. Anti-neutrophil cytoplasmic autoantibodies with specificity for myeloperoxidase in patients with systemic vasculitis and idiopathic necrotizing and crescentic glomerulonephritis. *N Engl J Med* 1988;318:1651–1657.

42. Tervaert JWC, Limburng PC, Elema JD, et al. Detection of autoantibodies against myeloid lysosomal enzymes: a useful adjunct to classification of patients with biopsy-proven necrotizing arteritis. *Am J Med* 1991;91:59–65.

43. Cochrane CG. Studies on the localization of circulating antigen-antibody complexes and other macromolecules in vessels. I. Structural studies. *J Exp Med* 1963;118: 489–502.

44. Cochrane CG. Studies on the localization of circulating antigen-antibody complexes and other macromolecules in vessels. II. Pathogenic and pharmacodynamic studies. *J Exp Med* 1963;118:503–513.

45. Cochrane CG, Weigle WO. The cutaneous reaction to soluble antigen-antibody complexes. A comparison with the Arthus phenomenon. *J Exp Med* 1958;108:591–604.

46. Mannik M. Pathophysiology of circulating immune complexes. *Arthritis Rheum* 1982;25:783–787.

47. Henson PM, Johnston RB Jr. Tissue injury in inflammation. Oxidants, proteinases, and cationic proteins. *J Clin Invest* 1987;79:669–674.

48. Kniker WT, Cochrane CG. The localization of circulating immune complexes in experimental serum sickness. The role of vasoactive amines and hydrodynamic forces. *J Exp Med* 1968;127:119–136.

49. Cochrane CG. Mechanisms involved in the deposition of immune complexes in tissues. *J Exp Med* 1971;134: 75s–89s.

50. Fligiel SEG, Ward PA, Johnson KJ, Till GO. Evidence for a role of hydroxyl radical in immune-complex-induced vasculitis. *Am J Pathol* 1984;115:375–382.

51. Fabry Z, Fitzsimmons KM, Herlein JA, et al. Production of the cytokines interleukin 1 and 6 by murine brain microvessel endothelium and smooth muscle pericytes. *J Neuroimmunol* 1993;47:23–34.

52. Prober JS, Gimbrone MA Jr, Cotran RS, et al. Ia expression by vascular endothelium is inducible by activated T cells and by human γ-interferon. *J Exp Med* 1983;157: 1339–1353.

53. Wong GHW, Bartlett PF, Clark-Lewis I, et al. Inducible expression of H-2 and Ia antigens on brain cells. *Nature* 1984;310:688–691.

54. Pober JS, Collins T, Gimbrone MA Jr, et al. Inducible expression of class II major histocompatibility complex antigens and the immunogenicity of vascular endothelium. *Transplantation* 1986;41:141–146.

55. Fabry Z, Waldschmidt MM, Hendrickson D, et al. Adhesion molecules on murine brain microvascular endothelial cells; expression and regulation of ICAM-1 and Lgp 55. *J Neuroimmunol* 1992;36:1–11.

56. Hickey WF, Kimura H. Perivascular microglial cells are bone marrow-derived and present antigens in vivo. *Science* 1988;234:290–292.

57. Cross AH, Cannella B, Brosnan CF, Raine CS. Homing to central nervous system vasculature by antigen-specific lymphocytes. *Lab Invest* 1990;63:162–169.

58. Fabry Z, Raine CS, Hart MN. Nervous tissue as an immune compartment: the dialect of the immune response in the CNS. *Immunol Today* 1994;15:218–224.

59. Hickey WF. Migration of hematogenous cells through the blood-brain barrier and the initiation of CNS inflammation. *Brain Pathol* 1991;1:97–105.

60. Hart MN, Zsuzsanna F, Waldschmidt M, Sandor M. Lymphocyte interacting adhesion molecules on brain microvascular cells. *Mol Immunol* 1990;27:1355–1359.

61. Bevilacqua MP, Pober JS, Majeau GR, et al. Interleukin 1 (IL-1) induces biosynthesis and cell surface expression of procoagulant activity in human vascular endothelial cells. *J Exp Med* 1984;160:618–623.

62. Rossi V, Breviario F, Ghezzi P, et al. Prostacyclin synthesis induced in vascular cells by interleukin-1. *Science* 1985;229:174–176.

63. Stern DM, Bank I, Nawroth PP, et al. Self-regulation of procoagulant events on the endothelial cell surface. *J Exp Med* 1985;162:1223–1235.

64. Bevilacqua MP, Pober JS, Majeau GR, et al. Recombinant tumor necrosis factor induces procoagulant activity in cultured human vascular endothelium: characterization and comparison with the actions of interleukin 1. *Proc Natl Acad Sci USA* 1986;83:4533–4537.

65. Goligorsky MS, Tsukahara H, Magazine H, et al. Termination of endothelin signaling: role of nitric oxide. *J Cell Physiol* 1994;158:485–494.

66. Brenner BM, et al. Endothelium-dependent vascular responses. *J Clin Invest* 1989;84:1373–1377.

67. Hallenbeck JM, Dutka AJ. Background review and current concepts of reperfusion injury. *Arch Neurol* 1990;47:1245–1254.

68. Yamasaki Y, Matsuura N, Shozuhara H, et al. Interleukin-1 as a pathogenetic mediator of ischemic brain damage in rats. *Stroke* 1995;26:676–681.

69. Zhang ZG, Chopp M, Zaloga C, et al. Cerebral endothelial nitric oxide synthase expression after focal cerebral ischemia in rats. *Stroke* 1993;24:2016–2021.

70. Luscher TF, Boulanger CM, Yang Z, et al. Interactions between endothelium-derived relaxing and contracting factors in health and cardiovascular disease. *Circulation* 1993;87:36–44.

71. Hamann GF, del Zoppo GJ. Leukocyte involvement in vasomotor reactivity of the cerebral vasculature. *Stroke* 1994;25:2117–2119.

72. Brenner BM, Troy JL, Ballermann BJ. Endothelium-dependent vascular responses. *J Clin Invest* 1989;84: 1373–1378.

73. Gibbons GH, Dzau VJ. The emerging concept of vascular remodeling. *N Engl J Med* 1994;330:1431–1438.

74. Lightfoot RW Jr, Michel BA, Bloch DA, et al. The American College of Rheumatology 1990 criteria for the classification of polyarteritis nodosa. *Arthritis Rheum* 1990;33:1088–1093.

75. Scott DGI, Bacon PA, Elliot PJ, et al. Systemic vasculitis in a district general hospital 1972–1980; clinical and laboratory features, classification, and prognosis in 80 cases. *Q J Med* 1982;51:292–311.

76. Ronco P, Verroust P, Mignon F, et al. Immunopathological studies of polyarteritis nodosa and Wegener's granulomatosis: a report of 43 patients and 51 renal biopsies. *Q J Med* 1983;52:212.

77. Guillevin L, Le Thi Huong D, Godeau P, et al. Clinical findings and prognosis of polyarteritis nodosa and Churg Strauss angiitis: a study in 165 patients. *Br J Rheumatol* 1988;27:258–264.

78. Savage COS, Winearls CG, Evans DJ, et al. Microscopic polyarteritis: presentation, pathology and prognosis. *Q J Med* 1985;220:467–483.

79. Li JT. Illustrated histopathologic classification criteria for selected vasculitis syndrome. *Arthritis Rheum* 1990;33:1074–1087.

80. Moore PM, Fauci AS. Neurologic manifestations of systemic vasculitis. A retrospective and prospective study of the clinicopathologic features and responses to therapy in 25 patients. *Am J Med Sci* 1981;71:517–524.

81. Lovshin LL, Kernohan JW. Peripheral neuritis in periarteritis nodosa: a clinicopathologic study. *Arch Intern Med* 1948;82:321–338.

82. Chang RW, Bell CL, Hallett M. Clinical characteristics and prognosis of vasculitic mononeuropathy multiplex. *Arch Neurol* 1984;41:618–621.

83. Bouche P, Leger JM, Travers MA, et al. Peripheral neuropathy in systemic vasculitis: clinical and electrophysiologic study of 22 patients. *Neurology* 1986;36:1598–1602.

84. Sunderland S. Blood supply of the nerves of the upper limb in man. *Arch Neurol Psychiatry* 1945;53:91–115.

85. Said G, Lacrois-Ciaudo C, Fujimura H. The peripheral neuropathy of necrotizing arteritis: a clinicopathologic study. *Ann Neurol* 1988;23:461–465.

86. Cid M, Grau JM, Casademont J, et al. Immunochemical characterization of inflammatory cells and immunologic markers in muscle and nerve biopsy specimens from patients with systemic polyarteritis nodosa. *Arthritis Rheum* 1994;37:1055–1061.

87. Parker HL, Kernohan JW. The central nervous system in periarteritis nodosa. *Mayo Clin Proc* 1949;24:43–48.

88. Ford RG, Siekert RG. Central nervous system manifestation of periarteritis nodosa. *Neurology* 1965;15:114–122.

89. Tervaert JW, Kallenberg C. Neurologic manifestations of systemic vasculitis. *Rheum Dis Clin North Am* 1993;19:913–940.

90. Goldsmith J. Periarteritis nodosa with involvement of the choroidal and retinal arteries. *Am J Pathol* 1946;29:435–446.

91. Kinyoun JL, Kalina RE, Klein ML. Choroidal involvement in systemic necrotizing vasculitis. *Arch Ophthalmol* 1987;105:939–942.

92. Akova YA, Jabbur NS, Foster CS. Ocular presentation of polyarteritis nodosa. *Ophthalmology* 1993;100:1775–1781.

93. Goldstein I, Wexler D. Bilateral atrophy of the optic nerve in periarteritis nodosa. *Arch Ophthalmol* 1937;18:767–773.

94. Kirkali P, Topaloglu R, Kansu T, Baddaloglu A. Third nerve palsy and internuclear ophthalmoplegia in periarteritis nodosa. *J Pediatr Ophthalmol Strabismus* 1991;1:45–46.

95. Topaloglu R, Besbas N, Saatci U, et al. Cranial nerve involvement in childhood polyarteritis nodosa. *Clin Neurol Neurosurg* 1992;94:11–13.

96. Churg J, Strauss L. Allergic granulomatosis, allergic angiitis, and periarteritis nodosa. *Am J Pathol* 1951;27:277–301.

97. Chumbley LC, Harris EG, DeRemee RA. Allergic granulomatosis and angiitis (Churg-Strauss syndrome). Report and analysis of 30 cases. *Mayo Clin Proc* 1977;52:477–484.

98. Aupy M, Vital C, Deminiere C, et al. Angeite granulomateuse allergique (syndrome de churg et strauss) revelee par une multinevrite. *Rev Neurol (Paris)* 1983;139:651–656. Abstract.

99. Masi AT, Hunder GG, Lie JT, et al. The American College of Rheumatology 1990 criteria for the classification of Churg-Strauss syndrome (allergic granulomatosis and angiitis). *Arthritis Rheum* 1990;33:1094–1100.

100. Lanham JG, Elkon KB, Pusey CD, Hughes GR. Systemic vasculitis with asthma and eosinophilia; a clinical approach to the Churg-Strauss syndrome. *Medicine* 1984;63:65–81.

101. Lichtig C, Ludatscher R, Eisenberg E, Bental E. Small blood vessel disease in allergic granulomatous angiitis (Churg-Strauss syndrome). *J Clin Pathol* 1989;42:1001–1002.

102. Sehgal M, Swanson J, DeRemee R, Colby T. Neurologic manifestations of Churg-Strauss syndrome. *Mayo Clin Proc* 1995;70:337–341.

103. Chang Y, Karga S, Goates J, Horoupian D. Intraventricular and subarachnoid hemorrhage resulting from necrotizing vasculitis of the choroid plexus in a patient with Churg-Strauss syndrome. *Clin Neuropathol* 1993;12:84–87.

104. Kok J, Bosseray A, Brion J, Micoud M. Chorea in a child with Churg Strauss syndrome. *Stroke* 1993;24:1263–1264.

105. Weinstein JM, Chui H, Lane S, et al. Churg Strauss syndrome (allergic granulomatous angiitis). Neuroophthalmologic manifestations. *Arch Ophthalmol* 1983;101:1217–1220.

106. Acheson JF, Cockerell OC, Bentley CR, Sanders MD. Churg Strauss vasculitis presenting with severe visual loss due to bilateral sequential optic neuropathy. *Br J Ophthalmol* 1993;77:118–119.

107. Liou H, Yip P, Chang Y, Liu H. Allergic granulomatosis and angiitis (Churg-Strauss syndrome) presenting as prominent neurologic lesions and optic neuritis. *J Rheumatol* 1994;21:2380–2384.

108. O'Donovan CA, Keogan M, Staunton H, et al. Peripheral neuropathy in Churg-Strauss syndrome associated with IgA-C3 deposits. *Ann Neurol* 1992;32:411.

109. Sams WM Jr, Thorne EG, Small P, et al. Leukocytoclastic vasculitis. *Arch Dermatol* 1976;112:219–226.

110. Hodge SJ, Callen JP, Ekenstam E. Cutaneous leukocytoclastic vasculitis: correlation of histopathological changes with clinical severity and course. *J Cutan Pathol* 1987;14:279–284.

111. Zax RH, Hodge SJ, Callen JP. Cutaneous leukocytoclastic vasculitis. *Arch Dermatol* 1990;126:69–72.

112. Parish WE. Studies on vasculitis. I. Immunoglobulins BIC, C reactive protein, and bacterial antigens in cutaneous vasculitic lesions. *Clin Allergy* 1971;1:97–109.

113. Parish WE, Rhodes EL. Bacterial antigens and aggregated gamma globulin in the lesions of nodular vasculitis. *Br J Dermatol* 1967;79:131–147.

114. Ong ACM, Handler CE, Walker JM. Hypersensitivity vasculitis complicating intravenous streptokinase therapy in acute myocardial infarction. *Int J Cardiol* 1988;21:71–73.

115. Mullick FG, McAllister HA, Wagner BM, Fenoglio JJ Jr. Drug related vasculitis. Clinicopathologic correlations in 30 patients. *Hum Pathol* 1979;10:313–325.

116. Mills JA, Michel BA, Bloch DA, et al. The American Col-

lege of Rheumatology 1990 criteria for the classification of Henoch-Schönlein purpura. *Arthritis Rheum* 1990;33: 1114–11121.

117. Park AM, Richardson JC. Cerebral complications of serum sickness. *Neurology* 1953;3:227–283.

118. Lawley TJ, Bielory L, Gascon P, et al. A prospective clinical and immunologic analysis of patients with serum sickness. *N Engl J Med* 1984;311:1407–1413.

119. Lewis IC, Philpott MG. Neurological complications in the Schönlein-Henoch syndrome. *Arch Dis Child* 1956; 31:369–371.

120. Leavitt RY, Fauci AS, Bloch DA, et al. The American College of Rheumatology 1990 criteria for the classification of Wegener's granulomatosis. *Arthritis Rheum* 1990;33:1101–1107.

121. Miller K, et al. Wegener's granulomatosis presenting as a primary seizure disorder with brain lesions demonstrated by magnetic resonance imaging. *Chest* 1993;103: 316–318.

122. Bullen CL, Liesegang TJ, McDonald TJ, DeRemee RA. Ocular complications of Wegener's granulomatosis. *Am J Ophthalmol* 1989;90:279–290.

123. Stern GM, Hoffbrand AV, Urich H. The peripheral nerves and skeletal muscles in Wegener's granulomatosis: a clinico-pathological study of four cases. *Brain* 1989; 58:151–164.

124. Nishino H, Rubino FA, DeRemee RA, et al. Neurological involvement in Wegener's granulomatosis: an analysis of 324 consecutive patients at the Mayo Clinic. *Ann Neurol* 1993;33:4–9.

125. Hoffman GS, Kerr GS, Leavitt RY, et al. Wegener granulomatosis: an analysis of 158 patients. *Ann Intern Med* 1992;116:488–498.

126. Gross WL, Csernok E, Flesch BK. 'Classic' antineutrophil cytoplasmic autoantibodies (cANCA), 'Wegener's autoantigen' and their immunopathogenic role in Wegener's granulomatosis. *J Autoimmun* 1993;6:171–184.

127. Cupps TR, Moore PM, Fauci AS. Isolated angiitis of the central nervous system. Prospective diagnostic and therapeutic experience. *Am J Med* 1983;74:97–105.

128. Moore PM. Diagnosis and management of isolated angiitis of the central nervous system. *Neurology* 1989;39: 167–173.

129. Kolodny EH, Rebeiz JJ, Caviness VS Jr, Richardson EP Jr. Granulomatous angiitis of the central nervous system. *Arch Neurol* 1968;19:510–524.

130. Hughes JT, Brownell B. Granulomatous giant-celled angiitis of the central nervous system. *Neurology* 1966; 16:293–298.

131. Jellinger K. Giant cell granulomatous angiitis of the central nervous system. *J Neurol* 1977;215:175–190.

132. Crane R, Kerr LD, Spiera H. Clinical analysis of isolated angiitis of the central nervous system. A report of 11 cases. *Arch Intern Med* 1991;151:2290–2294.

133. Kristoferitsch W, Jellinger K, Bock F. Cerebral granulomatous angiitis with atypical features. *Neurology* 1984;231:38–40.

134. Miller DH, Ormerod IE, Gibson A, et al. MR brain scanning in patients with vasculitis: differentiation from multiple sclerosis. *Neuroradiology* 1987;29:226–231.

135. Hellman DB, Roubenoff R, Healy RA, Wang H. Central nervous system angiography: safety and predictors of a positive result in 125 consecutive patients evaluated for possible vasculitis. *J Rheumatol* 1992;19:568–572.

136. Stein RL, Martino CR, Weinert DM, et al. Cerebral angiography as a guide for therapy in isolated central nervous system vasculitis. *JAMA* 1987;257:2193–2195.

137. Alhalabi M, Moore PM. Serial angiography in isolated angiitis of the central nervous system. *Neurology* 1994;44:1221–1226.

138. Kissel JT, Slivka AP, Warmolts JR, Mendell JR. The clinical spectrum of necrotizing angiopathy of the peripheral nervous system. *Ann Neurol* 1985;18:251–257.

139. Harati Y, Niakan A. The clinical spectrum of inflammatory angiopathic neuropathy. *J Neurol Neurosurg Psychiatry* 1986;49:1313–1316.

140. Hawke SH, Davies L, Pamphlett R, et al. Vasculitis neuropathy. A clinical and pathologic study. *Brain* 1991;114: 2175–2190.

141. Engelhardt A, Lorler H, Neundorfer B. Immunohistochemical findings in vasculitic neuropathies. *Acta Neurol Scand* 1993;87:318–321.

142. Fabian RH, Petroff G. Intraneuronal IgG in the central nervous system: uptake by retrograde axonal transport. *Neurology* 1987;37:1780–1784.

143. Miller DH, Haas LF, Teague C, Neale TJ. Small vessel vasculitis presenting as neurological disorder. *J Neurol Neurosurg Psychiatry* 1984;47:791–794.

144. Bogousslavsky J, Gaio JM, Caplan LR, et al. Encephalopathy, deafness and blindness in young women: a distinct retinocochleocerebral arteriolopathy? *J Neurol Neurosurg Psychiatry* 1989;52:43–46.

145. Cheson BD, Bluming AZ, Alroy J. Cogan's syndrome: a systemic vasculitis. *Am J Pathol* 1976;60:549–555.

146. Haynes BF, Kaiser-Kupfer MI, Mason P, Fauci AS. Cogan syndrome: studies in thirteen patients, long-term follow-up, and review of the literature. *Medicine* 1980; 59:426–441.

147. Dodge PR, Swartz MN. Bacterial meningitis—a review of selected aspects. II. Special neurologic problems, postmeningitic complications and clinicopathological correlations (concluded). *N Engl J Med* 1965;272:1003–1010.

148. Lyons EL, Leeds NE. The angiographic demonstration of arterial vascular disease in purulent meningitis. Report of a case. *Radiology* 1967;88:935–938.

149. Igarashi M, Gilmartin RC, Gerald B, et al. Cerebral arteritis and bacterial meningitis. *Arch Neurol* 1984;41: 531–535.

150. Walsh TJ, Hier DB, Caplan LR. Aspergillosis of the central nervous system: clinicopathological analysis of 17 patients. *Ann Neurol* 1985;18:574–582.

151. Schigenaga K, Okabe M, Ethon K. An autopsy case of aspergillus infection of the brain. *Kumamoto Med J* 1975;28:135–144.

152. Wheat LJ, Batteiger BE, Sathapatayavongs B. *Histoplasma capsulatum* infections of the central nervous system; a clinical review. *Medicine* 1990;69:244–260.

153. Tija D, Yeow UK, Tan CB. Cryptococcal meningitis. *J Neurol Neurosurg Psychiatry* 1985;48:853–858.

154. Williams PL, Johnson R, Pappagianis D. Vasculitic and encephalitic complications associated with *Coccidioides immitis* infection of the central nervous system in humans: report of 10 cases and review. *Clin Infect Dis* 1992;14:673–682.

155. Koeppen AH, Lansing LS, Peng S, Smith RS. Central nervous system vasculitis in cytomegalovirus infection. *J Neurosci* 1981;51:395–410.

156. Martin FP, Lukeman JM, Ranson RF, Geppert LJ. Mucormycosis of the central nervous system associated with thrombosis of the internal carotid artery. *J Pediatr* 1954;44:437–444.

157. de la Torre FE, Gorraez MT. Toxoplasma-induced occlusive hypertrophic arteritis as the cause of discrete coagulative necrosis in the CNS. *Hum Pathol* 1989;20:604.

158. Kobayashi RM, Coel M, Niwayama G, Trauner D. Cerebral vasculitis in coccidioidal meningitis. *Ann Neurol* 1977;1:281–284.

159. Meurers B, Kohlepp W, Gold R, et al. Histopathologic findings of the central and peripheral nervous system in neuroborreliosis: a report of three cases. *J Neurol* 1990;237:113–116.

160. Miklossy J, Kuntzer T, Bogousslavsky J, et al. Meningovascular form of neuroborreliosis: similarities between neuropathological findings in a case of Lyme disease and those occurring in tertiary neurosyphilis. *Acta Neuropathol (Berl)* 1990;80:568–572.

161. Lehrer H. The angiographic triad in tuberculous meningitis. A radiographic and clinicopathologic correlation. *Radiology* 1966;87:829–835.

162. Teoh R, Humphries MJ, Chan JC, et al. Intranuclear ophthalmoplegia in tuberculous meningitis. *Tubercle* 1989;70:61–64.

163. Rabinov KR. Angiographic findings in a case of brain syphilis. *Radiology* 1968;80:622–624.

164. Linnemann CC Jr, Alvira MM. Pathogenesis of varicella-zoster angiitis in the CNS. *Arch Neurol* 1980;37:239–340.

165. Powers JM. Herpes zoster maxillaris with delayed occipital infarction. *J Clin Neuroophthalmol* 1986;6:113–115.

166. Hirose S, Hamashima Y. Morphological observations on the vasculitis in the mucocutaneous lymph syndrome. *Eur J Pediatr* 1978;129:17–27.

167. Walker RJ III, Gammel TE, Allen MB. Cranial arteritis associated with herpes zoster. Case report with angiographic findings. *Radiology* 1973;107:109–110.

168. Hilt DC, Buchholz D, Krumholz A, et al. Herpes zoster ophthalmicus and delayed contralateral hemiparesis caused by cerebral angiitis: diagnosis and management approaches. *Ann Neurol* 1983;14:543–553.

169. Huang TE, Chou SM. Occlusive hypertrophic arteritis as the cause of discrete necrosis in CNS toxoplasmosis in the acquired immunodeficiency syndrome. *Hum Pathol* 1988;19:1210–1214.

170. Citron BP, Halpern M, McCarron M, et al. Necrotizing angiitis with drug abuse. *N Engl J Med* 1970;283:1003–1011.

171. Reichlin M. Clinical and immunological significance of antibodies to Ro and La in systemic lupus erythematosus. *Arthritis Rheum* 1982;25:767–772.

172. Rumbaugh CL, Bergeron RT, Fang HC, McCormick R. Cerebral angiographic changes in the drug abuse patient. *Radiology* 1971;101:335–344.

173. Krendel DA, Ditter SM, Frankel MR, Ross WK. Biopsy-proven cerebral vasculitis associated with cocaine abuse. *Neurology* 1990;40:1092–1094.

174. Rubenstein MK. Mononeuritis in association with malignancy. *Bull Los Angeles Neurol Soc* 1966;31:157–163.

175. Johnson PC, Rolak LA, Hamilton RH, Laguna JF. Paraneoplastic vasculitis of nerve: a remote effect of cancer. *Ann Neurol* 1979;5:437–444.

176. Petito CK, Gottlieb GJ, Dougherty JH, Petito FA. Neoplastic angioendotheliosis: ultrastructural study and review of the literature. *Ann Neurol* 1978;3:393–399.

177. Greer JM, Longley S, Edwards NL, et al. Vasculitis associated with malignancy. Experience with 13 patients and literature review. *Medicine* 1988;67:220–230.

178. Roux S, Grossin M, De Brandt M, et al. Angiotropic large cell lymphoma with mononeuritis multiplex mimicking systemic vasculitis. *J Neurol Neurosurg Psychiatry* 1995;58:363–366.

179. Estey E, Lieberman A, Pinto R, et al. Cerebral arteritis in scleroderma. *Stroke* 1979;10:595–599.

180. Watson P. Intracranial hemorrhage with vasculitis in rheumatoid arthritis. *Arch Neurol* 1979;36:58.

181. Skowronski T, Gatter RA. Cerebral vasculitis associated with rheumatoid disease: a case report. *J Rheumatol* 1974;1:473.

182. Ramos M, Mandybur TI. Cerebral vasculitis in rheumatoid arthritis. *Arch Neurol* 1975;32:271–275.

183. Peyronnard JM, Charron L, Beaudet F, Couture F. Vasculitic neuropathy in rheumatoid disease and Sjögren syndrome. *Neurology* 1982;32:839–845.

184. Scott DGI, Bacon PA, Tribe CR. Systemic rheumatoid vasculitis: a clinical and laboratory study of 50 cases. *Medicine* 1981;60:288–297.

185. Koo EH, Solbrig N, Massey EW. Granulomatous angiitis: its protean manifestations and response to treatment. *Neurology* 1984;34(S1):202.

186. Pallis CP, Scott JT. Peripheral neuropathy in rheumatoid arthritis. *BMJ* 1965;1:1141–1147.

187. Alexander EL, Arnett FC, Provost TT, Stevens MB. Sjögren's syndrome: association of anti-Ro (SS-A) antibodies with vasculitis, hematological abnormalities, and serologic hyperreactivity. *Ann Intern Med* 1983;98:155–159.

188. Malinow K, Yannakakis GD, Glusman SM. Subacute sensory neuronopathy secondary to dorsal root ganglionitis in primary Sjögren's syndrome. *Ann Neurol* 1986;20:535–537.

189. Harris KG, Tran DD, Sickels WJ, et al. Diagnosing intracranial vasculitis: the roles of MR and angiography. *Am J Neuroradiol* 1994;15:317–330.

190. Sole-Llenas J, Pons-Tortella E. Cerebral angiitis. *Neuroradiology* 1978;15:1–11.

191. Ferris EJ, Levine HL. Cerebral arteritis: classification. *Radiology* 1973;109:327–441.

192. Travers RL, Allison DJ, Brettle RP, Hughes GRV. Polyarteritis nodosa. A clinical and angiographic analysis of 17 cases. *Semin Arthritis Rheum* 1979;8:184–189.

193. Garner BF, Burns P, Bunning RD, Laureno R. Acute blood pressure elevation can mimic arteriographic appearance of cerebral vasculitis (a postpartum case with relative hypertension). *J Rheumatol* 1990;17:93–97.

194. Carcassi MU. Cytotoxic drugs in systemic autoimmune diseases. *Clin Exp Rheumatol* 1989;7:181–186.

195. Kissel JT, Rammohan KW. Pathogenesis and therapy of nervous system vasculitis. *Clin Neuropharmacol* 1991;14:28–48.

196. De Vita S, Ner R, Bombardieri S. Cyclophosphamide pulses in the treatment of rheumatic diseases: an update. *Clin Exp Rheumatol* 1991;9:179–193.

197. De Jesus, Talal N. Practical use of immunosuppressive drugs in autoimmune rheumatic diseases. *Crit Care Med* 1990;18:132–137.

198. Omdal R, Husby G, Koldingsnes W. Intravenous and oral cyclophosphamide pulse therapy in rheumatic diseases: side effects and complications. *Clin Exp Rheumatol* 1993;11:283–288.

199. Morand EF, Goulding NJ. Glucocorticoids in rheumatoid arthritis—mediators and mechanisms. *Br J Rheumatol* 1993;32:816–819.

200. Goulding NJ, Guyre PM. Regulation of inflammation by lipocortin 1. *Immunol Today* 1992;13:295–297.

201. Conn DL, Tompkins RB, Nichols WL. Glucocorticoids in the management of vasculitis—a double edge sword? *J Rheumatol* 1988;15:1181–1183.

202. Conn DL. Update on systemic necrotizing vasculitis. *Mayo Clin Proc* 1989;64:535–543.

203. Newcomer JW, Craft S, Hershey T, et al. Glucocorticoid-induced impairment in declarative memory perfor-

mance in adult humans. *J Neurosci* 1994;14:2047–2053.

204. McCune WJ, Golbus J, Zeldes W, et al. Clinical and immunologic effects of monthly administration of intravenous cyclophosphamide in severe systemic lupus erythematosus. *N Engl J Med* 1988;318:1423–1431.

205. Scott DGI, Bacon PA. Intravenous cyclophosphamide plus methylprednisolone in treatment of systemic rheumatoid vasculitis. *Am J Med* 1984;76:377–384.

206. Hoffman GS, Leavitt RY, Fleisher TA, et al. Treatment of Wegener's granulomatosis with intermittent high-dose intravenous cyclophosphamide. *Am J Med* 1990;89:403–410.

207. Kahan BD. Drug therapy. *N Engl J Med* 1989;321:1725–1738.

208. Campion EW. Desperate diseases and plasmapheresis. *N Engl J Med* 1992;326:1425–1427.

209. Guillevin L, Jarrousse B, Lok C, et al. Longterm followup after treatment of polyarteritis nodosa and Churg-Strauss angiitis with comparison of steroids, plasma exchange and cyclophosphamide to steroids and plasma exchange. A prospective randomized trial of 71 patients. *J Rheumatol* 1991;18:567–574.

210. Sessa A, Meroni M, Battini G. Treatment and prognosis of renal and systemic vasculitis. *Contrib Nephrol* 1993;94:72–80.

211. Lockwood CM, Worlledge S, Nicholas A, et al. Reversal of impaired splenic function in patients with nephritis or vasculitis (or both) by plasma exchange. *N Engl J Med* 1979;300:524.

212. Schwartz SA. Intravenous immunoglobulin (IVIG) for the therapy of autoimmune disorders. *J Clin Immunol* 1990;10:81–89.

213. Jayne DRW, Lockwood CM. High-dose pooled immunoglobulin in the therapy of systemic vasculitis. *J Autoimmun* 1993;6:207–219.

214. Tuso P, Moudgil A, Hay J, et al. Treatment of antineutrophil cytoplasmic autoantibody-positive systemic vasculitis and glomerulonephritis with pooled intravenous gammaglobulin. *Am J Kidney Dis* 1992;20:504–508.

215. Brooks PM, Day RO. Nonsteroidal antiinflammatory drugs—differences and similarities. *N Engl J Med* 1991;324:1716–1725.

216. Hauptman HW, Ruddy S, Robert WN. Reversal of the vasospastic component of lupus vasculopathy by infusion of prostaglandin E. *J Rheumatol* 1991;18:1747–1752.

217. Isaacs JD, Clark MR, Greenwood J, Waldmann H. Therapy with monoclonal antibodies. *J Immunol* 1992;148:3062–3071.

218. Mathieson PW, Cobbold SP, Hale G, et al. Monoclonal-antibody therapy in systemic vasculitis. *N Engl J Med* 1990;323:250–254.

219. Durand JM, Kaplanski G, Telle H, et al. Beneficial effects of interferon-α2b in Behçet's disease. *Arthritis Rheum* 1993;36:1025.

Chapter 17

Inflammatory Cytokines, Astrocytes, and the Regeneration of the Central Nervous System

Voon Wee Yong, Abbas F. Sadikot, and Gordon H. Baltuch

Following insults to the central nervous system (CNS), the regeneration of damaged neurons and their axons and of injured oligodendrocytes and their myelin is limited. A more successful degree of regeneration depends both on *intrinsic* neuronal or oligodendrocyte determinants, such as the proper expression of growth-related genes and the synthesis of molecules critical to the structural changes and function of the cell, and on *extrinsic* environmental influences, which include the presence of permissive substrates, growth-promoting trophic factors, and the neutralization of growth inhibitory or toxic molecules.

The requirement for intrinsic cell determinants is demonstrated by the observation that older neurons do not grow as well as younger ones in the same environment (1,2). Similarly, for oligodendrocytes, the regeneration of processes in vitro depends on the age of the animal from which the cells are derived; neonatal cells have the best regenerative capability and this is progressively reduced with aging (3).

The importance of extrinsic influences is best illustrated by the experiments of David and Aguayo (4). They inserted a sciatic nerve graft as a bridge between the dorsolateral region of the spinal cord, at the site of laminectomy, and the lower medulla of adult rats. After 22 to 30 weeks, the sciatic nerve graft contained regenerated fibers from both CNS regions that traversed the entire 35 mm of the graft but then terminated within 2 mm after re-entering the CNS environment. In the converse experiments, optic nerve was grafted onto the lesioned sciatic nerve; very limited regeneration occurred through the optic nerve graft and many peripheral axons regenerated around the graft or avoided it completely (5). Nonpermissive substrates for axonal regeneration that are present within the CNS environment are thought to be expressed primarily in white rather than gray matter (6,7) and they include proteins that are present on oligodendrocytes and myelin which can cause the collapse of neuronal growth cones (8–10).

The role of astrocytes as extrinsic impediments to neural regeneration is complex and controversial. Scars formed by astrocytes are thought to prevent axonal elongation (11,12), and some of the astrocyte proteins contributing to the inhibitory activity include chondroitin sulfate proteoglycan and tenascin (13–16). However, there is also ample evidence that reactive astrocytes have many neurotrophic properties; in lower vertebrates such as the fish and amphibia, glial scars are not impediments to regenerating neurites.

It has been known for sometime that neurotrophic molecules are secreted around the locus of traumatic lesions (17–21). The maximal levels are reached some 9 to 15 days after the onset of trauma and decline thereafter. The suggestion has been made that the sources of these factors are reactive astrocytes because the locus of lesions contains such cells and because the implantation of astrocytes into adult rats with medial frontal cortex ablation can result in recovery of T-maze learning behavior (22). Other neurotrophic properties of astrocytes are discussed later.

Another cell type that can influence successful regeneration of the CNS is the microglial cell. There is an abundance of evidence that neurons can be destroyed by toxins elaborated by microglia (23–28); in some experimental situations, the toxicity of microglia to neurons can be reduced by astrocytes (26,27). Giulian and Robertson (23) previously described the suppression of mononuclear phagocytes after ischemic injury, with consequent improved recovery from the ischemic episode. The use of receptor antagonists to interleukin (IL)-1, a microglia/macrophage product, markedly inhibited the neurodegeneration that was induced by focal cerebral ischemia in rats (29).

With regards to oligodendrocyte-microglia interactions, Merrill et al (30) reported that rat microglia are toxic to rat oligodendrocytes. We found that adult human oligodendrocytes in vitro are also susceptible to toxicity by microglia, whereas astrocytes afford protection (31); similarly, the free radical–mediated damage to oligodendrocytes can be prevented by astrocytes (32). Nonetheless, the role of microglia cells or blood-derived macrophages in CNS regeneration is controversial since trophic properties of microglia for neurons have also been reported (33–35). Regarding oligodendrocytes, microglia have been observed to stimulate their myelinogenic program (36,37).

Another extrinsic determinant for successful CNS regeneration, and an alternative source of the aforementioned neurotrophic factors that are found after injury, may be provided by inflammatory cytokines produced either by endogenous neural cells or by inflammatory mononuclear cells that infiltrate into the CNS upon injury. These inflammatory cytokines can have direct neurotrophic activity, or they may influence the neurotrophic activity of neural cells, particularly astrocytes. In the following section, we discuss the evidence that 1) inflammatory cytokines are elevated in the CNS following various types of insults, 2) inflammatory cytokines have neurotrophic activity, 3) astrocytes have neurotrophic activity, and 4) inflammatory cytokines can modulate the neurotrophic activity of astrocytes. Finally, we discuss the evidence that in some circumstances, inflammatory cytokines can be detrimental.

Inflammatory Cytokines Are Elevated in the CNS Following Various Types of Insults

Various types of injuries to the adult CNS result in the activation of parenchymal microglia as well as the recruitment of systemic inflammatory mononuclear cells that include monocytes, natural killer (NK) cells, and T lymphocytes (38–40). These inflammatory cells are sources of cytokines and the levels of IL-1, IL-2, IL-6, transforming growth factor (TGF)-β, tumor necrosis factor (TNF)-α, and several others are known to be elevated following CNS insults (41–46). We determined the time course of the increase of TNF-α messenger RNA (mRNA) following acute trauma (stab) in adult mice and found that very high levels are found within 3 hours after the injury and are maintained for 24 hours (unpublished observations, 1996).

The potential role of *neural cells* as cellular sources of cytokines following CNS injury also needs to be considered, as a multitude of reports now indicate that astrocytes in vitro can produce IL-1, IL-3, IL-6, macrophage colony-stimulating factor (M-CSF), interferon (IFN), TNF-α, and TGF-β1 either under basal culture conditions or when stimulated with viruses or other cytokines (47–55). Similarly, in vivo, astrocytes can produce IFN-γ, IL-1, IL-2, IL-3, and TGF (56–59). Reports are emerging that *neurons* can produce IL-1, IL-2, IL-3, IFN-γ (or a closely related molecule), M-CSF, TGF-α, and TNF-α (60–66).

Thus, the existing evidence shows that the levels of inflammatory cytokines increase following insults to the CNS, and that their potential effects on cells of the CNS need to be addressed.

Inflammatory Cytokines Have Neurotrophic Activity

In the peripheral nervous system, the infiltration of macrophages into the site of injury appears to be critical to the capability of peripheral nerves to regenerate. Using C57 BL/Ola mice in which the regeneration of peripheral nerves following wallerian degeneration is reduced, Brown et al (67) found that the recruitment of macrophages is much lower when compared to that in C57BL/6J and BALB/c mice with impressive rates of regeneration. Conversely, Lu and Richardson (68) demonstrated that by provoking inflammation in rat dorsal root ganglia, regeneration of the associated dorsal root following a crush injury is increased fourfold when compared to the noninflamed crushed dorsal root ganglia. The requirement for macrophages appears to be due to IL-1, a macrophage product, stimulating the production of nerve growth factor (NGF) and its receptor (69,70). Similarly, in the aforementioned experiments of Brown et al (67) in C57BL/Ola mice, the levels of mRNAs for both NGF and its receptor are raised only slightly above basal levels, in contrast to the large increase seen in other mouse strains.

In the CNS, the requirement for inflammation in regeneration is also increasingly being appreciated. Thus, at sites of *anisomorphic injury*, where the blood-brain barrier is disrupted and inflammatory cells accumulate, the implantation of grafts results in extensive axonal outgrowth from the grafts. In contrast, isomorphic sites where the blood-brain barrier is intact do not allow the grafts to extend neurites (71). In the rat optic nerve following a crush injury, Hirschberg et al (72) observed that daily intraperitoneal injection of dexamethasone prior to the injury reduced the permissiveness of the injured nerves to neural adhesion and regrowth in vitro, indicating that inflammation is favorable for regeneration.

In vitro, the expression of certain neurotransmitters or neuropeptides by sympathetic ganglia can be regulated by factors elaborated by activated lymphocytes (73) and by IL-1β (74). Furthermore, certain cytokines have direct neurotrophic activity in vitro. Thus, TGF-β1, TGF-α, IFN-γ, IL-1, and IL-6 improve the survival of various populations of neurons in culture (Table 17-1) (75–85). IL-2, IL-6, and IFN-γ also facilitate neurite ex-

Table 17-1.
In Vitro Evidence That Cytokines Have Neurotrophic Activity: Effects on Neuronal Survival and Neurite Extension

Effect	Cytokine	Cells	Reference
Neuronal survival	IL-1α	E12 mouse SC neurons	75
	IL-2	E17 rat neurons	76
	IL-6	E17 or P10 rat septum	29, 77
		E20 rat hippocampus	78
	IFN-γ	E15 mouse hippocampus	79
	TGF-β1	E14 rat SC neurons	80
		Neonatal olfactory neuron	81
	TGF-α	Neonatal rat DRG	82
Neurite extension	IL-2	Chick E9–11 SG	83
	IL-3	E15 mouse, E17 rat septum	84
	IL-6	PC12 cells	85
	IFN-γ	E15 mouse hippocampus	79

IL = interleukin; IFN = interferon; TGF = transforming growth factor; E = embryonic age; P = postnatal day age; SC = spinal cord; DRG = dorsal root ganglion; SG = sympathetic ganglia.

tension in vitro (see Table 17-1). David et al (35) showed that the nonpermissive nature of the isolated rat optic nerve can become permissive to ingrowth of neurites from dorsal root ganglia if the optic nerve sections are treated with macrophages isolated from injured brains. Finally, several inflammatory cytokines have the ability to cause the maturation of progenitor cells into hippocampal neurons (86).

In vivo, the application of TNF-α to the injured adult rabbit optic nerve produces a regeneration of axons that traverse the site of injury (87). When the lesioned optic nerve is treated in vivo with TNF-α, and then explanted in vitro, it becomes more permissive for PC12 cell adhesion when compared to non-TNF-α–treated nerves (88). Administration of IL-3 in vivo after fimbria-fornix transection in rats results in about twofold more acetylcholinesterase-positive cells in the lesioned septum when compared to lesioned control animals (84); similarly, the in vivo administration of granulocyte-macrophage colony-stimulating factor (GM-CSF) promotes the survival of septal cholinergic neurons in adult rats that had undergone fimbria-fornix transections (89). The coinfusion of IL-6 with the excitotoxin *N*-methyl-D-aspartate (NMDA) into the rat striatum reduces the neurotoxic effects of the latter (90).

Finally, the story of IFN-γ in regeneration is intriguing. Olsson et al (64) reported the appearance of IFN-γ–like immunoreactivity (by 2 days) in the cytoplasm of facial motor neurons following interruption (cut or crush injury) of the facial nerve. While this IFN-γ–like product is not identical to immune IFN-γ (91), its immunoreactivity subsides in the crush injury as the target muscles are reinnervated (when rats regain movements of their whiskers) but persist when nerve regeneration is prevented after the cut injury. Olsson et al (64) speculated that the neuron-derived IFN-γ–like molecule could be involved with reinnervation, a contention that finds support in the observation that NGF-treated PC12 cells (which differentiate into cells with many of the properties of sympathetic neurons) have an early response gene (PC4) that encodes a protein homologous to IFN-γ; the PC4 gene is also found in the developing spinal cord (92).

In summary, several lines of evidence demonstrate that inflammatory cytokines have neurotrophic activity. CNS neural cells, including neurons, are potential sources of cytokines under certain conditions, and these neuron-derived cytokines may be participating in the general context of CNS recovery following injury.

Astrocytes Have Trophic Activity for Neurons and Oligodendrocytes

The concept that astrocytes, and reactive astrocytes, have many neurotrophic functions has evolved from several lines of observations. Firstly, astrocytes are excellent tissue culture substrates for the survival and growth of many populations of neurons in vitro (93,94). Fibroblasts have less of this neurotrophic activity and, indeed, when growing CNS neurons encounter a boundary between astrocytes and fibroblasts, they stay

on astrocytes and do not encroach on the fibroblasts (95). The neurite-promoting effects of astrocytes are partially due to the production of basic fibroblast growth factor (bFGF) (96), N-cadherin, and extracellular matrix proteins (97,98). Furthermore, the neurite-promoting effect of astrocytes decreases with the age of the astrocytes (99). Indeed, Geisert et al (100) noted that on neonatal astrocytes, neurites have a pronounced tendency to lie parallel to the processes of astrocytes, maximizing contact. On adult astrocytes, however, the majority of neurites appear to cross the astrocytic processes orthogonally, minimizing contact with astrocytes.

The second line of evidence that astrocytes have neurotrophic activity comes from reports that neurotrophic factors are produced around the locus of a CNS lesion, as described already, and that the source of these appears to be reactive astrocytes (17–21). Ip et al (18) demonstrated that the soluble extracts collected from around a lesioned CNS site in adult mice contain neurotrophic activity for cultured neurons; this trophic action can be completely abolished by an antiserum to ciliary neurotrophic factor (CNTF). Furthermore, Northern blot analyses showed that levels of mRNA for CNTF increase in cortical areas following injury, and results of in situ hybridization studies suggest that the cells responsible for the increased CNTF production are likely reactive astrocytes.

In addition to CNTF, other neurotrophic factors found to be elevated around lesion sites include NGF, fibroblast growth factors (FGFs), brain-derived neurotrophic factor (BDNF), and neurotrophin-3 (NT-3); the source of these factors appears to be astrocytes or neurons (101–104).

Interestingly, in brain transplant studies, the survival of grafts is enhanced by cotransplanting extracts from injured brains, or by creating a lesion and then waiting for a few days before the implant surgery (105,106). Both cases presumably allow for astrocytes to undergo reactive changes and to produce neurotrophic factors. As mentioned, the implantation of astrocytes into adult rats after medial frontal cortex ablation results in the recovery of T-maze learning behavior (22); recently this observation was confirmed independently (107). The implantation of astrocytes into the hemisected adult rat spinal cord also reduces scarring and increases the intensity of neurofilament labeling at the lesion site (108).

In further support of the postulate that astrocytes have neurotrophic activity are the observations that implants of perinatal astrocytes provide a terrain suitable for axons to regrow in vivo (109–111). Kawaja and Gage (112) implanted primary fibroblasts genetically engineered to express NGF into the striatum of adult rats. Cholinergic neurons arising from the nucleus basalis grew toward and penetrated these grafts, but not into non-NGF-producing control fibroblasts. Significantly, axons grew into grafts of NGF-producing cells only on reactive astrocytic processes.

Finally, enriched populations of astrocytes in vitro produce a range of neurotrophic factors that include CNTF, acidic or basic FGF, EGF, insulin-like growth factors (IGFs), and the neurotrophins NGF, NT-3, and BDNF (Table 17-2). Indeed, it has become increasingly difficult to find a trophic factor that is not produced by astrocytes in vitro.

Certain characteristics of cells of the oligodendrocyte lineage are also dependent on astrocyte function. Thus, growth factors from astrocytes cause the proliferation of oligodendrocyte precursors and modulate their survival and differentiation into oligodendrocytes (reviewed elsewhere (122)). Astrocytes are also conducive substrates for the extension of processes from adult human oligodendrocytes (Fig 17-1), by providing bFGF and an unidentified component of the astrocyte extracellular matrix (31). Rome et al (123,124) demonstrated that oligodendrocytes adhere well to an astrocyte matrix via integrin-dependent mechanisms. In lesion areas of multiple sclerosis, oligodendrocytes are observed to be invested within hypertrophic astrocytes (125–127); the role of such glial associations remains controversial and may represent a protective mechanism for oligodendrocytes by astrocytes (126) or destruction of oligodendrocytes by astrocytes (127).

The role of astrocytes in myelin formation by oligodendrocytes has been the subject of few studies, and some of the results are conflicting. Bhat and Pfeiffer (128) reported that soluble extracts from astrocyte cultures increase myelin proteins of oligodendrocytes. However, astrocytes can inhibit the myelination of dorsal root ganglion axons by adult rat oligodendrocytes (129) and can prevent the translocation of myelin basic protein mRNA from soma into the processes of oligodendrocytes (130). Nonetheless, in the ethidium bromide model of demyelination, transplants of astrocytes improve remyelination by oligodendrocytes (131). In vivo, astrocytic processes are closely associated with the oligodendrocyte soma and fibers (132), suggestive of intimate interactions. Further evidence to suggest that the astrocyte-oligodendrocyte interactions in vivo are beneficial include the observations of Komoly et al (133) that reactive astrocytes produce IGF-1 during demyelination in a mouse cuprizone model, which may then act to activate remyelination; recently, the same group demonstrated that IGF-1 treatment of mice with experimental allergic encephalomyelitis (EAE) reduced demyelination and also upregulated their expression of myelin-related genes (134). As mentioned, the extension of oligodendroglial processes by adult human oligodendrocytes, an early event in myelinogenesis, is facilitated by astrocytes (see Fig 17-1).

How then may we reconcile the many reports of neurotrophic effects of astrocytes to the observations that astrocytic scars are impediments to neurite regeneration (11,12) and remyelination, and may be the sites of genesis of electrical instability and epilepsy (135)? The most probable explanation lies in the period of astrocytic reactivity, with the early phases being neurotrophic and the subsequent longer-term "scars" having lost this activity. As alluded to earlier, neurotrophic activity that occurs around the sites of acute traumatic lesions (e.g., stab injury or corticectomy) rises gradually following an insult, peaks between 9 to 15 days, but thereafter declines to control levels.

The Neurotrophic Actions of Astrocytes Can Be Modulated by Inflammatory Cytokines

The simultaneous presence of cytokines, reactive astrocytes, and neurotrophic factors around the locus of a CNS lesion suggests the possibility for interactions; in addition to their role in mediating astrogliosis (136–138), it has become evident that cytokines can influence the production of neurotrophic factors by astrocytes. Several reports showed that the synthesis of NGF by astrocytes in vitro is enhanced by treatment with IL-1, IL-4, IL-5, IL-6, and TNF-α; this also appears to be the case for other trophic factors (see Table 17-2). As discussed already, astrocytes can synthesize various cytokines, which raises the possibility of autocrine control of neurotrophic factor production by astrocytes through cytokines.

Receptors for several cytokines (e.g., IL-1, IL-6, IL-7, TNF-α, IFNs, and colony-stimulating factors) have been identified on astrocytes (139–142), highlighting the postulate that many actions of inflammatory cytokines may be mediated through astrocytes.

In other studies, Erkman et al (143) found that IFN-γ can increase the activity of choline acetyltransferase (marker of cholinergic neurons) in human fetal spinal cord cultures but only when astrocytes are present. Johnson-Green et al (144) demonstrated that astrocyte-conditioned medium, when coated onto an appropriate substrate, increases the neurite extension of chick sensory neurons; however, when astrocytes are treated with IL-1 or lipopolysaccharide, or with medium conditioned from peritoneal macrophages, then the resultant astrocyte-conditioned medium loses some of its

Table 17-2.
The Production of Neurotrophic Factors by Astrocytes and Its Regulation In Vitro by Inflammatory Cytokines

Neurotrophic Factor	Cytokines That Enhance Production	Reference
Nerve growth factor (NGF)	IL-1β, IL-5, TNF-α, and TGF-β	113–117
Ciliary neurotrophic factor	IFN-γ but not IL-1	118
Brain-derived neurotrophic factor	Not increased by cytokines that elevate NGF mRNA (IL-1, TGF-β)	119
Basic fibroblast growth factor	Increased by IL-1 and IL-6	120
Neurotrophin-3	Not known	121

IL = interleukin; TNF = tumor necrosis factor; TGF = transforming growth factor; IFN = interferon.

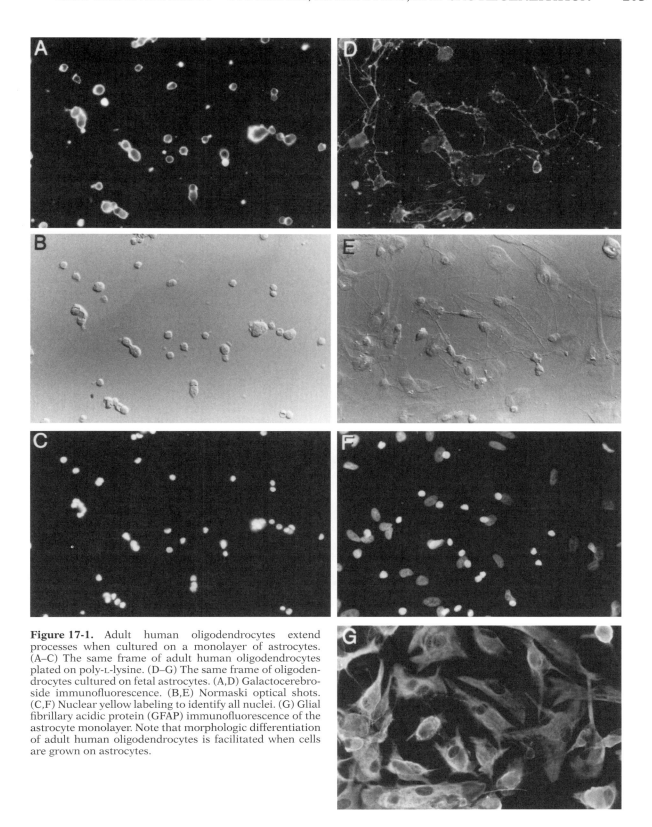

Figure 17-1. Adult human oligodendrocytes extend processes when cultured on a monolayer of astrocytes. (A–C) The same frame of adult human oligodendrocytes plated on poly-L-lysine. (D–G) The same frame of oligodendrocytes cultured on fetal astrocytes. (A,D) Galactocerebroside immunofluorescence. (B,E) Normaski optical shots. (C,F) Nuclear yellow labeling to identify all nuclei. (G) Glial fibrillary acidic protein (GFAP) immunofluorescence of the astrocyte monolayer. Note that morphologic differentiation of adult human oligodendrocytes is facilitated when cells are grown on astrocytes.

neurite-extending activity. Miller et al (145) reported that the treatment of astrocytes in vitro with IL-1β– or macrophage-conditioned medium results in the astrocytes promoting the growth of long neurites by cerebellar neurons.

In summary, as the list of neurotrophic properties of astrocytes increases, the capability of inflammatory cytokines in regulating these neurotrophic activities becomes more evident.

Effects of Inflammatory Cytokines

While inflammatory cytokines have neurotrophic effects, as discussed previously, in certain circumstances, inflammatory cytokines also have nonbeneficial effects. This is typified by TNF-α, whose beneficial properties have been described; in contrast, in multiple sclerosis and its animal model, EAE, TNF-α appears to be pathogenic.

In the serum or cerebrospinal fluid of patients with multiple sclerosis, levels of TNF-α correlate with disease activity (146–148). In brain lesions of patients with multiple sclerosis, TNF-α protein or mRNA levels are elevated (149–151). The elevation of TNF-α in multiple sclerosis is considered by some to be pathogenetic, because in vitro, TNF-α can cause the death of oligodendrocytes through apoptotic mechanisms (152–155). Similarly, in vitro, TNF-α reduces the content of myelin basic protein in myelinated rat brain aggregate cultures (37). The in vivo intravitreal injection of TNF-α causes demyelination of mouse optic nerve axons (156,157). Furthermore, the differential susceptibility of rat strains to the development of EAE has been ascribed to the corresponding ease at which TNF-α gene expression can be regulated in astrocytes (158). Finally, in concordance with a pathogenetic role for TNF-α, the administration of anti–TNF-α or -β antibodies, or soluble TNF-α receptor, prevents the transfer of EAE and abrogates subsequent autoimmune demyelination (159–161).

Final Comments

If inflammatory cytokines, reactive astrocytes, and growth factors, all of which appear to have neurotrophic activity, are present around the locus of a lesion, why then does regeneration of CNS neurons or oligodendrocytes ultimately fail? Many possibilities exist, and these highlight the early infancy of our understanding of factors that facilitate CNS regeneration. Thus, neurotrophic factors may not be produced in adequate amounts to facilitate regeneration. Furthermore, while some characteristics of cytokines or reactive astrocytes are permissive, others may be detrimental under different conditions; this was discussed in relation to TNF-α, which in some situations enhances regeneration but in other conditions causes CNS destruction. In addition, many negative influences to CNS regeneration have to be overcome and these include some inhibitory properties of astrocytes as mentioned, and axon inhibitory molecules expressed by oligodendrocytes and myelin. Finally, while macro-

phages/microglia have some neurotrophic functions as discussed, activated macrophages/microglia can also produce toxins detrimental to neurons. The need to identify those cytokines with negative actions, or to unravel the conditions under which cytokines become unfavorable for regeneration, seems compelling.

In summary, several inflammatory cytokines are elevated in the CNS following many types of pathology. These cytokines have the potential to be central players in influencing CNS regeneration, either by direct neurotrophic actions or by causing astrocytes to become reactive and also by affecting the neurotrophic activity of astrocytes. Under certain conditions, cytokines become impairments to the recovery of the CNS. A key step toward understanding CNS regeneration is thus the determination of the many roles of inflammatory cytokines within the CNS, and how each action of cytokines can be regulated or controlled.

References

1. Fawcett JW. Intrinsic neuronal determinants of regeneration. *Trends Neurosci* 1992;15:5–8.
2. Shewan D, Berry M, Cohen J. Extensive regeneration in vitro by early embryonic neurons on immature and adult CNS tissue. *J Neurosci* 1995;15:2057–2062.
3. Yong VW, Cheung JCB, Uhm JH, Kim SU. Age-dependent decrease of process formation by cultured oligodendrocytes is augmented by protein kinase C stimulation. *J Neurosci Res* 1991;29:87–99.
4. David S, Aguayo AJ. Axonal elongation into peripheral nervous system "bridges" after central nervous system injury in adult rats. *Science* 1981;214:931–933.
5. Giftochristos N, David S. Immature optic nerve glia of rat do not promote axonal regeneration when transplanted into a peripheral nerve. *Brain Res* 1988;467: 149–153.
6. Carbonetto S, Evans D, Cochard P. Nerve fiber growth in culture on tissue substrate from central and peripheral nervous system. *J Neurosci* 1987;7:610–620.
7. Savio T, Schwab ME. Rat CNS white matter, but not gray matter, is nonpermissive for neuronal cell adhesion and fiber outgrowth. *J Neurosci* 1989;9:1126–1133.
8. Caroni P, Schwab ME. Two membrane protein fractions from rat central myelin with inhibitory properties for neurite growth and fibroblast spreading. *J Cell Biol* 1988;106:1281–1288.
9. McKerracher L, David S, Jackson DL, et al. Identification of myelin-associated glycoprotein as a major myelin-derived inhibitor of neurite outgrowth. *Neuron* 1994;13:805–811.
10. Luo Y, Raible D, Raper JA. Collapsin: a protein in brain that induces the collapse and paralysis of neuronal growth cones. *Cell* 1993;75:217–227.
11. Reier PJ, Stensaas LJ, Guth L. The astrocytic scar as an impediment to regeneration in the central nervous system. In: Kao CC, Bunge RP, Reier PJ, eds. *Fundamentals of spinal cord reconstruction.* New York: Raven, 1983: 163–196.
12. Liuzzi FJ, Lasek RJ. Astrocytes block axonal regeneration in mammals by activating the physiological stop pathway. *Science* 1987;237:642–645.
13. McKeon RJ, Schreiber RC, Rudge JS, Silver J. Reduction of neurite outgrowth in a model of glial scarring following CNS injury is correlated with the expression of

inhibitory molecules on reactive astrocytes. *J Neurosci* 1991;11:3398–3411.

14. Grierson JP, Petroski RE, Ling DSF, Geller HM. Astrocyte topography and tenascin/cytotactin expression: correlation with the ability to support neuritic outgrowth. *Dev Brain Res* 1990;55:11–19.

15. Ohira A, Matsui F, Katoh-Semba R. Inhibitory effects of brain chondroitin sulfate proteoglycans on neurite outgrowth from PC12D cells. *J Neurosci* 1991;11:822–827.

16. Snow DM, Lemmon V, Carrino DA, et al. Sulfated proteoglycans in astroglial barriers inhibit neurite outgrowth in vitro. *Exp Neurol* 1990;109:111–130.

17. Nieto-Sampedro M, Lewis ER, Cotman CW. Brain injury causes a time-dependent increase in neurotrophic activity at the lesion site. *Science* 1982;217:860–861.

18. Ip NY, Wiegand SJ, Morse J, Rudge JS. Injury induced regulation of ciliary neurotrophic factor mRNA in the adult rat brain. *Eur J Neurosci* 1993;5:25–33.

19. Nieto-Sampedro M, Manthrope M, Barbin G, et al. Injury-induced neuronotrophic activity in adult rat brain: correlation with survival of delayed implants in the wound cavity. *J Neurosci* 1983;3:2219–2229.

20. Whittemore SR, Nieto-Sampedro M, Needels DL, Cotman CW. Neuronotrophic factors for mammalian brain neurons: injury induction in neonatal, adult and aged rat brain. *Dev Brain Res* 1985;20:169–178.

21. Needels DL, Nieto-Sampedro M, Cotman CW. Induction of a neurite-promoting factor in rat brain following injury or deafferentation. *Neuroscience* 1986;18:517–526.

22. Kesslak JP, Nieto-Sampedro M, Globus J, Cotman CW. Transplants of purified astrocytes promote behavioral recovery after frontal cortex ablation. *Exp Neurol* 1986; 92:377–390.

23. Giulian D, Robertson C. Inhibition of mononuclear phagocytes reduce ischemic injury in the spinal cord. *Ann Neurol* 1990;27:33–42.

24. Piani D, Frei K, Do KQ, et al. Murine brain macrophages incude NMDA receptor mediated neurotoxicity in vitro by secreting glutamate. *Neurosci Lett* 1991;133:159–162.

25. Chao CC, Hu S, Molitor TW, et al. Activated microglia mediate neuronal cell injury via a nitric oxide mechanism. *J Immunol* 1992;149:2736–2741.

26. Vaca K, Wendt E. Divergent effects of astroglial and microglial secretions on neuron growth and survival. *Exp Neurol* 1992;118:62–72.

27. Giulian D, Vaca K, Corpuz M. Brain glia release factors with opposing actions upon neuronal survival. *J Neurosci* 1993;13:29–37.

28. Thanos S, Mey J, Wild M. Treatment of the adult retina with microglia-suppressing factors retards axotomy-induced neuronal degradation and enhances axonal regeneration in vivo and in vitro. *J Neurosci* 1993;13: 455–466.

29. Rothwell NJ, Hopkins SJ. Cytokines and the nervous system. II: actions and mechanisms of action. *Trends Neurosci* 1995;18:130–136.

30. Merrill JE, Ignarro LJ, Sherman MP, et al. Microglial cell cytotoxicity of oligodendrocytes is mediated through nitric oxide. *J Immunol* 1993;151:2132–2141.

31. Oh LYS, Yong VW. Astrocytes promote process outgrowth by adult human oligodendrocytes in vitro through interaction between bFGF and astrocyte extracellular matrix. *Glia* 1996;17:237–253.

32. Noble PG, Antel JP, Yong VW. Astrocytes and catalase prevent the toxicity of catecholamines to oligodendrocytes. *Brain Res* 1994;633:83–90.

33. Nagata K, Takei N, Nakajima K, et al. Microglial conditioned medium promotes survival and development of

cultured mesencephalic neurons from embryonic rat brain. *J Neurosci Res* 1993;34:357–363.

34. Chamak B, Morandi V, Mallat M. Brain macrophages stimulate neurite growth and regeneration by secreting thrombospondin. *J Neurosci Res* 1994;38:221–233.

35. David S, Bouchard C, Tsatas O, Giftochristos N. Macrophages can modify the nonpermissive nature of the adult mammalian central nervous system. *Neuron* 1990; 5:463–469.

36. Hamilton SP, Rome LH. Stimulation of in vitro myelin synthesis by microglia. *Glia* 1994;11:326–335.

37. Loughlin AJ, Honeggar P, Woodroofe MN, et al. Myelin basic protein content of aggregating rat brain cell cultures treated with cytokines and/or demyelinating antibody: effects of macrophage enrichment. *J Neurosci Res* 1994;37:647–653.

38. Giulian D. Ameboid microglia as effectors of inflammation in the central nervous system. *J Neurosci Res* 1987;18:155–171.

39. Perry VH, Anderson PB, Gordon S. Macrophage and inflammation in the central nervous system. *Trends Neurosci* 1993;16:268–273.

40. Woodroofe MN, Sarna GS, Wadhwa, M et al. Detection of interleukin-1 and interleukin-6 in adult rat brain, following mechanical injury, by in vivo microdialysis: evidence of a role for microglia in cytokine production. *J Neuroimmunol* 1991;33:227–236.

41. da Cunha A, Jefferson JJ, Tyor WR, et al. Control of astrocytosis by interleukin-1 and transforming growth factor-beta 1 in human brain. *Brain Res* 1993;631:39–45.

42. Nieto-Sampedro M, Chandy KG. Interleukin-2 like activity in the injured rat brain. *Neurochem Res* 1987;12: 723–727.

43. Nieto-Sampedro M, Berman MA. Interleukin-1 like activity in rat brain: sources, targets, and effect of injury. *J Neurosci Res* 1987;17:214–219.

44. Yan HQ, Banos MA, Herregodts P, et al. Expression of interleukin (IL)-1β, IL-6 and their respective receptors in the normal rat brain and after injury. *Eur J Immunol* 1992;22:2963–2971.

45. Logan A, Frautschy SA, Gonzalez AM, et al. Enhanced expression of transforming growth factor β1 in the rat brain after a localized cerebral injury. *Brain Res* 1992; 587:216–225.

46. Quan N, Sundar SK, Weiss JM. Induction of interleukin-1 in various brain regions after peripheral and central injections of lipopolysaccharide. *J Neuroimmunol* 1994; 49:125–134.

47. Fontana A, Kristensen F, Dubs R, et al. Production of prostaglandin E and an interleukin-1 like factor by cultured astrocytes and C_6 glioma cells. *J Immunol* 1982; 129:2413–2419.

48. Lieberman AP, Pitha PM, Shin HS, Shin ML. Production of tumor necrosis factor and other cytokines by astrocytes stimulated with lipopolysaccharide or a neurotropic virus. *Proc Natl Acad Sci USA* 1989;86:6348–6352.

49. Frei K, Bodmer S, Schwerdel C, Fontana A. Astrocytes of the brain synthesize interleukin 3–like factors. *J Immunol* 1985;135:4044–4047.

50. Frei K, Malipiero UV, Leist TP, et al. On the cellular source and function of interleukin 6 produced in the central nervous system in viral diseases. *Eur J Immunol* 1989;19:689–694.

51. Benveniste EN, Sparacio SM, Norris JG, et al. Induction and regulation of interleukin-6 gene expression in rat astrocytes. *J Neuroimmunol* 1990;30:201–212.

52. Hao C, Guilbert LJ, Fedoroff S. Production of colony-

stimulating factor-1 (CSF-1) by mouse astroglia in vitro. *J Neurosci Res* 1990;27:314–323.

53. Tedeschi B, Barrett JN, Keane RW. Astrocytes produce interferon that enhances the expression of H-2 antigens on a subpopulation of brain cells. *J Cell Biol* 1986;102: 2244–2253.

54. da Cunha A, Vitkovic L. Transforming growth factor-beta 1 (TGF-β1) expression and regulation in rat cortical astrocytes. *J Neuroimmunol* 1992;36:157–169.

55. Aloisi F, Care A, Borsellino G, et al. Production of hemolymphopoietic cytokines (IL-6, IL-8, colony stimulating factors) by normal human astrocytes in response to IL-1β and tumor necrosis factor-α. *J Immunol* 1992;149: 2358–2366.

56. Lindholm D, Castren E, Keifer R, et al. Transforming growth factor-β1 in the rat brain: increase after injury and inhibition of astrocyte proliferation. *J Cell Biol* 1992;117:395–400.

57. Traugott U, Lebon P. Multiple sclerosis: involvement of interferons in lesion pathogenesis. *Ann Neurol* 1988;24: 243.

58. Schmidt B, Stoll G, Toyka KV, Hartung H-P. Rat astrocytes express interferon-γ immunoreactivity in normal optic nerve and after nerve transection. *Brain Res* 1990;515:347.

59. Eizenberg O, Faberelman A, Lotan A, Schwartz M. Interleukin-2 transcripts in human and rodent brains—possible expression by astrocytes. *J Neurochem* 1995; 64:1928–1936.

60. Farrar WL, Vinocour M, Hill JM. In situ hybridization histochemistry localization of interleukin-3 mRNA in mouse brain. *Blood* 1989;73:137–140.

61. Breder CD, Tsujimoto M, Terano Y, et al. Distribution and characterization of tumor necrosis factor-α–like immunoreactivity in the murine central nervous system. *J Comp Neurol* 1993;337:543–567.

62. Tchelingerian J-L, Quinonero J, Booss J, Jacque C. Localization of TNFα and IL-1α immunoreactivities in striatal neurons after surgical injury of the hippocampus. *Neuron* 1993;10:213–224.

63. Lapchak PA, Araujo DM, Quirion R, Beaudet A. Immunoautoradiographic local ization of interleukin 2–like immunoreactivity and interleukin 2 receptors (Tac antigen-like immunoreactivity) in the rat brain. *Neuroscience* 1991;44:173–184.

64. Olsson T, Kristensson K, Ljungdahl Å, et al. Gamma-interferon-like immunoreactivity in axotomized rat motor neurons. *J Neurosci* 1989;9:3870–3875.

65. Nohava K, Malipiero U, Frei K, Fontana A. Neurons and neuroblastoma as a source of macrophage colony-stimulating factor. *Eur J Immunol* 1992;22:2539–2545.

66. Junier MP, Coulpier M, Forestier NL, et al. Transforming growth factor α (TGFα) in degenerating motoneurons of the murine mutant wobbler: a neuronal signal for astrogliosis? *J Neurosci* 1994;14:4206–4216.

67. Brown MC, Perry VH, Lunn ER, et al. Macrophage dependence of peripheral sensory nerve regeneration: possible involvement of nerve growth factor. *Neuron* 1991;6:359–370.

68. Lu X, Richardson PM. Inflammation near the nerve cell body enhances axonal regeneration. *J Neurosci* 1991;11: 972–978.

69. Lindholm D, Heumann R, Meyer M, Thoenen H. Interleukin-1 regulates synthesis of nerve growth factor in nonneuronal cells of rat sciatic nerve. *Nature* 1987;330: 658–659.

70. Heumann R, Lindholm D, Bandtlow C, et al. Differential regulation of mRNA encoding nerve growth factor and its receptor in rat sciatic nerve during development, degeneration, and regeneration: role of macrophages. *Proc Natl Acad Sci USA* 1987;84:8735–8739.

71. Mansour H, Asher R, Dahl D, et al. Permissive and non-permissive reactive astrocytes: immunofluorescence study with antibodies to the glial hyaluronate-binding protein. *J Neurosci Res* 1990;25:300–311.

72. Hirschberg DL, Yoles E, Belkin M, Schwartz M. Inflammation after axonal injury has conflicting consequences for recovery of function: rescue of spared axons is impaired but regeneration is supported. *J Neuroimmunol* 1994;50:9–16.

73. Barbany G, Friedman WJ, Persson H. Lymphocyte-mediated regulation of neurotransmitter gene expression in rat sympathetic ganglia. *J Neuroimmunol* 1991; 32:97–104.

74. Freidin M, Kessler JA. Cytokine regulation of substance P expression in sympathetic neurons. *Proc Natl Acad Sci USA* 1991;88:3200–3203.

75. Brenneman DE, Schultzberg M, Bartfai T, Gozes I. Cytokine regulation of neuronal survival. *J Neurochem* 1992;58:454–460.

76. Awatsuji H, Furukawa Y, Nakajima M, et al. Interleukin-2 as a neurotrophic factor for supporting the survival of neurons cultured from various regions of fetal rat brain. *J Neurosci Res* 1993;35:305–311.

77. Hama T, Miyamoto M, Tsukui H, et al. Interleukin-6 as a neurotrophic factor for promoting the survival of cultured basal forebrain cholinergic neurons from postnatal rats. *Neurosci Lett* 1989;104:340–344.

78. Yamada M, Hatanaka H. Interleukin-6 protects cultured rat hippocampal neurons against glutamate-induced cell death. *Brain Res* 1994;643:173–180.

79. Barish ME, Mansdorf NB, Raissdana SS. γ-Interferon promotes differentiation of cultured cortical and hippocampal neurons. *Dev Biol* 1991;144:412–423.

80. Martinou J-C, Le Van Thai A, Valette A, Weber MJ. Transforming growth factor β1 is a potent survival factor for rat embryo motoneurons in culture. *Dev Brain Res* 1990;52:175–181.

81. Mahanthappa NK, Schwarting GA. Peptide growth factor control of olfactory neurogenesis and neuron survival in vitro: roles of EGF and TGF-βs. *Neuron* 1993;10:293–305.

82. Chalazonitis A, Kessler JA, Twardzik DR, Morrison RS. Transforming growth factor α, but not epidermal growth factor, promotes the survival of sensory neurons in vitro. *J Neurosci* 1992;12:583–594.

83. Haugen PK, Letourneau PC. Interleukin-2 enhances chick and rat sympathetic, but not sensory, neurite outgrowth. *J Neurosci Res* 1990;25:443–452.

84. Kamegai M, Niijima K, Kunishita T, et al. Interleukin 3 as a trophic factor for central cholinergic neurons in vitro and in vivo. *Neuron* 1993;2:429–436.

85. Satoh T, Nakamura S, Taga T, et al. Induction of neuronal differentiation in PC12 cells by B-cell stimulatory factor 2/interleukin 6. *Mol Cell Biol* 1988;8:3546–3549.

86. Mehler MF, Rozental R, Dougherty M, et al. Cytokine regulation of neuronal differentiation of hippocampal progenitor cells. *Nature* 1993;362:62–65.

87. Schwartz M, Solomon A, Lavie V, et al. Tumor necrosis factor facilitates regeneration of injured central nervous system axons. *Brain Res* 1993;545:334–338.

88. Lotan M, Solomon A, Ben-bassat SB, Schwartz M. Cytokines modulate the inflammatory response and change permissiveness to neuronal adhesion in injured mammalian central nervous system. *Exp Neurol* 1994; 126:284–290.

89. Konishi Y, Chui DH, Hirose H, et al. Trophic effect of erythropoietin and other hematopoietic factors on central cholinergic neurons in vitro and in vivo. *Brain Res* 1993;609:29–35.

90. Toulmond S, Vige X, Fage D, Benavides J. Local infusion of interleukin-6 attenuates the neurotoxic effects of NMDA on rat striatal cholinergic neurons. *Neurosci Lett* 1992;144:49–52.

91. Kiefer R, Haas CA, Kreutzberg GW. Gamma interferon-like immunoreactive material in rat neurons: evidence against a close relationship to gamma interferon. *Neuroscience* 1991;45:551–560.

92. Tirone F, Shooter EM. Early gene regulation by nerve growth factor in PC12 cells: induction of an interferon-related gene. *Proc Natl Acad Sci USA* 1989;86:2088–2092.

93. Noble M, Fok-Seang J, Cohen J. Glia are a unique substrate for the in vitro growth of central nervous system neurons. *J Neurosci* 1984;4:1892–1903.

94. Lindsay RM. Adult rat brain astrocytes support survival of both NGF-dependent and NGF-insensitive neurones. *Nature* 1979;282:80–82.

95. Fallon JR. Preferential outgrowth of central nervous system neurites on astrocytes and Schwann cells as compared with nonglial cells in vitro. *J Cell Biol* 1985;100:198–207.

96. Hatten ME, Lynch M, Rydel RE, et al. In vitro neurite extension by granule neurons is dependent upon astroglial-derived fibroblast growth factor. *Dev Biol* 1988;125:280–289.

97. Neugebauer KM, Tomaselli KJ, Lilien J, Reichardt LF. N-Cadherin, NCAM and integrins promote retinal neurite outgrowth on astrocytes in vitro. *J Cell Biol* 1988;107:1177–1187.

98. Tomaselli KJ, Neugebauer KM, Bixby JL, et al. N-Cadherin and integrins: two receptor systems that mediate neuronal process outgrowth on astrocyte surfaces. *Neuron* 1988;1:33–43.

99. Wang LC, Baird DH, Hatten ME, Mason CA. Astroglial differentiation is required for support of neurite outgrowth. *J Neurosci* 1994;14:3195–3207.

100. Geisert EE, Stewart AM. Changing interactions between astrocytes and neurons during CNS maturation. *Dev Biol* 1991;143:335–345.

101. Finklestein SP, Apostolides PJ, Caday CG, et al. Increased basic fibroblast growth factor (bFGF) immunoreactivity at the site of focal brain wounds. *Brain Res* 1988;460:253–259.

102. Ernfors P, Henschen A, Olson L, Persson H. Expression of nerve growth factor receptor mRNA is developmentally regulated and increased after axotomy in rat spinal cord motoneurons. *Neuron* 1989;2:1605–1613.

103. Lindvall O, Ernfors P, Bengzon J, et al. Differential regulation of mRNAs for nerve growth factor, brain-derived neurotrophic factor, and neurotrophin 3 in the adult rat brain following cerebral ischemia and hypoglycemia coma. *Proc Natl Acad Sci USA* 1992;89:648–652.

104. Ishikawa R, Nishikori K, Furukawa S. Appearance of nerve growth factor and acidic fibroblast growth factor with different time courses in the cavity-lesioned cortex of the rat brain. *Neurosci Lett* 1991;127:70–72.

105. Nieto-Sampedro M, Whittemore SR, Needels DL,et al. The survival of brain transplants is enhanced by extracts from injured brain. *Proc Natl Acad Sci USA* 1984;81:6250–6254.

106. Nieto-Sampedro M, Kesslak JP, Gibbs R, Cotman CW. Effects of conditioning lesions on transplant survival, connectivity, and function. *Ann NY Acad Sci* 1987;495:108–119.

107. Bradbury EJ, Kershaw TR, Marchbanks RM, Sinden JD. Astrocyte transplants alleviate lesion induced memory deficits independently of cholinergic recovery. *Neuroscience* 1995;65:955–972.

108. Wang JJ, Chuah MI, Yew DTW, et al. Effects of astrocyte implantation into the hemisected adult rat spinal cord. *Neuroscience* 1995;65:973–981.

109. Silver J, Ogawa MY. Postnatally induced formation of the corpus callosum in acallosal mice on glia-coated cellulose bridges. *Science* 1983;220:1067–1069.

110. Smith GM, Miller RH, Silver J. Changing role of forebrain astrocytes during development, regenerative failure, and induced regeneration upon transplantation. *J Comp Neurol* 1986;251:23–43.

111. Kliot M, Smith GM, Siegal JD, Silver J. Astrocyte-polymer implants promote regeneration of dorsal root fibers into the adult mammalian spinal cord. *Exp Neurol* 1990;109:57–69.

112. Kawaja MD, Gage FH. Reactive astrocytes are substrates for the growth of adult CNS axons in the presence of elevated levels of nerve growth factor. *Neuron* 1991;7:1019–1030.

113. Yoshida K, Gage FH. Fibroblast growth factors stimulate nerve growth factor synthesis and secretion by astrocytes. *Brain Res* 1991;538:118–126.

114. Gradient RA, Cron KC, Otten U. Interleukin-1β and tumor necrosis factor-α synergistically stimulate nerve growth factor (NGF) release from cultured rat astrocytes. *Neurosci Lett* 1990;117:335–340.

115. Carman-Krzan M, Vige X, Wise BC. Regulation by interleukin-1 of nerve growth factor secretion and nerve growth factor mRNA expression in rat primary astroglial cultures. *J Neurochem* 1991;56:636–643.

116. Awatsuji H, Furukawa Y, Hirota M, et al. Interleukin-4 and -5 as modulators of nerve growth factor synthesis/secretion in astrocytes. *J Neurosci Res* 1993;34:539–545.

117. Hattori A, Iwasaki S, Murase K, et al. Tumor necrosis factor is markedly synergistic with interleukin 1 and interferon-gamma in stimulating the production of nerve growth factor in fibroblasts. *FEBS Lett* 1994;340:177–180.

118. Carroll P, Sendtner M, Meyer M, Thoenen H. Rat ciliary neurotrophic factor (CNTF): gene structure and regulation of mRNA levels in glial cell cultures. *Glia* 1993;9:176–187.

119. Zafra F, Linholm D, Castren E, et al. Regulation of brain-derived neurotrophic factor and nerve growth factor mRNA in primary cultures of hippocampal neurons and astrocytes. *J Neurosci* 1992;12:4793–4799.

120. Araujo DM, Cotman CW. Basic FGF in astroglial, microglial, and neuronal cultures: characterization of binding sites and modulation of release by lymphokines and trophic factors. *J Neurosci* 1992;12:1668–1678.

121. Rudge JS, Alderson RF, Pasnikowski E, et al. Expression of ciliary neurotrophic factor and the neurotrophins—nerve growth factor, brain-derived neurotrophic factor and neurotrophin 3—in cultured rat hippocampal astrocytes. *Eur J Neurosci* 1992;4:459–471.

122. McLaurin J, Yong VW. Oligodendrocytes and myelin. In: Antel JP, ed. *Neurologic clinics of North America: multiple sclerosis*. Vol. 13. Philadelphia: WB Saunders, 1995:23–49.

123. Cardwell CC, Rome LH. Evidence that an RGD-dependent receptor mediates the binding of oligodendrocytes to a novel ligand in a glial-derived matrix. *J Cell Biol* 1988;107:1541–1549.

124. Malek-Hedayat S, Rome LH. Expression of beta 1-relat-

ed integrin by oligodendroglia in primary culture: evidence for a functional role in myelination. *J Cell Biol* 1994;124:1039–1046.

125. Ghatak NR. Occurrence of oligodendrocytes within astrocytes in demyelinating lesions. *J Neuropathol Exp Neurol* 1992;51:40–46.

126. Wu E, Raine CS. Multiple sclerosis: interactions between oligodendrocytes and hypertrophic astrocytes and their occurrence in other non-demyelinating conditions. *Lab Invest* 1992;67:88–99.

127. Prineas JW, Kwon EE, Goldenberg PZ, et al. Interaction of astrocytes and newly formed oligodendrocytes in resolving multiple sclerosis lesions. *Lab Invest* 1990;63:624–636.

128. Bhat S, Pfeiffer SE. Stimulation of oligodendrocytes by extracts from astrocyte-enriched cultures. *J Neurosci Res* 1986;15:19–27.

129. Rosen CL, Bunge RP, Ard MD, Wood PM. Type 1 astrocytes inhibit myelination by adult rat oligodendrocytes in vitro. *J Neurosci* 1989;9:3371–3379.

130. Amur-Umarjee S, Phan T, Campagnoni AT. Myelin basic protein mRNA translocation in oligodendrocytes is inhibited by astrocytes in vitro. *J Neurosci Res* 1993;36:99–110.

131. Franklin RJM, Crang AJ, Blakemore WF. The role of astrocytes in the remyelination of glia-free areas of demyelination. *Adv Neurol* 1993;59:125–133.

132. Butt AM, Ibrahim M, Ruge FM, Berry M. Biochemical subtypes of oligodendrocyte in the anterior medullary velum of the rat as revealed by the monoclonal antibody Rip. *Glia* 1995;14:185–197.

133. Komoly S, Hudson LD, deF Webster H, Bondy CA. Insulin-like growth factor I gene expression is induced in astrocytes during experimental demyelination. *Proc Natl Acad Sci USA* 1992;89:1894–1898.

134. Yao DL, Liu X, Hudson LD, deF Webster H. Insulin-like growth factor I treatment reduces demyelination and up-regulates gene expression of myelin-related proteins in experimental autoimmune encephalomyelitis. *Proc Natl Acad Sci USA* 1995;92:6190–6194.

135. Pollen DA, Trachtenberg MC. Neuroglia: gliosis and focal epilepsy. *Science* 1970;167:1252.

136. Yong VW, Moumdjian R, Yong FP, et al. γ-Interferon promotes proliferation of adult human astrocytes in vitro and reactive gliosis in the adult mouse brain in vivo. *Proc Natl Acad Sci USA* 1991;88:7016–7020.

137. Balasingam V, Tejada-Berges T, Wright E, et al. Reactive astrogliosis in the neonatal mouse brain and its modulation by cytokines. *J Neurosci* 1994;14:846–856.

138. Yong VW, Balasingam V. Determining the contribution of cytokines as mediators astrogliosis. In: Pillips MI, Evans D, eds. *Neuroimmunology*. San Diego: Academic, 1995:220–235.

139. Rubio N, de Felipe C. Demonstration of the presence of a specific interferon-γ receptor on murine astrocyte cell surface. *J Neuroimmunol* 1991;35:111–117.

140. Ban EM, Sarlieve LL, Haour FG. Interleukin-1 binding sites on astrocytes. *Neuroscience* 1993;52:725–733.

141. Sawada M, Itoh Y, Suzumura A, Marunouchi T. Expression of cytokine receptors in cultured neuronal and glial cells. *Neurosci Lett* 1993;160:131–134.

142. Tada M, Diserens AC, Desbaillets I, de Tribolet N. Analysis of cytokine receptor messenger RNA expression in human glioblastoma cells and normal astrocytes by reverse-transcription polymerase chain reaction. *J Neurosurg* 1994;80:1063–1073.

143. Erkman L, Wuarin L, Cadelli D, Kato AC. Interferon induces astrocyte maturation causing an increase in cholinergic properties of cultured human spinal cord cells. *Dev Biol* 1989;132:375–388.

144. Johnson-Green PC, Dow KE, Riopelle RJ. Neurite growth modulation associated with astrocyte proteoglycans: influence of activators of inflammation. *Glia* 1992;5:33–42.

145. Miller C, Tsatas O, David S. Dibutyryl cAMP, interleukin-1β, and macrophage conditioned medium enhance the ability of astrocytes to promote neurite outgrowth. *J Neurosci Res* 1994;38:56–63.

146. Sharief MK, Hentges R. Association between TNF-α and disease progression in patients with multiple sclerosis. *N Engl J Med* 1991;325:467–472.

147. Mokhtarian F, Shi Y, Shirazian D, et al. Defective production of anti-inflammatory cytokine, TGF-beta by T cell lines of patients with active multiple sclerosis. *J Immunol* 1994;152:6003–6010.

148. Reickmann P, Albrecht M, Kitze B, et al. Tumor necrosis factor-α messenger RNA expression in patients with relapsing-remitting multiple sclerosis is associated with disease activity. *Ann Neurol* 1995;37:82–88.

149. Hofman FM, Hinton DR, Johnson K, Merrill JE. Tumor necrosis factor identified in multiple sclerosis brain. *J Exp Med* 1989;170:607-612.

150. Selmaj K, Raine CS, Cannella B, Brosnan CF. Identification of lymphotoxin and tumor necrosis factor in multiple sclerosis lesions. *J Clin Invest* 1991;87:949–954.

151. Brosnan CF, Cannella B, Battistini L, Raine CS. Cytokine localization in multiple sclerosis lesions. *Neurology* 1995;45(suppl 6):S16–S21.

152. Selmaj K, Raine CS, Farooq M, et al. Cytokine cytotoxicity against oligodendrocytes: apoptosis induced by lymphotoxin. *J Immunol* 1991;147:1522–1529.

153. Louis J-C, Magal E, Takayama S. CNTF protection of oligodendrocytes against natural and tumor necrosis factor α–induced death. *Science* 1993;259:689.

154. Wilt SG, Milward E, Zhou JM, et al. In vitro evidence for a dual role of tumor necrosis factor-α in human deficiency virus type I encephalopathy. *Ann Neurol* 1995;37:381–394.

155. D'Souza S, Alinauska K, McCrea E, et al. Differential susceptibility of human CNS-derived cell populations to TNF-dependent and independent immune-mediated injury. *J Neurosci* 1995;15:7293–7300.

156. Butt AM, Jenkins HG. Morphological changes in oligodendrocytes in the intact mouse optic nerve following intravitreal injection of tumor necrosis factor. *J Neuroimmunol* 1994;51:27–33.

157. Jenkins HG, Ikeda H. Tumor necrosis factor causes an increase in axonal transport of protein and demyelination in the mouse optic nerve. *J Neurol Sci* 1992;108:99–104.

158. Chung IY, Norris JG, Benveniste EN. Differential tumor necrosis factor-α gene expression by astrocytes from experimental allergic encephalomyelitis-susceptible and -resistant strains. *J Exp Med* 1991;173:801–811.

159. Ruddle NH, Bergman CM, McGarth KM, et al. An antibody to lymphotoxin and tumor necrosis factor prevents transfer of experimental allergic encephalomyelitis. *J Exp Med* 1990;172:1193–1200.

160. Selmaj K, Raine CS, Cross AH. Anti-tumor necrosis factor therapy abrogates autoimmune demyelination. *Ann Neurol* 1991;30:694–700.

161. Selmaj KW, Raine CS. Experimental autoimmune encephalomyelitis: immunotherapy with anti-tumor necrosis factor antibodies and soluble tumor necrosis factor receptors. *Neurology* 1995;45(suppl 6):S44–S49.

Chapter 18

Immunology of Central Nervous System Grafts

Abbas F. Sadikot and Voon Wee Yong

Understanding the immune interactions between graft and host is critical to the development of successful transplantation strategies for the damaged central nervous system (CNS). Besides the obvious clinical importance, study of graft-host interactions in the CNS provides valuable insight into the developmental mechanisms and immunology of the CNS. A successful graft survives in the host environment, has functional capacity, and is free of harmful side effects. Fetal allografts recently were used for the treatment of Parkinson's disease in limited trials (1). Neural grafts are also of potential use in other neurodegenerative diseases, cerebrovascular disease, traumatic neural injury, autoimmune inflammatory disease, and epilepsy (for review, see (2)). In this chapter, we discuss the general mechanisms of transplant antigen recognition, the mechanisms of CNS graft rejection, the pathology of CNS graft rejection, and the methods that may be helpful in attenuating the transplant rejection response.

Following successful graft harvest and transplantation to an appropriate target, the principal determinant of functional graft survival is host acceptance. Syngeneic grafts, transplants where the host and donor are homozygotic twins or of the same inbred strain, are usually accepted without signs of rejection. Allogeneic grafts are transplants where the host and donor are of the same species but not heavily inbred. Allograft acceptance is variable, and depends in part on the degree of genetic disparity and the site of transplantation. Allografts usually show at least a partial immune rejection response. Xenografts, transplants between individuals of different species, are almost invariably rejected in the immunocompetent host (for review, see (3)). Xenograft survival depends on modification of the rejection response.

Presentation of Transplant Antigens to the Host Immune System

The major histocompatibility complex (MHC) encodes the main immune system antigens responsible for recognition of self and nonself. The MHC comprises three gene loci that are members of the immunoglobulin gene superfamily. Class I and II gene loci show the greatest capacity for individual polymorphism in their cell surface glycoprotein products, and are considered the main determinants of graft rejection or acceptance (for reviews, see (4,5)). The presence or absence of MHC molecules on a cell determines whether it can present foreign antigens as peptide fragments to T lymphocytes. MHC class I molecules are widely distributed on nucleated cells, with the notable exception of the CNS where constitutive expression is low (5–8). MHC class II molecules have a more restricted distribution than class I molecules, and they are expressed mainly on cells of monocyte/macrophage lineage (6–8).

Graft-derived transplantation antigens can be presented to host cytotoxic T cells in association with MHC class I antigens. However, class I–mediated presentation is likely less efficient than class II–mediated presentation, owing to the absence of amplification by cytokines produced by helper T cells. Prior sensitization would allow cytotoxic T cells to take on more importance in graft rejection (9). Although the importance of minor, non-MHC transplantation antigens is emphasized in some cases, they generally are thought to be less important in graft rejection than are MHC products (10,11). For example, minor histocompatibility antigen disparities may play a role in the rejection of some HLA-matched kidney allografts. In mice, male antigen disparities can induce acute rejection of skin allografts (12). With respect to mammalian CNS grafts, membrane-bound glycoproteins such as Thy-1, and the adhesion molecule neural cell adhesion molecule (NCAM) display interindividual polymorphism and may play a role in transplant rejection (10,13–16).

Factors that determine the character and intensity of the immune response include the level of baseline and inducible expression of transplantation antigens, transplant antigen access to the host immune system, host immune competence, degree of graft-host transplant antigen disparity, and permissibility of the graft site to host immune effector mechanisms (3,10,17–21).

The conventional immune response to graft tissue requires activation of the host immune system by graft-derived soluble antigens or graft-derived immunostimulatory cells that have gained access to the host spleen or lymph nodes (afferent phase). In addition to peripheral activation, antigen presentation and host T-cell activation may also occur at the graft site, provided inactive immune effector cells are able to gain access (22). In CNS grafts, such local mechanisms of antigen presentation may be important owing to limited access of transplantation antigens to the peripheral immune system (23). However, as discussed later, the trauma of transplantation may expose graft antigens to the host immune system. Once activated, T cells are readily able to access the CNS (18).

T cells are able to recognize alloantigens by either direct or indirect pathways (12,24). Direct presentation involves activation of host T cells by alloantigen, obviating the need for antigen processing and presentation by host-derived antigen-presenting cells (APCs). This form of T-cell activation may be the result of cross-reactivity of host T-cell receptors with graft MHC-antigen complex (24–26). Removal of passenger leukocytes prior to transplantation of renal allografts results in the reduction of acute rejection responses, illustrating the importance of direct mechanisms of allograft MHC-antigen complex recognition by host effector cells. Addition of donor dendritic cells restores immunogenicity (25,27). Indirect presentation involves activation of host T cells by host-derived APCs after endocytosis of graft-derived peptide fragments. This mode of transplant recognition may be of relevance to xenograft rejection (21) and chronic allograft rejection (27), thought to be unresponsive to immunosuppressive agents such as cyclosporine (24). The relative importance of direct and indirect mechanisms of T-cell activation in the context of CNS grafts has not been characterized (see below).

Classification of Graft Rejection

The conventional graft rejection response is best characterized with respect to solid-organ grafts, and may be classified as hyperacute, acute, or chronic (20). Hyperacute rejection typically occurs within the first 24 to 48 hours after transplantation. Acute rejection occurs in the first days to weeks after transplantation. Chronic rejection is characterized by a slow, progressive loss of graft function over months or years (20).

Hyperacute rejection is mediated by preformed host antibodies to donor-derived MHC, ABO blood group antigens, or other glycoprotein antigens such as endothelial cell surface glycoproteins (20). The antigen-antibody complex activates the classic complement pathway. Direct cell lysis and formation of massive intravascular platelet thrombi occur in a procoagulant environment and result in ischemic necrosis. This form of humoral reaction is especially prominent in xenografts between distantly related species, although cell-mediated mechanisms also play an important role in xenograft rejection (17).

Although the xenograft rejection response has similarities to cell-mediated rejection occurring in allografts, the xenograft cell response is usually more vigorous. In acute cell-mediated rejection occurring in allografts, both direct and indirect mechanisms of antigen presentation appear important (21,25,26). Acute rejection may occur early when the host is sensitized to donor MHC antigens as a result of previous transplan-

tation, pregnancy or blood transfusions. At a later date, acute rejection may also be due to a strong primary rejection response. Clinically acute rejection often occurs in renal or cardiac transplant patients, and manifests as functional deterioration (20). Biopsy confirms the diagnosis in clinical cases. The mononuclear cell infiltrate comprises mainly helper and cytotoxic T lymphocytes, with a smaller component of B lymphocytes, natural killer (NK) cells, neutrophils, and eosinophils (20). Such rejection usually responds to immunosuppressive drug therapy. In the context of brain grafts, biopsy is not a viable option in determining graft rejection. Functional testing, functional imaging, or postmortem examination help in determining the viability of brain grafts.

Delayed or chronic rejection manifests as insidious deterioration of graft function over months to years. It appears to be due to a progressive obliterative arteriopathy, possibly initiated by immunoglobulin deposition. Chronic rejection is characterized by progressive endothelial and intimal smooth muscle injury; subintimal smooth muscle proliferation; infiltration by lymphocytes, macrophages, neutrophils, and eosinophils; proliferative fibrosis; and occlusion of blood vessels (28). This form of rejection is difficult to reverse with presently available immunosuppressive drugs. Optimal immunosuppressive therapy with reduction of episodes of acute rejection may prevent its development (29,30). T-cell populations capable of mediating acute rejection of kidney grafts after direct pathway sensitization appear incapable of mediating late graft rejection, suggesting differences in the mechanism of acute and chronic rejection (27). Studies of CNS tissue transplantation are as yet too preliminary for adequate characterization of a chronic rejection equivalent. Since an arterial pedicle with smooth muscle does not directly supply brain grafts, it is difficult to draw homologies between chronic rejection of CNS grafts and that of solid-organ transplants.

Factors Determining Graft Acceptance in the CNS

The CNS, the anterior chamber of the eye, and the testis are examples of immunologically privileged sites. Although the phrase *immune privilege* appears in the literature at a later date, Medewar (31) introduced the concept in reference to skin allografts transplanted to the brain or the anterior chamber of the eye (for reviews, see (32–34)). Survival of MHC-incompatible allografts transplanted to immunologically privileged sites may occur as a result of a muted afferent arc with failure of antigen presentation. Alternatively, immune privilege may be due to an impaired efferent response, with defective ability of sensitized lymphocytes to mount a rejection response at the graft site. In the cornea, immune privilege is mainly due to an impaired afferent arm resulting from lack of corneal lymphatic drainage and absence of MHC class II APCs (33,35).

Immune privilege in the CNS is readily evidenced by tissue transplants in the brain surviving longer as compared to similar tissues grafted at other sites (33). However, immune privilege in the CNS is not absolute. The degree of immune acceptance of neural CNS transplants depends on diverse factors, including genetic disparity between host and graft, limited expression of transplantation antigens, graft composition, transplantation technique, site of transplantation, host immunocompetence, tissue trauma, and host sensitization (23,36–39).

Influence of Genetic Disparity Between Host and Graft

The degree of genetic disparity between host and graft is an important determinant of immune acceptance (13,14,38,40–42). With some exceptions (43), xenografts of brain tissue are promptly rejected in the absence of immune suppression (13). Allografts have greater longevity in the brain as compared to other transplant sites (33). Syngeneic grafts adapt to the brain environment with little evidence of rejection (13,44–48).

Brain allografts between inbred members of a given strain survive better than grafts between outbred members of the same strain. Allografts between outbred members of the same rat strain fare better than those between distantly related rat strains (for reviews, see (19,47)). Brain grafts with donor-host disparity in either major or minor histocompatibility antigens survive better than do brain grafts with differences in both major and minor histocompatibility antigens (13,14,23). This observation emphasizes the importance of so-called "minor" transplantation antigens. Certain donor-host strain combinations may allow for better survival of allogeneic grafts owing to factors that are poorly understood (37,41,49). Although genetic disparity is important in determining graft survival, the degree of destruction of different allografts, or even xenografts, can be variable (43). The unpredictability may be in part due to variability in MHC antigen induction to a level sufficient to provoke a sufficient host immune response (13,43,44).

Limited Expression and Presentation of Transplantation Antigens in the CNS

Expression of MHC molecules within normal brain is generally very low to absent (for reviews, see (5–8)). Astrocytes and microglia are potential APCs in the CNS under pathologic conditions and in transplant models (16,50). Both glial types can be induced to express MHC class I and II antigens, produce cytokines, and act as APCs in culture after exposure to cytokines such as interferon-γ (5,51–53). Recent studies emphasize the role of microglia rather than astrocytes as "professional" APCs (54–56). The two glial types may, however, act in concert. For example, microglial interleukin (IL)-1 can stimulate astrocyte proliferation (57) and astrocyte-derived IL-3 can in turn stimulate microglial proliferation (58).

Influence of Graft Composition on Immune Acceptance

The susceptibility of neural grafts to immunogenic attack varies based on cell composition. Neuron-rich grafts appear less susceptible to immune rejection than do grafts that contain both astrocytes and neurons, perhaps owing to the relative lack of major transplantation antigens (59). Rejection of astrocytes within neural grafts may occur prior to rejection of neural tissue, further suggesting that donor astrocytes may be especially susceptible to graft rejection (60,61).

Embryonic neural tissue is better accepted than adult neural tissue in part because of sparse expression of transplantation antigens (16,62). However, other factors such as an abundance of neurotrophic factors in the developing CNS and the neuroblastic nature of embryonic tissue undoubtedly play an important role in functional graft survival (for review, see (2)). The ontogeny of MHC expression is important in the context of transplantation of embryonic neural tissue. MHC expression is absent in CNS tissue of developing mouse embryos (16). However, numerous studies documented induction of class I and II MHC antigens in immature CNS tissue in vitro (51,58,63). The immunogenic potential of immature fetal tissue is of course clearly demonstrated by immune rejection of histoincompatible fetal grafts.

Influence of Transplant Site and the Effect of Tissue Trauma

Minimization of trauma during transplantation and maintenance of a relatively intact blood-brain barrier appears to correlate with better functional and anatomic graft survival (39,64). Both host and graft astrocytes likely respond to the trauma of transplantation by producing a wide variety of cytokines including interferon-γ, different ILs, and tumor necrosis factor-α (see Chapter 17). Local production of inflammatory cytokines may enhance the immune response in different circumstances. For example, the production of cytokines such as interferon-γ or tumor necrosis factor-α may disrupt the blood-brain barrier and also induce production of transplantation antigens (51,52,58,65–67). On the other hand, since inflammatory cytokines have demonstrated neurotrophic activity (see Chapter 17), astrocytes and microglia may be important to graft survival. Local concentration and time of production of different cytokines and neurotrophic factors are likely critical to determining whether graft survival is enhanced or hindered.

Site of transplantation also influences graft rejection. For example, intraventricular grafts of neonatal cortex or striatum appear to fare worse and show a greater immune rejection response than do similar intraparenchymal grafts (38,43,68). Such site-specific effects may be related to differences in induction of transplantation antigens on the graft tissue, variations in the character of the afferent and efferent phases of the immune response, or differential availability of neuro-trophic factors and other substrates for neuronal regeneration.

Effect of Host Immunocompetence

Host immunocompetence has a significant influence on neural graft survival. Immunosuppressants have an important effect on the survival of a variety of neural xenografts and allografts (see below). Neural xenografts survive for prolonged periods in immunodeficient rodents such as athymic nude mice (13,69). Furthermore, thymectomized mice rendered immunodeficient in T-cell populations using intravenous antibody to T-cell subsets show diminished rejection of fetal neocortical allografts (70). Host age is also an important determinant of graft survival (19,33,71). Xenografts are better accepted in neonatal animals than in adult counterparts. This is likely due to immunodeficiency, relative resistance to induction of MHC antigens, and increased availability of neurotrophic factors in neonates (19,71–73).

Medewar (31) documented the effect of previous sensitization of the host by donor antigens. More recent studies showed that neural tissue transplanted homotopically, or even orthotopically under the kidney capsule, is rapidly rejected in previously sensitized hosts (13,38,49). Sensitization by orthotopically placed skin grafts results in rapid rejection of previously well-accepted neural brain grafts (38,42,74,75).

Although systemic sensitization almost always causes an increase in cell infiltration, certain host-donor strain combinations allow allogeneic grafts to survive despite subsequent sensitization (37,41,49). Implantation of a second intracerebral neural allograft after previous intracerebral neural allograft transplantation does not result in rejection of either the first or the second graft (47,76). Lack of rejection in this model may be due to the weak systemic immunogenicity of neural allografts (49,76,77).

Immunology and Pathology of CNS Graft Rejection

Immune Mechanisms of CNS Graft Rejection

To elicit a rejection response, grafted cells must be identified as foreign by the host, effector cells must be generated, and activated effector cells must gain access to the graft (Fig. 18-1). Antigen presentation by more classic means requires detection of transplantation antigens by the peripheral host lymphoid system (see Fig. 18-1A). The paucity of lymphatic drainage within the normal CNS may contribute to CNS immune privilege (78). Lack of lymphatic drainage would impair the access of APCs or MHC molecules to lymphatic tissues, thus impairing activation of host effector cells. However, more recent studies demonstrated that large molecules injected into the cerebrospinal fluid (CSF) are transported to deep cervical lymph nodes. This transport likely occurs via periolfactory subarachnoid spaces

found in close association with nasal mucosal interstitial spaces (79–81). Injection of radioactive sheep red blood cells as T cell–dependent antigens into the mouse caudate nucleus results in the appearance of antibody-secreting cells in deep cervical lymph nodes in less than a week, further supporting a role for cerebral lymphatic drainage. On the other hand, injections into the lateral ventricles result in the detection of antibody-producing cells in the spleen and not the cervical lymphatics. This suggests that arachnoid villi draining CSF into the systemic circulation may also play a role in antigen transfer outside the CNS (82). Lymphocytes, macrophages, and red blood cells injected into the CNS are also detected in the periphery (78,81,83). Clearly the host lymphoid system is able to sample non-self-antigens within the CNS to a limited extent (81). The importance of peripheral activation is emphasized by the studies outlined above demonstrating that even well-accepted brain grafts are rejected upon peripheral sensitization.

As an alternative, graft antigens may be presented within the host CNS itself (see Fig. 18-1A). CNS tissue, with the exception of neurons and possibly oligodendrocytes, is capable of expressing MHC antigens under a variety of stimulated conditions including trauma and inflammation (5). T cells may access the CNS, either as part of a normal immune surveillance function, or more likely, across a breached blood-brain barrier (see Fig. 18-1A) (84–86). Trauma following transplantation results in breakdown of the blood-brain barrier, potentially providing inactive host T cells and other immune effector cells access to the graft (39). However, the blood-brain barrier reconstitutes within 1 to 2 weeks after placement of healthy neural allografts and xenografts (39,45,87–90). Thus, in the presence of CNS inflammation or trauma, a short temporal window exists for in situ presentation of graft antigens to host effector cells. Restriction of trauma upon graft implantation or use of immunosuppression (64,91,92) limits T-cell activation and may decrease induction of MHC class II antigens.

At the graft site, antigen presentation of graft antigens to host-derived perivascular T cells may be mediated by indirect presentation by host microglia/macrophages or less likely by astrocytes or endothelial cells (52,54,57,58,93–95). Alternatively, this central mode of antigen presentation may take place by direct presentation of donor antigens by graft-derived APCs (24,46,96–98).

The predominant cell types seen with xenograft and allograft rejection are T lymphocytes and microglia/macrophages (see Fig. 18-1B) (13,45,46,48,99–101). In xenografts, the cytotoxic T-cell population density may equal or exceed that of helper T cells, suggesting a significant role for MHC class I–restricted T cells in xenograft rejection (44,46,48,49,100). The predominant T-cell population associated with the initial phases of allograft rejection is composed of helper T cells (13,14,37,42,101,102). Some reports, however, suggested that both helper and cytotoxic T-cell populations are equally abundant or cytotoxic T-cell responses are more important (44,49,99). The observation that certain rat strain combinations allow for cytotoxic T-cell activation independent of helper T cells may help explain discrepancies (37). Acceleration of allograft rejection using extraneural sensitization or highly histoincompatible allografts appears to increase the relative numerical density of the cytotoxic T-cell population (19,37,46).

Pathology of CNS Graft Rejection

The pathology of the immune response to CNS transplantation of immature neural tissue has been extensively studied in the last decade (13,14,36–38,41,42, 44–46,48,49,60,70,76,97,99,100,103–105). The immune response to solid fetal grafts is qualitatively different compared to that to suspension grafts, but the fundamental mechanisms of graft rejection are likely similar. Cell suspensions are vascularized as a result of capillary ingrowth from the host, whereas the vascular supply of solid grafts develops from intrinsic, donor-derived vessels that anastomose with host vessels (87,90,106,107). Accessibility of activated host lymphocytes to donor antigens on vascular endothelium may render solid graft tissue more susceptible to immune attack (90). Both solid and suspension neural grafts develop a blood-brain barrier 1 to 2 weeks after transplantation (45,87,90,106,107). As discussed already, prior to the development of an effective blood-brain barrier, a potential window of time exists shortly after transplantation. This period allows for exposure of graft antigens to systemic host immune mechanisms, with resulting lymphocyte activation. Once the rejection response begins, blood-brain barrier integrity is once again compromised (see Fig. 18-1) (108).

Finsen et al (41) performed detailed studies of the cellular response to xenografts of solid hippocampal embryonic tissue transplanted into the hippocampus of adult rats. Grafts were examined at 3 days, 7 to 14 days, 21 days, and 35 days. The cellular infiltrate was initially composed of microglia/macrophages, and later of a heavy concentration of microglia/macrophages and T cells. Induction of MHC class II antigens was less prominent than class I induction. Class II activation occurred predominantly in infiltrating leukocytes at early phases, with later time periods showing expression mainly in microglial cells within host tissue and in leukocytes within graft tissue. Lymphocytes in this study were composed of comparable numbers of helper T cells and cytotoxic T cells (41). In contrast, a study of fetal mesencephalic cell suspension xenografts implicated cytotoxic T cells as the predominant lymphocytes (48). In the context of xenograft rejection, the relative abundance of cytotoxic T cells correlates with their capacity for lysis of xenogeneic class I–positive cells, and emphasizes the importance of MHC class I expression (46,96–98).

Lawrence et al (44) performed a detailed study of the immune response to syngeneic and allogeneic rat embryonic hippocampal primordia grafted to adult hippocampus as fragments of solid tissue. They divided the cellular immune response into an immune induction phase, a phase of immune attack, and a quiescent phase. According to their findings, the immune induction phase is similar in both allogeneic and syngeneic grafts. It lasts up to 6 days after transplantation, and is characterized by partial graft necrosis likely occurring as a result of trauma or ischemia. Within 1 to 2 days after transplantation, both syngeneic and allogeneic grafts show edema and formation of capillary vessels composed of both host- and graft-derived endothelial cells. In addition, perigraft host tissue, but not healthy graft tissue, is invaded by perivascular foamy macrophages. Early MHC class I antigen expression is seen in host tissue along the needle tract and in perigraft tissue. Although scattered MHC class II antigen–positive cells are seen in host tissue, they are absent at this stage in both syngeneic and allogeneic grafts.

The phase of immune attack extends from 1 to 7 weeks after transplantation. Both syngeneic and allogeneic grafts show a reduction in edema and histologic signs of reconstitution of an effective blood-brain barrier (88,106–108). Perivascular cuffs, which partially resemble peripheral lymph nodes, accumulate in allogeneic grafts. Syngeneic grafts show only a minor lymphocytic response. On electron microscopy, host lymphocytes are seen at first at the luminal surface, and then progress by diapedesis through the endothelial wall to the perivascular cuffs. Perivascular cuffs initially contain helper and cytotoxic T cells, and later contain an additional minor population of B cells (see Fig. 18-1B). Immunostaining with donor allospecific antibody to MHC class I antigen shows expression throughout the transplant, except in perivascular cuffs, where staining is pale. MHC class II antigen expression shows a complementary pattern. Staining is dense in perivascular tissue within the allograft and less intense in the rest of the allograft, and only occasional points of induction are seen in perivascular host tissue. MHC class II–positive perivascular cuffs include a heterogeneous cell population of macrophages, perivascular microglia, lymphocytes, lymphoblasts, and dendritic cells. Syngeneic grafts initially stain for MHC class I and II antigens both in peritransplant host tissue and within the graft, but immunostaining is not persistent. MHC class II antigen staining appears associated mainly with cells of microglial lineage rather than astrocytes (44). By 4 weeks after transplantation, syngeneic transplants are almost indistinguishable from host tissue and MHC class I and II expression has diminished.

Some allografts go on to a phase of immune destruction. In this phase, lymphocytes, dendritic cells, macrophages, and microglia migrate from their initial perivascular location and intermingle with allograft tissue. Macrophages/microglia form perineuronal nets around neurons that may still appear healthy. Host astrocytes in both syngeneic and allogeneic cases are hypertrophic. In allogeneic tissue, donor astrocytes also appear hypertrophic. The duration of the immune destruction phase can be quite variable (44). The final quiescent phase is characterized by a reduction of injury-induced MHC class I expression within host tissue, diminished perivascular cuffing, and gradual abating of

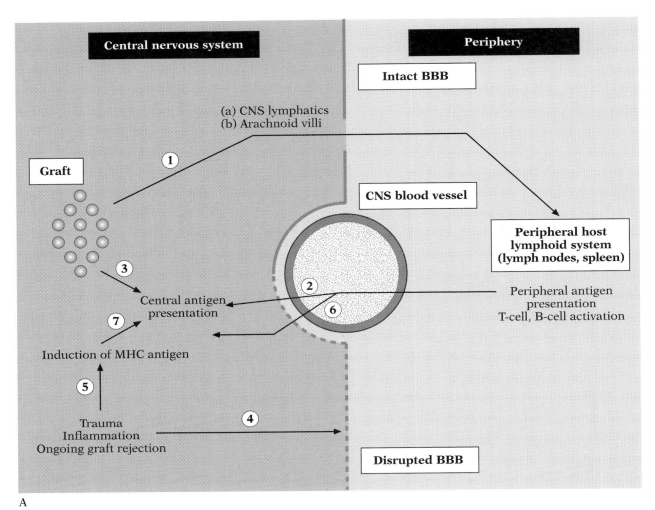

A

Figure 18-1.   (A) Afferent phase of the immune response to CNS allografts, resulting in allograft antigen presentation to host lymphocytes. 1) Graft antigens are transported to the host lymphoid system via CNS lymphatics or arachnoid villi. 2) Host lymphocytes, once sensitized in the periphery, gain access to the CNS, even across an intact blood-brain barrier (BBB). 3) Graft antigens may be presented to host T cells at the perivascular cuff or at the graft site. 4) Initial antigen presentation may occur after blood-brain barrier breakdown due to trauma or inflammation. 5) Trauma and inflammation also contribute to the induction of MHC antigens necessary for antigen presentation. 6) Inactive host lymphoid cells may be transported to the brain across a breached blood-brain barrier, allowing in situ presentation. 7) Indirect presentation involves use of host-derived antigen-presenting cells, whereas direct antigen presentation involves graft-derived antigen-presenting cells.

the immune response as MHC-incompatible grafts are destroyed (44).

Possible Mechanisms of CNS Graft Rejection

Studies demonstrating induced rejection of previously well-integrated xenografts illustrated the importance of MHC induction in graft rejection. Embryonic mouse retinal grafts transplanted into the mesencephalon of neonatal rats have a low incidence of spontaneous rejection. However, rejection can be induced in these grafts by disruption of the blood-brain barrier (103,108), remote injury resulting in neural degenera-

tion in the vicinity of the graft (109), or systemic sensitization (103). A common feature of induced rejection under these diverse circumstances is induction of MHC antigens. In a recent study using the same neonatal model, systemic administration of interferon-gamma, a cytokine known to induce MHC expression in the CNS, resulted in induction of graft rejection (67). MHC induction occurs prior to lymphocyte infiltration and graft destruction, and is especially prominent on cells with a microglial morphology. However, Subramanian et al (67) cautioned that the evidence is suggestive but not conclusive for a causal role of the MHC in graft rejection. Interferon-γ is known to have diverse effects in

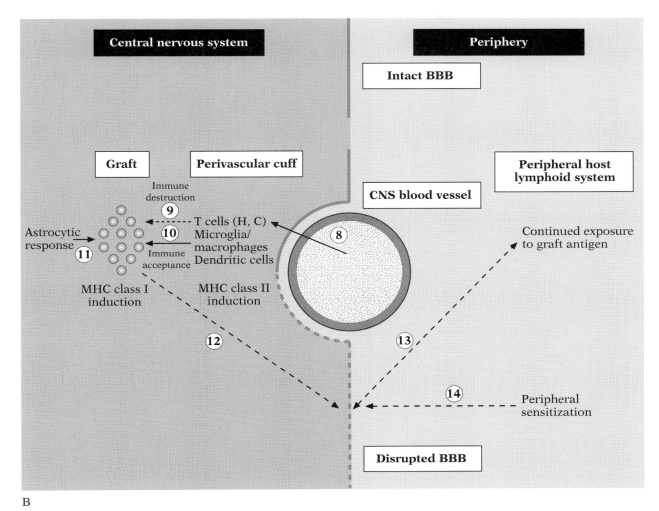

B

Figure 18-1 (*continued*).   (B) Efferent phase of the immune response to CNS allografts, resulting in variable degrees of allograft destruction. 8) T cells (helper and cytotoxic), microglia/macrophages, and dendritic cells accumulate at the perivascular cuff, resulting in a CNS "lymphoid station." MHC class II induction is noted to be especially prominent at the perivascular site and is mainly associated with microglia/macrophages. 9) There is immune destruction of the graft with loss of neurons by "bystander mechanisms." 10) There is immune acceptance associated with a quiescent phase, with a progressive reduction of the cellular response and downregulation of MHC antigen expression. 11) The astrocytic response may be beneficial or harmful to graft survival. 12) Immune destruction results in reopening of the blood-brain barrier, 13) with continued central/peripheral exchange of graft antigens and host lymphoid cells. 14) Peripheral sensitization after initial graft acceptance may rekindle the rejection response with breakdown of the blood-brain/graft barrier.

addition to induction of MHC expression. Interferon-γ induces breakdown of the blood-brain barrier (66), and activation of macrophages, cytotoxic T cells, and NK cells (67) may contribute to graft rejection.

Lawrence et al (44,110) suggested that the histologic picture of allograft rejection within the brain shares similarities to that of rejection of allografts of other tissues such as skin, kidney, and heart, and to the brain response to autoantigens seen in multiple sclerosis or experimental allergic encephalomyelitis (38). They hypothesized that perivascular microglia are activated by nonspecific tissue damage, and contribute to inflam-

matory changes in endothelial cells. This facilitates passage of a few lymphocytes through the blood-brain barrier and allows local antigen presentation by dendritic cells at the perivascular site. Alternatively, T-cell activation may occur as a result of contact with small amounts of alloantigen.

The in situ mode of antigen presentation within perivascular cuffs represents an alternative to antigen presentation at peripheral sites, obviating the necessity for transplant antigen access to extraneural lymph node sites (see Fig. 18-1A). Initially, only weak local T-cell activation occurs as a result of presentation of small amounts of graft-derived major or minor histocompatibility antigens. Activated lymphocytes entering the perivascular cuffs come in contact with trauma-activated microglia, which express class I and II antigens. The initial lymphocyte population may be of mixed specificity. Accumulation of perivascular lymphocytes at the allograft site is associated with a major increase in allotypic MHC antigens, likely mediated by cytokines. In syngeneic grafts, MHC expression increases as a result of initial trauma, but is not as amplified as in allografts since lymphocytes do not detect allotypic antigen. In allografts, amplification results in the induction of MHC class II antigen expression on lymphocytes, dendritic cells, macrophages, microglia, and also perhaps astrocytes and endothelial cells (44,110). Perivascular microglia with high MHC class II density (54) and phagocytic capacity process transplant antigens and present them to the T-cell population, resulting in more allospecific T cells (44,110). Activated astrocytes and endothelial cells may also contribute to antigen presentation and further activation of lymphocytes (111,112).

Perineuronal accumulation of MHC class I and II antigen-positive microglia may result in alloantigen presentation to helper and cytotoxic T cells in the vicinity of neurons, with direct destruction of MHC-expressing glia (see Fig. 18-1B). Neurons themselves may be destroyed by an as yet poorly understood bystander mechanism (110,113). Although cell death in grafts is classically considered necrotic, results of recent studies of fetal ventral mesencephalon grafts suggest that neuronal cell death may also occur by apoptosis (114).

Methods Used To Abrogate the Graft Rejection Response

Conventional immunosuppressive agents used in clinical practice were introduced prior to more precise delineation of humoral and cellular components of the immune response. Corticosteroids depress immunity in a relatively nonselective manner, with wide-ranging effects on immune function and the inflammatory response. Such nonselective depression results in increased allograft survival, but has the disadvantage of increased host susceptibility to undesirable effects such as infections.

Compared to the relative nonspecificity and toxicity of steroids and cytotoxic agents, the newer immunosuppressants cyclosporine, FK 506, and rapamycin are more specific and better tolerated. Cyclosporine is a cyclic peptide that inhibits protein synthesis (115) and exerts its immunosuppressive action mainly by inhibition of T cell–mediated mechanisms (116). Cyclosporine inhibits cytotoxic T-cell activity in vitro in the allogeneic mixed lymphocyte reaction (117), suppresses helper T-cell activity, and inhibits NK-cell activity indirectly by inhibition of interferon-γ (115). In the context of CNS grafts, cyclosporine has been systematically investigated in animal models (39,91,92); it convincingly reduces xenograft rejection. Little information is available on the effect of FK 506 and rapamycin on CNS grafts. In human trials of CNS grafts, up to three immunosuppressants have been used (1). However, the utility of immunosuppressants to prevent allograft rejection, including human allografts, requires further study.

Antibodies to different immune system components have been investigated as an alternative to immunosuppressive drugs (118). Thymectomy followed by elimination of T-cell subpopulations results in improved survival of neocortical allografts (15). Immunosuppression using antibodies to CD4 helper T-cell antigens enhances the survival of neural xenografts (119). Furthermore, systemic injections of antibodies to IL-2 receptors found on activated T cells are effective in promoting survival of neural xenografts (120) and allografts (105).

Pretreatment of embryonic porcine striatum cell suspensions with F(ab')$_2$ antigen–binding fragments of monoclonal antibodies to porcine MHC class I molecules results in enhanced graft survival as compared to nonimmunosuppressed controls (121–123). Low levels of MHC class I antigens are detected in embryonic porcine neural tissue prior to transplantation. Protection provided by masking prior to transplantation suggests a role for MHC class I antigens in xenograft rejection (123).

Because neurons are unable to express MHC antigens under constitutive or induced states, use of neuron-enriched grafts may represent an important method for cell transplantation (59,124). Transplantation of neuron-rich cell populations using antibody-based selection methods for sorting of neurons from glia in embryonic tissue (59) appears to markedly diminish the host rejection response, with reduced expression of MHC antigens. However, the lack of trophic effects from glia may counterbalance enhanced survival from reduced immune rejection (124).

Immunologic Issues Relevant to Human Transplantation

Catecholamine-rich tissues have been transplanted into the dopamine-denervated striatum in limited numbers of patients with Parkinson's disease or 1-methyl-4-phenyl-1,2,3,6-tetrahydropyridine (MPTP)–induced parkinsonism. Autografts of adrenal medulla have been abandoned in favor of fetal ventral mesencephalon (1). HLA typing is generally not practical owing to the unpredictable availability of donor tissues. Immunologic issues of relevance to clinical transplantation include 1) the efficacy of immunosuppressant drugs in preventing the rejection of allografts, 2) whether the presence of multiple donors contributing a pool of alloantigens enhances allograft rejection, and 3) whether placement of multiple grafts at separate sessions results in rejection of previous grafts.

Immunosuppressants have not been used consistently in different clinical trials. Whereas some groups do not use immunosuppressive therapy, others use one or multiple immunosuppressants for variable periods (1,125–132). Most human trials used some form of immunosuppression (1), although one trial that included a heterogeneous population of immunosuppressed and nonimmunosuppressed patients did not show a significant difference in clinical outcome between the two groups (131). Furthermore, studies of survival of embryonic substantia nigra allografts in monkeys with MPTP-induced lesions did not usually include immunosuppression (133–135).

Arguments in favor of immunosuppression include the following: Varying degrees of immune rejection of fetal CNS allografts occur upon transplantation; immunosuppression may reduce the risk of host sensitization to the graft and may be advantageous in case a sequential graft is needed; and the risk of spurious autoimmune reactions may be reduced (1,90). Cyclosporine may be given alone, or in combination with steroids or azathioprine or both. The required duration of immunosuppressive treatment has not been determined, although limited patient studies suggest that drug withdrawal at 12 to 31 months does not result in graft dysfunction over the subsequent year (125,136). Given the relatively low toxicity of these drugs, it seems prudent to administer them for at least the initial year after transplantation. However, more definitive recommendations require randomized trials in patients and nonhuman primates.

Whereas initial clinical trials used only one allograft, recent trials favor use of multiple donors due to the limited 5% to 10% survival rate of dopaminergic neurons in experimental grafts (1,137). In patients with Parkinson's disease, grafts of embryonic mesencephalon from multiple human fetal donors appear to provide superior results to single grafts (1). Due to the use of multiple HLA-incompatible donors, it is important to determine whether pooling results in an increased rejection response. There is no difference in dopaminergic neuron survival in ventral mesencephalon allografts obtained from pooling of embryos from different mouse strains as compared to pooled allografts from embryos of the same strain (43).

Lack of sufficient donors at the time of one session may require that human transplant tissue be grafted at several sessions. A sequential graft may be rejected as a result of peripheral sensitization. However, sequential grafting of rat fetal allograft tissue at different time points did not result in loss of function of either the first or the subsequent graft (73). Furthermore, there is a lack of a detectable systemic humoral or cellular allogeneic immune response in human and nonhuman primate recipients of embryonic mesencephalic allografts for Parkinson's disease (77). These data suggest that sequential grafting may be performed in clinical cases provided an atraumatic technique is used (47,76).

Conclusions

In the last 15 years, the science of tissue grafting to the CNS has progressed from limited experience in rodent models to clinical trials. Review of the basic science of neural transplantation suggests that our knowledge of host-graft immune interactions is still at an early phase, and clinical trials should proceed with caution. Understanding the immunology of grafts is critical to optimizing functional survival of transplants placed in the damaged nervous system. Figures 18-1A and 18-1B provide a schematic summary of the immune response to CNS grafts. Further investigations important to the development of rational transplantation strategies include study of mechanisms of transplant antigen expression; further characterization of mechanisms by which microglia and other APCs participate in the graft rejection response; distinguishing salutary or destructive effects of graft-derived glial elements; clarifying mechanisms of lymphocyte activation by transplant antigens; and exploring better methods for abrogating the rejection response. Knowledge of the immunology of fetal grafts will also serve as a basis for studying rejection of novel alternative transplants such as genetically modified cells, microencapsulated cells, or stem cells.

References

1. Lindvall O. Neural transplantation in Parkinson's disease. In: Dunnett SB, Björklund A, eds. *Functional neural transplantation.* New York: Raven, 1994:103–137.
2. Björklund A. Dopaminergic transplants in experimental parkinsonism: cellular mechanisms of graft-induced functional recovery. *Curr Opin Neurobiol* 1992;2:683–689.
3. Abbas AK, Lichtman AH, Pober JS. *Cellular and mole immunology.* 2nd ed. Philadelphia: WB Saunders, 1994.
4. Williams AF. A year in the life of the immunoglobulin gene superfamily. *Immunol Today* 1987;8:296–303.
5. Yong VW, JP Antel. Major histocompatibility complex molecules on glial cells. *Semin Neurosci* 1992;4:231–240.
6. Hart DA, Fabre JW. Demonstration and characterization of Ia-positive dendritic cells in the interstitial connective tissues of rat, heart and other tissues, but not brain. *J Exp Med* 1981;154:347–361.
7. Daar A, Fuggle S, Fabre J, et al. The detailed distribution of HLA ABC in normal human organs. *Transplantation* 1984;38:287–292.
8. Daar AS, Fuggle SV, Fabre JW, et al. The detailed distribution of class II in normal human organs. *Transplantation* 1984;38:293.
9. Stepkowski SM, Duncan WR. The role of T_{DTH} and T_c populations in organ graft rejection. *Transplantation* 1986;42:406–412.
10. Loveland B, Simpson E. The non-MHC transplantation antigens: neither weak nor minor. *Immunol Today* 1986;7:223–229.
11. Steinmuller D. Tissue-specific and tissue-restricted histocompatibility antigens. *Immunol Today* 1984;5:234–240.
12. Stepkowski SM. Transplantation immunobiology. An update. Horizons in organ transplantation. *Surg Clin North Am* 1994;75:991–1013.
13. Mason DW, Charlton HM, Jones AJ, et al. The fate of allogeneic and xenogeneic neuronal tissue transplanted into the third ventricle of rodents. *Neuroscience* 1986;19:685–694.
14. Nicholas MK, Antel JP, Stefansson K, Arnason BGW. Rejection of fetal neocortical neural transplants by H-2 incompatible mice. *J Immunol* 1987;139:2275–2283.
15. Nicholas MK, Chenelle AG, Brown MM, et al. Prevention of neural allograft rejection in the mouse following in vivo depletion of L3T4+ but not LYT-2+ T-lymphocytes. *Prog Brain Res* 1990;82:161–167.

16. Lampson LA, Grabowska A, Whelan JP. Class I and II MHC expression and its implications for regeneration in the nervous system. *Prog Brain Res* 1994;103:307–317.
17. Calne RY. Organ transplantation between widely disparate species. *Transplant Proc* 1970;2:550–553.
18. Hickey WF, Hsu BL, Kimura H. T-lymphocyte entry into the central nervous system. *J Neurosci Res* 1991;28:254–260.
19. Lund RD, Banerjee R. Immunological considerations in neural transplantation. In: Dunnett SB, Björklund A, eds. *Neural transplantation: a practical approach.* Oxford: Oxford University, 1992:57–78.
20. Kahan BD, Clark JH III. Transplantation of solid organs. In: Frank MM, Austen KF, Claman HW, Unanue ER, eds. *Samter's immunologic disease.* 5th ed. Boston: Little, Brown, 1995:1495–1511.
21. Kaufman CL, Gaines BA, Ildstad ST. Xenotransplantation. *Annu Rev Immunol* 1995;13:339–367.
22. Geppert TD, Lipksy PE. Antigen presentation at the inflammatory site. *Crit Rev Immunol* 1989;9:313–362.
23. Head JR, Griffin WST. Functional capacity of solid tissue transplants in the brain: evidence for immunological privilege. *Proc R Soc Lond Biol Sci* 1985;224:375–387.
24. Shoskes DA, Wood KJ. Indirect presentation of MHC antigens in transplantation. *Immunol Today* 1994;15:32–38.
25. Lechler RI, Batchelor JR. Restoration of immunogenicity to passenger cell-depleted kidney allografts by the addition of donor strain dendritic cells. *J Exp Med* 1982;155:31–41.
26. Stock PG, Ascher NL, Chen S, et al. Evidence for the direct and indirect pathways in the generation of the alloimmune response against pancreatic islets. *Transplantation* 1991;52:704–709.
27. Braun MY, McCormick A, Webb G, Batchelor JR. Mediation of acute but not chronic rejection of MHC-incompatible rat kidney grafts by alloreactive CD4 T cells activated by the direct pathway of sensitization. *Transplantation* 1993;55:177–182.
28. Beckingham IJ, Stubington SR, Dennis MJ, et al. Experimental studies of the pathogenesis of chronic allograft rejection. *Transplant Proc* 1995;27:2129–2130.
29. Sketris I, Yatscoff R, Keown P, et al. Optimizing the use of cyclosporine in renal transplantation. *Clin Biochem* 1995;28:195–211.
30. Paul LC. Experimental models of chronic renal allograft rejection. *Transplant Proc* 1995;27:2126–2128.
31. Medewar PB. Immunity to homologous grafted skin. III. The fate of skin homografts transplanted to the brain, to subcutaneous tissue and to the anterior chamber of the eye. *Br J Exp Pathol* 1948;29:58–69.
32. Billingham RE, Boswell T. Studies on the problem of corneal homografts. *Proc Roy Soc Ser B* 1953;141:392–406.
33. Barker CF, Billingham RE. Immunologically privileged sites. *Adv Immunol* 1977;23:1–54.
34. Brent L. Immunologically privileged sites. In: Johansson BB, Owman CH, Widner H, eds. *Long term consequences of barrier dysfunction for the brain. (Proceedings of Erik K. Fernström symposium on pathophysiology of the blood-brain barrier.)* Amsterdam: Elsevier 1990:383–402.
35. Streilein JW, Toews GB, Bergstresser PR. Corneal grafts fail to express Ia antigens. *Nature* 1979;282:326–327.
36. Poltorak M, Freed WJ. Immunological reactions induced by intracerebral transplantation: evidence that host microglial but not astroglia are the antigen-presenting cells. *Exp Neurol* 1989;103:222–233.
37. Isono M, Poltorak M, Kulaga H, et al. Certain host-donor rat strain combinations do not reject brain allografts after systemic sensitization. *Exp Neurol* 1993;122:48–56.
38. Sloan DJ, Baker BJ, Puklavec M, Charlton HM. The effect of site of transplantation and histocompatibility differences on the survival of neural tissue transplanted to the CNS of defined inbred rat strains. *Prog Brain Res* 1990;82:141–152.
39. Brundin P, Widner H, Nilsson OG, et al. Intracerebral xenografts of dopamine neurons: the role of immunosuppression and the blood-brain barrier. *Exp Brain Res* 1989;75:195–207.
40. Geyer SJ, Gill TJ, Kunz HW, Moody E. Immunogenetic aspects of transplantation in the rat brain. *Transplantation* 1985;39:244–247.
41. Poltorak M, Freed WJ. BN rats do not reject F344 brain allografts even after systemic sensitization. *Ann Neurol* 1991;29:377–388.
42. Nicholas MK, Stefansson K, Antel JP, Arnason BGW. An in vivo and in vitro analysis of systemic immune function in mice with histologic evidence of neural transplant rejection. *J Neurosci Res* 1987;18:245–257.
43. Widner H, Brundin P. Immunological aspects of grafting in the mammalian central nervous system. A review and speculative synthesis. *Brain Res* 1988;472:287–324.
44. Lawrence JM, Morris RJ, Wilson DJ, Raisman G. Mechanisms of allograft rejection in the rat brain. *Neuroscience* 1990;37:431–462.
45. Finsen B, Pedersen EB, Sørensen T, et al. Immune reactions against intracerebral murine xenografts of fetal hippocampal tissue and cultured cortical astrocytes in the adult rat. *Prog Brain Res* 1990;82:111–128.
46. Finsen BR, Sørensen T, Castellano B, et al. Leukocyte infiltration and glial reactions in xenografts of mouse brain tissue undergoing rejection in the adult rat brain. A light and electron microscopic study. *J Neuroimmunol* 1991;32:159–183.
47. Widner H, Brundin P. Sequential intracerebral transplantation of allogeneic and syngeneic fetal dopamine-rich neuronal tissue in adult rats: will the first graft be rejected? *Cell Transplant* 1993;2:307–317.
48. Duan WM, Widner H, Brundin P. Temporal pattern responses against intrastriatal grafts of syngeneic, allogeneic or xeno-embryonic neuronal tissue in rats. *Exp Brain* 1995;104:227–242.
49. Duan W-M, Widner H, Frodl EM, Brundin P. Immune reactions following systemic immunization prior or subsequent to intrastriatal transplantation of allogeneic mesencephalic tissue in adult rats. *Neuroscience* 1995;64:629–641.
50. Fabry Z, Raine CS, Hart MN. Nervous tissue as an immune compartment: the dialect of the immune response in the CNS. *Immunol Today* 1994;15:218–224.
51. Wong GHW, Bartlett PF, Clark-Lewis I, et al. Inducible expression of H-2 and Ia antigens on brain cells. *Nature* 1984;310:688–691.
52. Fierz J, Endler B, Reske K, et al. Astrocytes as antigen-presenting cells. I. Induction of Ia antigen expression on astrocytes by T cells via immune interferon and its effect on antigen presentation. *J Immunol* 1985;134:3785–3793.
53. Yong VW, Yong FP, Ruis TCG, et al. Expression and modulation of HLA-DR on cultured human adult astrocytes. *J Neuropathol Exp Neurol* 1991;50:16–28.
54. Streit WJ, Graeber MB, Kreutzberg GW. Functional plasticity of microglia: a review *Glia* 1988;1:301–307.
55. Hickey WF, Kimura H. Perivascular microglial cells of the CNS are bone marrow-derived and present antigen in vivo. *Science* 1988;239:290–292.
56. Matsumoto Y, Ohmori K, Fujiwara M. Immune regula-

tion by brain cells in the central nervous system: microglia but not astrocytes present myelin basic protein to encephalitogenic T cells under in situ mimicking conditions. *Immunology* 1992;76:209–216.

57. Guilian D. Ameboid microglia as effectors of inflammation in the central nervous system. *J Neurosci Res* 1987;18:155–171.

58. Frei K, Siepl C, Grosweth P, et al. Antigen presentation and tumor cytotoxicity by interferon-gamma treated microglial cells. *Eur J Immunol* 1987;17:1271–1278.

59. Bartlett PF, Rosenfeld, J, Bailey KA, et al. Allograft rejection overcome by immunodetection of neuron precursor cells. *Prog Brain Res* 1990:153–160.

60. Backes M, Lund RD, Lagenaur CF, et al. Cellular events associated with peripherally induced rejection of mature neural xenografts placed into neonatal rat brains. *J Comp Neurol* 1990;295:428–437.

61. Lund RD, Banerjee R, Rao K. Microglia, MHC expression and graft rejection. *Neuropathol Appl Neurobiol* 1994;20:202–203.

62. Kerr RSC, Bartlett PF. The immune response to intraparenchymal fetal CNS transplants. *Transplant Proc* 1989;21:3166–3168.

63. Fontana A, Kristensen F, Dubs R, et al. Production of prostaglandin E and an interleukin-1 like factor by cultured astrocytes and C6 glioma cells. *J Immunol* 1982;129:2413–2419.

64. Nikkah G, Cunningham MG, Jodicke A, et al. Improved graft survival and striatal reinnervation by microtransplantation of fetal nigral cell suspensions in the rat Parkinson model. *Brain Res* 1994;633:133–143.

65. Lavi E, Suzumura A, Murasko DM, et al. Tumor necrosis factor induces MHC class I antigen expression on mouse astrocytes. *J Neuroimmunol* 1988;18:245–253.

66. Steineger B, Van der Meide PH. Rat ependyma and microglia cells express class II MHC antigens after intravenous infusion of recombinant gamma interferon. *J Neuroimmunol* 1988;19:111–118.

67. Subramanian T, Pollack IF, Lund RD. Rejection of mesencephalic retinal xenografts in the rat induced by systemic administration of systemic recombinant interferon-gamma. *Exp Neurol* 1995;131:157–162.

68. Murphy JB, Sturm E. Conditions determining the transplantability of tissue in the brain. *J Exp Med* 1923;38:183–197.

69. Stromberg I, Almqvist P, Bygdeman M, et al. Intracerebral xenografts of human mesencephalic tissue into athymic rats: immunochemical and in vivo electrochemical studies. *Proc Natl Acad Sci USA* 1988;85:8331–8334.

70. Nicholas MK, Arnason BGW. A role for CD8+ T lymphocytes in the late rejection of intraventricular fetal neocortical fragment allografts in the mouse. In: *Long term consequences of barrier dysfunction for the brain (Proceedings of Eric K. Fernström symposium on pathophysiology of the blood brain barrier).* Amsterdam: Elsevier, 1990.

71. Lund RD, Rao K, Kunz HW, Gill TJ III. Transplantation of retina and visual cortex to rat brain of different ages: maturation, connection patterns, and immunologic consequences. *Ann NY Acad Sci* 1987;495:227–241.

72. Steinmuller D. Transplantation immunity in the newborn rat. I. The response at birth and maturation of response capacity. *J Exp Zool* 1961;147:233–258.

73. Yee KT, Smetanka AM, Lund RD, Rao K. Differential expression of class I and class II major histocompatibility complex antigen in early postnatal rats. *Brain Res* 1990;530:121–125.

74. Freed WJ. Functional brain tissue transplantation: reversal of lesion-induced rotation by intraventricular substantia nigra and adrenal medulla grafts, with a note on intracranial retinal grafts. *Biol Psychiatry* 1983;18:1205–1267.

75. Lund RD, Rao K, Kunz HW, Gill TJ III. Instability of neural xenografts placed in neonatal rat brains. *Transplantation* 1988;46:216–223.

76. Duan W-M, Widner H, Brundin P. Sequential intrastriatal grafting of allogeneic embryonic dopamine-rich neuronal tissue in adult rats: will a second graft be rejected? *Neuroscience* 1993;57:261–274.

77. Ansari AA, Mayne A, Freed CR, et al. Lack of a detectable systemic humoral/cellular allogeneic response in human and nonhuman primate recipients of embryonic mesencephalic allografts for the therapy of Parkinson's disease. *Transplant Proc* 1995;27:1401–1405.

78. Yoffey JM, Courtice FC. *Lymphatics, lymph and the lymphomyeloid complex.* New York: Academic, 1970.

79. Cserr HF, Cooper DN, Milhorat TH. Flow of cerebral interstitial fluid as indicated by the removal of extracellular markers from the rat caudate nucleus. *Exp Eye Res* 1977;25(suppl):461–473.

80. Bradbury MWB, Westrop RJ. Factors influencing the exit of substances from cerebrospinal fluid into deep cervical lymph of the rabbit. *J Physiol* 1981;339:519–534.

81. Cserr HF, Knopf PM. Cervical lymphatics, the blood-brain barrier and the immunoreactivity of the brain: a new view. *Immunol Today* 1992;13:507–512.

82. Widner H, Møller G, Johansson BB. Immune response in deep cervical lymph nodes and spleen in the mouse after antigen deposition in different intracerebral sites. *Scand J Immunol* 1988;28:563–571.

83. Oehmichen M, Wietholter H, Gruninger H, Gencic M. Destruction of intracerebrally applied red blood cells in cervical lymph nodes. Experimental investigations. *Forensic Sci Int* 1983;21:43–57.

84. Cross AH, Canella B, Brosnan CF, Raine CS. Homing to central nervous system vasculature by antigen-specific lymphocytes. I. Localization of ^{14}C-labeled cells during acute and chronic-relapsing experimental allergic encephalitis. *Lab Invest* 1990;63:162–170.

85. Wekerle H, Linington C, Lassmann H, Meyermann R. Cellular immune reactivity within the CNS. *Trends Neurosci* 1986;9:271–277.

86. Wekerle H, Engelhardt B, Risau W, Meyermann R. Passage of lymphocytes across the blood-brain barrier in health and disease. In: Johansson BB, Owman CH, Widner H, eds. *Long-term consequences of barrier dysfunction for the brain. (Proceedings of the Erik K. Fernström symposium on pathophysiology of the blood-brain barrier.)* Amsterdam: Elsevier, 1990:439–446.

87. Broadwell RD, Charlton HM, Balin BJ, Salcman M. Angioarchitecture of the CNS, pituitary gland, and intracerebral grafts revealed with peroxida cytochemistry. *J Comp Neurol* 1987;260:47–62.

88. Broadwell RD. Absence of a blood-brain barrier within transplanted tissue? *Science* 1988;241:473–474.

89. Dusart I, Nothias F, Roudier F, Pechanski M. Role possible de l'environment neuronal dans las vascularisation d'une greffe intracerebrale. *CR Acad Sci III* 1987;305:277–283.

90. Widner H, Brundin P, Lindvall O. Clinical trials with allogeneic fetal neural grafts in Parkinson's disease: theoretical and practical immunological aspects. In: Johansson BB, Owman C, Widner H, eds. *Long-term consequences of barrier disfuntion for the brain. (Proceedings of the Eric K. Fernström symposium on pathophysiology*

of the blood-brain barrier.) Amsterdam: Elsevier Science, 1990:593–608.

91. Brundin P, Nilsson OG, Gage FH, Björklund A. Cyclosporin A increases survival of cross-species intrastriatal grafts of embryonic dopamine-containing neurons. *Exp Brain Res* 1985;60:204–208.

92. Inoue H, Kohsaka S, Yoshida K, et al. Cyclosporin A enhances the survivability of mouse cerebral cortex grafted into the third ventricle of rat brain. *Neurosci Lett* 1985;54:85–90.

93. Fabry Z, Waldschmidt MM, Moore SA, Hart MN. Antigen presentation by brain microvessel smooth muscle and endothelium. *J Neuroimmunol* 1990;28:63–71.

94. Gehrmann J, Banati RB, Kreutzberg GW. Microglia in the immune surveillance of the brain: human microglia constitutively express HLA-DR molecules. *J Neuroimmunol* 1993;48:189–198.

95. Gehrmann J. Microglia: intrinsic immunoeffector of the brain. *Brain Res Rev* 1995;20:269–287.

96. Bluestone JA, Pescovitz MD, Frels WI, et al. Cytotoxic T lymphocyte recognition of a xenogeneic major histocompatibility complex antigen expressed in transgenic mice. *Eur J Immunol* 1987;17:1035–1041.

97. Nakashima H, Kawamura K, Date I. Immunological reaction and blood-brain barrier in mouse-rat cross-species neural graft. *Brain Res* 1988;475:232–243.

98. Kievets F, Wijfels J, Lockhorst W, Ivanyi P. Recognition of xeno-(HLA,SLA) major histocompatibility antigens by mouse cytotoxic T cells is not H-2 restricted: a study with transgenic mice. *Proc Natl Acad Sci USA* 1989;86:617–620.

99. Date I, Kawamura K, Nakashima H. Histological signs of reactions against allogeneic solid fetal neural grafts in the cerebellum depend on the MHC locus. *Exp Brain Res* 1988;73:15–22.

100. Finsen B, Oteruelo F, Zimmer J. Immunocytochemical characterization of the cellular response to intracerebral xenografts of brain tissue. *Prog Brain Res* 1988;78:261–270.

101. Nicholas MK, Sagher O, Hartley JP, et al. A phenotypic analysis of T lymphocytes isolated from the brains of mice with allogeneic neural transplants. *Prog Brain Res* 1988;78:249–259.

102. Hall BM. Cells mediating allograft rejection. *Transplantation* 1991;51:1141–1151.

103. Pollack H, Lund RD, Rao K. MHC antigen expression and cellular response in spontaneous and induced expression of neuronal xenografts. *Prog Brain Res* 1990;82:129–140.

104. Rao K, Lund RD, Kunz HW, Gill TJ III. The role of MHC and non-MHC antigens in the rejection of intracerebral allogeneic neural grafts. *Transplantation* 1989;48:1018–1021.

105. Wood MJA, Sloan DJ, Dallman MJ, Charlton HM. A monoclonal antibody to the interleukin-2 receptor enhances the survival of neural allografts: a time-course study. *Neuroscience* 1992;49:409–418.

106. Broadwell RD, Charlton HM, Ganong WF, et al. Allografts of CNS tissue possess a blood-brain barrier. I. Grafts of medial preoptic area in hypogonadal mice. *Exp Neurol* 1989;105:135–151.

107. Broadwell RD, Baker BJ, Ebert P, et al. Intracerebral grafting of solid tissues and cell suspensions: the blood-brain barrier and the host immune response. *Prog Brain Res* 1992;91:95–102.

108. Young MJ, Rao K, Lund RD. Integrity of the blood-brain barrier in retinal xenografts is correlated with the immunological status of the host. *J Comp Neurol* 1989;283:107–117.

109. Rao K, Lund RD. Optic nerve degeneration induces the expression of MHC antigens in the rat visual system. *J Comp Neurol* 1989;336:613–627.

110. Lawrence JM, Morris RJ, Raisman G. Anatomical evidence that microglia are involved in both the immune presenting and immune attack phases of intracerebral allograft rejection. *Neuropathol Appl Neurobiol* 1994;20:203–205.

111. Wekerle H, Sun D, Oropeza-Wekerle RL, Meyermann R. Immune reactivity in the nervous system: modulation of T-lymphocyte activation by glial cells. *J Exp Biol* 1987;132:43–57.

112. Takei K, Nakano Y, Shinozaki T, et al. Immunological rejection of grafted tissue in xenogeneic neural transplantation. *Prog Brain Res* 1990;82:103–109.

113. Banati RB, Gehrmann J, Schubert P, Kreutzberg GW. Cytotoxicity microglia. *Glia* 1993;7:111–118.

114. Mahalik et al. Programmed cell death in developing grafts of fetal substantia nigra. *Exp Neurol* 1994;129:27–36.

115. Sigal NH, Dumont FJ. Cyclosporin A, FK-506, and rapamycin: pharmacologic probes of lymphocyte signal transduction. *Annu Rev Immunol* 1992;10:519–560.

116. Britton S, Palacios R. Cyclosporin A—usefulness, risks, and mechanism of action. *Immunol Rev* 1982; 65:5–22.

117. Horsburgh T, Wood P, Brent L. Suppression of in vitro lymphocyte reactivity by cyclosporin A: existence of a population of drug-resistant cytotoxic lymphocytes. *Nature* 1980;286:609–611.

118. Walmann H. Manipulation of T cell responses with monoclonal antibodies. *Annu Rev Immunol* 1989;7:407–444.

119. Honey CR, Charlton HM, Wood KJ. Rat brain xenografts reverse hypogonadism in mice immunosuppressed with anti-CD4 monoclonal antibody. *Exp Brain Res* 1991;85:149–152.

120. Honey CR, Clarke DJ, Dallman MJ, Charlton HM. Human neural graft function in rats treated with anti-interleukin II receptor antibody. *Neuroreport* 1990;1:247–249.

121. Faustman D, Coe C. Prevention of xenograft rejection by masking donor HLA class I antigens. *Science* 1991;252:1700–1702.

122. Osorio RW, Ascher NL, Stock PG. Prolongation of in vivo mouse islet allograft survival by modulation of MHC class I antigen. *Transplantation* 1994;57:783–788.

123. Pakzaban P, Deacon TW, Burns LH, et al. A novel mode of immunoprotection of neural xenotransplants: masking of donor major histocompatibility complex class I enhances transplant survival in the central nervous system. *Neuroscience* 1995;65:983–996.

124. Sadikot AF, Alonso-Vanegas M, Faure MP, et al. Characterization of in vivo survival of embryonic dopaminergic cells after selective sorting using a fluorescent neurotensin derivative. In: *Society for Neuroscience abstracts*. Washington, DC: 1996.

125. Widner H, Tetrud J, Rehncrona S, et al. Bilateral fetal mesencephalic grafting in two patients with parkinsonism induced by 1-methyl-4-phenyl-1,2,3,6-tetrahydropyridine (MPTP). *N Engl J Med* 1992;327:1556–1563.

126. Lindvall O, Rehncrona S, Brundin P, et al. Human fetal dopamine neurons grafted into the striatum in two patients with severe Parkinson's disease: a detailed account of methodology and a 6 month follow-up. *Arch Neurol* 1989;46:615–631.

127. Lindvall O, Widner H, Rehncrona S, et al. Transplantation of fetal dopamine neurons in Parkinson's disease: 1-year clinical and neurophysiological observations in two patients with putaminal implants. *Ann Neurol* 1992;31:155–165.

128. Henderson BTH, Clough CG, Hughes RC, et al. Implan-

tation of human fetal ventral mesencephalon to the right caudate nucleus in advanced Parkinson's disease. *Arch Neurol* 1991;48:822–827.

129. Molina H, Quinones R, Alvarez L, et al. Transplantation of human fetal mesencephalic tissue in caudate nucleus as treatment for Parkinson's disease: the Cuban experience. In: Lindvall O, Björklund A, Widner H, eds. *Intracerebral transplantation in movement disorders: experimental basis and clinical experiences.* Amsterdam: Elsevier, 1991:99–110.

130. Madrazo I, Franco-Bourland R, Aguilera M, et al. Fetal ventral mesencephalon brain homotransplantation in Parkinson's disease: the Mexican experience. In: Lindvall O, Björklund A, Widner H, eds. *Intracerebral transplantation in movement disorders: experimental basis and clinical experiences.* Amsterdam: Elsevier, 1991: 123–129.

131. Freed CR, Breeze RE, Rosenberg NL, et al. Survival of implanted fetal dopamine cells and neurologic improvement 12 to 46 months after transplantation for Parkinson's disease. *N Engl J Med* 1992;327:1549–1555.

132. Spencer DD, Robbins RJ, Naftolin F, et al. Unilateral transplantation of human fetal mesencephalic tissue into the caudate nucleus of patients with Parkinson's disease. *N Engl J Med* 1992;327:1541–1548.

133. Fine A, Hunt SP, Oertel WH, et al. Transplantation of embryonic marmosets dopaminergic neurons to the corpus striatum of marmosets rendered parkinsonian by 1-methyl-4-phenyl-1,2,3,6-tetrahydropyridine. *Prog Brain Res* 1988;78:479–489.

134. Taylor JR, Elsworth JD, Roth RH, et al. Grafting of fetal substantia nigra to striatum reverses behavioral deficits induced by MPTP in primates: a comparison with other types of grafts as controls. *Exp Brain Res* 1991;85:335–348.

135. Taylor JR, Elsworth JD, Sladek JR Jr, et al. Sham surgery does not ameliorate MPTP-induced behavioral deficits in monkeys. *Cell Transplant* 1995;4:13–26.

136. Lindvall O, Sawle G, Widner H, et al. Evidence for long-term survival and function of dopaminergic grafts in progressive Parkinson's disease. *Ann Neurol* 1994;35: 172–180.

137. Boyer KL, Bakay RA. The history, theory, and present status of brain transplantation. *Neurosurg Clin North Am* 1995;6:113–125.

Chapter 19

Guillain-Barré Syndrome and Chronic Inflammatory Demyelinating Polyradiculoneuropathy

Hans-Peter Hartung, Klaus V. Toyka, and John W. Griffin

Guillain-Barré syndrome (GBS) and chronic inflammatory demyelinating polyradiculoneuropathy (CIDP) are prototypic neuropathies resulting from disordered immunity. These immune-mediated neuropathies differ, among other features, by the tempo of evolution and clinical course. GBS is the most common cause of acute neuromuscular paralysis and represents a neurologic emergency (1). In most instances, relatively symmetric weakness develops within days to some weeks and the disease reaches its nadir by 4 weeks, when after a plateau phase most patients start to recover. Infrequently, complete tetraplegia evolves within a matter of hours. Outside specialized centers, mortality still approximates 10% and only 15% of all patients make a complete recovery. Two thirds will have some neurologic deficits and in 3% to 5%, relapses, months or years apart, can develop. Death is due to respiratory failure, autonomic dysfunction, and secondary complications of immobilization. CIDP, by arbitrary definition, evolves subacutely over a time interval of at least 8 weeks, but much more frequently chronically over months and years. In younger patients, the disease tends to follow a relapsing-remitting or relapsing-progressive course, whereas with onset in middle and old age a progressive evolution of disabling sensorimotor deficits is more common (2).

Guillain-Barré Syndrome—A Heterogeneous Disease

Evidence collected in the past decade indicates that GBS truly is a syndrome involving a common clinical phenotype shared by a group of variant forms of the neuropathy. This notion is based on careful clinical-pathologic correlations of single cases with a particularly severe course observed in the Western Hemisphere and analysis of epidemic clusters of the disease occurring in China and elsewhere. Feasby et al (3,4) were the first to draw attention to a primary axonal variant of GBS when they studied five extremely severely afflicted patients with inexcitable nerves and denervation on electrophysiologic examination. Recovery was poor and autopsy of one patient who died within 4 weeks of disease onset revealed marked axonal degeneration of roots and nerves with little or no evidence of demyelination and absence of inflammatory infiltrates. The issue was clouded by subsequent reports of patients with a similar clinical course and electrophysiologic findings in whom conduction block was noted before electrophysiologic features of axonal damage developed (5). Motor neuron inexcitability and low compound muscle action potential in the initial stages of GBS were electrophysiologically shown to result from either distal conduction block or axonal degeneration (6). Further autopsy studies of patients with a similar explosive onset and clinical course revealed widespread demyelination with admixed axonal degeneration as the key underlying pathologic process (7–9). Another autopsy series (10) revealed a spectrum of demyelinative and axonal changes. The fiercely disputed notion of the existence of a primarily axonal form of GBS received support from clinical, electrophysiologic, and pathologic observations of summer epidemics of an acute paralytic disease in rural China that turned out to represent a particular variant of GBS (11,12).

Pathology

According to a recently proposed classification, GBS can be subdivided into the classic acute demyelinating variant that represents the great majority of cases in the Western world; the acute motor axonal neuropathy (AMAN) initially described as Chinese paralytic syndrome and the most prevalent form of GBS in China (11); the acute motor and sensory axonal neuropathy (AMSAN), which is distinguished by significant sensory involvement and apparently associated with a more severe cause and poorer prognosis; and the Miller Fisher syndrome (13–15).

Concepts of the underlying pathology in GBS in the Western Hemisphere have been based on relatively few biopsy and autopsy studies on small numbers of patients (16). In their landmark study, Asbury et al (17) considered multifocal demyelination associated with perivascular mononuclear cell infiltrates distributed ubiquitously in the peripheral nervous system (PNS) the pathologic hallmark of the disorder. They called attention to an intimate association of invading lymphocytes and early focal myelin breakdown. A more recent large autopsy series of GBS patients in the United Kingdom revealed a spectrum of pathologic alterations ranging from focal demyelination with or without attendant invasion of nerves by T cells and macrophages, to extensive demyelination with only few or no inflammatory infiltrates, to widespread axonal degeneration with or without appreciable demyelination or cellular infiltrates (10). Pathologic changes can be prominent at the spinal root level involving both ventral and dorsal roots or either in isolation, or may affect the most distal part of the motor nerves, the intramuscular arborizations where not only demyelinative changes, but also axonal damage have been noted (18–20). In some patients, vesicular disintegration of myelin in proximity to macrophages situated within the basement membrane of affected fibers and widening of the nodes of Ranvier are early features. Characteristically, myelin is predominantly lost at and around the nodes of Ranvier where macrophages cluster. Electron microscopically, these cells strip and phagocytose compact myelin (16,21,22). Hughes et al (21) stressed that in many instances macrophages attacking the myelin sheath are numerous in the absence of T cells.

Maier et al (23) recently reported intriguing findings of central nervous system (CNS) pathology in the majority of 13 autopsy cases of clinically typical GBS. In addition to changes such as central chromatolysis of spinal anterior horn cells and degeneration of posterior columns considered secondary to the pathologic process in the PNS (4,7,10,13), they observed perivascular cuffing of lymphocytes within the spinal cord and medulla oblongata, macrophages apposed to motor neurons of the anterior horn, and neurons of the olive, in clusters, in a perivascular distribution or diffusely scattered. In addition, they found CD4+ and CD8+ T cells. A prominent feature was activation of microglia, particularly in the gray matter of the spinal cord. The involvement of the CNS described in this study may reflect remote immune activation in the absence of the relevant antigen, as described in experimental allergic neuritis (EAN) (24), or mirror predominantly T cell–driven responses to a shared myelin protein. In this context, it is noteworthy that in EAN, autoimmune pathology can be induced with myelin basic protein (MBP)–reactive T cells (25,26).

In a recent autopsy of a patient with "classic demyelinating" GBS who died 3 days after onset, pathologic changes in the spinal cords were very mild and only few lymphocytes were identified. Activated complement was found deposited on the outermost surface of the Schwann cell (the abaxonal Schwann cell plasmalemma) and electron microscopy provided evidence for vesicular dissolution of the myelin sheaths (27). Activation products of complement (C3a, C5a, C3c, C5b-9)

have been detected in the serum, plasma, and cerebrospinal fluid of Western GBS patients (28–32). Earlier immunohistochemical studies in this population showed that C3d was localized to myelin sheaths in sural nerve biopsy specimens and C5b-9 deposits were observed in one biopsy sample from a patient with classic GBS (31,33,34).

The earliest changes noted in well-preserved autopsy samples of AMAN were found at the nodes of Ranvier in motor fibers where nodal gaps were lengthened and the nodes decorated with activation products of the complement cascade (13,15,27). Macrophages overlay the node of Ranvier and penetrated the outer basal lamina of the Schwann cell to eventually enter the periaxonal space of the internode. Activated complement components (C3d, C9 neoantigen) could be localized to the adaxonal Schwann cell plasmalemma. Despite invasion of the periaxonal space by macrophages, the axons were intact. Wallerian degeneration was observed in the most severe cases. Based on these observations, the authors raised the possibility that antibodies to GM_1 or related glycoconjugates would bind to the axolemma.

Ensuing complement activation would provide a chemotactic signal for macrophages to invade the periaxonal space. Binding of such antibodies to the nodes of Ranvier could produce partial and reversible conduction block. Two groups showed that GM_1 antibody–containing sera from patients with multifocal motor neuropathies and those with GBS and GQ_{1b} antibody–containing sera from Miller Fisher syndrome patients can block conduction and reduce or eliminate end-plate potentials in the mouse phrenic nerve hemidiaphragm preparation (35–38). Whether this clear pathologic distinction between "axonal" and "demyelinating" cases holds up remains to be seen. It is certainly conceivable that axonal degeneration results from specific immune-mediated injury or is consequent to bystander damage caused by an intense inflammatory response. Evidence in support of this notion comes from EAN where axonal degeneration is proportional to the dose of neuritogenic antigen or the number of neuritogenic T cells transferred. With a vigorous inflammatory response, endoneurial fluid pressure is markedly increased and may result in ischemic nerve damage with subsequent wallerian degeneration of affected fibers (39–41).

Humoral Immune Responses

Complement fixing IgM antibodies to human myelin were originally identified in 90% of patients with classic GBS (42–44). On serial determinations no immunoglobulin isotype switching to IgG was noted, which would be compatible with the (auto)antigen being a thymus-independent antigen (43,45). These IgM antibodies were claimed to bind to carbohydrate residues similar to those of the Forssman antigen, a ceramide with five carbohydrate residues distributed widely in many mammalian species and infectious agents (45). The specificity of these findings was questioned by Ilyas et al (46) who studied a large series of 54 GBS patients.

More recently, attention has focused on humoral immune responses to the glycoconjugate family of antigens. The reported frequency of antiglycolipid antibodies ranged from as low as 5% in one study to 60% in another, which may reflect the variable sensitivity of assays to detect these antibodies (47) and problems with classifying low-titer antibodies (48). Antibodies were frequently directed to one or more of the gangliosides GM_1, GD_{1a}, GD_{1b}, GT_{1b}, asialo-GM_1, and LM_1 (reviewed by Hartung et al (49)). These antibodies commonly recognize the Gal(β1-3)GalNac carbohydrate moiety. Titers of these glycolipid antibodies tend to decline after the acute phase of the disease. Several investigators found an association of GM_1 antibodies with a more severe and predominantly axonal type of GBS, and some reported that these antibodies occurred more frequently in patients in whom the neuropathy was preceded by an infection with *Campylobacter jejuni* (50–58), although this association has been disputed (59–61). The lacking correlation with clinical features of the disease was confirmed in a large prospective case-control study (62). Yuki et al (63) claimed that high-titer GD_{1a} antibodies of the IgG or IgM class are associated with more severe disease. They never observed in serial determinations isotype class switching in the IgM anti-GD_{1a}–positive group (63). Some GBS patients have antibodies against rare ganglioside species; for example, as recently reported, sera from 6 of 50 GBS patients in one series and from 8 of 58 in another contained antibodies to *N*-acetylgalactosaminyl-GD_{1a} (64,65). Most of the Japanese patients with severe GBS, ganglioside antibodies, and evidence of a preceding *C. jejuni* infection reported by Yuki et al (52,66,67) had the HLA-B35 haplotype, whereas Kuroki et al (68) noted this particular haplotype association in only 25% of their stool culture–positive Japanese patients, making an immunogenetic basis of the variations reported unlikely. Rees et al (56), looking at major histocompatibility complex (MHC) class II alleles in 97 patients with GBS, noted a significant association between HLA-DQB1*03 and preceding *C. jejuni* infection.

Fredman et al (69) found antibody activity, mostly of the IgG isotype, predominantly to LM_1, not only in 43% of GBS patients but also in 20% of blood donors. Anti-sulfatide antibodies of the IgG isotype were detected in 65% of GBS patients. IgM and IgA class antibodies have also been observed (46,70–74). Anti-SGPG (sulfate-3-glucuronyl paragloboside) antibodies of the IgM or IgG class were detected in 13 (25%) of 53 GBS serum samples in one series (72), but in only 1 of 21 GBS serum samples in another (75). Five of 96 acute demyelinating GBS serum samples were found to harbor high-titer IgG antibodies to sialosyl paragloboside (SPG) (76).

Antibodies to galactocerebroside were not found more frequently in GBS patients (77) compared to control subjects, but were detected in five patients who developed GBS after infection with *Mycoplasma pneumoniae* (78).

Ho et al (79) determined antiglycolipid antibodies in the serum of Chinese patients with GBS. They found IgG anti-GM_1 antibodies with a frequency of 42%, versus 6% in controls. Seventeen percent had antibodies to GM_2, 26% to GD_{1a}, and 18% to GD_{1b}. Antibodies to LM_1 notably occurred less frequently in GBS patients than in control subjects, and were markedly less common in those GBS patients who had evidence of an antecedent *C. jejuni* infection. There was no significant correlation with the pattern of the disease (AMAN vs "classic" GBS) or with the presence of *C. jejuni* antibodies.

In most patients with the Miller Fisher variant of GBS, serum contains IgG antibodies to the minor ganglioside GQ_{1b} (80–82). Such antibodies can also be detected in some GBS patients with pronounced ophthalmoplegia (83). The antibodies to GQ_{1b} usually cross-react with GT_{1a} and in about 50% with GD_{1b} or GD_3 (84,85). Two groups reported that the serum GQ_{1b} antibodies were of IgG1 and IgG3 isotypes invoking a primary T cell–dependent immune response (86,87).

The regional distribution and function of glycolipids in different areas of the human nervous system may play a role in defining the pathophysiologic features of their autoantibody-associated diseases. For example, GQ_{1b} is enriched in human ocular muscle nerves compared with other sites, which may account for the vulnerability of these nerves to immune-mediated attack in the anti-GQ_{1b} antibody–associated neuropathy, Miller Fisher syndrome (80–83). A similar explanation may hold for other regional or fiber-selective syndromes; for example, in the myelin sheaths GM_1 is enriched in motor nerves compared to sensory nerves, although the data in the literature are conflicting (88–91). However, clearly other factors such as antibody access and glycolipid membrane topography are also important. The fine specificity of antibodies will also have an influence on their ability to bind a particular antigen in a physiologic membrane.

Table 19-1 shows the structure of the glycolipids discussed above.

The Origin of Antiglycolipid Antibodies

Antiglycolipid IgM antibodies of differing specificities are frequently found at low levels in normal sera (92). In addition, umbilical cord B cells, which are naive to foreign antigen, and adult peripheral blood and tonsillar B cells can be induced to secrete anti-GM_1 IgM antibodies from donors with low or absent serum antibody titers (93,94). These data suggest that some anticarbohydrate antibodies form part of the naturally occurring autoantibody repertoire that comprises low-affinity, polyreactive IgM antibodies encoded by immunoglobulin variable-region genes in germline configuration. Such IgM antibodies may have an immunoregulatory role in shaping immune maturation and may act as a first-line defense against invading microorganisms. Microbial polysaccharide antigens such as lipopolysaccharide (LPS) containing repeating sugar sequences can activate B cells, particularly those of the CD5 subset, by cross-linking their surface immunoglobulin receptors in a T cell–independent (type 1

Table 19-1.
Structure of Glycolipids

	Carbohydrate Sequences
GM1b	Gal (β1-3) GalNAc (β1-4) Gal (β1-4) Glc (β1-1) Ceramide (α 2-3) NeuNAc
GM1	Gal (β1-3) GalNAc (β1-4) Gal (β1-4) Glc (β1-1) Ceramide (α 2-3) NeuNAc
GM2	GalNAc (β1-4) Gal (β1-4) Glc (β1-1) Ceramide (α2-3) NeuNAc
GM3	Gal (β1-4) Glc (β1-1) Ceramide (α2-3) NeuNAc
GD1a	Gal (β1-3) GalNAc (β1-4) Gal (β1-4) Glc (β1-1) Ceramide (α2-3) (α2-3) NeuNAc NeuNAc
GD1b	Gal (β1-3) GalNAc (β1-4) Gal (β1-4) Glc (β1-1) Ceramide (α2-3) NeuNAc (α2-8) NeuNAc
GT1b	Gal (β1-3) GalNAc (β1-4) Gal (β1-4) Glc (β1-1) Ceramide (α2-3) (α2-3) NeuNAc NeuNAc (α2-8) NeuNAc
GT1a	Gal (β1-3) GalNAc (β1-4) Gal (β1-4) Glc (β1-1) Ceramide (α2-3) (α2-3) NeuNAc NeuNAc (α2-8) NeuNAc
GQ1b	Gal (β1-3) GalNAc (β1-4) Gal (β1-4) Glc (β1-1) Ceramide (α2-3) (α2-3) NeuNAc NeuNAc (α2-8) (α2-8) NeuNAc NeuNAc
GD3	Gal (β1-4) Glc(β1-1) Ceramide (α2-3) NeuNAc (α2-8) NeuNAc
Asialo-GM1	Gal (β1-3) GalNAc (β1-4) Gal (β1-4) Glc (β1-1) Ceramide
LM1 (= SPG)	Gal (β1-4) GlcNAc (β1-3) Gal (β1-4) Glc (β1-1) Ceramide (α2-3) NeuNAc
SGPG	Gal (β1-4) GlcNAc (β1-3) Gal (β1-4) Glc (β1-1) Ceramide (β1-3) SO$_4$3GlcUA

TI) but antigen-specific manner or alternatively can polyclonally activate B cells. This results in the predominant production of long-lived IgM responses. Affinity maturation, class switching from IgM to IgG, and recruitment of B cells into the memory compartment are typical features of cognate, T cell–dependent interactions. Traditional immunologic thinking has it that complex carbohydrate molecules such as gangliosides cannot be processed by antigen-presenting cells in this way (95). More recently, evidence has surfaced that some bacterial lipid and glycolipid antigens can be presented to T cells by professional antigen-presenting cells endowed with the CD1b protein (96). One can only speculate whether such a CD1-restricted presentation of glycoconjugate antigens could directly trigger a response of T cells to deliver help to B lymphocytes for antibody production. However in GBS, high-affinity IgG subclass 1 and 3 antiganglioside antibody responses are seen, suggesting that T-cell help has been recruited in the immune response; the mechanism by which this takes place is unknown (87,97,98). Whether the B-cell subset that gives rise to the chronically elevated IgM antibodies is CD5 positive and distinct from that which gives rise to the IgG antibodies is not known (99).

Evidence suggests that the source of the carbohydrate complex that drives the antiglycolipid response in many patients with GBS is bacterial LPS. In approximately 30% of patients it is possible to obtain serologic evidence of a preceding *C. jejuni* infection (49). Molecular mimicry, whereby infectious agents share antigenic epitopes common to host (i.e., neural) tissues, has been demonstrated for certain strains of *C. jejuni* LPS and gangliosides including GM_1, GD_{1a}, GT_{1a}, GD_3, and GQ_{1b}. In GBS and Miller Fisher syndrome following *C. jejuni* enteritis, the LPS fractions of the infecting bacteria have been shown to react with anti-GM_1 and anti-GQ_{1b} antibodies and to contain the appropriate oligosaccharide structures (68,86,100–108).

It is possible that other microorganisms may bear carbohydrate epitopes that mimic glycolipid structures (108–109). In contrast to the prediction that anti–glycolipid IgM antibodies, along with IgM antibodies in general, would be encoded by immunoglobulin variable-region genes in germline configuration, several sequencing studies showed that anti–glycolipid IgM antibodies contain extensive somatic mutation. This indicates that they have arisen through antigen-driven mechanisms, possibly stimulated by cross-reactive bacterial LPS (110,111,112). No specific or unifying patterns of V-gene usage have so far been described and it thus seems that antiglycolipid antibodies can be encoded by diverse V genes from different heavy- and light-chain families.

Another potential microbial trigger of a misguided immune response is infection with cytomegalovirus (CMV) (113–116). A few patients with IgM and IgG antibodies to CMV also have antibodies directed to GM_2, asialo-GM_2, and GD_2. Apparently, these antibodies recognize the terminal GalNac-Gal moiety and internal residues GalNac-Gal-Glc. Since glycoproteins of CMV contain *O*-glycosylated and sialylated sites, these findings suggest that anti-GM_2 antibodies cross-react with the glycosylated sites of CMV glycoproteins. Interestingly, CMV also contains sequences homologous to the P0 protein and therefore, apart from antibodies, T cells may also launch cross-reactive responses to peripheral nerve following CMV infection (117).

The Pathogenic Relevance of Antiglycolipid Antibodies

There is evidence from some studies, contradicted in others, in a variety of experimental animal models to support a direct role for antiganglioside antibodies in causing neuropathy. Two major contentious issues should be outlined. Firstly, once formed and present in the circulation, can antiglycolipid antibodies induce neuropathy in isolation or are other factors such as perturbations in cytokine profiles or T cells also required for full expression of the pathophysiology? Assuming that antiglycolipid antibodies are involved in causation, are their effects predominantly proinflammatory or are they capable of acting pharmacologically to block a ganglioside-mediated physiologic process? It is likely that there is some truth in all of these views but this is clearly a complex issue. Interpretation of data derived from animal studies is hampered by species differences in many areas including glycolipid function and distribution in nerve, immunologic background, and physiologic performance.

The motor nerve terminal and neuromuscular junction may be an important site of action of antiglycolipid antibodies, particularly since their position with the blood-nerve barrier allows for easy antibody access.

Anti-GM_1 antibody immunoreactive material is present at the nodes of Ranvier and motor nerve terminals, two sites crucial to efficient nerve function (18,118,119). Many studies have been performed to establish whether anti-GM_1–containing sera can cause neuropathic effects. Two studies (120,121) demonstrated conduction block with intraneural injection of anti-GM_1 antibody into rat sciatic and tibial nerve, with or without an additional source of complement. In an in vitro rat sciatic nerve preparation, both human and rabbit anti-GM_1 antibody–containing sera induced partial conduction block (122). Immunization of rabbits with GM_1 induced serum anti-GM_1 antibodies, immunoglobulin deposits at nodes of Ranvier, and conduction block in one study (123). Repeat therapeutic administration of ganglioside mixture can produce an axonal neuropathy associated with anti-GM_1 antibodies circulating in blood and deposited at the paranodal myelin sheaths and the motor terminals (124). Using the mouse hemidiaphragm preparation as a model system, Roberts et al (38) showed electrophysiologically both direct in vitro effects and passive transfer effects of anti-GM_1 antibody–containing sera. In the Miller Fisher variant of the disease, GQ_{1b} antibody–containing serum blocked neuromuscular transmission in this experimental model (35). In some of these studies the effects appeared to be complement independent (36,37); in others the converse was seen. The mechanism by which these effects are induced is unknown but has been speculated to involve sodium channels; in support of this Takigawa et al (125) showed that high-titer rabbit anti-GM_1 antisera can block Na^+ channels in an isolated single myelinated fiber preparation in the presence of complement. In contrast to studies reporting positive effects of anti-GM_1 antibodies in animal models, Harvey et al (126) failed to obtain any morphologic or electrophysiologic effects with IgG or IgM anti-GM_1 antisera when injected together with complement into rat tibial nerves, although immunoglobulin was deposited at the nodes of Ranvier in the experimental animals.

These issues cannot be reconciled easily. Differences in experimental design and conduct must be the major factors in producing these discrepancies: The choices of anti-GM_1 antisera, species, and electrophysiologic site to be studied seem to be critical. Further experimentation is clearly needed.

Recently, an animal model of neuropathy induced by *C. jejuni* became available. A paralytic neuropathy occurs in chickens living on farms of families in rural China where one member suffered from GBS. Inoculation of chickens with *C. jejuni* Penner O:19 cultured from the stools of an affected patient with AMAN produced weakness in about half of all animals. Pathologic changes in the peripheral nerve of diseased chickens included massive wallerian-like degeneration, lengthening of the nodes of Ranvier, and in rare instances, paranodal demyelination. Occasionally, macrophages overlay widened paranodes. Some macrophages had entered the periaxonal space of affected internodes, separating the inner myelin lamellae from the axon. Lymphocytic infiltration was scarce. Taken together, these changes were akin to those seen in the AMAN pattern of GBS in humans (127).

Cellular Immune Responses

The demonstration of inflammatory infiltrates in nerve and of the crucial pathogenic role of neuritogenic T cells in the animal model EAN (see Chapter 4) prompted the search for evidence of disordered cellular immunity in GBS. Systemic T-cell activation has been documented by an enhanced expression of HLA-DR, the interleukin (IL)-2 receptor, and the transferrin receptor on cells in the blood (128); by the occurrence with increased frequency of hypoxanthine guanine phosphor:basyltransferase (HPRT)-mutant T cells (129); and by raised levels of IL-2 (130) and the IL-2 receptor (131,132). Increased serum concentrations of neopterin, a macrophage product released in response to the Th1 cytokine interferon (IFN)-γ, and of the cytokine tumor necrosis factor (TNF)-α likewise reflect systemic activation (133–137). The CD4+ CD29+ helper/inducer subset was increased while the CD4+ CD45RA+ suppressor/cytotoxic subpopulation of T cells was decreased in number (138). Various attempts have been made to identify nerve antigen(s) to which aberrant T-cell responses are mounted. Many researchers employing the macrophage migration inhibition test, skin testing for hypersensitivity, or lymphocyte proliferation assays ex vivo failed to demonstrate a specific T-cell response to P2, the major neuritogen of EAN, while others succeeded (136,139–146). In one study it was possible to raise a P2-specific T-cell line from one GBS patient but with equal efficiency from three healthy control subjects (147). More recently it was shown that T cells given irradiated autologous mononuclear cells as antigen presenters underwent marked transformation in response to P2 and its peptides P2 14-25 and P2 58-81 in the first few days of GBS, and to P0 (P0 70-85, P0 180-199) in a minor proportion of patients (148,149). T-cell responses to P0 or its peptides were detectable before those against P2 and P2 peptides and were clearly transient, subsiding within 2 to 3 weeks while the response to P2 persisted for months. There were no apparent clinical correlations other than onset of disease to any of these responses. A note of caution is in order. All these studies employed bovine proteins. There is evidence that T cells reacting to bovine P2 or P0 may not recognize the human proteins (150–152).

Results obtained with the P0 protein and its peptides are of particular importance since the extracellular domain of P0 (residues 1-124) is readily available for T-cell recognition in contrast to the cytoplasmically located protein P2. The relevance of these observations is strengthened by findings in EAN. Immunization with P0 or adoptive transfer of T-cell lines raised against extracellular portions of P0 produces an inflammatory neuropathy characterized by primary demyelination with preservation of axons (153,154).

Analysis of T-cell receptor (TCR) Vβ-gene usage in short-term T-cell lines reactive to P2, P0, and P0AA194-208 retrieved from a patient with classic demyelinating GBS disclosed heterogeneity with biased utilization of Vβ15 in the cell line responsive to the P0 peptide (155). TCR Vβ-gene usage by freshly isolated activated T cells was broad in four patients with acute inflammatory demyelinating polyradiculoneuropathy although there was some enhanced Vβ15 usage. Interestingly, activated and nonactivated T cells from a patient with AMSAN exhibited Vβ-gene usage similar to that of healthy controls (155). While it is difficult to extrapolate from studies on a few patients, these results of a somewhat focused repertoire of TCR Vβ genes may suggest a restricted response to a common antigen like P0 or indicate a role for an as yet undefined superantigen in the pathogenesis of GBS.

T-cell lines established from sural nerve biopsy samples in four of six patients failed to undergo proliferation on in vitro exposure to a peripheral myelin protein extract. Interestingly, the γδ T-cell line was isolated from the nerve of a patient who developed GBS after *C. jejuni* infection. Since many antigen-specific γδ T cells recognize their antigen with non-MHC, but CD1-mediated restriction, the possibility arises that they may have been activated by bacterial antigens, in particular of *C. jejuni*, that share homology with ganglioside antigens of peripheral nerve (156).

T-cell Migration

To generate an inflammatory lesion in the nerve, activated T cells circulating in blood need to enter the PNS. The complex process of homing, adhesion, and migration has been analyzed in detail in EAN (see Chapter 4). In this experimental model of GBS, the key functional importance of the adhesion molecules intercellular adhesion molecule (ICAM)-1, vascular cellular adhesion molecule (VCAM)-1, very late activation antigen (VLA)-4, and leukocyte function–associated antigen (LFA)-1 is well established. In GBS, patient sera contain increased levels of soluble E-selectin released from cytokine-activated endothelial cells serving as a fingerprint of the migratory process (157,158). T cells, as well as antibodies, may have unrestricted access at the most proximal and most distal parts of the nerve, that is, the spinal roots and the motor end plate. T-cell penetration of the blood-nerve barrier may permit circulating antibodies and inflammatory mediators access to the nerve (159,160). Importantly, neural antigen specificity is not required for such T cells (161,162).

The role conceivably played by T lymphocytes in GBS is manyfold. By issuing differentiation and proliferation signals such as IL-4, IL-5, and IL-6, T cells could help B cells to engineer antibodies; through the release of proinflammatory Th1 cytokines (TNF-α, IFN-γ) they could render immigrating or resident macrophages activated to augment generation and stimulate discharge of an array of toxic molecules or to engage in heightened phagocytic activity (29,108); they could inflict cytotoxic damage on Schwann cells as demonstrated in EAN (163). Finally, one has to consider that specialized populations of T lymphocytes may terminate the acute immunoinflammatory process in this mostly monophasic disorder. Such a function could be subserved by CD4 Th2 cells via synthesis of downregulatory cytokines such as IL-4, IL-10, and transforming growth factor (TGF)-β (see Chapter 4) or by CD8+ suppressor T cells. Evidence from studies in EAN suggests that apoptosis of autoreactive T cells in situ may also be involved in shutting off the acute immunoinflammatory response (164).

Macrophages featured prominently in the nerve lesion of GBS (16,165) may be derived from circulating monocytes that invade the peripheral nerve or represent endoneurial macrophages or their progeny (166). They act as professional antigen presenters and are of pivotal importance in the amplification and effector phase of immune-mediated demyelination (146). Mechanisms that are operative include phagocytosis and the release of proinflammatory cytokines (such as IL-1 and TNF-α) and other highly active mediators that act at short range (proteases, complement components, oxygen radicals, nitric oxide eicosanoids) (29). Monocytes/macrophages are activated in GBS. Monocytes isolated from the peripheral blood of GBS patients in the early phase of their disease produce increased amounts of toxic oxygen species when stimulated with phorbol diester, and elevated levels of neopterin, a biosynthetic product generated in response to IFN-γ, have been detected in GBS sera (133,136).

Therapy

Controlled trials have established the therapeutic efficacy of plasma exchange and high-dose intravenous immunoglobulin (IVIG) in patients requiring support for walking (54,108,167–169). The combined use of plasma exchange and a subsequent course of high-dose IVIG apparently offers no significantly increased benefit (167). The Dutch group (170) reported that recovery of patients with anti-GM$_1$ antibodies and preceding *C. jejuni* infections was not as good after plasma exchange compared with recovery after high-dose IVIG. A trial is ongoing in the Netherlands to verify preliminary data on a synergistic therapeutic action of IVIG and methylprednisolone. A significant proportion of GBS patients, in particular those with major axonal involvement, do not benefit from currently available therapies. Studies in EAN would suggest that immunomodulatory intervention with antibodies to or competitive ligands of adhesion molecules, matrix metalloproteinase inhibitors, TNF-α blockers, or antigen should be explored

(171–173). In addition, administration of neurotrophic factors may be used to enhance regeneration.

Chronic Inflammatory Demyelinating Polyradiculoneuropathy

The clinical features of this chronic relapsing-remitting or progressive neuropathy and currently used diagnostic criteria have been summarized elsewhere (174–177).

Pathology

In this disorder, the peripheral nerve can be affected at any level from within spinal roots to the distal ends of motor nerves. Commonly, one or more of the following changes are found: endoneurial or subperineurial edema; demyelinative nerve fibers; macrophage-mediated phagocytosis of myelin: myelin stripping and vesicular dissolution in the presence of mononuclear cells; thinly myelinated fibers; onion bulb formation following repeated episodes of demyelination and remyelination; and axonal degeneration (2). Immunocytochemically T cells of both CD4 and CD8 phenotypes and macrophages have been identified within the endoneurium. MHC class I and II antigens have been localized to Schwann cells and macrophages (165,178,179). There is also evidence that at least in a proportion of patients T cells actively cross the blood-nerve barrier, as mirrored by increased levels of circulating E-selectin (157,158).

Humoral Immune Responses

Interest in exploring possible aberrant humoral immune responses in CIDP was stimulated by the efficacy of plasmapheresis in many patients with this neuropathy and the possibility to produce demyelination by interneural injection of whole serum or the IgG fraction from CIDP patients, although the latter finding could not be confirmed (reviewed by Pollard (2)). The strongest evidence derives from a model of CIDP inducible in rabbits by prolonged immunization with galactocerebroside. The demyelinating activity of EAN serum was carried by antigalactocerebroside antibodies (180–184).

In CIDP, however, identification of the target antigens for the humoral immune responses has not been achieved. Reports on a high incidence of antibodies to the glycolipid LM$_1$ (>60%) by Freedman et al (69) have not been confirmed. Melendez-Vasquez et al (185) found IgM antibodies to LM$_1$ in only 5% and to GM$_1$ in only 15% of CIDP patients. In 9 of 30 CIDP patients studied, Yuki et al (76) detected IgM antibodies to the sialosyl lactoseaminyl paragloboside (SLPG). With enzyme-linked immunosorbent assay, IgG or IgM isotype antibodies to chondroitin sulfate C and sulfatide were detected in up to 7.5% of patients (185). In view of the associations described in GBS, these authors also sought serologic evidence of infection with *C. jejuni* (10% of all patients were positive) and CMV (none were positive). They concluded that CIDP is not commonly associated with either of these infections or with a significant antibody-mediated response to glycolipids or myelin protein autoantigens.

Antibodies to peripheral nerve proteins P0 and P2 have been detected only in a small proportion of patients (139,185,186). Finally, reports on the presence of high-titer antibodies to the cytoskeletal protein tubulin (187) have been refuted (188).

Elevated serum levels of the soluble membrane attack complex of complement were detected in six of seven CIDP patients (31) and C3d was shown to decorate the outer portion of the myelin sheath in nerve biopsy specimens (34).

Cellular Immune Responses

CIDP patients have increased percentages of activated circulating T lymphocytes and raised serum concentrations of both IL-2 and soluble IL-2 receptors (128–131). In one single study, primary T-cell proliferative responses to P2 and P0 protein or peptides were recorded in almost half of the patients studied (149). Levels of TNF-α, a potentially myelinotoxic Th1 cytokine, were not different from control levels.

Therapy

A series of open randomized, double-blind randomized, placebo-controlled, and cross-over studies provided evidence that a number of immunotherapies are beneficial in CIDP: corticosteroids, plasma exchange, and high-dose IVIG (189–192). Long-term immunosuppression with azathioprine or cyclosporine is also used and pulsed cyclophosphamide therapy has been advocated for rapidly progressive disease (192). Trials of recombinant interferon beta are under way.

References

1. Ropper AH. The Guillain-Barré syndrome. *N Engl J Med* 1992;326:1130–1136.
2. Pollard JD. Chronic inflammatory demyelinating polyradiculoneuropathy. *Baillieres Clin Neurol* 1994;3:107–127.
3. Feasby TE. Axonal Guillain-Barré syndrome. *Muscle Nerve* 1994;17:678–679.
4. Feasby TE, Gilbert JJ, Brown WF, et al. An acute axonal form of Guillain-Barré polyneuropathy. *Brain* 1986;109:1115–1126.
5. van der Meché FGA, Meulstee J, Kleyweg RP. Axonal damage in Guillain-Barré syndrome. *Muscle Nerve* 1991;14:997–1002.
6. Triggs WJ, Cros D, Gominak SC, et al. Motor nerve inexcitability in Guillain-Barré syndrome. *Brain* 1992;115:1291–1302.
7. Kanda T, Hayashi H, Tanabe H, et al. A fulminant case of Guillain-Barré syndrome: topographic and fibre size related analysis of demyelinating changes. *J Neurol Neurosurg Psychiatry* 1989;52:857–864.
8. Berciano J, Coria F, Monton F, et al. Axonal form of Guillain-Barré syndrome: evidence for macrophage-associated demyelination. *Muscle Nerve* 1993;16:744–751.
9. Fuller GN, Jacobs JM, Lewis PD, Lane RJ. Pseudoaxonal Guillain-Barré syndrome: severe demyelination mimicking axonopathy. A case with pupillary involvement. *J Neurol Neurosurg Psychiatry* 1992;55:1079–1083.
10. Honavar M, Tharakan JK, Hughes RAC, et al. A clinicopathological study of the Guillain-Barré syndrome. Nine cases and literature review. *Brain* 1991;114:1245–1269.
11. McKhann GM, Cornblath DR, Ho T, et al. Clinical and electrophysiological aspects of acute paralytic disease of children and young adults in northern China. *Lancet* 1991;338:593–597.
12. McKhann GM, Cornblath DR, Griffin JW, et al. Acute motor axonal neuropathy: a frequent cause of acute flaccid paralysis in China. *Ann Neurol* 1993;33:333–342.
13. Griffin JW, Li CY, Ho TW, et al. Pathology of the motor-sensory axonal Guillain-Barré syndrome [see comments]. *Ann Neurol* 1996;39:17–28.
14. Hughes RAC. The concept and classification of Guillain-Barré syndrome and related disorders. *Rev Neurol (Paris)* 1995;151:291–294.
15. Griffin JW, Li CY, Ho TW, et al. Guillain-Barré syndrome in northern China. The spectrum of neuropathological changes in clinically defined cases. *Brain* 1995;118:577–595.
16. Prineas JW. Pathology of inflammatory demyelinating neuropathies. *Baillieres Clin Neurol* 1994;3:1–24.
17. Asbury AK, Arnason BG, Adams RD. The inflammatory lesion in idiopathic polyneuritis. Its role in pathogenesis. *Medicine (Baltimore)* 1969;48:173–215.
18. Ho TW, Hsieh S, Nachamkin I, et al. Motor nerve terminal degeneration provides a potential mechanism for rapid recovery in acute motor axonal neuropathy after *Campylobacter* infection. *Neurology* 1997;48:717–724.
19. Ho TW, Li CY, Cornblath DR, et al. Patterns of recovery in the Guillain-Barré syndromes. *Neurology* 1997;48:695–700.
20. Hall SM, Hughes RAC, Atkinson PF, et al. Motor nerve biopsy in severe Guillain-Barré syndrome. *Ann Neurol* 1992;31:441–444.
21. Hughes RAC, Atkinson P, Braheny SL, et al. Sural nerve biopsies in Guillain-Barré syndrome: axonal degeneration and macrophage associated demyelination and absence of cytomegalovirus genome. *Muscle Nerve* 1992;15:568–575.
22. Brechenmacher C, Vital C, Deminiere C, et al. Guillain-Barré syndrome: an ultrastructural study of peripheral nerve in 65 patients. *Clin Neuropathol* 1987;6:19–24.
23. Maier H, Schmidbauer M, Pfausler B, et al. Central nervous system pathology in patients with the Guillain-Barré syndrome. *Brain* 1997;120:451–464.
24. Gehrmann J, Gold R, Linington C, et al. Spinal cord microglia in experimental allergic neuritis. Evidence for fast and remote activation. *Lab Invest* 1992;67:100–113.
25. Weilbach FX, Jung S, Hartung H-P, et al. T-cell receptor V β-element expression in peripheral nerves of Lewis rats suffering from experimental autoimmune neuritis. *J Neuroimmunol* (submitted).
26. Abromson-Leeman S, Bronson R, Dorf ME. Experimental autoimmune peripheral neuritis induced in BALB/c mice by myelin basic protein-specific T cell clones. *J Exp Med* 1995;182:587–592.
27. Hafer-Macko CE, Sheikh KA, Li CY, et al. Immune attack on the Schwann cell surface in acute inflammatory demyelinating polyneuropathy. *Ann Neurol* 1996;39:625–635.
28. Koguchi Y, Yamachi T, Kuwabara, S, et al. Increased CSF C4d in demyelinating neuropathy indicates radicular involvement. *Acta Neurol Scand* 1995;91:58–61.

29. Hartung HP, Jung S, Stoll G, et al. Inflammatory mediators in demyelinating disorders of the CNS and PNS. *J Neuroimmunol* 1992;40:197–210.

30. Hartung HP, Schwenke C, Bitter-Suermann D, Toyka KV. Guillain-Barré syndrome: activated complement components C3a and C5a in CSF. *Neurology* 1987;37: 1006–1009.

31. Koski CL, Sanders ME, Swoveland PT, et al. Activation of terminal components of complement in patients with Guillain-Barré syndrome and other demyelinating neuropathies. *J Clin Invest* 1987;80:1492–1497.

32. Sanders ME, Koski CL, Robbins D, et al. Activated terminal complement in cerebrospinal fluid in Guillain-Barré syndrome and multiple sclerosis. *J Immunol* 1986;136:4456–4459.

33. Koski CL. Characterization of complement-fixing antibodies to peripheral nerve myelin in Guillain-Barré syndrome. *Ann Neurol* 1990;27(suppl):S44–S47.

34. Hays AP, Lee SS, Latov N. Immune reactive C3d on the surface of myelin sheaths in neuropathy. *J Neuroimmunol* 1988;18:21–44.

35. Roberts M, Willison H, Vincent A, Newsom-Davis J. Serum factor in Miller-Fisher variant of Guillain-Barré syndrome and neurotransmitter release [see comments]. *Lancet* 1994;343:454–455.

36. Buchwald B, Weishaupt A, Toyka KV, Dudel J. Pre- and postsynaptic blockade of synaptic transmission by Miller-Fisher syndrome IgG a mouse motor nerve terminals. *Eur J Neurosci* 1997 (in press).

37. Buchwald BM, Weishaupt A, Toyka KV, Dudel J. Immunoglobulin G from a patient with Miller-Fisher syndrome rapidly and reversibly depresses evoked quantal release at the neuromuscular junction of mice. *Neurosci Lett* 1995;201:163–166.

38. Roberts M, Willison H, Vincent A, Newsom-Davis J. Multifocal motor neuropathy human sera block distal motor nerve conduction in mice. *Ann Neurol* 1995;38:111–118.

39. Hartung HP, Stoll G, Toyka KV. Immune reactions in the peripheral nervous system. In: Dyck PJ, Thomas PK, Griffin JW, et al, eds. *Peripheral neuropathy*. 3rd ed. Philadelphia: WB Saunders, 1993:418–444.

40. Feasby TE, Hahn AF, Brown WF, et al. Severe axonal degeneration in acute Guillain-Barré syndrome: evidence of two different mechanisms? *J Neurol Sci* 1993;116: 185–192.

41. Powell HC, Myers RR. The axon in Guillain-Barré syndrome: immune target or innocent bystander? *Ann Neurol* 1996;39:4–5. Editorial.

42. Latov N, Gross BB, Kastelman J, et al. Complement fixing antiperipheral nerve myelin antibodies in patients with inflammatory polyneuritis and with polyneuropathy and paraproteinemia. *Neurology* 1981;31:1530–1534.

43. Koski CL, Humphrey R, Shin ML. Anti-peripheral myelin antibody in patients with demyelinating neuropathy: quantitative and kinetic determination of serum antibody by complement component 1 fixation. *Proc Natl Acad Sci USA* 1985;82:905–909.

44. Koski CL, Gratz E, Sutherland J, Mayer RF. Clinical correlation with anti-peripheral-nerve myelin antibodies in Guillain-Barré syndrome. *Ann Neurol* 1986;19:573–577.

45. Koski CL, Chou DK, Jungalwala FB. Anti-peripheral nerve myelin antibodies in Guillain-Barré syndrome bind a neutral glycolipid of peripheral myelin and cross-react with Forssman antigen. *J Clin Invest* 1989;84: 280–287.

46. Ilyas AA, Mithen FA, Chen ZW, Cook SD. Search for antibodies to neutral glycolipids in sera of patients with Guillain-Barré syndrome. *J Neurol Sci* 1991;102:67–75.

47. Svennerholm L, Fredman P. Antibody detection in Guillain-Barré syndrome. *Ann Neurol* 1990;27(suppl): S36–S40.

48. Zielasek J, Ritter G, Magi S, et al. A comparative trial of anti-glycoconjugate antibody assays: IgM antibodies to GM1. *J Neurol* 1994;241:475–480.

49. Hartung H-P, Pollard JD, Harvey GK, Toyka KV. Immunopathogenesis and treatment of the Guillain-Barré syndrome. Part I. *Muscle Nerve* 1995;18:137–153.

50. Kornberg AJ, Pestronk A, Bieser K, et al. The clinical correlates of high-titer IgG anti-GM$_1$ antibodies [see comments]. *Ann Neurol* 1994;35:234–237.

51. Visser LH, van der Meche FGA, van Doorn PA, et al. Guillain-Barré syndrome without sensory loss (acute motor neuropathy). A subgroup with specific clinical, electrodiagnostic and laboratory features. *Brain* 1995;118: 841–848.

52. Yuki N, Yoshino H, Sato S, Miyatake T. Acute axonal polyneuropathy associated with anti-GM1 antibodies following *Campylobacter* enteritis. *Neurology* 1990;40: 1900–1902.

53. Walsh FS, Cronin M, Koblar S, et al. Association between glycoconjugate antibodies and *Campylobacter* infection in patients with Guillain-Barré syndrome. *J Neuroimmunol* 1991;34:43–51.

54. van der Meché FGA, Schmitz PIM, Dutch Guillain-Barré Syndrome Study Group. High-dose intravenous immunoglobulin versus plasma exchange in Guillain-Barré syndrome. *N Engl J Med* 1992;326:1123–1129.

55. van den Berg LH, Marrink J, De Jager AE, et al. Anti-GM1 antibodies in patients with Guillain-Barré syndrome. *J Neurol Neurosurg Psychiatry* 1992;55:8–11.

56. Rees JH, Vaughan RW, Kondeatis E, Hughes RAC. HLA-class II alleles in Guillain-Barré syndrome and Miller Fisher syndrome and their association with preceding *Campylobacter jejuni* infection. *J Neuroimmunol* 1995;62:53–57.

57. Nobile-Orazio E, Carpo M, Meucci N, et al. Guillain-Barré syndrome associated with high titers of anti-GM1 antibodies. *J Neurol Sci* 1992;109:200–206.

58. Gregson NA, Koblar S, Hughes RAC. Antibodies to gangliosides in Guillain-Barré syndrome: specificity and relationship to clinical features. *QJM* 1993;86:111–117.

59. Vriesendorp FJ, Mishu B, Blaser MJ, Koski CL. Serum antibodies to GM$_1$, GD$_{1b}$, peripheral nerve myelin, and *Campylobacter jejuni* in patients with Guillain-Barré syndrome and controls: correlation and prognosis [see comments]. *Ann Neurol* 1993;34:130–135.

60. Enders U, Karch H, Toyka KV, et al. The spectrum of immune responses to *Campylobacter jejuni* and glycoconjugates in Guillain-Barré syndrome and in other neuro-immunological disorders. *Ann Neurol* 1993;34: 136–144.

61. Simone IL, Annunziata P, Maimone D, et al. Serum and CSF anti-GM1 antibodies in patients with Guillain-Barré syndrome and chronic inflammatory demyelinating polyneuropathy. *J Neurol Sci* 1993;114:49–55.

62. Rees JH, Gregson NA, Hughes RAC. Anti-ganglioside GM$_1$ antibodies in Guillain-Barré syndrome and their relationship to *Campylobacter jejuni* infection. *Ann Neurol* 1995;38:809–816.

63. Yuki N, Yoshino H, Sato S, et al. Severe acute axonal form of Guillain-Barré syndrome associated with IgG anti-GD1a antibodies. *Muscle Nerve* 1992;15:899–903.

64. Yuki N, Taki T, Handa S. Antibody to GalNAc-GD1a and GalNAc-GMlb in Guillain-Barré syndrome subsequent

to *Campylobacter jejuni* enteritis. *J Neuroimmunol* 1996;71:155–161.

65. Kusunoki S, Chiba A, Kon K, et al. *N*-Acetylgalactosaminyl CD1a is a target molecule for serum antibody in Guillain-Barré syndrome. *Ann Neurol* 1994;35:570–576.

66. Yuki N, Sato S, Fujimoto S, et al. Serotype of *Campylobacter jejuni*, HLA, and the Guillain-Barré syndrome. *Muscle Nerve* 1992;15:968–969. Letter.

67. Yuki N, Sato S, Itoh T, Miyatake T. HLA-B35 and acute axonal polyneuropathy following *Campylobacter* infection. *Neurology* 1991;41:1561–1563.

68. Kuroki S, Saida T, Nukina M, et al. *Campylobacter jejuni* strains from patients with Guillain-Barré syndrome belong mostly to Penner serogroup 19 and contain beta-N-acetylglucosamine residues. *Ann Neurol* 1993;33:243–247.

69. Freedman MS, Ruijs TC, Selin LK, Antel JP. Peripheral blood gamma-delta T cells lyse fresh human brain-derived oligodendrocytes [see comments]. *Ann Neurol* 1991;30:794–800.

70. Ilyas AA, Mithen FA, Chen ZW, Cook SD. Anti-GM1 IgA antibodies in Guillain-Barré syndrome. *J Neuroimmunol* 1992;36:69–76.

71. Ilyas AA, Mithen FA, Dalakas MC, et al. Antibodies to acidic glycolipids in Guillain-Barré syndrome and chronic inflammatory demyelinating polyneuropathy. *J Neurol Sci* 1992;107:111–121.

72. Ilyas AA, Mithen FA, Dalakas MC, et al. Antibodies to sulfated glycolipids in Guillain-Barré syndrome. *J Neurol Sci* 1991;105:108–117.

73. Ilyas AA, Willison HJ, Quarles RH, et al. Serum antibodies to gangliosides in Guillain-Barré syndrome. *Ann Neurol* 1988;23:440–447.

74. Fredman P, Vedeler CA, Nyland H, et al. Antibodies in sera from patients with inflammatory demyelinating polyradiculoneuropathy react with ganglioside LM1 and sulphatide of peripheral nerve myelin. *J Neurol* 1991;238:75–79.

75. van den Berg LH, Lankamp CLAM, DeJager AEJ, et al. Anti-sulphatide antibodies in peripheral neuropathy. *J Neurol Neurosurg Psychiatry* 1993;56:1164–1168.

76. Yuki N, Tagawa Y, Handa S. Autoantibodies to peripheral nerve glycosphingolipids SPG, SLPG, and SGPG in Guillain-Barré syndrome and chronic inflammatory demyelinating polyneuropathy. *J Neuroimmunol* 1996;70:1–6.

77. Rostami A, Burns JB, Eccleston PA, et al. Search for antibodies to galactocerebroside in the serum and cerebrospinal fluid in human demyelinating disorders. *Ann Neurol* 1987;22:381–383.

78. Kusunoki S, Chiba A, Hitoshi S, et al. Anti-Gal-C antibody in autoimmune neuropathies subsequent to mycoplasma infection. *Muscle Nerve* 1995;18:409–413.

79. Ho TW, Mishu B, Li CY, et al. Guillain-Barré syndrome in northern China. Relationship to *Campylobacter jejuni* infection and anti-glycolipid antibodies. *Brain* 1995;118:597–605.

80. Yuki N, Sato S, Tsuji S, et al. Frequent presence of anti-GQ1b antibody in Fisher's syndrome. *Neurology* 1993;43:414–417.

81. Willison HJ, Veitch J, Paterson G, Kennedy PG. Miller Fisher syndrome is associated with serum antibodies to GQ1b ganglioside. *J Neurol Neurosurg Psychiatry* 1993;56:204–206.

82. Chiba A, Kusunoki S, Shimizu T, Kanazawa I. Serum IgG antibody to ganglioside GQ_{1b} is a possible marker of Miller Fisher syndrome. *Ann Neurol* 1992;31:677–679.

83. Chiba A, Kusunoki S, Obata H, et al. Serum anti-GQ-1b IgG antibody is associated with ophthalmoplegia in Miller-Fisher syndrome and Guillain-Barré syndrome: clinical and immunohistochemical studies. *Neurology* 1993;43:1911–1918.

84. Salloway S, Mermel LA, Seamans M, et al. Miller-Fisher syndrome associated with *Campylobacter jejuni* bearing lipopolysaccharide molecules that mimic human ganglioside GD3. *Infect Immun* 1996;64:2945–2949.

85. Willison HJ, Almemar A, Veitch J, Thrush D. Acute ataxic neuropathy with cross-reactive antibodies to GD1b and GD3 gangliosides. *Neurology* 1994;44:2395–2397.

86. Yuki N, Ichihashi Y, Taki T. Subclass of IgG antibody to GM1 epitope-bearing lipopolysaccharide of *Campylobacter jejuni* in patients with Guillain-Barré syndrome. *J Neuroimmunol* 1995;60:161–164.

87. Willison HJ, Veitch J. Immunoglobulin subclass distribution and binding characteristics of anti-GQ1b antibodies in Miller Fisher syndrome. *J Neuroimmunol* 1994;50:159–165.

88. Svennerholm L, Boström K, Fredman P, et al. Gangliosides and allied glycosphingolipids in human peripheral nerve and spinal cord. *Biochim Biophys Acta* 1994;1214:115–123.

89. Thomas PK, Claus D, Jaspert A, et al. Focal upper limb demyelinating neuropathy. *Brain* 1996;119:765–774.

90. Ogawa-Goto K, Funamoto N, Ohta Y, et al. Myelin gangliosides of human peripheral nervous system: an enrichment of GM1 in the motor nerve myelin isolated from cauda equina. *J Neurochem* 1992;59:1844–1849.

91. Ogawa-Goto K, Funamoto N, Abe T, Nagashima K. Different ceramide compositions of gangliosides between human motor and sensory nerves. *J Neurochem* 1990;55:1486–1493.

92. Mizutamari RK, Wiegandt H, Nores GA. Characterization of anti-ganglioside antibodies present in normal human plasma. *J Neuroimmunol* 1994;50:215–220.

93. Heidenreich F, Leifeld L, Jovin T. T cell-dependent activity of ganglioside GM1-specific B cells in Guillain-Barré syndrome and multifocal motor neuropathy in vitro. *J Neuroimmunol* 1994;49:97–108.

94. Willison HJ, Kennedy PGE. Gangliosides and bacterial toxin in Guillain-Barré syndrome. *J Neuroimmunol* 1993;46:105–112.

95. Ishioka GY, Lamont AG, Thomson D, et al. MHC interaction and T cell recognition of carbohydrates and glycopeptides. *J Immunol* 1992;148:2446–2451.

96. Jullien D, Stenger S, Ernst WA, Modin RL. CD1 presentation of microbial nonpeptide antigens to T cells. *J Clin Invest* 1997;99:2071–2074.

97. Yuki N, Ichihashi Y, Taki T. Subclass of IgG antibody to GM1 epitope-bearing lipopolysaccharide of *Campylobacter jejuni* in patients with Guillain-Barré syndrome. *J Neuroimmunol* 1995;60:161–164.

98. Ogino M, Orazio N, Latov N. IgG anti-GM1 antibodies from patients with acute motor neuropathy are predominantly of the IgG1 and IgG3 subclasses. *J Neuroimmunol* 1995;58:77–80.

99. Graves MC, Ravindranath RM. Do CD5+ B cells secrete antiasialoGM1 antibodies in motor neuron disease? *Ann NY Acad Sci* 1992;651:570–571.

100. Yuki N, Handa S, Tai T, et al. Ganglioside-like epitopes of lipopolysaccharides from *Campylobacter jejuni* (PEN 19) in three isolates from patients with Guillain-Barré syndrome. *J Neurol Sci* 1995;130:112–116.

101. Yuki N, Taki T, Takahashi M, et al. Penner's serotype 4 of *Campylobacter jejuni* has a lipopolysaccharide that

bears a GM1 ganglioside epitope as well as one that bears a GD1a epitope. *Infect Immun* 1994;62:2101–2103.

102. Jacobs BC, Endtz H, van der Meché FGA, et al. Serum anti-GQ$_{1b}$ IgG antibodies recognize surface epitopes on *Campylobacter jejuni* from patients with Miller Fisher syndrome. *Ann Neurol* 1995;37:260–264.

103. Yuki N, Taki T, Takahashi M, et al. Molecular mimicry between GQ$_{1b}$ ganglioside and lipopolysaccharides of *Campylobacter jejuni* isolated from patients with Fisher's syndrome. *Ann Neurol* 1994;36:791–793.

104. Yuki N, Taki T, Inagaki F, et al. A bacterium lipopolysaccharide that elicits Guillain-Barré syndrome has a GM1 ganglioside-like structure. *J Exp Med* 1993;178:1771–1775.

105. Aspinall GO, McDonald AG, Pang H. Lipopolysaccharides of *Campylobacter jejuni* serotype O:19: structures of O antigen chains from the serostrain and two bacterial isolates from patients with the Guillain-Barré syndrome. *Biochemistry* 1994;33:250–255.

106. Oomes PG, Jacobs BC, Hazenberg MPH, et al. Anti-GM$_1$ IgG antibodies and *Campylobacter* bacteria in Guillain-Barré syndrome: evidence of molecular mimicry. *Ann Neurol* 1995;38:170–175.

107. Griffin JW. Antiglycolipid antibodies and peripheral neuropathies: links to pathogenesis. *Prog Brain Res* 1994;101:313–326.

108. Hartung HP, Pollard TD, Harvey GK, Toyka KV. Immunopathogenesis and treatment of the Guillain-Barré syndrome. Part II. *Muscle Nerve* 1995;18:154–164.

109. O'Leary CO, Willison HJ. Immunological investigation. *Curr Opin Neurol* 1995;8:349–353.

110. Mariette X, Tsapis A, Brouet JC. Nucleotidic sequence analysis of the variable domains of four human monoclonal IgM with an antibody activity to myelin-associated glycoprotein. *Eur J Immunol* 1993;23:846–851.

111. Weng NP, Yu Lee LY, Sanz I, et al. Structure and specificities of anti-ganglioside autoantibodies associated with motor neuropathies. *J Immunol* 1992;149:2518–2529.

112. Paterson G, Wilson G, Kennedy PGE, Willison HJ. Analysis of anti-GM1 ganglioside antibodies cloned from motor neuropathy patients demonstrates diverse V region gene usage with extensive somatic mutation. *J Immunol* 1995;155:3049–3059.

113. Visser LH, van der Meché FGA, Meulstee J, et al. Cytomegalovirus infection and Guillain-Barré syndrome: the clinical, electrophysiologic, and prognostic features. *Neurology* 1996;47:668–673.

114. Irie S, Saito T, Nakamura K, et al. Association of anti-GM2 antibodies in Guillain-Barré syndrome with acute cytomegalovirus infection. *J Neuroimmunol* 1996;68:19–26.

115. Boucquey D, Sindic CJ, Lamy M, et al. Clinical and serological studies in a series of 45 patients with Guillain-Barré syndrome. *J Neurol Sci* 1991;104:56–63.

116. Winer JB, Hughes RAC, Anderson MJ, et al. A prospective study of acute idiopathic neuropathy. II. Antecedent events. *J Neurol Neurosurg Psychiatry* 1988;51:613–618.

117. Adelmann M, Linington C. Molecular mimicry and the autoimmune response to the peripheral nerve myelin PO glycoprotein. *Neurochem Res* 1992;17:887–891.

118. Thomas FP. Antibodies to GM1 and Gal(β1-3)GalNAc at the nodes of Ranvier in human and experimental autoimmune neuropathy. *Microsc Res Tech* 1996;34:536–543.

119. Corbo M, Quattrini A, Latov N, Hays AP. Localization of GM1 and Gal(β1-3)GalNAc antigenic determinants in peripheral nerve. *Neurology* 1993;43:809–814.

120. Santoro M, Uncini A, Corbo M, et al. Experimental conduction block induced by serum from a patient with anti-GM$_1$ antibodies. *Ann Neurol* 1992;31:385–390.

121. Uncini A, Santoro M, Corbo M, et al. Conduction abnormalities induced by sera of patients with multifocal motor neuropathy and anti-GM1 antibodies. *Muscle Nerve* 1993;16:610–615.

122. Arasaki K, Kusunoki S, Kudo N, Kanazawa I. Acute conduction block in vitro following exposure to antiganglioside sera. *Muscle Nerve* 1993;16:587–593.

123. Thomas FP, Trojaborg W, Nagy C, et al. Experimental autoimmune neuropathy with anti-GM1 antibodies and immunoglobulin deposits at the nodes of Ranvier. *Acta Neuropathol (Berl)* 1991;82:378–383.

124. Illa I, Ortiz N, Gallard E, et al. Acute axonal Guillain-Barré syndrome with IgG antibodies against motor axons following parenteral gangliosides. *Ann Neurol* 1995;38:218–224.

125. Takigawa T, Yasuda H, Kikkawa R, et al. Antibodies against GM$_1$ ganglioside affect K+ and Na+ currents in isolated rat myelinated nerve fibers. *Ann Neurol* 1995;37:436–442.

126. Harvey GK, Toyka KV, Zielasek J, et al. Failure of anti-GM1 IgG or IgM to induce conduction block following intraneural transfer. *Muscle Nerve* 1995;18:388–394.

127. Li CY, Xue P, Tian WQ, et al. Experimental *Campylobacter jejuni* infection in the chicken: an animal model of axonal Guillain-Barré syndrome. *J Neurol Neurosurg Psychiatry* 1996;61:279–284.

128. Taylor WA, Hughes RAC. T lymphocyte activation antigens in Guillain-Barré syndrome and chronic idiopathic demyelinating polyradiculoneuropathy. *J Neuroimmunol* 1989;24:33–39.

129. van den Berg LH, Mollee I, Wokke JH, Logtenberg T. Increased frequencies of HPRT mutant T lymphocytes in patients with Guillain-Barré syndrome and chronic inflammatory demyelinating polyneuropathy: further evidence for a role of T cells in the etiopathogenesis of peripheral demyelinating diseases. *J Neuroimmunol* 1994;58:37–42.

130. Hartung HP, Reiners K, Schmidt B, et al. Serum interleukin-2 concentrations in Guillain-Barré syndrome and chronic idiopathic demyelinating polyradiculoneuropathy: comparison with other neurological diseases of presumed immunopathogenesis. *Ann Neurol* 1991;30:48–53.

131. Hartung HP, Hughes RAC, Taylor WA, et al. T cell activation in Guillain-Barré syndrome and in MS: elevated serum levels of soluble IL-2 receptors. *Neurology* 1990;40:215–218.

132. Bansil S, Mithen FA, Cook SD, et al. Clinical correlation with serum-soluble interleukin-2 receptor levels in Guillain-Barré syndrome. *Neurology* 1991;41:1302–1305.

133. Bansil S, Mithen FA, Singhal BS, et al. Elevated neopterin levels in Guillain-Barré syndrome. Further evidence of immune activation. *Arch Neurol* 1992;49:1277–1280.

134. Exley AR, Smith N, Winer JB. Tumour necrosis factor-alpha and other cytokines in Guillain-Barré syndrome. *J Neurol Neurosurg Psychiatry* 1994;57:1118–1120.

135. Sharief MK, McLean B, Thompson EJ. Elevated serum levels of tumor necrosis factor-alpha in Guillain-Barré syndrome. *Ann Neurol* 1993;33:591–596.

136. Hartung HP, Toyka KV. T-cell and macrophage activation in experimental autoimmune neuritis and Guillain-Barré syndrome. *Ann Neurol* 1990;27(suppl):S57–S63.

137. Créange A, Bélec L, Clair B, et al. Circulating tumor necrosis factor (TNF)-α and soluble TNF-α receptors in patients with Guillain-Barré syndrome. *J Neuroimmunol* 1996;68:95–99.

138. Dahle C, Vrethem M, Ernerudh J. T lymphocyte subset abnormalities in peripheral blood from patients with the Guillain-Barré syndrome. *J Neuroimmunol* 1994;53: 219–225.

139. Zweiman B, Rostami A, Lisak RP, et al. Immune reactions to P2 protein in human inflammatory demyelinative neuropathies. *Neurology* 1983;33:234–237.

140. Ohno R, Hamaguchi K, Nomura K, et al. Cellular hypersensitivity to nervous antigens in Guillain-Barré syndrome. *Neurochem Pathol* 1986;4:119–126.

141. Linington C, Brostoff SW. Peripheral nerve antigens. In: Dyck PJ, Thomas PK, Griffin JW, et al, eds. *Peripheral neuropathy*. 3rd ed. Philadelphia: WB Saunders, 1993: 404–417.

142. Korn-Lubetzkii I, Abramsky O. Acute and chronic demyelinating inflammatory polyradiculoneuropathy. Association with autoimmune diseases and lymphocyte response to human neuritogenic protein. *Arch Neurol* 1986;43:604–608.

143. Iqbal A, Oger JJF, Arnason BW. Cell-mediated immunity in idiopathic polyneuritis. *Ann Neurol* 1981;9(suppl):65–69.

144. Hughes RAC, Gray IA, Gregson NA, et al. Immune responses to myelin antigens in Guillain-Barré syndrome. *J Neuroimmunol* 1984;6:303–312.

145. Geczy C, Raper R, Roberts IM, et al. Macrophage procoagulant activity as a measure of cell-mediated immunity to P2 protein of peripheral nerves in the Guillain-Barré syndrome. *J Neuroimmunol* 1985;9:179–191.

146. Arnason BGW, Soliven B. Acute inflammatory demyelinating polyradiculoneuropathy. In Dyck PJ, Thomas PK, Griffin JW, et al, eds. *Peripheral neuropathy*. 3rd ed. Philadelphia: WB Saunders, 1993:1437–1497.

147. Burns J, Krasner LJ, Rostami A, Pleasure D. Isolation of P2 protein-reactive T-cell lines from human blood. *Ann Neurol* 1986;19:391–393.

148. Taylor WA, Brostoff SW, Hughes RAC. P2 specific lymphocyte transformation in Guillain-Barré syndrome and chronic idiopathic demyelinating polyradiculoneuropathy. *J Neurol Sci* 1991;104:52–55.

149. Khalili-Shirazi A, Hughes RAC, Brostoff SW, et al. T cell responses to myelin proteins in Guillain-Barré syndrome. *J Neurol Sci* 1992;111:200–203.

150. Pette M, Linington C, Gengaroli C, et al. T lymphocyte recognition sites on peripheral nerve myelin P0 protein. *J Neuroimmunol* 1994;54:29–34.

151. Weishaupt A, Giegerich G, Jung S, et al. T cell antigenic and neuritogenic activity of recombinant human peripheral myelin P2 protein. *J Neuroimmunol* 1995;63: 149–156.

152. Pette M, Gengaroli C, Hartung HP, et al. Human T lymphocytes distinguish bovine from human P2 peripheral myelin protein: implications for immunological studies on inflammatory demyelinating neuropathies. *J Neuroimmunol* 1994;52:47–52.

153. Milner P, Lovelidge CA, Taylor WA, Hughes RAC. P0 myelin protein produces experimental allergic neuritis in Lewis rats. *J Neurol Sci* 1987;79:275–285.

154. Linington C, Lassmann H, Ozawa K, et al. Cell adhesion molecules of the immunoglobulin supergene family as tissue-specific autoantigens: induction of experimental allergic neuritis (EAN) by P0 protein-specific T cell lines. *Eur J Immunol* 1982;22:1813–1817.

155. Khalili-Shirazi A, Gregson NA, Hall MA, et al. T cell receptor Vβ gene usage in Guillain-Barré syndrome. *J Neurol Sci* 1997;145:169–176.

156. Ben-Smith A, Gatson JSH, Barber PC, Winer JB. Isolation and characterization of T lymphocytes from sural nerve biopsies in patients with Guillain-Barré syndrome and chronic inflammatory demyelinating polyneuropathy. *J Neurol Neurosurg Psychiatry* 1996;61:362–368.

157. Oka N, Akiguchi I, Kawasaki T, et al. Elevated serum levels of endothelial leukocyte adhesion molecules in Guillain-Barré syndrome and chronic inflammatory demyelinating polyneuropathy. *Ann Neurol* 1994;35: 621–624.

158. Hartung HP, Reiners K, Michels M, et al. Serum levels of soluble E-selectin (ELAM-1) in immune-mediated neuropathies. *Neurology* 1994;44:1153–1158.

159. Hahn AF, Feasby TE, Wilkie L, Lovegren D. Antigalactocerebroside antibody increases demyelination in adoptive transfer experimental allergic neuritis. *Muscle Nerve* 1993;16:1174–1180.

160. Spies JM, Westland KW, Bonner JG, Pollard JD. Intraneural activated T cells cause focal breakdown of the blood-nerve barrier. *Brain* 1995;118:857–868.

161. Pollard JD, Westland KW, Harvey GK, et al. Activated T cells of nonneural specificity open the blood-nerve barrier to circulating antibody. *Ann Neurol* 1995;37:467–475.

162. Harvey GK, Gold R, Hartung H-P, Toyka KV. Nonneural-specific T lymphocytes can orchestrate inflammatory peripheral neuropathy. *Brain* 1995;118:1263–1272.

163. Argall KG, Armati PJ, Pollard JD, Bonner J. Interactions between CD4+ T-cells and rat Schwann cells in vitro. 2. Cytotoxic effects of P2-specific CD4+ T-cell lines on Lewis rat Schwann cells. *J Neuroimmunol* 1992;40: 19–29.

164. Gold R, Hartung H-P, Lassmann H. T cell apoptosis in autoimmune diseases: termination of inflammation in the nervous system and other sites with specialized immune-defense mechanisms. Trends Neurosci 1997 (in press).

165. Schmidt B, Toyka KV, Kiefer R, et al. Inflammatory infiltrates in sural nerve biopsies in Guillain-Barré syndrome and chronic inflammatory demyelinating neuropathy. *Muscle Nerve* 1996;19:474–487.

166. Griffin JW, George R, Ho T. Macrophage systems in peripheral nerves. A review. *J Neuropathol Exp Neurol* 1993;52:553–560.

167. Plasma Exchange/Sandoglobulin Guillain-Barré Syndrome Trial Group. Randomised trial of plasma exchange, intravenous immunoglobulin, and combined treatments in Guillain-Barré syndrome. *Lancet* 1997; 349:225–230.

168. French Cooperative Group of Plasma Exchange in Guillain-Barré Syndrome. Efficiency of plasma exchange in Guillain-Barré syndrome: role of replacement fluids. *Ann Neurol* 1987;22:753–761.

169. Guillain-Barré Syndrome Study Group. Plasmapheresis and acute Guillain-Barré syndrome. *Neurology* 1985;35: 1096–1104.

170. Jacobs BC, van Doorn PA, Schmitz PI, et al. *Campylobacter jejuni* infections and anti-GM$_1$ antibodies in Guillain-Barré syndrome. *Ann Neurol* 1996;40:181–187.

171. Stoll G, Jung S, Jander S, et al. Tumor necrosis factor-alpha in immune-mediated demyelination and wallerian degeneration of the rat peripheral nervous system. *J Neuroimmunol* 1993;45:175–182.

172. Archelos JJ, Maurer M, Jung S, et al. Suppression of experimental allergic neuritis by an antibody to the intracellular adhesion molecule ICAM-1. *Brain* 1993; 116:1043–1058.

173. Redford EJ, Smith KJ, Gregson NA, et al. A combined inhibitor of matrix metalloproteinase activity and tumour necrosis factor alpha processing attenuates experimental autoimmune neuritis. *Brain* 1997 (in press).

174. Cornblath DR, Asbury AK, Albers JW. Research criteria for diagnosis of chronic inflammatory demyelinating polyneuropathy (CIDP). *Neurology* 1991;41:617–618.

175. Gorson K, Allam G, Ropper AH. Chronic inflammatory demyelinating polyneuropathy: clinical features and response to treatment in 67 consecutive patients with and without a monoclonal gammopathy. *Neurology* 1997;48:321–328.

176. McCombe PA, Pollard JD, McLeod JG. Chronic inflammatory demyelinating polyradiculoneuropathy. A clinical and electrophysiological study of 92 cases. *Brain* 1987;110:1617–1630.

177. Barohn RJ, Kissel JT, Warmolts JR, Mendell JR. Chronic inflammatory demyelinating polyradiculoneuropathy. Clinical characteristics, course, and recommendations for diagnostic criteria. *Arch Neurol* 1989;46: 878–884.

178. Mancardi GL, Cadoni A, Zicca A, et al. HLA-DR Schwann cell reactivity in peripheral neuropathies of different origins. *Neurology* 1988;38:848–851.

179. Pollard JD, McCombe PA, Baverstock J, et al. Class II antigen expression and T lymphocyte subsets in chronic inflammatory demyelinating polyneuropathy. *J Neuroimmunol* 1986;13:123–134.

180. Stoll G, Schwendemann G, Heininger K, et al. Relation of clinical, serological, morphological, and electrophysiological findings in galactocerebroside-induced experimental allergic neuritis. *J Neurol Neurosurg Psychiatry* 1986;49:258–264.

181. Harvey GK, Pollard JD, Schindhelm K, Antony J. Chronic experimental allergic neuritis. An electrophysiological and histological study in the rabbit. *J Neurol Sci* 1987;81:215–225.

182. Saida K, Saida T, Kayama H, Nishitani H. Rapid alterations of the axon membrane in antibody-mediated demyelination. *Ann Neurol* 1984;15:581–589.

183. Saida T, Saida K, Dorfman SH, et al. Experimental allergic neuritis induced by sensitization with galactocerebroside. *Science* 1994;204:1103–1106.

184. Saida T, Saida K, Silberberg DH, Brown MJ. Transfer of demyelination with experimental allergic neuritis serum by intraneural injection. *Nature* 1978;272:629–641.

185. Meléndez-Vasquez C, Redford J, Choudhary PP, et al. Immunological investigation of chronic inflammatory demyelinating polyradiculoneuropathy. *J Neuroimmunol* 1997;73:124–134.

186. Khalili-Shirazi A, Atkinson P, Gregson N, Hughes RA. Antibody responses to P0 and P2 myelin proteins in Guillain-Barré syndrome and chronic idiopathic demyelinating polyradiculoneuropathy. *J Neuroimmunol* 1993;46:245–251.

187. Connolly AM, Pestronk A, Trotter JL, et al. High titer selective serum anti-β-tubulin antibodies in chronic inflammatory demyelinating polyneuropathy. *Neurology* 1993;43:557–562.

188. Manfredini E, Nobile-Orazio E, Allaria S, Scarlato G. Anti-alpha- and beta-tubulin IgM antibodies in dysimmune neuropathies. *J Neurol Sci* 1995;133:79–84.

189. Dyck PJ, Litchy WJ, Kratz KM, et al. A plasma exchange versus immune globulin infusion trial in chronic inflammatory demyelinating polyradiculoneuropathy. *Ann Neurol* 1994;36:838–845.

190. Hahn AF, Bolton CF, Pillay N, et al. Plasma-exchange therapy in chronic inflammatory demyelinating polyneuropathy (CIDP): a double-blind, sham-controlled, cross-over study. *Brain* 1996;119:1055–1066.

191. Hahn AF, Bolton CF, Zochodne D, Feasby TE. Intravenous immunoglobulin treatment (IVIG) in chronic inflammatory demyelinating polyneuropathy (CIDP): a double-blind placebo-controlled cross-over study. *Brain* 1996;119:1067–1077.

192. Toyka KV, Hartung H-P. Chronic inflammatory polyneuritis and related neuropathies. *Curr Opin Neurol* 1996;9:240–250.

Chapter 20
Dysglobulinemic Neuropathies

G. C. Miescher, N. Latov, and A. J. Steck

A circulating monoclonal immunoglobulin is found in about 10% of patients with peripheral neuropathies of unknown etiology (1), whereas it is found in about 1% of the general population. However, this prevalence increases with age. In subjects older than 70 years it is between 3% and 6% as measured by cellulose acetate electrophoresis (2,3) and around 10% as determined by a more sensitive high-resolution agarose gel electrophoresis and immunofixation technique (2).

Dysglobulinemia is a general term that covers the existence of biclonal or oligoclonal gammopathies and also takes into account the observation that clonally restricted autoantibodies directed against peripheral nerve components such as myelin-associated glycoprotein (MAG) may be detected some years before a paraprotein is found by serum electrophoresis. As dysglobulinemia, by itself, is fairly common, it is clearly important to exclude independently occurring neuropathies. A vasculitic autoimmune disease or systemic disease such as diabetes should be excluded.

Theoretically, a chronic neuropathic process could provide continuing antigenic stimulation and favor the emergence of a gammopathy. Such a scenario where the autoantibodies' specificity might or might not have a pathogenic role for the neuropathy has been discussed (4). In particular, IgG and IgA dysglobulinemic neuropathies show considerable similarities to chronic inflammatory demyelinating polyneuropathy (CIDP). However, in many patients the gammopathy may have developed prior to any neuropathy. Autoantibodies are often directed against bacterial lipopolysaccharide antigens that mimic carbohydrate determinants present on myelin and axons (5). Thus, the self-reactive B-cell clone may have originated during an antibacterial immune response. Present evidence suggests that an age-related dysregulation of B-cell clones leads to an accumulation of antibody-producing plasma cells (6).

The potential for malignant progression of these gammopathies has been appreciated variously, and in 1978 Kyle (7) introduced the designation *monoclonal gammopathy of unknown significance*, or MGUS, to allow for variable outcomes of this condition. Hospital-based studies report an actuarial probability of malignant transformation of close to 20% at 10 years (8) and 33% at 20 years (9). An outpatient study conducted over a 14-year period documented a cumulative incidence of

malignant transformation of 11% (10). A long-term survey of a healthy population, however, identified 62 patients with a monoclonal gammopathy, with malignant evolution occurring in only 2 patients during 20 years of follow-up (11). The corresponding figures in patients with neuropathy and gammopathy are likely to be within these extremes, but only a minority of these patients show evidence of a malignant disorder such as Waldenström's macroglobulinemia, amyloidosis, lymphoma, osteosclerotic myeloma, or Castleman's disease.

The designation *MGUS* may be unfortunate as it tends to obscure the pathogenetic significance of some of these antibodies' specificities. Indeed, there is mounting evidence that neuropathy may be directly caused by some of these autoantibodies. We therefore prefer to describe these conditions as malignant or nonmalignant dysglobulinemic neuropathies.

This chapter emphasizes the pathogenetic links between dysglobulinemia and peripheral neuropathy syndromes. For neuropathy associated with monoclonal IgM antibodies directed against the MAG, there is now considerable evidence for a causal relationship. Other antibody specificities, most of which are restricted to monoclonal IgM antibodies, have also been associated with different neuropathy syndromes. IgG and IgA paraproteins are less common than IgM paraproteins in patients with neuropathy, and IgA monoclonal gammopathies are seen most infrequently.

IgM Dysglobulinemic Neuropathies

Clinical Aspects

The association of Waldenström's macroglobulinemia and peripheral neuropathy was well established by 1958 (12). We now understand that the varied clinical presentations of neuropathy in this condition are due to numerous immune and nonimmune pathogenic mechanisms. Typical causes of multiple mononeuropathy in macroglobulinemia patients are plasma cell infiltration of peripheral nerves, amyloid deposition, and vascular disorders such as microhemorrhages and microinfarcts (9). Interestingly in some patients, particularly those with a distal sensorimotor neuropathy, the neurologic symptoms precede other manifestations of Waldenström's disease by several years. In due course it became apparent that there is a considerable number of patients with nonmalignant IgM gammopathies and similar neuropathies of otherwise unknown etiology. This association stands out on the basis of epidemiologic data. While monoclonal IgM gammopathies represent between 11% and 27% of all gammopathies (13), they are found in over half of the patients with paraproteinemic neuropathy (1).

Early on, an unusual series of such patients conveyed the impression of a relatively homogeneous clinical presentation (14). These patients were identified by serum protein electrophoresis of 14,000 serum samples from patients admitted to a large neurologic referral hospital. Fifty-six patients had nonmalignant paraproteinemia. Twelve of the 56 had an associated neuropathy without an apparent etiology; 7 of these 12 patients had an IgM paraprotein and presented with a sensorimotor neuropathy, slow motor conduction velocities, segmental demyelination, and high-titer antimyelin immunoreactivity of the paraprotein (14,15).

In general, over half of such IgM paraproteins were directed against MAG (16,17). Initially, studies could not find statistically significant differences in clinical and electrophysiologic parameters between paraproteinemic neuropathies with and those without anti-MAG antibodies (1,4). Subsequently, a larger study of 75 patients with IgM monoclonal gammopathy and neuropathy reported a clear association between anti-MAG immunoreactivity and a predominantly sensory neuropathy, marked reduction of motor nerve conduction velocity, and segmental demyelination; these parameters were much more heterogeneous in the patients without anti-MAG antibodies (18). A further study of 64 patients with sensorimotor neuropathies identified 13 patients with elevated anti-MAG IgM levels, and only 5 of them had paraproteins (19).

Neuropathy Associated with Anti-MAG IgM

The annual incidence of neuropathy associated with anti-MAG IgM paraproteins has been estimated at 1 to 5 per 10,000 adults (20). Among these patients, there is a sevenfold excess of men over women (18,21). More than 80% present with predominantly sensory symptoms (21). Physical examination and testing generally reveal a distally pronounced and symmetric sensory deficiency. Footdrop and steppage gait are common. A minority of patients, however, have a predominantly motor neuropathy and are severely disabled. Pain is an infrequent symptom. Nearly half the patients have marked or severe ataxia, a manifestation of the disease that may be linked to the slowing of nerve conduction and not be of central origin (22).

Paresthesias in the lower limbs are a consistent first symptom. At onset, the ankle jerk is generally absent and there is a mild impairment of balance as judged by Romberg's test. These neurologic manifestations usually precede the detection of the gammopathy (23). After a few years the patients may complain of paresthesias and numbness in the hands and may develop some tremor. In addition, they may experience increasing ataxia, motor impairment, and muscle atrophy. In a series with 33 patients and a mean follow-up period of nearly 5 years, 7 patients died, 2 as a direct consequence of the neuropathy and 1 owing to the development of a fatal B-cell cerebral lymphoma secreting the IgM paraprotein (21). In an unusual case, a patient with amyotrophy and fasciculations progressed to tetraplegia and died within 19 months (24).

The electrophysiologic findings generally indicate a predominantly demyelinating neuropathy and in 90% of patients the motor peroneal conduction velocity is less than 35 m/sec (18). as a distinguishing feature of this neuropathy, there is a marked distal accentuation of conduction slowing, which is consistent with the distally pronounced impairment of predominantly sensory functions (25). Cranial nerves remain unaffected but electrophysiologic studies may reveal subclinical involvement.

The neurologic manifestations of Waldenström's macroglobulinemia with anti-MAG specificity are essentially the same as those of benign IgM gammopathy and will not be considered separately. Occasionally, patients with anti-MAG antibodies may present initially as a CIDP, with the anti-MAG IgM gammopathy remaining undetected for a considerable time (26). We also observed a patient with a sensorimotor demyelinating neuropathy and anti-MAG IgM antibodies but no manifestations of paraproteinemia (Gabriel JM, et al, unpublished data, 1996).

Neuropathies Associated with Other IgM Specificities

Nobile-Orazio et al (18) investigated 75 patients with neuropathies and IgM paraproteins. They found 4 patients with antisulfatide, 4 with anti–200-kd neurofilament, 1 with anti-GD$_{1b}$ ganglioside, and 1 with anti–chondroitin sulfate C antibodies; over half of their patients had anti-MAG IgM and about one third had undetermined specificities.

Patients with increased titers of antisulfatide antibodies comprise a heterogeneous group and generally present with a predominantly sensory neuropathy (19). Several of these patients have a small-fiber sensory neuropathy or a syndrome resembling ganglioneuritis with electrophysiologic or nerve biopsy evidence of axonal degeneration in some patients and demyelination in others. Immunocytochemical studies reveal that the antibodies bind to the surface of rat dorsal root ganglia neurons but their pathogenetic importance remains unclear (27). Antisulfatide antibodies have a variety of cross-reactivities, which may explain the absence of correlation with a particular neurologic syndrome. Some antibodies are highly specific for sulfatide, and others also recognize MAG. A considerable number of antisulfatide antibodies have broad cross-reactivities to MAG, P0, chondroitin sulfate A, chondroitin sulfate C, GM$_1$ ganglioside, and asialo-GM$_1$ ganglioside (19).

IgM paraproteins with predominantly anti-GM$_1$ specificities are rare and may define a separate syndrome (18). High titers of anti-GM$_1$ antibodies—irrespective of whether they are due to polyclonal or mono-clonal antibody production—correlate with symptoms of either a motor neuropathy or a motor neuron–like disease frequently associated with conduction blocks and only occasionally with evidence of demyelination (28–30). GM_1 gangliosides are enriched in the nodes of Ranvier and may represent the antigenic target. In some patients with monoclonal anti-GM_1 IgM neuropathy, a cross-reactivity to lipopolysaccharides of *Campylobacter jejuni* strains is demonstrated, suggesting that the B-cell clone might develop following an infection (31).

A different group of patients has a predominantly sensory neuropathy and circulating monoclonal IgM antibodies that recognize ganglioside containing disialosyl groups such as GD_3, GD_{1b}, GD_{1a}, or GQ_{1b} (32). Most of these patients have large-fiber sensory loss with areflexia, gait ataxia, elevated protein concentrations in the cerebrospinal fluid (CSF), and a demyelinating neuropathy. This association of antibodies directed against GQ_{1b} with chronic sensory neuropathies characterized by prominent ataxia and sometimes ophthalmoplegia resembles the Miller Fisher syndrome, in which antibodies against GQ_{1b} arise transiently, generally following an infection (33).

Immunopathologic Findings

Routine Diagnostic Procedures

Segmental demyelinating lesions and endoneural IgM deposits in the absence of inflammatory infiltrates are the most obvious features seen in sural nerve biopsy specimens from patients with neuropathy and monoclonal anti-MAG IgM. For routine clinical diagnosis, a nerve biopsy is generally not required in the presence of a sensorimotor neuropathy with anti-MAG IgM antibodies, prolonged nerve conduction times, and electrophysiologic evidence of segmental demyelination. The demonstration of high-titer IgM antibodies reacting with the 100-kd MAG band by Western blot analysis using crude myelin protein preparations is sufficient and reliable for diagnosis. Enzyme-linked immunosorbent assays (ELISAs) either using purified MAG or taking advantage of the cross-reactivity of the anti-MAG paraprotein to sulfate 3-glucuronyl paragloboside (SGPG) have been developed but do not always have satisfactory specificity for diagnosis (34,35). More recently developed ELISAs, which are now available commercially, use affinity-purified MAG and achieve a similar high specificity of diagnosis as the immunoblot assay. Additionally, they provide a convenient quantification of anti-MAG titers.

Immunopathogenesis of Anti-MAG Neuropathy

The pathogenetic role of the anti-MAG IgM antibodies has been a matter of considerable debate. Their affinities to MAG, which can be variable, or their titers do not correlate with the severity of the disease (36,37). These antibodies recognize carbohydrate determinants on MAG that are very similar to those detected with the HNK-1 murine monoclonal antibody (38). There is a variable cross-reactivity to similar carbohydrates present on the P0 and peripheral myelin protein (PMP)22 myelin glycoproteins as well as glycolipids (39–43). A neural crest-specific glucuronyl transferase is presumed to be responsible for this type of glycosylation (44). Compared to the HNK-1 monoclonal antibody, the IgM paraproteins in patients have a higher affinity for MAG, have relatively weak and varying cross-reactivities with the other myelin glycoproteins, and do not react with some of the other molecules recognized by HNK-1 such as neural cellular adhesion molecule (NCAM). This marked preference of the anti-MAG IgM antibodies is due to the relatively low intrinsic affinity of the antibodies to the monovalent oligosaccharides and to cooperative binding of the multimeric IgM with up to eight HNK-1 epitopes per MAG molecule, resulting in dissociation constants of around 10^{-10} M (45,46).

Adoptive transfer experiments have now convincingly shown that the anti-MAG IgM antibodies are sufficient to elicit most of the hallmarks of the human neuropathy in an animal model (47). HNK-1 determinants are not expressed in rodents; however, they are prominently expressed in chickens. Hatchling chicks injected repeatedly over an 8-week period with purified anti-MAG IgM develop a neuropathy, slowing of nerve conduction, demyelination with widening of myelin lamellae, and typical deposition of IgM in myelin (47). The features of a chronic human disease are inducible in chicks presumably because of the high rate of myelin synthesis at this time in development. Therefore, it is possible that anti-MAG antibodies in adult humans interfere with MAG turnover and in particular remyelination. Surprisingly, marked myelin edema with large vacuole formation at the internode is seen in the chick model but not in humans, suggesting dramatic but transient alterations of electrolyte transport not apparent in the chronic human neuropathy. It remains to be seen whether MAG plays a role in maintaining the electrolyte homeostasis of myelin.

The effects of anti-MAG autoantibodies in patients with neuropathy are not presumably mediated by complement activation, as evidenced by the lack of C3 deposition and the absence of cellular infiltrates in areas of antibody deposition. However, there are conflicting reports on in situ fixation of complement components, including terminal membrane attack complex (48–51).

The structural features of anti-MAG IgM antibodies provide some clues about the pathogenesis of this autoimmune condition. The DNA sequencing data indicate that the IgM V genes are not shared and that they are hypermutated as seen following a T cell–dependent process such as an acute infection (52–54). This may seem surprising as most B cells expressing monoclonal anti-MAG IgM bear a CD5 cell surface antigen characteristic of so-called natural B cells, which typically produce antibodies directed against carbohydrate antigens and were believed to be incapable of somatic mutation (55). It is now well accepted that such CD5+ B cells respond to cytokines produced by helper T cells (56) and it has been suggested that they undergo hypermutation of their immunoglobulin genes (57). Evidence in support of molecular mimicry of MAG carbohydrates with bacterial antigens was reported recently (5). Conceivably, anti-MAG B cells might remain quiescent until an age-dependent dysfunction of the idiotypic network somehow triggers clonal expansion (6).

There is evidence suggesting that in benign gammopathies, B cells are dependent on the autocrine production of interleukin (IL)-6 whereas in Waldenström's macroglobulinemia B-cell proliferation is independent of growth factors (58). Indeed, the age distribution, male preponderance, and preferred use of κ light chains in anti-MAG neuropathy are similar as those of other benign gammopathies (18). The possibility that there may also be genetic predisposing factors has been raised by the observation of an unusual case with a hereditary motor and sensory neuropathy, a Charcot-Marie-Tooth disease type 1A, preceding anti-MAG paraproteinemic neuropathy arising in the fourth decade of life (59).

Ultrastructural Findings and Expression of Myelin Proteins

Ultrastructural studies in the 1980s noted a characteristic widening of the outer myelin lamellae. In place of the intraperiod line, there is a spacing of 23 nm between the outer leaflets of the Schwann cell plasma membrane (60,61). This feature is fairly typical of anti-MAG neuropathy but may be seen in only a small minority of fibers in a nerve biopsy specimen. Conversely, this characteristic widening of the myelin lamellae was observed in a majority of myelinated fibers in a patient with sensorimotor demyelinating paraproteinemic neuropathy associated with a specificity distinct from MAG (62). Another ultrastructural feature observed in the setting of anti-MAG paraproteinemic neuropathy is the widening of myelin lamellae at additional sites such as the Schmidt-Lanterman incisures and paranodal loops (61). Also, granular material may be deposited in the areas of loosening of myelin architecture as well as in occasionally increased gaps between the axolemma and inner Schwann cell membrane. Finally, an abnormal spiraling of the whole myelin sheath, so-called tomaculous bodies, and, as an expression of inadequate remyelination, onion bulb formation can be seen (61). These features are not to be confused with the typical "uncompacted" myelin lamellae seen in POEMS syndrome and consisting of a loss of the major dense line in inner and median parts of the myelin sheaths (63).

To better understand the pathogenesis of the demyelinating process, we compared by quantitative immunohistochemistry the levels of different myelin components in affected nerves (64). We found a coordinate reduction of most HNK-1–positive and HNK-1–negative myelin proteins that corresponded to the degree of demyelination but did not correlate with the serum titers of the anti-MAG IgM antibodies. MAG, however, was disproportionately reduced and a large proportion of myelinated fibers demonstrated a selective lack of

MAG. Also, the relative distribution of MAG compared to that of either P0 or myelin basic protein showed a highly significant inverse correlation to the anti-MAG antibody titers and may therefore represent an index of disease activity. This observation is consistent with MAG being an important functional target of the autoimmune process.

The preceding study was extended with a two-color immunofluorescence analysis of MAG and IgM localization in nerve biopsy specimens from patients with anti-MAG neuropathy (Erne B, Gabriel JM, unpublished data, 1996). Variable colocalization of MAG and IgM deposits was observed almost exclusively in MAG-positive uncompacted myelin at Schmidt-Lanterman incisures and nodes of Ranvier (see Plates III and IV). Loss of periaxonal MAG was not directly associated with localized IgM deposits. Another intriguing observation was the colocalization of IgM with collagen IV in the basal lamina of myelinated but not of unmyelinated fibers. The identity of the putative HNK-1–positive sites in the basal lamina of myelinated fibers is not clear but they might include MAG degradation products (65,66). Our results suggest that the anti-MAG IgM antibodies gain access to the myelin sheaths at the nodes of Ranvier and Schmidt-Lanterman incisures. Conceivably MAG can disappear from myelin following antibody-mediated modulation or cellular signaling events. Old but not young transgenic mice with disrupted MAG genes appear to develop similar clinical and pathologic features as patients with anti-MAG neuropathy (67). This observation suggests that a chronic lack of MAG can result in long-term myelin instability.

Therapeutic Considerations

The symptoms of patients with neuropathies and monoclonal IgM antibodies are often mild and the disease progression slow enough that only symptomatic treatment is needed. In patients with more severe symptoms or rapid progression, however, an immunosuppressive treatment should be considered. Unfortunately, of all dysglobulinemic neuropathies, those associated with monoclonal IgM antibodies and in particular those with anti-MAG antibodies are most refractory to therapy (9). It is important to distinguish progression of the neuropathy from malignant progression of the B-cell clone, the latter justifying cytostatic therapies including alkylating agents. Quantitation of the M protein concentration in serum is a useful parameter. Further prognostic parameters for malignant progression are β_2-microglobulin levels in serum and the bone marrow plasma cell labeling index (9). Morphologic examination of bone marrow is often inconclusive, however, and immunofluorescent phenotyping and analysis of short-term bone marrow cultures may be more sensitive parameters of the proliferative potential of the B-cell clone (68,69).

The optimal treatment of the neuropathies associated with monoclonal IgM is not definitively established. Plasma exchange has been used sporadically (70) but a controlled trial showed no clinical improvement in patients with neuropathy and IgM paraproteinemia (71). Plasma exchange is obviously indicated for patients with hyperviscosity syndrome (usually Waldenström's macroglobulinemia) or associated cryoglobulinemia. A study using chlorambucil showed marginal clinical effect, with no additional benefit from the combination with plasma exchange (72). Objective improvement of symptoms was noted in anti-MAG neuropathy patients following immunotherapy with monthly plasma exchange and intravenous cyclophosphamide (73). Clinical improvement was also noted in a few isolated patients following treatment with intravenous immunoglobulin (74). Preliminary results from a randomized study with 20 patients with anti-MAG IgM neuropathy showed only a transient improvement in 1 patient treated with intravenous immunoglobulin, whereas 8 of 10 patients improved under treatment with interferon-alfa (75). Confirmation of these results is awaited with much interest.

IgG and IgA Dysglobulinemic Neuropathies

Clinical Aspects

Neuropathy in Myeloma

Neuropathy is estimated to occur in 1% to 13% of all patients with myeloma (76–78), particularly with osteosclerotic myeloma. Osteosclerosis is found in less than 3% of all patients with myeloma, but approximately 50% of the patients have peripheral neuropathy, which is frequently the presenting manifestation (77,79). The neuropathy in osteosclerotic myeloma patients is typically distal, symmetric, and slowly progressive and involves both sensory and motor fibers. The serum M proteins are IgG or IgA, and almost always λ. Occasionally the myeloma is nonsecretory without a detectable serum M protein. The CSF protein concentration is usually elevated. Electrophysiologic and pathologic studies typically show axonal degeneration and demyelination (80). Therapy, utilizing radiation for solitary plasmocytomas, or chemotherapy using alkylating agents and corticosteroids for widespread disease, may result in improvement of the neuropathy (81,82). Tamoxifen may be helpful in some patients (83).

The cause of the neuropathy in the presence of osteosclerotic myeloma is unknown; it might be due to the monoclonal immunoglobulins, or to cytokines or other factors with biologic activity secreted by the monoclonal B cells or plasma cells. The close association with λ light chains suggests a role for the immunoglobulin molecule, possibly through neuronal uptake of light chains (84). Neuropathy has also been observed with experimental myeloma (85), and following passive transfer of human myeloma antibodies in the mouse (86). Secretion of biologically active factors including osteoclastic factors (87), calcitonin (88), and lymphotoxin (89) and accelerated conversion of androgen to estrogen with elevated serum estrogen levels have also been documented in isolated patients (90).

In other patients with multiple myeloma, neuropathy may result from nerve compression by bony fractures or plasmacytomas, or from infiltrations of nerves by plasma cells, and present as cranial nerve palsies, mononeuritis, or mononeuritis multiplex (91,92). Patients with sensory neuritis or with CIDP have also been described (76). In later stages of multiple myeloma, complicating factors such as renal failure or cachexia could contribute to or be responsible for the development of neuropathy.

Neuropathy in Nonmalignant IgG or IgA Dysglobulinemia

The neuropathy in patients with nonmalignant IgG or IgA monoclonal gammopathies may be caused by some of the same mechanisms responsible for the neuropathy in myeloma. The neuropathy in many of these patients improves following plasmapheresis, suggesting that the monoclonal gammopathy is indicative of an underlying inflammatory disease that is responsive to immunotherapy, regardless of the specific mechanisms (71). However, the association can be coincidental as we have also seen IgG or IgA monoclonal gammopathies in patients with other causes for neuropathy including human immunodeficiency virus (HIV)-1 infection, familial amyloidosis, and vasculitis without cryoglobulinemia, in whom the neuropathy was unlikely to be related to the monoclonal gammopathy. Patients with nonmalignant IgG or IgA dysglobulinemia may also present with a CIDP-like syndrome (71,93–95). Occasionally, a nonmalignant monoclonal gammopathy progresses to overt myeloma (7).

The POEMS Syndrome

Some of the patients with neuropathy and IgG or IgA nonmalignant gammopathy or myeloma have a peculiar syndrome, named the *Crow-Fukase* or *POEMS syndrome*, in which there is *p*olyneuropathy; *o*rganomegaly; *e*ndocrine abnormalities such as gynecomastia, anasarca, or hirsuitism; *m*onoclonal gammopathy; and *s*kin changes including hyperpigmentation and hypertrichosis (78,96,97). This syndrome is frequently associated with osteosclerotic myeloma, but also occurs in patients with osteolytic myeloma, extramedullary plasmacytomas, lymphatic hyperplasia, or monoclonal and polyclonal gammopathies without evidence for myeloma. Antibody activity against pituitary tissue was described in one patient with the POEMS syndrome (98). An intriguing example of POEMS syndrome in nonmalignant cases is the association with Castleman's disease, which is a rare condition characterized by angiofollicular lymph node hyperplasia and cytokine abnormalities such as elevated levels of IL-6, IL-1, and tumor necrosis factor (TNF)-α (99–101). In one patient with Castleman's disease and a relapsing but nonprogressive CIDP, Epstein-Barr virus genomes were identified in a lymph node as a possible etiology (102). In Castleman's disease without POEMS syndrome, IL-6 may be produced in the lymph nodes themselves and may be responsible for clinical symptoms such as fever, anemia, and hypergammaglobulinemia (99,103). In patients with Castleman's disease presenting with POEMS syndrome, IL-1 messenger RNA (mRNA) but not IL-6 mRNA was demonstrated in lymph node biopsy samples (104). In POEMS syndrome, as yet uncharacterized plasma cell clone–derived mediators may be responsible for endothelial stimulation resulting in angio-endotheliomatosis of the skin, thrombotic microangiopathy, and mesangioproliferative glomerulonephritis (105). In such a patient with renal insufficiency, endothelial cells in the kidney have been identified as a secondary source of IL-6 (106). The cause of neuropathy in these cases remains unclear.

Neuropathy in Primary Systemic Amyloidosis

It is estimated that up to 25% of patients with monoclonal gammopathy and neuropathy have amyloidosis (107–109). Initial symptoms usually consist of numbness or painful paresthesias distally in the hands or feet that progress proximally in a symmetric fashion. Patients then develop motor weakness, and autonomic symptoms of orthostatic hypotension, bowel and bladder dysfunction, and impotence. Neuropathy is frequently the initial presentation in systemic amyloidosis, but other presentations include cardiomyopathy, nephrotic syndrome, or gastrointestinal symptoms. In almost all affected patients, a monoclonal gammopathy can be discovered in the serum or blood. Amyloid neuropathy is more common with IgG or IgA monoclonal gammopathies than with IgM monoclonal gammopathies. The disease is thought to be caused by the deposition of fragments of immunoglobulin light chains in peripheral nerve and other tissues. The mechanism of light-chain deposition in amyloid formation is unknown. The response to therapy is generally poor, although autologous bone marrow transplantation is a promising new treatment (110).

Laboratory Investigations

If myeloma is suspected, as in the case of IgG or IgA monoclonal gammopathies or light-chain proteinuria, one or multiple bony lesions can be identified by skeletal survey or bone scan. Osteosclerotic myelomas are usually more reliably detected by plain films than by scans. Bony lesions may be present in the absence of serum M proteins if the myeloma is nonsecretory, or if the serum M protein concentration is below the limits of detection. The diagnosis of myeloma is confirmed by bone marrow biopsy of the affected region.

Therapeutic Considerations

In patients with myeloma, radiotherapy of solitary lesions can sometimes be curative (81), and alkylating agents plus prednisone are used to treat disseminated disease (82). The neuropathies associated with non-malignant IgG and IgA monoclonal gammopathies are heterogeneous, but in the absence of other identified causes for neuropathy, immunotherapy using plasmapheresis (71), or with intravenous immunoglobulin, prednisone, or a chemotherapeutic agent, may be effective.

References

1. Suarez GA, Kelly JJ. Polyneuropathy associated with monoclonal gammopathy of undetermined significance: further evidence that IgM-MGUS neuropathies are different than IgG-MGUS. *Neurology* 1993;43:1304–1308.
2. Crawford J, Eye MK, Cohen HJ. Evaluation of monoclonal gammopathies in the "well" elderly. *Am J Med* 1987;82:39–45.
3. Kyle RA. Monoclonal gammopathy of undetermined significance. *Blood Rev* 1994;8:135–141.
4. Gosselin S, Kyle RA, Dyck PJ. Neuropathy associated with monoclonal gammopathies of undetermined significance. *Ann Neurol* 1991;30:54–61.
5. Brouet JC, Mariette X, Gendron MC, Dubreuil ML. Monoclonal IgM from patients with peripheral demyelinating neuropathies cross-react with bacterial polypeptides. *Clin Exp Immunol* 1994;96:466–469.
6. Barbouche MR, Guilbert B, Makni S, et al. Common idiotypes expressed on human, monoclonal, abnormal immunoglobulins and cryoglobulins with polyreactive autoantibody activities. *Clin Exp Immunol* 1993;91:196–201.
7. Kyle RA. Monoclonal gammopathy of undetermined significance: natural history of 241 cases. *Am J Med* 1978;64:814–826.
8. Blade J, Lopez-Guillermo A, Rozman C, et al. Malignant transformation and life expectancy in monoclonal gammopathy of undetermined significance. *Br J Haematol* 1992;81:391–394.
9. Kyle RA, Dyck PJ. Neuropathy associated with the monoclonal gammopathies. In: Dyck PJ, Thomas PK, Griffin JW, et al, eds. *Peripheral neuropathy*. Vol. 2. 3rd ed. Philadelphia: WB Saunders, 1993:1275–1287.
10. van de Poel MH, Coebergh JW, Hillen HF. Malignant transformation of monoclonal gammopathy of undetermined significance among out-patients of a community hospital in southeastern Netherlands. *Br J Haematol* 1995;91:121–125.
11. Axelsson U. A 20-year follow-up study of 64 subjects with M-components. *Acta Med Scand* 1986;219:519–522.
12. Garcin R, Mallarmé J, Rondot P. Forme nevritique de la macroglobulinémie de Waldenström. *Bull Soc Med Hop Paris* 1958;74:562–573.
13. Latov N. Pathogenesis and therapy of neuropathies associated with monoclonal gammopathies. *Ann Neurol* 1995;37(suppl 1):32–42.
14. Kahn SN, Riches PG, Kohn J. Paraproteinaemia in neurological disease: incidence, association and classification of monoclonal immunoglobulins. *J Clin Pathol* 1980;33:617–621.
15. Smith IS, Kahn SM, Lacey BW, et al. Chronic demyelinating neuropathy associated with benign IgM paraproteinaemia. *Brain* 1983;106:169–195.
16. Latov N, Sherman WH, Nemmi R, et al. Plasma cell dyscrasia and peripheral neuropathy with a monoclonal antibody to peripheral nerve myelin. *N Engl J Med* 1980;303:521–618.
17. Braun PE, Frail DE, Latov N. Myelin-associated glycoprotein is the antigen for a monoclonal IgM in polyneuropathy. *J Neurochem* 1982;39:1261–1265.
18. Nobile-Orazio E, Manfredini E, Carpo M, et al. Fre-

quency and clinical correlates of anti-neural IgM antibodies in neuropathy associated with IgM monoclonal gammopathy. *Ann Neurol* 1994;36:416–424.

19. Pestronk A, Li F, Griffin J, et al. Polyneuropathy syndromes associated with serum antibodies to sulfatide and myelin associated glycoprotein. *Neurology* 1991;41:357–362.

20. Latov N, Hays AP, Sherman WH. Peripheral neuropathy and anti-MAG antibodies. *Crit Rev Neurobiol* 1988;3:301–332.

21. Ellie E, Vital A, Steck A, et al. Neuropathy associated with "benign" anti-myelin-associated glycoprotein IgM gammopathy: clinical, immunological, neurophysiological, pathological findings and response to treatment in 33 cases. *J Neurol* 1995;243:34–43.

22. Sindic CJ, Boucquey D, Bisteau M, et al. Monoclonal IgM gammopathy with anti-myelin associated glycoprotein (MAG) activity and polyneuropathy. A study of three cases. *Acta Neurol Belg* 1989;89:331–345.

23. Steck AJ, Murray N, Meier C, et al. Demyelinating neuropathy and monoclonal IgM antibody to myelin-associated glycoprotein. *Neurology* 1983;33:19–23.

24. Antoine J-C, Steck A, Michel D. Fatal peripheral neuropathy with predominant motor involvement associated with anti-MAG IgM monoclonal gammapathy. *Rev Neurol* 1993;149:496–499.

25. Kaku DA, England JD, Sumner AJ. Distal accentuation of conduction slowing in polyneuropathy associated with antibodies to myelin-associated glycoprotein and sulphated glucuronyl paragloboside. *Brain* 1994;117:941–947.

26. Valldeoriola F, Graus F, Steck AJ, et al. Delayed appearance of anti-myelin-associated glycoprotein antibodies in a patient with chronic demyelinating polyneuropathy. *Ann Neurol* 1993;34:394–396.

27. Quattrini A, Corbo M, Dhaliwal SK, et al. Anti-sulfatide antibodies in neurological disease: binding to rat dorsal root ganglia neurons. *J Neurol Sci* 1992;112:152–159.

28. Kinsella LJ, Lange DJ, Trojaborg W, et al. Clinical and electrophysiologic correlates of elevated anti-GM1 antibody titers. *Neurology* 1994;44:1278–1282.

29. Steck AJ, Adams D. Motor neuron syndromes and monoclonal IgM antibodies to gangliosides. *Adv Neurol* 1991;56:421–425.

30. Zielasek J, Ritter G, Magi S, et al. A comparative trial of anti-glyconjugate antibody assays: IgM antibodies to GM1. *J Neurol* 1994;241:475–480.

31. Wirguin I, Suturkova Milosevic L, Della Latta P, et al. Monoclonal IgM antibodies to GM$_1$ and asialo-GM$_1$ in chronic neuropathies cross-react with *Campylobacter jejuni* lipopolysaccharides. *Ann Neurol* 1994;35:698–703.

32. Ilyas AA, Quarles RH, Dalakas MC, et al. Monoclonal IgM in a patient with paraproteinemic polyneuropathy binds to gangliosides containing disialosyl groups. *Ann Neurol* 1985;18:655–659.

33. Willison H. Antiglycolipid antibodies in peripheral neuropathy: fact or fiction? *J Neurol Neurosurg Psychiatry* 1994;57:1303–1307.

34. Burger D, Perruisseau G, Steck AJ. Anti-myelin-associated glycoprotein antibodies in patients with a monoclonal IgM gammopathy and polyneuropathy, and a simplified method for the preparation of glycolipid antigens. *J Immunol Methods* 1991;140:31–36.

35. Pestronk A, Li F, Bieser K, et al. Anti-MAG antibodies: major effects of antigen purity and antibody cross-reactivity on ELISA results and clinical correlation. *Neurology* 1994;44:1131–1137.

36. Baldini L, Nobile Orazio E, Guffanti A, et al. Peripheral neuropathy in IgM monoclonal gammopathy and Waldenström's macroglobulinemia: a frequent complication in elderly males with low MAG-reactive serum monoclonal component. *Am J Hematol* 1994;45:25–31.

37. Brouet JC, Mariette X, Chevalier A, Hauttecoeur B. Determination of the affinity of monoclonal human IgM for myelin-associated glycoprotein and sulfated glucuronic paragloboside. *J Neuroimmunol* 1992;36:209–215.

38. Abo T, Blach CM. A differentiation antigen of human NK and K cells identified by a monoclonal antibody (HNK-1). *J Immunol* 1981;127:1024–1029.

39. Kruse J, Mailhammer R, Wernecke H, et al. Neural cell adhesion molecules and myelin-associated glycoprotein share a common carbohydrate moiety recognized by monoclonal antibodies L2 and HNK-1. *Nature* 1984;311:153–155.

40. Ariga T, Kohiriyama T, Freddo L, et al. Characterization of sulfated glucuronic acid containing glycolipids reacting with IgM M-proteins in patients with neuropathy. *J Biol Chem* 1987;262:848–853.

41. Bollensen E, Steck AJ, Schachner M. Reactivity with the peripheral myelin glycoprotein P0 in serum from patients with monoclonal IgM gammopathy and polyneuropathy. *Neurology* 1988;38:1266–1270.

42. Burger D, Perruisseau G, Simon M, Steck AJ. Comparison of the N-linked oligosaccharide structures of the two major human myelin glycoproteins MAG and P0: assessment of the structures bearing the epitope for HNK-1 and human monoclonal immunoglobulin M found in demyelinating neuropathy. *J Neurochem* 1992;58:854–861.

43. Hammer JA, O'Shannessy DJ, De-Leon M, et al. Immunoreactivity of PMP-22, P0, and other 19 to 28 kDa glycoproteins in peripheral nerve myelin of mammals and fish with HNK1 and related antibodies. *J Neurosci Res* 1993;35:546–558.

44. Oka S, Terayama K, Kawashima C, Kawasaki T. A novel glucuronyltransferase in nervous system presumably associated with the biosynthesis of HNK-1 carbohydrate epitope on glycoproteins. *J Biol Chem* 1992;267:22711–22714.

45. Ogino M, Tatum AH, Latov N. Affinity studies of human anti-MAG antibodies in neuropathy. *J Neuroimmunol* 1994;52:41–46.

46. Burger D, Pidoux L, Steck AJ. Identification of the glycosylated sequons of human myelin-associated glycoprotein. *Biochem Biophys Res Commun* 1993;197:457–464.

47. Tatum AH. Experimental paraprotein neuropathy, demyelination by passive transfer of human IgM anti-myelin-associated glycoprotein. *Ann Neurol* 1993;33:502–506.

48. Koski CL, Sanders ME, Swoveland PT, et al. Activation of terminal components of complement in patients with Guillain-Barré syndrome and other demyelinating neuropathies. *J Clin Invest* 1987;80:1492–1497.

49. Mendell JR, Sahenk Z, Whitaker JN, et al. Polyneuropathy and IgM monoclonal gammopathy: studies on the pathogenetic role of anti-myelin-associated glycoprotein antibody. *Ann Neurol* 1985;17:243–254.

50. Monaco S, Bonetti B, Ferrari S, et al. Complement-mediated demyelination in patients with IgM monoclonal gammopathy and polyneuropathy. *N Engl J Med* 1990;322:649–652.

51. Monaco S, Ferrari S, Bonetti B, et al. Experimental induction of myelin changes by anti-MAG antibodies and terminal complement complex. *J Neuropathol Exp Neurol* 1995;54:96–104.

52. Mihaesco E, Ayadi H, Congy N, et al. Multiple mutations in the variable region of the kappa light chains of three monoclonal human IgM with anti-myelin-associated glycoprotein activity. *J Biol Chem* 1989;264:21481–21485.

53. Spatz LA, Williams M, Brender B, et al. DNA sequence analysis and comparison of the variable heavy and light chain regions of two IgM, monoclonal, anti-myelin associated glycoprotein antibodies. *J Neuroimmunol* 1992;36:29–39.

54. Murray N, Page N, Steck AJ. The human anti-myelin-associated glycoprotein IgM system. *Ann Neurol* 1986; 19:473–478.

55. Lee KW, Inghirami G, Spatz L, et al. The B-cells that express anti-MAG antibodies in neuropathy and non-malignant IgM monoclonal gammopathy belong to the CD5 subpopulation. *J Neuroimmunol* 1991;31:83–88.

56. Nisitani S, Tsubata T, Murakami M, Honjo T. Administration of interleukin-5 or -10 activates peritoneal B-1 cells and induces autoimmune hemolytic anemia in anti-erythrocyte autoantibody-transgenic mice. *Eur J Immunol* 1995;25:3047–3052.

57. Murakami M, Honjo T. Involvement of B-1 cells in mucosal immunity and autoimmunity. *Immunol Today* 1995;16:534–539.

58. Levy Y, Fermand J-P, Navarro S, et al. Interleukin 6 dependence of spontaneous in vitro differentiation of B cells from patients with IgM gammopathy. *Proc Natl Acad Sci USA* 1990;87:3309–3313.

59. Gregory R, Thomas PK, King RH, et al. Coexistence of hereditary motor and sensory neuropathy type Ia and IgM paraproteinemic neuropathy. *Ann Neurol* 1993;33:649–652.

60. Vital A, Vital C, Julien J, et al. Polyneuropathy associated with IgM monoclonal gammopathy. Immunological and pathological study in 31 patients. *Acta Neuropathol (Berl)* 1989;79:160–167.

61. Jacobs JM, Scadding JW. Morphological changes in IgM paraproteinaemic neuropathy. *Acta Neuropathol (Berl)* 1990;80:77–84.

62. Lach B, Rippstein P, Atack D, et al. Immunoelectron microscopic localization of monoclonal IgM antibodies in gammopathy associated with peripheral demyelinative neuropathy. *Acta Neuropathol (Berl)* 1993;85:298–307.

63. Vital C, Gherardi R, Vital A, et al. Uncompacted myelin lamellae in polyneuropathy, organomegaly, endocrinopathy, M-protein and skin changes syndrome. Ultrastructural study of peripheral nerve biopsy from 22 patients. *Acta Neuropathol (Berl)* 1994;87:302–307.

64. Gabriel J-M, Erne B, Miescher GC, et al. Selective loss of myelin-associated glycoprotein from myelin correlates with anti-MAG antibody titer in demyelinating paraproteinaemic polyneuropathy. *Brain* 1996;119:775–787.

65. Fahrig T, Landa C, Pesheva P, et al. Characterization of binding properties of the myelin-associated glycoprotein to extracellular matrix constituents. *EMBO J* 1987;6:2875–2883.

66. Martini R, Schachner M. Immunoelectron microscopic localization of neural cell adhesion molecules (L1, N-CAM, and myelin-associated glycoprotein) in regenerating adult mouse sciatic nerve. *J Cell Biol* 1988;106:1735–1746.

67. Fruttiger M, Montag D, Schachner M, Martini R. Crucial role for the myelin-associated glycoprotein in the maintenance of axon-myelin integrity. *Eur J Neurosci* 1995;7:511–515.

68. Menke DM, Greipp PR, Colon-Otero G, et al. Bone marrow aspirate immunofluorescent and bone marrow biopsy immunoperoxidase staining of plasma cells in histologically occult plasma cell proliferative marrow disorders. *Arch Pathol Lab Med* 1994;118:811–814.

69. Bezwoda WR, Gordon V, Bagg A, Mendelow B. Light chain restriction analysis of bone marrow plasma cells in patients with MGUS or 'solitary' plasmacytoma: diagnostic value and correlation with clinical course. *Br J Haematol* 1990;74:420–423.

70. Dyck PJ, Low PA, Windebank AJ, et al. Plasma exchange in polyneuropathy associated with monoclonal gammopathy of undetermined significance. *N Engl J Med* 1991;325:1482–1486.

71. Hoang-Xuan K, Leger JM, Ben Younes Chennoufi A, et al. Treatment of immune deficient neuropathies with intravenous polyvalent immunoglobulins. An open study of 16 cases. *Rev Neurol* 1993;149:385–392.

72. Oksenhendler E, Chevret S, Léger J, et al. Plasma exchange and chlorambucil in polyneuropathy associated with monoclonal IgM gammopathy. IgM-associated Polyneuropathy Study Group. *J Neurol Neurosurg Psychiatry* 1995;59:243–247.

73. Blume G, Pestronk A, Goodnough LT. Anti-MAG antibody-associated polyneuropathies: improvement following immunotherapy with monthly plasma exchange and IV cyclophosphamide. *Neurology* 1995;45:1577–1580.

74. Cook D, Dalakas M, Galdi A, et al. High-dose intravenous immunoglobulin in the treatment of demyelinating neuropathy associated with monoclonal gammopathy [see comments]. *Neurology* 1990;40:212–214.

75. Mariette X, Oksenhendler E. Traitement des neuropathies périphériques associées à une gammopathie IgM monoclonale anti-myéline. *Rev Neurol Paris* 1996; 152(5):413–416.

76. Kelly JJ, Kyle RA, Miles JM, et al. The spectrum of peripheral neuropathy in myeloma. *Neurology* 1981;31: 24–31.

77. Driedger H, Pruzanski W. Plasma cell neoplasia with peripheral polyneuropathy. *Medicine* 1988;59:301–310.

78. Miralles GD, O'Fallon JR, Talley NJ. Plasma-cell dyscrasia with polyneuropathy. The spectrum of POEMS syndrome. *N Engl J Med* 1992;327:1919–1923.

79. Kelly JJ, Kyle RA, Miles JM, Dyck PJ. Osteosclerotic myeloma and peripheral neuropathy. *Neurology* 1983; 33:202–210.

80. Ohi T, Kyle RA, Dyck PJ. Axonal attenuation and secondary segmental demyelination in myeloma neuropathies. *Ann Neurol* 1985;17:255–261.

81. Donofrio PD, Albers JW, Greenberg HS, Mitchell BS. Peripheral neuropathy in osteosclerotic myeloma: clinical and electrophysiologic improvement with chemotherapy. *Muscle Nerve* 1984;7:137–141.

82. Alexanian R, Dimopoulos M. The treatment of multiple myeloma. *N Engl J Med* 1994;330:484–486.

83. Enevoldson TP, Harding AE. Improvement in the POEMS syndrome after administration of tamoxifen. *J Neurol Neurosurg Psychiatry* 1992;55:71–72.

84. Borges LF, Busis NA. Intraneuronal accumulation of myeloma proteins. *Arch Neurol* 1985;42:690–694.

85. Dayan AD, Stokes MI. Peripheral neuropathy and experimental myeloma in the mouse. *Nature* 1972;236: 117–118.

86. Bessinger VA, Toyka KV, Anzil AP, et al. Myeloma neuropathy: passive transfer from man to mouse. *Science* 1981;213:1027–1030.

87. Mundy GR, Raisz LG, Cooper RA, et al. Evidence for the secretion of an osteoclast stimulating factor in myeloma. *N Engl J Med* 1974;291:1041–1046.

88. Rousseau JJ, Franck G, Grisar T, et al. Osteosclerotic myeloma with polyneuropathy and ectopic secretion of calcitonin. *Eur J Cancer* 1978;14:133–140.

89. Garrett IR, Durie BGM, Nedwin GE, et al. Production of lymphotoxin, a bone resorbing cytokine, by cultured human myeloma cells. *N Engl J Med* 1987;317:526–532.

90. Matsumine H. Accelerated conversion of androgen to estrogen in plasma cell dyscrasia associated with polyneuropathy, anasarca, and skin pigmentation. *N Engl J Med* 1985;313:1025–1026.

91. Hesselvik M. Neuropathological studies on myelomatosis. *Acta Neurol Scand* 1969;45:95–108.

92. Silverstein A, Doniger DE. Neurological complication of myelomatosis. *Arch Neurol* 1963;9:534–544.

93. Read DJ, Vanhegan RI, Matthews WB. Peripheral neuropathy and benign IgG paraproteinemia. *J Neurol Neurosurg Psychiatry* 1978;41:215–219.

94. Noring L, Kjellin KG, Siden A. Neuropathies associated with disorders of plasmacytes. *Eur Neurol* 1980;19:224–230.

95. Bromberg MB, Feldman EL, Albers JW. Chronic inflammatory demyelinating polyradiculoneuropathy: comparison of patients with and without an associated monoclonal gammopathy. *Neurology* 1992;42:1157–1163.

96. Bardwick PA, Zvaifler NJ, Gill GN, et al. Plasma cell dyscrasia with polyneuropathy, organomegaly, endocrinopathy, M protein, and skin changes: the POEMS syndrome; report on two cases and a review of the literature. *Medicine* 1980;59:311–322.

97. Nakanishi T, Sobue I, Toyokura Y, et al. The Crow-Fukase syndrome: a study of 102 cases in Japan. *Neurology* 1984;34:712–720.

98. Reulecke M, Dumas M, Meier C. Specific antibody activity against neuroendocrine tissue in a case of POEMS syndrome with IgG gammopathy. *Neurology* 1988;38:614–616.

99. Yoshizaki K, Matsuda T, Nishimoto N, et al. Pathogenic significance of interleukin-6 (IL-6/BSF-2) in Castleman's disease. *Blood* 1989;74:1360–1367.

100. Mandler RN, Kerrigan DP, Smart J, et al. Castleman's disease in POEMS syndrome with elevated interleukin-6. *Cancer* 1992;69:2696–2703.

101. Gherardi RK, Chouaib S, Malapert D, et al. Early weight loss and high serum tumor necrosis factor-alpha levels in polyneuropathy, organomegaly, endocrinopathy, M protein, skin changes syndrome. *Ann Neurol* 1994;35:501–505.

102. Vingerhoets F, Kuntzer T, Delacretaz F, et al. Chronic relapsing neuropathy associated with Castleman's disease (angiofollicular lymph node hyperplasia). *Eur Neurol* 1995;35:336–340.

103. Leger-Ravet MB, Peuchmaur M, Devergne O, et al. Interleukin-6 gene expression in Castleman's disease. *Blood* 1991;78:2923–2930.

104. Gherardi RK, Belec L, Fromont G, et al. Elevated levels of interleukin-1 beta (IL-1 beta) and IL-6 in serum and increased production of IL-1 beta mRNA in lymph nodes of patients with polyneuropathy, organomegaly, endocrinopathy, M protein, and skin changes (POEMS) syndrome. *Blood* 1994;83:2587–2593.

105. Judge MR, McGibbon DH, Thompson RP. Angioendotheliomatosis associated with Castleman's lymphoma and POEMS syndrome. *Clin Exp Dermatol* 1993;18:360–362.

106. Fukatsu A, Ito Y, Yuzawa Y, et al. A case of POEMS syndrome showing elevated serum interleukin 6 and abnormal expression of interleukin 6 in the kidney. *Nephron* 1992;62:47–51.

107. Trotter JL, Engel WK, Ignaszak TF. Amyloidosis with plasma cell dyscrasia: an overlooked cause of adult onset sensorimotor neuropathy. *Arch Neurol* 1977;34:209–214.

108. Kelly JJ Jr, Kyle RA, O'Brien PC, Dyck PJ. The natural history of peripheral neuropathy in primary systemic amyloidosis. *Ann Neurol* 1979;6:1–7.

109. Kyle RA, Greipp PR. Amyloidosis (AL): clinical and laboratory features of 229 cases. *Mayo Clin Proc* 1983;58:665–683.

110. Bergethon PR, Skinner M, Simms RW, Comenzo RL. Reversal of the neuropathy in primary (AL) amyloidosis following treatment with high dose melphalan and stem cell rescue. *Neurology* 1996;46:A449.

Chapter 21
Vasculitic Neuropathies

Michael P. Collins, John T. Kissel, and Jerry R. Mendell

Vasculitis is a clinicopathologic entity that encompasses a heterogeneous group of relatively uncommon diseases characterized by inflammation and structural damage of blood vessel walls, leading to ischemic, hemorrhagic, and thrombotic events (1). Single or multiple organ systems may be involved, resulting in a wide variety of clinical manifestations. Peripheral neuropathy is common in many vasculitic syndromes, reflecting inflammation and occlusion of the vasa nervorum that produces ischemic damage to nerve fascicles. Vasculitic neuropathy may herald a life-threatening systemic immunologic disorder or be the sole manifestation of vasculitic involvement, with less severe prognostic implications. It is important for the clinician to make a timely and accurate diagnosis because of the potential stabilizing or reversing effects of treatment on the disease.

Historical Background and Epidemiology

Credit for the first description of systemic necrotizing vasculitis is given to Kussmaul and Maier (2) and their report of 1866, although Rokitansky and others (3) had previously recognized a similar disease. Kussmaul and Maier (2) reported a patient with a rapidly progressive neuropathy and multisystem illness whose autopsy revealed widespread nodular inflammation of small and medium-sized arteries, a disease they called *periarteritis nodosa*. The term *polyarteritis* was introduced by Ferrari (4) in 1903 to recognize the fact that inflammatory infiltrates could be found in all layers of the vessel wall and were not confined to the periarterial region. For the next five decades, most vasculitis was referred to as polyarteritis nodosa (PAN), despite many differentiating features. Little attention was paid to peripheral nerve pathology until 1938 when Kernohan and Woltman (5) reported a unique case of PAN limited to peripheral nerve, a concept that lay dormant until the 1980s.

A seminal work on vasculitic neuropathy was published in 1972 by Dyck et al (6), who painstakingly analyzed the histopathology of 15,000 sections from limb nerves removed at autopsy from a patient with rheumatoid vasculitis and correlated the three-dimensional morphology of nerve fiber degeneration with sites of vascular pathology. This study provided persuasive evidence that ischemia accounts for the observed fiber damage in vasculitic neuropathy. Several large series of patients with vasculitic neuropathy were subsequently studied, and the clinical and immunopathologic spectrum of these disorders better defined (7–18). Many of these series described patients with vasculitis restricted to the peripheral nervous system.

Precise figures on the incidence and prevalence of vasculitic neuropathy are not available because of the relative rarity of these disorders and the difficulty in establishing diagnostic criteria. In addition, the published studies originated from tertiary referral centers and therefore are confounded by referral bias and uncertain sample populations. Nevertheless, a reasonable estimate can be obtained by focusing on the most common type of systemic vasculitic neuropathy—PAN. Population-based studies from Olmsted County, Minnesota, found an annual PAN incidence of 9.0 cases per million population (19). Since 60% of patients with PAN develop a peripheral neuropathy, about 5 new cases of PAN-related vasculitic neuropathy annually per million population would be expected.

Classification

Although many classification systems for the necrotizing vasculitides have been proposed since Zeek's benchmark categorization in 1952 (3), none have proved adequate owing to the numerous variations in the clinical syndromes and the ignorance of etiologic and immunopathogenic mechanisms. Most systems distinguish between primary vasculitides, unrelated to any other disease process, and the secondary vasculitides, which accompany a known underlying disease or have a specific etiology. It is useful to compare the proposed classifications.

In 1990, the American College of Rheumatology (ACR) Subcommittee on Classification of Vasculitis published diagnostic criteria for vasculitis (20). Before their deliberations were completed, data were analyzed from 1000 cases collected from 48 centers. The criteria developed by the ACR subcommittee provide useful guidelines for classification of patients with vasculitis. However, a major shortcoming of the proposal is that the final recommendations addressed only seven forms of vasculitis (PAN, Churg-Strauss syndrome, Wegener's granulomatosis, Takayasu's arteritis, hypersensitivity vasculitis, Henoch-Schönlein purpura, and temporal arteritis). The system, therefore, suffers from a lack of comprehensiveness. In addition, the published diagnostic criteria do not absolutely require pathologic confirmation for any of the entities, and for two of the diseases (Churg-Strauss syndrome and Wegener's granulomatosis), pathologic evidence of vasculitis is not even included as one of the diagnostic criteria.

In 1994, an alternative nomenclature was proposed by the Chapel Hill Consensus Conference on the Nomenclature of Systemic Vasculitis (Table 21-1) (21). The size and histopathology of the involved vessels serve as the backbone for this system. This scheme has the advantage of providing nonambiguous, standardized definitions, but like the ACR approach, it lacks comprehensiveness. Moreover, the system is inflexible, forcing patients with otherwise classic PAN or Kawasaki disease into one of the small-vessel vasculitis groups should any small-vessel involvement be manifested, such as glomerulonephritis in PAN. In addition, the

clinically useful concept of hypersensitivity vasculitis is, unjustifiably, deleted from the nomenclature.

A categorization that we have found useful combines some of the best features of the above systems and incorporates them into the vasculitis classification outlined in Table 21-2 and presented in the discussion to follow. Two large groups comprise this classification scheme: infectious and immune-mediated. The system is both comprehensive and allows for overlap groups. In addition, the approach is especially well adapted for patients with neurologic disorders, providing separate categories for vasculitides restricted to the nervous system, either central or peripheral.

Vasculitides Resulting from Direct Infection

It is well documented that infectious organisms can produce vasculitis by direct invasion of blood vessel walls or by generation of immune complexes. Nervous system vasculitis due to infection with a wide range of bacterial, fungal, rickettsial, and viral agents has been

Table 21-1.
Names and Definitions of Vasculitides Adopted by the Chapel Hill Consensus Conference on the Nomenclature of Systemic Vasculitis

Large-vessel vasculitis	
Giant-cell (temporal) arteritis	Granulomatous arteritis of the aorta and its major branches, with a predilection for the extracranial branches of the carotid artery. *Often involves the temporal artery. Usually occurs in patients older than 50 and often is associated with polymyalgia rheumatica.*
Takayasu's arteritis	Granulomatous inflammation of the aorta and its major branches. *Usually occurs in patients younger than 50.*
Medium-sized vessel vasculitis	
Polyarteritis nodosa (classic polyarteritis nodosa)	Necrotizing inflammation of medium-sized or small arteries without glomerulonephritis or vasculitis in arterioles, capillaries, or venules.
Kawasaki disease	Arteritis involving large, medium-sized, and small arteries, and associated with mucocutaneous lymph node syndrome. *Coronary arteries are often involved. Aorta and veins may be involved. Usually occurs in children.*
Small-vessel vasculitis	
Wegener's granulomatosis*	Granulomatous inflammation involving the respiratory tract, and necrotizing vasculitis affecting small to medium-sized vessels (e.g., capillaries, venules, arterioles, and arteries). *Necrotizing glomerulonephritis is common.*
Churg-Strauss syndrome*	Eosinophil-rich and granulomatous inflammation involving the respiratory tract, and necrotizing vasculitis affecting small to medium-sized vessels, and associated with asthma and eosinophilia.
Microscopic polyangiitis*	Necrotizing vasculitis, with few or no immune deposits, affecting small vessels (i.e., capillaries, venules, or arterioles). *Necrotizing arteritis involving small and medium-sized arteries may be present. Necrotizing glomerulonephritis is very common. Pulmonary capillaritis often occurs.*
Henoch-Schönlein purpura	Vasculitis with IgA-dominant immune deposits, affecting small vessels (i.e., capillaries, venules, or arterioles). *Typically involves skin, gut, and glomeruli, and is associated with arthralgias or arthritis.*
Essential cryoglobulinemic vasculitis	Vasculitis, with cryoglobulin immune deposits, affecting small vessels (i.e., capillaries, venules, or arterioles), and associated with cryoglobulins in serum. *Skin and glomeruli are often involved.*
Cutaneous leukocytoclastic angiitis	Isolated cutaneous leukocytoclastic angiitis without systemic vasculitis or glomerulonephritis.

*Strongly associated with anti–neutrophil cytoplasmic autoantibodies.

Table 21-2.
Classification of Vasculitides

A. Vasculitides resulting from direct infection
   1. Bacterial (e.g., syphilis, tuberculous, ?Lyme)
   2. Fungal (e.g., cryptococcus, aspergillus)
   3. Rickettsial (e.g., Rocky Mountain spotted fever)
   4. Viral (e.g., herpes zoster, CMV, ?HIV)
B. Vasculitides resulting from immunologic mechanisms
   1. Systemic necrotizing vasculitis
      a. Classic polyarteritis nodosa (PAN)
      b. Anti–neutrophil cytoplasmic antibody
         (ANCA)–associated
         i.   Wegener's granulomatosis
         ii. Churg-Strauss syndrome
         iii. Microscopic polyangiitis
      c. Vasculitis with connective tissue disease (CTD)
      d. PAN related to hepatitis B virus
      e. Polyangiitis overlap syndrome
   2. Hypersensitivity vasculitis
      a. Primary
         i. Henoch-Schönlein purpura
         ii. Cutaneous leukocytoclastic angiitis
      b. Secondary*
         i.   Vasculitis associated with infections
         ii. Vasculitis associated with malignancy
         iii. Drug-induced vasculitis (e.g., ampheta-
              mines, cocaine)
         iv. Vasculitis with CTD
         v.   Essential mixed cryoglobulinemia
   3. Giant-cell arteritis
      a. Temporal arteritis
      b. Takayasu's arteritis
   4. Localized vasculitis
      a. Isolated peripheral nerve vasculitis (nonsystemic
         vasculitic neuropathy)
      b. Isolated central nervous system vasculitis
      c. Localized vasculitis of other organs (e.g., GI
         tract, testicles, uterus, retina, skin, kidney)

---

*Each of these entities can also produce a systemic necrotizing vasculitis less commonly.

reported (22,23). Cytomegalovirus (CMV) and herpes zoster can cause vasculitis by direct vascular invasion of the peripheral vasa nervorum (24,25). In contrast, direct evidence is lacking for human immunodeficiency virus (HIV) propagation within the endothelium of the vasa nervorum. The presence of HIV p24 antigen and HIV RNA in the blood vessel walls of the peripheral nerve (26,27) is most likely related to HIV within mononuclear phagocytes and extracellular immune complexes (28).

Vasculitis associated with HIV occurs as a multiple mononeuropathy (CD4+ count > 200/μL) during the early symptomatic stage (28–31). This is usually an isolated peripheral nerve vasculitis, but constitutional symptoms, Raynaud's phenomenon, arthritis, and cutaneous or gastrointestinal (GI) involvement are occasionally associated (32). Patients typically present with facial weakness, footdrop, hand weakness, or multifocal patches of sensory loss and the condition may then evolve into a more confluent asymmetric or symmetric

polyneuropathy. For patients with CD4+ counts higher than 200/μL and a limited neuropathy, the deficits usually improve or resolve over months irrespective of treatment. Sural nerve biopsy reveals axonal degeneration with perivascular inflammation, or less commonly, frank necrotizing arteritis (29–31).

Other HIV-infected patients present with mononeuropathy multiplex late in their illness, usually with CD4+ counts lower than 50/μL and when already diagnosed with acquired immunodeficiency syndrome (AIDS). In these patients, the neuropathy is more extensive and rapidly progressive. CMV infection is almost always the cause of this syndrome, typically preceded by signs of CMV involvement of the retina and GI tract (33). Nerve infiltration by lymphoma, toxoplasmosis, and herpes zoster should also be considered in the setting of HIV infections (28–31).

Recent interest has also focused on the peripheral neuropathy in Lyme disease. The clinical spectrum of peripheral nerve involvement in Lyme disease is varied and includes pressure palsies, painful monoradiculopathies or polyradiculopathies, plexopathies, multifocal neuropathies, symmetric sensory or sensorimotor polyneuropathies, and even Guillain-Barré syndrome (GBS) (30,31,34,35). Involvement of the cranial nerves, especially the facial nerve, is also common. Patients can show rapid improvement with antibiotic treatment although additional immunosuppressive therapy is sometimes required. Necrotizing vasculitis is only rarely seen in sural nerve biopsy specimens, and there are no reports of *Borrelia* organisms being isolated from the peripheral nerve of patients proved to have Lyme disease (30,31). Therefore, although an ischemic neuropathy is suggested by the clinical profile, direct evidence of *Borrelia burgdorferi* infection of the vasa nervorum is lacking.

Systemic Necrotizing Vasculitis (Group 1)

The systemic necrotizing vasculitides represent a diverse group of conditions characterized by involvement of multiple organs. The peripheral and, less commonly, central nervous systems can be affected in any of these disorders (36). This group includes classic PAN, allergic angiitis and granulomatosis (Churg-Strauss syndrome), Wegener's granulomatosis, microscopic polyangiitis, and vasculitis secondary to underlying connective tissue disease (CTD) such as systemic rheumatoid vasculitis (37). Each disorder has distinguishing anatomic, pathologic, pathogenic, or clinical features. With the exception of classic PAN, these entities involve small arteries, arterioles, capillaries, and venules, with less frequent spread to medium-sized arteries (21,38). Three of these conditions (Wegener's granulomatosis, Churg-Strauss syndrome, and microscopic polyangiitis) can be grouped together in a subcategory known as the anti-neutrophil cytoplasmic antibody (ANCA)–associated vasculitides based on the finding of these antibodies in the serum (39,40).

Classic Polyarteritis Nodosa

Classic PAN has traditionally represented one of the most common forms of systemic necrotizing vasculitis and the one most liable to cause neuropathy (3,41). It is a multisystem disease of small and medium-sized arteries that affects peripheral nerves, skin, skeletal muscles, kidney, GI tract, liver, and testes (42). Abdominal angiography shows microaneurysms in the renal, hepatic, and visceral arteries in two thirds of patients. Laboratory studies reveal elevations in sedimentation rate and other inflammatory signs in most patients but the abnormalities are not specific (42). ANCAs are found in only 10% to 20% (43). Peripheral nerve involvement occurs in 60% of patients, based on a combination of data from various series (7,41,44–49).

PAN develops in association with hepatitis B surface antigenemia in approximately 30% of patients (10%–75% range) (50,51). In some patients, there is evidence of immune complex disease, suggesting that PAN is an infectious vasculitis triggered by the hepatitis B surface antigen. Clinical manifestations are similar to those in patients with PAN unrelated to hepatitis B, although neuropathy may be more common in the hepatitis B group (51).

Microscopic Polyangiitis

Microscopic polyangiitis is a systemic vasculitis that affects arterioles, capillaries, and venules primarily without granulomas or immune deposits in pathologic specimens (21). The clinical presentation is similar to that of PAN, but there is a nearly constant association with rapidly progressive glomerulonephritis, and pulmonary involvement occurs in 50% of patients (42). Palpable purpura is more common than in classic PAN, while hypertension is less frequent. Both hepatitis B surface antigenemia and visceral aneurysms are rare in microscopic polyangiitis. ANCA titers are positive in 80% to 90% of patients, the majority of ANCAs being antimyeloperoxidase (see below) (39,42). Based on recent series, the frequency of peripheral nerve involvement in microscopic polyangiitis is 20%, significantly less than that in classic PAN (52–54).

Churg-Strauss Syndrome

Churg-Strauss syndrome is an uncommon disorder characterized by necrotizing small-vessel vasculitis of the pulmonary and systemic circulations associated with asthma and eosinophilia (55). It occurs one third less frequently than PAN (56). The prodromal phase of this illness consists of asthma, often preceded by allergic rhinitis, lasting several years. The second phase is marked by peripheral blood eosinophilia and chronic eosinophilic pneumonia and gastroenteritis. Systemic vasculitis represents the third and final phase (55). Characteristic pathologic findings are eosinophilic tissue infiltration, necrotizing vasculitis, and extravascular granulomas (57). Only 40% of autopsies, however, reveal granulomas or eosinophilic infiltration and only

25% contain all three abnormalities (55). Similarly, just 10% to 20% of tissue biopsy specimens contain granulomas (58). Nerve biopsy specimens commonly show changes typical of PAN, but eosinophils and granulomas are only rarely observed (59,60). Peripheral neuropathy occurs in 65% of patients (55,58,61,62) and ANCAs are found in up to 75% (39,43).

Wegener's Granulomatosis

Wegener's granulomatosis is characterized by granulomatous inflammation of the upper and lower respiratory tracts and disseminated necrotizing vasculitis affecting small to medium-sized vessels (63,64). Necrotizing glomerulonephritis is a frequent accompaniment but may be absent in the "limited" form of the disease (64). Cytoplasmic-pattern ANCAs (c-ANCAs), with specificity for proteinase 3, are found in over 90% of patients with active disease (vide infra) (65). Peripheral neuropathies are present in approximately 15% of affected individuals (66–69). Cranial neuropathies, often multiple and most commonly involving nerves II, VI, or VII, occur in 10% of patients, but these are usually produced by contiguous extension from nasal or paranasal granulomas rather than vasculitis (66).

The diagnostic yield of head and neck biopsies is relatively low, with true granulomatous vasculitis found in just 20% of specimens. Open lung biopsy yields vasculitis or granulomatous inflammation in 90% of patients (69). Information on nerve pathology is sparse. In one series of 54 patients, 7.5% of postmortem examinations revealed peripheral nerve necrotizing arteriolitis (70); granulomatous inflammation is very rare, however (71). We saw three patients with Wegener's granulomatosis whose sural nerve biopsies revealed nongranulomatous vasculitis.

Polyangiitis Overlap Syndromes

This subgroup of systemic necrotizing vasculitis was proposed by Fauci et al to encompass patients exhibiting clinical features characteristic of more than one type of vasculitis, such as PAN with Churg-Strauss syndrome, PAN with hypersensitivity vasculitis, or temporal arteritis with Wegener's granulomatosis (72,73). Under the Chapel Hill nomenclature, where vasculitis types are determined in part by the presence or absence of small-vessel involvement, the preceding vasculitides would all be defined as the smaller-vessel form of the overlapping pair (Churg-Strauss syndrome, microscopic polyangiitis, and Wegener's granulomatosis, respectively) (21). In the clinical arena, however, the size of the affected vessels in particular cases of vasculitis is occasionally difficult to measure, preserving polyarteritis overlap as a practically useful concept.

Vasculitis Associated with Connective Tissue Disease

"Secondary" forms of systemic vasculitis, occurring in association with a CTD, can be contrasted with the "primary" forms of vasculitis just described. Secondary vasculitis is seen most commonly in rheumatoid arthritis (RA), less frequently in systemic lupus erythematosus (SLE) and Sjögren's syndrome, and rarely in scleroderma (74). The clinical and histopathologic features of the neuropathy and multiorgan involvement in these disorders closely resemble those in PAN, but a wider variety of blood vessels may be affected in CTD-related vasculitis, ranging from capillaries to large arteries (75).

Rheumatoid Arthritis

Autopsy series of RA patients consistently revealed a 25% prevalence of vasculitis (76). Since 40% to 50% of rheumatoid vasculitis patients develop peripheral nerve involvement (77,78), roughly 10% of RA patients will develop vasculitic neuropathy. Clinical studies of RA patients report a 1% to 10% incidence of peripheral neuropathy (74), permitting the inference that most of these neuropathies are vasculitic in origin. Despite these relatively low frequencies, RA is such a common disorder (affecting 1% of the population) (79) that rheumatoid vasculitis is the third most common cause of vasculitic neuropathy. While most rheumatoid patients with mononeuropathy multiplex have necrotizing vasculitis as shown by nerve biopsy (80), the findings in patients with the more common syndrome of chronic, distal, symmetric, sensory-predominant polyneuropathy are variable, and can include vasculitis (80), proliferative endarteritis (81), and normal vessels with demyelination-remyelination of the nerve (82). Intimal proliferation of small vessels producing obliterative endarteritis probably represents healing rheumatoid vasculitis.

Rheumatoid vasculitis–associated neuropathy typically occurs in the setting of long-standing (>10 years), seropositive RA with rheumatoid nodules and other extra-articular features (75,77,78,83). Conversely, arthritis and synovitis are usually not active. IgG rheumatoid factors (RFs) are strongly associated. The neuropathy is commonly preceded by cutaneous changes such as chronic nonhealing leg ulcers and nailfold infarcts. Other organs frequently affected are the spleen and eyes, with less consistent involvement of the heart, lungs, and bowels. While isolated cutaneous lesions and a sensory polyneuropathy can go on for years without additional evidence of multisystem vasculitis, widespread motor involvement is a poor prognostic sign demanding aggressive treatment (75).

Sjögren's Syndrome

Sjögren's syndrome is a chronic autoimmune polyexocrinopathy. The lacrimal and sweat glands are characteristically affected, producing keratoconjunctivitis sicca and xerostomia, but glands in the skin and other mucous membranes can also be targeted. If it occurs as an isolated phenomenon, the sicca syndrome is referred to as *primary Sjögren's syndrome;* it is classified as sec-

ondary when accompanied by features of another CTD such as RA (84). Proposed diagnostic criteria for primary Sjögren's syndrome were recently published by the European Community Study Group. These criteria require some combination of the following: appropriate ocular and oral symptoms, positive serologic markers (anti-Ro or anti-La), objective evidence of keratoconjunctivitis sicca by Schirmer's test or rose bengal staining, salivary gland biopsy showing at least one focal accumulation of lymphocytes, and objective findings of salivary gland dysfunction (scintigraphy, sialography, sialometry) (85). About 20% of patients develop vasculitis, either a small-vessel hypersensitivity type or a systemic necrotizing form simulating PAN (86). Vasculitis most frequently involves the skin, but bowels and kidneys are also commonly affected. Forty percent of vasculitic patients had a peripheral neuropathy in one series, typically a sensory-predominant polyneuropathy (87).

In series unselected for vasculitis, peripheral neuropathy occurred in approximately 20% of patients (88–90). A sensory-predominant, distal, symmetric polyneuropathy is most common, but asymmetric sensorimotor polyneuropathies or mononeuropathy multiplex occur in 15% (89). A more recently recognized syndrome is an ataxic, large-fiber, sensory neuronopathy (91). Five percent of patients will develop unilateral or bilateral trigeminal sensory neuropathies (88). Several pathologic series have intimated that most of the neuropathies are vasculitic in origin (88,89), but the sensory neuropathies can also result from infiltration of the dorsal root ganglia (91).

Systemic Lupus Erythematosus

In SLE, autoantibodies and circulating immune complexes are produced, and they activate complement and induce tissue damage (92). A systemic vasculitis is uncommon, however, with an approximately 15% incidence over the length of the illness (93). Lupus vasculitis can affect the skin, GI tract, nervous system, myocardium, lungs, kidney, and rarely, the pancreas, liver, and reproductive organs (75).

The frequency of neuropathy in large series of SLE patients is approximately 10% (94,95), but this increases to 20% when electrophysiologic criteria are used (96). The typical presentation is a subacute-to-chronic, distal, symmetric polyneuropathy that is sensory predominant (74). Asymmetric polyneuropathies and multiple mononeuropathies can account for one third of patients (95). Neuropathic symptoms are usually mild and obscured by those due to the extraneurologic involvement. Pathologic analysis of sural nerve biopsy specimens revealed necrotizing vasculitis in relatively few reports (8,11,14,15,97,98). More commonly, nonspecific fiber loss, axonal degeneration, and occasional perivascular inflammation are seen (97–99). Immune staining of epineurial and perineurial blood vessels for immunoglobulin and complement deposits is usually negative (98).

Systemic Sclerosis

Systemic sclerosis, or scleroderma, is a chronic, multisystem, inflammatory disorder caused by abnormal deposition of collagen in skin structures, blood vessels, and visceral organs, including the kidneys, lungs, GI tract, and heart (100). Although vascular involvement characterized by intimal thickening of arteries and arterioles is common (75), true vasculitis is rare: Only 7 of 832 patients reviewed by Oddis et al (101) had vasculitis (4 with peripheral neuropathy). Necrotizing vasculitis of the nerve has been shown pathologically on rare occasions (14,15,101). On the other hand, peripheral neuropathy occurs in a more robust 10% to 20% of patients with scleroderma (102,103) and isolated trigeminal neuropathy occurs in approximately 5% (104).

Hypersensitivity Vasculitis (Group 2)

As originally conceived, hypersensitivity vasculitis refers to a vasculitis involving small vessels, with skin as the primary target organ (1,105). Exposure to a precipitating antigen is implied (usually an infectious organism or drug) and immune complex deposition is the presumed pathogenic mechanism. Biopsy specimens classically show leukocytoclastic vasculitis. Clinical manifestations develop 7 to 14 days after antigen exposure and consist of palpable purpura, arthralgias, myalgias, constitutional symptoms, and rarely, symptoms referable to other organ involvement. The course is usually self-limited. Henoch-Schönlein purpura and serum sickness are classic examples of this syndrome.

Over the past 10 years, the concept of hypersensitivity vasculitis as a distinct entity has been challenged for several reasons (36,106). First, the precipitating antigens are often never identified, leaving a large "primary" or "idiopathic" group. Second, the spectrum of antigens that can trigger vasculitis now includes a variety of endogenous proteins as well as the traditional exogenous agents. Third, vasculitis secondary to a CTD or malignancy can produce a variable clinicopathologic picture, sometimes matching hypersensitivity vasculitis and at other times resembling PAN, creating overlap between groups 1 and 2 (107). Finally, many otherwise typical cases of hypersensitivity vasculitis progress to affect multiple organ systems, necessitating immunosuppressive treatment (108). Despite these ambiguities, hypersensitivity vasculitis is retained as a separate diagnostic entity in most current classification systems.

Drugs

A small-vessel vasculitis has been associated with many commonly used therapeutic agents, including sulfonamides, penicillin, ciprofloxacin, ofloxacin, erythromycin, isoniazid, hydralazine, trimethoprim-sulfamethoxazole, acyclovir, zidovudine, cyclophosphamide, methotrexate, and biologic agents such as interferon (IFN)-alpha and granulocyte colony-stimulating factor (22,109,110). Drugs of abuse, notably the amphetamines, cocaine, and heroin, can also cause a systemic vasculitis although neuropathy is uncommon (110,111).

Infections

A hypersensitivity vasculitis has been associated with infections by virtually all common bacterial, viral, fungal, mycobacterial, and parasitic microorganisms (22,23). Among bacteria, the gram-positive cocci predominate. Viruses most commonly implicated include hepatitis B and C viruses, CMV, HIV, and parvovirus B19. *Strongyloides stercoralis*, microfilariae, and *Ascaris* species are rarely reported parasitic causes of the syndrome. The two most common infectious causes of neuropathy—*B. burgdorferi* and HIV—have already been discussed.

Malignancy

Hypersensitivity vasculitis in the setting of hematologic malignancies is well described (107,112,113). The strongest association is for hairy cell leukemia where a leukocytoclastic angiitis or, less frequently, a systemic necrotizing vasculitis similar to PAN has been described (107,112). Although normally restricted to skin, peripheral nerve involvement occurs rarely as a multiple mononeuropathy. The angiitis often antedates the diagnosis of malignancy except in hairy cell leukemia, where it commonly appears after splenectomy.

A number of cases incriminate solid tumors in the development of vasculitis, most commonly a non-small-cell lung cancer (114–116). In a recent review of 37 such patients, muscle and nerve microvasculitis was identified in 24% of those presenting with a clinical profile of asymmetric sensorimotor polyneuropathy (116). Some of these patients responded to immunosuppressive therapy (117). Given the rarity of these reports in the face of the high prevalence of cancer, the possibility of a chance association cannot be excluded.

Essential Mixed Cryoglobulinemia

Cryoglobulinemia is a clinical syndrome associated with serum immunoglobulin proteins that precipitate in the cold and dissolve at higher temperatures (118,119). Common features include palpable purpura, arthralgias, Raynaud's phenomenon, skin ulcers, glomerulonephritis, and bleeding tendencies. Variable organ involvement occurs related to vascular and parenchymal deposits of circulating immune complexes. Three types of cryoglobulins have been described. Type I are monoclonal proteins, usually IgM, in patients with plasma cell dyscrasias. Type II are a mixture of IgM monoclonal immunoglobulins having RF activity and polyclonal IgG. Type III are a mixture of polyclonal RFs and polyclonal IgG. Type II and III cryoglobulinemias, also referred to as *mixed*, are associated with CTDs, chronic infections, chronic liver diseases, and plasma cell dyscrasias. Mixed cryoglobulinemia without a specific cause is termed *essential*.

Peripheral neuropathy occurs in approximately 50% of patients with essential mixed cryoglobulinemia (119–121). The neuropathy is usually a painful, distal, symmetric, sensorimotor polyneuropathy or, less commonly, an overlapping multiple mononeuropathy. The predominant pathogenesis, based on examination of sural nerve biopsy specimens, appears to be vasculitis of the vasa nervorum (121,122), although intravascular deposition of cryoglobulins causing occlusive microangiopathy (123) and IgM binding to the myelin sheath producing demyelination may contribute in rare patients (124).

The importance of essential mixed cryoglobulinemia–related vasculitis is its increased incidence of peripheral nerve involvement compared with other forms of hypersensitivity vasculitis and its potential for treatment. Conventional therapy has consisted of plasma exchange, usually in conjunction with prednisone and a cytotoxic agent (119,125). However, a new avenue of treatment has emerged with the realization that 80% of patients with essential mixed cryoglobulinemia have circulating antibodies against hepatitis C virus or express hepatitis C virus RNA in serum (125,126). Many such patients have now been successfully treated with the antiviral agent IFN alfa (see below).

Giant-Cell Arteritis (Group 3)

The term *giant-cell arteritis* refers to two entities, temporal arteritis and Takayasu's arteritis, both of which are necrotizing vasculitides involving large and medium-sized arteries characterized by granulomatous infiltration and giant-cell formation in affected vessels (127). As giant cells and granulomas are demonstrated in less than 50% of temporal artery biopsy specimens, their presence is not mandatory for diagnosis (127,128). The two arteritides are distinguished by unique clinical syndromes and differing but partially overlapping arterial distributions. Takayasu's disease is not reported to cause vasculitic neuropathies and will not be discussed further (129).

Temporal arteritis has a predilection for branches of the carotid artery and other aortic arch vessels, but a systemic disease can develop and involve arteries in many locations. The disorder is rare before age 50. An elevated erythrocyte sedimentation rate is an almost constant accompaniment. The illness is self-limited, usually following a 1- to 2-year course, with a very low fatality rate (128,130). Morbidity arises from the 10% to 20% risk of visual loss (131).

Several large series initially suggested that the incidence of peripheral nerve involvement is low (132). However, in a large population-based series from the Mayo Clinic, 12% of patients with temporal arteritis had peripheral neuropathic syndromes (excluding entrapments) (133). No nerve biopsy data were presented in this article, but two patients underwent arteriography, which demonstrated widespread arteritis in the lower limbs, and pathologic examination of an above-the-knee amputation specimen showed diffuse vasculitis of medium-sized and large arteries with sparing of the vasa nervorum. The authors speculated that the neuropathies resulted from nutrient artery vasculitis. In another report, sural nerve biopsy of a treated patient with a sensory polyneuropathy revealed changes consistent with healing arteritis in epineurial vessels, suggesting that both epineurial and nutrient artery involvement may contribute to the ischemic neuropathy of temporal arteritis (134).

Isolated Peripheral Nerve Vasculitis/Nonsystemic Vasculitic Neuropathy (Group 4)

A syndrome of nonsystemic vasculitis restricted to peripheral nerves has been increasingly recognized since the initial series of seven patients reported by Kissel et al in 1985 (11). Similar patients have now been reported by other investigators (13–18,31), establishing the condition as a specific nosologic entity with the following characteristics: 1) objective clinical evidence of peripheral neuropathy confirmed by electrodiagnostic studies; 2) sensory nerve biopsy showing pathologic features diagnostic of or highly suspicious for necrotizing vasculitis involving the arteries of the vasa nervorum (see Plate V); 3) no historical, examination, or laboratory evidence of organ involvement outside the peripheral nervous system (with the exception of skeletal muscle (see below)); and 4) no clinical or laboratory evidence of a CTD, exogenous agent, malignancy, or other condition known to be associated with necrotizing vasculitis. The relative incidence of nonsystemic vasculitic neuropathy is on the order of 25%, just behind PAN as the second most common reported cause of vasculitis affecting the peripheral nerve (Table 21-3).

The precise nature of the nonsystemic vasculitic neuropathy is uncertain. Similar forms of organ-specific vasculitis have been described for the central nervous system, GI tract (small bowel, colon, appendix, gallbladder, pancreas), skin, retina, and reproductive organs, and most of these conditions remain self-limited (36,135–138). Nonsystemic vasculitic neuropathy, therefore, may be one of a number of vasculitic diseases that are tissue specific and, thus, fundamentally different from the systemic necrotizing vasculitides. This is supported by the fact that isolated peripheral nerve vasculitis has a more indolent course and favorable prognosis than neuropathies complicating systemic vasculitis. In the series of Dyck et al (14), no patient with nonsystemic vasculitic neuropathy died of their disease during a mean follow-up of 11 years. In contrast, of the 41 patients with a systemic vasculitis affecting the nerves, 12 died over a shorter follow-up period.

On the other hand, the neurologic presentation of nonsystemic vasculitic neuropathy and the associated nerve biopsy findings are similar to those seen in classic PAN (11,14,15). Moreover, subclinical involvement of skeletal muscle is common (see Plate VI). Among 32 patients with isolated vasculitic neuropathy, Said et al (15) found necrotizing arteritis in 81% of muscle specimens,

Table 21-3.
Prevalence of Vasculitis Types in Vasculitic Neuropathy

Series	Vasculitis Type (No. of Patients)						
	CPAN or MPA	CSS	RV	NSVN	SLE	CTD NOS	Other*
Wees et al, 1981 (8)	11	0	5	0	1	0	0
Chang et al, 1984 (10)	8	0	9	1	0	0	1
Kissel et al, 1985 (11)	3	0	0	7	1	5	0
Bouche et al, 1986 (12)	16	6	0	0	0	0	0
Harati and Niakan, 1986 (13)	2	0	2	21	0	4	3
Dyck et al, 1987 (14)	32	4	2	20	1	0	6
Said et al, 1988 (15)	19	6	25	32	1	3	14
Panegyres et al, 1990 (16)	0	3	5	7	0	0	5
Hawke et al, 1991 (17) McCombe et al, 1987 (98)	11	3	7	2	3	8	3
Nicolai et al, 1995 (18)	2	4	1	2	0	7	4
Midroni and Balbao, 1995 (31)	3	3	8	4	2	10	2
Total (no. of patients (%))	107 (28)	29 (7.5)	64 (17)	96 (25)	9 (2.5)	37 (10)	

*This category includes cases associated with cryoglobulinemia, HIV, hypereosinophilic syndrome, hypersensitivity vasculitis, malignancy, monoclonal gammopathy of undetermined significance, polymyositis, Raynaud's phenomenon, sarcoidosis, scleroderma, Sjögren's syndrome, temporal arteritis, and Wegener's granulomatosis.
CPAN = classic polyarteritis nodosa; CSS = Churg-Strauss syndrome; CTD NOS = connective tissue disease not otherwise specified; MPA = microscopic polyangiitis; NSVN = nonsystemic vasculitic neuropathy; RV = rheumatoid vasculitis; SLE = systemic lupus erythematosus.

a finding supported by others (16). Therefore, isolated peripheral nerve vasculitis might best be conceptualized as a localized and more indolent form of PAN.

Clinical Presentation

The clinical manifestations of peripheral nerve vasculitis depend on the distribution and tempo of the vasculitic process. Whereas the signs and symptoms are similar whether the patient has a systemic vasculitis or nonsystemic vasculitic neuropathy, the accompanying extraneurologic features vary. Constitutional symptoms such as fever, weight loss, anorexia, myalgias, and arthralgias occur in at least 80% of patients with a systemic necrotizing vasculitis and approximately 50% of patients with nonsystemic vasculitis. Symptoms of multiorgan involvement—typically skin, joints, kidneys, lung/respiratory tract, and GI tract—should alert the clinician to the possibility of a systemic disorder (8–12,15,16,18,74).

The mean age at onset of vasculitic neuropathy is 55 to 60 years. The classic distribution, produced by a succession of ischemic insults to individual peripheral nerve trunks, is a multifocal neuropathy (multiple mononeuropathy), which occurs in about 45% of patients (7,8,11,12,14,17,18,31,46). Patients present with pain of acute or subacute onset, sensory loss, and weakness in the distribution of a single-named peripheral or cranial nerve. The neuropathy progresses in a stepwise fashion, migrating from one nerve territory to the next in a random fashion. The nerves most commonly involved include the proximal peroneal nerve in the leg and the proximal ulnar nerve in the arm (10,14,15). Both sensory and motor fibers are affected, except for rare patients with a pure sensory syndrome, usually seen with RA or Sjögren's syndrome (7,14). Pain is typical (50%–80% of patients), beginning with a deep, aching discomfort in the proximal limb that evolves into a burning, dysesthetic pain in the cutaneous distribution of the affected nerves (11,15,17,18).

In approximately 25% of patients, there is a steadily progressive deterioration that is accentuated in the distribution of particular peripheral nerves. This "overlapping," "extensive," or "confluent" multiple mononeuropathy pattern is also referred to as an *asymmetric polyneuropathy*. In these patients, examination always reveals significant side-to-side asymmetries.

The final and most difficult distribution to recognize is a slowly progressive, distal, symmetric, and typically sensorimotor polyneuropathy that occurs in 30% to 35% of patients (7–18,44). This results from widespread multifocal and random ischemic events occurring at many levels of the nerve trunk which, when summated, yield a distally accentuated and symmetric pattern. While some of the symmetrically evolving patients will provide a history of an asymmetric onset or a stuttering progression of deficits, others will have a symmetric and steadily progressing neuropathy from onset. Extensive electrodiagnostic testing in these patients is invaluable, exposing asymmetries or non-length-dependent properties atypical for a generalized polyneuropathy.

Vasculitis patients with a multiple mononeuropathy tend to present earlier (mean, 9.2 weeks) than patients with a symmetric polyneuropathy (mean, 20.4 weeks) (17). The progression is highly variable, however. The condition in some patients with rapidly progressive areflexic paralysis over 1 to 2 weeks can mimic GBS, while others may have a chronic, indolent course for years before diagnosis (11). These many clinical variants can confuse the most accomplished diagnostician and demand a high index of suspicion for accurate diagnosis. Any neuropathy with features of pain, asymmetric or non-length-dependent findings, constitutional symptoms, skin and other organ-system dysfunction, or an underlying autoimmune disorder should be investigated for a possible vasculitic basis.

Diagnostic Investigation

The diagnostic work-up of suspected vasculitic neuropathy involves laboratory studies, electrodiagnostic evaluation, and cutaneous nerve biopsy (often with simultaneous muscle biopsy). Serologic studies are useful to detect multiorgan involvement and can help diagnose a primary systemic vasculitis or CTD. Routine blood tests should include a complete blood cell count; eosinophil count; erythrocyte sedimentation rate; coagulation battery; urinalysis; renal and liver function tests; fasting glucose measurement; evaluations for antinuclear antibody (ANA), extractable nuclear antigen antibodies, RF, serum complements, cryoglobulins, and hepatitis B surface antigen; and serum immunofixation electrophoresis. Although 20% to 35% of patients with vasculitic neuropathies exhibit elevated protein levels in the cerebrospinal fluid, lumbar puncture contributes little to the diagnosis unless the patient has concurrent central nervous system dysfunction (9,12–14,16–18). Studies to be performed under the appropriate clinical circumstances include measurements of HIV and Lyme titers, circulating immune complexes, and serum angiotensin-converting enzymes; chest x-ray films; and determination of ANCA titers.

ANCAs have recently emerged as serologic markers for certain forms of systemic necrotizing vasculitis (38–40). Two ANCA patterns may be seen with indirect immunofluorescence of alcohol-fixed neutrophils: a cytoplasmic pattern (c-ANCA) and an artifactual perinuclear pattern (p-ANCA). c-ANCA is a very specific and sensitive marker for active Wegener's granulomatosis (65). p-ANCAs demonstrate reasonable sensitivity for microscopic polyangiitis and Churg-Strauss syndrome but lack specificity because positive results occur in a wide diversity of diseases. This fact was borne out by the only prospective study of ANCA testing for the diagnosis of vasculitic neuropathy, which showed a high p-ANCA false-positive rate, making p-ANCA too nonspecific for routine use in diagnosing de novo neuropathy patients (139).

In patients with nonsystemic vasculitic neuropathy, laboratory testing is usually normal except for the sedimentation rate which can be mildly elevated (<60 mm/hr) in about 50% (11,14–16). For patients with systemic vasculitic neuropathies, laboratory abnormalities are common and include an elevated sedimentation rate (85%), leukocytosis (70%), mild anemia (45%), positive ANA titer (30%), positive RF (40%), hypocomplementemia (50%), and hepatitis B surface antigenemia (30%) (8–12,15–18,44). None of these tests are specific for a single entity and correlation with the clinical profile is mandatory.

Nerve conduction studies and needle electrode examination provide crucial information in the work-up of a patient. Electrodiagnostic studies can reveal involvement of clinically unaffected nerves, allowing diagnosed distal symmetric polyneuropathies to be reclassified as overlapping multifocal neuropathies (12,140,141). The studies can also establish a baseline for the degree and pattern of axon loss to serve as a reference in monitoring the patient's future course. Perhaps most importantly, they provide guidance in the determination of which sensory nerve to biopsy (8).

The electrodiagnostic findings in vasculitic neuropathies reflect the underlying neuropathology of multifocal axonal degeneration (7–14,17,18,74,141). On standard nerve conduction studies, the amplitudes of compound sensory and motor action potentials are reduced (or absent), while distal latencies and conduction velocities are normal or nearly so. Sensory responses are more pervasively affected than motor conductions and abnormalities are usually more prominent in the lower extremities, especially in the peroneal and sural nerves. Sural responses are typically absent or of low amplitude. In the upper extremities, the ulnar nerve is most commonly affected, with the median nerve more often involved than the radial. H-reflexes are either low in amplitude or unelicitable with a normal latency, similar to the F-wave findings.

Nerve conduction study results supporting the presence of a multifocal axon-loss process include a more than twofold difference in amplitude between the right and left motor or sensory compound action potentials of homologous nerves, a significant amplitude reduction in one nerve but not others in the same limb, or a low-amplitude response in an upper-extremity nerve while amplitudes are normal in the lower extremities (74,142). Transient conduction block can occasionally be identified if a patient is studied in the first week after an ischemic lesion has developed. As acute axonal degeneration evolves, the distal nerve segment remains capable of conducting impulses for about 6 days with motor fibers and 9 to 10 days with sensory fibers. This so-called axon noncontinuity conduction block will disappear over the course of a week as the distal stump degenerates (74,141).

Needle electrode examination usually demonstrates active partial denervation, with fibrillations and positive sharp waves in about half of the patients and markedly decreased motor unit recruitment in clinically affected muscles (8,11,17,18,74,141). Chronic neurogenic or reinnervational motor unit potentials can be seen with long-standing disease. Proximal muscles may show as much denervation as distal muscles, clear evidence that the process is not length dependent (11,18,142).

While electrodiagnostic findings in vasculitic neuropathy predominantly reflect axon loss, demyelinating features can infrequently be encountered (11,14,17,143), most likely due either to transient metabolic failure or to secondary paranodal and segmental demyelination (144,145). Nevertheless, *persistent* conduction block and demyelinating-range slowing of conduction velocities should always provoke reconsideration of the diagnosis.

Definitive diagnosis of vasculitic neuropathy requires

pathologic confirmation, obtained through biopsy of a cutaneous sensory nerve, usually the sural or superficial peroneal (8,15,31). If the lower limbs are not involved, a rarity in vasculitic syndromes, the superficial radial nerve is the next choice for pathologic examination (146). The yield for vasculitis is enhanced if the sensory nerve in question is involved both clinically and electrodiagnostically. Biopsy of the superficial peroneal nerve is usually preferred because a simultaneous peroneus brevis muscle biopsy can be obtained through the same incision, increasing the diagnostic yield. In a report by Said et al (15), vasculitis was revealed more frequently in the peroneous brevis muscle than the superficial peroneal nerve in 83 patients with biopsy-proved systemic or nonsystemic vasculitic neuropathies. The muscle biopsy study was diagnostic in 80% and the nerve biopsy study in 55% of these patients (15). We, too, found the superficial peroneal nerve/peroneus brevis muscle biopsy to be a useful procedure in diagnosing vasculitis of the nerve because muscle occasionally revealed vasculitis not seen in the nerve. In our experience, however, the relative yield of muscle and nerve biopsy is reversed from that reported by Said et al (15), nerve being diagnostic in 90% and muscle in 50%.

The sensitivity of nerve biopsy for detection of nerve vasculitis is not known. Dyck et al (14) reported that in 45 patients with systemic necrotizing vasculitis and neuropathy, sural nerve biopsy was diagnostic in 26 (58%), suggestive in 13 (29%), and negative in 6 (13%). While useful, these figures do not provide a true sensitivity because of the lack of a "gold standard" (31). Similar data do not exist for superficial peroneal nerve/peroneus brevis muscle biopsy.

The diagnosis of vasculitis requires the finding of inflammatory cell infiltration within the blood vessel wall along with evidence of vascular destruction such as fibrinoid necrosis, thrombosis, hemorrhage, or endothelial cell disruption (see Plate VII) (31,99,129,147). Perivascular or transmural inflammation without accompanying structural damage is not sufficient but can be suggestive in the proper clinical context. Transmural inflammation with karyorrhexis of the infiltrating cells, the so-called leukocytoclastic reaction, can also indicate vasculitis. If no active lesion is identified, a presumptive diagnosis can still be made if signs of a remote or healing vasculitis are present, such as intimal hyperplasia with luminal narrowing or thrombosis, vascular sclerosis with recanalization, or periadventitial hemosiderin-filled macrophages (see Plate VIII) (31,129).

Vasculitis of the nerve has a predilection for small epineurial arteries with diameters in the 75- to 250-μm range (6,11,14,17,44). The nerve fascicles themselves almost always show a reduction in myelinated nerve fibers, and the fiber loss is characteristically asymmetric between and within fascicles (see Plate IX). A central fascicular or peripheral sector pattern of fiber loss is highly suggestive of ischemia (6,11,14,31,148). Larger myelinated fibers (>7 μm in diameter) are more vulnerable to ischemia than smaller fibers, and myelinated fibers in general are more susceptible than unmyelinated fibers (122,148). Teased fibers reveal acute

axonal degeneration with minimal evidence of demyelination/remyelination (14,148).

While pathologic changes in nerve biopsy specimens are similar in all forms of vasculitis, detailed analysis of the caliber of the involved vessels and the nature of the inflammatory infiltrates can reveal some characteristic predilections (14,31,129). The larger epineurial arteries (100–250 μm) are most typically affected in PAN, rheumatoid vasculitis, Churg-Strauss syndrome, and Wegener's granulomatosis, while smaller epineurial vessels (<100 μm) are more commonly involved in nonsystemic vasculitic neuropathy, Sjögren's syndrome, and SLE. Endoneurial vessels are characteristically inflamed in hypersensitivity vasculitis, but might also be involved in microscopic polyangiitis, Churg-Strauss syndrome, Wegener's granulomatosis, and the CTDs. A marked eosinophilic infiltration suggests Churg-Strauss syndrome (31,59). Granulomatous angiitis appears very infrequently in peripheral nerve specimens; when present, Wegener's granulomatosis or Churg-Strauss syndrome is the most likely diagnosis (60,71), but granulomas have also been reported in PAN, lupus, and rheumatoid vasculitis (31,147).

Immunohistochemical characterization of the cellular infiltrates in nerve biopsy specimens from patients with vasculitic neuropathies has shown a predominance of T lymphocytes (50%–70% of cells) distributed throughout the vessel wall (see Plate X) (16,149–151). Macrophages are less prominent, comprising about 30% of the inflammatory cells. B lymphocytes and polymorphonuclear leukocytes have been sparse in most studies. Immunofluorescent staining with antisera against IgG, IgA, IgM, and complement is positive in epineurial blood vessel walls in 70% of patients (16,17,149), a finding that, in our experience, is specific for vasculitic neuropathy; it is not found in normal and nonvasculitic neuropathy control subjects (see Plate XII) (152).

Pathogenesis

Although the systemic vasculitides are assumed to be autoimmune disorders, the pathogenic mechanisms involved remain poorly understood, and the antigens that trigger the immunologic cascades are unknown except for a few of the secondary syndromes such as hepatitis B virus–related PAN. While significant progress has been made over the past 10 years in understanding the effector phase of the vasculitic immune response, our knowlege of the initiation phase is still primitive. The factors determining which particular organs and blood vessel types will be affected are also poorly understood. In view of the clinicopathologic diversity of the many vasculitic syndromes, multiple triggering events, antigens, immunologic responses, and perpetuating mechanisms probably exist (38,153,154).

The pathogenesis of vasculitis can be conceptualized using a common paradigm which begins with antigen recognition by the host that initiates a humoral or cellular immune response. The evolving immune response then disrupts the homeostasis between circulating leukocytes and endothelial cells, resulting in the adherence of selected leukocyte populations to the endothelial surface, a process that depends on a complex network of cellular adhesion molecules and soluble mediators that alter their expression (153–155). Subsequently, an equally complex array of cytokines, chemotactic agents, and other inflammatory regulators are produced and mediate leukocyte and endothelial cell activation, adherence of additional effector cells (neutrophils, eosinophils, monocytes, or T lymphocytes), and transendothelial migration of leukocytes (156,157). The effector cells damage the vessel wall by several mechanisms, including degradative enzyme release, respiratory burst–induced production of toxic oxygen free radicals, phagocytosis, perforin- or complement membrane attack complex–mediated cytolysis, or enzyme-induced apoptosis (38,158,159). The recruited inflammatory cells continue to manufacture and release new cytokines that recruit new effector and regulatory immune cells to the site, promote procoagulant tendencies, and induce local connective tissue reactions. Eventually, anti-inflammatory cytokines and regulatory growth factors gain supremacy and the inflammatory cells either die, emigrate into the tissues, or recirculate, while endothelial cells, fibroblasts, and smooth muscle cells proliferate. The final result is a thickened, scarred, and thrombosed or occluded blood vessel (154,160,161).

Central to the process of vascular inflammation is a dramatic upregulation, in both endothelial cells and leukocytes, of the surface expression of molecules that support intercellular adhesion. Before this can develop, however, a primary immunologic event must occur to send out signals to "prime" the circulating leukocytes and stimulate the involved endothelial cells (38). Three large families of cellular adhesion molecules have been characterized: the selectins, integrins, and immunoglobulin superfamily (162–166). Chemoattractant molecules, including the recently recognized family of chemoattractant cytokines, or chemokines, are also integral mediators of the leukocyte–endothelial cell interaction (157,167,168).

The adhesion molecules control and regulate leukocyte emigration from the vasculature at sites of inflammation in at least four sequential steps (Fig 21-1) (165,169,170). Leukocytes first attach to the vessel wall in a rolling fashion and remain tethered there by selectin-carbohydrate and α_4 integrin–ligand interactions. The second step requires activation of the tethered leukocyte, a process mediated by the chemoattractant molecules. The rolling leukocytes then arrest, spread, and firmly adhere, owing to integrin–immunoglobulin superfamily molecule interactions. Predominant molecular adhesion pairs are very late antigen (VLA)-4/vascular cell adhesion molecule (VCAM)-1, leukocyte function–associated antigen (LFA)-1/intercellular adhesion molecule (ICAM)-1, and LFA-1/ICAM-2.

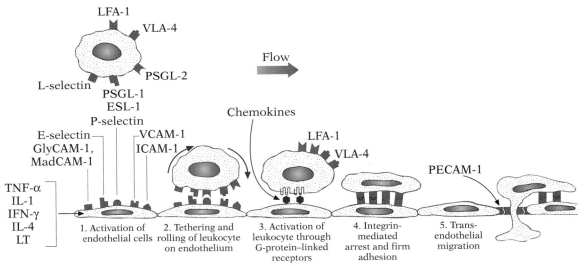

Figure 21-1. Multistep model of leukocyte emigration in inflammation. Endothelial cells are activated by inflammatory cytokines such as tumor necrosis factor (TNF)-α, interleukin (IL)-1, interferon (IFN)-γ, IL-4, and lymphotoxin (LT) to increase surface expression of E- and P-selectins, intercellular adhesion molecule (ICAM)-1, and vascular cell adhesion molecule (VCAM)-1. Circulating leukocytes then attach to the endothelium and roll on this surface by means of the selectins, α_4 integrins such as very late antigen (VLA)-4, and their ligands. Leukocyte integrin activation next occurs, producing higher-affinity VLA-4 and lymphocyte function–associated antigen (LFA)-1 molecules, with G protein–linked chemokine receptors as the putative signal. The leukocyte-endothelial interaction is then strengthened, leading to leukocyte arrest, firm adhesion, and flattening, mediated by integrin–immunoglobulin superfamily member pairings (LFA-1/ICAM-1; VLA-4/VCAM-1). The same molecules participate in the final step, transendothelial migration, complemented by platelet–endothelial cell adhesion molecule (PECAM)-1 found on both leukocytes and the intercellular junctions of endothelial cells. GlyCAM = glycosylation-dependent cell adhesion molecule; MadCAM = mucosal addressin cell adhesion molecule; PSGL = P-selectin glycoprotein ligand; ESL = E-selectin ligand.

Transendothelial migration, the final step, is dependent on continued activation by chemoattractants and the formation of new adhesion contacts at the migration front. The adhesion force is modulated by the transience of the augmented integrin function and by shedding of adhesion molecules such as L-selectin, E-selectin, and ICAM-1. Diapedesis is also dependent on an interaction between leukocyte and endothelial cell platelet–endothelial cell adhesion molecule (PECAM)-1, an immunoglobulin superfamily member concentrated at endothelial tight junctions.

Soluble forms of the adhesion molecules are produced by proteolytic cleavage in situ or by alternatively spliced transcripts missing the transmembrane region (165). Assays for these circulating molecules in patients with systemic vasculitis have revealed consistently elevated levels of soluble(s) ICAM-1 and sVCAM-1 and variable increases in sE-selectin (154,171,172). In the only series devoted to vasculitic neuropathy, there was a significant elevation of sE-selectin in patients with systemic or nonsystemic vasculitis of the nerve compared with healthy control subjects and patients with other neurologic diseases (173). Increased levels of circulating adhesion molecules are considered a sign of endothelial cell activation in response to cytokines and other inflammatory stimuli. An in situ study of muscle and nerve biopsy specimens in seven patients with vasculitic neuropathies demonstrated increased endothelial expression of ICAM-1 in all patients, while E-selectin was present in only one patient (174).

The "pathogenic" features of the endothelial-leukocyte interactions are those induced by cytokines and other inflammatory mediators. The specific patterns of cytokine release and function pertinent to the vasculitides have been difficult to decipher, although pioneering work has begun. Most investigations to date evaluated serum levels of soluble cytokines or expression by circulating leukocytes (154,175–177). These have detected elevated levels or expression of interleukin (IL)-1, tumor necrosis factor (TNF)-α, IL-2, IL-6, soluble IL-2 receptor (sIL-2r), IL-8, lymphotoxin, transforming growth factor-β, IFN-α, and IFN-γ. The elevations of IL-2 and IFN-α were most significant and correlated with treatment in one study (176).

Within this framework of antigen-specific immunity progressing to an effector phase marked by vascular inflammation and destruction, four predominant intermediary mechanisms have been proposed, three involving humoral or antibody-mediated processes and the fourth a T cell–mediated process (38,153,154). Of the three humoral schemes, passive deposition of circulating immune complexes has undergone the most extensive study (Fig 21-2) (178,179). In this model, antibodies interact with circulating antigens under conditions of slight antigen excess to form complexes of varying size (37,178). These complexes activate complement, becoming coated with C3b and C4b and priming circulating leukocytes. Under normal circumstances, the erythrocyte C3b receptors bind the antigen-complement complexes and transport them to the liver for clearance (178,180). Pathogenic deposition in vessel walls occurs if the host's clearance mechanisms are overcome (or flawed), the immune complexes acquire certain physical properties (medium sized and cationic), or the vessel walls are abnormally permeable (178,180). Local deposition of immune complexes activates the complement cascade, generating the neutrophil chemotaxin C5a and other inflammatory mediators. Neutrophils are recruited to the site, interact with the complexed immunoglobulins by engagement of their Fc receptors, and undergo phagocytosis (38,153). The final effector pathway, outlined above, is then implemented.

This mechanism is believed to subserve most types of

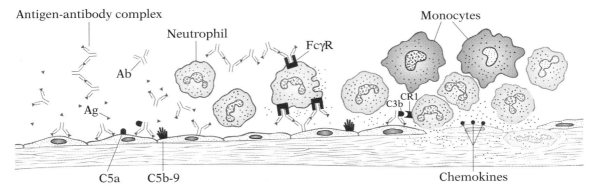

Figure 21-2. Schematic representation of immune complex–mediated vascular damage. Circulating antigen (Ag)-antibody (Ab) complexes form in antigen excess and deposit in blood vessel walls. Complement components are then activated, generating chemoattractants (C3a, C5a) that recruit neutrophils to the site. Further complement activation leads to assembly of the C5b-9 membrane attack complex, promoting cellular lysis, and opsonization of the immune complexes with C3b fragments. Neutrophils bind to C3b-coated complexes via specific complement receptors such as CR1 as well as Fc receptors for IgG (FcγR). Activated neutrophils release proteolytic enzymes and reactive oxygen metabolites that damage the vessel wall. Subsequently formed chemokines (e.g., interleukin-8, monocyte chemoattractant protein-1) and other chemoattractants secondarily recruit and activate monocytes and additional neutrophils. This cascade amplifies vascular destruction and promotes vessel thickening, thombosis, and occlusion.

hypersensitivity vasculitis related to infections, drugs, malignancy, and cryoglobulinemia, and also hepatitis B–associated PAN (37,180). In addition, many of the secondary vasculitides related to CTDs may be mediated by immune complex mechanisms triggered by endogenous antigens (75,180). Circulating immune complexes, however, are not typically found in many other vasculitic disorders, including Wegener's granulomatosis, Churg-Strauss syndrome, non–hepatitis B–associated PAN, microscopic polyangiitis, and temporal arteritis (21,181), for which a second potential mechanism of humorally mediated vasculitis may apply: in situ immune complex formation within the vessel wall due to anti–endothelial cell antibodies (182). Target antigens could be constitutive components of the blood vessel wall or foreign antigens, but none have been identified. An immune response would be facilitated by the antigen-presenting ability of endothelial cells (183). Numerous studies documented the presence of anti–endothelial cell antibodies in 40% to 80% patients with systemic vasculitis, including Wegener's granulomatosis, microscopic polyangiitis, Churg-Strauss syndrome, rheumatoid vasculitis, and Sjögren's syndrome (184). In the only study of patients with vasculitis of the peripheral nerve and muscle, anti–endothelial cell antibodies were present in only 2 of 12 patients, raising questions about their pathogenic significance in vasculitic neuropathies (174).

ANCAs, which react against specific proteins in the cytoplasm of neutrophils and monocytes, represent a third potential mechanism of humorally mediated vascular damage in the vasculitides (38–40). Almost all c-

ANCAs recognize proteinase 3 (PR3) and most p-ANCAs are directed against myeloperoxidase (MPO). PR3 and MPO are constituents of the neutrophil's azurophilic granules and can also be found in the peroxidase-positive lysosomes of monocytes. Based on in vitro data, ANCAs may cause vasculitis by activating primed neutrophils to adhere to endothelial cells, undergo degranulation and respiratory burst, and lyse the adherent cells (185,186). An alternative mechanism derives from data showing that endothelial cells can be upregulated by TNF-α, IL-1, and IFN-γ to express PR3 both in the cytoplasm and in the cell membrane (187). ANCAs specific for PR3, when bound to their antigen in the endothelial cell membrane, induce membrane expression of E-selectin and VCAM-1, thereby enhancing endothelial adhesion of leukocytes, and also lyse those endothelial cells via an antibody-dependent cellular cytotoxicity mechanism (188). A third proposal suggests that ANCA binding to target antigens inhibits inactivation of those antigens by natural inhibitors (α_1-antitrypsin in the case of PR3), prolonging their tissue-damaging capability (189).

Although antibody-mediated mechanisms appear important in some forms of vasculitis, there are compelling data to support a crucial role for cellular immunity as well (Fig 21-3) (153,154). The occurrence of granulomas in Wegener's granulomatosis, Churg-Strauss syndrome, and temporal arteritis is prima facie evidence that T-cell and macrophage responses are involved in these disorders, confirmed by phenotypic analyses of pulmonary and renal cellular infiltrates in patients with Wegener's granulomatosis and temporal

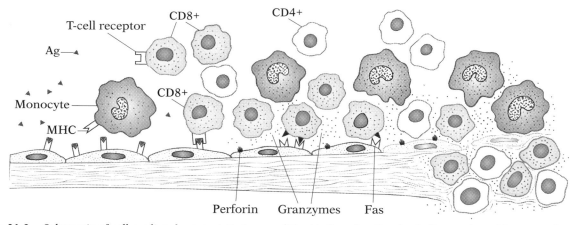

Figure 21-3.   Schematic of cell-mediated cytotoxicity in vasculitis. At sites of antigenic challenge, chemokines are released and enhance recruitment of circulating monocytes and T lymphocytes. CD8+ T cells recognize antigens (Ag) presented by major histocompatibility complex (MHC) class I–bearing endothelial cells and monocytes, while CD4+ T cells recognize antigens in the context of MHC class II molecules. Antigenic signals transform the T cells into activated cytotoxic (predominantly CD8+) and helper/inducer (CD4+) subsets. Cytokines generated by the stimulated mononuclear inflammatory cells recruit additional lymphocytes and monocytes to the area. Activated monocytes secrete degradative enzymes and reactive oxygen species, damaging the vessel wall nonspecifically. Cytotoxic T cells destroy antigen-bearing cells specifically via two independent pathways. In the first, cytoplasmic granules are secreted toward the target cell. Perforin aggregates form membrane pores through which proteolytic granzymes enter the cell, triggering DNA fragmentation and apoptosis. In the second, nonsecretory pathway, upregulated Fas ligand on the surface of the cytotoxic T cell interacts with Fas antigen on the target cell, resulting in the delivery of a separate apoptotic signal.

artery infiltrates in patients with temporal arteritis showing a predominance of T cells and macrophages with variable CD4+/CD8+ ratios (190–192). Studies of the cellular infiltrates of patients with vasculitic neuropathy revealed similar findings (16,149–151), with most T cells being of the CD8+ cytotoxic/suppressor subset in our series (149). B cells are rare and immune deposits are seen only in heavily infiltrated vessels. These findings suggest that cell-mediated cytotoxicity, perhaps directed against the endothelium, is an important pathogenic mechanism in systemic and nonsystemic peripheral nerve vasculitis. Another observation implicating T cells in the pathogenesis of systemic necrotizing vasculitis is the therapeutic response shown by some patients to cyclosporine, a drug with T-cell actions, and to monoclonal antibodies directed against T-cell antigens (193,194). Moreover, a recent study of cytokine messenger RNA (mRNA) expression in temporal artery biopsy specimens from patients with temporal arteritis found a predominance of IL-2 and IFN-γ, a profile typical of the Th1 subset of helper T cells that mediate delayed-type hypersensitivity reactions (195).

Regardless of which immunologic mechanism is operant in any particular case of vasculitis, the final common pathway of nonvascular tissue damage is regional ischemia due to occlusion of the involved blood vessels. Peripheral nerve has a very rich anastomotic blood supply composed of two functionally distinct and partially independent vascular systems (31,196). The extrinsic system comprises the regional nutrient arteries along with the epineurial vasculature, while the intrinsic system consists of the longitudinal microvessels within the fascicles themselves. These two systems are linked by a complex pattern of interconnecting vessels that provide a relatively high blood flow in the baseline state (197). This rich blood supply, coupled with the ability of the nerve to tolerate anaerobic conditions, helps the peripheral nerve resist the effects of chronic ischemia (196). Only with extensive involvement of the vasa nervorum, as occurs in vasculitis, does ischemia-induced axonal degeneration result. Nerve injury is most prominent in the "watershed" zones of poor perfusion (6,129). In the upper limb, the median and ulnar nerves frequently receive no nutrient arteries between the axilla and elbow, while in the lower limb, the sciatic nerve receives few feeding vessels between the inferior gluteal and popliteal arteries. Hence, major nerve trunks are most vulnerable to peripheral nerve vasculitis in the mid-upper-arm and mid-thigh levels, matching the clinical data presented previously.

Treatment and Outcome

Once a patient's diagnosis has been confirmed by biopsy, an appropriate therapeutic regimen can be planned. Unfortunately, therapy based on an in-depth understanding of underlying pathogenic mechanisms is not yet possible for the primary vasculitides and treatment decisions must still be grounded on predominantly anecdotal empiric data. Because no prospective treatment trials for peripheral nerve vasculitis exist, management of vasculitic neuropathy depends on information available for the systemic vasculitis syndromes, much of which is retrospective (108,198,199). Four therapeutic principles should be considered: 1) removal of any inciting antigens, 2) institution of immunosuppressive therapy, 3) management of vaso-occlusive disease, and 4) provision of appropriate supportive care.

Antigen Removal

Identifiable antigens are infrequent in most vasculitic syndromes, classically occurring only in hypersensitivity vasculitis caused by drugs and infections. In these instances, removal of the implicated drug or treatment of the infectious process can result in resolution of the vasculitis (Fig 21-4) (22,108,199). The same principle applies to vasculitis associated with malignancy, although the vasculitic response to treatment of the cancer is variable and often negative (112). More recently, it has been recognized that hepatitis B virus–associated PAN and hepatitis C virus–associated mixed cryoglobulinemia respond well to antiviral therapy. Specifically, in several studies, patients with hepatitis B virus–related PAN were successfully treated using a short course of prednisone and prolonged courses of plasma exchange plus an antiviral agent, either vidarabine or INF alfa-2b (51,200). Thirty-three (80%) of 41 patients recovered from PAN and 45% were cured of the hepatitis B infection. Similarly, cryoglobulinemic vasculitis associated with hepatitis C virus has been managed successfully with INF alfa-2a (201). Recent reports indicated a 70% response rate, although the neuropathy is more refractory than the skin manifestations and treatment discontinuation has uniformly led to a relapse of both the viremia and the clinical syndrome (202,203).

Immunosuppression

In most patients with vasculitic neuropathy, the inciting antigen is unknown and an immunosuppressive regimen must be implemented (see Fig 21-4). The classification system employed for patients with peripheral nerve vasculitis (see Table 21-2) can be used to assist with this treatment decision. For patients with a systemic necrotizing vasculitis and peripheral nerve involvement (group 1), therapy usually involves a combination of glucocorticoids (usually prednisone) and a cytotoxic agent (usually cyclophosphamide) because of the established effectiveness of this regime in Wegener's granulomatosis, PAN, and isolated CNS angiitis (67,199,204). In patients with hypersensitivity vasculitis (group 2) and widespread or severe involvement (visceral ischemia, glomerulonephritis, or progressive neuropathy), treatment is usually initiated with glucocorticoids alone, with cytotoxic drugs added only for lack of response or steroid-sparing effect (108). Vasculitic neuropathies resulting from temporal arteritis (group 3) will generally respond to corticosteroid monotherapy (130,198). In patients with a nonsystemic vasculitic neuropathy (group 4), treatment should be modified from that utilized for group 1 vasculitides be-

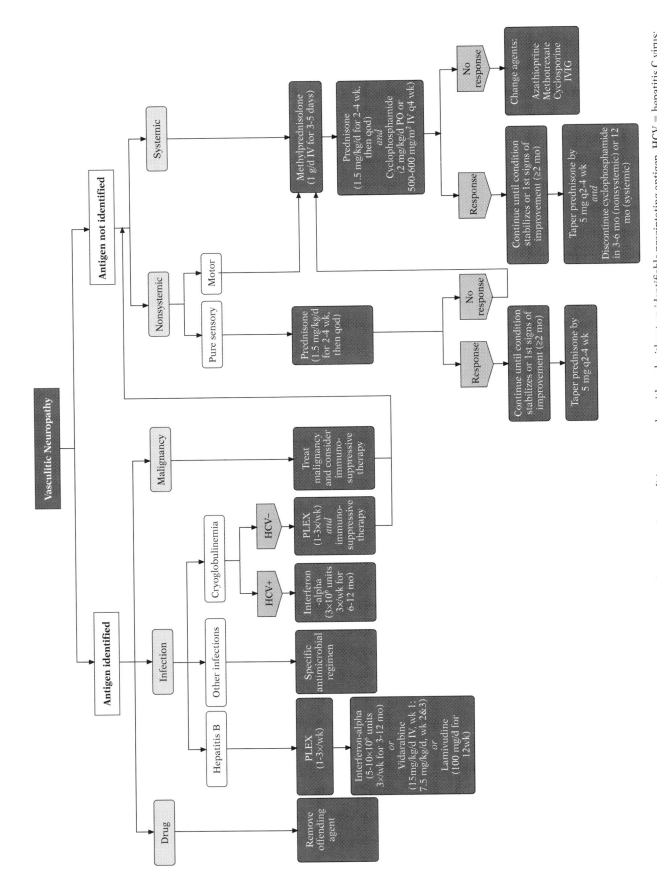

Figure 21-4. Algorithm for the treatment of systemic and nonsystemic vasculitic neuropathy with and without an identifiable precipitating antigen. HCV = hepatitis C virus; PLEX = plasma exchange; IVIG = intravenous immunoglobulin.

cause the condition is not immediately life-threatening and the neurologic prognosis is less ominous (14,17). For patients with mild, sensory-predominant symptoms, treatment is usually initiated with prednisone alone, while severe, rapidly progressive, or motor neuropathies are best managed with a combination of glucocorticoids and a cytotoxic agent (as in group 1), but the cytotoxic drug can be discontinued as soon as 3 months if an early response is shown.

A standard immunosuppressive regimen for systemic vasculitis consists of prednisone, 1.5 mg/kg/day, and cyclophosphamide, 1.5 to 2.5 mg/kg/day, both administered in a single-morning dose. In fulminant cases, intravenous methylprednisolone can be used for induction, 1000 mg every other day for six total doses or 15 mg/kg/day over 3 to 5 consecutive days (108,146,205). Higher induction doses of oral cyclophosphamide (up to 5 mg/kg/day for 2–5 days) can also be employed in life-threatening situations (64).

Following 2 to 4 weeks of daily therapy, the prednisone is switched to an every-other-day schedule at the same dose, while cyclophosphamide is continued without change. This regimen is then maintained for at least 3 months. Neurologic recovery is typically extremely slow since it depends on axonal regeneration. The first signs of improvement will usually be increased strength in proximal muscles. Once the clinical condition has stabilized, the prednisone can be slowly tapered, usually at a rate of 5 mg every 2 to 3 weeks. If the disease relapses, a re-bolus with prednisone or methylprednisolone is indicated, at doses equivalent to the initial therapy. Cyclophosphamide is continued for at least 1 year after disease stabilization and then stopped.

Corticosteroids are known to have a broad range of immunosuppressive and anti-inflammatory effects, influencing virtually every humoral and cellular immune mechanism (206–209). At standard doses, corticosteroids have a greater impact on T lymphocytes than B lymphocytes, including a stronger inhibition of T-cell proliferation and differentiation in response to antigens and IL-2 (206–209). Low doses do not affect B cell–mediated antibody synthesis. Daily high-dose therapy will suppress antibody production and the humoral response after a 2- to 4-week delay. Mononuclear phagocytes are also prominently antagonized by glucocorticoids; chemotaxis, ability to process and present antigens, stimulated release of cytokines, and phagocytic capabilities are all inhibited. In addition, steroids block endothelial cell activation and upregulation of adhesion molecules, reduce production of various cytokines, and decrease synthesis of proinflammatory eicosanoids (207–209).

Cyclophosphamide is an alkylating agent that acts by cross-linking DNA, thereby interfering with DNA replication and RNA transcription, reducing cell division and clonal expansion of both B and T lymphocytes. It has wide-ranging effects and influences nearly every component of the cellular and humoral immune response (210–212). Acute intravenous doses are most toxic to B cells and suppressor T cells (210). While responses to chronic low-dose therapy are mixed, there appears to be a preferential suppression of B-cell function, as cell-mediated reactions are not consistently inhibited (212,213). Macrophage cytotoxicity is also reduced by cyclophosphamide.

Immunosuppressive treatment with steroids and cytotoxic agents has had a dramatic impact on the natural history of systemic vasculitis. Prior to the introduction of immunosuppressives, the prognosis for PAN was extremely poor, with a 5-year survival rate of about 10% (47,48). With the advent of corticosteroid monotherapy, the 5-year survival rate increased to 50% to 70% (47,48), further improving to 75% to 80% with steroid/cytotoxic combination chemotherapy (204). Equally impressive results have been reported for Wegener's granulomatosis, a disease that untreated is associated with a 5-month mean survival time. Glucocorticoid treatment alone improves the outcome only marginally whereas combination therapy results in a 90% complete remission or even "cure" rate (67).

Unfortunately, extended follow-up studies have identified several problems with the standard combination regimen, including a higher relapse rate, less complete efficacy, greater disease morbidity, and more prevalent drug toxicity than had previously been appreciated. In a 24-year follow-up study of 158 patients with Wegener's granulomatosis, most treated with daily cyclophosphamide and corticosteroids, only 75% achieved complete remission and 50% had a relapse (68). Permanent disease-related morbidity occurred in 86% while 43% had serious drug-induced side effects such as hemorrhagic cystitis (43%), cataracts (21%), osteoporosis-related fractures (11%), aseptic necrosis (3%), bladder cancer (2.8%), and myelodysplasia (2%). There was a 2.4-fold overall increase in malignancy compared with the rate in the general population, including a 33-fold increase in bladder cancer and an 11-fold increase in lymphoma. Half of the patients experienced at least one serious infection. Another study of 150 consecutive patients on combination therapy confirmed the high relapse rate in systemic vasculitis: 42% for Wegener's granulomatosis, 42% for classic PAN, and 25% for microscopic polyangiitis (214). These findings suggest that systemic vasculitis is not routinely curable using current therapeutic strategies, emphasizing the need for safer and more effective alternative treatments.

An alternative protocol that has received much recent attention is pulse cyclophosphamide. Intravenous cyclophosphamide pulses have been administered in doses ranging from 350 to 1000 mg/m², or 15 mg/kg, at frequencies of every 1 to 4 weeks (209,215–218). The results are conflicting. While uncontrolled studies on patients with Wegener's granulomatosis yielded sustained responses in less than 50% and high relapse rates (215,216), several controlled trials involving patients with PAN, microscopic polyangiitis, Wegener's granulomatosis, or rheumatoid vasculitis showed that pulse cyclophosphamide is equally efficacious to continuous oral therapy (217,218). In all reports, periodic intravenous cyclophosphamide had a less serious side effect profile than did conventional oral cyclophosphamide, especially regarding the incidence of bladder toxicity.

When treatment with cyclophosphamide fails, azathioprine (AZA) has generally been the second cytotoxic drug of choice (209). AZA inhibits purine metabolism, interfering with DNA synthesis. While B-, T-, and NK-cell functions are all affected, several lines of evidence suggest that AZA has a predominant action on T cells (219). The typical dose is 2 to 3 mg/kg/day. While AZA has a slower onset of action than cyclophosphamide, it is better tolerated, suggesting a role in maintaining remissions induced by cyclophosphamide (209). The efficacy of this agent in vasculitis cannot be ascertained from the available data, which are all retrospective and anecdotal in nature (48).

Methotrexate (MTX) is another immunosuppressive agent that has drawn recent attention in the treatment of vasculitis. MTX is a folate antagonist that blocks the synthesis of purines and pyrimidines, and thus, DNA and RNA. It inhibits the production of IL-1, IL-6, and IL-8 and has additional anti-inflammatory properties (198,220). In an open-label study of 29 patients with refractory Wegener's granulomatosis, oral MTX combined with a corticosteroid resulted in an initially promising 70% complete remission rate (221). However, 40% of the responders had a relapse after a median follow-up of 2 years (222).

Cyclosporine preferentially suppresses T-cell activation and proliferation by inhibiting the transcription of IL-2 and other cytokines in T cells and downregulating the expression of IL-2 receptors. CD4+ helper/inducer T cells and CD8+ cytolytic T cells are affected at concentrations that still permit suppressor T-cell activity (223). Anecdotes testify to successful outcomes obtained with cyclosporine in treating refractory PAN or Wegener's granulomatosis at doses up to 5 mg/kg/day (194,198). Pending further study, cyclosporine should be considered in patients refractory to other agents or with tenuous bone marrow function.

Plasma exchange has been tried as treatment for vasculitides assumed to be mediated by immune complex deposition. Prospective controlled studies of plasma exchange added to standard therapy in patients with PAN and Churg-Strauss syndrome showed no improvement in overall disease control (205). On the other hand, plasma exchange in combination with antiviral therapy was effective in hepatitis B virus–associated PAN, with an 80% recovery rate, but no control group was recruited (51,200). Apheresis has been used for many years to treat symptomatic cryoglobulinemia, but no controlled trials have been performed (108). In a controlled randomized study of patients with renal insufficiency due to microscopic polyangiitis, Wegener's granulomatosis, and idiopathic rapidly progressive glomerulonephritis, plasma exchange added to oral immunosuppressive drugs improved outcome in patients who were dialysis dependent (224). In summary, plasma exchange is not routinely indicated for the initial treatment of systemic vasculitis but may be useful for selected indications such as cryoglobulinemia or hepatitis B infections and for patients with refractory disease.

Interest in intravenous immunoglobulin (IVIG) for the treatment of systemic vasculitis was spurred by its effectiveness in preventing coronary artery aneurysms in Kawasaki disease (225). There are now anecdotal reports of dramatic therapeutic successes in ANCA-associated vasculitis, hepatitis B virus–related PAN, isolated central nervous system vasculitis, childhood PAN, and systemic vasculitis associated with parvovirus B19 infection (209,226). Jayne and Lockwood (227) treated 26 patients with ANCA-positive microscopic polyangiitis or Wegener's granulomatosis refractory to conventional therapy in an open-label trial of IVIG, which resulted in prompt improvement in all patients and a complete remission in 19 patients (mean follow-up time, 12 months). Mean doses of cyclophosphamide and prednisone decreased significantly (227). Other studies, however, did not confirm these encouraging results (228).

Vaso-occlusion

Treatment of vaso-occlusive disease is an often-neglected principle in patients with vasculitis. The endothelium reacts to vasculitic injury with the release of cytokines and growth factors that promote vasospasm, proliferation of endothelial and smooth muscle cells, and procoagulant tendencies, all of which serve to precipitate occlusive changes in the involved vessel (154). In vitro observations suggest that glucocorticoids in therapeutic doses block prostaglandin I_2 synthesis in the endothelium but not thromboxane in platelets. Hence, thromboxane-induced vasoconstriction, thrombogenesis, and platelet activation might proceed unopposed by the counterregulatory prostaglandin I_2, accelerating the development of vessel stenosis (229). Antiplatelet agents such as low-dose aspirin should be considered in any patient with signs of progressive neurologic injury in the face of aggressive immunosuppression (199). Calcium channel blockers and other vasodilators might also be useful additions. Comorbid cardiovascular risk factors may potentiate vessel occlusion in patients with vasculitis. Diabetes, hypertension, and hyperlipidemia should also be rigorously controlled and tobacco use halted (229).

Supportive Care

Supportive care is particularly important in patients with severe vasculitic neuropathies complicated by extensive axon loss, where prolonged recovery periods are anticipated. Patients treated with prednisone must be carefully monitored for side effects including hypertension, weight gain, glucose intolerance, electrolyte imbalance, cataracts, glaucoma, osteoporosis, myopathy, and aseptic necrosis of the hip (207,208). All patients should undergo tuberculin skin testing prior to immunosuppression, with antituberculosis prophylaxis administered to positive responders. Single-morning dosage and alternate-day regimens minimize side effects (207). A low-sodium, low-simple-sugar, calorie-restricted diet will limit weight gain in most patients. Bone densitometry should be considered for all patients at baseline, especially postmenopausal women and others at risk for osteoporosis, with yearly follow-up studies (230). Osteoporosis can be minimized by participation in a regular weight-bearing program that includes resistance exercises (230) and by supplementation with 1000 to 1500 mg of elemental calcium daily along with 50,000 units of vitamin D twice weekly or 0.25 µg of calcitriol daily (231). Estrogen replacement is also important in postmenopausal women with no contraindications. In patients with reduced bone mass at baseline, fractures, or progressive osteopenia, ancillary agents such as calcitonin, bisphosphonates, or fluoride should be added to the regimen (230).

Chronic low-dose cyclophosphamide therapy carries a 40% risk of hemorrhagic cystitis and a 16% incidence of bladder cancer at 15 years after the initial exposure (232). Hematologic malignancies are also increased, GI symptoms are common, gonadal dysfunction can be expected, and temporary alopecia occurs in 15% (68,209,211). Bladder toxicity, which is caused by acrolein, a toxic metabolite of cyclophosphamide, can be minimized by aggressive oral hydration and frequent urination. Mesna is an intravenous medication that detoxifies acrolein in the bladder. It can be administered with pulse cyclophosphamide therapy to decrease the risk of hemorrhagic cystitis (209). Complete blood cell counts and urinalyses should be performed every 4 to 6 weeks during treatment with cyclophosphamide. Lifelong surveillance for bladder and hematologic cancers with periodic urinalyses is indicated (232).

Aggressive physical therapy is important for patients with significant neurologic impairment so as to maintain range of motion and strength, improve functional status, minimize osteoporosis, and reduce the risk of steroid myopathy (233). Orthotic devices, especially custom-fit ankle-foot orthoses in patients with footdrop, can be essential to maintaining ambulation. Occupational therapy can assist patients in their recovery of upper-limb function, reacquisition of daily living skills, and proper use of splints. Occupational and physical therapists are also key participants in the management of neuropathic pain, a feature of vasculitic neuropathy that can be debilitating. Chronic pain medications such as tricyclic antidepressants, selective serotonin-reuptake inhibitors, anticonvulsants, mexiletine, clonazepam, topical lidocaine cream, and transdermal clonidine may also be required (234). Short-term use of scheduled opioids is sometimes necessary.

Future Modalities

Newer and more specific strategies of immunotherapy for systemic vasculitis are under investigation and may soon enter the clinical realm (235). Anti–T cell monoclonal antibodies (MAbs) are one of these approaches. The first clinical use of MAb therapy in vasculitis was reported in 1990 for a patient with refractory microscopic polyangiitis treated with CAMPATH-1H, a "humanized" rat MAb directed against the CD52 glycoprotein complex found on lymphocytes, followed by anti-CD4 MAbs (193). This combination produced a dramatic remission that was sustained for more than 3

years. The same investigators have now treated 11 patients, 6 with Wegener's granulomatosis or microscopic polyangiitis and 5 with ANCA-negative small-vessel vasculitis. Anti-CD52 MAbs alone induced remissions in all patients, although 7 patients had a relapse and had to be retreated with anti-CD52 plus anti-CD4 (235).

An outgrowth of recombinant DNA technology has been the production of MAbs and purified proteins that interfere with the production, expression, and function of proinflammatory cell adhesion molecules and cytokines. Many of these biologic agents are under investigation as potential therapies for a variety of immunologic and inflammatory conditions, including vasculitis, although no human trials in vasculitis have yet been reported (155,198,236–238). A modulatory rather than curative role is envisioned, geared toward suppressing disease activity and thereby minimizing patient exposure to toxic immunosuppressive drugs (198). Problems with this form of therapy may include antigenicity and immune complex disease, short-lasting effects, need for intravenous administration, and unexpected proinflammatory or immunostimulatory effects (155,236,237). The most promising agents at present are anti–ICAM-1 Mabs, anti–TNF-α Mabs, soluble TNF-α receptors, soluble IL-1 receptors, and the natural receptor antagonist for IL-1 (198,236,238).

Two older drugs with anticytokine actions, pentoxifylline and thalidomide, may also soon augment the antivasculitic armamentarium. Both have anti-inflammatory properties mediated by the inhibition of TNF-α production and both also selectively inhibit the Th1 subset of CD4+ helper T cells (239–241). For pentoxifylline, successful treatment, as monotherapy or in combination with other agents, of cutaneous PAN, cutaneous leukocytoclastic angiitis, and Kawasaki disease has been reported (239). Vasculitic conditions with documented responsiveness to thalidomide include Behçet's disease and erythema nodosum leprosum (242).

References

1. Fauci AS, Haynes BF, Katz P. The spectrum of vasculitis: clinical, pathological, immunologic, and therapeutic considerations. *Ann Intern Med* 1978;89:660–676.
2. Kussmaul A, Maier R. Ueber eine bisher nicht beschriebene eigenthumliche Arterienerkrankung (Periarteritis nodosa), die mit Morbus Brightii und rapid fortschreitender allgemeiner Muskellahmung einhergeht. *Dtsch Arch Klin Med* 1866;1:484–517.
3. Zeek PM. Periarteritis nodosa: a critical review. *Am J Clin Pathol* 1952;22:777–790.
4. Ferrari E. Ueber polyarteritis acuta nodosa (sogenannte Periarteritis nodosa) und ihre Beziehungen zur Polymyositis und Polyneuritis acuta. *Beitr Pathol Anat* 1903;34:350–386.
5. Kernohan JW, Woltman HW. Periarteritis nodosa: a clinicopathological study with special reference to the nervous system. *Arch Neurol Psychiatry* 1938;39:655–686.
6. Dyck PJ, Conn DL, Ozaki H. Necrotizing angiopathic neuropathy: three-dimensional morphology of fiber degeneration related to sites of occulated vessels. *Mayo Clin Proc* 1972;47:461–475.
7. Moore PN, Fauci AS. Neurologic manifestations of sys-

temic vasculitis: a retrospective study of the clinico-pathologic features and responses to therapy in 25 patients. *Am J Med* 1981;71:517–524.

8. Wees SJ, Sunwoo IN, Oh SJ. Sural nerve biopsy in systemic necrotizing vasculitis. *Am J Med* 1981;71:525–532.

9. Castaigne P, Brunet P, Hauw JJ, et al. Systeme nerveux peripherique et panarterite nodeuse: revue de 27 cas. *Rev Neurol (Paris)* 1984;140:343–352.

10. Chang RN, Bell CC, Hallett M. Clinical characteristics and prognosis of vasculitic mononeuropathy multiplex. *Arch Neurol* 1984;41:618–621.

11. Kissel JT, Slivka AP, Warmolts JR, Mendell JR. The clinical spectrum of necrotizing angiopathy of the peripheral nervous system. *Ann Neurol* 1985;18:251–257.

12. Bouche P, Leger JM, Travers MA, et al. Peripheral neuropathy in systemic vasculitis: clinical and electrophysiologic study of 22 patients. *Neurology* 1986;36:1598–1602.

13. Harati Y, Niakan E. The clinical spectrum of inflammatory-angiopathic neuropathy. *J Neurol Neurosurg Psychiatry* 1986;49:1313–1316.

14. Dyck PJ, Benstead TJ, Conn DL, et al. Nonsystemic vasculitic neuropathy. *Brain* 1987;110:843–854.

15. Said G, Lacroix-Ciaudo C, Fujimura H, et al. The peripheral neuropathy of necrotizing arteritis: a clinicopathological study. *Ann Neurol* 1988;23:461–465.

16. Panegyres PK, Blumbergs PC, Leong AS-Y, Bourne AJ. Vasculitis of peripheral nerve and skeletal muscle: clinicopathological correlation and immunopathogenic mechanisms. *J Neurol Sci* 1990;100:193–202.

17. Hawke SHB, Davies L, Pamphlett R, et al. Vasculitic neuropathy: a clinical and pathological study. *Brain* 1991;114:2175–2190.

18. Nicolai A, Bonetti B, Lazzarino LG, et al. Peripheral nerve vasculitis: a clinico-pathological study. *Clin Neuropathol* 1995;14:137–141.

19. Kurland LT, Chuang TY, Hunder G. The epidemiology of systemic arteritis. In: Lawrence RC, Shulman LE, eds. *The epidemiology of the rheumatic diseases*. New York: Gower, 1984:196–205.

20. Hunder GG, Arend WP, Bloch DA, et al. The American College of Rheumatology 1990 criteria for the classification of vasculitis: introduction. *Arthritis Rheum* 1990;33:1101–1107.

21. Jennette JC, Falk AJ, Andrassy K, et al. Nomenclature of systemic vasculitides: proposal of an international consensus conference. *Arthritis Rheum* 1994;37:187–192.

22. Somer T, Finegold SM. Vasculitides associated with infections, immunization, and antimicrobial drugs. *Clin Infect Dis* 1995;20:1010–1036.

23. Cupps TR. Infections and vasculitis: mechanisms considered. In: LeRoy EC, ed. *Systemic vasculitis. The biological basis*. New York: Marcel Dekker, 1992:483–503.

24. Said G, Lacroix C, Chemouilli P, et al. Cytomegalovirus neuropathy in acquired immunodeficiency syndrome: a clinical and pathological study. *Ann Neurol* 1991; 29:139–146.

25. Chretien F, Gray E, Lescs MC, et al. Acute varicella-zoster virus ventriculitis and meningo-myelo-radiculitis in acquired immunodeficiency syndrome. *Acta Neuropathol (Berl)* 1993;86:659–665.

26. Said G, Lacroix C, Andriev JN, et al. Necrotizing arteritis in patients with inflammatory neuropathy and human immunodeficiency virus (HIV-III) infection. *Neurology* 1987;37(suppl 1):176.

27. Gherardi R, Lebargy F, Gaulard P, et al. Necrotizing vasculitis and HIV replication in peripheral nerves. *N Engl J Med* 1989;321:685–686. Letter.

28. Cornblath DR, McArthur JC, Parry GJG, Griffin JW. Peripheral neuropathy in human immunodeficiency virus infection. In: Dyck PJ, Thomas PK, Griffin JW, et al, eds. *Peripheral neuropathy*. 3rd ed. Philadelphia: WB Saunders, 1993:1343–1353.

29. Simpson DM, Olney RK. Peripheral neuropathies associated with human immunodeficiency virus infection. *Neurol Clin* 1992;10:685–711.

30. Said G. Inflammatory neuropathies associated with known infections (HIV, leprosy, Chagas' disease, Lyme disease). *Baillieres Clin Neurol* 1994;3:149–171.

31. Midroni G, Bilboa JM. *Biopsy diagnosis of peripheral neuropathy*. Boston: Butterworth-Heinemann, 1995.

32. Gherardi R, Belec L, Mhiri C, et al. The spectrum of vasculitis in human immunodeficiency virus-infected patients. *Arthritis Rheum* 1993;36:1164–1174.

33. Roullet E, Assuerus V, Gozlan J, et al. Cytomegalovirus multifocal neuropathy in AIDS: analysis of 15 consecutive cases. *Neurology* 1994;44:2174–2182.

34. Halperin J, Luft BJ, Volkman DJ, Dattwyler RJ. Lyme neuroborreliosis: peripheral nervous system manifestations. *Brain* 1990;113:1207–1221.

35. Garcia-Monco JC, Benach JL. Lyme neuroborreliosis. *Ann Neurol* 1995;37:691–702.

36. Moore PM, Calabrese LH. Neurologic manifestations of systemic vasculitides. *Semin Neurol* 1994;14:300–306.

37. Fauci AS. The vasculitis syndromes. In: Isselbacher KJ, Braunwald E, Wilson JD, et al, eds. *Harrison's principles of internal medicine*. 13th ed. New York: McGraw-Hill, 1994:1670–1679.

38. Jennette JC, Falk RJ. Update on the pathobiology of vasculitis. In: Schoen FJ, Gimbrone MA, eds. *Cardiovascular pathology, clinicopathologic correlations and pathogenetic mechanisms*. Baltimore: Williams & Wilkins, 1995:156–172.

39. Kallenberg CGM, Brouwer E, Weening JJ, Cohen Tervaert JW. Anti-neutrophil cytoplasmic antibodies: current diagnostic and pathophysiological potential. *Kidney Int* 1994;46:1–15.

40. Gross WL. Antineutrophil cytoplasmic autoantibody testing in vasculitides. *Rheum Dis Clin North Am* 1995;21:987–1011.

41. Lightfoot RW, Michel BA, Bloch DA, et al. The American College of Rheumatology 1990 criteria for the classification of polyarteritis nodosa. *Arthritis Rheum* 1990;33: 1088–1093.

42. Lhote F, Guillevin L. Polyarteritis nodosa, microscopic polyangiitis, and Churg-Strauss syndrome: clinical aspects and treatment. *Rheum Dis Clin North Am* 1995;21:911–947.

43. Guillevin L, Visser H, Noel LH, et al. Antineutrophil cytoplasm antibodies in systemic polyarteritis nodosa with and without hepatitis B virus infection and Churg-Strauss syndrome—62 patients. *J Rheumatol* 1993;20: 1345–1349.

44. Lovshin LL, Kernohan JW. Peripheral neuritis in periarteritis nodosa: a clinicopathologic study. *Arch Intern Med* 1948;82:321–338.

45. Nuzum JW. Polyarteritis nodosa: statistical review of one hundred seventy-five cases from the literature and report of a "typical" case. *Arch Intern Med* 1954;94:942–955.

46. Ford RG, Siekert RG. Central nervous system manifestations of periarteritis nodosa. *Neurology* 1965;15: 114–122.

47. Frohnert PP, Sheps SG. Long-term follow-up study of periarteritis nodosa. *Am J Med* 1967;43:8–14.

48. Leib ES, Restivo C, Paulus HE. Immunosuppressive and

corticosteroid therapy of polyarteritis nodosa. *Am J Med* 1979;67:941–947.

49. Guillevin L, Le Thi Huong D, Godeau P, et al. Clinical findings and prognosis of polyarteritis nodosa and Churg-Strauss angiitis: a study in 165 patients. *Br J Rheumatol* 1988;27:258–264.

50. Marcellin P, Calmus Y, Takahushi H, et al. Latent hepatitis B virus (HBV) infection in systemic necrotizing vasculitis. *Clin Exp Rheumatol* 1991;9:23–28.

51. Guillevin L, Lhote F, Cohen P, et al. Polyarteritis nodosa related to hepatitis B virus: a prospective study with long-term observation of 41 patients. *Medicine* 1995;74:238–253.

52. Serra A, Cameron JS, Turner DR. Vasculitis affecting the kidney: presentation, histopathology and long-term outcome. *Q J Med* 1984;53:181–207.

53. Savage COS, Winearls CG, Evans DJ, et al. Microscopic polyarteritis: presentation, pathology, and prognosis. *Q J Med* 1985;56:467–483.

54. Adu D, Howie AJ, Scott DGI, et al. Polyarteritis and the kidney. *Q J Med* 1987;62:221–237.

55. Lanham JG, Elkon KB, Pusey CD, Hughes GR. Systemic vasculitis with asthma and eosinophilia: a clinical approach to the Churg-Strauss syndrome. *Medicine* 1984;63:65–81.

56. Guillevin L, Lhote F, Gayrand M, et al. Prognostic factors in polyarteritis nodosa and Churg-Strauss syndrome: a prospective study in 342 patients. *Medicine* 1996;75:17–28.

57. Churg J, Strauss L. Allergic granulomatosis, allergic angiitis, and periarteritis nodosa. *Am J Pathol* 1951;27: 277–301.

58. Masi AT, Hunder GG, Lie JT, et al. The American College of Rheumatology 1990 criteria for the classification of Churg-Strauss syndrome (allergic granulomatosis and angiitis). *Arthritis Rheum* 1990;33:1094–1100.

59. Oh SJ, Herrara GA, Spalding DM. Eosinophilic vasculitic neuropathy in the Churg-Strauss syndrome. *Arthritis Rheum* 1986;29:1173–1175. Letter.

60. Inoue A, Koh C-S, Tsukada N, Yanagisawa N. Allergic granulomatosis angiitis and peripheral nerve lesion. *Intern Med* 1992;31:989–993.

61. Guillevin L, Guittard T, Bletry O, et al. Systemic necrotizing angiitis with asthma: causes and precipitating factors in 43 cases. *Lung* 1987;165:165–172.

62. Sehgal M, Swanson JW, DeRemee RA, Colby TV. Neurologic manifestations of Churg-Strauss syndrome. *Mayo Clin Proc* 1995;70:337–341.

63. Godman GC, Churg J. Wegener's granulomatosis: pathology and review of the literature. *Arch Pathol* 1954;58:533–553.

64. Duna GF, Galperin C, Hoffman GS. Wegener's granulomatosis. *Rheum Dis Clin North Am* 1995;21:949–986.

65. Rao JK, Weinberger M, Oddone EZ, et al. The role of antineutrophil cytoplasmic antibody (c-ANCA) testing in the diagnosis of Wegener granulomatosis: a literature review and meta-analysis. *Ann Intern Med* 1995;123: 925–932.

66. Anderson JM, Jamieson DG, Jefferson JM. Non-healing granuloma and the nervous system. *Q J Med* 1975;44: 309–323.

67. Fauci AS, Haynes BF, Katz P, Wolff SM. Wegener's granulomatosis: prospective clinical and therapeutic experience with 85 patients for 21 years. *Ann Intern Med* 1983;98:76–85.

68. Hoffman GS, Kerr GS, Leavitt RY, et al. Wegener granulomatosis: an analysis of 158 patients. *Ann Intern Med* 1992;116:488–498.

69. Nishino H, Rubino FA, DeRemee RA, et al. Neurological involvement in Wegener's granulomatosis: an analysis of 324 consecutive patients at the Mayo Clinic. *Ann Neurol* 1993;33:4–9.

70. Walton EW. Giant cell granuloma of the respiratory tract (Wegener's granulomatosis). *BMJ* 1958;2:265–270.

71. Finkelman R, Munsat T, Mandell H, et al. Neuromuscular manifestations of Wegener's granulomatosis: a case report. *Neurology* 1993;43:617–618.

72. Leavitt RY, Fauci AS. Polyangiitis overlap syndrome: classification and prospective clinical experience. *Am J Med* 1986;81:79–85.

73. Nishino H, DeRemee RA, Rubino FA, Parisi JE. Wegener's granulomatosis associated with vasculitis of the temporal artery: report of five cases. *Mayo Clin Proc* 1993;68:115–121.

74. Olney RK. AAEM minimonograph #38: neuropathies in connective tissue disease. *Muscle Nerve* 1992;15: 531–542.

75. Bacon PA, Carruthers DM. Vasculitis associated with connective tissue disorders. *Rheum Dis Clin North Am* 1995;21:1077–1096.

76. Cruickshank B. The arteritis of rheumatoid arthritis. *Ann Rheum Dis* 1954;13:136–145.

77. Scott DGI, Bacon PA, Tribe CR. Systemic rheumatoid vasculitis: a clinical and laboratory study of 50 cases. *Medicine* 1981;60:288–297.

78. Vollertson RS, Conn DL, Ballard DJ, et al. Rheumatoid vasculitis: survival and associated risk factors. *Medicine* 1986;65:365–375.

79. Harris ED. Rheumatoid arthritis: pathophysiology and implications for therapy. *N Engl J Med* 1990;322:1277–1289.

80. Puechal X, Said G, Hilliquin P, et al. Peripheral neuropathy with necrotizing vasculitis in rheumatoid arthritis: a clinicopathologic and prognostic study of thirty-two patients. *Arthritis Rheum* 1995;38:1618–1629.

81. Weller RO, Bruckner FE, Chamberlain MA. Rheumatoid neuropathy: a histological and electrophysiological study. *J Neurol Neurosurg Psychiatry* 1970;33: 592–604.

82. Beckett VL, Dinn JJ. Segmental demyelination in rheumatoid arthritis. *Q J Med* 1972;61:71–80.

83. Voskuyl AE, Zwinderman AH, Westedt ML, et al. Factors associated with the development of vasculitis in rheumatoid arthritis: results of a case-control study. *Ann Rheum Dis* 1996;55:190–192.

84. Fox RI, Kang H-I. Sjögren's syndrome. In: Kelley WN, Harris ED, Ruddy S, Sledge CB, eds. *Textbook of rheumatology*. 4th ed. Philadelphia: WB Saunders, 1991: 931–942.

85. Vital C, Bombardieri S, Moutsopoulos HM, et al. Preliminary critieria for the classification of Sjögren's syndrome. *Arthritis Rheum* 1993;36:340–347.

86. Tsokos M, Lazaron SA, Moutsopoulos HM. Vasculitis in Sjögren's syndrome: histologic classification and clinical presentation. *Am J Clin Pathol* 1987;88:26–31.

87. Molina R, Provost TI, Alexander EL. Peripheral inflammatory vascular disease in Sjögren's syndrome: association with nervous system complications. *Arthritis Rheum* 1985;28:1341–1347.

88. Kaltreider HB, Talal N. The neuropathy of Sjögren's syndrome: trigeminal nerve involvement. *Ann Intern Med* 1969;70:751–762.

89. Mellgren SI, Conn DL, Stevens JC, Dyck PJ. Peripheral neuropathy in primary Sjögren's syndrome. *Neurology* 1989;39:390–394.

90. Gemignani F, Marbini A, Pavesi G, et al. Peripheral neu-

ropathy associated with Sjögren's syndrome. *J Neurol Neurosurg Psychiatry* 1994;57:983–986.

91. Griffin JW, Cornblath DR, Alexander E, et al. Ataxic sensory neuropathy and dorsal root ganglionitis associated with Sjögren's syndrome. *Ann Neurol* 1990;27:304–315.

92. Belmont HM, Abramson SB, Lie JT. Pathology and pathogenesis of vascular injury in systemic lupus erythematosus: interactions of inflammatory cells and activated endothelium. *Arthritis Rheum* 1996;39:9–22.

93. Font J, Cervera R, Navarro M, et al. Systemic lupus erythematosus in men: clinical and immunological characteristics. *Ann Rheum Dis* 1992;51:1050–1052.

94. Dubois EL, Tuffanelli DL. Clinical manifestations of systemic lupus erythematosus: computer analysis of 520 cases. *JAMA* 1964;190:104–111.

95. Feinglass EJ, Arnett FC, Dorsch CA, et al. Neuropsychiatric manifestations of systemic lupus erythematosus: diagnosis, clinical spectrum, and relationship to other features of the disease. *Medicine* 1976;55:323–339.

96. Omdal R, Mellgren SI, Husby G, et al. A controlled study of peripheral neuropathy in systemic lupus erythematosus. *Acta Neurol Scand* 1993;88:41–46.

97. Hughes RAC, Cameron JC, Hall SM, et al. Multiple mononeuropathy as the initial presentation of systemic lupus erythematosus—nerve biopsy and response to plasma exchange. *J Neurol* 1982;228:239–247.

98. McCombe PA, McLeod JG, Pollard JD, et al. Peripheral sensorimotor and autonomic neuropathy associated with systemic lupus erythematosus: clinical, pathological and immunologic features. *Brain* 1987;110:533–549.

99. Richardson EP, DeGirolami U. *Pathology of the peripheral nerve*. Philadelphia: WB Saunders, 1995.

100. Seibold JR. Scleroderma. In: Kelly WN, Harris ED, Ruddy S, Sledge CB, eds. *Textbook of rheumatology*. 4th edition. Philadelphia: WB Saunders, 1993:1113–1143.

101. Oddis CV, Eisenbeis CH, Reidbord HE, et al. Vasculitis in systemic sclerosis: association with Sjögren's syndrome and the CREST syndrome variant. *J Rheumatol* 1987;14:942–948.

102. Schady W, Sheard A, Hassell A, et al. Peripheral nerve dysfunction in scleroderma. *Q J Med* 1991;80:661–675.

103. Hietaharju A, Jaaskelainen S, Kalimo H, Hietarintu M. Peripheral neuromuscular manfestations in systemic sclerosis (scleroderma). *Muscle Nerve* 1993;16:1204–1212.

104. Farrell DA, Medsger TA. Trigeminal neuropathy in progressive systemic sclerosis. *Am J Med* 1982;73:57–62.

105. Conn DL, Hunder GG, O'Duffy JD. Vasculitis and related disorders. In: Kelley WN, Harris ED, Ruddy S, Sledge CB, eds. *Textbook of rheumatology*. 4th ed. Philadelphia: WB Saunders, 1993:1071–1102.

106. Calabrese LH, Michel BA, Bloch DA, et al. The American College of Rheumatology 1990 criteria for the classification of hypersensitivity vasculitis. *Arthritis Rheum* 1990;33:1108–1113.

107. Mertz LE, Conn DL. Vasculitis associated with malignancy. *Curr Opin Rheumatol* 1992;4:39–46.

108. Calabrese LH, Hoffman GS, Guillevin L. Therapy of resistant systemic necrotizing vasculitis: polyarteritis, Churg-Strauss syndrome, Wegener's granulomatosis, and hypersensitivity vasculitis group disorders. *Rheum Dis Clin North Am* 1995;21:41–57.

109. Dubost JJ, Souteyrand P, Sauvezie B. Drug-induced vasculitides. *Baillieres Clin Rheumatol* 1991;5:119–138.

110. Calabrese LH, Duna GF. Drug-induced vasculitis. *Curr Opin Rheumatol* 1996;8:34–40.

111. Stafford CR, Bogdanoff BM, Green L, Spector HB. Mononeuropathy multiplex as a complication of amphetamine angiitis. *Neurology* 1975;25:570–572.

112. Greer JM, Longley S, Edwards NL, et al. Vasculitis associated with malignancy: experience with 13 patients and literature review. *Medicine* 1988;67:220–230.

113. Sanchez-Guerrero J, Gutierrez-Urena S, Vidaller A, et al. Vasculitis as a paraneoplastic syndrome. Report of 11 cases and review of the literature. *J Rheumatol* 1990;17:1458–1462.

114. Johnson PC, Rolak LA, Hamilton RH, Laguna JF. Paraneoplastic vasculitis of nerve: a remote effect of cancer. *Ann Neurol* 1979;5:437–444.

115. Vincent D, Dubas F, Hauw JJ, et al. Nerve and muscle microvasculitis in peripheral neuropathy: a remote effect of cancer? *J Neurol Neurosurg Psychiatry* 1986;49:1007–1010.

116. Kurzrock R, Cohen PR, Markowitz A. Clinical manifestations of vasculitis in patients with solid tumors: a case report and review of the literature. *Arch Intern Med* 1994;154:334–340.

117. Matsumuro K, Izumo S, Umehara F, et al. Paraneoplastic vasculitic neuropathy: immunohistochemical studies on a biopsied nerve and post-mortem examination. *J Intern Med* 1994;236:225–230.

118. Meltzer M, Franklin EC, Elias K, et al. Cryoglobulins with rheumatoid factor activity. *Am J Med* 1966;40:837–856.

119. Gorevic PD, Kassab HJ, Levo Y, et al. Mixed cryoglobulinemia: clinical aspects and long-term follow-up of 40 patients. *Am J Med* 1980;69:287–308.

120. Ferri C, LaCivita L, Cirafisi C, et al. Peripheral neuropathy in mixed cryoglobulinemia: clinical and electrophysiologic investigations. *J Rheumatol* 1992;19:889–895.

121. Gemignani F, Pavesi G, Manganelli P, et al. Peripheral neuropathy in essential mixed cryoglobulinemia. *J Neurol Neurosurg Psychiatry* 1992;55:116–120.

122. Nemni R, Corbo M, Fazio R, et al. Cryoglobulinemic neuropathy. A clinical, morphological and immunocytochemical study of 8 cases. *Brain* 1988;111:541–552.

123. Prior R, Schober R, Scharffeter K, Wechsler W. Occlusive microangiopathy by immunoglobulin (IgM-kappa) precipitation: pathogenic relevance in paraneoplastic cryoglobulinemic neuropathy. *Acta Neuropathol (Berl)* 1992;83:423–426.

124. Chad D, Pariser K, Bradley WG, et al. The pathogenesis of cryoglobulinemic neuropathy. *Neurology* 1982;32:725–729.

125. Agnello V, Romain PL. Mixed cryoglobulinemia secondary to hepatitis C infection. *Rheum Dis Clin North Am* 1996;22:1–21.

126. Monti G, Galli M, Invernizzi F, et al. Cryoglobulinemias: a multi-centre study of the early clinical and laboratory manifestations of primary and secondary disease. *Q J Med* 1995;88:115–126.

127. Lie JT. The classification and diagnosis of vasculitis in large and medium-sized blood vessels. *Pathol Annu* 1987;22:125–162.

128. Huston KA, Hunder GG, Lie JT, et al. Temporal arteritis: a 25-year epidemiologic, clinical, and pathological study. *Ann Intern Med* 1978;88:162–167.

129. Chalk CH, Dyck PJ, Conn DL. Vasculitic neuropathy. In: Dyck PJ, Thomas PK, Griffin JW, et al, eds. *Peripheral neuropathy*. 3rd ed. Philadelphia: WB Saunders, 1993:1424–1436.

130. Nordborg E, Nordborg C, Malmvall B-E, et al. Giant cell arteritis. *Rheum Dis Clin North Am* 1995;21:1013–1126.

131. Caselli RJ, Hunder GG. Neurologic complications of giant cell (temporal) arteritis. *Semin Neurol* 1994;14:349–353.

132. Hollenhorst RW, Brown JR, Wagener HP, Shick RM. Neurologic aspects of temporal arteritis. *Neurology* 1960;10:490–498.

133. Caselli RJ, Daube JR, Hunder GG, Whisnant JP. Peripheral neuropathic syndromes in giant cell (temporal) arteritis. *Neurology* 1988;38:685–689.

134. Bridges AJ, Porter J, England D. Lower extremity peripheral neuropathy and ischemic ulcers associated with giant cell arteritis. *J Rheumatol* 1989;16:1366–1369.

135. Moreland LW, Ball GV. Cutaneous polyarteritis nodosa. *Am J Med* 1990;88:426–430.

136. Vine AK. Retinal vasculitis. *Semin Neurol* 1994;14:354–360.

137. Warfield AT, Lee SJ, Phillips SMA, Pall AA. Isolated testicular vasculitis mimicking a testicular neoplasm. *J Clin Pathol* 1994;47:1121–1123.

138. Burke AP, Sobin LH, Virmani R. Localized vasculitis of the gastrointestinal tract. *Am J Surg Pathol* 1995;19:338–349.

139. Chalk CH, Homburger HA, Dyck PJ. Anti-neutrophil cytoplasmic antibodies in vasculitic peripheral neuropathy. *Neurology* 1993;43:1826–1827.

140. Battaglia M, Mitsumoto H, Wilbourn AJ, Estes ML. Utility of electromyography in the diagnosis of vasculitic neuropathy. *Neurology* 1990;40(suppl 1):427. Abstract.

141. Wilbourn AJ, Levin KH. Ischemic neuropathy. In: Brown WF, Bolton CF, eds. *Clinical electromyography*. 2nd ed. Boston: Butterworth-Heinemann, 1993:369–390.

142. Parry GJG. AAEE case report #11: mononeuropathy multiplex. *Muscle Nerve* 1985;8:493–498.

143. Jamieson PW, Giuliani MJ, Martinez AJ. Necrotizing angiopathy presenting with multifocal conduction blocks. *Neurology* 1991;41:442–444.

144. Nukada H, Dyck PJ. Acute ischemia causes axonal stasis, swelling, attenuation and secondary demyelination. *Ann Neurol* 1987;22:311–318.

145. Parry GJ, Linn DJ. Conduction block without demyelination following acute nerve infarction. *J Neurol Sci* 1988;84:265–273.

146. Kissel JT, Mendell JR. Vasculitic neuropathy. *Neurol Clin* 1992;101:761–781.

147. Lie JT. Histopathological specificity of systemic vasculitis. *Rheum Dis Clin North Am* 1995;21:883–909.

148. Fujimura H, LaCroix C, Said G. Vulnerability of nerve fibers to ischaemia: a quantitative light and electron microscopic study. *Brain* 1991;114:1929–1942.

149. Kissel JT, Riethman JL, Omerza J, et al. Peripheral nerve vasculitis: immune characterization of the vascular lesions. *Ann Neurol* 1989;25:291–297.

150. Engelhardt A, Lorler H, Neundorfer B. Immunocytochemical findings in vasculitic neuropathies. *Acta Neurol Scand* 1993;87:318–321.

151. Cid M-C, Grau JM, Casademont J, et al. Immune histochemical characterization of inflammatory cells and immunologic activation markers in muscle and nerve biopsy specimens from patients with systemic polyarteritis nodosa. *Arthritis Rheum* 1994;37:1055–1061.

152. Schenone A, DeMartini I, Tabaton M, et al. Direct immunofluorescence in sural nerve biopsies. *Eur Neurol* 1988;28:262–269.

153. Sundy JS, Haynes BF. Pathogenic mechanisms of vessel damage in vasculitic syndromes. *Rheum Dis Clin North Am* 1995;21:861–881.

154. Cid MC. New developments in the pathogenesis of systemic vasculitis. *Curr Opin Rheumatol* 1996;8:1–11.

155. Albelda SM, Smith CM, Ward PA. Adhesion molecules and inflammatory injury. *FASEB J* 1994;8:504–512.

156. Pober JS, Cotran RS. Cytokines and endothelial cell biology. *Physiol Rev* 1990;70:427–451.

157. Ben-Baruch A, Michiel DF, Oppenheim JJ. Signals and receptors involved in recruitment of inflammatory cells. *J Biol Chem* 1995;270:11703–11706.

158. Pike MC. The role of the monocyte and macrophage in the pathogenesis of vasculitis. In: LeRoy EC, ed. *Systemic vasculitis: the biological basis*. New York: Marcel Dekker, 1992:129–147.

159. Takayama H, Kojima H, Shinohara N. Cytotoxic T lymphocytes: the newly identified Fas (CD95)-mediated killing mechanism and a novel aspect of their biological functions. *Adv Immunol* 1995;60:289–321.

160. Border WA, Noble NA. Transforming growth factor β in tissue fibrosis. *N Engl J Med* 1994;331:1286–1292.

161. Wu KK, Thiagarajan P. Role of endothelium in thrombosis and hemostasis. *Annu Rev Med* 1996;47:315–331.

162. Bevilacqua MP. Endothelial-leukocyte adhesion molecules. *Annu Rev Immunol* 1993;11:767–804.

163. Rosen SD, Bertozzi CR. The selectins and their ligands. *Curr Opin Cell Biol* 1994;6:663–673.

164. Dianzani U, Malavasi F. Lymphocyte adhesion to endothelium. *Crit Rev Immunol* 1995;15:167–200.

165. Imhof BA, Dunon D. Leukocyte migration and adhesion. *Adv Immunol* 1995;58:345–416.

166. Stewart M, Thiel M, Hogg N. Leukocyte integrins. *Curr Opin Cell Biol* 1995;7:690–696.

167. Prieschl EE, Kulmburg PA, Baumruker T. The nomenclature of chemokines. *Int Arch Allergy Immunol* 1995;107:475–483.

168. Bacon KB, Schall TJ. Chemokines as mediators of allergic inflammation. *Int Arch Allergy Immunol* 1996;109:97–109.

169. Springer TA. Traffic signals for lymphocyte recirculation and leukocyte emigration: the multistep paradigm. *Cell* 1994;76:301–314.

170. Butcher EC, Picker LJ. Lymphocyte homing and homeostasis. *Science* 1996;272:60–66.

171. Stegeman CA, Cohen Tervaert JW, Huitema MG, et al. Serum levels of soluble adhesion molecules intercellular adhesion molecule 1, vascular cell adhesion molecule 1, and E-selectin in patients with Wegener's granulomatosis. *Arthritis Rheum* 1994;37:1228–1235.

172. Voskuyl AE, Martin S, Melchers I, et al. Levels of circulating intercellular adhesion molecule-1 and -3 but not circulating endothelial leucocyte adhesion molecule are increased in patients with rheumatoid vasculitis. *Br J Rheumatol* 1995;34:311–315.

173. Hartung H-P, Reiners K, Michels M, et al. Serum levels of soluble E-selectin (ELAM-1) in immune-mediated neuropathies. *Neurology* 1994;44:1153–1158.

174. Panegyres PK, Faull RJ, Russ GR, et al. Endothelial cell activation in vasculitis of peripheral nerve and skeletal muscle. *J Neurol Neurosurg Psychiatry* 1992;55:4–7.

175. Haskard DO. Cytokines, growth factors, and interferons. In: Le Roy EC, ed. *Systemic vasculitis: the biological basis*. New York: Marcel Dekker, 1992:223–247.

176. Grau GE, Roux-Lombard P, Gysler C, et al. Serum cytokine changes in systemic vasculitis. *Immunology* 1989;68:196–198.

177. Kekow J, Szymkowiak CH, Sticherling M, et al. Pro- and anti-inflammatory cytokines in primary systemic vasculitis. In: Gross WL, ed. *ANCA-associated vasculitides: immunological and clinical aspects*. New York: Plenum, 1993:341–344.

178. Cochrane CG, Koffler D. Immune complex disease in experimental animals and man. *Adv Immunol* 1973;16:185–264.

179. Gauthier VJ, Mannik M. Immune complexes in the pathogenesis of vasculitis. In: LeRoy EC, ed. *Systemic vasculitis: the biological basis*. New York: Marcel Dekker, 1992:401–420.

180. Haynes BF. Vasculitis: pathogenic mechanisms of vessel damage. In: Gallin JI, Goldstein IM, Snyderman R, eds. *Inflammation: basic principles and clinical correlates*. New York: Raven, 1992:921–941.

181. Van Vollenhaven RF. Adhesion molecules, sex steroids, and the pathogenesis of vasculitis syndromes. *Curr Opin Rheumatol* 1995;7:4–10.

182. Palacios-Boix A, Alarcon-Segovia D. Antibodies to endothelial cells: new clues for the study of vascular damage in the autoimmune diseases. In: Cervera R, Khamashta MA, Hughes GRV, eds. *Antibodies to endothelial cells and vascular damage*. Boca Raton, FL: CRC, 1994:1–15.

183. Hirschberg H, Bergh OJ, Thorsby E. Antigen presenting properties of human vascular endothelial cells. *J Exp Med* 1980;52:249S–255S.

184. Meroni PL, Khamashta MA, Youinou P, Shoenfeld Y. Conference report. Mosaic of anti-endothelial antibodies. Review of the first international workshop on anti-endothelial antibodies: clinical and pathological significance. *Lupus* 1995;4:95–99.

185. Falk RJ, Terrell RS, Charles LA, Jennette JC. Anti-neutrophil cytoplasmic autoantibodies induce neutrophils to degranulate and produce oxygen radicals *in vitro*. *Proc Natl Acad Sci USA* 1990;87:4115–4119.

186. Ewart BH, Jennette JC, Falk RJ. Anti-myeloperoxidase antibodies stimulate neutrophils to damage human endothelial cells. *Kidney Int* 1992;41:375–383.

187. Mayet WJ, Csernok E, Szymkowiak C, et al. Human endothelial cells express proteinase 3, the target antigen of autocytoplasmic antibodies in Wegener's granulomatosis. *Blood* 1993;82:1221–1229.

188. Mayet WJ, Schwarting A, Orth T, et al. Antibodies to proteinase 3 mediate expression of vascular cell adhesion molecule-1 (VCAM-1). *Clin Exp Immunol* 1996;103:259–267.

189. van de Wiel BA, Dolman KM, van der Meer-Gerritsen CH, et al. Interference of Wegener's granulomatosis antibodies with neutrophil proteinase 3 activity. *Clin Exp Immunol* 1992;90:409–414.

190. Gephardt GN, Ahmad M, Tubbs RR. Pulmonary vasculitis (Wegener's granulomatosis): immunohistochemical study of T and B cell markers. *Am J Med* 1983;74:700–704.

191. Ten Berge I, Wilmink J, Meyer C, et al. Clinical and immunologic follow up of patients with severe renal disease in Wegener's granulomatosis. *Am J Nephrol* 1985;5:21–29.

192. Shiki H, Shimokama T, Watanabe T. Temporal arteritis: cell composition and the possible pathogenic role of cell-mediated immunity. *Hum Pathol* 1989;20:1057–1064.

193. Mathieson PW, Cobbold SP, Hale G, et al. Monoclonal antibody therapy in systemic vasculitis. *N Engl J Med* 1990;323:250–254.

194. Allen NB, Caldwell DS, Rice JR, McCallum RM. Cyclosporin A therapy for Wegener's granulomatosis. In: Gross WL, ed. *ANCA-associated vasculitides: immunological and clinical aspects*. New York: Plenum, 1993:473–476.

195. Weyand CM, Hicok KC, Hunder GG, Goronzy JJ. Tissue cytokine patterns in patients with polymyositis rheumatica and giant cell arteritis. *Ann Intern Med* 1994;121:484–491.

196. McManis PG, Low PA, Lagerlund JD. Microenvironment of nerve: blood flow and ischemia. In: Dyck PJ, Thomas PK, Griffin JW, et al, eds. *Peripheral neuropathy*. 3rd ed. Philadelphia: WB Saunders, 1993:453–473.

197. Beggs J, Johnson PC, Olafsen A, et al. Transperineurial arterioles in human sural nerve. *J Neuropathol Exp Neurol* 1991;50:704–718.

198. Duna GF, Hoffman GS. Immunosuppression: new perspectives in the treatment of the systemic vasculitides. *Ann Med Interne (Paris)* 1994;145:581–594.

199. Moore PM. Vasculitis: diagnosis and therapy. *Semin Neurol* 1994;14:159–167.

200. Guillevin L, Lhote F, Leon A, et al. Treatment of polyarteritis nodosa related to hepatitis B virus with short term steroid therapy associated with antiviral agents and plasma exchange: a prospective trial in 33 patients. *J Rheumatol* 1993;20:289–298.

201. Khella SL, Frost S, Hermann GA, et al. Hepatitis C virus infection, cryoglobulinemia, and vasculitic neuropathy. Treatment with interferon-alpha: case report and literature review. *Neurology* 1995;45:407–411.

202. Ferri C, Marzo E, Longombardo G, et al. Interferon-alpha in mixed cryoglobulinemia patients: a randomized, crossover-controlled trial. *Blood* 1993;81:1132–1136.

203. Misiani R, Bellavita P, Fenili D, et al. Interferon alpha-2a therapy in cryoglobulinemia associated with hepatitis C virus. *N Engl J Med* 1994;330:751–756.

204. Fauci AS, Katz P, Haynes BF, Wolff SM. Cyclophosphamide therapy of severe systemic necrotizing vasculitis. *N Engl J Med* 1979;301:235–238.

205. Guillevin L, Lhote F, Cohen P, et al. Corticosteroids plus pulse cyclophosphamide and plasma exchanges versus corticosteroids plus pulse cyclophosphamide alone in the treatment of polyarteritis nodosa and Churg-Strauss syndrome patients with factors predicting poor prognosis. *Arthritis Rheum* 1995;38:1638–1645.

206. Bach JF, Strom TB. *The mode of action of immunosuppressive agents. Corticosteroids*. 2nd edition. New York: Elsevier, 1985:21–103.

207. Axelrod L. Glucocorticoids. In: Kelly WN, Harris ED, Ruddy S, Sledge CB, eds. *Textbook of rheumatology*. 4th ed. Philadelphia: WB Saunders, 1993:779–796.

208. Boumpas DT. Glucocorticoid therapy for immune diseases: basic and clinical correlates. *Ann Intern Med* 1993;119:1198–1208.

209. Lhote F, Guillevin L. Treatment of polyarteritis nodosa and microscopic polyangiitis. *Ann Med Interne (Paris)* 1994;145:550–565.

210. Bach JF, Strom TB. *The mode of action of immunosuppressive agents. Alkylating agents*. 2nd ed. New York: Elsevier, 1985:175–239.

211. Denman AM, Denman DJ, Palmer RG. Alkylating agents. In: Rugstad HE, Endresen L, Forre O, eds. *Immunopharmacology in autoimmune diseases and transplantation*. New York: Plenum, 1992:139–158.

212. Fauci AS, Young KR. Immunoregulatory agents. In: Kelly WN, Harris ED, Ruddy S, Sledge CB, eds. *Textbook of rheumatology*. 4th ed. Philadelphia: WB Saunders, 1993:797–821.

213. Zhu L-P, Cupps TR, Whalen G, Fauci AS. Selective effects of cyclophosphamide on activation, proliferation, and differentiation of human B cells. *J Clin Invest* 1987;79:1082–1090.

214. Gordon M, Luqmani RA, Adu D, et al. Relapses in patients with a systemic vasculitis. *Q J Med* 1993;86:779–789.

215. Hoffman GS, Leavitt RY, Fleisher TA, et al. Treatment of Wegener's granulomatosis with intermittent high-dose

intravenous cyclophosphamide. *Am J Med* 1990;89: 403–410.

216. Reinhold-Keller E, Kekow J, Schnabel A, et al. Influence of disease manifestation and antineutrophil cytoplasmic antibody titer on the response to pulse cyclophosphamide therapy in patients with Wegener's granulomatosis. *Arthritis Rheum* 1994;37:919–924.

217. Luqmani RA, Pall A, Adu D, et al. Controlled trial of pulse vs continuous cyclophosphamide (CY) and prednisolone (P) in the treatment of systemic vasculitis. *Arthritis Rheum* 1993;36(suppl):S96. Abstract.

218. Guillevin L, LeClerc P, Jarrousee B, et al. Treatment of severe Wegener's granulomatosis: a prospective trial in 58 patients comparing prednisone (CS), pulse cyclophosphamide (CY) versus CS and oral CY. *Arthritis Rheum* 1994;37(suppl):S352. Abstract.

219. Bach JF. Mode of action of thiopurines. In: Rugstad HE, Endresen L, Foree O, eds. *Immunopharmacology in autoimmune diseases and transplantation*. New York: Plenum, 1992:123–126.

220. Weinblatt ME. Methotrexate. In: Kelly WN, Harris ED, Ruddy S, Sledge CB, eds. *Textbook of rheumatology*. 4th ed. Philadelphia: WB Saunders, 1993:767–778.

221. Hoffman GS, Leavitt RY, Kerr GS, Fauci AS. The treatment of Wegener's granulomatosis with glucocorticoids and methotrexate. *Arthritis Rheum* 1992;35:1322–1329.

222. Sneller MC, Talar-Williams C, Hallahan C, et al. Analysis of 42 patients with Wegener's granulomatosis treated with low dose methotrexate plus glucocorticoids. *Arthritis Rheum* 1994;37(suppl):S353. Abstract.

223. Faulds D, Goa KL, Benfield P. Cyclosporin: a review of its pharmacodynamic and pharmacokinetic properties, and therapeutic use in immunoregulatory disorders. *Drugs* 1993;45:953–1040.

224. Pusey CD, Rees AJ, Evans DJ, et al. Plasma exchange in focal necrotizing glomerulonephritis without anti-GBM antibodies. *Kidney Int* 1991;40:757–763.

225. Newburger J, Takahashi M, Burns J, et al. The treatment of Kawasaki syndrome with intravenous gamma globulin. *N Engl J Med* 1986;315:341–347.

226. Boman S, Ballen JL, Seggev JS. Dramatic responses to intravenous immunoglobulin in vasculitis. *J Intern Med* 1995;238:375–377.

227. Jayne DRW, Lockwood CM. Pooled intravenous immunoglobulin in the management of systemic vasculitis. In: Gross WL, ed. *ANCA-associated vasculitides: immunological and clinical aspects*. New York: Plenum, 1993:469–472.

228. Richter C, Schnabel A, Csernok E, et al. Treatment of ANCA-associated systemic vasculitis with high-dose intravenous immunoglobulin. *Arthritis Rheum* 1994; 37(suppl):S353. Abstract.

229. Conn DL. Overview of therapy and management of systemic vasculitis. In: Le Roy EC, ed. *Systemic vasculitis: the biological basis*. New York: Marcel Dekker, 1992: 547–574.

230. LeBoff MS, Wade JP. Osteoporosis and rheumatic disorders. In: Weisman MH, Weinblatt ME, eds. *Treatment of the rheumatic diseases*. Philadelphia: WB Saunders, 1995:349–364.

231. Sambrook P, Birmingham J, Kelly P, et al. Prevention of corticosteroid osteoporosis: a comparison of calcium, calcitriol, and calcitonin. *N Engl J Med* 1993;328:1747–1752.

232. Talar-Williams C, Hijazi YM, Walther MM, et al. Cyclophosphamide-induced cystitis and bladder cancer in patients with Wegener granulomatosis. *Ann Intern Med* 1996;124:477–484.

233. Dalakas M. Pharmacologic concerns of corticosteroids in the treatment of patients with immune-related neuromuscular diseases. *Neurol Clin* 1990;8:93–118.

234. Galer BS. Neuropathic pain of peripheral origin: advances in pharmacologic treatment. *Neurology* 1995; 45(suppl 9):S17–S25.

235. Jayne DRW, Lockwood CM. New strategies in the treatment of systemic vasculitis. *Ann Med Interne (Paris)* 1994;145:595–600.

236. Arend WP. Inhibiting the effects of cytokines in human diseases. *Adv Intern Med* 1995;40:365–394.

237. Barrera P, Boerbooms AMT, van de Putte LBA, van der Meer JWM. Effects of antirheumatic agents on cytokines. *Semin Arthritis Rheum* 1996;25:234–253.

238. McMurray RW. Adhesion molecules in autoimmune diseases. *Semin Arthritis Rheum* 1996;25:215–233.

239. Anaya J-M, Espinoza LR. Phosphodiesterase inhibitor pentoxifylline: an anti-inflammatory/immunomodulatory drug potentially used in some rheumatic diseases. *J Rheumatol* 1995;22:595–597.

240. Rott O, Cash E, Fleischer B. Phosphodiesterase inhibitor pentoxifylline, a selective suppressor of T helper type 1- but not type 2-associated lymphokine production, prevents induction of experimental autoimmune encephalomyelitis in Lewis rats. *Eur J Immunol* 1993;23:1745–1751.

241. McHugh SM, Rifkin IR, Deighton J. The immunosuppressive drug thalidomide induces T helper cell type 2 (Th2) and concomitantly inhibits Th1 cytokine production in mitogen- and antigen-stimulated human peripheral blood mononuclear cell cultures. *Clin Exp Immunol* 1995;99:160–167.

242. Schuler U, Ehninger G. Thalidomide: rationale for renewed use in immunological disorders. *Drug Saf* 1995;12:364–369.

The views expressed herein are those of the authors and do not necessarily reflect the views of the United States Air Force or the Department of Defense.

Chapter 22

Antibody-Mediated Disorders of the Neuromuscular Junction and Myasthenia Gravis

Angela Vincent

The neuromuscular junction (NMJ) has long been considered the archetypal synapse, being both relatively simple in its function and easy to study. It remains the most accessible synapse in the nervous system and is very susceptible to circulating factors, notably neurotoxins and specific autoantibodies.

In this chapter, I briefly describe the structure and function of the NMJ, and then discuss the clinical, pathologic, and immunologic features of myasthenia gravis (MG), an autoimmune disease caused by antibodies to muscle acetylcholine receptor (AChR). In the next chapter, I discuss two other autoimmune diseases and the role of antibodies to gangliosides. These topics have been reviewed many times, and the emphasis here is mainly on the current thinking and new areas of research.

Neuromuscular Junction

To understand the pathophysiology of autoimmune disorders of the NMJ, it is necessary to be familiar with its molecular structure and function (see (1)). The terminal portions of the motor nerve axons are devoid of myelin sheath and expand into "boutons," as illustrated in Figure 22-1A. These lie in close apposition to infoldings on the muscle membrane surface called *postsynaptic or junctional folds*. Schwann cell extensions form a protective layer around the boutons. The presynaptic nerve terminal is distinguished by the large number of mitochondria and small spherical vesicles (synaptic vesicles) that contain the neurotransmitter acetylcholine (ACh). These are mainly concentrated just inside the presynaptic membrane, particularly close to "active zones" (AZs) (see Fig 22-1B). AZs are defined by the presence, in freeze-fracture representations, of double parallel rows of particles that are thought to be voltage-gated calcium channels (VGCCs) (see Chapter 23). The AZs are opposite the entrance to the secondary synaptic clefts between the junctional folds. Around the synaptic vesicles are cytoplasmic densities that are thought to represent a network of filaments and specific proteins involved in exocytosis (for a recent review, see (2)). Between the presynaptic and postsynaptic membranes is a gap of 500 Å filled with a deceptively amorphous-looking basal lamina. This contains collagen IV, heparin sulfate, laminin, and other specific components, and is where the enzyme acetylcholinesterase (AChE) is anchored (see Fig 22-1B).

The peaks of the postsynaptic folds are electron dense corresponding to the distribution of the highly concentrated (10,000/m²) AChRs. On the cytoplasmic face of the AChR-containing membrane, postsynaptic densities represent the web of proteins that anchor the AChR and other functional proteins.

The nerve action potential is propagated along the nerve by the opening of voltage-gated sodium channels at the nodes of Ranvier. When it invades the motor nerve terminals, the depolarization opens the VGCCs at the AZs, resulting in a transient and very localized increase in cytoplasmic Ca^{2+}. This causes fusion of synaptic vesicles with the motor nerve terminal membrane by mechanisms that are still poorly understood, and release of ACh into the synaptic space by exocytosis. ACh diffuses rapidly to the postsynaptic membrane and binds to the AChRs, leading to opening of the AChR-associated ion channel (see Fig 22-1C). Cations, mainly Na^+, diffuse through the channel, leading to a localized depolarization called the *end-plate potential* (EPP). If the depolarization exceeds a certain threshold, voltage-gated sodium channels that may lie at the bottom of the postsynaptic folds are opened (see Fig 22-1B). This generates the muscle action potential that propagates along the muscle fiber and activates contraction. The action of ACh is terminated by its dissociation from the AChR; the AChR ion channel closes spontaneously after 1 to 4 msec, and ACh is hydrolyzed by AChE.

The action potential in nerve and muscle is terminated by the spontaneous inactivation of sodium channels and the opening of several different kinds of potassium channels. Efflux of potassium from the cell through these channels brings the membrane potential back to resting values (around −80 mV). The ouabain-sensitive Na^+/K^+ exchanger is responsible for maintaining the concentration gradient for Na^+ and K^+.

Spontaneous release of single vesicles or "quanta" of ACh occurs in the absence of nerve impulses and results in a small depolarization called the *miniature end-plate potential* (MEPP). The number of quanta released per

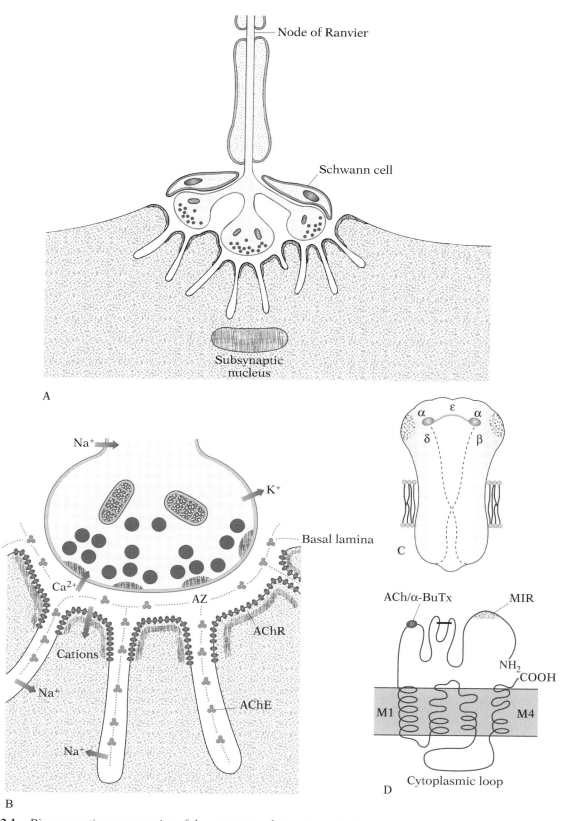

Figure 22-1. Diagrammatic representation of the neuromuscular junction (A), the motor nerve terminal and postsynaptic membrane (B), and the acetylcholine receptor (C). (D) The topology of the α subunit, which has a main immunogenic region (MIR) and acetylcholine (ACh)/α-bungarotoxin (BuTx) binding site. Each of the subunits has a similar topology. AChR = acetylcholine receptor; AChE = acetylcholinesterase; AZ = active zone.

nerve impulse, the *quantal content* (QC), can be calculated by measuring the amplitude of the EPP and dividing this by the amplitude of the MEPPs (with correction for nonlinear summation). The QC is very sensitive to changes in extracellular Ca^{2+} or the effect of drugs or other substances on the VGCCs. The amplitude of the MEPPs is sensitive to substances that affect the function of the postsynaptic AChRs, or to those that increase the concentration and duration of action of ACh. AChE inhibitors, for instance, increase the amplitude and prolong the time course of both the MEPP and the EPP. In MG, when there are reduced numbers of AChRs, leading to small MEPPs and EPPs, the increase in EPP amplitude achieved with AChE inhibitors can be sufficient to achieve the threshold depolarization required to restore neuromuscular transmission.

Although neuromuscular transmission is apparently a simple, one-way process, recent evidence indicates that there are several autoregulatory and exogenous substances that can increase or reduce ACh release from the motor nerve terminal, or modulate postsynaptic AChR activity (3).

Neurotoxins with Specificity for Neuromuscular Transmission

The venom of many species of snake, scorpion, spiders, fish, fish-eating snails, and other creatures contains alkaloid and polypeptide toxins that bind with high affinity to specific proteins at the NMJ and can cause paralysis, respiratory failure, and death within a short period of time in their prey. These neurotoxins have provided us with a unique library of tools for investigation and purification of the proteins involved in neuromuscular transmission (NMT) (4). For instance, α-bungarotoxin (BuTx) binds irreversibly to muscle AChRs, blocking the ACh-binding site (see Fig 22-1C). Radioiodinated α-BuTx can be used to label AChRs in whole tissue and to tag AChR after detergent extraction for use in immunoprecipitation assays; neurotoxins specific for calcium and potassium channels are used in a similar manner (see below).

Vulnerability of the Neuromuscular Junction to Circulating Factors

The accessibility of the NMJ to serum factors is well illustrated by the rapid, potentially fatal, respiratory failure produced by some of the venomous species mentioned above, particularly in smaller mammals, but also in humans. There is ample evidence that circulating autoantibodies can bind to antigenic targets at the NMJ, as illustrated by the studies of MG discussed in this chapter and of the Lambert-Eaton syndrome (see Chapter 23). The accessibility of antigens located in the nerve axons, nodes of Ranvier, and nerve roots is not so clear. Direct application and passive transfer studies in peripheral nerve disorders, described in Chapter 23, make it likely that these antigens are also accessible to antibodies in vivo and in vitro.

Myasthenia Gravis

Clinical and Pathophysiologic Features

MG is an acquired autoimmune disorder in which autoantibodies to the postsynaptic AChRs are reduced in number or function, leading to muscle fatigue and weakness. The weakness often starts in the eye muscles, resulting in double vision and ptosis (drooping eyelids), but may involve any muscle group. Typically, the weakness varies in distribution and severity from day to day, is often worse at the end of the day, increases with stress, and tends to improve with rest. For a comprehensive review of the clinical features, see the publications by Oosterhuis (5,6). MG is frequently associated with thymic abnormalities, thymitis, or thymic hyperplasia in about 60% and thymoma in around 10% of patients.

The diagnosis is made by a positive anti-AChR antibody titer (7,8), which is present in 85% to 90% of patients. Patients also show a transient clinical response to the intravenous AChE inhibitor edrophonium. A decrement in the compound muscle action potential is typically revealed on low-frequency nerve stimulation studies and, in virtually all patients, increased "jitter" is apparent on single-fiber studies (for details of these methods, see the article by Drachman (9)).

Treatment

Anti-AChE drugs are the first line of treatment, but most patients require further help. Plasma exchange by removing circulating antibodies provides short-term improvement. Thymectomy is performed in most seropositive patients who were young (<40 years) at disease onset, resulting in remission in about 25% and improvement in 50%. Removal of thymoma is essential, because of the risk of local infiltration, but seldom leads to clinical improvement, and immunosuppression with corticosteroids or azathioprine, or both, is usually required. Immunosuppression is often the treatment of choice in older patients (see works by others (5,9)).

Autoimmunity

The occurrence of MG in young females, its association with other autoimmune diseases, the presence of thymic pathology, and the transfer of MG from mothers to their neonates, "neonatal MG," led Simpson (10) to propose that MG is an autoimmune disease with antibodies directed against "end-plate" protein. Nastuk et al (11,12) also proposed an autoimmune basis. In a recent study, 9% of patients had other autoimmune disorders, mostly thyroid and rheumatoid arthritis, and these patients had more severe MG (13).

Simpson's theory was validated in 1973 when Patrick and Lindstrom (14) showed that immunization against affinity-purified AChRs could induce weakness and paralysis in rabbits that, like MG, was responsive to edrophonium. This condition, termed *experimental au-*

toimmune myasthenia gravis (EAMG), has since been induced in many species by immunization with affinity-purified AChRs from a variety of sources (see below).

The Acetylcholine Receptor

The AChR is an oligomeric membrane protein that consists of five subunits: α_2, β, γ, and δ in embryonic or denervated muscle, and α_2, β, δ, and ϵ at the adult end plate (see Fig 22-1C). Each subunit has four transmembrane domains (see Fig 22-1D). Each of the two α subunits has a binding site for ACh that is shared with the neurotoxin α-BuTx (see Fig 22-1C) (15). Isolated α subunits, and synthetic peptides representing α185-199, bind α-BuTx but the binding is several orders of magnitude less than that to the native molecule, suggesting that other sequences and tertiary structures are essential for the high-affinity neurotoxin binding. The same applies to most of the antibody binding sites (see below).

In human muscle there are two isoforms of the α subunit expressed in roughly equal amounts. The P3A+ isoform contains an extra 25–amino acid sequence between α58 and 59 (16). However, it does not appear to contribute to a functional AChR and its role in normal or MG muscle function is not yet clear (17).

Antibodies to Acetylcholine Receptor

Anti-AChR is measured by immunoprecipitation of ^{125}I-α-BuTx–labeled AChR extracted from ischemic human muscle (7,8) or from the rhabdomyosarcoma cell line, TE671 (18). The latter gives about 5% to 7% false-negative results because it contains only the extrajunctional or embryonic form of the AChR (see above). Amputated-leg muscle from patients with ischemic disease is a good source of both types. With either source, anti-AChR titers are highly variable among MG patients, ranging from 0 to more than 1000 nm/L (Fig 22-2), and between individuals titers do not correlate well with clinical severity. However, positive values are extremely rare in healthy subjects, and the level of antibody within an individual correlates well with clinical scores in serial studies after plasma exchange (19), thymectomy (20,21), or immunosuppressive treatment.

Antibodies to Other Muscle Antigens

More than 90% of patients with thymoma, and many patients older than 40 years at disease onset, have antibodies to antigens of striated and cardiac muscle (22). These include myosin, actin, α actinin, ryanodine receptor, and a particular epitope on the giant structural protein titin (23–25). The antibodies are mostly IgG1 and IgG3 (26). Cross-reactivity has been demonstrated between AChR and myosin heavy chain (27) and fast troponin I (28). Although there is no evidence that anti-AChR in MG is derived from cross-reaction with any of these proteins, within individual patients, antimuscle antibodies correlate well with anti-AChR and, like anti-AChR, they may first appear after removal of a thy-

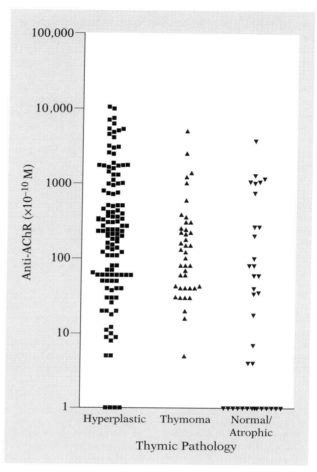

Figure 22-2. Anti–acetylcholine receptor (AChR) antibody levels in myasthenia gravis (MG) patients before thymectomy or immunosuppressive therapy, shown in relation to the subsequently demonstrated thymic pathology. Note that a proportion of patients did not have detectable anti-AChR ($<2 \times 10^{-10}$ M), and those are mainly the patients who had a normal or atrophic thymus.

moma (29–31). Thus, understanding the origin of these antibodies and their relationship with thymoma may throw light on the origin of the anti-AChR response. IgM monoclonal antimyosin and antititin antibodies, with a specificity similar to the patients' IgG antibodies, have been successfully raised by immortalizing lymphocytes from thymoma tissue (32,33).

Pathophysiology

In MG, MEPPs are substantially reduced (34) owing to a reduction in the number of functional AChRs at the NMJ, as measured by binding of ^{125}I-, peroxidase-, or fluoresceinated-labeled α-BuTx (35,36). The EPP is moderately reduced in amplitude but the QC is normal or even raised. In fact, a recent study suggested that a compensatory increase in QC results from a positive feedback mechanism in both MG and EAMG (37).

Electron microscopy shows an essentially normal nerve terminal (38). By contrast, the postsynaptic membrane lacks junctional folds and has reduced areas of contact between the presynaptic nerve terminal and the muscle membrane. There is also considerable debris within the synaptic cleft (Fig 22-3).

Pathologic Role and Pathogenic Mechanisms of Anti-AChR Antibodies

The presence of anti-AChR antibody is diagnostic for MG, and the levels reflect the severity of the disease within an individual, but by itself this does not prove that the antibodies cause the disease. However, several approaches illustrate the pathogenic role of anti-AChR. Firstly, EAMG can be induced by the immunization of rabbits with purified AChR from the electric organ of the electric ray (14). Secondly, MG can be passively transferred to experimental animals by injection of MG IgG (39), and EAMG can be transferred to naive litter mates by injection of EAMG serum (40) or monoclonal anti-AChR antibodies (41). Thirdly, Engel et al showed that IgG and complement components are present at the NMJ, both on the postsynaptic membrane and in the synaptic debris (see Fig 22-3) (42); the distribution of IgG corresponds well to the distribution of AChRs as shown by peroxidase α-BuTx binding; and the amount of membrane attack complex is inversely related to the number and density of AChRs (43). Thus, MG fulfills the

criteria of Witbesky: the presence of antibodies to a defined antigen, the ability to induce the disease experimentally by immunization with the purified antigen and to transfer it by experimental and patients' serum, and the demonstration that these antibodies are involved in the pathology of the human disease (44). The beneficial effects of plasma exchange and immunosuppression provide further confirmation.

Complement-mediated damage to the NMJ is not the only mechanism by which anti-AChR reduces the numbers of AChRs. Drachman et al (45,46) clearly demonstrated cross-linking of AChRs by divalent antibodies. This results in a change in the rate of internalization and degradation of the AChRs, reducing the half-life for AChRs from about 10 days to about 5 days. This in itself would be sufficient to reduce the numbers of AChR by about 40%. However, there may be a compensatory increase in AChR synthesis, as shown in experimental studies of AChR turnover (47) and in raised messenger RNA (mRNA) levels for AChR subunits in MG (48) and in EAMG (49). Thus, the importance of this mechanism in ongoing disease is not clear.

Direct inhibition of AChR function by antibodies appears to be less common. Only a few investigators described direct functional effects of serum or an IgG preparation on the amplitudes of MEPPs in vitro (50), although serum reduced AChR function in cultured cells (51). Antibodies specifically inhibiting fetal AChRs were found in two mothers with a history of recurrent fetal arthrogryposis (see below).

Clinical Heterogeneity and Immunogenetics

It is now generally accepted that MG is not a single disease entity. Characteristics of the main groups of patients are summarized in Table 22-1. Patients with generalized myasthenia without anti-AChR antibodies are considered below.

Ocular Myasthenia Gravis

Ocular MG, defined by symptoms that remain restricted to extraocular muscles for at least 2 years, has often been considered a distinct condition (although there may be electrophysiologic defects in other muscle groups). Anti-AChR levels are generally low or undetectable in about 50% of affected patients. The thymus gland is often normal, in the few patients examined, and most studies show no apparent HLA association. In Taiwan, a large proportion of MG patients present with ocular symptoms before the age of 10 (52). These patients show an association with HLA Bw46 and DR9 (53).

It has been suggested that ocular muscle AChR is antigenically different from the AChR of other muscles; it is known that ocular muscle contains some multiply-innervated fibers of the slow twitch type, and serum antibodies from patients with ocular MG bind to multiply-innervated end plates as demonstrated by immunohistochemistry (54). However, radioimmunoassays reveal no preference for ocular muscle AChR over adult leg muscle AChR (55), suggesting that the

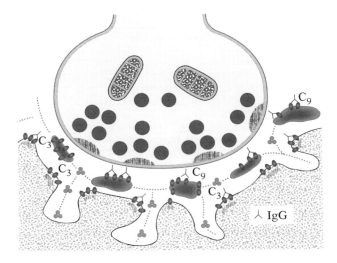

Figure 22-3. Diagrammatic representation of the neuromuscular junction in MG. Note the essentially normal nerve terminal but grossly simplified postsynaptic folds and debris in the synaptic cleft. Acetylcholine receptor numbers are reduced, IgG and C3 are found on the postsynaptic membrane, and AChR, IgG, C3, and C9 are found in the synaptic debris.

Table 22-1.
HLA Type, Thymic Pathology, and Anti–Acetylcholine Receptor (AChR) Antibody Status in Myasthenia Gravis Patients*

| | No. of Males/Females | Typical HLA | Thymic Pathology | | |
			Thymoma	Hyperplastic	Involuted
Seropositive					
General disease					
Onset <40 yr	60/206	B8DR3	—	160	28
Onset ≥40 yr	54/37	B7DR2	—	6	9
Thymoma	40/39	—	63	—	—
Ocular disease	24/16	—	1	0	1
Seronegative					
General	20/24	—	0	3	17
Ocular	25/8	—	0	1	3

Thymoma is usually associated with generalized disease, and is always anti-AChR positive; also there are relatively more seronegative patients with involuted thymuses. Anti-AChR antibody status was determined before immunosuppressive treatment or thymectomy.
*All patients were seen by Prof. J. Newsom-Davis.

two forms are not antigenically distinct. Horton et al (56) showed that ocular muscle contains the fetal-specific γ subunit of the AChR, but the adult-specific ε subunit is expressed more strongly (57). Moreover, a healthy woman with high levels of antibodies directed against fetal AChR shows no clinical evidence of ocular involvement (see below). Since ocular weakness is often the presenting symptom in neurotoxin poisoning (e.g., botulism, *Bungarus krait* envenoming) it may be that physiologic factors or accessibility of the end plates to circulating factors underlie their susceptibility to clinical involvement.

Generalized Myasthenia Gravis

In the majority of white MG patients, generalized weakness develops after puberty, without obvious precipitating factors, and the levels of anti-AChRs are increased; patients are divided into three groups on the basis of their thymic pathology and age at onset (see Table 22-1). There are only subtle differences in the characteristics of the anti-AChR between the patients (58), and it seems likely that the distinguishing clinical and pathologic features reflect a difference in the factors involved in the initiation of the disease, rather than an intrinsic difference in the patients' immune responses to a single precipitating factor. An association between a Km-3 κ light-chain immunoglobulin allotype and high serum anti-AChR titers in MG was recently shown, but the clinical subgroup of the patients was not reported (59). Involvement with a particular AChR α-subunit microsatellite, that is, a noncoding region of the gene, has also been reported (60). Therefore, it is possible that polymorphisms in gene regulatory sequences alter AChR expression and disease susceptibility.

An important provoking factor in a minority of patients is treatment with D(-)-penicillamine, usually for rheumatoid arthritis. About 2% of treated patients develop anti-AChR antibodies and clinical signs of MG that usually resolve after they stop taking the drug. This interesting form of MG is associated with HLA-DR1

rather than DR4 (61), as expected in rheumatoid arthritis, or DR3 as typical in MG patients. The antibodies are of slightly lower avidity and less heterogeneous, but this may reflect their relative short duration (62).

Early Onset
There is a 3:1 female-male ratio for patients who develop MG in early adult life. The thymus gland is usually hyperplastic (see below) and the patients respond well to thymectomy. In Northern Europeans, there is a very strong association with the HLA-A1 B8 DRB1*0301 DRB3*0101 DQB1*0201 DQA1*0501 ancestral haplotype (63–65).

Although the pathogenic autoantibodies depend on class II–restricted helper T cells, the associations are stronger with B8 than with DR3 (63,65). This suggests that some other predisposing gene between the class II and class I region may be responsible. Various possibilities, such as genes for tumor necrosis factor (TNF), heat shock proteins, and transporter proteins associated with antigen processing (TAP), have been considered (Janer M, Demaine A, Willcox N, unpublished data, 1994). On the other hand, class I–restricted cytotoxic T-cell responses might be directly involved in initiating the anti-AChR response. There are at least some potential class I epitopes on the AChR α subunit (66) and the role of cytotoxic/suppressor T cells in MG needs to be addressed. Interestingly, however, in Chinese and Japanese patients, the associations are stronger with class II than class I. In Japanese patients, DRw53, DQB1*03, and DPB1*0201 (67) and DR9 (68) associations have been documented in young-onset MG patients.

Late Onset
In patients who present with symptoms of MG after the age of 40 years, the thymus is mainly atrophic or involuted and there are weak biases toward males and HLA-B7, DR2 (65) or DR4, DQw8 (64). Although the overall prevalence of late onset MG is lower than that of early onset MG the annual incidence is actually higher (based

on the age at which patients are being referred for assays (Vincent A, Jacobson L, unpublished observations, 1996)). Anti-AChR levels are quite variable, and some are low or negative. There is a significant association with a polymorphic marker on the switch region of the immunoglobulin heavy-chain gene, *Sm* (69), suggesting that the existence of a particular humoral immune response, not necessarily against the AChR, may be involved in the development of this form of MG.

Thymoma-Associated Myasthenia Gravis

Thymoma, present in about 10% of patients, can arise at any age, although most patients present between the ages of 30 and 60 years. The thymus gland is usually removed, but the myasthenia rarely improves (70,71), anti-AChR levels seldom fall (21), and immunosuppressive therapy is often required. An HLA association has been difficult to demonstrate, although a lower than normal incidence of HLA-B8 and -DR3, and an association with DQB1*0604 (63) and with Drw15 Dw2 in female patients (64) have been found. Immunoglobulin allotypes have not generally been informative in MG, but associations in Japanese thymoma patients (72) and in white patients (73) have been reported. The role of the thymus in MG is discussed further later.

Neonatal Myasthenia Gravis and Arthrogryposis Multiplex Congenita

A proportion of babies born to MG mothers have transient respiratory and feeding difficulties, owing to transplacental transfer of maternal anti-AChR (74). These problems may be more common in the offspring of mothers who have a high proportion of antibodies reactive with fetal-type AChR (75), although the fetal form is thought to be replaced by the adult form from around 33 weeks' gestation. Occasionally neonatal MG occurs without maternal disease, or when the mother is anti-AChR negative.

Recently, two cases of severe arthrogryposis multiplex congenita, a condition consisting of fixed joint contractures associated with inadequate development of the jaws and lungs, were found in successive pregnancies. One mother was diagnosed as having MG only after her fourth affected pregnancy (76); the other remains clinically normal (77). Maternal anti-AChR antibodies that even at high dilution completely inhibited the function of fetal AChR in an in vitro assay, but had no effect on adult AChR function, were present in both mothers. These antibodies appeared to be responsible for the complete loss of fetal movement in utero and deformities that were incompatible with survival after birth. Both women also had anti-AChR binding to other sites on adult receptors, so the relationship between their symptoms and anti-AChR antibodies is not so clear.

Anti-AChR Characteristics

Anti-AChR antibodies are heterogeneous in light chain and IgG subclass and are highly specific for the intact human autoantigen. The high affinity (around 10^{-10} M)

and specificity of MG anti-AChRs indicate that the MG antibodies, at least those detected in the assay, are induced by some form of the native AChR molecule (58).

The antibodies show little ability to bind to denatured or recombinant polypeptides. Therefore, it has been difficult to define directly the epitopes for MG antibodies on human AChRs. However, in many patients, a high proportion of the anti-AChR antibody competes with monoclonal antibodies directed toward the main immunogenic region (MIR) on the α subunits. This is the dominant epitope defined by sera and monoclonal antibodies derived from animals immunized with purified AChR (78). Although the MIR is a conformational epitope, mapping studies with synthetic peptides and site-directed mutagenesis show that the sequence α67-76 makes an important contribution toward it (for a review, see (79)).

Many patients also have antibodies that compete with monoclonal antibodies directed against other epitopes (80) (Jacobson L, Vincent A, unpublished data, 1996). One of these may be on the δ subunit, but overlaps the MIR. Another is specific to fetal AChR (58) and is on the γ subunit; antibodies to this region may be induced by expression of the fetal AChR in thymic myoid cells (see below) but would not be expected to cause symptoms of MG because the γ subunit is not found at the normal adult NMJ. A minority of antibodies overlap a monoclonal antibody site on the β subunit. Antibodies to the ACh/α-BuTx binding site are a minority in most MG patients (81), in contrast to mothers with arthrogrypotic babies (see above) (77), but can displace α-BuTx from its binding site in the immunoprecipitation assay (82). Antibodies to α125-148 are found in 52% of MG patients but their contribution to the total anti-AChR is not clear (83).

Synthesis of Anti-AChR

Anti-AChR can be synthesized spontaneously in vitro by plasma cells from hyperplastic MG thymus or bone marrow, though cells from the latter make more total immunoglobulin (84). This spontaneous synthesis is rarely found in lymphocytes from thymoma or from atrophic tissue (85). Anti-AChR can also be synthesized in vitro by peripheral blood and lymph node cells, but this usually requires pokeweed mitogen stimulation (86,87).

Monoclonal Anti-AChR Antibodies

There have been few reports of monoclonal antibodies derived from immortalized AChR-specific MG cells, owing to low precursor frequencies and to the difficulty in obtaining stable IgG-secreting, rather than IgM-secreting, hybrids or Epstein-Barr virus (EBV)–transformed lines. Those that have been produced do not appear to recognize AChR in solution, suggesting that they may not be representative of the patients' anti-AChRs. Some bind to *Torpedo* (fish electric organ) AChR or to recombinant or chimeric AChR (88). One of these antibodies has been sequenced (89).

Phage display techniques offer the opportunity to

identify specific antibodies in an MG patient library. Some preliminary success has been achieved using TE671 cells for panning (90) or ^{125}I-α-BuTx–labeled AChR to identify plaques containing specific Fabs (91). It will now be necessary to establish that these antibodies are representative of those found in the individual's serum. If that can be confirmed, the sequencing and other characterization of these antibodies should be highly informative regarding the clonal origin and degree of somatic mutation that the anti-AChR–producing B cells undergo.

Anti-AChR, Idiotypes, and Bacterial Antigens

Antibodies against human or mouse anti-AChR idiotypes have been identified by several groups using enzyme-linked immunosorbent assay (ELISA) techniques (92,93). Most were of IgM class and their ability to inhibit anti-AChR binding to AChR was not demonstrated, suggesting that the binding was not necessarily idiotypic (see also (94)). Dwyer et al (95) described an extensive network of idiotype/anti-idiotypes. The network included antibodies specific for bacterial α1-3 dextrans, and they found antidextran antibodies in about 40% of MG patients, suggesting that anti-AChR antibodies might arise as a secondary result of an antibacterial response. In experimental rats, however, injection of an antidextran monoclonal antibody reduces the subsequent antibody response to AChR (96).

Other evidence for involvement of microorganisms is the cross-reaction between the *Torpedo* AChR α subunit and microbial proteins (97), and between human AChR α157-170 and herpes simplex glycoprotein D (98). However, it seems unlikely that cross-reacting antibodies could demonstrate the heterogeneity, high affinity, and specificity that characterize MG anti-AChR (58), and it is noteworthy that no further developments in this area have been reported. Nevertheless, such a cross-reaction could be an initiating event that leads subsequently to autosensitization against the muscle AChR by a process of determinant spreading (see below).

The Thymus in Myasthenia Gravis

Young-Onset Myasthenia Gravis

In young-onset MG the thymus gland is often hyperplastic with many T-cell areas in the medulla, some containing lymphoid follicles (Fig 22-4A, B). (For reviews see other publications (99–102).) The expression of accessory molecules like CD28/B7 is normal in hyperplastic thymus (103), but a recent report claims that the expression of the apoptosis-related antigen, Fas, is reduced in these lymphoid follicles, suggesting that the regulation of lymphocyte survival may be abnormal (104). Interleukin (IL)-1 production is increased in the hyperplastic MG thymus (105), and expression of IL-2, IL-6, and interferon (IFN)-γ is upregulated in perifollicular areas (106). It is not clear whether any of these changes are causative or merely a predictable feature of a lymph node–type infiltrate.

Lymphocytes cultured from the thymus gland synthesize anti-AChR antibody (84), and serum anti-AChR levels frequently decline slowly after the operation (20). Germinal centers of the MG thymus contain polyclonal activated B cells expressing a range of V_H and V_K genes, similar to that in the peripheral blood lymphocyte (107). AChR has been demonstrated in muscle-like cells grown from thymus (108,109) or "myoid" cells found in situ between the epithelial cells in both normal and MG thymic medullae (110) (see Fig 22-4C, D); myoid cells are clearly not in the lymph node–type areas. Some workers (111) found myoid cells to be the focus of antigen-presenting cells (APCs) and T cells in MG, but other workers did not (110); therefore, it is not clear whether this is a primary event in MG.

The presence of AChR in the thymus suggests that it may be involved in inducing T-cell tolerance in normal individuals or in breaking tolerance in MG (see (100,102)). However, the origin and significance of AChR expression in the thymus are quite controversial. Several groups reported the presence of mRNA for α subunit in whole tissue from normal and MG (112) or mouse thymus (113), and some workers found mRNA for α, β, γ, and δ subunits but little for the ε subunit (114); these results are consistent with the reported expression of fetal-type AChR on (presumably noninnervated) myoid cells in the thymic medulla (110). However, a problem with many of these studies is the use of sensitive polymerase chain reaction (PCR) techniques on mRNA from whole thymus; a more quantitative or in situ study of AChR expression would clarify the amount and localization of individual subunits of AChR in myoid cells or in the cortical epithelium of the thymus. A report that the P3A+ isoform of the human α subunit is expressed not only in thymus but also in other visceral tissues (115) has not been confirmed (116).

Thymoma

Thymomas associated with MG are epithelial in origin, perhaps derived from a stem cell common to both cortical and subcapsular epithelium (see (117)). A well-differentiated thymic carcinoma of low-grade malignancy is associated with MG in 77% of patients (118). A full description of these tumors and their classification can be found elsewhere (119,120). Medullary thymomas that contain spindle cells are more often associated with red cell aplasia. The typical MG thymoma contains large numbers of polyclonal developing T lymphocytes, many double positive for CD4 and CD8 and others with the single markers of maturing T cells (121). The number of T cells is often drastically depleted owing to preceding steroid therapy (122). The remaining lymphocytes might either escape deletion in the grossly disorganized cortex, or be specifically sensitized to antigens presented and expressed by the thymoma epithelium. The adjacent thymus is typically hyperplastic, though not in thymoma patients without MG (123), and a few B cells are present in thymoma tissue (124). However, anti-AChR synthesis by thymoma cells is rare (see above).

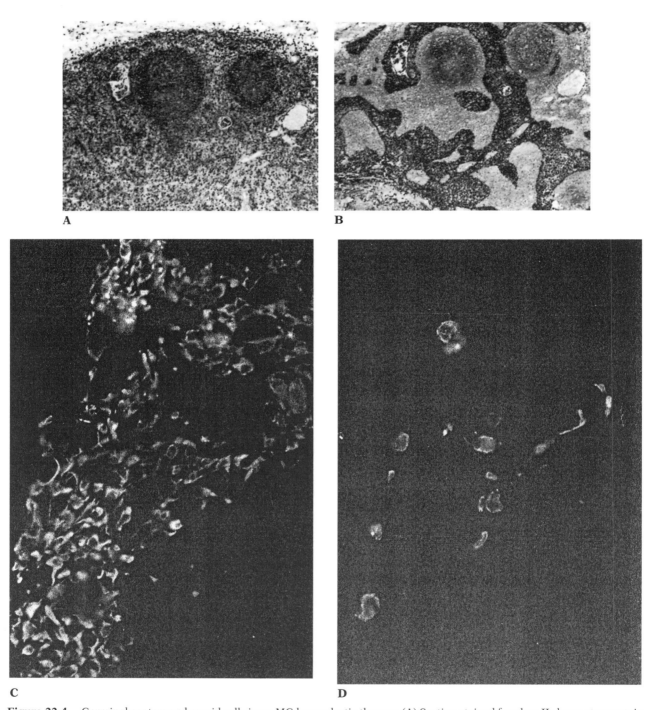

Figure 22-4. Germinal centers and myoid cells in an MG hyperplastic thymus. (A) Section stained for class II shows strong staining of B and T cells in the germinal center, and of interdigitating cells in the medulla. (B) Staining for a medullary epithelial marker shows compression of epithelial tissue into characteristic bands. Immunofluorescent staining (rhodamine) (C) for medullary epithelium shows myoid cells within the medulla. Immunofluorescent staining for acetylcholine receptor (fluorescein) (D) also shows myoid cells within the medulla. (A and B are reproduced with permission from Willcox N. The thymus in myasthenia gravis patients, and the *in vivo* effects of corticosteroids on its cellularity, histology and functions. *Thymus Update* 1989;2:105–124. C and D are reproduced by kind permission of Dr. N. Willcox of John Radcliffe Hospital, Oxford, England.)

Cultured neoplastic epithelial cells express epidermal growth factor receptor and Ki67, indicative of their growth potential (125). There is no increased expression of p53 or bcl-2. Interestingly, CD28/B7 expression is high in thymoma epithelial cells in comparison with those in normal cortex, indicating the potential for these cells to activate T-cell responses (102).

The AChR α subunit is present only at very low levels in the thymoma tissue itself, as identified by PCR (126,127), but an AChR-like epitope on a 153-kd cytoplasmic protein in cortical epithelium was identified by binding of monoclonal antibodies specific for AChR α373-380 (128). Its presence correlates well with MG or the cortical epithelial tumor with which it associates (see above); however, neither T-cell nor antibody responses in thymoma patients are directed against this epitope (Nagvekar N, Jacobson L, Willcox N, Vincent A, unpublished observations, 1994), making it unlikely that it is involved in initiating MG. It now appears that an epitope that cross-reacts with α370-380 is expressed on neurofilament protein in cortical epithelium (129). This epitope is also shared by striated muscle antigens such as myosin and titin. It is possible that future work on the neurofilament expression in thymoma may point to the importance of responses to this epitope in the initiation of MG.

Cultured cortical epithelial cells show no evidence of functional AChR, although sodium and potassium channels are detectable (130). These cells can process and present antigens to class II–restricted T cells (131), indicating that they express both the appropriate class II molecule and the necessary processing apparatus and accessory molecules. Whether they can also present endogenous antigens is not yet reported.

Lymphocyte Function

Early studies noticed some changes in peripheral blood lymphocyte function and cell markers (see (132)). The number CD5+ B cells does not appear to differ between MG patients and healthy control subjects, in spite of some earlier reports (133). Levels of soluble IL-2 receptor are increased in MG patients, and appear to correlate with clinical state but not with anti-AChR levels (134), and they fall after thymectomy (135).

Results of experimental studies in animals suggest that a wide range of animal species are able to respond to immunization with xenogeneic, and even allogeneic or syngeneic, AChR (see below), indicating that there is little "self-tolerance" to AChR. Over the last few years several groups characterized specific T cells from MG patients and control subjects. The methods employed ranged from short-term stimulation with *Torpedo* AChR or synthetic peptides, to raising cell lines and clones with recombinant human AChR α subunit, or with pools of synthetic peptides. Some studies identified the epitope specificity and class II restrictions. Each method has its advantages and can be informative, but some caution has to be exercised regarding the conclusions (136). Two important criteria of the pathogenicity of T cells would be their ability to respond to AChRs processed and presented by autologous presenting cells, and to provide specific help for antibody production. The former is not always convincing, and the latter has not yet been achieved with any human T-cell line.

Initial work used *Torpedo* AChR and synthetic peptides representing parts of the human α subunit to look for specific responses of fresh T cells in MG patients and control subjects (137–139). Subsequently, responses to recombinant mouse AChR subunit suggested that the epitopes recognized by MG patients differ from those recognized by control subjects (140). Table 22-2 provides the characteristics of some T-cell lines raised against human recombinant AChR. These lines are highly specific for the AChR sequence and for the class II–restricting element; most recognize different AChR sequences, in the context of different class II–restricting elements (Fig 22-5A, B). One of the five T-cell lines was raised from a normal healthy individual (as were some raised against *Torpedo* AChR) (141). Importantly, they all recognize very small amounts of purified human AChR, often best presented by capture on immunomagnetic particles (142). However, one DQ-restricted line specific for part of the sequence coded for by the α-subunit isoform sequence, P3A, only recognized AChR when some proteolysis had occurred after purification (139), suggesting either that this is not a natural epitope or that unusual processing may be involved in its generation. Another feature of importance is that the T cells appear to be of the Th1 subclass; that is, they secrete

Table 22-2.
T-Cell Lines Selected with Recombinant Acetylcholine Receptor (AChR) α Subunit: HLA Restriction and Response to Purified Human AChR*

Line or Clone	Source	HLA Restriction	Core Epitope	Response to AChR (% response to recombinant antigen)
PM-A (151)	MG thymus	DR4	α149-156	50–100
KB-L1	MG thymoma	DR52a	α149-156	25–50
MBu	MG thymoma	DPB 1401	α73-90	25–50
GD (139)	MG PBL	DQw5	P3A17′-25	25–50
BA-C	Healthy control PBL	DR53	α51-65	25–50

*By contrast, T cells selected with synthetic peptides did not respond to naturally processed whole AChR; see (147).
MG = myasthenia gravis; PBL = peripheral blood lymphocyte.
Sources: Data from (139,147,151).

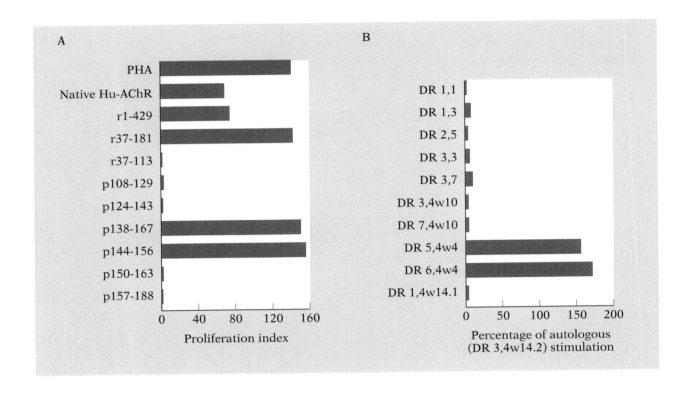

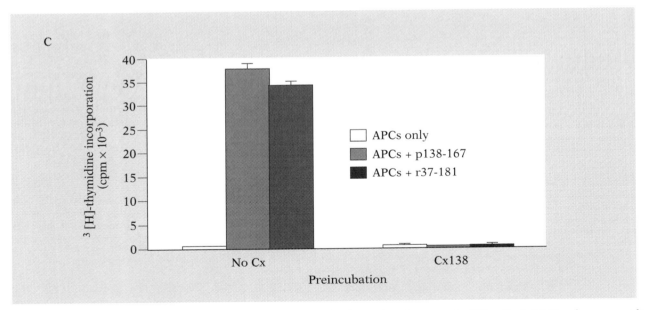

Figure 22-5. Responses of a T-cell clone (PM-A) obtained from the thymic lymphocytes of a MG patient. (A) The clone responds to recombinant acetylcholine receptor (AChR) α subunit (r1-429) and a smaller fragment (37-181), but not to r37-113. The epitope was further mapped with synthetic peptides to p144-156. This clone also responds strongly to purified human AChR (but not to *Torpedo* AChR, not shown). (B) Class II restriction demonstrated by using different class II–sharing antigen-presenting cells (APCs) to present the antigen. (C) Anergy induced in the clone by preincubation overnight with a complex (Cx138) made of DR4.w4.2 and p138-167. Cells that had been preincubated in medium responded to APCs and p138-167 or r37-181; cells that had been preincubated with Cx138 were completely unresponsive. (A and B are modified from Ong B, Willcox N, Wordsworth P, et al. Critical role for the Val/Gly[86] HLA-DRβ dimorphism in autoantigen presentation to human T cells. *Proc Natl Acad Sci USA* 1991;88:7343. C is reproduced with permission from Nicolle MW, Nag B, Sharma SD, et al. Specific tolerance to an acetylcholine receptor epitope induced *in vitro* in myasthenia gravis CD4+ lymphocytes by soluble major histocompatibility complex class II–peptide complexes. *J Clin Invest* 1994;93:1361–1369.)

IL-2 and IFN-γ, but little of the IL-4 or IL-5 characteristic of the Th2 cells involved in T-cell help for antibody production (see (136)) (Hawke S, Nicolle M, Willcox N, unpublished data, 1995). This raises the important question of whether these T cells are capable of providing T-cell help for antibody production, whether they have some other role in vivo such as T cell–mediated lysis of AChR-expressing cells, or whether they have undergone a phenotypic switch during their selection in the laboratory. Few T-cell lines/clones have been raised from thymoma patients, though the thymoma appears to be enriched for AChR-reactive cells (143,144).

It has been easier to raise cell lines against synthetic peptides. Pools of overlapping peptides corresponding to the sequences of each AChR subunit have been used (for a review, see articles by Protti et al (145,146)). The T-cell lines were class II and MG patient specific; for each subunit, many different peptides were recognized, although some stimulated several different lines. Sequence homology between some of these peptides and bacterial antigens was demonstrated. With the γ subunit, some of the specific T cells responded modestly to AChR purified from embryonic mammalian muscle, but there have been no analogous tests of responses to adult AChR. Furthermore, it is not clear to what extent any of these lines represent cells that might be pathogenic in vivo (see (136, 147)). In particular, T cells raised against synthetic peptides often require large doses of peptide and rarely recognize the native antigen after natural processing by APCs.

Another approach to look for specific T cells in MG is to use the ELISA spot technique. Link and his colleagues have (148,149) reported an increased incidence of AChR-specific cells in MG, though this was using the homologous but antigenically distinct *Torpedo* AChR, and Yi et al (150) used human AChR bound to ELISA plates to show antigen-specific production of IL-4, IFN-γ, and IL-2 by cells from MG patients.

It seems clear that the AChR-specific T cells are not unique to MG patients; they can also be found in healthy individuals (see Table 22-2), emphasizing that MG probably does not occur as a result of a lack of T-cell tolerance to the AChR. Whether the T cells in MG patients prove to differ, in terms of their antigenic specificity, cytokine profile, or ability to provide B-cell help, from those in healthy individuals will require much careful study. It is interesting that one DR4.Dw14.2-restricted T-cell clone derived from a hyperplastic MG thymus (151) recognizes the same core epitope, α146-162, that is immunodominant in C57Bl6 mice with EAMG (see below).

A novel approach to specific immunotherapy has been demonstrated using this clone. Preincubation of the T cells with a soluble complex of DR4.Dw4.2:α138-167 induces apoptosis in a high proportion and anergy in the surviving cells (152). The unresponsiveness persists during several cycles of restimulation. The cells can be "rescued" from the effects of the complex by co-incubation with fresh APCs, suggesting that it acts by engaging the T-cell receptor in the absence of accessory signals (see Fig 22-5C).

Antigen Processing and Presentation

Muscle does not normally express class II, but there is evidence that class II can be induced by viral infections in vivo (153) or by IFN gamma in vitro (154). Indeed, class II expression in vitro does not always require IFN (155). It is possible that the ability to upregulate class II on the muscle is controlled by genes within the MHC, and that once MHC is expressed, the muscle could present autoantigens to specific T cells. For instance, presentation of exogenously added peptides and recombinant polypeptides has been demonstrated in thymic epithelial cells (156).

To be relevant to the induction of MG, the muscle cell would need to process and present its own AChR to the relevant T cells. The T-cell clone specific for AChR α144-163 can recognize AChR endogenously presented by the TE671 muscle cell line after it is transfected with DNA for the α and β chains of DR4.Dw4.2. The responding T cells show only modest proliferation, but bind to and kill the presenting TE671 cells (157) (Fig 22-6). By this mechanism these cells can cause release of antigen from muscle or myoid cells and further stimulate the autoimmune response.

Seronegative Myasthenia Gravis

About 10% to 15% of all MG patients with generalized symptoms do not have detectable anti-AChRs by current laboratory methods; they appear to represent a distinct population from the majority of MG patients. Seronegative MG (SNMG) patients have symptoms and distribution of weakness similar to those of patients with seropositive generalized MG, but proportionately more develop MG before the age of puberty (158). There are some T-cell areas in the thymic medulla, but lymphoid follicles are few, and thymus histology is "normal" (158,159). Thymoma is never found, and no HLA association has been identified. Thus on clinical and pathologic grounds, the disease appears to have several unusual features.

SNMG is associated with some reduction in ^{125}I-α-BuTx binding to AChRs at the NMJ and reduced MEPP amplitudes, as typically found in seropositive MG. However, these features may be caused by antibodies to some other neuromuscular determinant(s) that indirectly affect AChR number or function. Seronegative immunoglobulin passively transfers a defect in neuromuscular transmission to mice without substantially reducing the numbers of AChRs, as measured by ^{125}I-α-BuTx binding; seronegative MG plasma, and IgM-containing fractions, inhibit AChR function in the TE671 cell line, again without reducing ^{125}I-α-BuTx binding (160); and SNMG plasma reduces ACh-induced currents in whole-cell clamped TE671 (Fig 22-7) cells by a mechanism that appears to be partly calcium dependent (161). AChR function can be reduced in TE671 cells by activation of second messenger systems via β-adrenergic receptors, binding of cholera toxin, or cross-linking of membrane proteins with multivalent lectins (162), and we have proposed that antibodies may indi-

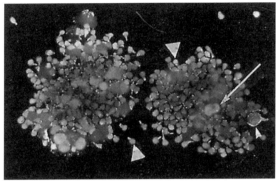

A

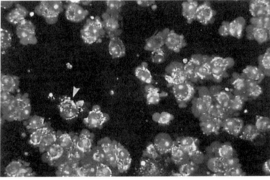

B

Figure 22-6. Presentation of endogenous acetylcholine receptor (AChR) epitopes by a class II–expressing muscle cell line. PM-A T cells (see Fig 22-5) bound to AChR-expressing TE671 cells that had been transfected with DR4.w4.2 (A), but not to untransfected TE671 (B). (Reproduced with permission from Baggi F, Nicolle M, Vincent A, et al. Presentation of endogenous acetylcholine receptor epitope by an MHC class II-transfected human muscle cell line to a specific CD4+ T cell clone from a myasthenia gravis patient. *J Neuroimmunol* 1993;46:57–66.)

rectly affect AChR function by binding to another receptor at the NMJ, leading, via signal transduction, to a modification of AChR function.

Experimental Autoimmune Myasthenia Gravis as a Model

The induction of EAMG in experimental animals was a major contribution to demonstrating the role of anti-AChR antibodies in MG, and the model has been helpful in elucidating the pathogenic mechanisms of the disease. The model is only reviewed briefly here (for comprehensive reviews, see (163,164)). The proportion of antibodies that cross-react between the immunizing protein and the recipient's muscle AChR depends on the closeness of the species, being only about 1% between *Torpedo* and rodent AChR. Nevertheless, the animals have reduced AChR numbers at the muscle end plates, have reduced MEPPs and EPPs, and show either overt

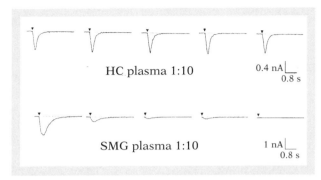

Figure 22-7. Effect of seronegative MG plasma on acetylcholine receptor function in TE671 cells. Whole-cell voltage clamp was used to look at acetylcholine-induced (arrowheads) currents in TE671 cells. Healthy control plasma had no effect; seronegative MG plasma completely inhibited the currents. This effect was not seen when the cells were depleted of calcium. (Reproduced with permission from Barrett-Jolley R, Byrne N, Vincent A, Newsom-Davis J. Seronegative myasthenia gravis plasmas reduce acetylcholine-induced currents in TE671 cells. *Pflugers Arch* 1994;428:492–498.)

signs of weakness or marked sensitivity to the neuromuscular blocking drug *d*-tubocurarine. The clinical effects of immunization depend partly on the susceptibility of the immunized strain to changes in AChR numbers. For instance, whereas New Zealand white rabbits become severely weak within 4 to 6 weeks of a single immunization, rats or mice are much more varied in their response. The AChR is very immunogenic. Rats (165) and mice (166) can show an immune response to syngeneic AChR, even in the absence of adjuvant (166).

The role of antibodies in EAMG was confirmed by the passive transfer of serum to naive litter mates, or of monoclonal anti-AChR antibodies, as mentioned already (40,41). Monoclonal antibodies against the α-BuTx binding site produce a hyperacute form of EAMG by directly inhibiting ACh binding to the AChR (167). However, most antibodies are directed against other sites on the AChR and lead to a reduction in AChR numbers by downregulation and complement-dependent lysis (see (163,164)). Antibodies induced by the purified AChR bind mainly to the extracellular determinants such as the MIR that are very conformation dependent (78,79). Only a proportion of anti-MIR antibodies bind to recombinant α subunit on Western blots, or to the synthetic peptide α67-76. Monoclonal antibodies against *Torpedo*, rat, or human AChR have been used extensively to characterize the binding sites for MG anti-AChR (58,79).

Determinant Spreading

When animals are immunized against denatured α subunits, the antibody response to the cytoplasmic region of the AChR usually dominates the response. However, a few investigators demonstrated production of anti-AChR antibodies in experimental animals immunized with peptides representing extracellular sequences of the AChR α subunit or recombinant α subunit, although few animals showed clinical signs of EAMG (see (168)). Three peptides representing human AChR α138-199 induced antipeptide antibodies, followed in most rabbits by the presence of anti-AChRs and severe muscle weakness. The anti-AChR antibodies were directed against the MIR and α-BuTx binding site on rabbit AChRs, and could be separated from the antipeptide antibodies, suggesting that they arose as a result of determinant spreading (168). It is possible that this represents a mechanism by which low-affinity, perhaps cross-reacting, antibodies lead to secondary high-affinity anti-AChRs.

Several investigators (169) found only minimal thymic changes in EAMG. These observations suggest that thymic changes in MG are not the secondary result of the immune response against the AChR.

T- and B-Cell Responses

It is relatively easy to measure T-cell responses to *Torpedo* AChR, which can be purified in milligram quantities, and to map the responses using synthetic peptides (see (170)). A large number of epitopes, some specific to particular mouse strains, have been identified. Similarly, anti-AChR antibodies can be shown to bind to synthetic peptides. However, these approaches do not define the epitopes that are crucial in the auto anti-AChR response.

In Lewis rats, the main T-cell epitope is α100-116. B cells from rats primed with native AChR induce T-cell proliferative responses to intact AChR, and in turn can be stimulated to produce anti-AChR (171). Thus, this epitope fulfills the criteria for pathogenicity (see Lymphocyte Responses). This epitope is also a useful target for specific immunosuppression via class II–peptide complex (172), similar to that with MG T cells described previously.

T- and B-cell reactivity toward AChR can also be detected via ELISA spot assays based on IFN-γ or IgG secretion, respectively (173,174), and such reactivity is reduced in rats orally tolerized toward AChR (175). Transforming growth factor (TGF)-β secretion is increased. Depletion of CD8+ T cells may suppress EAMG in Lewis rats, associated with lower proliferative responses and lower anti-AChR titers (176). An effect of class I is also found in mice (177). Thus, class I genes may make a substantial contribution to the induction or maintenance of the immune response, as proposed for MG (see above).

Immunogenetics

Studies on inbred rodents demonstrated the importance of immunogenetic factors in the susceptibility to EAMG. C57Bl/6 mice and AKR mice are the most susceptible laboratory mouse strain correlating with H-2^b and Ig-1^b, whereas BALB/c strains are relatively resistant (178,179). Lewis rats are much more likely to become weak after immunization than are Wistar Furth

rats (180). The basis for these differences in susceptibility, however, is still not clear. It does not relate to the serum antibody levels (178), or to intrinsic muscle factors. The I-A^{bm12} mutation in C57Bl/6 mice confers resistance to EAMG, probably by changing the T-cell repertoire and preventing recognition of α146-162, a dominant T-cell epitope (181,182). Detailed analysis of the role of class II and T-cell receptor genes in EAMG is provided elsewhere (183).

There have been few studies of IgG genes in EAMG. A study of 19 monoclonal antibodies derived from BALB/c and C57Bl/6 mice immunized with *Torpedo* or human AChR showed a relation to PC7183 germline genes and some sharing of V$_H$ gene sequences between three pathogenic antibodies (184).

Severe Combined Immunodeficient Mice and a Transgenic Model

Schönbeck et al (185) found that injection of dissociated MG thymic cells into severe combined immunodeficient (SCID) mice led to transient anti-AChR production, but implantation of thymus tissue beneath the kidney capsule produced a more sustained anti-AChR response (185), perhaps because myogenesis was evident in the thymic transplants (186). IgG was identified at the NMJ of the mice, indicating that the antibody was able to react with AChRs in situ. Martino et al (187) reported a similar model.

Recently Gu et al (188) induced a form of myasthenia in transgenic mice by expressing IFN-γ at the NMJ using the mouse ε-subunit promoter. The mice showed some signs of disease, antibodies to a 87-kd protein, but no anti-AChR. Reactivity with the 87-kd band was shown in MG sera, including those that were seronegative. These results suggest that the 87-kd protein may be involved in the early stages of determinant spreading, and could be one of the targets for seronegative MG.

As a Model for Experimental Immunotherapy

The experimental model is ideal for testing therapy, and many different approaches have been used. These are reviewed by Drachman et al (189). Further developments combining the SCID mouse model with specific immunotherapy directed at human anti-AChR responses should be particularly informative, and may eventually lead to real advances in the treatment of MG.

Conclusions

MG is an autoantibody-mediated disease of unknown etiology. The autoantigen, muscle nicotinic AChR, has been cloned and sequenced, and a great deal is known about its localization and expression. The antibodies are of high affinity and specific for human AChR, suggesting that sensitization against the AChR itself has taken place. Whether this is primary or whether it follows, by determinant spreading, a separate initiating event is unclear. The role of antibodies to other antigens at the NMJ or in muscle, particularly those shared with thymoma tissue, needs to be investigated. Much work has gone into investigating the etiologic factors in MG, particularly the role of the thymus, and in cloning and characterizing T cells from MG patients that may be involved in T-cell help for antibody production. There is an animal model induced by immunization against AChR that faithfully reproduces many aspects of the disease, but no spontaneous model in laboratory animals. In spite of the enormous amount of research that has led to these insights, the etiology of the disease and the goal of specific immunotherapy are still elusive.

References

1. Vincent A, Wray D, eds. *Neuromuscular transmission; basic and applied aspects*. Oxford, England: Pergamon, 1992.
2. Hall ZW, Sanes JR. Synaptic structure and development: the neuromuscular junction. *Cell* 1993;72:99–121.
3. Van der Kloot W, Molgo J. Quantal acetylcholine release at the vertebrate neuromuscular junction. *Physiol Rev* 1994;74:900–991.
4. Harvey AL, ed. *Natural and synthetic neurotoxins. Neuroscience perspectives*. San Diego, CA: Academic, 1993.
5. Oosterhuis HJGH. The natural course of myasthenia gravis: a long term follow up study. *J Neurol Neurosurg Psychiatry* 1989;52:1121–1127.
6. Oosterhuis HJGH. Myasthenia gravis. *Clinical neurology and neurosurgery monographs*. Edinburgh: Churchill Livingstone, 1984.
7. Lindstrom JM, Seybold ME, Lennon VA, et al. Antibody to acetylcholine receptor in myasthenia gravis. Prevalence, clinical correlates and diagnostic value. *Neurology* 1976;26:1054–1059.
8. Vincent A, Newsom-Davis J. Acetylcholine receptor antibody as a diagnostic test for myasthenia gravis: results in 153 validated cases and 2967 diagnostic assays. *J Neurol Neurosurg Psychiatry* 1985;48:1246–1252.
9. Drachman DB. Myasthenia gravis. *N Engl J Med* 1994;330:1797–1810.
10. Simpson JA. Myasthenia gravis: a new hypothesis. *Scott Med J* 1960;5:419–439.
11. Nastuk WL, Strauss AJL, Osserman KE. Search for a neuromuscular blocking agent in the blood of patients with myasthenia gravis. *Am J Med* 1959;26:394–409.
12. Nastuk WL, Plescia O, Osserman KE. Changes in serum complement activity in patients with myasthenia gravis. *Proc Soc Exp Biol Med* 1960;105:177–184.
13. Christensen PB, Jensen TS, Tsiropoulos I, et al. Associated autoimmune diseases in myasthenia gravis. A population-based study. *Acta Neurol Scand.* 1995;91:192–195.
14. Patrick J, Lindstrom J. Autoimmune response to acetylcholine receptor. *Science* 1973;180:871–872.
15. Karlin A, Akabas MH. Toward a structural basis for the function of nicotinic acetylcholine receptors and their cousins. *Neuron* 1995;15:1231–1244.
16. Beeson D, Morris A, Vincent A, Newsom-Davis J. The human muscle nicotinic acetylcholine receptor alpha-subunit exists as two isoforms: a novel exon. *EMBO J* 1990;9:2101–2106.
17. Newland CF, Beeson D, Vincent A, Newsom-Davis J. Functional and non-functional isoforms of the human muscle acetylcholine receptor. *J Physiol (Lond)* 1995;489:767–778.
18. Somnier F. Anti-acetylcholine receptor (AChR) antibod-
ies measurement in myasthenia gravis: the use of cell line TE671 as a source of AChR antigen. *J Neuroimmunol* 1994;51:63–68.
19. Newsom-Davis J, Pinching AJ, Vincent A, Wilson SG. Function of circulating antibody to acetylcholine receptor in myasthenia gravis: investigation by plasma exchange. *Neurology* 1978;28:266–272.
20. Vincent A, Newsom-Davis J, Newton P, Beck N. Acetylcholine receptor antibody and clinical response to thymectomy in myasthenia gravis. *Neurology* 1983;33:1276–1282.
21. Kuks JB, Oosterhuis HJ, Limburg PC, The TH. Anti-acetylcholine receptor antibodies decrease after thymectomy in patients with myasthenia gravis. Clinical correlations. *J Autoimmun* 1991;4:197–211.
22. Aarli JA, Lefvert AK, Tonder O. Thymoma-specific antibodies in sera from patients with myasthenia gravis demonstrated by indirect haemagglutination. *J Neuroimmunol* 1981;1:421–427.
23. Ohta M, Ohta K, Itoh N, et al. Anti-skeletal muscle antibodies in the sera from myasthenic patients with thymoma: identification of anti-myosin, actomyosin, and alpha-actinin antibodies by a solid-phase radioimmunoassay and a Western blotting analysis. *Clin Chem Acta* 1990;187:255–264.
24. Mygland A, Tysnes O-B, Matre R, et al. Ryanodine receptor autoantibodies in myasthenia gravis patients with a thymoma. *Ann Neurol* 1992;32:589–591.
25. Gautel M, Lakey A, Barlow DP, et al. Titin antibodies in myasthenia gravis: identification of a major immunogenic region of titin. *Neurology* 1993;43:1581–1585.
26. Mygland A, Tysnes OB, Aarli JA, et al. IgG subclass distribution of ryanodine receptor autoantibodies in patients with myasthenia gravis and thymoma. *J Autoimmun* 1993;6:507–515.
27. Mohan S, Babohn RJ, Krolick KA. Unexpected cross-reactivity between myosin and a main immunogenic region (MIR) of the acetylcholine receptor by antisera obtained from myasthenia gravis patients. *Clin Immunol Immunopathol* 1992;64:218–226.
28. Osborn M, Marx A, Kirchner T, et al. A shared epitope in the acetylcholine receptor-α subunit and fast troponin I of skeletal muscle. *Am J Pathol* 1992;140:1215–1223.
29. Kuks JB, Limburg PC, Horst G, et al. Antibodies to acetylcholine receptors in myasthenia gravis. Part 1. Diagnostic value for the detection of thymoma. *J Neurol Sci* 1993;119:183–188.
30. Kuks JB, Limburg PC, Horst G, Oosterhuis HJ. Antibodies to skeletal muscle in myasthenia gravis. Part 2. Prevalence in non-thymoma patients. *J Neurol Sci* 1993;120:78–81.
31. Kuks JB, Limburg PC, Horst G, Oosterhuis HJ. Antibodies to skeletal muscle in myasthenia gravis. Part 3. Relation with clinical course and therapy. *J Neurol Sci* 1993;120:168–173.
32. Williams CL, Lennon VA. Thymic B lymphocyte clones from patients with myasthenia gravis secrete monoclonal striational autoantibodies reacting with myosin, α actinin, or actin. *J Exp Med* 1986;164:1043–1059.
33. Williams CL, Hay JE, Huiatt TW, Lennon VA. Paraneoplastic IgG striational autoantibodies produced by clonal thymic B cells and in serum of patients with myasthenia gravis and thymoma react with titin. *Lab Invest* 1992;66:331–336.
34. Elmqvist D, Hofmann WW, Kugelberg J, Quastel DMJ. An electrophysiological investigation of neuromuscular transmission in myasthenia gravis. *J Physiol (Lond)* 1964;174:417–434.

35. Fambrough DM, Drachman DB, Satyamurti S. Neuromuscular junction in myasthenia gravis: decreased acetylcholine receptors. *Science* 1973;182:293–295.

36. Ito Y, Miledi R, Vincent A, Newsom-Davis J. Acetylcholine receptors and end-plate electrophysiology in myasthenia gravis. *Brain* 1978;101:345–368.

37. Plomp JJ, Van-Kempen GTH, De Baets M, et al. Acetylcholine release in myasthenia gravis: regulation at single end-plate level. *Ann Neurol* 1995;37:627–636.

38. Engel AG. Myasthenia gravis and myasthenic syndromes. *Ann Neurol* 1984;16:519–534.

39. Toyka KV, Drachman DB, Griffin DE, et al. Myasthenia gravis: study of humoral immune mechanisms by passive transfer to mice. *N Engl J Med* 1977;296:125–131.

40. Lindstrom JM, Lennon VA, Seybold ME, et al. Experimental autoimmune myasthenia gravis and myasthenia gravis: biochemical and immunochemical aspects. *Ann NY Acad Sci* 1976;274:254–274.

41. Lennon VA, Lambert EH. Myasthenia gravis induced by monoclonal antibodies to acetylcholine receptors. *Nature* 1980;285:238–240.

42. Engel AG, Lambert EH, Howard FM. Immune complexes (IgG and C3) at the motor endplate in myasthenia gravis. Ultrastructural and light microscopic localization and electrophysiologic correlations. *Mayo Clin Proc* 1977;52:267–280.

43. Engel AG, Arahata K. The membrane attack complex of complement at the endplate in myasthenia gravis. *Ann NY Acad Sci* 1987;505:326–332.

44. Rose NR, Bona C. Defining criteria for autoimmune diseases. *Immunol Today* 1993;14:426–430.

45. Drachman DB, Angus DW, Adams RN, et al. Myasthenia antibodies cross-link acetylcholine receptors to accelerate degradation. *N Engl J Med* 1978;198:1116–1122.

46. Stanley EF, Drachman DB. Effect of myasthenic immunoglobulin on acetylcholine receptors of intact mammalian neuromuscular junctions. *Science* 1978;200:1285–1287.

47. Wilson S, Vincent A, Newsom-Davis J. Acetylcholine receptor turnover in mice with passively transferred myasthenia gravis. II. Receptor synthesis. *J Neurol Neurosurg Psychiatry* 1983;46:383–387.

48. Guyon T, Lavasseru P, Truffault F, et al. Regulation of acetylcholine receptor alpha subunit variants in human myasthenia gravis: quantification of steady-state levels of messenger RNA in muscle biopsy using the polymerase chain reaction. *J Clin Invest* 1994;94:16–24.

49. Asher O, Neumann D, Witzemann V, Fuchs S. Acetylcholine receptor gene expression in experimental autoimmune myasthenia gravis. *FEBS Lett* 1990;267:231–235.

50. Burges J, Wray DW, Pizzighella S, et al. A myasthenia gravis plasma immunoglobulin reduces miniature endplate potentials at human endplates *in vitro*. *Muscle Nerve* 1990;13:407–413.

51. Drachman DB, Adams RN, Josifek LF, Self SG. Functional activities of autoantibodies to acetylcholine receptors and the clinical severity of myasthenia gravis. *N Engl J Med* 1982;307:769–775.

52. Chiu HC, Vincent A, Newsom-Davis J, et al. Myasthenia gravis: population differences in disease expression and acetylcholine receptor antibody titers between Chinese and Caucasians. *Neurology* 1987;37:1854–1857.

53. Chiu HC, Hsieh RP, Hsieh KH. Association of HLA antigens with myasthenia gravis in Chinese on Taiwan. *Chung Hua Min Kuo Wei Sheng Wu Chi Mien I Hsueh Tsa Chih* 1990;23:12–18.

54. Oda K, Shibasaki H. Antigenic difference of acetylcholine receptor between single and multiple form endplates of human extraocular muscle. *Brain Res* 1988;449:337–340.

55. Vincent A, Newsom-Davis J. Acetylcholine receptor antibody characteristics in myasthenia gravis. III. Patients with low anti-AChR antibody levels. *Clin Exp Immunol* 1985;60:631–636.

56. Horton RM, Manfredi AA, Conti-Tronconi B-M. The "embryonic" gamma subunit of the nicotinic acetylcholine receptor is expressed in adult extraocular muscle. *Neurology* 1993;43:983–985.

57. MacLennan C, Beeson D, Buijs A-M, et al. Acetylcholine receptor expression in human extraocular muscles and their susceptibility to myasthenia gravis. *Ann Neurol* 1997;41:423–431.

58. Vincent A, Whiting PJ, Schluep M, et al. Antibody heterogeneity and specificity in myasthenia gravis. *Ann NY Acad Sci* 1987;505:326–332.

59. Dondi E, Gajdos P, Bach J-F, Garchon H-J. Association of Km-3 allotype with increased serum levels of autoantibodies against muscle acetylcholine receptor in myasthenia gravis. *J Neuroimmunol* 1994;51:221–224.

60. Garchon HJ, Djabiri F, Viard J-P, et al. Involvement of human muscle acetylcholine receptor alpha-subunit gene (CHRNA) in susceptibility to myasthenia gravis. *Proc Natl Acad Sci USA* 1994;91:4668–4672.

61. Garlepp MH, Dawkins RI, Christiansen FT. HLA antigens and acetylcholine receptor antibodies in penicillamine-induced myasthenia gravis. *Br Med J* 1983;286:338–340.

62. Vincent A, Newsom-Davis J. Acetylcholine receptor antibody characteristics in myasthenia gravis. II. Patients with penicillamine-induced myasthenia or idiopathic myasthenia of recent onset. *Clin Exp Immunol* 1982;49:266–272.

63. Vieira ML, Caillat Zucman S, Gajdos P, et al. Identification by genomic typing of non-DR3 HLA class II genes associated with myasthenia gravis. *J Neuroimmunol* 1993;47:115–122.

64. Carlsson B, Wallin J, Pirskanen R, et al. Different HLA DR-DQ associations in subgroups of idiopathic myasthenia gravis. *Immunogenetics* 1990;31:285–290.

65. Compston DAS, Vincent A, Newsom-Davis J, Batchelor JR. Clinical, pathological, HLA antigen and immunological evidence for disease heterogeneity in myasthenia gravis. *Brain* 1980;103:579–601.

66. Baggi F, Mantegazza R, Vincent A, Newsom-Davis J. HLA-A2 restricted T cell line recognizing an epitope of the human acetylcholine receptor. *Ann NY Acad Sci* 1993;681:276–279.

67. Horiki T, Inoko H, Moriuchi J, et al. Combinations of HLA-DPB1 and HLA-DQB1 alleles determine susceptibility to early-onset myasthenia gravis in Japan. *Autoimmunity* 1994;19:49–54.

68. Matsuki K, Juji T, Tokunaga K, et al. HLA antigens in Japanese patients with myasthenia gravis. *J Clin Invest* 1990;86:392–399.

69. Demaine A, Willcox N, Janer M, et al. Immunoglobulin heavy chain gene associations in myasthenia gravis: new evidence for disease heterogeneity. *J Neurol* 1992;238:53–56.

70. Palmisani MT, Evoli A, Batocchi AP, et al. Myasthenia gravis associated with thymoma:clinical characteristics and long-term outcome. *Eur Neurol* 1994;34:78–82.

71. Somnier FE. Exacerbation of myasthenia gravis after removal of thymomas. *Acta Neurol Scand* 1994;90:56–66.

72. Nakao Y, Matsumoto H, Miyazaki T, et al. IgG heavy chain allotypes (Gm) in autoimmune diseases. *Clin Exp Immunol* 1980;42:20–26.

73. Gilhus NE, Pandey JP, Gaarder PI, Aarli JA. Immunoglobulin allotypes in myasthenia gravis patients with a thymoma. *J Autoimmun* 1990;3:299–305.

74. Morel E, Eymard B, Vernet-Der Garabedian B, et al. Neonatal myasthenia gravis; a new clinical and immunologic appraisal on 30 cases. *Neurology* 1988;38: 138–142.

75. Vernet Der Garabedian B, Lacokova M, Eymard B, et al. Association of neonatal myasthenia gravis with antibodies against the fetal acetylcholine receptor. *J Clin Invest* 1994;94:555–559.

76. Barnes PRJ, Kanabar DJ, Brueton L, et al. Recurrent congenital arthrogryposis leading to a diagnosis of myasthenia gravis in an initially asymptomatic mother. *Neuromuscul Disord* 1995;5:59–65.

77. Vincent A, Newland C, Brueton L, et al. Arthrogryposis multiplex congenita with maternal autoantibodies specific for a fetal antigen. *Lancet* 1995;346:24–25.

78. Tzartos SJ, Lindstrom JM. Monoclonal antibodies used to probe acetylcholine receptor structure: localization of the main immunogenic region and detection of similarities between subunits. *Proc Natl Acad Sci USA* 1990;77:755–759.

79. Tzartos SJ, Barkas T, Cung MT, et al. The main immunogenic region of the acetylcholine receptor: structure and role in myasthenia gravis. *Autoimmunity* 1991;8:259–270.

80. Whiting PJ, Vincent A, Newsom-Davis J. Myasthenia gravis: monoclonal antihuman acetylcholine receptor antibodies used to analyze antibody specificities and responses to treatment. *Neurology* 1986;36:612–617.

81. Vincent A, Newsom-Davis J. Acetylcholine receptor antibody characteristics in myasthenia gravis. I. Patients with generalised myasthenia or disease restricted to ocular muscles. *Clin Exp Immunol* 1982;49:257–265.

82. Hara H, Hayashi K, Ohta K, et al. Detection and characterization of blocking-type anti-acetylcholine receptor antibodies in sera from patients with myasthenia gravis. *Clin Chem* 1993;39:2053–2057.

83. Ohta M, Ohta K, Itoh N, et al. Antibodies to synthetic peptide (125-148) of the alpha-subunit of human nicotinic acetylcholine receptor in sera from patients with myasthenia gravis. *Neurology* 1990;40:1776–1778.

84. Scadding GK, Vincent A, Newsom-Davis J, Henry K. Acetylcholine receptor antibody synthesis by thymic lymphocytes: correlation with thymic histology. *Neurology* 1981;31:935–943.

85. Fujii Y, Monden Y, Hashimoto J, et al. Acetylcholine receptor antibody–producing cells in thymus and lymph nodes in myasthenia gravis. *Clin Immunol Immunopathol* 1985;34:141–146.

86. Newsom-Davis J, Willcox HNA, Calder L. Thymus cells in myasthenia gravis selectively enhance production of anti–acetylcholine receptor antibody by autologous blood lymphocytes. *N Engl J Med* 1981;305:1313–1318.

87. Kuks JB, Limburg PC, Oosterhuis HJ. The TH antibodies to acetylcholine receptors in myasthenia gravis. *In vitro* synthesis by peripheral blood lymphocytes before and after thymectomy. *Clin Exp Immunol* 1992;87: 246–250.

88. Cardona A, Garchon HJ, Vernet-der-Garabedian B, et al. Human IgG monoclonal autoantibodies against muscle acetylcholine receptor: direct evidence for clonal heterogeneity of the antiself humoral response in myasthenia gravis. *J Neuroimmunol* 1994;53:9–16.

89. Serrano M, Cardona A, Vernet-der-Garabedian B, et al. Nucleotide sequence of variable regions of a human anti-acetylcholine receptor autoantibody derived from a myasthenic patient. *Mol Immunol* 1994;31:413.

90. Grauss YF, de Baets MH, Parren PWH, et al. Human anti-nicotinic acetylcholine receptor recombinant Fab fragments isolated from thymus-derived phage display libraries from myasthenia gravis patients reflect predominant specificities in serum and block the action of pathogenic serum antibodies. *J Immunol* 1997;158: 1919–1929.

91. Farrar J, Portolano S, Willcox N, et al. Diverse Fabs specific for acetylcholine receptor epitopes from a myasthenia gravis thymus combinatorial library. *Int Immunol* (in press).

92. Dwyer DS, Bradley RJ, Urquhart CK, Kearney JF. Naturally occurring anti-idiotypic antibodies in myasthenia gravis patients. *Nature* 1983;301:611–614.

93. Lefvert A-K. Anti-idiotypic antibodies against the receptor antibodies in myasthenia gravis. *Scand J Immunol* 1981;13:493–497.

94. Vincent A. Are spontaneous anti-idiotypic antibodies against anti-acetylcholine receptor antibodies present in myasthenia gravis? *J Autoimmun* 1981;1:131–142.

95. Dwyer DS, Vakil M, Kearney JF. Idiotypic network connectivity and a possible cause of myasthenia gravis. *J Exp Med* 1986;164:1310–1318.

96. Tong Z, Dwyer DS. Monoclonal antibody against $\alpha(1{\rightarrow}3)$ dextran transfers suppression of the immune response to the acetylcholine receptor. *Eur J Immunol* 1990;20: 1635–1639.

97. Stefansson K, Dieperink ME, Richman DP, et al. Sharing of antigenic determinants between the nicotinic acetylcholine receptor and proteins in *E. coli, Proteus vulgaris* and *Klebsiella pneumoniae;* passive role in the pathogenesis of myasthenia gravis. *N Engl J Med* 1985;312:221–225.

98. Schwimmbeck PL, Dyrberg T, Drachman DB, Oldstone MBA. Molecular mimicry and myasthenia gravis. *J Clin Invest* 1989;840:1174–1180.

99. Levine GD, Rosai J. Thymic hyperplasia and neoplasia: a review of current concepts. *Prog Hum Pathol* 1978;9: 495–515.

100. Hohlfeld R, Wekerle H. The role of the thymus in myasthenia gravis. *Adv Neuroimmunol* 1994;4:373–386.

101. Schluep M, Willcox N, Ritter MA, et al. Myasthenia gravis thymus: clinical, histological and culture correlations. *J Autoimmun* 1988;1:445–467.

102. Willcox N, Vincent A. Myasthenia gravis as an example of organ-specific autoimmune disease. In: Bird G, Calvert JE, eds. *B lymphocytes in human disease.* Oxford, England: Oxford University, 1988:469–506.

103. Marx A, Schoemig D, Schultz A, et al. Distribution of molecules mediating thymocyte-stroma interactions in human thymus, thymitis and thymic epithelial tumours. *Thymus* 1994;23:83–93.

104. Masunaga A, Arai T, Yoshitake T, et al. Reduced expression of apoptosis-related antigens in thymuses from patients with myasthenia gravis. *Immunol Lett* 1994;39: 169–172.

105. Aime C, Cohen-Kaminsky S, BerihAknin S. *In vitro* interleukin-1 (IL-1) production in thymic hyperplasia and thymoma from patients with myasthenia gravis. *J Clin Immunol* 1991;11:268–278.

106. Emilie D, Crevon MC, Cohen-Kaminsky S, et al. In situ production of interleukins in hyperplastic thymus from myasthenia gravis patients. *Hum Pathol* 1991;22: 461–468.

107. Guigou V, Emilie D, Berrih-Aknin S, et al. Individual

germinal centres of myasthenia gravis human thymuses contain polyclonal activated B cells that express all the Vh and Vk families. *Clin Exp Immunol* 1991;83: 262–266.

108. Wekerle H, Ketelsen U-P. Intrathymic pathogenesis and dual genetic control of myasthenia gravis. *Lancet* 1977;1:678–680.

109. Kao I, Drachman DB. Thymic muscle cells bear acetylcholine receptors: possible relation to myasthenia gravis. *Science* 1977;195:74–75.

110. Schluep M, Willcox N, Vincent A, et al. Acetylcholine receptors in human thymic myoid cells in situ: an immunohistological study. *Ann Neurol* 1987;22:212–222.

111. Kirchner T, Hoppe F, Schalke B, Muller-Hermelink HK. Microenvironment of thymic myoid cells in myasthenia gravis. *Virch Arch B Cell Pathol* 1988;54:295–302.

112. Kornstein MJ, Asher O, Fuchs S. Acetylcholine receptor alpha-subunit and myogenin mRNAs in thymus and thymomas. *Am J Pathol* 1995;146:1320–1324.

113. Hara H, Hayashi K, Ohta K, et al. Nicotinic acetylcholine receptor mRNAs in myasthenic thymuses. *Biochem Biophys Res Commun* 1993;194:1269–1275.

114. Kaminski HJ, Fenstermaker RA, Abdul Karim FW, et al. Acetylcholine receptor subunit gene expression in thymic tissue. *Muscle Nerve* 1993;16:1332–1337.

115. Talib S, Okarma TB, Lebkowski JS. Differential expression of human nicotinic acetylcholine receptor α subunit variants in muscle and non-muscle tissues. *Nucleic Acids Res* 1993;21:233–237.

116. MacLennan C, Beeson D, Vincent A, Newsom-Davis J. Human nicotinic acetylcholine receptor α-subunit isoforms: origins and expression. *Nucleic Acids Res* 1993;21:5463–5467.

117. Willcox N, Schluep M, Ritter MA, et al. Myasthenic and nonmyasthenic thymoma. An expansion of a minor cortical epithelial cell subset? *Am J Pathol* 1987;127: 447–460.

118. Kirchner T, Schalke B, Buchwald J, et al. Well-differentiated thymic carcinoma. *Am J Surg Pathol* 1992;16: 1153–1169.

119. Willcox HNA. Thymic tumours with myasthenia gravis or bone marrow dyscrasias. In: Peckham M, ed. *Oxford textbook of oncology.* Oxford, UK: Oxford University Press, 1994:1562–1568.

120. Kirchner T, Muller Hermelink HK. New approaches to the diagnosis of thymic epithelial tumours. *Prog Surg Pathol* 1989;10:167–189.

121. Fujii Y, Hayakawa M, Inada K, Nakahara K. Lymphocytes in thymoma: association with myasthenia gravis is correlated with increased number of single-positive cells. *Eur J Immunol* 1990;20:2355–2358.

122. Willcox N. The thymus in myasthenia gravis patients, and the *in vivo* effects of corticosteroids on its cellularity, histology and functions. *Thymus Update* 1989;2: 105–124.

123. Yoshitake T, Masunaga A, Sugawara I, et al. A comparative histological and immunohistochemical study of thymomas with and without myasthenia gravis. *Surg Today* 1994;24:1044–1049.

124. Kornstein MJ, Kay S. B cells in thymomas. *Mod Pathol* 1990;3:61–63.

125. Gilhus NE, Jones M, Turley H, et al. Oncogene proteins and proliferation antigens in thymomas: increased expression of epidermal growth factor receptor and Ki67 antigen. *J Clin Pathol* 1995;48:447–455.

126. Hara Y, Useno S, Uemichi T, et al. Neoplastic epithelial cells express α-subunit of muscle nicotinic acetylcholine receptor in thymomas from patients with myasthenia gravis. *FEBS Lett* 1991;279:137–140.

127. Geuder KI, Marx A, Witzemann V, et al. Genomic organization and lack of transcription of the nicotinic acetylcholine receptor subunit genes in myasthenia gravis-associated thymoma. *Lab Invest* 1992;66:452–458.

128. Marx A, Kirchner T, Hoppe F, et al. Proteins with epitopes of the acetylcholine receptor in epithelial cell cultures of thymomas in myasthenia gravis. *Am J Pathol* 1989;134:865–877.

129. Marx A, Kirchner T, Greiner A, et al. Neurofilament epitopes in thymoma and antiaxonal autoantibodies in myasthenia gravis. *Lancet* 1992;339:707–708.

130. Marx A, Siara J, Rudel R. Sodium and potassium channels in epithelial cells from thymus glands and thymomas of myasthenia gravis patients. *Pflugers Arch* 1991; 417:537–539.

131. Gilhus NE, Willcox N, Harcourt G, et al. Antigen presentation by thymoma epithelial cells from myasthenia gravis patients to potentially pathogenic T cells. *J Neuroimmunol* 1995;56:65–76.

132. Newsom-Davis J, Vincent A. Myasthenia gravis. In: Lachman PJ, Peters DK, eds. *Clinical aspects of immunology.* 4th ed. London: Blackwell Scientific, 1982:1011–1068.

133. Yi Q, Ahlberg R, Pirskanen R, Lefvert AK. Levels of CD5+ B lymphocytes do not differ between patients with myasthenia gravis and healthy individuals. *Neurology* 1992;42:1081–1084.

134. Confalonieri P, Antozzi C, Cornelio F, et al. Immune activation in myasthenia gravis; soluble interleukin-1 receptor, interferon gamma and tumor necrosis factor-alpha levels in patients' serum. *J Neuroimmunol* 1993;48: 33–36.

135. Cohen-Kaminsky S, Jacques-Y, Aime C, et al. Follow-up of soluble interleukin-2 receptor levels after thymectomy in patients with myasthenia gravis. *Clin Immunol Immunopathol* 1992;62:190–198.

136. Hawke S, Matsuo H, Nicolle M, et al. Autoimmune T cells in myasthenia gravis; heterogeneity and potential for specific immunotargeting. *Immunol Today* 1996;17: 307–311.

137. Hohlfeld R, Toyka KV, Heininger K, et al. Autoimmune human T lymphocytes specific for acetylcholine receptor. *Nature* 1984;310:244–246.

138. Brocke S, Brautbar C, Steinman L, et al. *In vitro* proliferative responses and antibody titers specific to human acetylcholine receptor synthetic peptides in patients with myasthenia gravis and relation to HLA class II genes. *J Clin Invest* 1988;82:1894–1900.

139. Harcourt GC, Sommer N, Rothbard J, et al. A juxtamembrane epitope on the human acetylcholine receptor recognized by T cells in myasthenia gravis. *J Clin Invest* 1988;82:1295–1300.

140. Zhang Y, Schluep M, Frutiger S, et al. Immunological heterogeneity of autoreactive T lymphocytes against the nicotinic acetylcholine receptor in myasthenic patients. *Eur J Immunol* 1990;20:2577–2583.

141. Sommer N, Harcourt GC, Willcox N, et al. Acetylcholine receptor–reactive T lymphocytes from healthy subjects and myasthenia gravis patients. *Neurology* 1991;41: 1270–1276.

142. Hawke S, Willcox N, Harcourt G, et al. Stimulation of human T cells by sparse antigens captured on immunomagnetic particles. *J Immunol Methods* 1992;155:41–48.

143. Melms A, Malcherek G, Gern U, et al. T cells from normal and myasthenic individuals recognize the human

acetylcholine receptor: heterogeneity of antigenic sites on the α-subunit. *Ann Neurol* 1992;31:311–318.

144. Sommer N, Willcox N, Harcourt GC, Newsom-Davis J. Myasthenic thymus and thymoma are selectively enriched in acetylcholine receptor-reactive T cells. *Ann Neurol* 1990;28:312–319.

145. Protti P, Manfredi AA, Horton RM, et al. Myasthenia gravis: recognition of a human autoantigen at the molecular level. *Immunol Today* 1993;14:363–368.

146. Protti MP, Manfredi AA, Straub C, et al. Use of synthetic peptides to establish anti-human acetylcholine receptor CD4-positive cell lines from myasthenia gravis patients. *J Immunol* 1990;144:1711–1720.

147. Matsuo H, Batocchi A-P, Hawke S, et al. Recognition of unnatural epitopes by peptide-selected T cell lines in myasthenia gravis patients and controls. *J Immunol* 1995;155:3683–3692.

148. Sun J-B, Harcourt G, Wang Z-Y, et al. T cell responses to human recombinant acetylcholine receptor–α subunit in myasthenia gravis and controls. *Eur J Immunol* 1992;22:1553–1559.

149. Link H, Olsson O, Sun J, et al. Acetylcholine receptor–reactive T and B cells in myasthenia gravis and controls. *J Clin Invest* 1991;87:2191–2196.

150. Yi Q, Ahlberg R, Pirskanen R, Lefvert AK. Acetylcholine receptor-reactive T cells in myasthenia gravis: evidence for the involvement of different subpopulations of T helper cells. *J Neuroimmunol* 1994;50:177–186.

151. Ong B, Willcox N, Wordsworth P, et al. Critical role for the Val/Gly^{86} HLA-DRβ dimorphism in autoantigen presentation to human T cells. *Proc Natl Acad Sci USA* 1991;88:7343.

152. Nicolle MW, Nag B, Sharma SD, et al. Specific tolerance to an acetylcholine receptor epitope induced *in vitro* in myasthenia gravis CD4$^+$ lymphocytes by soluble major histocompatibility complex class II–peptide complexes. *J Clin Invest* 1994;93:1361–1369.

153. Bao S, King NJC, Dos Remedio CG. Flavivirus induces MHC antigen on human myoblasts: a model of autoimmune myositis? *Muscle Nerve* 1992;15:1271–1277.

154. Hohlfeld R, Engel A. Induction of HLA-DR expression on human myoblasts with interferon-gamma. *Am J Pathol* 1990;136:503–508.

155. Cifuentes-Diaz C, Delaporte C, Dautreaux B, et al. Class II MHC antigens in normal human skeletal muscle. *Muscle Nerve* 1992;15:295–302.

156. Gilhus NE, Willcox N, Harcourt G, et al. Antigen presentation by thymoma epithelial cells from myasthenia gravis patients to potentially pathogenic T cells. *J Neuroimmunol* 1995;56:65–76.

157. Baggi F, Nicolle M, Vincent A, et al. Presentation of endogenous acetylcholine receptor epitope by an MHC class II-transfected human muscle cell line to a specific CD4$^+$ T cell clone from a myasthenia gravis patient. *J Neuroimmunol* 1993;46:57–66.

158. Vincent A, Li Z, Hart A, et al. Seronegative myasthenia gravis; evidence for plasma factor(s) interfering with acetylcholine receptor function. *Ann NY Acad Sci* 1993;681:529–538.

159. Verma PK, Oger JJ. Seronegative generalized myasthenia gravis: low frequency of thymic pathology [see comments]. *Neurology* 1992;42:586–589.

160. Yamamoto T, Vincent A, Ciulla TA, et al. Seronegative myasthenia gravis: a plasma factor inhibiting agonist–induced acetylcholine receptor function copurifies with IgM. *Ann Neurol* 1991;30:550–557.

161. Barrett-Jolley R, Byrne N, Vincent A, Newsom-Davis J. Seronegative myasthenia gravis plasmas reduce acetyl-choline-induced currents in TE671 cells. *Pflugers Arch* 1994;428:492–498.

162. Li Z, Forester N, Vincent A. Modulation of acetylcholine receptor function in TE671 (rhabdomyosarcoma) cells by non-AChR ligands; a role in seronegative myasthenia gravis? *J Neuroimmunol* 1996;64:179–183.

163. Vincent A. Experimental autoimmune myasthenia gravis. In: Cohen IR, Miller A, eds. *Autoimmune disease models: a guidebook.* San Diego, CA: Academic, 1994: 83–106.

164. Lindstrom J, Shelton D, Fujii Y. Myasthenia gravis. *Adv Immunol (NY)* 1988;42:233–284.

165. Lindstrom JM, Einarson BL, Lennon VA, Seybold ME. Pathological mechanisms in experimental autoimmune myasthenia gravis. 1. Immunogenicity of syngeneic muscle acetylcholine receptor and quantitative extraction of receptor and antibody-receptor complexes from muscles of rats with experimental autoimmune myasthenia gravis. *J Exp Med* 1976;144:726–738.

166. Jermy A, Beeson D, Vincent A. Pathogenic autoimmunity to affinity-purified mouse acetylcholine receptor induced without adjuvant in BALB/c mice. *Eur J Immunol* 1993;23:973–976.

167. Gomez CM, Richman DP. Monoclonal anti–acetylcholine receptor antibodies with differing capacities to induce experimental autoimmune myasthenia gravis. *J Immunol* 1985;135:234–235.

168. Vincent A, Jacobson L, Shillito P. Response to human acetylcholine receptor α138-199: determinant spreading initiates autoimmunity to self-antigen in rabbits. *Immunol Lett* 1994;39:269–275.

169. Meinl E, Klinkert WE, Wekerle H. The thymus in myasthenia gravis. Changes typical for the human disease are absent in experimental autoimmune myasthenia gravis of the Lewis rat. *Am J Pathol* 1991;139:995–1008.

170. Pachner AR, Kantor FS, Mulac-Jericevic B, Atassi MZ. An immunodominant site of acetylcholine receptor in experimental myasthenia mapped with T lymphoctye clones and synthetic peptides. *Immunol Lett* 1989;20: 199–204.

171. Fujii Y, Lindstrom J. Regulation of antibody production by helper T cell clones in experimental autoimmune myasthenia gravis. *J Immunol* 1988;141:3361–3369.

172. Spack EG, McCutcheon M, Corbellatta N, et al. Induction of tolerance in experimental autoimmune myasthenia gravis with solubilized MHC class II:acetyl-choline receptor peptide complexes. *J Autoimmun* 1995;8:787–808.

173. Wang ZY, Link H, Qiao J, et al. B cell autoimmunity to acetylcholine receptor and its subunits in Lewis rats over the course of experimental autoimmune myasthenia gravis. *J Neuroimmunol* 1993;45:103–112.

174. Wang ZY, Link H, Huang WX. T-cell immunity to acetylcholine receptor and its subunits in Lewis rats over the course of experimental autoimmune myasthenia gravis. *Scand J Immunol* 1993;37:615–622.

175. Wang ZY, Qiao J, Melms A, Link H. T cell reactivity to acetylcholine receptor in rats orally tolerized against experimental autoimmune myasthenia gravis. *Cell Immunol* 1993;152:394–404.

176. Zhang GX, Ma CG, Xiao BG, et al. Depletion of CD8+ T cells suppresses the development of experimental autoimmune myasthenia gravis in Lewis rats. *Eur J Immunol* 1995;25:1191–1198.

177. Shenoy M, Kaul R, Goluzko E, et al. Effect of MHC class I and CD8 cell deficiency on experimental autoimmune myasthenia gravis pathogenesis. *J Immunol* 1994;153: 5330–5335.

178. Berman PW, Patrick J. Experimental myasthenia gravis: a murine system. *J Exp Med* 1980;151:204–223.

179. Christadoss P, Lennon VA, David C. Genetic control of experimental autoimmune myasthenia gravis in mice. *J Immunol* 1979;123:2540–2543.

180. Biesecker G, Koffler D. Resistance to experimental autoimmune myasthenia gravis in genetically inbred rats. *J Immunol* 1988;140:3406–3410.

181. Christadoss P, David CS, Keve S. 1-Aα^κ transgene pairs with 1-Aβ^β gene and protects C57BL 10 mice from developing autoimmune myasthenia gravis. *Clin Immunol Immunopathol* 1992;62:235–239.

182. Bellone M, Ostlie N, Lei S, et al. The I-A^bm12 mutation, which confers resistance to experimental myasthenia gravis, drastically affects the epitope repertoire of murine CD4+ cells sensitized to nicotinic acetylcholine receptor. *J Immunol* 1991;147:1484–1491.

183. Kaul R, Shenoy M, Christadoss P. The role of major histocompatibility complex genes in myasthenia gravis and experimental autoimmune myasthenia gravis pathogenesis. *Adv Neuroimmunol* 1994;4:387–402.

184. Graus YMF, Meng F, Vincent A, et al. Sequence analysis of anti-AChR antibodies in experimental autoimmune myasthenia gravis. *J Immunol* 1995;154:6382–6396.

185. Schönbeck S, Padberg F, Hohlfeld R, Wekerle H. Transplantation of thymic autoimmune microenvironment to severe combined immunodeficiency mice. A new model of myasthenia gravis. *J Clin Invest* 1992;90:245–250.

186. Spuler S, Marx A, Kirchner T, et al. Myogenesis in thymic transplants in the severe combined immunodeficient mouse model of myasthenia gravis. Differentiation of thymic myoid cells into striated muscle cells. *Am J Pathol* 1994;145:766–770.

187. Martino G, DuPont BL, Wollman RL, et al. The human severe combined immunodeficiency myasthenic mouse model: a new approach for the study of myasthenia gravis. *Ann Neurol* 1993;34:48–56.

188. Gu D, Wogensen L, Calcutt NA, et al. Myasthenia gravis-like syndrome induced by expression of interferon gamma at the neuromuscular junction. *J Exp Med* 1995;181:547–557.

189. Drachman DB, McIntosh KR, Reim J, Balcer L. Strategies for treatment of myasthenia gravis. *Ann NY Acad Sci* 1993;681:515–527.

Chapter 23

Antibody-Mediated Disorders of the Neuromuscular Junction: The Lambert-Eaton Myasthenic Syndrome, Acquired Neuromyotonia, and Conditions Associated with Antiglycolipid Antibodies

Angela Vincent

The way in which the autoimmune basis of myasthenia gravis (MG) was elucidated, and the many studies that sought to understand its etiology are outlined in Chapter 22. MG is not the only autoimmune disorder of neuromuscular transmission. In this chapter, two other diseases associated with antibodies to neuronal ion channels and studies investigating the pathologic role of antibodies to gangliosides are described. The reader is referred to the Chapter 22 for a description of the role of ion channels and gangliosides in neuronal function and neuromuscular transmission.

Figure 23-1 illustrates the relative positions of some of these functional molecules. The voltage-gated sodium channels are highly concentrated at the nodes of Ranvier, and at the motor nerve terminal they are probably restricted to the region close to the last heminode (1). Voltage-gated potassium channels (VGKCs) are located in the paranodal areas and on the motor nerve terminal itself. Voltage-gated calcium channels (VGCCs) are concentrated at the active zones, where they are intimately involved with the process of neurotransmitter release (2).

The Lambert-Eaton Myasthenic Syndrome

In 1957 Lambert and Eaton described a myasthenic syndrome that was electrophysiologically distinct from MG (3). There was a greatly reduced compound muscle action potential (CMAP) amplitude following supramaximal nerve stimulation that became smaller at low rates of repetitive nerve stimulation (< 10/sec), but that increased during stimulation at higher rates, or following a few seconds of voluntary contraction. These findings contrasted with those in MG where the CMAP is not usually reduced initially and fails to show an increment following high-frequency stimulation.

Five of Lambert's six original patients had direct or radiologic evidence of lung tumor; two of these were subsequently shown to be small-cell lung cancer (SCLC). These early studies established Lambert-Eaton myasthenic syndrome (LEMS) as an archetypal paraneoplastic neurologic disorder, associated with SCLC. Subsequently it became clear that the syndrome could also arise without an associated cancer.

Clinical Features

A full review of the clinical and electrophysiologic features of LEMS can be found elsewhere (4,5). LEMS is more common in males than females (6). Weakness involves predominantly proximal muscles of the limbs and nearly always affects the legs first. Strength may increase during the first few seconds of a voluntary contraction. Ocular symptoms are far less common than in MG. Reflexes are absent or depressed but can show posttetanic potentiation. The disease can occur at any age but the age at onset is lower in patients without detectable cancer (NCD-LEMS). Autonomic symptoms (dry mouth, constipation, impotence) are present in many patients, suggesting that the target antigen may be common to certain autonomic systems (6).

SCLC is found in about 50% of patients (CD-LEMS), but the neurologic symptoms may be evident for up to 5 years before the tumor is evident. Other tumors including lymphoproliferative disorders (7) and thymoma (8) may also associate with LEMS; LEMS with thymoma has been observed in the setting of MG (9). LEMS has also been observed in the presence of paraneoplastic cerebellar degeneration (10) and para-

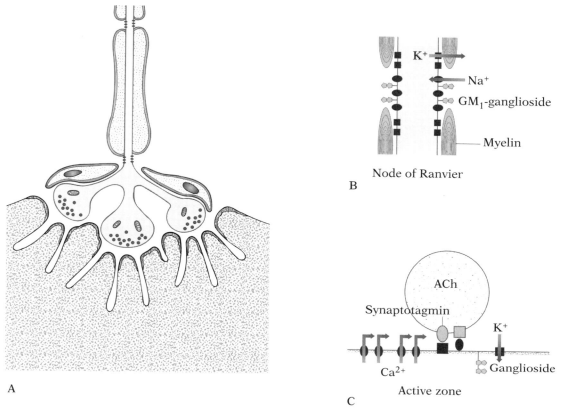

Figure 23-1. Representation of the motor nerve and motor nerve terminal (A), showing the approximate distribution of voltage-gated sodium at the nodes of Ranvier (B). GM$_1$ ganglioside is also concentrated at the nodes of Ranvier, and voltage-gated potassium channels are found in the paranodal regions. The calcium channels involved in neurotransmitter release (C) are intimately associated with components of the release mechanism at the active zones (see (1)), and GQ$_{1b}$ and other polysialosylated gangliosides are also found on the motor nerve terminal. Voltage-gated potassium channels are probably distributed throughout the motor nerve terminal membrane. ACh = acetylcholine.

neoplastic encephalomyelitis (11). Thus, LEMS is a member of the expanding family of paraneoplastic autoimmune conditions (see Chapter 10).

Diagnosis

LEMS is diagnosed by the combination of weakness, reduced tendon reflexes, improvement following voluntary contraction, and the typical electromyographic (EMG) findings mentioned already. The diagnosis can now be confirmed by identification of serum anti-VGCC antibodies, which are positive in more than 90% of patients (see below).

Treatment

Pharmacologic treatment includes antiacetylcholinesterase drugs that prolong the action of acetylcholine (ACh), and aminopyridines that increase the release of ACh by prolonging the depolarization of the motor nerve terminal (12). In CD-LEMS, treatment of the pri-

mary cancer often leads to clinical improvement (13). In both CD- and NCD-LEMS, neurologic symptoms can be temporarily ameliorated by plasma exchange, and long-term improvement achieved with immunosuppression using prednisolone or azathioprine, or both (14). Intravenous immunoglobulin therapy resulted in the improvement of several parameters of strength, and an associated decline in specific antibody, in a double blind crossover trial in 8 LEMS patients (15).

Electrophysiologic Abnormalities

In vitro recordings from biopsied intercostal muscle revealed normal miniature end-plate potentials (MEPPs) but very small end-plate potentials (EPPs), indicating that the quantal content (the number of packets of ACh released per nerve impulse) was reduced (16,17). The EPPs increased during repetitive stimulation, and also in response to increases in extracellular calcium concentration. This was the first indication that reduced calcium entry might underlie the defect in ACh release.

It is now clear that during high-frequency stimulation, Ca^{2+} accumulates in the nerve terminal, overcoming the reduced Ca^{2+} entry (16,17).

Morphologic Abnormalities

Freeze-fracture electron microscopic studies of motor nerve terminals in healthy human muscle biopsy samples reveal, as in other species, double parallel rows of intramembranous particles (each about 10–12 nm in diameter). These particle arrays are associated with the presynaptic active zones that are known to be close to the site of exocytosis of the transmitter (see Fig 23-1C). The particles themselves (active zone particles) appear to represent VGCCs. Fukunaga et al (18) found a highly significant reduction in the number of active zone particles and the number of particles per active zone in LEMS patients, and an increase in the number of clusters of particles (reviewed elsewhere (19)).

Clinical Immunologic Associations

Many LEMS patients have other autoimmune disorders. In the 50 LEMS patients of O'Neill et al (4), there were cases of thyroid disease, vitiligo, pernicious anemia, celiac disease, and juvenile-onset diabetes mellitus. Lennon et al (20) found one or more organ-specific autoantibodies in almost half of their series of 64 patients. The incidence was higher in patients without tumor. A study of 30 LEMS patients found an increased association with HLA-B8, particularly in the NCD-LEMS group, in whom there was also an increased frequency of IgG heavy-chain markers (21,22). Taken together, these clinical studies strongly suggest involvement of the immune system in the etiology of LEMS.

Clinical Evidence for a Humoral Factor

It was suggested that the SCLC secretes a biologically active peptide that interferes with neuromuscular transmission (23). However, Lambert and Lennon (24) found no evidence of impaired neuromuscular transmission in nude mice transplanted with SCLC tumors. The evidence for an antibody-mediated pathogenesis is now overwhelming. Plasma exchange, a procedure that removes circulating factors including autoantibodies (14,25,26), leads to clinical improvement associated with an increase in CMAP amplitudes (14), with the maximal response occurring about 10 days after the treatment. Moreover, as mentioned already, most patients respond to immunosuppressive drugs or intravenous immunoglobulin therapy.

Passive Transfer of Immunoglobulins

Physiologic Effects

The combination of autoimmune and immunogenetic associations with evidence for a circulating factor in LEMS is strongly reminiscent of observations in MG. The "passive transfer" of patient's plasma or immunoglobulins into experimental animals was crucial in leading to the recognition that MG is an antibody-mediated disorder (27). This approach also successfully elucidated the autoimmune mechanism in LEMS (25,28–30). Daily injection of plasma, or its IgG fraction, into mice reproduced the principal neurophysiologic changes of LEMS: reduced EPP amplitudes (by 40%–60%) that increased during short trains of high-frequency stimulation (20 or 40 Hz) (28,30). Interestingly, complement did not seem to be involved as C5-deficient mice were as susceptible as normal mice (31), and IgG was as effective as plasma. None of the mice showed signs of weakness, probably because the extent to which the EPP normally exceeds the threshold for activation of the muscle action potential ("the safety factor"; see Chapter 22), is very high in rodents so that even a substantial reduction would not necessarily prevent transmission in many muscle fibers.

The reduction in quantal content followed the level of human IgG in the mouse serum during long-term daily injections (31), with the time to half-maximal effect being about 36 hours for both the "on" effect and the "off" effect; however, in most cases acute incubation in LEMS sera or IgG (1–3 hours) did not affect quantal content (31,32).

Morphologic Effects

Quantitative freeze-fracture electron microscopy in mice injected daily for 52 to 69 days with LEMS IgG showed reductions in the number of active zones (33) that were very similar to those seen at the nerve terminals of LEMS patients (18). These studies lent support to the view that LEMS IgG interferes with ACh release by targeting the channels themselves or structures very closely related to them. The clustering of the active zone particles was preceded by a reduction in the distance between particles, suggesting that the divalent antibodies were acting by cross-linking adjacent particles (34). Motor nerve terminals exposed to monovalent F(ab') LEMS IgG showed no changes, whereas F(ab')$_2$ was as effective as the native molecule in demonstrating morphologic and electrophysiologic changes. Because the F(ab')$_2$ molecule does not fix complement, these results provide further evidence that the morphologic and electrophysiologic effects of LEMS IgG do not require the complement system.

Using a sensitive immunoelectron microscopy technique, Engel et al (35,36) localized IgG at the sites of presynaptic active zones in mice that had received multiple intraperitoneal doses of LEMS IgG. The amount and distribution of IgG were small, reflecting the low number of active zone particles and their restricted localization.

Functional Effects of Immunoglobulins on Cultured Cells

The physiologic and morphologic passive transfer studies clearly point to an effect of LEMS IgG on nerve terminal VGCCs or to structures closely associated with them. Studies by several groups using cell lines, primary cell cultures, or synaptosomes provided further supportive evidence for anti-VGCC activity in LEMS IgG.

SCLC cells can generate Ca^{2+} spikes that are blocked by calcium channel blockers (37,38). Roberts et al (39) established an assay for VGCC function by using K^+ to depolarize the cells and thus open the VGCCs. Depolarization-dependent calcium influx, measured by $^{45}Ca^{2+}$, was sensitive to dihydropyridine calcium channel blockers (39). The $^{45}Ca^{2+}$ flux into a SCLC cell line (derived from a non-LEMS patient) was markedly reduced by growing the cells for 2 to 4 days in LEMS IgG, either from CD- or NCD-LEMS patients. IgG from SCLC patients without LEMS had no effect. Thus, LEMS IgG appears to interfere with the function of VGCCs in SCLC cell lines. Others obtained similar results in SCLC lines raised from non-LEMS and from LEMS patients (40), and in rat cortical synaptosomes at 37°C (41).

Calcium-dependent release processes are common to many neuroendocrine cells, and Login et al (42) showed that spontaneous release of prolactin and growth hormone by rat pituitary cells was significantly reduced after incubation for 48 hours with LEMS IgG at 4 mg/mL. Interestingly, this effect was also seen within 30 minutes of exposure, suggesting that this particular IgG can directly block calcium channel function.

There are several types of calcium channels (see below). Kim and Neher (43), using a microelectrode electrophysiologic approach, showed that LEMS IgG reduces calcium currents in bovine adrenal chromaffin cells by interfering with L-type VGCCs. Similarly, Peers et al (44) demonstrated that LEMS IgG causes functional loss of L-type VGCCs in the murine hybrid neuroblastoma cell line NG108, but has no effect on T-type VGCCs.

Defining the Target Calcium Channel Type

VGCC subtypes are transmembrane proteins comprising α1, β, and α2/δ subunits. The α1 subunit is thought to contain the central Ca^{2+} conducting channel, and appears to be the principal determinant of the functional properties of the particular subtype, and to contain the ligand-binding sites. Several VGCC subtypes are known and may be present within a single neuron (45), making it difficult to identify in any one cell the VGCC subtypes being targeted by LEMS autoantibodies.

The use of ω-toxins derived from snail and spider venoms has made it possible to define the subtype of VGCC present in intact neurons, in cell lines, and at the neuromuscular junction. The cone snail–derived toxin ω-Conotoxin (ω-CmTx) MVIIC and the spider venom–derived toxin ω-Agatoxin (ω-Aga) IVA (46) interfere with the EPP at the mouse neuromuscular junction, indicating that P- or Q-type VGCCs mediate ACh release. There is evidence for several different subtypes of VGCCs in SCLC cell lines. The N-type VGCC antagonist ω-CgTx GVIA reportedly inhibits K^+-stimulated influx into an SCLC line (40), and polymerase chain reaction (PCR) demonstrated different subtypes of VGCCs (47). Johnston et al (48), using an SCLC cell line (MB) derived

from a patient with LEMS, found that ω-Aga IVA and ω-CmTx MVIIC inhibited flux by about 80%, suggesting that the dominant VGCC in this SCLC cell line was the P or Q type. Since preincubation of the SCLC cell line in LEMS IgG (2 mg/mL) produced a 46% to 78% inhibition of stimulated Ca^{2+} flux, these channels are probably a major target in LEMS.

Antibodies to Calcium Channels

Several attempts were made to identify LEMS antibodies binding to VGCCs on Western blots of VGCC-containing tissues. However, this approach has not been successful with either SCLC cell membranes (49) or chromaffin cell fractions (50), probably because only very small amounts of antigen were available in these preparations.

The antibody assays now used in LEMS are based on the same approach as that used in MG. Solubilized VGCCs are prelabeled with ^{125}I-neurotoxins and immunoprecipitated with LEMS serum. Sher et al (51) used as the source of VGCCs the human neuroblastoma cell line IMR32, labeled with ^{125}I-ω-CgTx GVIA which binds to N-type channels. Antibodies were found at raised titers in 90% of the patients, but positivity was also found in 42% of SCLC patients without LEMS. Lennon and Lambert (52) used an SCLC line labeled with ω-CgTx GVIA and reported raised titers in 27 (52%) of 52 patients, and in none of a large group of healthy and other neurologic disease control subjects. Similar results were found with a human neuroblastoma cell line (SKN-SH), 46% of patients being positive (53). Antibodies to L-type VGCCs, using rat brain as antigen, were detected using a labeled dihydropyridine (L-type antagonist) as the ligand (54). The IgG fractions also stained a 55-kd band, probably the β subunit, in immunoblots of the purified skeletal muscle dihydropyridine receptor.

Since P/Q-type VGCCs appear to mediate transmitter release at the mammalian neuromuscular junction, and LEMS sera inhibit the P/Q-type channels in an SCLC line, ^{125}I-ω-CmTx MVIIC or ^{125}I-agatoxin, which labels P/Q-type channels, should provide a much better label for detecting anti-VGCC antibodies in LEMS sera. Motomura et al (55) found that 56 (85%) of 66 LEMS serum samples gave results significantly above the range for healthy control subjects. The results in 40 other disease control subjects including 10 patients with SCLC without LEMS and 10 patients with MG were negative. The incidence of positivity was 90% in those with histologically proved SCLC and 76% in those without tumor who had been followed for more than 5 years (Fig 23-2). Lennon et al (56) reported very similar results, but also found positive results in a proportion of patients with paraneoplastic disorders without LEMS. The incidence and significance of the antibodies in other paraneoplastic conditions are not yet clear.

An inverse relationship between the anti-VGCC antibody titer and clinical severity was found in a longitudinal study on individuals receiving immunosuppressive therapy (57), and after intravenous

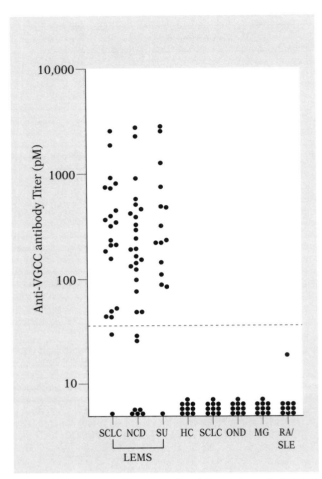

Figure 23-2. Anti–voltage-gated calcium channel (VGCC) antibodies in Lambert-Eaton myasthenic syndrome (LEMS) measured by immunoprecipitation of ^{125}I-ω-conotoxin MVIIC–labeled VGCCs extracted from human cerebellar cortex. Results are based on 66 LEMS patients and various control subjects including healthy ones (HC), patients with small-cell lung cancer without LEMS (SCLC), other neurological controls (OND), patients with myasthenia gravis (MG), and patients with rheumatoid arthritis and systemic lupus erythematosus (RA/SLE). The dotted line represents the mean ± 3 standard deviations of the controls. SU = cancer status uncertain; NCD = no cancer detected. (Reproduced by permission from Motomura M, Johnston I, Lang B, et al. An improved diagnostic assay for Lambert-Eaton myasthenic syndrome. *J Neurol Neurosurg Psychiatry* 1995;58:85–87.)

immunoglobulin treatment. In a double-blind crossover trial of eight LEMS patients, intravenous immunoglobulin reduced anti-VGCC levels by about 40%. The effect was not seen at 1 week but was evident at 2 weeks, by which time total serum IgG levels were within the normal range. The decline in specific antibody persisted until 6 to 8 weeks (15).

Because N-type channels appear to be the dominant VGCC subtype in the autonomic nervous system, it will be interesting to see whether anti–N-type antibodies, detected by binding to VGCCs labeled with ^{125}I-ω-conotoxin GVIA, associate particularly with those patients in whom autonomic nervous system symptoms are prominent. Preliminary observations indicate that autonomic function is markedly reduced in mice injected with LEMS IgG (58).

The binding sites of the anti-VGCC antibodies have not yet been mapped. Since the α_1 subunit appears to determine the channel subtype, antibodies that interfere with neuromuscular transmission presumably recognize this subunit. However, three of seven LEMS sera recognized a fusion protein that was encoded by the β subunit of the human VGCC in Western blots (59). These antibodies are not likely to initiate the autoimmune process as this subunit appears to have no extracellular domain. Antibodies binding to synaptotagmin, a synaptic vesicle protein (see Fig 23-1C), have also been detected, mainly in patients with high levels of anti–N-type VGCC (60). It may be that antibodies to N-type VGCC, β subunit, and synaptotagmin are associated, and represent a secondary antibody response following the primary attack on VGCC-containing cells.

Anti-VGCC Antibodies in Motor Neuron Disease

Antibodies to L-type VGCCs, purified from rabbit muscle, were detected in patients with motor neuron disease (61) using an enzyme-linked immunosorbent assay (ELISA), and it was proposed that these antibodies lead to increased Ca^{2+} influx resulting in neuronal cell death. Antibodies to P/Q-type VGCCs were detected in about 25% of motor neuron disease patients in one study (56), but this finding was not confirmed (62).

Mechanisms of Action of LEMS Antibodies

The studies summarized above imply that the main mechanism by which LEMS antibodies interfere with calcium channel function is through cross-linking and internalization, causing a reduction in the number of functional channels. There seems to be no evidence for a complement-mediated effect; if complement is activated on the motor nerve terminals, one might expect to find abnormalities in spontaneous as well as nerve-evoked transmitter release, but this has not been described. Nor is there any evidence for denervation as would be expected if motor nerve terminals are being destroyed by a complement-dependent process. The effects of LEMS IgG on VGCC function in cell lines have generally not addressed the question of a direct block of VGCC function. Only one study showed such an effect and this was stated to be the exception (32). An effect within 24 hours of direct application was probably due to cross-linking and downregulation, because monovalent Fab fragments were ineffective (63) (Fig 23-3). However, some LEMS sera do inhibit binding of ω-conotoxin to solubilized VGCCs, and it may transpire that these sera contain antibodies that can directly inhibit function.

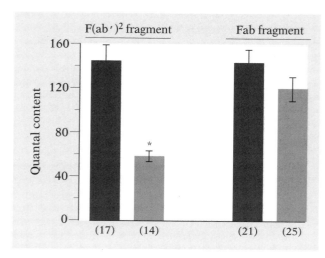

Figure 23-3. The quantal content in mouse diaphragms after 24 hours of incubation with divalent or monovalent Fab fragments. Only the divalent Fab produced a significant effect. (Reproduced by permission from Peers C, Johnston I, Lang B, Wray D. Cross-linking of presynaptic calcium channels: a mechanism of action for Lambert-Eaton myasthenic syndrome antibodies at the mouse neuromuscular junction. *Neurosci Lett* 1993;153:45–48.)

Small-Cell Lung Cancer and LEMS

LEMS is an excellent example of a paraneoplastic disorder (see Chapter 10). There is good circumstantial evidence that SCLC can provoke the neurologic disorder: the high incidence of SCLC in LEMS, expression by SCLC cells of neural antigens including VGCCs, and the presence of anti-VGCC antibodies. Moreover, the degree to which LEMS IgG inhibits K^+-stimulated (voltage-gated) Ca^{2+} influx into SCLC cells correlates with disease severity (64). In addition, selective tumor therapy (chemotherapy, radiotherapy, or surgery) can result in remission of the neurologic features (3,13). This improvement develops within 6 to 12 months of the initiation of treatment (13).

An immunocytochemical analysis of SCLC in patients with LEMS showed a greater infiltration of activated macrophages (implying an active immune response), compared to tumors from patients without LEMS (65), and an excess of less well-differentiated cells as indicated by reduced expression of the 200-kd neurofilament antigen and of class I antigens. These findings were interpreted as being due to loss of the well-differentiated tumor cells as a consequence of an autoimmune response by the host. Using tumor size, mass, and doubling times in a small series of SCLC patients, Geddes (66) calculated the times from malignant change to the earliest diagnosis as 2.4 years, to the usual time of diagnosis as 2.8 years, and to death as 3.2 years. It seems likely that the immune response against VGCCs begins early in the life of the tumor in most patients (66,67). This immune response may be beneficial to the patient since those with LEMS and SCLC survive longer than do those with SCLC alone.

It is entirely unclear what provokes the anti-VGCC response in noncancer patients. As mentioned already, the association with class I and class II immune response genes suggests an immunogenetic susceptibility. In a recent study, 22 (61%) of 36 NCD-LEMS patients (61%) were HLA-B8 and -DR3 positive, whereas in a similar number of CD-LEMS patients the frequency of positivity did not differ from that in control subjects (Willcox N, Janer M, Newsom-Davis J, unpublished data, 1994). The increased frequency of HLA-B8 and -DR3 is similar to that in young-onset MG where the autoimmune stimulus is also unknown.

Animal Models

One of the criteria for establishing the autoimmune nature of a disease is the induction of an experimental form of the disease by immunization of experimental animals with the purified antigen (as shown for MG using affinity-purified acetylcholine receptor (AChR); see Chapter 22). Chapman et al (68) immunized rats with cholinergic synaptosomes from *Torpedo* electric organ and detected antibodies by ELISA. No clinical abnormalities were observed in the rats, but EMG studies showed a reduced muscle action potential with some facilitation at high frequency. A humoral response to neuronal antigens in these rabbits may have included anti-VGCC antibodies, but no specific assay was employed. Takamori et al (69) proposed an alternative model. They immunized rats with synthetic peptides from the N-terminus of synaptotagmin, a synaptic vesicle protein to which antibodies have been found in LEMS (see above). The animals did not become weak, but there were reduced EPP amplitudes with normal MEPP amplitudes. Since synaptotagmin is only exposed on the surface of the motor nerve terminal following exocytosis and release of ACh, one might expect antibodies to synaptotagmin to interfere with the recycling of synaptic vesicles. The physiologic evidence in this study was insufficient to define the mechanism involved.

Conclusions

LEMS is an autoimmune disease in which antibodies to the P/Q-type VGCCs that are involved in the control of neurotransmitter release at the motor nerve terminal lead to a reduction in the number of channels and reduced calcium-dependent ACh release. The antibodies can be measured by a radioimmunoprecipitation assay employing ^{125}I-ω-conotoxin as a radioactive label for solubilized calcium channel protein. LEMS is associated with SCLC and is thus one of a growing number of paraneoplastic disorders in which an autoantibody response against a tumor leads to neuronal dysfunction.

Acquired Neuromyotonia

Neuromyotonia (NMT), or Isaacs' syndrome (70), is a syndrome of spontaneous and continuous muscle fiber contraction resulting from hyperexcitability of motor nerves. The diagnosis largely rests on a combination of clinical and EMG findings. Only about 100 cases of NMT have been reported and the clinical presentation is heterogeneous not only in terms of features and severity, but also in its association with a variety of other diseases (70,71).

There are genetic and acquired forms of NMT. One, associated with paroxysmal ataxia, is linked to the gene for a voltage-gated potassium channel (VGPC) on chromosome 12 (72). The acquired form, however, is the most prevalent and until recently has been regarded as idiopathic. However, there is now good evidence for a pathogenic role of antibodies to VGPCs.

Clinical Features

These include muscle stiffness, cramps, myokymia (visible undulation of the muscle), and weakness, most prominent in the limbs and trunk. Increased sweating is common. Myokymia characteristically continues during sleep and general anesthesia. Pseudomyotonia, a slow relaxation of muscles after contraction, may also be present. The syndrome usually follows a chronic course although spontaneous remissions have been reported. The acquired form most commonly presents between the ages of 25 and 35 years. For detailed reviews of the clinical and electrophysiologic findings, see other publications (71,73). A minority of patients have sensory symptoms, including transient or continuous paresthesia, dysesthesia, and numbness, that may be present even when there is no peripheral neuropathy. Central nervous system symptoms such as insomnia, hallucinations, delusions, and personality change may also be present.

The abnormal muscle activity may be generated at different sites throughout the length of the nerve (70). In most cases these sites are principally distal, but in others they may be proximal, perhaps even including the anterior horn cell (see (73)). Diagnosis of NMT is confirmed by EMG. The pathognomonic finding is the occurrence of spontaneous motor unit discharges that occur in distinctive doublets, triplets, or longer runs (70,74). These neuromyotonic discharges have a high (40–300 sec^{-1}) intraburst frequency usually occurring at irregular intervals of 1 to 30 seconds. In one third of patients there may also be evidence of damage to nerve fibers. Occasionally, the characteristic physiologic abnormalities are associated with either acute or chronic inflammatory demyelinating polyneuropathy.

To date there have been no studies of motor nerve conduction or neuromuscular transmission in muscle biopsy specimens from NMT patients.

Treatment

At present the symptoms of NMT can be improved by use of the anticonvulsant drugs carbamazepine (70) and phenytoin (75). Their mechanism of action may be related to their ability to reduce maximal sodium conductance in axonal membranes. Plasma exchange should be considered in the minority of patients with disabling symptoms that fail to respond to drugs. Five patients treated this way showed useful improvement in symptoms lasting about 3 weeks, and confirmed by serial EMG studies (71). There is little experience with the use of intravenous immunoglobulin.

Data on the use of immunosuppressive drugs are limited. The results of a pilot study, in which three patients who responded to plasma exchange were given azathioprine (2.5 mg/kg/day) and prednisolone (up to 80 mg on alternate days) for up to 8 months, were inconclusive. Further trials are needed to determine the usefulness of long-term immunosuppressive therapy.

Morphologic Studies

Some morphologic studies have been performed on sural nerve, although this is mainly a sensory nerve. There may be axonal damage or myelin degeneration or loss of large myelinated axons. Intramuscular nerve biopsy specimens may show sprouting (76), probably due to nerve degeneration. Muscle biopsy specimens show some fiber size variability and type II atrophy. No IgG deposits were found in the few patients examined.

Pathogenesis

Autoimmunity

As in MG and LEMS, NMT may be associated with other autoimmune diseases or other autoantibodies (71). In patients with acquired NMT, cerebrospinal fluid analysis occasionally shows a raised total IgG level or oligoclonal bands, suggesting that there is intrathecal IgG synthesis (71). There is one report of a patient with rheumatoid arthritis who developed NMT after treatment with penicillamine; the muscle overactivity stopped after this drug was withdrawn (77). Penicillamine can precipitate MG and the production of anti-AChR antibodies, and has also been implicated in triggering other autoimmune diseases including dermatomyositis (78).

NMT was found in 10 patients with thymoma, equivalent to about 20% of all of the patients with NMT reported in the past 20 years (71,73). Thymoma has long been associated with MG (see Chapter 22) and with other immunologically mediated conditions (79). Seven of the NMT patients with thymoma had MG and 2 others had raised anti-AChR antibody titers (80). In addition, three patients with bronchial carcinoma developed NMT, one with and two without peripheral neuropathy (81,82). At least one tumor was a SCLC (see section on LEMS).

There is now clinical evidence that a humoral factor is involved in the pathogenesis of acquired NMT. In five patients, plasma exchange, which depletes circulating immunoglobulins, resulted in clinical improvement and a reduction in the frequency of the abnormal muscle discharges on EMG (71,83,84). Experimental evidence that this humoral factor is an IgG autoantibody is provided by studies where plasma or IgG from patients with NMT was injected into mice. The mice did not have any signs of muscle overactivity, nor was there any evidence of spontaneous nerve discharges. However, phrenic nerve–diaphragm preparations dissected from animals treated with NMT IgG, when compared with those from control-injected mice, showed increased *d*-tubocurarine resistance at the neuromuscular junction (84), and a moderate increase in the quantal content of the EPP (i.e., there were more ACh quanta released per nerve impulse) (85). The simplest explanation for these findings is that an IgG autoantibody is mediating an increase in nerve excitability on the motor nerve or at the motor nerve terminal.

The Antigen

The most likely target for an autoantibody is a neuronal ion channel. After generation of a nerve action potential, the sodium channels are inactivated and the nerve is repolarized, and the resting membrane potential restored, through the action of VGPCs. Drugs that lead to delayed inactivation of sodium channels can cause repetitive activity in the nerve. Alternatively, if the potassium channel currents are blocked, by drugs such as 4-aminopyridine (4-AP) and tetraethylammonium (86), or specific toxins such as α-dendrotoxin (87), the axon membrane becomes more excitable and generates spontaneous bursts of action potentials. In either case, the quantal content of the EPP might be increased due

to prolongation of the action potential at the nerve terminal. In fact, a low concentration of 4-AP or 3,4-diamino pyridine (DAP) in vitro mimics changes in the nerve-diaphragm preparation that are seen after injection of NMT IgG (85). A functional VGPC consists of four transmembrane α subunits that combine as homomultimeric and heteromultimeric (88) tetramers to interact with intracellular β subunits (89), which are also thought to group as a tetramer. Six different VGPC α subunits have been cloned from human brain, and each is encoded by a different gene; there may well be others. Nothing is yet known about the region-specific expression of any of these subunits in the human nervous system.

Immunoprecipitation of VGPCs by Neuromyotonia Sera

Antibodies to VGPCs can be detected in a proportion of NMT patients by immunoprecipitation of ^{125}I-α-dendrotoxin VGPCs extracted with digitonin from human frontal cortex (85), and the level of this antibody is reduced by immunosuppressive treatment (Fig 23-4). Only 5 of 10 sera were positive in this assay and the titers (picomoles of α-dendrotoxin binding sites/L) were low; this assay is now being evaluated as a diagnostic test. To test for binding of antibodies to other forms of

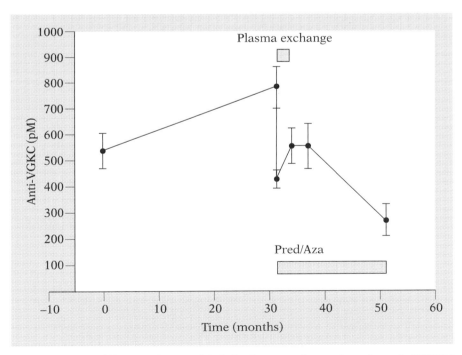

Figure 23-4. Levels of antibodies to ^{125}I-α-dendrotoxin–labeled voltage-gated potassium channels (VGKCs) extracted from human frontal cortex in a patient with acquired neuromyotonia. Control sera gave results of less than 100 pM. The anti-VGKC levels are reduced by plasma exchange and following immunosuppression with prednisolone (Pred) and azathioprine (Aza). (Reproduced by permission from Shillito P, Molenaar PC, Vincent A, et al. Acquired neuromyotonia: evidence for autoantibodies against K+ channels of peripheral nerves. *Ann Neurol* 1995;38:714–722.)

VGPCs, several different recombinant human brain VGPC α-subunit proteins were expressed individually in *Xenopus* oocytes by injection with the relevant subunit chromosomal RNA (cRNA). Results using ^{125}I-α-dendrotoxin–labeled recombinant HBK2 (*KCNA6*) α-subunit protein were very similar to those with labeled VGPCs from whole frontal cortex. These findings confirm the presence of raised antibody titers to VGPCs in NMT, and suggest that these antibodies may bind to more than one type of VGPC α-subunit protein. However, the results of these assays in a significant number of patients are negative, prompting the search for a more sensitive technique (90).

Binding of Neuromyotonia Sera to Recombinant VGPCs Expressed in *Xenopus* Oocytes

A novel immunohistochemical assay that uses recombinant VGPC subunits expressed in *Xenopus* oocytes has been developed (90). Oocytes are injected with the cRNA for a particular VGPC subunit, and after a 3-day period during which protein expression occurs, frozen sections are incubated in serum dilutions and IgG binding is detected with anti-IgG/biotin-steptavidin/horseradish peroxidase. The advantages of this method are the high concentration of the individual subunit that can be expressed in the oocyte cytoplasm, and the lack of solubilization or labeling required. Antibodies to the ligand-binding site should be detected as efficiently as those to other domains on the protein.

With this assay, antibodies to HBK2 α-subunit proteins were detected in 13 of 14 NMT sera (90). Some sera also bound to a VGPC α-subunit protein cloned from a SCLC cDNA library. The amino acid sequence of this SCLC α subunit is more than 99% homologous with the HuK1 (*KCNA1*) α-subunit protein that in mutated form was implicated as the cause of the autosomal dominant episodic ataxia/myokymia syndrome (72). Therefore, it appears that antibodies binding to HuK1 α subunits in acquired NMT, by reducing the number or function of individual VGPCs, have a similar physiologic effect to the point mutations in HuK1 in the inherited syndrome.

Conclusions

NMT is a condition in which muscle hyperactivity stems from peripheral nerve hyperexcitability. Some patients have other immunologic disorders and at least two tumors frequently associated with autoimmune disease. Recent findings suggest that patients with acquired NMT have autoantibodies that bind to some subtypes of VGPC and that these antibodies may play an important role in the pathogenesis of the nerve hyperexcitability that characterizes NMT. Further electrophysiologic and immunologic characterization of the effect of these antibodies and identification of the region-specific expression of VGPCs may eventually throw light on the clinical diversity of the condition.

Antiganglioside Antibodies and Motor Nerve Function

Gangliosides are sialic acid–containing glycosphingolipids. They are sited in the extracellular leaflet of the cell membrane, anchored in the lipid bilayer by their hydrophobic ceramide moiety with the sialylated oligosaccharide core exposed extracellularly. They are widely distributed but particularly highly concentrated in the nervous system. Gangliosides are also present in high concentrations in peripheral nerve axons and myelin (91–95) and studies using both antibodies and bacterial toxins that bind to gangliosides (96,97) indicate that GM_1 and polysialylated gangliosides are present at the nodes of Ranvier and neuromuscular junctions (see also (98)).

Antibodies to Gangliosides

Antibodies to gangliosides have been found at significantly increased levels in several neuropathies, as described elsewhere in this book. Many reviews of these disorders are available (for example, see (99)). This section describes these conditions briefly and focuses on recent evidence that supports a pathogenic role for antiganglioside antibodies.

Miller Fisher syndrome (MFS) is a postinfectious polyneuropathy comprising ataxia and areflexia, with motor manifestations restricted to weakness of the eye muscle (ophthalmoplegia) (100,101). It is believed to be a variant of Guillain-Barré syndrome (GBS), in which motor symptoms are more evident, and overlap syndromes with features of both illnesses may occur. In MFS, anti-GQ_{1b} antibodies are found in over 90% of patients at clinical presentation, and disappear over the course of 2 to 3 months as the patient recovers. The antibodies are predominantly IgG (subclass IgG1 or IgG3) although IgM and IgA antibodies may also be found early in the course of the disease (102). MFS-associated anti-GQ_{1b} antibodies also react with GT_{1a} in most patients, and with other gangliosides bearing disialosyl epitopes (GD_3 and GD_{1b}) in about half of the patients.

A chronic peripheral neuropathy associated with IgM paraproteinemia and red cell agglutination (termed *CANOMAD*) has clinical features quite similar to MFS. The syndrome is largely sensory with prominent ataxia and areflexia, and little clinical evidence of limb weakness. However, some patients have intermittent or partial ophthalmoplegia (103), and motor nerve conduction may be reduced. The close relevance of this syndrome to MFS is reinforced by the reactivity of the IgM paraprotein with all gangliosides bearing disialosyl groups including GQ_{1b}, GT_{1a}, GT_{1b}, GD_{1b}, and GD_3 (reviewed in (104)).

Some patients with GBS have antibodies to GM_1 ganglioside; these patients tend to have prominent motor axon involvement (105,106) and often have had preceding *Campylobacter jejuni* infection that may induce the antiganglioside response (107–109). In these patients there is a significant association with HLA-DQB1*03 (110). In GBS, standard clinical electrophysiologic analysis detects nerve conduction abnormalities, and changes in neuromuscular transmission have not been reported.

Multifocal motor neuropathy (MMN) is a chronic neuropathy resembling motor neuron disease (111). Affected patients typically have focal motor nerve conduction block, and IgM deposits have been identified at the nodes of Ranvier (112,113). *Campylobacter* infection may also be an important finding in some of these patients (114).

Functional Effects of Antiganglioside Antibodies

Several studies showed that antiganglioside antibodies may be affecting motor nerve function, but the results have not been conclusive. Injection of serum from rabbits hyperimmunized with galactocerebrosides caused a reduction in nerve-evoked muscle action potentials and morphologic changes (115). Lafontaine et al (116) applied serum topically to rat ventral root nerves and found slowing of conduction that was not due to a block of sodium channels, but associated with a change in nodal capacitance assumed to be the result of focal demyelination. More recently, Uncini et al (117) reported that injection of MMN sera into rat tibial nerves induced dispersion and reduction in amplitude of the nerve action potential after proximal nerve stimulation. From these studies it was inferred that demyelination contributes to the physiologic effects. Arasaki et al (118) showed some reduction in the compound nerve action potential after application of anti-GM_1–positive human serum to rat sciatic nerve, but a direct effect of the antiganglioside antibodies was not confirmed, and injection of IgG fractions of anti-GM_1–positive sera into rat nerves, even with complement, had no effect on the action potential (119). However, Na^+ currents were reduced after application of serum positive for anti-GM_1 ganglioside antibodies, demonstrated by patch clamp of axonal membranes (120). The effect was abolished by heating the serum, suggesting the involvement of complement, although this was not demonstrated directly. There was also a marked increase in potassium currents. Both of these effects might be expected to lead to a reduction in nerve conduction.

Physiologic Effects of Antiganglioside Antibody–Containing Sera at the Neuromuscular Junction

The neuromuscular junction offers a particularly suitable site at which to investigate the effect of serum antibodies on neuronal function, because the distal motor nerve terminal is not myelinated and is exposed to the extracellular environment. Moreover, rather than measuring neuronal action potentials between two points on the surface of the nerve trunk, the conduction in *individual* motor nerves can be investigated by looking for the presence of nerve-evoked EPPs at each motor end plate.

The direct effect of serum (or plasma) from patients with antiganglioside antibody–associated peripheral neuropathies has been demonstrated by applying serum, diluted in Ringer's solution, to the mouse phrenic nerve–diaphragm preparation. μ-Conotoxin, which blocks the muscle action potential without affecting neuronal conduction, was used in some experiments to prevent muscle contraction during nerve stimulation so that EPPs could be measured directly. In other "passive transfer" studies, the plasma or purified IgG was injected intraperitoneally into the mice for 3 to 10 days. The mice were killed 24 hours later and the preparation examined in vitro.

Application of MFS sera (diluted 1:2) caused a variable but often striking increase in MEPP frequency, suggesting an effect on the motor nerve terminal membrane (121). This was followed by a decrease in MEPP frequency, often to values below control values (mean, 0.5–1.0/sec), sometimes leading to a complete absence of MEPPs in some or all of the muscle fibers. Early experiments (121) suggested that this was associated with complete block of nerve-evoked muscle contraction, but experiments with further sera did not always show such a dramatic effect. No effect on MEPP amplitudes was seen in any experiment, indicating that postsynaptic AChR function was not affected by MFS serum or plasma (121).

The IgG fraction of another MFS patient had a rapid-onset and reversible inhibitory effect on evoked quantal release of transmitter (122). These experiments were performed under conditions of reduced quantal release, and the relationship with the previous results (121) is not clear. However, the IgM antidisialosyl antibodies found in the CANOMAD syndrome can be affinity purified on red blood cells. Purified antibody, identical in electrophoretic and ganglioside-binding pattern to a cloned IgM antibody from the same patient, was tested on the mouse phrenic nerve–diaphragm preparation. The effects of direct application were minimal, but passive transfer for 10 days produced a substantial reduction in the EPP amplitudes in the treated muscles (123) (Fig 23-5).

The direct application of GBS sera or plasma to the preparation produced variable results. Many sera had no effect (Roberts M, Tang T, Vincent A, Willison MJ, unpublished data, 1995). However, one anti-GM_1–positive serum sample, from a GBS patient with preceding *C. jejuni* infections, altered nerve conduction after passive transfer for 3 to 5 days (Roberts M, et al, unpublished observations, 1997). The MEPP frequencies were not altered substantially, but the EPP amplitude was decreased. Similar results were found with IgM anti-GM_1–positive sera from patients with multifocal motor neuropathies (124).

Conclusions

Antiganglioside antibodies are associated with particular clinical neuropathies. Although in the past there has been skepticism regarding their pathogenic role, recent results using in vitro and in vivo applications show that antiganglioside antibody–containing sera from patients

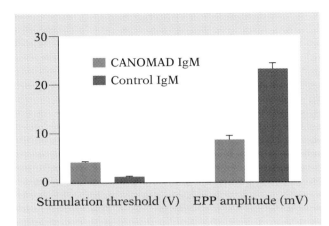

Figure 23-5. Electrophysiologic findings in mice injected with affinity-purified IgM antibody for 10 days from a patient with CANOMAD syndrome. The voltage that had to be applied to the nerve to evoke end-plate potentials (EPP) (stimulus threshold) was increased, and the amplitude of the EPPs decreased. (Data from Willison HJ, O'Hanlon GM, Paterson G, et al. A somatically mutated human anti-ganglioside IgM antibody that induces experimental neuropathy in mice is encoded by the variable region heavy chain gene, V1-18. *J Clin Invest* 1996;97:1155–1164.)

have effects on motor nerve function. In the CANOMAD syndrome, the purified IgM, specific for disialosylated gangliosides, produced physiologic changes in mice, indicating that the antiganglioside antibodies themselves can induce these effects, although the contribution of host factors, such as complement, has not been excluded. Gangliosides are highly concentrated in the nervous system, including the nodes of Ranvier and the motor nerve terminal, and it remains to be seen by what mechanisms the binding of antibodies to gangliosides leads to physiologic effects.

General Conclusions

The motor nerve appears to be an important target in several different antibody-mediated conditions, and at least some of the antibodies involved bind to specific functional molecules such as VGCCs in LEMS and VGPCs in acquired NMT. Other antibodies are specific for gangliosides in in vitro assays, and probably bind to gangliosides in vivo. However, the exact target and distribution of the binding sites for antiganglioside antibodies that cause functional effects on the motor nerve and motor nerve terminal remain to be determined.

References

1. Waxman S, Ritchie JM. Molecular dissection of the myelinated axon. *Ann Neurol* 1993;33:121–136.
2. Van der Kloot W, Molgo J. Quantal acetylcholine release at the vertebrate neuromuscular junction. *Physiol Rev* 1994;74:899–991.
3. Eaton LM, Lambert EH. Electromyography and electric stimulation of nerves in diseases of motor unit. Observations on myasthenic syndrome associated with malignant tumors. *JAMA* 1957;163:1117–1124.
4. O'Neill JH, Murray NM, Newsom-Davis J. The Lambert-Eaton myasthenic syndrome. A review of 50 cases. *Brain* 1988;111:577–596.
5. Newsom-Davis J, Lang B. The Lambert Eaton myasthenic syndrome. In: Engel AE, ed. *Myasthenia gravis and myasthenic syndromes. Contemporary topics in neurology.* CA: Davis, 1997 (in press).
6. Oh SJ. The Eaton-Lambert syndrome. *Arch Neurol* 1972;27:91–94.
7. Argov Z, Shapira Y, Wirguin I. Lambert-Eaton myasthenic syndrome (LEMS) in lymphoproliferative disorders (LPD). *J Neurol* 1994;241:S36.
8. Lauritzen M, Smith T, Fischer-Hansen B, et al. Eaton-Lambert syndrome and malignant thymoma. *Neurology* 1980;30:634–638.
9. Tabbaa MA, Leshner RT, Campbell WW. Malignant thymoma with dysautonomia and disordered neuromuscular transmission. *Arch Neurol* 1986;43:955–957.
10. Clouston PD, Saper CB, Arbizu T, et al. Paraneoplastic cerebellar degeneration. III. Cerebellar degeneration, cancer and the Lambert-Eaton myasthenic syndrome. *Neurology* 1992;42:1944–1950.
11. Pou Serradell A, Fueyo J, Gomez C, et al. Paraneoplastic encephalomyelitis and Lambert-Eaton syndrome. *Rev Neurol (Paris)* 1992;148:605–609.
12. Murray NMF, Newsom-Davis J. Treatment with oral 4-aminopyridine in disorders of neuromuscular transmission. *J Physiol (Lond)* 1990;421:293–308.
13. Chalk CH, Murray NM, Newsom-Davis J, et al. Response of the Lambert-Eaton myasthenic syndrome to treatment of associated small-cell lung carcinoma. *Neurology* 1990;40:1552–1556.
14. Newsom-Davis J, Murray NM. Plasma exchange and immunosuppressive drug treatment in the Lambert-Eaton myasthenic syndrome. *Neurology* 1984;34:480–485.
15. Bain PG, Motomura M, Newsom-Davis J, et al. Effects of intravenous immunoglobulin on muscle weakness and calcium-channel autoantibodies in the Lambert-Eaton syndrome. *Neurology* 1996;47:678–683.
16. Elmqvist D, Lambert EH. Detailed analysis of neuromuscular transmission in a patient with the myasthenic syndrome sometimes associated with bronchogenic carcinoma. *Mayo Clin Proc* 1968;43:689–713.
17. Lambert EH, Elmqvist D. Quantal components of end-plate potentials in the myasthenic syndrome. *Ann NY Acad Sci* 1971;183:183–199.
18. Fukunaga H, Engel AG, Osame M, Lambert EH. Paucity and disorganisation of presynaptic membrane active zones in the Lambert-Eaton myasthenic syndrome. *Muscle Nerve* 1982;5:686–697.
19. Engel AG. Review of evidence for loss of motor nerve terminal calcium channels in Lambert-Eaton myasthenic syndrome. *Ann NY Acad Sci* 1991;635:246–258.
20. Lennon VA, Lambert EH, Whittingham S, Fairbanks V. Autoimmunity in the Lambert-Eaton myasthenic syndrome. *Muscle Nerve* 1982;5:S21–S25.
21. Demaine A, Willcox N, Welsh K, Newsom-Davis J. Associations of the autoimmune myasthenias with genetic markers in the immunoglobulin heavy chain region. *Ann NY Acad Sci* 1988;540:266–268.
22. Willcox N, Demaine AG, Newsom-Davis J, et al. Increased frequency of IgG heavy chain marker Glm(2) and of HLA-B8 in Lambert-Eaton myasthenic syndrome with and without associated lung carcinoma. *Hum Immunol* 1985;14:29–36.
23. Ishikawa K, Engelhardt JK, Fujisawa T, et al. A neuro-

muscular transmission block produced by a cancer tissue extract derived from a patient with the myasthenic syndrome. *Neurology* 1987;27:140–143.

24. Lambert EH, Lennon VA. Neuromuscular transmission in nude mice bearing oat cell tumors from Lambert-Eaton myasthenic syndrome. *Muscle Nerve* 1982;5:S39–S45.

25. Lang B, Newsom-Davis J, Wray D, et al. Autoimmune aetiology for myasthenic (Eaton-Lambert) syndrome. *Lancet* 1981;2:224–226.

26. Dau PC, Denys EH. Plasmapheresis and immunosuppressive drug therapy in the Eaton-Lambert syndrome. *Ann Neurol* 1982;11:570–575.

27. Toyka KV, Drachman DB, Griffin DE, et al. Myasthenia gravis: study of humoral immune mechanisms by passive transfer to mice. *N Engl J Med* 1977;296:125–131.

28. Lang B, Newsom-Davis J, Prior C, Wray D. Antibodies to motor nerve terminals: an electrophysiological study of a human myasthenic syndrome transferred to mouse. *J Physiol (Lond)* 1983;344:335–345.

29. Kim YI. Passive transfer of the Lambert-Eaton myasthenic syndrome: neuromuscular transmission in mice injected with plasma. *Muscle Nerve* 1985;8:162–172.

30. Kim YI. Passively transferred Lambert-Eaton syndrome in mice receiving purified IgG. *Muscle Nerve* 1986;9:532–530.

31. Prior C, Lang B, Wray D, Newsom-Davis J. Action of Lambert-Eaton myasthenic syndrome IgG at mouse motor nerve terminals. *Ann Neurol* 1985;17:587–592.

32. Kim YI, Sanders DB, Johns TR, et al. Lambert-Eaton myasthenic syndrome: the lack of short-term *in vitro* effects of serum factors on neuromuscular transmission. *J Neurol Sci* 1988;87:1–13.

33. Fukunaga H, Engel AG, Lang B, et al. Passive transfer of Lambert-Eaton myasthenic syndrome with IgG from man to mouse depletes the presynaptic membrane active zones. *Proc Natl Acad Sci USA* 1983;80:7636–7640.

34. Nagel A, Engel AG, Lang B, et al. Lambert-Eaton myasthenic syndrome IgG depletes presynaptic membrane active zone particles by antigenic modulation. *Ann Neurol* 1988;24:552–558.

35. Fukuoka T, Engel AG, Lang B, et al. Lambert-Eaton myasthenic syndrome: II. Immunoelectron microscopy localization of IgG at the mouse motor end-plate. *Ann Neurol* 1987;22:200–211.

36. Engel AG, Nagel A, Fukuoka T, et al. Motor nerve terminal calcium channels in Lambert-Eaton myasthenic syndrome. Morphologic evidence for depletion and that the depletion is mediated by autoantibodies. *Ann NY Acad Sci* 1989;560:278–290.

37. Tischler AS, Dichter MA, Biales B. Electrical excitability of oat cell carcinoma. *J Pathol* 1977;122:153–156.

38. McCann FV, Pettengill OS, Cole JJ, et al. Calcium spike electrogenesis and other electrical activity in continuously cultured small cell carcinoma of the lung. *Science* 1981;212:1155–1157.

39. Roberts A, Perera S, Lang B, et al. Paraneoplastic myasthenic syndrome IgG inhibits $^{45}Ca^{2+}$ flux in a human small cell carcinoma line. *Nature* 1985;317:737–739.

40. De Aizpurua HJ, Lambert EH, Griesmann GE, et al. Antagonism of voltage-gated calcium channels in small cell carcinomas of patients with and without Lambert-Eaton myasthenic syndrome by autoantibodies, ω-conotoxin and adenosine. *Cancer Res* 1988;48:4719–4724.

41. Meyer EM, Momol AE, Kramer BS, et al. Effects of serum fractions from patients with Eaton-Lambert syndrome on rat cortical synaptosomal (^{3}H)acetylcholine release. *Biochem Pharmacol* 1986;35:3412–3414.

42. Login IS, Kim YI, Judd AM, et al. Immunoglobulins of Lambert-Eaton myasthenic syndrome inhibit rat pituitary hormone release. *Ann Neurol* 1987;22:610–614.

43. Kim YI, Neher E. IgG from patients with Lambert-Eaton syndrome blocks voltage dependent calcium channels. *Science* 1988;239:405–408.

44. Peers C, Lang B, Newsom-Davis J, Wray DW. Selective action of myasthenic syndrome antibodies on calcium channels in a rodent neuroblastoma x glioma cell line. *J Physiol (Lond)* 1990;421:293–308.

45. Olivera BM, Miljanich GP, Ramachandran J, Adams ME. Calcium channel diversity and neurotransmitter release: the ω-conotoxins and ω-agatoxins. *Annu Rev Biochem* 1994;63:823–867.

46. Protti DA, Uchitel OD. Transmitter release and presynaptic Ca^{2+} currents blocked by the spider toxin ω-Aga-IVA. *Neuroreport* 1993;5:333–336.

47. Oguro-Okano M, Griesmann GE, Wieben ED, et al. Molecular diversity of neuronal-type calcium channels identified in small cell lung carcinoma. *Mayo Clin Proc* 1992;67:1150–1159.

48. Johnston I, Lang B, Leys K, Newsom-Davis J. Heterogeneity of calcium channel autoantibodies detected using a small cell lung cancer line derived from a Lambert-Eaton syndrome patient. *Neurology* 1994;44:334–338.

49. Chester KA, Lang B, Gill J, et al. Lambert-Eaton syndrome antibodies: reaction with membranes from a small cell lung cancer xenograft. *J Neuroimmunol* 1988;18:97–104.

50. Viglione MP, Creutz CE, Kim YI. Lambert-Eaton syndrome: antigen-antibody interaction and calcium current inhibition in chromaffin cells. *Muscle Nerve* 1994;15:1325–1333.

51. Sher E, Canal N, Piccolo G, et al. Specificity of calcium channel autoantibodies in Lambert-Eaton myasthenic syndrome. *Lancet* 1989;2:640–643.

52. Lennon VA, Lambert EH. Autoantibodies bind solubilized calcium channel-omega-conotoxin complexes from small cell lung carcinoma: a diagnostic aid for Lambert-Eaton myasthenic syndrome. *Mayo Clin Proc* 1989;64:1498–1504.

53. Leys K, Lang B, Johnston I, Newsom-Davis J. Calcium channel autoantibodies in the Lambert-Eaton myasthenic syndrome. *Ann Neurol* 1991;29:307–314.

54. El Far O, Marqueze B, Leveque C, et al. Antigens associated with N and L type calcium channels in Lambert-Eaton myasthenic syndrome. *J Neurochem* 1995;64:1696–1702.

55. Motomura M, Johnston I, Lang B, et al. An improved diagnostic assay for Lambert-Eaton myasthenic syndrome. *J Neurol Neurosurg Psychiatry* 1995;58:85–87.

56. Lennon VA, Kryzer TJ, Griesmann GE, et al. Calcium channel antibodies in the Lambert Eaton myasthenic syndrome and other paraneoplastic syndromes. *N Engl J Med* 1995;332:1467–1474.

57. Bird SJ. Clinical and electrophysiologic improvement in Lambert-Eaton syndrome with intravenous immunoglobulin therapy. *Neurology* 1992;42:1422–1423.

58. Waterman SA, Lang B, Newsom-Davis J. Effect of Lambert-Eaton myasthenic syndrome antibodies on autonomic neurons in the mouse. *Ann Neurol* 1997 (in press).

59. Rosenfeld MR, Wong E, Dalmau J, et al. Cloning and characterization of a Lambert-Eaton myasthenic syndrome antigen. *Ann Neurol* 1993;33:113–120.

60. Leveque C, Hoshino T, David P, et al. The synaptic vesicle protein synaptotagmin associates with calcium channels and is a putative Lambert-Eaton myas-

thenic syndrome antigen. *Proc Natl Acad Sci USA* 1992;89:3625–3629.

61. Smith RG, Hamilton S, Hofman P, et al. Serum antibodies to L-type calcium channels in patients with amyotrophic lateral sclerosis. *N Engl J Med* 1992;327:1721–1728.

62. Vincent A, Drachman DB. Amyotrophic lateral sclerosis and antibodies to voltage-gated calcium channels—new doubts. Editorial. *Ann Neurol* 1996;40:691–693.

63. Peers C, Johnston I, Lang B, Wray D. Cross-linking of presynaptic calcium channels: a mechanism of action for Lambert-Eaton myasthenic syndrome antibodies at the mouse neuromuscular junction. *Neurosci Lett* 1993;153:45–48.

64. Lang B, Vincent A, Murray NM, Newsom-Davis J. Lambert-Eaton myasthenic syndrome: immunoglobulin G inhibition of Ca^{2+} flux in tumor cells correlates with disease severity. *Ann Neurol* 1989;25:265–271.

65. Morris CS, Esiri MM, Marx A, Newsom-Davis J. Immunocytochemical characteristics of small cell lung carcinoma associated with the Lambert-Eaton myasthenic syndrome. *Am J Pathol* 1992;140:839–845.

66. Geddes DM. The natural history of lung cancer: a review based on rates of tumour growth. *Br J Dis Chest* 1979;73:1–17.

67. Elrington GM, Murray NMF, Spiro SG, Newsom-Davis J. Neurological paraneoplastic syndromes in patients with small cell lung cancer: a prospective survey of 150 patients. *J Neurol Neurosurg Psychiatry* 1991;54:764–767.

68. Chapman J, Rabinowitz R, Korczyn AD, Michaelson DM. Rats immunized with cholinergic synaptosomes: a model for Lambert-Eaton syndrome. *Muscle Nerve* 1990;13:726–733.

69. Takamori M, Hamada T, Komai K, et al. Synaptotagmin can cause an immune-mediated model of Lambert Eaton myasthenic syndrome in rats. *Ann Neurol* 1994;35:74–80.

70. Isaacs H. A syndrome of continuous muscle-fiber activity. *J Neurol Neurosurg Psychiatry* 1961;24:319–325.

71. Newsom-Davis J, Mills KR. Immunological associations of acquired neuromyotonia (Isaacs' syndrome). Report of five cases and literature review. *Brain* 1993;116:453–469.

72. Browne DL, Gancher ST, Nutt JG, et al. Episodic ataxia/myokymia syndrome is associated with point mutations in the human potassium channel gene KCNA1. *Nat Genet* 1994;8:136–140.

73. Hart I, Vincent A, Willison HJ. Disorders of the motor nerve and motor nerve terminal. In: Engel AG, ed. *Myasthenia gravis and myasthenic syndromes. Contemporary topics in neurology.* CA: Davis, 1997 (in press).

74. Denny-Brown D, Foley JM. Myokymia and the benign fasciculation of muscular cramps. *Trans Assoc Am Physicians* 1948;61:88–96.

75. Mertens HG, Zschocke S. Neuromyotonie. *Klin Wochenschr* 1965;43:917–925.

76. Coërs C, Telermann-Toppet N, Durdu J. Neurogenic benign fasciculations, pseudomyotonia and pseudotetany. A disease in search of a name. *Arch Neurol* 1981;38:282–287.

77. Reeback J, Benton S, Swash M, Schwartz MS. Penicillamine-induced neuromyotonia. *BMJ* 1979;279:1464–1465.

78. Fernandes L, Swinson DR, Hamilton EBD. Dermatomyositis complicating penicillamine treatment. *Ann Rheum Dis* 1977;36:94–95.

79. Souadjian JV, Enriquez P, Silverstein MN, Pepin J-M. The spectrum of diseases associated with thymoma. *Arch Intern Med* 1974;134:374–379.

80. Halbach M, Homberg V, Freund H-J. Neuromuscular, autonomic and central cholinergic hyperactivity associated with thymoma and acetylcholine receptor-binding antibody. *J Neurol (Berlin)* 1987;234:433–436.

81. Waerness E. Neuromyotonia and bronchial carcinoma. *Electromyogr Clin Neurophysiol* 1974;14:527–535.

82. Walsh JC. Neuromyotonia: an unusual presentation of intrathoracic malignancy. *J Neurol Neurosurg Psychiatry* 1976;39:1086–1091.

83. Bady B, Chauplannaz G, Vial C, Savet J-F. Autoimmune aetiology for acquired neuromyotonia. *Lancet* 1991;338:1330.

84. Sinha S, Newsom-Davis J, Mills K, et al. Autoimmune aetiology for acquired neuromyotonia (Isaacs' syndrome). *Lancet* 1991;338:75–77.

85. Shillito P, Molenaar PC, Vincent A, et al. Acquired neuromyotonia: evidence for autoantibodies against K+ channels of peripheral nerves. *Ann Neurol* 1995;38:714–722.

86. Black JA, Kocsis JD, Waxman SG. Ion channel organization of the myelinated fiber. *Trends Neurosci* 1990;13:48–54.

87. Harvey AL, Anderson AJ. Dendrotoxins: snake toxins that block potassium channels and facilitate neurotransmitter release. In: Harvey A, ed. *Snake toxins.* New York: Pergamon, 1991:131–164.

88. Wang H, Kunkel DD, Martin TM, et al. Heteromultimeric potassium channels in terminal and juxtaparanodal regions of neurons. *Nature* 1993;365:75–79.

89. Rettig J, Heinemann SH, Wunder F, et al. Inactivation properties of voltage-gated potassium channels altered by presence of β-subunit. *Nature* 1994;369:289–294.

90. Hart IK, Waters C, Vincent A, et al. Autoantibodies detected to human brain potassium channels expressed in *Xenopus* oocytes are implicated in neuromyotonia (Isaacs' syndrome). *Ann Neurol* 1997;41:238–246.

91. Merrill AH, Hannun YA, Bell RM. Introduction: sphingolipids and their metabolites in cell regulation. *Adv Lipid Res* 1993;25:1–21.

92. Hannun YA, Bell R. Functions of sphingolipids and sphingolipid breakdown products in cellular regulation. *Science* 1989;243:500–507.

93. Corbo M, Quattrino A, Lugaresi A, et al. Patterns of reactivity of human anti-GM$_1$ antibodies with spinal cord and motor neurons. *Ann Neurol* 1992;32:487–493.

94. Kotani M, Kawashima I, Ozawa H, et al. Differential distribution of major gangliosides in rat central nervous system detected by specific monoclonal antibodies. *Glycobiology* 1993;3:137–146.

95. Ogawa Goto K, Funamoto N, Abe T, Nagashima K. Different ceramide compositions of gangliosides between human motor and sensory nerves. *J Neurochem* 1990;55:186–193.

96. Ganser AL, Kirschner DA, Willinger M. Ganglioside localisation on myelinated nerve fibres by cholera toxin binding. *J Neurocytol* 1983;12:921–938.

97. Kitamura M, Iwamori M, Nagai Y. Interaction between *Clostridium botulinum* neurotoxin and gangliosides. *Biochem Biophys Acta* 1980;628:328–335.

98. Willison HJ, Kennedy PGE. Gangliosides and bacterial toxins in Guillain Barré syndrome. *J Neuroimmunol* 1993;46:105–112.

99. Hohlfeld R. *Immunology of neuromuscular disease.* Boston: Kluwer Academic, 1994.

100. Fisher M. An unusual variant of acute idiopathic polyneuritis (syndrome of ophthalmoplegia, ataxia and areflexia). *N Engl J Med* 1956;255:57–65.
101. Berlit P, Rakicky J. The Miller Fisher syndrome. Review of the literature. *J Clin Neuroophthalmol* 1992;12:57–63.
102. Willison HJ, Veitch J. Immunoglobulin subclass distribution and binding characteristics of anti-GQ_{1b} antibodies in Miller Fisher syndrome. *J Neuroimmunol* 1994;50:159–165.
103. Willison HJ, Paterson G, Veitch J,et al. Peripheral neuropathy associated with monoclonal IgM anti-Pr2 cold agglutinins. *J Neurol Neurosurg Psychiatry* 1993;56:1178–1184.
104. Willison HJ. Antiglycolipid antibodies in peripheral neuropathies: fact or fiction? *J Neurol Neurosurg Psychiatry* 1994;57:1303–1307.
105. Gregson NA, Jones D, Thomas PK, Willison HJ. Acute motor neuropathy with antibodies to GM1 ganglioside. *J Neurol* 1991;238:447–451.
106. Latov N. Antibodies to glycoconjugates in neurological disease. *Clin Aspects Autoimmun* 1990;4:18–29.
107. Kaldor J, Speed BR. GBS and *Campylobacter jejuni*: a serological study. *BMJ* 1984;288:1867–1870.
108. Yuki N, Taki T, Inagaki F, et al. A bacterium lipopolysaccharide that elicits Guillain-Barré syndrome has a GM1 ganglioside-like structure. *J Exp Med* 1993;178:1771–1775.
109. Rees JH, Soudain SE, Gregson NA, Hughes RAC. *Campylobacter jejuni* infection and Guillain-Barré syndrome. *N Engl J Med* 1995;333:1374–1379.
110. Rees JH, Vaughan RW, Kondeatis E, Hughes RAC. HLA-class II alleles in Guillain-Barré syndrome and Miller Fisher syndrome and their association with preceding *Campylobacter jejuni* infection. *J Neuroimmunol* 1995;62:53–57.
111. Lewis RA, Sumner AJ, Brown MJ, Asbury AK. Multifocal demyelinating neuropathy with persistent conduction block. *Neurology* 1982;32:958–964.
112. Pestronk A, Cornblath DR, Llyas AA, et al. A treatable multifocal neuropathy with antibodies to GM_1 ganglioside. *Ann Neurol* 1988;24:73–78.
113. Santoro M, Thomas FP, Fink ME, et al. IgM deposits at nodes of Ranvier in a patient with motor neuropathy, anti-GM_1 antibodies and multifocal motor conduction block. *Ann Neurol* 1990;28:373–379.
114. Wirguin I, Suturkova-Milsevic L, Della-Latta P, et al. Monoclonal IgM antibodies to GM_1 and asialo-GM_1 in chronic neuropathies cross-react with *Campylobacter jejuni* lipopolysaccharides. *Ann Neurol* 1994;35:698–703.
115. Saida K, Saida T, Brown MJ, Silberberg DH. *In vivo* demyelination induced by intraneural injection of anti-galactocerebroside serum. *Am J Pathol* 1979;95:99–116.
116. Lafontaine S, Rasminsky M, Saida T, Sumner AJ. Conduction block in rat myelinated fibres following acute exposure to anti-galactocerebroside serum. *J Physiol* 1982;323:287–306.
117. Uncini A, Santoro M, Corbo M, et al. Conduction abnormalities induced by sera of patients with multifocal motor neuropathy and anti-GM1 antibodies. *Muscle and Nerve* 1993;16:610–615.
118. Arasaka K, Kusonoki S, Kudo N, Kanazawa I. Acute conduction block *in vitro* following exposure to anti-ganglioside sera. *Muscle Nerve* 1993;16:587–593.
119. Harvey GK, Toyka KV, Zielasek J, et al. Failure of anti-GM1 IgG or IgM to induce conduction block following intraneural transfer. *Muscle Nerve* 1995;18:388–394.
120. Takigawa T, Yasuda H, Kikkawa R, et al. Antibodies against GM_1 ganglioside affect K^+ and Na^+ currents in isolated rat myelinated nerve fibers. *Ann Neurol* 1995;37:436–442.
121. Roberts M, Willison HJ, Vincent A, Newsom-Davis J. Serum factor in the Miller Fisher variant of Guillain-Barré syndrome and neurotransmitter release. *Lancet* 1994;343:454–455.
122. Buchwald B, Weishaupt A, Toyka KV, Dudel J. Immunoglobulin G from a patient with Miller-Fisher syndrome rapidly and reversibly depresses evoked quantal release at the neuromuscular junction. *Neurosci Lett* 1995;201:163–166.
123. Willison HJ, O'Hanlon GM, Paterson G, et al. A somatically mutated human anti-ganglioside IgM antibody that induces experimental neuropathy in mice is encoded by the variable region heavy chain gene, V1-18. *J Clin Invest* 1996;97:1155–1164.
124. Roberts M, Willison HJ, Vincent A, Newsom-Davis J. Multifocal motor neuropathy human sera block distal motor nerve conduction in mice. *Ann Neurol* 1995;38:111–118.

Chapter 24

Immunopathogenesis of Inflammatory Myopathies

Marinos C. Dalakas

The inflammatory myopathies comprise three major and distinct subsets: *polymyositis* (PM), *dermatomyositis* (DM), and *inclusion-body myositis* (IBM) (1–8). Although each subset retains characteristic clinical, immunopathologic, and morphologic features, they all have in common the presence of moderate to severe muscle weakness and inflammation of the muscles. The autoimmune origin of the inflammatory myopathies has been based on their association with other putative or definite autoimmune diseases or viral infections, the evidence for a T cell–mediated myocytotoxicity or complement-mediated microangiopathy, the presence of a variety of autoantibodies, and the varying responses to immunotherapies (1–8). Although in IBM the immune-mediated process is weaker and IBM patients do not readily respond to immunotherapies, there are convincing immunopathologic signs to suggest that a definite autoimmune component, similar to that seen in PM, plays a role in the cause of IBM. This chapter reviews the main clinical and histologic features of these diseases, their association with autoimmune conditions and viruses, the main immunologic characteristics including potential target antigens and unique features of the sensitized autoinvasive T cells, and the various immunotherapeutic interventions.

Clinical Features

Dermatomyositis

DM occurs in both children and adults. It is a distinct clinical entity identified by a characteristic rash accompanying, or more often, preceding the muscle weakness. The skin manifestations include a heliotrope rash (blue-purple discoloration) on the upper eyelids with edema, a flat red rash on the face and upper trunk, and erythema of the knuckles with a raised violaceous scaly eruption (*Gottron's rash*) that later results in scaling of the skin. The erythematous rash can also occur on other body surfaces, including the knees, elbows, malleoli, neck, and anterior part of the chest (often in a *V sign*), or back and shoulders (*shawl sign*), and may be exacerbated after exposure to the sun. Dilated capillary loops at the base of the fingernails are also characteristic of DM. The cuticles may be irregular, thickened, and distorted, and the lateral and palmar areas of the fingers

may become rough and cracked, with irregular, "dirty" horizontal lines, resembling *mechanic's hands*. The degree of weakness can be mild, moderate, or severe leading to quadriparesis. At times, the muscle strength appears normal, hence the term *dermatomyositis sine myositis*. In muscle biopsy specimens obtained from such patients, however, significant perivascular and perimysial inflammation is seen (9). In children, DM resembles the adult disease, except for more frequent extramuscular manifestations, as discussed later. A common early abnormality in children is *misery*, defined as an irritable child who feels uncomfortable, has a red flush on the face, is fatigued, does not feel well to socialize, and has a varying degree of proximal muscle weakness. A tiptoe gait due to flexion contracture of the ankles is also common.

DM usually occurs alone, but may overlap with systemic sclerosis and mixed connective tissue disease (1,2). Fasciitis and skin changes similar to those found in DM have occurred in patients with the eosinophilia-myalgia syndrome associated with the ingestion of contaminated L-tryptophan (1,2).

Polymyositis

In contrast with DM, PM has no unique clinical features, and its diagnosis is one of exclusion. It is best defined as an inflammatory myopathy that develops subacutely, usually over weeks to months, progresses steadily, and occurs in adults who *do not have* any of the following: rash, involvement of the eye and facial muscles, family history of neuromuscular disease, history of exposure to myotoxic drugs or toxins, endocrinopathy, neurogenic disease or dystrophy, and biochemical muscle disease or IBM as determined by muscle enzyme histochemistry and biochemistry.

Unlike in DM, in which the rash secures early recognition, the actual onset of PM cannot be easily determined, and the disease may exist for several months before the patient seeks medical advice.

PM can be viewed as a syndrome of diverse causes that can occur separately or in association with systemic autoimmune or connective tissue diseases and certain known viral or bacterial infections. Other than D-penicillamine and zidovudine, which can cause the myopathy involving endomysial inflammation, myotoxic drugs such as emetine, chloroquine, steroids, cimetidine, ipecac, and lovastatin do not cause PM. Instead, the latter drugs elicit a *toxic noninflammatory* myopathy that is histologically different from PM and does not require immunosuppressive therapy (1,2). Several animal parasites such as *protozoa* (*Toxoplasma, Trypanosoma*), *cestodes* (*cysticerci*), and *nematodes* (*trichinae*) can produce a focal or diffuse inflammatory myopathy known as *parasitic polymyositis.* A suppurative myositis, known as *tropical polymyositis* or *pyomyositis* can be produced by *Staphylococcus aureus, Yersinia* species, *Streptococcus* organisms, or other anaerobes. Pyomyositis, a previous rarity in the West, can now be seen in rare patients with acquired immunodeficiency syndrome (AIDS). Certain bacteria, such as *Borrelia burgdorferi* of Lyme disease and *Legionella pneumophila* of legionnaires' disease may infrequently be the cause of polymyositis.

Inclusion-Body Myositis

Although IBM is commonly suspected when a patient with presumed PM does not respond to therapy, involvement of distal muscles, especially foot extensors and deep finger flexors, in almost all the patients, may be a clue to the early clinical diagnosis (1–7,10). The weakness and atrophy can be asymmetric with selective involvement of the quadriceps, iliopsoas, triceps, biceps, and finger flexors in the forearm. Dysphagia is common, occurring in up to 60% of patients, especially late in the disease. Because of the distal and at times, asymmetric weakness and atrophy and the early loss of the patellar reflex owing to severe weakness of the quadriceps muscle, a lower motor neuron disease is often suspected, especially when the serum creatine kinase (CK) level is not elevated. Sensory examination generally reveals normal findings except for a mildly diminished vibratory sensation at the ankles, presumably related to the patient's age. Contrary to early suggestions, the distal weakness does not represent neurogenic involvement but is part of the distal myopathic process, as we confirmed with macroelectromyography (11). In contrast to PM and DM in which facial muscles are spared, we noted mild facial muscle weakness in 60% of IBM patients (10). Dysphagia is also common, especially late in the disease, occurring in up to 50% of our patients. The diagnosis is always made by the characteristic findings on the muscle biopsy specimens, as discussed later. Patients with IBM account for the majority of the patients older than 50 years referred to us as having "polymyositis unresponsive to therapy."

IBM can be associated with systemic autoimmune or connective tissue diseases in at least 20% of the patients. Hereditary IBM, most often recessive and less frequently dominant, with sparing of the quadriceps in some patients, may be found. At present, hereditary IBM includes various ill-defined vacuolar, distal more than proximal, myopathies with a clinical profile different from the one described for sporadic IBM (12). Hereditary IBM can occur in certain ethnic groups, especially Iranian Jews. There is also a subset of patients with familial IBM who have the typical phenotype of sporadic IBM with histologic and immunopathologic features identical to the sporadic form (12).

Progression of IBM is slow but steady. The degree of disability in relation to the duration of the disease has not been studied. Review of the course of 14 randomly chosen patients with symptoms for more than 5 years revealed that 10 of them required a cane or support for ambulation by the fifth year after onset of disease whereas 3 of 5 patients with symptoms for 10 years or more were using wheelchairs for ambulation. Using quantitative muscle strength testing, we found a 10% drop in muscle strength over 1½-year period.

Extramuscular Manifestations

In addition to the primary disturbance of the skeletal muscles, extramuscular manifestations may be prominent in patients with inflammatory myopathies. These include the following:

1. *Dysphagia,* most prominent in IBM and DM, due to involvement of the oropharyngeal striated muscles and distal esophagus.
2. *Cardiac* abnormalities consisting of atrioventricular conduction defects, tachyarrhythmias, low ejection fraction, and dilated cardiomyopathy either from the disease itself or from hypertension associated with long-term steroid use.
3. *Pulmonary* involvement, as the result of primary weakness of the thoracic muscles, drug-induced pneumonitis (e.g., from methotrexate), or interstitial lung disease. Interstitial lung disease may precede the myopathy or occur early in the disease and develops in up to 10% of patients with PM or DM, the majority of whom have anti–Jo-1 antibodies. Adult respiratory distress syndrome resulting in death can occur in PM patients with anti–Jo-1 antibodies (13), emphasizing the diagnostic importance of these antibodies. Pulmonary capillaritis with varying degrees of diffuse alveolar hemorrhage also has been described (14).
4. *Subcutaneous calcifications,* sometimes extruding on the skin and causing ulcerations and infections, are found in patients with DM, not only in children but also in some adults (15).
5. *Gastrointestinal ulcerations* seen more often in childhood DM, due to vasculitis and infection.
6. *Contractures* of the joints, especially in childhood DM.
7. *General systemic disturbances* such as fever, malaise, weight loss, arthralgia, and Raynaud's phenomenon, when the inflammatory myopathy is associated with a connective tissue disorder.
8. *Malignancies,* the incidence of which is increased in patients with DM, but not PM or IBM. Because tumors are usually uncovered not by a radiologic blind search, but by abnormal findings on medical history and physical examination, a complete *annual* physical examination with pelvic and rectal examinations, urinalysis, complete blood cell count,

blood chemistry tests, and a chest x-ray film are recommended.

Diagnosis

The clinically suspected diagnosis of PM, DM, or IBM is established or confirmed by examining the serum muscle enzymes, the electromyographic (EMG) findings, and the muscle biopsy specimen.

Serum Muscle Enzymes

The most sensitive enzyme is CK, which in the presence of active disease can be elevated as much as 50 times the normal level. Although the CK value usually parallels disease activity, it can be normal in active DM and rarely, in active PM. In IBM, the CK level is not usually elevated more than tenfold, and in some patients it may be normal even from the beginning of the illness. The level may also be normal in patients with untreated, even active, childhood DM and in some patients with PM or DM associated with a connective tissue disease, reflecting the concentration of the pathologic process in the intramuscular vessels and the perimysium. Along with the CK, the serum alanine aminotransferase, aspartate aminotransferase, lactate dehydrogenase, and aldolase levels may be elevated.

Electromyography

Needle EMG shows myopathic potentials characterized by short-duration, low-amplitude, polyphasic units on voluntary activation, and increased spontaneous activity with fibrillations, complex repetitive discharges, and positive sharp waves. This EMG pattern occurs in a variety of acute, toxic, and active myopathic processes and should not be considered diagnostic for the inflammatory myopathies. Mixed myopathic and neurogenic potentials (polyphasic units of short and long duration) are more often seen in IBM but they can be seen in both PM and DM as a consequence of muscle fiber regeneration and chronicity of the disease. Contrary to previous reports, our findings using macro-EMG failed to show a neurogenic pattern of involvement in IBM patients (11). EMG studies are generally useful for excluding neurogenic disorders and confirming either active or inactive myopathy.

Muscle Biopsy

Muscle biopsy is the definitive test not only for establishing the diagnosis of DM, PM, or IBM, but also for excluding other neuromuscular diseases. Although the presence of inflammation is the histologic hallmark for these diseases, there are additional unique histologic features characteristic for each group.

In DM the endomysial inflammation is predominantly perivascular or in the interfascicular septa and around rather than within the fascicles. The intramuscular blood vessels show endothelial hyperplasia with tubuloreticular profiles, fibrin thrombi, especially in children, and obliteration of capillaries (1–6). The muscle fibers undergo necrosis, degeneration, and phagocytosis often in groups involving a portion of a muscle fasciculus in a wedge-like shape, or at the periphery of the fascicle due to microinfarcts within the muscle. This results in perifascicular atrophy, characterized by 2 to 10 layers of atrophic fibers at the periphery of the fascicles. The presence of perifascicular atrophy is diagnostic of DM, *even in the absence of inflammation.*

In PM there is no perifascicular atrophy and the blood vessels are normal. The endomysial infiltrates are mostly within the fascicles surrounding individual, healthy muscle fibers, resulting in phagocytosis and necrosis. When the disease is chronic, the connective tissue is increased and often reacts positively with alkaline phosphatase.

The histologic hallmarks of IBM are as follows:

1. Basophilic granular inclusions distributed around the edge of slitlike vacuoles (rimmed vacuoles).
2. Angulated or round fibers, often in small groups.
3. Eosinophilic cytoplasmic inclusions.
4. Sparse to prominent endomysial inflammation in a pattern identical to that seen in PM.
5. Tiny deposits of Congo red– or crystal violet–positive amyloid within or next to some vacuoles. The amyloid, seen in 50% of our patients, immunoreacts with β-amyloid protein, the type of amyloid sequenced from the amyloid fibrils of blood vessels of patients with Alzheimer's disease (16–18).
6. Characteristic filamentous inclusions seen by electron microscopy in the cytoplasm or myonuclei, prominent in the vicinity of the rimmed vacuoles. Although demonstration of the filaments by electron microscopy was initially essential for the diagnosis of IBM, we do not believe that this is now necessary if all the characteristic clinical and light microscopic features are observed. Further, such filaments are not unique to IBM but they can be seen in other vacuolar myopathies. The vacuolated muscle fibers contain strong ubiquitin immunoreactivity localized to the cytoplasmic tubulofilaments (16).
7. Abnormal mitochondria seen as ragged-red fibers that are often negative for cytochrome oxidase and contain mitochondrial DNA deletions (19).

Immune-Mediated Mechanisms

Presence of Autoantibodies

Various *autoantibodies* against *nuclear* (*antinuclear antibodies*) and *cytoplasmic* antigens are found in up to 20% of patients with inflammatory myopathies (1–3,8,20). The antibodies to cytoplasmic antigens are directed against cytoplasmic ribonucleoproteins that are involved in translation and protein synthesis. They include antibodies against various *synthetases, translation factors,* and *proteins of the signal-recognition particles.* The antibody directed against the histidyl-transfer RNA synthetase, called *anti–Jo-1,* accounts for 75% of all the antisynthetases and is clinically useful because up to 80% of patients with anti–Jo-1 antibodies have interstitial lung disease. In general, these antibodies may be nonmuscle specific because a) they are directed against ubiquitous targets and may represent epiphenomena of no pathogenic significance; b) they occur in all three subtypes (PM, DM, and IBM), in spite of their clinical and immunopathologic differences; c) they are almost always associated with interstitial lung disease; and d) at times, we have seen them in patients with interstitial lung disease who do not have active myositis. Patients with the overlap syndrome of DM and systemic sclerosis may have a specific antinuclear autoantibody, the anti-PM/Scl, directed against a nucleolar protein complex.

Immunopathology of Dermatomyositis

The primary antigenic target in DM involves components of the vascular endothelium of the endomysial blood vessels and the capillaries. Banker (21) first demonstrated the signs of an ongoing angiopathy in DM, based on light and electron microscopic observations (21). Engel et al (22) showed that the earliest pathologic alterations in DM are changes in the endothelial cells consisting of pale and swollen cytoplasm with microvacuoles. Carpenter and Karpati (23) confirmed and expanded on these findings by demonstrating active focal destruction of capillaries consisting of undulating tubules in the smooth endoplasmic reticulum of the endothelial cells, along with obliteration, vascular necrosis, and thrombi.

The first indication that such alterations in the microvasculature are caused by an immune-mediated process was the demonstration of immune complexes on the endomysial blood vessels (24). These observations were reinforced by finding C5b-9 membranolytic attack complex (MAC), the lytic component of the complement pathway, on the endomysial capillaries early in the disease and before inflammatory or structural changes in the muscle fibers had taken place (25). We investigated further the role of the complement in DM patients utilizing an in vitro assay system that measures C3 consumption by sensitized erythrocytes on the basis of radiolabeled anti-C3 antibodies (26). Patients with active but not chronic DM had very high C3 uptake in the serum that correlated not only with disease activity but also with response to therapies. Further, MAC and the active fragments of the early complement components C3b and C4b were increased as shown by a radioimmunoassay (RIA). The neoantigen C3bNEO, which is complex specific because it gets exposed when the C3b is incorporated into an immune complex, was also deposited on the muscle capillaries along with the MAC (26).

Sequentially, the disease begins when antibodies in the circulation activate complement C3, forming C3b and C4b fragments that lead to the formation of C3bNEO and MAC, both of which are deposited in the endomysial microvasculature (see Plate XIII). The MAC deposition on the intramuscular capillaries, through os-

motic lysis of the endothelial cells, leads to necrosis of the capillaries (see Plate XIII), resulting in marked reduction in the number of capillaries per muscle fiber and dilatation of the remaining capillaries in an effort to compensate for the impaired perfusion. Larger intramuscular blood vessels are also affected in the same pattern, leading to muscle fiber destruction, often resembling microinfarcts, and inflammation. The perifascicular atrophy often seen in more chronic stages is a reflection of the endofascicular hypoperfusion that is prominent distally. (These stages are diagrammed in Plate XIV.)

The antibodies that fix complement are probably directed against endothelial cells, as determined by the immunocytochemical localization of the MAC (see Plate XIII) and supported by the presence of circulating anti–endothelial cell antibodies (27), which can be detected by enzyme-linked immunosorbent assay (ELISA) using human umbilical vein endothelial cells as antigen (28). These antibodies are probably pathogenic because they disappear after successful treatment with intravenous immunoglobulin (IVIg) (28). The antigenic target on the endothelial cells and the ability of the patients' IgG to cause endothelial cell destruction are under intense study in our laboratory. Systemic features, with involvement of myocardium, pericardium, lungs, and the gut, suggest that the MAC-mediated microvascular injury may be widespread and the target antigen a ubiquitous component of the endothelium of blood vessels. Consequently, identifying a specific autoantibody and its antigen would be of importance in elucidating the pathogenic mechanisms. The activation of complement by the putative anti–endothelial cell antibodies is believed to be responsible for the induction of cytokines (29), which in turn upregulate the expression of vascular cell adhesion molecule (VCAM)-1 and intercellular adhesion molecule (ICAM)-1 on the endothelial cells (30). These molecules serve as ligands for the integrins very late activation antigen (VLA)-4, leukocyte function–associated antigen (LFA)-1, and Mac-1 expressed on T cells and macrophages, and facilitate their exit through the blood vessel wall to the perimysial and endomysial spaces (as depicted in Plate XIV).

Immunophenotypic analysis of the lymphocytic infiltrates in the muscle biopsy specimens of patients with DM demonstrates that B cells and CD4+ cells are the predominant cells in the perimysial and perivascular regions, supporting a humoral mediated process, as described already (4,31). In the perifascicular areas, however, the infiltrates are mostly CD8+ cells and macrophages and invade major histocompatibility complex (MHC) class I antigen–expressing muscle fibers, a sign of a coexisting T cell–mediated and MHC class I–restricted cytotoxic process. The latter also appears to be of pathogenetic significance because after successful therapy, repeat biopsy fails to demonstrate such abnormalities, as described later.

An autoantibody, called *anti–Mi-2*, directed against a 220-kd nuclear protein found recently in the sera of 20% of patients with DM may shed light in identifying a candidate endothelial cell antigen (31,32). The complementary DNA (cDNA) and protein sequences of the autoantigens recognized by the anti–Mi-2 antibodies have been worked out by immunoscreening cDNA expression libraries and cDNA isolation alignment, followed by sequence analysis by Northern blotting and in situ hybridization techniques (31–33). A major antigen recognized by anti–Mi-2–positive sera from DM patients was found to constitute a 218-kd nuclear protein (218-kd Mi-2), encoded on chromosome 12, that belongs to the SNF2/RAD 54 helicase family. With the recombinant Mi-2 protein, these autoantibodies were detected by an ELISA (32). Whether this antibody is specific for DM and fixes complement causing capillary destruction remains to be determined.

Immunopathology of Polymyositis and Inclusion-Body Myositis

Cytotoxic T Cells, T-Cell Receptors, Macrophages, and NK Cells

In PM and IBM, there is evidence not of microangiopathy and muscle ischemia, as in DM, but of an *antigen-directed cytotoxicity mediated by cytotoxic T cells* (4,5). This conclusion is supported by the presence of CD8+ cells (see Plate XI), which along with macrophages initially surround healthy, but MHC class I–expressing, nonnecrotic muscle fibers (see Plate XI) that eventually invade and destroy.

Quantification of the endomysial infiltrates demonstrates that the majority consist of CD8+ cells followed by macrophages and CD4+ cells. The distribution of cells with the phenotypic markers noted above are proportionally equal in PM and IBM and identical in PM associated with human immunodeficiency virus (HIV) and human T-cell lymphotropic virus type I (HTLV-I) infection (34,35). These cells are activated as evidenced by their expression of ICAM-1 and MHC class I and II antigens. Further, there is convincing evidence of T cell–mediated cytotoxicity directed against muscle fibers based on the following:

1. Cell lines established from muscle biopsy samples from PM patients exert cytotoxicity to their autologous myotubules in vitro (36).
2. As shown by immunoelectron microscopy, CD8+ cells and macrophages send spikelike processes into nonnecrotic muscle fibers, which traverse the basal lamina and focally displace or compress the muscle fibers (37). This also can be seen by light microscopy in our immunocytochemical preparations where the trafficking of the CD8+ cells toward the muscle membrane can be traced and CD8+ spikes penetrating the plasmalemma can be visualized (38). The macrophages have cytotoxic rather than phagocytic properties because they contain only a few heterophagic vacuoles (4,37) and they are activated expressing complement and Fc receptors for IgG (39).
3. Some of the cytotoxic autoinvasive CD8+ T cells express cytotoxic granules containing perforin and granzyme, as shown by immunocytochemistry and polymerase chain reaction (PCR) (40). These enzymes in vitro have been shown to be proteolytic to many muscle proteins such as dystrophin and myosin. Although it has been traditionally thought that CD8+ T cells via their released cytotoxic granules induce killing of their targets through apoptosis, we have not been able to demonstrate apoptosis in the muscle fibers of PM patients, even in those infected with HIV (41). The fleeting nature of apoptosis might have been responsible for the inability to detect this form of cell death in vivo.
4. The γ/δ T cells, another subset of cytotoxic T cells, mediated the cytotoxicity in one patient with PM and appeared to recognize heat shock protein expressed intensely on the surface or the interior of nonnecrotic muscle fibers (42). A restricted profile of γ/δ T-cell receptor (TCR) gene expression was also demonstrated in this thoroughly studied patient (43). To investigate whether γ/δ T cells play a role in additional cases of PM as well as in DM and sporadic IBM, we utilized PCR to study TCR gene expression in 45 muscle biopsy samples from such patients. In 9 of 45 muscle specimens from clinically heterogeneous patients, γ/δ TCR gene was amplified (44). Analysis of the junctional sequences of Vγ3 and Vδ1 transcripts, however, failed to reveal amino acid sequence similarities within the Vγ-NDγ-N-γδ junctional domains. In patients with PM, DM, or IBM therefore, a primary cytotoxic role for the γ/δ T cells is, overall, unlikely. The few scattered γ/δ T cells found within the endomysial infiltrates of PM patients may be secondary, probably related to a nonspecific inflammatory response.
5. TCR analysis revealed that in PM there is clonal expansion of T cells with restricted usage of the TCR variable region of certain TCR gene families, notably Vα1, Vβ15, and Vβ6, indicating that in PM the T-cell response is driven by a common antigen (45,46). The combination of inverse PCR with double immunocytochemistry to analyze the TCR repertoire expressed by autoinvasive and nonautoinvasive T cells showed that in PM certain TCR Vβ families are overexpressed among the CD8+ autoinvasive T cells. Most importantly, there appears to be a dissociation of TCR usage between the nonautoinvasive and the autoinvasive T cells. Further, the autoinvasive T cells are clonally expanded expressing a predominance of certain Vβ elements in different patients (47). In contrast, in the muscle of IBM patients certain Vβ3 and Vβ6 families are predominantly overexpressed among the infiltrating T cells (46). Sequence analysis of Vβ clonotypes from the endomysial infiltrates demonstrated heterogeneity in the nucleotide sequence at the joining region of the TCR, suggesting that in IBM the T-cell response is not driven by a muscle-specific antigen. Because expansion of Vβ families without nucleotide restriction in their CD3 region suggests superantigenic stimulation, we hypothesized that a superantigen (virus, bacterial toxin) may be involved in triggering the inflammatory response in IBM patients (46). A superantigen-driven T-cell response would

suggest that the T-cell infiltrates are directed nonspecifically to the muscle, a notion that may provide clues as to resistance of the IBM to immunotherapies.

6. The CD45RO+ memory T cells predominate in the endomysial or perivascular sites in PM, DM, and IBM, exceeding the numbers in normal blood. Such a finding implies that in these diseases there exist memory cells primed to a putative muscle-specific target antigen (48).

7. In addition to CD8+ T cells and γ/δ T cells, NK cells and macrophages also participate in the myocytoxicity. In two patients with sporadic IBM and immunodeficiency, NK cells, defined as CD57+, CD56+, CD3-, CD8-, CD68- cells, accounted for up to 10% of the total infiltrating cells (49). These cells were positive for ICAM-1 and invaded MHC class I–negative muscle fibers. Because NK cell–mediated cytotoxicity is MHC class I independent, the finding provided convincing evidence that in these patients the autoinvasive NK cells may have been cytotoxic to the muscle fiber by using ICAM-1 as their ligand. The macrophages are also activated, as noted already, and when they invade nonnecrotic muscle fibers they have fewer heterophagic vacuoles, which are acid phosphatase negative (4,39).

8. In vivo kinetic studies of indium-labeled autologous lymphocytes in PM patients showed increased uptake in the major muscle groups when compared with control tissues or with other nonmuscle tissues such as liver, lung, or spleen (8). The lymphocyte trafficking in the muscle is also proportional to the degree of inflammation seen in concurrently obtained muscle biopsy specimens (1,8), supporting the view that circulating sensitized lymphocytes are directed abnormally and specifically to muscle, in proportion to disease activity.

9. The cytotoxicity mediated by the CD8+ cells appears to be antigen specific because, in addition to the clonal expansion of certain TCR gene families described above, the T cells invade muscle fibers expressing MHC class I antigen, a prerequisite for antigen recognition by the CD8+ cells. MHC class I antigen is not present on normal muscle fibers but is ubiquitously expressed on the sarcolemma of the muscle fibers in patients with PM or IBM (38,50). MHC class I expression is probably upregulated by cytokines secreted by activated T cells, macrophages, or viruses (in a setting of a viral infection). Although it is clear that in PM the CD8+ cell–mediated cytotoxicity is MHC class I antigen restricted, the antigenic peptides bound by MHC class I for presentation to the CD8+ cells are still unknown. It is assumed that such antigens could be either endogenous sarcolemmal or cytoplasmic self-proteins synthesized within the muscle fiber, or endogenous viral peptides (4). Because PCR has failed to amplify viruses within the muscle fibers not only in patients with a putative viral infection (38,51,52) but also in patients with classic PM associated with HIV-1 or HTLV-I infection (as discussed later), it is highly unlikely that this antigen represents peptides from any of the examined viruses. A diagram demonstrating the events leading to PM is shown in Plate XV.

Cytokines and Adhesion Molecules

The T cell–derived cytokines (interleukin (IL)-2, IL-4, IL-5, and interferon (IFN)-γ), the macrophage-derived cytokines (IL-1, IL-6, and tumor necrosis factor (TNF)-α), and cytokines that are either T cell or macrophage derived such as granulocyte-macrophage colony-stimulating factor (GM-CSF) and transforming growth factor (TGF)-β1 and -β2 have been explored in the tissues of patients with PM, DM ,and IBM using the reverse transcriptase-PCR method. In one study (29), among the proinflammatory cytokines, the messenger RNA (mRNA) of IL-4 was specifically, consistently, and strongly expressed in patients with PM but not in those with DM or IBM. In contrast, TNF-α mRNA was variably expressed, while GM-CSF was strongly expressed in most patients with PM, DM, or IBM but not in control subjects. Further, TGF-β1 and -β2 were strongly expressed in all patients including control patients with Duchenne's muscular dystrophy. The strong expression of the mRNA of IL-4, a Th2 cell–derived cytokine, in patients with active PM was in contrast to its weak expression in DM where endomysial B cells are thought to play a role in autoantibody production. An upregulation of IL-1α and -1β, IL-2, TNF-α, IL-4, and IFN-γ in the muscle fibers close to the sites of inflammatory exudates has been also suggested in PM (53,54). In our experience using PCR, the mRNA of the proinflammatory cytokines was variably expressed without a consistent pattern or differentiation between patients with PM, DM, or IBM, including those whose conditions were due to HIV infection. The most consistently found cytokines were TGF-β and GM-CSF. Such a variable expression of cytokines in inflammatory myopathies may represent a fleeting and elusive phenomenon. As in experimental systems, cytokines may be expressed transiently, and perhaps acutely, very early in the disease process, not allowing their capture with the methods used in the studied specimens. In this scenario, cytokines may play a role in triggering the immune response but not in sustaining the inflammatory process. Using the RNA-PCR method, IL-2 receptor expression was also seen in 92% of PM patients (54), suggesting ongoing T-cell and macrophage activation, as also seen by immunocytochemistry (55). The noted upregulation of TGF-β (27), a "good cytokine," may be responsible for downregulating the expression of the proinflammatory cytokines whose mRNA is weakly present, thereby preventing a more destructive process. (However, this hypothesis also may be weak; we could not find a correlation between TGF-β expression and disease activity.) In general, when an inflammatory reaction in the muscle has begun, the inflammation may be sustained through mechanisms unrelated to the continuous release of T cell–derived cytokines. However, the site of autosensitization is still unknown and it is unclear whether it takes place in the circulation or the muscle.

ICAM-1 and VCAM are also upregulated on the endothelial cells, fibroblasts, and infiltrating T cells in patients with PM, DM, or IBM (54) and may facilitate the exit of activated T cells from the circulation (as depicted in Plate XIV). In addition, varying amounts of VLA-4, SLe^x, and LFA-1α and -1β, the respective ligands for VCAM-1, extracellular leukocyte adhesion molecule (ELAM)-1, and ICAM-1, have been consistently found in all three types of inflammatory myopathies (54,56).

Association with Viral Infections

The following viruses have been associated directly or indirectly with the cause of inflammatory myopathies:

Coxsackieviruses

These viruses can cause chronic and acute myositis with convincing histologic features in mice inoculated with various coxsackievirus strains (57–59). Muscle cultures, especially immature myotubes, can be also infected with coxsackieviruses. In humans, however, the role of coxsackieviruses in the cause of PM has been indirect and, up to now, unconvincing (57,58). A possible molecular mimicry phenomenon has been proposed because of structural homology between Jo-1, a histidyl-transfer RNA synthetase (mentioned earlier), and the genomic RNA of an animal picornavirus, the encephalomyocarditis virus. This association was strengthened when in situ hybridization revealed the presence of enteroviral RNA within the muscle fibers of specimens from patients with myositis (60). However, our very sensitive PCR studies have repeatedly failed to confirm the presence of enteroviruses in these patients' muscle biopsy specimens (51,52). Therefore, it is unlikely, although not impossible, that replication of enteroviruses takes place within the muscles of patients with chronic inflammatory myopathies.

Influenza Virus

These orthomyxoviruses have been connected with inflammatory myopathy because of reports that myalgia, CK elevation, or rhabdomyolysis can follow infection with influenza (59). Further, the influenza B/Lee strain can infect the human rhabdomyosarcoma cell lines. Apart from these circumstantial observations, however, there has not been any clear evidence connecting these viruses with the cause of sporadic PM in humans.

Other Viruses

Paramyxoviruses (mumps) were initially implicated in the cause of IBM because the 15- to 20-nm microtubular filaments seen in IBM muscle specimens resembled viral nucleocapsids (61). A search by PCR conducted by two different laboratories revealed no mumps virus (51,62). PCR has also been used to search for the genome from other viruses in the muscles of patients with inflammatory myopathies. Specifically, our search in the RNA extracted from muscle specimens of 44 patients revealed no encephalomyocarditis virus, adenovirus, HIV, HTLV-I, or HTLV-II (51).

By in situ hybridization and PCR, cytomegalovirus (CMV) and Epstein-Barr virus (EBV) were investigated as a cause of the rapidly progressive interstitial pneumonitis associated with PM and DM (63). Although CMV and EBV were amplified from PM and DM patients, these viruses were also amplified from lung specimens of other disease control subjects, including patients with collagen vascular diseases. The theoretical implication of this finding is that immunosuppression may increase the pathogenic potential of these viruses.

Postviral Myositis

This rare condition occurs in children or adults (57–59). It is characterized by an acute onset of mild to severe muscle weakness with or without myoglobinuria and the elevated CK level that follows a viral infection. Although patients with mild weakness may recover spontaneously or respond to immunosuppressive drugs, patients with severe weakness often times respond poorly, or they are left with an incapacitating permanent disability. The viruses responsible for these cases are unknown and no indirect or direct association with any infectious agent has been identified. Further, no virus has been isolated from these patients' muscle and the immunopathology triggered by the responsible agent has not been characterized.

Retroviruses

The first evidence that retroviruses might be associated with inflammatory myopathy was in monkeys infected with the simian immunodeficiency virus (64,65). Almost the same year the first cases of HIV-associated myositis were reported (66). About 3 years later, the association of HTLV-I with myositis became apparent (67). Further, transgenic mice expressing a human foamy retrovirus gene developed a myopathy and the viral genome was detected in the muscle (68). Because PM occurs during an infection with at least four different retroviruses, it appears that retroviruses are, at the moment, the most reasonable candidates among viruses connected with the cause of PM, DM, and IBM.

HIV Myositis. In HIV-positive patients, an inflammatory myopathy (HIV PM) can occur either as an isolated clinical phenomenon, being the first clinical indication of HIV infection, or concurrently with other manifestations of AIDS (66,69–72). HIV seroconversion can also coincide with myoglobulinuria and acute myalgia, suggesting that myotropism for HIV may be symptomatic early in the infection.

Human T-Cell Lymphotropic Virus (HTLV-I) Myositis. HTLV-I can cause not only a myeloneuropathy—referred to as *tropical spastic paraparesis* (TSP)—but also PM, which may coexist with TSP or may be the only clinical manifestation of HTLV-I infection (67,70–73). Of interest, IBM can also occur with HIV or HTLV-I infection (74).

Using in situ hybridization, PCR, immunocytochemistry, and electron microscopy, we could not detect viral antigens within the muscle fibers of patients with HIV PM, HTLV-I PM, or HIV or HTLV IBM, but did detect them only in occasional endomysial macrophages (34,35,70–74). These observations led us to conclude that in HIV and HTLV-I PM and IBM, there is no evidence of persistent infection of the muscle fiber with the virus and that viral replication does not take place within the human muscle. The predominant endomysial cells in HIV and HTLV-1 PM and IBM are CD8+, non-viral-specific, cytotoxic T cells, which along with macrophages invade or surround MHC class I antigen–expressing nonnecrotic muscle fibers. Because this pattern is similar to the one described earlier for retroviral-negative PM and IBM, we proposed that a T cell–mediated and MHC class I–restricted cytotoxic process is a common pathogenetic mechanism in PM, IBM, and HIV or HTLV-I PM and IBM. The various cytokines or toxic lymphokines released by the retroviral-infected endomysial inflammatory cells may contribute to the development of PM by altering the antigenic expression of normal muscle fibers, generating a secondary autoimmune response. However, the mRNA of the cytokine profile in HIV-positive patients with PM did not differ from that seen in HIV-negative patients, except for the IFN-γ, which appeared to be more overexpressed (Dalakas MC, et al, unpublished observations).

Treatment

Because the specific target antigens in DM, PM, and IBM are unknown, the immunosuppressive therapies do not selectively target the autoreactive T cells or the complement-mediated process on the intramuscular blood vessels. Instead, they induce a nonselective immunosuppression or immunomodulation. Further, many of these therapies are empirical, and mostly uncontrolled.

The goal of therapy in inflammatory myopathies is to improve the function in activities of daily living as the result of improvement in muscle strength. Although when the strength improves, the serum CK falls concurrently, the reverse is not always true because most of the immunosuppressive therapies can result in a decrease in serum muscle enzyme levels without necessarily improving muscle strength. Unfortunately, this has been misinterpreted as "chemical improvement," and has formed the basis for the common habit of "chasing" or "treating" the CK level instead of the muscle weakness, a practice that has led to prolonged use of unnecessary immunosuppressive drugs and erroneous assessment of their efficacy. The prudence of discontinuing these drugs when after an adequate trial they have only led to a reduction in CK and not to an objective improvement in muscle strength has been repeatedly emphasized (1–3,75–78). The agents and therapies discussed in subsequent sections are used in the treatment of PM and DM.

Corticosteroids

Prednisone is the first-line drug of this *empirical* treatment. Its action is unclear but it may exert a beneficial effect by inhibiting the recruitment and migration of lymphocytes to the areas of muscle inflammation and interfering with the production of lymphokines. Its effect on the lymphokine IL-1 may be important because IL-1 is myotoxic (79) and it is secreted by the activated macrophages that invade the muscle fibers. Steroid-induced suppression of ICAM-1 may also be relevant because downregulation of ICAM-1 can prevent the trafficking of lymphocytes across the endothelial cell wall toward the muscle fibers (see Plates XIV and XV).

Because the effectiveness and relative safety of prednisone therapy will determine the future need for stronger immunosuppressive drugs, our preference has been to start with high-dose prednisone, *80 to 100* mg/day, early in the disease. After an initial period of 3 to 4 weeks, the prednisone dose is tapered over a 10-week period to 80- to 100-mg *single daily doses*, to *alternate-day* doses by gradually reducing an alternate "off day" dose by 10 mg/wk, or faster if necessitated by side effects, though this carries a greater risk of breakthrough of disease. If there is evidence of efficacy, and there are no serious side effects, the dosage is reduced gradually by 5 to 10 mg every 3 to 4 weeks until the lowest possible dose that controls the disease is reached. If by the time the dosage has been reduced to 80 to 100 mg every other day (approximately 14 weeks after initiating therapy), there is no objective benefit (defined as increased muscle strength), the patient may be considered unresponsive to prednisone and tapering is accelerated while the next-in-line immunosuppressive drug is started (75–79).

Immunosuppressive Agents

Although almost all the patients with bone fide PM or DM respond to steroids to *some degree and for some period of time*, a number of them fail to respond or become steroid resistant. The decision to start an immunosuppressive drug in PM or DM patients is based on the following factors: a) There is a need for its "steroid-sparing" effect, when in spite of steroid responsiveness the patient has developed significant complications; b) attempts to lower a high steroid dosage have repeatedly resulted in a new relapse; c) an adequate dose of prednisone for at least a 2- to 3-month period has been ineffective; and d) there is rapidly progressive disease with evolving severe weakness and respiratory failure. The preference for selecting the next-in-line immunosuppressive therapy is, however, empirical. The choice is usually based on our own prejudices, our personal experience with each drug, and our own assessment of the relative efficacy-safety ratio. The following immunosuppressive agents are then used.

Azathioprine

Azathioprine is a derivative of 6-mercaptopurine and is given orally. Although lower doses (1.5–2.0 mg/kg) are commonly used, we prefer higher doses, up to 3 mg/kg, for effective immunosuppression. This drug is well tolerated, has fewer side effects, and empirically appears to be as effective for long-term therapy as the other drugs.

Methotrexate

Methotrexate is an antagonist of folate metabolism. Although its superiority to azathioprine has not been established, it has a faster action. It can be given intravenously over 20 to 60 minutes at weekly doses of 0.4 mg/kg up to 0.8 mg/kg with sufficient fluids, or orally starting at 7.5 mg weekly for the first 3 weeks (given in a total of three doses, 2.5 mg every 12 hours), increasing it gradually by 2.5 mg/wk up to a total of 25 mg weekly. A relevant side effect is *methotrexate-induced pneumonitis,* which can be difficult to distinguish from the interstitial lung disease of the primary myopathy, often associated with Jo-1 antibodies, as described already.

Cyclophosphamide

This alkylating agent is given intravenously or orally, at doses of 2.0 to 2.5 mg/kg, usually 50 mg orally three times a day. Cyclophosphamide has been ineffective in our hands (80) in spite of occasional promising results reported by others (81).

Chlorambucil

Chlorambucil is an antimetabolite that has been tried in some patients, with variable results (82).

Cyclosporine

Although the toxicity of cyclosporine can now be monitored by measuring optimal trough serum levels (which vary between 100 and 250 ng/mL), its effectiveness in PM and DM is uncertain. A report that low doses of cyclosporine could be of benefit in children with DM needs confirmation (83). The advantage of cyclosporine is that it acts faster than azathioprine and methotrexate and the results (positive or negative) may be apparent early (84).

Other Treatments

Plasmapheresis was not helpful in a double-blind, placebo-controlled study that we conducted (85).

Total lymphoid irradiation has been helpful in rare patients and may have long-lasting benefit (86). The long-term side effects of this treatment, however, should be seriously considered before deciding on this experimental approach. Total lymphoid irradiation has been ineffective in IBM (87).

IVIg is a promising, but very expensive therapy. In uncontrolled studies, IVIg was reported to be effective (88–90). In the first double-blind study conducted for DM, we demonstrated that IVIg is effective in patients with refractory DM. Not only the strength improves but also the underlying immunopathology may resolve (91). The improvement begins after the first IVIg infu-

sion but it is clearly evident by the second monthly infusion. The benefit is short-lived (not more than 8 weeks), requiring repeated infusions every 6 to 8 weeks to maintain improvement.

The mechanism of action of IVIg in DM may be inhibition of the deposition of activated complement fragment on the capillaries (26), by suppressing cytokines, especially ICAM-1, or by saturating Fc receptors and interfering with the action of macrophages (91).

A controlled double-blind study for PM is still underway, although the drug has been effective in up to 80% of the patients in uncontrolled studies.

IVIg also exerted some benefit in up to 30% of patients with IBM in a controlled double-blind study (92,93). Although the improvement was not dramatic, it made a difference to these patients' life styles.

Treatment Recommendation

Until further control drug trials are completed, the following step-by-step empirical approach for the treatment of PM, DM, or IBM is suggested:

- Step 1: High-dose prednisone.
- Step 2: If the need for "steroid-sparing" effect arises, try azathioprine or methotrexate.
- Step 3: If step 2 fails, try high-dose IVIg.
- Step 4: If step 3 fails, consider a trial, with guarded optimism, of one of the following agents, chosen according to the patient's age, degree of disability, tolerance, and general health, and experience with the drug: cyclosporine, chlorambucil, or cyclophosphamide.

References

1. Dalakas MC. Polymyositis, dermatomyositis, and inclusion-body myositis. *N Engl J Med* 1991;325:1487–1498.
2. Dalakas MC. Inflammatory myopathies: pathogenesis and treatment. *Clin Neuropharmacology* 1992;5:327–351.
3. Dalakas MC, ed. *Polymyositis and dermatomyositis.* Boston: Butterworths, 1988.
4. Engel AG, Hohlfeld R, Banker BQ. The polymyositis and dermatomyositis syndrome. In: Engel AG, Franzini-Armstrong C, eds. *Myology.* New York: McGraw-Hill, 1994:1335–1383.
5. Hohlfeld R, Goebels N, Engel AG. Cellular mechanisms in inflammatory myopathies. *Baillieres Clin Neurol* 1993;2:617–636.
6. Karpati G, Carpenter S. Pathology of the inflammatory myopathies. *Baillieres Clin Neurol* 1993;2:527–556.
7. Dalakas MC. Inflammatory myopathies. *Curr Opin Neurol Neurosurg* 1990; 3:689–696.
8. Plotz PH, Dalakas M, Leff RL, et al. Current concepts in the idiopathic inflammatory myopathies: polymyositis, dermatomyositis and related disorders. *Ann Intern Med* 1989;111:143–157.
9. Otero C, Illa I, Dalakas MC. Is there dermatomyositis (DM) without myositis? *Neurology* 1992;42:388.
10. Sekul EA, Dalakas MC. Inclusion body myositis: new concepts. *Semin Neurol* 1993;13:256–263.
11. Luciano CA, Dalakas MC. A macro-EMG study in inclusion-body myositis: no evidence for a neurogenic component. *Neurology* 1997;48:29–33.

12. Sivakumar K, Dalakas MC. The spectrum of familial inclusion body myopathies in 13 families and description of a quadriceps sparing phenotype in non-Iranian Jews. *Neurology* 1996;47:977–984.

13. Clawson K, Oddis CV. Adult respiratory distress syndrome in polymyositis patients with the anti-Jo-I antibody. *Arthritis Rheum* 1995;38:1519–1523.

14. Schwarz MI, Sutarik JM, Nick JA, et al. Pulmonary capillaritis and diffuse alveolar hemorrhage: a primary manifestation of polymyositis. *Am J Respir Crit Care Med* 1995;151:2037–2040.

15. Dalakas MC. Calcifications in dermatomyositis. *N Engl J Med* 1995;333:978.

16. Askanas V, Serdaroglu P, Engel WK, Alvarez RB. Immunocytochemical localization of ubiquitin in inclusion body myositis allows its light-microscopic distinction from polymyositis. *Neurology* 1992;42:460–461.

17. Mendell JR, Sahenk Z, Gales T, Paul L. Amyloid filaments in inclusion body myositis. *Arch Neurol* 1991;48:1229–1234.

18. Askanas V, Engel WK, Alvarez RB, Glenner GG. β-Amyloid protein immunoreactivity in muscle of patients with inclusion-body myositis. *Lancet* 1992;339:560–561.

19. Santorelli FM, Sciacco M, Tanji K, et al. Multiple mitochondrial DNA deletions in sporadic inclusion body myositis: a study of 56 patients. *Ann Neurol* 1996;39:789–795.

20. Targoff IN. Immune mechanisms of myositis. *Curr Opin Rheumatol* 1990;2:882–888.

21. Banker BQ. Dermatomyositis of childhood. Ultrastructural alterations of muscle and intramuscular blood vessels. *J Neuropathol Exp Neurol* 1975;35:46–75.

22. Jerusalem F, Rakusa M, Engel AG, MacDonald RD. Morphometric analysis of skeletal muscle capillary ultrastructure in inflammatory myopathies. *J Neurol Sci* 1974;23:391–401.

23. Carpenter S, Karpati G, Rothman S, Walters G. The childhood type of dermatomyositis. *Neurology* 1976;26:952–962.

24. Whitaker J.N, Engel WK. Vascular deposits of immunoglobulin and complement in idiopathic inflammatory myopathy. *N Engl J Med* 1972;286:333–338.

25. Emslie-Smith AM, Engel AG. Microvascular changes in early and advanced dermatomyositis: a quantitative study. *Ann Neurol* 1990;27:343–356.

26. Basta M, Dalakas MC. High-dose intravenous immunoglobulin exerts its beneficial effect in patients with dermatomyositis by blocking endomysial deposition of activated complement fragments. *J Clin Invest* 1994;94:1729–1735.

27. Cervera R, Ramires G, Fernandez-Sola J, et al. Antibodies to endothelial cells in dermatomyositis: association with interstitial lung diseases. *BMJ* 1991;302:880–882.

28. Stein DP, Jordan SC, Toyoda M, et al. Anti-endothelial cell antibodies (AECA) in dermatomyositis (DM). *Neurology* 1993;43:356.

29. Lundberg I, Brengman JM, Engel AG. Analysis of cytokine expression in muscle in inflammatory myopathies, Duchenne's dystrophy and non-weak controls. *J. Neuroimmunol* 1995;63:9–16.

30. Stein DP, Dalakas MC. Intercellular adhesion molecule-1 expression is upregulated in patients with dermatomyositis (DM). *Ann Neurol* 1993;34:268.

31. Seelig HP, Moosbrugger I, Ehrfeld H, et al. The major dermatomyositis-specific Mi-2 autoantigen is a presumed helicase involved in transcriptional activation. *Arthritis Rheum* 1995;38:1389–1399.

32. Ge Q, Nilasena DS, O'Brien CA, et al. Molecular analysis of a major antigenic region of the 240-kD protein of Mi-

2 autoantigen. *J Clin Invest* 1995;96:1730–1737.

33. Dalakas MC, Sivakumar K. On the immunopathologic and inflammatory differences between polymyositis, inclusion body myositis and dermatomyositis. *Curr Opin Neurol Neurosurg* 1996;9:235–239.

34. Illa I, Nath A, Dalakas MC. Immunocytochemical and virological characteristics of HIV-associated inflammatory myopathies: similarities with seronegative polymyositis. *Ann Neurol* 1991;29:474–481.

35. Leon-Monzon M, Illa I, Dalakas MC. Polymyositis in patients infected with HTLV-I: the role of the virus in the cause of the disease. *Ann Neurol* 1994;36:643–649.

36. Hohlfeld R, Engel AG. Coculture with autologous myotubes of cytotoxic T cells isolated from muscle in inflammatory myopathies. *Ann Neurol* 1991;29:498–507.

37. Arahata K, Engel AG. Monoclonal antibody analysis of mononuclear cells in myopathies. III. Immunoelectron microscopy aspects of cell-mediated muscle fiber injury. *Ann Neurol* 1986;19:112–125.

38. Dalakas MC. Immunopathogenesis of inflammatory myopathies. *Ann Neurol* 1995;37:74–86.

39. Drosos AA, Dalakas MC. Expression of activation markers on endomysial macrophages in patients with inflammatory myopathies. *Arthritis Rheum* 1993;36:S256.

40. Goebels N, Michaelis D, Engelhardt M, et al. Differential expression of perforin in muscle-inflammatory T cells in polymyositis and dermatomyositis. *J Clin Invest* 1996;97:2905–2910.

41. Schneider C, Gold R, Dalakas MC, et al. MHC class I-mediated cytotoxicity does not induce apoptosis in muscle fibers nor in inflammatory T cells: studies in patients with polymyositis, dermatomyositis and inclusion body myositis. *J Neuropathol Exp Neurol* 1996;55:1205–1209.

42. Hohlfeld R, Engel AG, Kunio Li, Harper MC. Polymyositis mediated by T lymphocytes that express the gamma/delta receptor. *N Engl J Med* 1991;324:877–881.

43. Puschke G, Ruegg D, Hohlfeld R, Engel AG. Autoaggressive myocytotoxic T-lymphocytes expressing an unusual gamma delta T cell receptor. *J Exp Med* 1992;176:1785–1789.

44. O'Hanlon TP, Messersmith WA, Dalakas MC, et al. Gamma delta T cell receptor gene expression by muscle-infiltrating lymphocytes in the idiopathic inflammatory myopathies. *Clin Exp Immunol* 1995;100:519–528.

45. Mantegazza R, Andreette F, Bemasconi P, et al. Analysis of T cell receptor repertoire of muscle-infiltrating T lymphocytes in polymyositis. *J Clin Invest* 1993;91:2880–2886.

46. O'Hanlon TP, Dalakas MC, Plotz PH, Miller FW. The αβ T cell receptor repertoire in inclusion body myositis: diverse patterns of gene expression by muscle infiltrating lymphocytes. *J Autoimmun* 1994;7:321–333.

47. Bender A, Ernst N, Iglesias A, et al. T cell receptor in polymyositis: clonal expansion of autoaggressive CD8+ T cells. *J Exp Med* 1995;181:1863–1868.

48. De Bleecker JL, Engel AG. Immunocytochemical study of CD45 T cell isoforms in inflammatory myopathies. *Am J Pathol* 1995;146:1178–1187.

49. Dalakas MC, Illa I. Common variable immunodeficiency and inclusion body myositis: a distinct myopathy mediated by natural killer cells. *Ann Neurol* 1995;37:806–810.

50. Karpati G, Pouliot Y, Carpenter S. Expression of immunoreactive major histocompatibility complex products in human skeletal muscles. *Ann Neurol* 1988;23:64–72.

51. Leff RL, Love LA, Miller FW, et al. Viruses in the idiopathic inflammatory myopathies: absence of candidate viral genomes in muscle. *Lancet* 1992;339:1192–1195.

52. Leon-Monzon M, Dalakas MC. Absence of persistent in-

fection with enteroviruses in muscles of patients with inflammatory myopathies. *Ann Neurol* 1992;32:219–222.

53. Tews DS, Goebel HH. Cytokine expression profiles in idiopathic inflammatory myopathies. *J Neuropathol Exp Neurol* 1996;55:342–347.

54. Tews DS, Goebel HH. Expression of cell adhesion molecules in inflammatory myopathies. *J Neuroimmunol* 1995;59:185–194.

55. Drosos AA, Dalakas MC. Identification of macrophages in the muscle biopsy preparations: a comparative study using specific monoclonal antimacrophage antibodies. *Muscle Nerve* 1995;18:242–244.

56. De Bleecker JL, Engel AG. Expression of cell adhesion molecules in inflammatory myopathies and Duchenne dystrophy. *J Neuropathol Exp Neurol* 1994;53:369–376.

57. Dalakas MC. Infection of human muscle, nerve and motor neurons with polioviruses and other enteroviruses. In: Rotbard HA, ed. *Human enteroviral infections.* Washington, DC: American Society for Microbiology (ASM) Press, 1995:387–398.

58. Dalakas MC. Viral and retroviral myositis. In: Gilman S, Goldstein GW, Waxman SG, eds. *Neurobase.* La Jolla, CA: Arbor Publishing, 1995.

59. Hays AP, Gamboa ET. Acute viral myositis. In: Engel AG, Franzini-Armstong C, eds. *Myology.* NewYork: McGraw-Hill, 1994:1399–1418.

60. Yousef GE, Isenberg DA, Mowbray JF. Detection of enterovirus specific RNA sequences in muscle biopsy specimens from patients with adult onset myositis. *Ann Rheum Dis* 1990;49:310–315.

61. Chou SM. Inclusion body myositis: a chronic persistent mumps myositis. *Hum Pathol* 1986;17:765–777.

62. Nishino H, Engel AG, Rima BK. Inclusion body myositis: the mumps virus hypothesis. *Ann Neurol* 1989;25:260–264.

63. Hashimoto Y, Nawata Y, Kurasawa K, et al. Investigation of EB virus and cytomegalovirus in rapidly progressive interstitial pneumonitis in polymyositis/dermatomyositis by in situ hybridization and polymerase chain reaction. *Clin Immunol Immunopathol* 1995;77:298–306.

64. Dalakas MC, London WT, Gravell M, Sever JL. Polymyositis in an immunodeficiency disease in monkeys induced by a type D retrovirus. *Neurology* 1986;36:569–572.

65. Dalakas MC, Gravell M, London WT, et al. Morphological changes of an inflammatory myopathy in rhesus monkeys with simian acquired immunodeficiency syndrome (SAIDS). *Proc Soc Exp Biol Med* 1987;185:368–376.

66. Dalakas MC, Pezeshkpour GH, Gravell M, Sever JL. Polymyositis in patients with AIDS. *JAMA* 1986; 256:2381–2383.

67. Morgan OStC, Rodgers-Johnson P, Mora C, Char G. HTLV-I and polymyositis in Jamaica. *Lancet* 1989;2: 1184–1187.

68. Bothe K, Aguzzi A, Lassman H, et al. Progressive encephalopathy and myopathy in transgenic mice expressing human foamy virus gene. *Science* 1991;253:555–558.

69. Dalakas MC, Pezeshkpour GH. Neuromuscular diseases associated with human immunodeficiency virus infection. *Ann Neurol* 1988;23:38–48.

70. Dalakas MC. Retroviruses and inflammatory myopathies in humans and primates. *Baillieres Clin Neurol* 1993;2: 659–691.

71. Dalakas MC, Illa I, Leon-Monzon M. Retroviral related neuromuscular disorders. In: Hohlfeld R, ed. *Immunology of neuromuscular diseases.* Lancaster, UK: Kluwer Academic, 1994:255–288.

72. Dalakas MC. Retroviral myopathies. In: Engel AG,

Franzini-Armstrong C, eds. *Myology.* Vol. II. NewYork: McGraw-Hill, 1994:1419–1437.

73. Wiley CA, Nerenberg M, Cros D, Soto-Aguilar MC. HTLV-I polymyositis in a patient also infected with the human immunodeficiency virus. *N Engl J Med* 1989;320:992–995.

74. Cupler EJ, Leon-Monzon M, Miller J, et al. Inclusion body myositis in HIV-I and HTLV-I infected patients. *Brain* 1996;119:1887–1893.

75. Dalakas MC. Treatment of polymyositis and dermatomyositis. *Curr Opin Rheumatol* 1989;1:443–449.

76. Dalakas MC. How to diagnose and treat the inflammatory myopathies. *Semin Neurol* 1994;14:137–145.

77. Dalakas MC. Current treatment of the inflammatory myopathies. *Curr Opin Rheumatol* 1994;6;595–601.

78. Dalakas MC. Inflammatory myopathies: In: Rowland LP, DiMauro S, eds. *Handbook of clinical neurology.* Vol. 18 (62). *Myopathies.* Amsterdam: Elsevier Science, 1992: 369–390.

79. Leon-Monzon M, Dalakas MC. Interleukin-1 (IL-1) is toxic to human muscle. *Neurology* 1994;44(S):132.

80. Cronin ME, Miller FW, Hicks JE, et al. The failure of intravenous cyclophosphamide therapy in refractory idiopathic inflammatory myopathy. *J Rheumatol* 1989;16: 1225–1228.

81. Bombardieri S, Hughes GRV, Neri R, et al. Cyclophosphamide in severe polymyositis. *Lancet* 1989;1:1138–1139.

82. Sinoway TA, Callen JP. Chlorambucil: an effective corticosteroid-sparing agent for patients with recalcitrant dermatomyositis. *Arthritis Rheum* 1993;36:319–324.

83. Heckmatt J, Hasson N, Saunders C, et al. Cyclosporin in juvenile dermatomyositis. *Lancet* 1989;1:1063–1066.

84. Grau JM, Herrero C, Casademont J, et al. Cyclosporine A as first choice for dermatomyositis. *J Rheumatol* 1994;21:381–382.

85. Miller FW, Leitman SF, Cronin ME, et al. A randomized double-blind controlled trial of plasma exchange and leukapheresis in patients with polymyositis/dermatomyositis. *N Engl J Med* 1992;326:1380–1384.

86. Dalakas MC, Engel WK. Total body irradiation in the treatment of intractable polymyositis/dermatomyositis. In: Dalakas MC, ed. *Polymyositis/dermatomyositis.* Boston: Butterworths 1988:281–291.

87. Kelly JJ Jr, Madoc-Jones H, Adelman LS, et al. Total body irradiation not effective in inclusion body myositis. *Neurology* 1986;36:1264–1266.

88. Cherin P, Herson S, Wechsler B, et al. Efficacy of intravenous immunoglobulin therapy in chronic refractory polymyositis and dermatomyositis. An open study with 20 adult patients. *Am J Med* 1991;91:162–168.

89. Lang B, Laxer RM, Murphy G, et al. Treatment of dermatomyositis with intravenous immunoglobulin. *Am J Med* 1991;91:169–172.

90. Jan S, Beretta S, Moggio M, et al. High-dose intravenous human immunoglobulin in polymyositis resistant to treatment. *J Neurol Neurosurg Psychiatry* 1992;55:60–64.

91. Dalakas MC, Illa I, Dambrosia JM, et al. A controlled trial of high-dose intravenous immunoglobulin infusions as treatment for dermatomyositis. *N Engl J Med* 1993; 329:1993–2000.

92. Soueidan SA, Dalakas MC. Treatment of inclusion-body myositis with high-dose intravenous immunoglobulin. *Neurology* 1993;43:876–879.

93. Dalakas MC, Dambrosia JM, Sekul EA, et al. The efficacy of high-dose intravenous immunoglobulin (IVIg) in patients with inclusion-body myositis (IBM). *Neurology* 1995;45(S):208.

Chapter 25

Neural-Immune Interactions During Axonal Degeneration and Regeneration

John W. Griffin and Hsing-Fei Chien

The focus of this chapter is on the interactions between cells of the immune system and cells of the nervous system during nerve fiber degeneration and regeneration in the peripheral nervous system (PNS). Currently, lymphocytes and polymorphonuclear leukocytes appear to play little or no role in these processes. In contrast, the cell types of increasing interest are the resident macrophages of the PNS and the hematogenous macrophages that enter after nerve injury. Mast cells and endothelial cells also undergo well-documented changes. Finally, the behavior of Langerhans' cells of the epidermis merit comment. The differences among these cell responses indicate that selective mechanisms of recruitment and activation are involved.

Regeneration includes the restoration of full original function in an altered nervous system as a consequence of axonal sprouting, outgrowth, reinnervation, and maturation. The term is loosely applied in reference to any fragment of the complete process (such as outgrowth and sprout extension). Axonal regeneration has been most extensively studied following axonal interruption (axotomy) (1). Important insights, however, have come from models in which terminal and ultra-terminal sprouting of nerve fibers occurs. For example, motor nerve fiber terminals sprout in response to denervation of neighboring muscle fibers or to agents that block neuromuscular transmission, such as botulinum toxin (2,3). Collateral sprouting can occur from an intact parent axon in the setting of chronic partial degeneration of a nerve. Finally, there is increasing interest in new neuronal generation as seen in the olfactory system following olfactory nerve injury.

Wallerian Degeneration

The events during wallerian degeneration following axotomy set the stage for the success or failure of subsequent regeneration. In the PNS, the axon distal to the site of transection undergoes few changes during the latent period. The length of this latent period varies. In rodents the latent period is usually 24 to 48 hours (4–6), whereas in humans it is 5 to 11 days (7,8). At the end of the latent period, the axoplasm undergoes a characteristic change, granular degeneration of the cytoskeleton (9–11), which occurs abruptly and, along any segment of an individual fiber, in an "all or none" fashion. The spatiotemporal sequence of axonal breakdown has been extensively studied. In general, degeneration proceeds from proximal (near the site of axotomy) to distal with time, moving at a relatively rapid rate (4–6). For example, in dorsal root fibers of the rat the advance of degeneration is of the order of 3 to 4 mm/hr after the end of the latent period (6). Reynolds et al (12) used a confocal microscopic technique to demonstrate the proximal-distal degeneration of individual fibers. However, the spatiotemporal sequence is complicated by the early degeneration of synaptic terminals. This has been well documented in motor nerve fibers of the PNS (13), and recently demonstrated in the gracile nucleus in the dorsal column as well (6).

The mechanism initiating granular degeneration of the cytoskeleton is unknown, but it involves the entry of calcium (9,11,14), and in tissue culture axonal degeneration can be delayed by the presence of low calcium concentrations in the medium, ion channel–active agents, and some other metal ions including cobalt that serve to block calcium channels (14). Calcium-activated proteases (calpains) are involved in the proteolysis of the axonal cytoskeleton, and calpain inhibitors can also retard the sequence (14). At present the precise mechanisms leading to calcium entry remain incompletely understood (14).

As the axon breaks down, there are prompt changes in the surrounding Schwann cell. In myelinated fibers the myelin sheath is interrupted and divided into a series of closed-end segments (ovoids) (1,4). The length of each ovoid decreases with time as the myelin debris is cleared. Beginning on day 3 in the rat, the Schwann cells of the distal stumps enter the cell cycle and undergo a series of divisions (15,16), all within the basal lamina of the original fiber, to produce a longitudinal column of daughter Schwann cells (Büngner's band). This column serves as an ideal scaffolding for subsequent regeneration of nerve fibers. It provides several features that are supportive for regenerating sprouts. The Schwann cell basal lamina of the Schwann cell column is a favored structural substrate for growing axons, and because it remains in continuity with the target, it provides optimal "contact guidance."

The distal stump produces abundant neurotrophins, including nerve growth factor (NGF), brain-derived neurotrophic factor (BDNF), and neurotrophin-3 (NT3). In addition, the Schwann cells produce a low-affinity NGF (p75) and locate this on their plasmalemma (17). This in turn binds NGF, creating an enriched local environment on the plasmalemma directly beneath the basal lamina. The extending axonal sprout, containing the high-affinity NGF receptor trkA, can compete off the NGF from the Schwann cell plasmalemma. Finally, in the PNS there are few "stop" signals for regenerating sprouts. This is in contrast to the central nervous system (CNS), where specific glycoproteins in myelin debris act as contact inhibitors of elongation of regenerating sprouts (18,19).

Recent studies of motor nerve terminal sprouting in models of chronic partial denervation produced surprising new insights into the role of Schwann cells. It has been long known that terminal sprouts extend from intact motor nerve endings to neighboring denervated muscle fibers and establish functional neuromuscular junctions (20,21). Using double labeling immunocytochemical techniques, Son and Thompson (2,3) showed that Schwann cell processes lead the regenerating axon to the neighboring neuromuscular junctions. Strikingly, nerve sprouting appears to be both induced and guided by the Schwann cell processes that extend from the denervated neuromuscular junction.

In contrast to the PNS with its highly supportive Schwann cells, the denervated mammalian CNS is not supportive of regeneration. The structural substrate is inimical. A meshwork of interlaced astrocytic processes provides a poor substrate for regeneration. This appears to represent active remodeling of the glycoconjugates present on the astrocyte surface (22). In addition, there are numerous desmosomal junctions and no clear "pathway" among these interlaced processes. As noted below, macrophages fail to enter the degenerating CNS from the circulation, and myelin debris remains for long periods of time (23,24). CNS myelin debris provides a "stop" signal for regenerating sprouts and its presence is highly inimical to regeneration (18,19), as amplified below.

Axonal Regeneration

General Principles of Nerve Fiber Regeneration in the PNS

The following nine principles provide a framework for the subsequent discussion.

1. The axon is *dependent* on material received from the nerve cell body, both for normal maintenance and for regeneration.
2. This dependence is not "hour to hour" but week by week—all the constituents necessary for regeneration are present within the normal axon, and

sprouting can start with no participation of the nerve cell body.
3. Neither the normal axonal nor the regenerating axon can be considered by itself–the axon with its ensheathing and glial cells form a *interdependent multicellular unit.*
4. Regeneration does not recapitulate development at a cellular level, but the regenerating nervous system takes advantage of many of the same strategies used by the developing nervous system.
5. The successive regeneration varies enormously among species, among regions of the nervous system, and with age of the animals. These differences reflect both intrinsic axonal capabilities and differences in the "landscape" into which sprouts extend.
6. Axonal outgrowth is a local phenomenon occurring at the *growth cone*—most longitudinal growth during development occurs at the growing tip. (Note that this is a little-recognized contrast with developmental growth, in which most elongation of the axon occurs segment by segment during centrifugal displacement of innervated structures.)
7. *Neurotropism* (1) and *contact guidance* (25) are complementary rather than alternative mechanisms.
8. During regeneration the responses of the neuronal perikarya are altered in ways consistent with promoting outgrowth and elongation at the expense of neurotransmission or maintenance of mature structures.
9. In mammals, the CNS is less effective in providing a "prepared way" for regenerating sprouts—CNS neurons have a similar intrinsic capacity to extend sprouts as PNS neurons, but the CNS environment is inimical to regeneration.

Cellular Features of Axonal Regeneration

Transection of an axon is promptly followed by sealing of the distal end of the proximal stump (26). Vesicular organelles rapidly accumulate, forming a "pellet" (26,27). From this organelle-filled terminal swelling, rudimentary outgrowth begins within a few hours, and recognizable regenerating sprouts are present within 24 to 48 hours in mammals (26). The rate of subsequent extension varies widely. In the young rat following nerve crush injury, it is about 4.5 mm/day (28), whereas in humans the rate averages 0.1 mm/day (8,29).

In regeneration the site of elongation is the growth cone (1). The growth cone is a bulbous structure containing numerous vesicular organelles and a predominantly microtubule cytoskeleton with an extensive subplasmalemmal meshwork of microfilaments (30). Extension appears to be the result of coordinated addition of soluble tubulin monomer to the "plus" ends of the microtubules and motile expansions of membrane, the lamellipodia, as well as highly motile spikelike processes, the filopodia, pushing forward by an actin-based mechanism. New membrane is added to the growth cone from the vesicular organelles present within it. The phosphorylation substrate, growth-associated protein-43 (GAP43), is involved in membrane expansion, and may be a necessary constituent for growth cone extension (31).

In the preterminal axon of effectively growing fibers, the axonal shafts just proximal to the growth cones are cytologically simple, containing low concentrations of vesicular organelles and a predominantly microtubular cytoskeleton. Some maturation of the axon occurs before the growing tip has reached an appropriate target. Maturation includes an increase in axonal diameter with an increasing proportion of neurofilaments, as well as maturation of the axon-glial unit. In the PNS the Schwann cell segregates into a 1:1 relationship with regenerating sprouts, and then begins myelination in appropriate fibers (for review see (32)).

Following axotomy there are appropriate changes in the proximal stump and in the nerve cell body. At early times after axotomy the proximal stump appears normal. However, near the site of axotomy the axon decreases in caliber (33,34). In addition, the highly characteristic and highly orderly process of atrophy begins near the nerve cell body and advances down the axon. This is associated with a decrease in the content of neurofilaments within the axon (33,34). The typical changes in the nerve cell body include dispersion of the large blocks of granular endoplasmic reticulum (Nissl substance), an increased content of polyribosomes, and variable morphologic changes such as eccentric displacement of the nucleus and somal enlargement. These changes, termed the *axon reaction* or *chromatolysis*, are seen in both successful and frustrated regeneration.

Responses of Immune-Relevant Cells During Degeneration and Regeneration

Endothelial Cell Responses

One of the most striking consequences of axotomy in the PNS is the early and massive opening of the blood-nerve barrier. Normally, the endoneurial contents are isolated from circulating macromolecules behind a barrier comparable to the blood-brain barrier (35–38). In the CNS the blood-brain barrier is formed by tight junctions between endothelial cells; these tight junctions in turn appear to be formed in response to signals from the astrocytic foot processes that surround the vessels. In the PNS comparable tight junctions are found in the endoneurial vessels. In this instance there is of course no surrounding cell layer comparable to the astrocytes, so the stimulus for tight junction formation in endoneurial vessels is unknown. The endoneurial space is isolated from the epineurium by tight junctions between the perineurial cells that surround each nerve fascicle. It is noteworthy that the blood-nerve barrier is not as strict a barrier as the blood-brain barrier; circulating macromolecules enter to a somewhat greater degree, as described below.

When a peripheral nerve is transected, the blood-nerve barrier opens at relatively early times. For example, when the rat sciatic nerve is transected, the barrier opens and edema is present within the nerve between 24 and 48 hours after injury (36,37). Thus, it is one of the earliest structural changes in the PNS. Whether there is a spatial gradient—from proximal to distal, or from distal to proximal—remains unexplored. Injury to only a portion of nerve fibers is sufficient to open the blood-nerve barrier throughout the whole fascicle. Edema is observed in nerve fascicles in which only sensory nerve fibers were degenerating (as a consequence of dorsal root ganglionectomy). Whether degeneration of unmyelinated fibers alone is sufficient to produce this change is uncertain.

There are differing descriptions of the duration of opening of the blood-nerve barrier after axotomy. All authors agree that the barrier "reseals" after regeneration. Bouldin et al (36,37,39) presented evidence that macromolecules enter with less facility as regenerating sprouts invade a given region of nerve. A correlate of this observation is that repair of the blood-nerve barrier during nerve regeneration is likely to advance from proximal to distal with time. Weerasuriya (38) found that the blood-nerve barrier in the frog is open for a few weeks after sciatic axotomy and then is repaired even in the absence of regeneration, whereas Bouldin et al (36,37,39) found that in the rat the barrier remains open until reinnervation has occurred.

The mechanism of opening of the blood-nerve barrier is uncertain. It is often ascribed to degranulation of endoneurial mast cells (40), with consequent release of histamine and other agents with vasoactive properties. However, we observed endoneurial edema in degenerating sciatic nerves from mast cell–deficient mouse strains (George R, Griffin JW, unpublished observation). Thus, it seems likely that other mechanisms must participate as well. An attractive but so far untested possibility is that chemokines are produced by Schwann cells at very early times following nerve fiber injury, and that these chemokines are sufficient to alter the blood-nerve barrier at the endothelial cell level.

Macrophages

The extensive resident macrophage population of the normal peripheral nerve (35,41,42) undoubtedly participates during the process of peripheral nerve degeneration, but the specific responses remain incompletely studied. An effective way of examining this issue has been by using organ cultures of degenerating peripheral nerve (43,44). Samples of peripheral nerve have been transferred into short-term culture conditions. In the absence of additional macrophages, the resident cell population is insufficient to achieve rapid removal of the debris of degenerating fibers, particularly myelin debris. When exogenous macrophages are added to such cultures, as done by Beuche and Friede (43,44), myelin debris is efficiently removed. In line with these observations, we (Lobato C, Griffin JW, unpublished observations) identified a population of normal-appearing macrophages within the endoneurium at intervals after initiation of organ cultures. Goodrum and Novicki

(45) demonstrated that a population of these resident macrophages migrates out from the cut end of the nerve into the culture dish. Relatively few appear to be transformed into large phagocytic macrophages in the few days in which these cultures are maintained.

The major phagocyte of the degenerating peripheral nerve is unquestionably the hematogenous macrophage, which enters in large numbers. In the rat sciatic nerve some macrophages enter by 48 hours; in many fibers they appear to arrange themselves along the perinuclear region of the early degenerating fiber. By 4 days their numbers have increased markedly, and continue to increase during the subsequent 2 weeks (41,42,46). These macrophages migrate selectively to degenerating fibers; in preparations in which only 1 per 1000 fibers in a nerve is degenerating, macrophages seek out that nerve and arrange themselves along its outer surface (46). Macrophages then pass through the Schwann cell basal lamina of degenerating fibers and dissect into the degenerating fiber, where Schwann cell nuclei are interposed between nuclei of macrophages (46). The macrophages that adhere to and enter degenerating fibers bear a number of activation markers, including major histocompatibility complex (MHC) class II (42,46). They rapidly become phagocytic cells, ingesting myelin debris and forming large, clear, lipid droplets containing cholesterol ester (44,47,48). In time these cells become spherical "foamy" macrophages resembling the gitter cells of the CNS. Such cells congregate around endoneurial vessels and the subperineurial space. Whether they enter vessels to leave the PNS has been questioned, but the relatively modest numbers of these foamy cells at any one time suggest that many must have left by mechanisms other than local death and degeneration.

The mechanism by which macrophages are attracted into the degenerating PNS is not understood, but the signals must be highly selective, and it is likely that multiple signals are involved. As noted below, neither polymorphonuclear leukocytes nor lymphocytes enter degenerating nerves, and lymphokines are not involved in macrophage recruitment, as demonstrated by the fact that macrophages enter degenerating nerves in abundant numbers in the interferon-α knockout mouse (George R, Griffin JW, unpublished data). In addition, during wallerian-like degeneration of sensory axons in patients with acquired immunodeficiency syndrome (AIDS)–associated sensory neuropathy, macrophages are attracted in numbers that appear at least comparable to those in seronegative individuals with comparable sensory neuropathies, even though the individuals with AIDS have almost no CD4 cells remaining (49). Similarly, local activation of complement has been proposed to produce chemoattractants responsible for macrophage recruitment in vitro (44,47), but macrophages enter normally in animals that have been decomplementized by cobra venom, or that are congenitally complement deficient (C5-deficient mice, C3-deficient dogs) (George R, Griffin JW, unpublished data).

Two recent lines of evidence suggest potentially relevant molecules. Banner and Patterson (50) found that initial macrophage recruitment is deficient in a leukemia-inhibitory factor (LIF) knockout mouse line, suggesting that LIF produced in the distal stump may indirectly lead to production of macrophage chemoattractants. Chien, Griffin, and Ransohoff (unpublished data) identified an induction of MCP-1 in the distal stump. This chemokine is an attractive candidate to play a prominent role in macrophage recruitment. It may be produced by the denervated Schwann cell.

Polymorphonuclear Leukocytes and Lymphocytes

It is useful to devote a section to these cells, to emphasize the meager evidence of their participation in nerve fiber degeneration or regeneration. Occasional polymorphonuclear leukocytes enter injured or regenerating peripheral nerves (51), but they are very infrequent (46), and their numbers are overwhelmed by the large numbers of macrophages that enter (42,46,51). Similarly, lymphocytes do not appear in significant numbers within the degenerating nerve in either rodents or humans (23,52,53). The selective access of macrophages to the endoneurial space points to the highly selective signals involved. The two most likely signals are generation of specific chemokines and elaboration of specific adhesion molecules on endothelial cell surfaces.

Langerhans' Cells of the Epidermis

Langerhans' cells are bone marrow–derived cells of a macrophage lineage that migrate to the skin, mature within the dermis, and enter the epidermis where they are highly ramified, constitutively class II–positive cells. They are capable of taking up, processing, and presenting a wide variety of antigens. After a variable interval within the epidermis they migrate to draining lymph nodes, where they are found within follicles as dendritic cells.

Nerve fibers within the epidermis were long considered to be exceptional, but highly sensitive immunocytochemical techniques recently identified abundant C fibers within the normal epidermis. These fibers disappear following dorsal root ganglionectomy.

Hosoi et al (54) first observed the presence of contacts between terminal C fibers and Langerhans' cells (54). The innervating fibers appear to be particularly positive for calcitonin gene–related peptide (CGRP). That CGRP might alter antigen presentation by Langerhans' cells was suggested by in vitro experiments (54). Following denervation of the epidermis, the numbers of Langerhans' cells appear little changed, but Hsieh et al (55) showed that Langerhans' cells within the epidermis increase expression of a neuronal form of ubiquitin carboxy-terminal hydrolase (PGP9.5), as reflected in both elevated messenger RNA and protein levels. The significance of these phenotypic changes in Langerhans' cell markers is at present unknown.

Contributions of Macrophages to Nerve Regeneration

Within the nerve, macrophages make important contributions to subsequent regeneration. They are responsible for the production of interleukin-1β and probably other cytokines that are required for the production of growth factors such as NGF from cells of the injured nerve (56,57). The cells that produce NGF in response to interleukin-1 include endoneurial fibroblasts (56,57) and almost certainly Schwann cells. The mechanisms of gene regulation are incompletely understood, but in astrocytes the transcription factor Nfκb is involved. The possible roles of cytokines in the production of more recently recognized growth factors such as BDNF and NT3 from the distal stump remain incompletely understood.

Increasingly it appears that the differences between the CNS and the PNS in effectiveness of nerve regeneration depend in part on the activities of macrophages in the PNS.

References

1. Ramon y Cajal S. *Degeneration and regeneration of the nervous system* (May RM, transl.). London: Oxford University Press, 1928.
2. Son Y-J, Thompson WJ. Schwann cell processes guide regeneration of peripheral axons. *Neuron* 1995;14:125–132.
3. Son Y-J, Thompson WJ. Nerve sprouting in muscle is induced and guided by processes extended by Schwann cells. *Neuron* 1995;14:133–141.
4. Lubinska L. Early course of wallerian degeneration in myelinated fibers of the rat phrenic nerve. *Brain Res* 1977;130:47–63.
5. Lubinska L. Patterns of wallerian degeneration of myelinated fibres in short and long peripheral stumps and in isolated segments of rat phrenic nerve. Interpretation of the role of axoplasmic flow of the trophic factor. *Brain Res* 1982;233:227–240.
6. George R, Griffin JW. The proximo-distal spread of axonal regeneration in the dorsal columns of the rat. *J Neurocytol* 1994;23:657–667.
7. Chaudhry V, Cornblath DR. Wallerian degeneration in human nerves: serial electrophysiological studies. *Muscle Nerve* 1992;15:687–693.
8. Chaudhry V, Glass JD, Griffin JW. Wallerian degeneration in peripheral nerve disease. *Neurol Clin* 1992;10:613–627.
9. Glass JD, Schryer BL, Griffin JW. Calcium-mediated degeneration of the axonal cytoskeleton in the Ola mouse. *J Neurochem* 1994;62:2472–2475.
10. Griffin JW, George EB, Hsieh S-T, et al. Axonal degeneration and other disorders of the axonal cytoskeleton. In: Waxman S, Kocsis J, Stys P, eds. *The axon: structure, function, and pathophysiology.* New York: Oxford University Press, 1995:375–390.
11. Schlaepfer WW, Bunge RP. Effects of calcium ion concentration on the degradation of amputated axons in tissue culture. *J Cell Biol* 1973;59:456–470.
12. Reynolds RJ, LIttle GJ, Lin M, Heath JW. Imaging myelinated nerve fibres by confocal fluorescence microscopy: individual fibres in whole nerve trunks traced through multiple consecutive internodes. *J Neurocytol* 1994;23:555–564.
13. Miledi R, Slater CK. On the degeneration of rat neuromuscular junctions after nerve section. *J Physiol* 1970;207:507–528.
14. George EB, Glass J, Griffin JW. Axotomy-induced axonal degeneration is mediated by calcium influx through ion-specific channels. *J Neurosci* 1995;15:6445–6452.
15. Friede RL, Johnstone MA. Response of thymidine labeling of nuclei in gray matter and nerve following sciatic transection. *Acta Neuropathol (Berl)* 1967;7:218–231.
16. Pellegrino RG, Spencer PS. Schwann cell mitosis in response to regenerating peripheral axons in vivo. *Brain Res* 1985;341:16–25.
17. Taniuchi M, Clark HB, Schweitzer JB, Johnson EM. Expression of nerve growth factor receptors by Schwann cells of axotomized peripheral nerves: ultrastructural location, suppression by axonal contact, and binding properties. *J Neurosci* 1988;8:664–681.
18. Schwab ME. Myelin-associated inhibitors of neurite growth and regeneration in the CNS. *Trends Neurosci* 1990;13:452–456.
19. Schnell L, Schwab ME. Axonal regeneration in the rat spinal cord produced by an antibody against myelin-associated neurite growth inhibitors. *Nature* 1990;343:269–272.
20. Duchen LW, Strich SJ. The effects of botulinum toxin on the pattern of innervation of skeletal muscle in the mouse. *Q J Exp Physiol* 1968;53:84–89.
21. Pestronk A, Drachman DB, Griffin JW. Effect of botulinum toxin on trophic regulation of acetylcholine receptors. *Nature* 1976;264:787–789.
22. Silver J, Lorenz SE, Wahlsten D, Coughlin J. Axonal guidance during development of the great commissures: description and experimental studies, in vivo, on the role of preformed glial pathways. *J Comp Neurol* 1982;210:10–29.
23. George R, Griffin JW. Delayed macrophage responses and myelin clearance during wallerian degeneration in the central nervous system: the dorsal radiculotomy model. *Exp Neurol* 1994;129:225–236.
24. Miklossy J, Van der Loos H. The long-distance effects of brain lesions: visualization of myelinated pathways in the human brain using polarizing and fluorescence microscopy. *J Neuropathol Exp Neurol* 1991;50:1–15.
25. Weiss P, Taylor AC. Further experiments against "neurotropism" in nerve regeneration. *J Exp Zool* 1944;95:233.
26. Zelena J, Lubinska L, Gutmann E. Accumulation of organelles at the ends of interrupted axons. *Z Zellforsch Mikrosk Anat* 1968;91:200–219.
27. Griffin JW, Price DL, Spencer PS. Fast axonal transport through giant axonal swellings in hexacarbon neuropathy. *J Neuropathol Exp Neurol* 1977;36:603. Abstract.
28. Pestronk A, Drachman DB, Griffin JW. Effects of aging on nerve sprouting and regeneration. *Exp Neurol* 1980;70:65–82.
29. Sunderland S. *Nerves and nerve injuries*. Edinburgh: Churchill LIvingstone, 1991.
30. Bunge MB, Williams AK, Wood PM. Further evidence that neurons are required for the formation of basal lamina around Schwann cells. *J Cell Biol* 1972;83:130. Abstract.
31. Skene JHP. Axonal growth–associated proteins. *Annu Rev Neurosci* 1989;12:127–156.
32. Griffin JW, Hoffman PN. Degeneration and regeneration in the peripheral nervous system. In: Dyck PJ, Thomas PK, Griffin JW, et al, eds. *Peripheral neuropathy*. Philadelphia: WB Saunders, 1992:361–376.
33. Hoffman PN, Griffin JW, Price DL. Control of axonal cal-

iber by neurofilament transport. *J Cell Biol* 1984; 99:705–714.

34. Hoffman PN, Cleveland DW, Griffin JW, et al. Neurofilament gene expression: a major determinant of axonal caliber. *Proc Natl Acad Sci USA* 1987;84:3472–3476.

35. Arvidson B. Cellular uptake of exogenous horseradish peroxidase in mouse peripheral nerve. *Acta Neuropathol (Berl)* 1977;37:35–41.

36. Bouldin TW, Earnhardt TS, Goines ND. Sequential changes in the permeability of the blood-nerve barrier over the course of ricin neuronopathy in the rat. *Neurotoxicology* 1990;11:23–34.

37. Bouldin TW, Earnhardt TS, Goines ND. Restoration of blood-nerve barrier in neuropathy is associated with axonal regeneration and remyelination. *J Neuropathol Exp Neurol* 1991;50:719–728.

38. Weerasuriya A. Patterns of change in endoneurial capillary permeability and vascular space during nerve regeneration. *Brain Res* 1990;510:135–139.

39. Bouldin TW, Earnhardt TS, Goines ND, Goodrum J. Temporal relationship of blood-nerve barrier breakdown to the metabolic and morphologic alterations of tellurium neuropathy. *Neurotoxicology* 1989;10:79–90.

40. Powell HC, Myers RR, Lampert PW. Edema in neurotoxic injury. In: Spencer PS, Schaumburg HH, eds. *Experimental and clinical neurotoxicology*. Baltimore: Williams & Wilkins, 1980:118–138.

41. Griffin JW, George R, Lobato C, et al. Macrophage responses and myelin clearance during wallerian degeneration: relevance to immune-mediated demyelination. *J Neuroimmunol* 1992;40:153–166.

42. Monaco S, Gehrmann J, Raivich G, Kreutzberg GW. MHC-positive, ramified macrophages in the normal and injured rat peripheral nervous system. *J Neurocytol* 1992;21:623–634.

43. Beuche W, Friede RL. The role of non-resident cells in wallerian degeneration. *J Neurocytol* 1984;13:767–796.

44. Beuche W, Friede RL. Myelin phagocytosis in wallerian degeneration depends on silica-sensitive, bg/bg-negative and Fc-positive monocytes. *Brain Res* 1986;378:97–106.

45. Goodrum JF, Novicki DL. Macrophage-like cells from explant cultures of rat sciatic nerve produce apolipoprotein E. *J Neurosci Res* 1988;20:457–462.

46. Stoll G, Griffin JW, Li CY, Trapp BD. Wallerian degeneration in the peripheral nervous system: participation of both Schwann cells and macrophages in myelin degradation. *J Neurocytol* 1989;18:671–683.

47. Freeman JA, Bock S, Deaton M, et al. Axonal and glial proteins associated with the development and response to injury in the rat and goldfish optic nerve. *Exp Brain Res* 1986;(suppl 13):34–47.

48. Popko B, Goodrum JF, Bouldin TW, et al. Nerve regeneration occurs in the absence of apolipoprotein E in mice. *J Neurochem* 1993;60:1155–1158.

49. Griffin JW, Crawford TO, Tyor WR, et al. Sensory neuropathy in AIDS. 1997 (in press).

50. Banner LR, Patterson PH. Major changes in the expression of the mRNAs for cholinergic differentiation factor/leukemia inhibitory factor and its receptor after injury to adult peripheral nerves and ganglia. *Proc Natl Acad Sci USA* 1994;91:7109–7113.

51. Perry VH, Brown MC, Gordon S. The macrophage response to central and peripheral nerve injury: a possible role for macrophages in regeneration. *J Exp Med* 1987;165:1218–1223.

52. Griffin JW, Li CY, Ho TW, et al. Guillain-Barré syndrome in northern China: the spectrum of neuropathologic changes in clinically defined cases. *Brain* 1995; 118:577–595.

53. Griffin JW, Li CY, Ho TW, et al. Pathology of the motor-sensory axonal Guillain-Barré syndrome. *Ann Neurol* 1996;39:17–28.

54. Hosoi J, Murphy GF, Egan CL, et al. Regulation of Langerhans cell function by nerves containing calcitonin gene–related peptide. *Nature* 1993;363:159–163.

55. Hsieh S-T, Choi S, Lin W-M, et al. Epidermal denervation and its effects on keratinocytes and Langerhans cells. *J Neurocytol* 1996;25:513–524.

56. Lindholm D, Heumann R, Meyer M, Thoenen H. Interleukin-1 regulates synthesis of nerve growth factor in non-neuronal cells of rat sciatic nerve. *Nature* 1987;330:658–659.

57. Lindholm D, Heumann R, Hengerer B, Thoenen H. Interleukin-1 increases stability and transcription of mRNA encoding nerve growth factor in cultured rat fibroblasts. *J Biol Chem* 1988;263:16348–16351.

Chapter 26
Historical Perspective and Overview

Byron H. Waksman

The first neuroimmunologic observation, made over a century ago, was of paralytic encephalomyelitis in patients receiving injections of Pasteur's new rabies vaccine. This established that immune responses might play a causative role in human neurologic disease. Rivers and his colleagues in 1932 produced a similar disease by repeated injections of neural tissue into monkeys and rabbits. This animal model became known as experimental allergic (or autoimmune) encephalomyelitis (EAE) and served for 40 years as the principal subject of investigations on immunologically mediated disease of the nervous system.

More fundamental investigations of nervous system–immune system interactions began with attempts, at the turn of the century, to discriminate antigenic tissue components by their ability to elicit antibodies. Characteristic protein and glycolipid antigens were found in the brain, eye, and other organs. Crystallin, a protein of the ocular lens, was obtainable in almost pure form and was used by Verhoeff in 1922 in the first investigation of the pathogenesis of the autoimmune disorder phakogenic uveitis, an inflammatory eye disease that follows cataract extraction, when there has been accidental leakage of immunogenic lens contents. Skin tests with lens crystallin elicited typical delayed (tuberculin-type) skin reactions (delayed-type hypersensitivity (DTH)) in patients with the disease and not in control subjects. Burky produced a rabbit model for phakogenic uveitis in 1934, following Rivers' discovery of EAE and Verhoeff's clinical demonstration.

Investigators sought to develop additional disease models in animals that could be easily studied and provided reproducible representations of uncommon human disorders; new autoimmune models, affecting both the nervous system (Table 26-1) and other organs, were described in a steady stream over the years. The concept of autoimmunity, however, was not quickly accepted, in part because of Ehrlich's widely quoted dictum about the immune system's "horror autotoxicus." Only after 1960, when studies of experimental autoimmune thyroiditis and of chronic thyroiditis in humans had established the astonishing degree of similarity between the human and experimental conditions, was there widespread acceptance of this idea.

Immunologic knowledge before 1960 was too limited to permit sophisticated research, either on animal models or on their human counterparts, beyond what was possible with basic morphologic, serologic, and simple protein separation techniques (Table 26-2). The model diseases described before this time proved to be mediated primarily by cell-mediated immunity (CMI); they presented inflammatory, destructive lesions that could not be missed, even by skeptical pathologists. Antibody-mediated conditions were first studied after 1970, when myasthenia gravis (MG) and its animal model became dominant paradigms of autoimmune neurologic disease. The changes that characterized these new models were more subtle, often requiring careful neurophysiologic investigation; the identification and quantification of experimental autoimmune myasthenia gravis (EAMG) in mice, for example, could only be achieved by the use of electromyography. The expanded range of new investigative methods in the 1980s (and the expanded pool of investigators who regarded autoimmune disease as a fruitful field of investigation) enormously accelerated the pace of new research. More was learned about MG and EAMG in 5 to 10 years than had been learned about EAE in its first 40 years.

Neuroimmunologic Diseases

Experimental Autoimmune Encephalomyelitis

EAE must serve, in this brief review, as the paradigm of research on animal models with autoimmune disease that depends primarily on the induction of CMI; that is, a CD4+ Th1 cell-mediated response directed to an autoantigen. The course of EAE research (Table 26-3) has followed the evolution of immunologic concepts and techniques. Between the end of World War II and 1960, the basic biologic and pathologic features of EAE were established and the disease was assigned to the class of cell-mediated immune reactions. Chemical and histochemical studies of EAE during this time can be viewed (with hindsight) as studies of the chemistry of myelin breakdown, largely within phagocytic macrophages.

Between 1960 and 1970, the assignment of EAE to the CMI class was confirmed and the cells found in the lesions were characterized as hematogenous T cells and macrophages. Traditionally, the macrophages had been viewed simply as microglia that responded to tissue

Table 26-1.
Autoimmune Neurologic and Related Diseases in
Experimental Animals

1933	Experimental autoimmune encephalomyelitis (EAE)
1934	Phakogenic uveitis
1949	Experimental autoimmune uveitis (EAU)
1955	Experimental autoimmune neuritis (EAN)
1965, 1991	Experimental autoimmune autonomic neuropathy
1965	Experimental autoimmune myositis
1967	Experimental autoimmune adenohypophysitis
1972	Myeloma associated with neuropathy (mice)
1973	Experimental autoimmune myasthenia gravis (EAMG)
1981	Lambert-Eaton syndrome (LEMS) in mice (serum transfer from patients)
1981	POEMS syndrome in mice (serum transfer from patients)
1982	Retinal ganglion cell blindness
1986	Experimental autoimmune motor neuron disease (EAMND)
1986	Experimental autoimmune gray matter disease (EAGMD)
1988	Sulfate glucuronyl paragleboside (SGPG) model of peripheral neuropathy
1990, 1992	CNS lesions of systemic lupus erythematosus (SLE) (NZB, MRL mice)
1991	Rat narcolepsy (genetic model)
1994	LEMS in rats (immunization with synaptotagmin)

Table 26-2.
Immunology: Conceptual Highlights over Half a Century

Before 1950	Role of antibody in immunity and in anaphylaxis
	Antibody made by plasma cells
	CMI recognized only by skin test DTH and by adoptive transfer with living mononuclear cells
1950–60	Immunoglobulin isotypes distinguished
	CMI recognized as distinct class of reactions
	Lymphocytes recognized as the central cells of immunology
1960–70	Role of thymus in lymphocyte differentiation
	T and B lymphocytes distinguished
	Lymphocyte stimulation in vitro, cytotoxicity
	First cytokines identified (bioassay only)
	First use of T-cell markers
1970–80	CD4+ and CD8+ subsets of T cells
	MHC (HLA) restriction of T-cell responses (dual recognition)
	Network concept and idiotypes
	"Suppressor cells" and downregulation
	Molecular mimicry
After 1980	Sequence and steric structure of MHC class I and MHC class II, later of T-cell receptor
	Structure and function of cytokines, adhesion molecules, growth factors, and their receptors
	Signaling, transduction pathways, gene regulation and expression
	α/β and γ/δ T cells
	Cytokine profiles and CD4+ T-cell subsets: Th1 and Th2
	Similar CD8+ T-cell subsets (Tc1 and Tc2)
	Thymus deletion, clonal anergy, or deletion in periphery
	Apoptosis and programmed cell death
	Downregulation by cytokines: IL-4, IL-10, TGF-β
	Interactions among CNS; HPA, HPT, HPG; and immune system

CMI = cell-mediated immunity; DTH = delayed-type hypersensitivity; IL = interleukin; TGF = transforming growth factor; CNS = central nervous system; HPA = hypothalamic-pituitary-adrenal; HPT = hypothalamic-pituitary-thyroid; HPG = hypothalamic-pituitary-gonadal.

damage by becoming activated and cleaning up debris, not as the primary agents of tissue destruction. Therefore, these new insights constituted a fundamental "paradigm shift." Shiraki's observation in 1957 that EAE can be followed by typical MS in human subjects of Japanese origin (i.e., a particular racial background), was an insufficiently appreciated forerunner of studies on genetic determinants of EAE and MS susceptibility.

Beginning in 1955–1956 with myelin proteolipid (PLP) and myelin basic protein (MBP), single homogenous proteins of myelin were found to be effective encephalitogens. MBP, because of its water-solubility, became the antigen of choice for more refined studies of encephalitogenicity over the following decades. Subsequently, with improvements in technique, many additional encephalitogenic proteins were identified; the total approaches ten at the present time. The study of peptides, begun by Eylar, Hashim, Kibler, and others around 1970, became an essential feature of all later EAE studies. A key technology, exploited by Linington, Wekerle, and their collaborators since 1990, is the generation in vitro of T-cell lines/clones against individual proteins and their peptides for the rapid identification of specific epitopes that induce clones with pathogenic potential. Using this technique, investigators have shown that certain astrocytic components produce new types of EAE with unusual differences in lesion distribution and character.

Genetic studies of EAE, first undertaken in the 1970s,

identified major histocompatibility complex (MHC) II as a major susceptibility gene. The encephalitogenicity of specific MBP or PLP peptides was shown, not surprisingly, to be MHC-restricted. Later, the genes encoding TCR peptide polymorphisms were also incriminated, as were genes governing the level of expression of MHC, the preferential production of particular CK and the Th1/Th2 balance, and various aspects of inflammation (e.g., the sensitivity of vascular endothelium to vasoamines). As yet, the genetic determinants of immune regulation remain largely unknown.

The 1980s saw a wide diversification of studies on the cells and soluble factors (antibody, cytokine (CK), complement components) contributing to EAE pathogenesis. The chronic phase of EAE was recognized as presenting different problems from the chronic phases

Table 26-3.
Experimental Autoimmune Encephalomyelitis (EAE)

Neurologic and Immunopathologic Studies		
1933	Rivers et al	EAE is first demonstrated (monkeys, rabbits).
1940s	Ferraro, Cazzullo, Roizin	EAE can take many forms, including hyperacute (hemorrhagic) and chronic (MS-like).
1947	Kabat; Morgan	Freund's complete adjuvant intensifies EAE.
1949	Waksman, Morrison	EAE is correlated with DTH vs homologous (and presumably autologous) CNS tissue.
1957	Uchimura, Shiraki	Postvaccinal encephalomyelitis (EAE in humans) may be followed by typical MS (in Japanese).
1958	Waksman	Character of early lesion indicates typical CMI: perivenous mononuclear cell infiltrate, invasive-destructive lesion of parenchyma.
1960	Paterson	Adoptive transfer of EAE with living lymphoid cells suggests EAE is expression of CMI.
1961	Arbouys	EAE is prevented by antilymphocyte serum—disease is mediated by circulating lymphocytes.
1962	Arnason, Janković	EAE is prevented by neonatal thymectomy—disease-producing cells are thymus derived.
1962	Waksman	EAE is model for two classes of human disease: monophasic after immunizing event (PVE, PIE, ADEM) and chronic progressive or relapsing-remitting (MS).
1963–65	Berg, Källén; Kornguth, Thompson; David	EAE lymphocytes perform typical CMI functions in vitro: proliferation, cytotoxicity, secretion of cytokines.
1963	Kosunen et al	Cells in lesions of EAE are hematogenous, mostly macrophages (^{3}H-thymidine labeling).
1965	Stone, Lerner	Chronic relapsing EAE is produced in guinea pigs.
1968	Lubaroff	Macrophages in EAE lesions are nonspecific, bone marrow derived (LexDA rat chimeras, cell transfer).
Encephalitogenic Antigens and Peptides		
1948	Kabat	Autologous brain can induce EAE.
1955	Waksman, Folch-Pi	Myelin proteolipid (PLP) is an effective EAE antigen.
1956	Kies; Roboz-Einstein	Myelin basic protein (MBP) is an EAE antigen.
1970	Eylar; others	Peptides of MBP as short as 9 or 10 amino acid residues are encephalitogenic.
1982	Fritz	Different "immunodominant" peptides of MBP in different mouse strains are restricted by MHC class II alleles.
1990	Tuohy, Lees	Encephalitogenic peptides of PLP and their relation to MHC class II are established.
1990s	Kojima, Linington, Wekerle	MAG, MOG, S100-β, and GFAP are encephalitogenic and may contribute to EAE.
1990s	Wekerle, Lassmann	Distribution and character of lesions differ with different encephalitogens.
1994	Martin; Braun	Cyclic nucleotide phosphohydrolase of myelin is also a potential encephalitogen.
1994	Van Noort	B-crystallin (HSP25) is also a potential encephalitogen.
Immunogenetic Studies		
1960s 1970s	Levine; Stone	Susceptible and resistant strains of inbred rats and guinea pigs are produced. Congenic and backcross strains are developed.
1973	Williams, Moore	Study of LexBN rat backcrosses demonstrates a single dominant susceptibility gene: MHC class II.
1977	Teitelbaum, Arnon; Bernard	In guinea pigs and mice the dominant susceptibility gene is MHC class II.
1980s	Lublin	Congenic backcross strains of mice differ in frequency and severity of exacerbations.
1982	Linthicum, Frelinger	EAE susceptibility genes govern vascular sensitivity to vasoamines.
1985	Ben-Nun	MBP epitopes are related to specific TCR peptide polymorphisms.
1986	Korngold	Study of interstrain chimeras shows that multiple immunologic and nonimmunologic factors (genes) underlie susceptibility/resistance.
1988	Heber-Katz	$V_\beta 8.2$ is overrepresented in mouse and rat autoimmune diseases: the "V region disease" theory.
1987, 1988	Goldowitz, Lublin; Nicholas, Arnason	Heterotopic brain grafts provide a finer analysis of factors underlying susceptibility/resistance.
1991	J. Miller	In transgenic mice, H-2K^b placed under control of MBP promoter results in "Wonky" (hypomyelinated) mice.
Cell and Molecular Immunobiology of EAE		
1977, 1979	McFarlin; Kies	Adoptive transfer of EAE requires "activated" CD4+ T cells (antigen, mitogen).
1981	Ben-Nun, Cohen	MBP-specific T cells are cloned. On adoptive syngeneic transfer, they produce EAE.
1984	Mokhtarian, McFarlin	Chronic EAE after transfer of a single clone is accompanied by successive recruitment of T cells vs new epitopes, also vs new antigens and their epitopes, with new MHC restrictions.

Table 26-3. *Continued*

Cell and Molecular Immunobiology of EAE (cont.)

1984	Lassmann, Linington	Simultaneous transfer of MBP-specific T cells (clone) and of antibody vs MOG in various ratios leads to full spectrum of MS lesions.
1988	Lassmann; Hickey	Perivascular macrophages ("microglia") act as site of antigen presentation in elicitation of EAE.
1990	Pender; Lassmann; Mason	Apoptosis of specific T cells in CNS terminates acute attack of EAE: Due to steroids? "Suppressor" cytokine?
1990	Selmaj, Brosnan	Recruitment of γ/δ T cells into EAE lesions is demonstrated.
1992	Selmaj, Brosnan	There is increased HSP60 expression in EAE lesions.
1993	Jones et al	SCID mice cannot be restored with hemopoietic and lymphoid cells from MS patients.
1994	Prabhu-Das, Kuchroo	Th1 vs Th2 cell lines vs PLP peptides express distinct effector end regulatory functions.
1995	Chen, Weiner	Use of transgenic mice expressing a unique TCR facilitates studies of tolerance.

Diffusible Mediators in EAE Pathogenesis

1983	Shin	Normal myelin induces complement activation and lysis (enhanced by specific antibody).
1984	Compston	Oligodendrocyte lysis by complement in vivo is demonstrated.
1988	Hartung, Toyka	Free radicals (ROS and NO) from activated macrophages damage neural parenchyma.
1988	Selmaj, Raine; Brosnan et al	TNF damages tissue directly; IL-1, IL-2, and TNF damage vascular endothelium.
1993	Piddlesden	Role of complement in antibody-mediated demyelination of MBP/MOG lesion is delineated.
1994	Berman, Ransohoff	Chemokines play an essential role in lesion pathogenesis.
1995	Ruddle	Production of LT and/or TNF is essential for encephalitogenicity of T cells.
1990	Several laboratories	Upregulatory and downregulatory CK play a major role in both induction and elicitation of EAE lesions.

Immune Regulation in Acute and Chronic EAE

1949	Cazzullo	Myelin in incomplete Freund's adjuvant intraperitoneally prevents EAE.
1970, 1994	Ellison; Khoury	Injection of MBP into the thymus (rats) prevents EAE.
1977	Swanborg	Two types of suppressor T cell paly a role in termination of first attack and in resistance to relapse.
1981	Ben Nun, Wekerle, Cohen	Vaccination with inactivated MBP-specific T-cell clones prevents EAE.
1985	Lyman, Brosnan	MBP-specific "suppressor" cells are present in spleen during remission phase of relapsing EAE.
1988	Sun, Wekerle	CD8+ idiotype-specific "suppressor" cells in animals vaccinated with CD4+ MBP clone are CTLs.
1988	Whitacre	Oral tolerance to MBP is demonstrated.
1989	Karpus, Swanborg	CD4+ "suppressor" cells in recovery phase of EAE are idiotype specific and produce IL-4 and TGF-β.
1989	S. D. Miller	Tolerization with MBP or PLP-membrane conjugates is associated with clonal anergy of effector T cells.
1990	Pender	Low-dose cyclosporine in MBP-immunized rats results in chronic EAE; may work by eliminating a "suppressor" cell population.
1992	Mak; Pernis	CD8 knockout mice (transgenic; use of Mab) show marked increase in EAE relapses and decrease of severity.
1992	Lider, Miller, Weiner	Oral tolerance to MBP in rats is mediated by CD8+ epitope-specific "suppressor" cells producing TGF-β.
1995	Prabhu-Das, Kuchroo	CD4+ Th2-cell clones vs PLP peptides make IL-4 and IL-10 and suppress EAE on transfer.
1995	Chen, Weiner	Oral tolerance to MBP peptides in mice is mediated by CD4+ epitope-specific cells producing high levels of TGF-β.
1995	Ware, Pernis	CD8+ T cells (resistance to relapse) kill CD4+ epitope-specific T cells and are restricted by Qa-1.

EAE = experimental autoimmune encephalomyelitis; MS = multiple sclerosis; DTH = delayed-type hypersensitivity; CNS = central nervous system; CMI = cell-mediated immunity; PVE = postvaccinal encephalomyelitis; PIE = postinfectious encephalomyelitis; MAG = myelin-associated glycoprotein; GFAP = glial fibrillary acidic protein; TCR = T-cell receptor; ROS = reactive oxygen species; NO = nitric oxide; TNF = tumor necrosis factor; IL = interleukin; CTLs = cytotoxic T lymphocytes; TGF = transforming growth factor.

associated with initiation of the disease process, among them the so-called "epitope spreading," the recruitment of γ/δ T cells, and the induction of regulatory responses associated with remission and relapse. The blackout on studies of "suppressor" mechanisms throughout the 1980s hampered research on immune regulation in EAE, but in the 1990s, the discovery of the regulatory capacities of IL-12 (up) and of IL-4, IL-10, and TGF-β (down) and interest in responses to idiotypes (of effector cells) have led to new initiatives in this area.

Multiple Sclerosis

An immunologic theory of multiple sclerosis (MS) was put forward in the 1930s by Pette, Schaltenbrand, and others, primarily on morphologic grounds. The combined presence of inflammation and parenchymal damage, in the absence of a known toxic or infectious agent, argued for an underlying immunologic process. The discovery of the EAE model provided support for this idea.

Starting in the mid-1970s, the increasingly refined immunohistochemical and electron microscope studies of Prineas and later of Raine, Wisniewski, Lassmann, Sobel, Brosnan, and others demonstrated the early presence of MS lesions of both CD4+ and CD8+ α/β and later γ/δ T cells (and concurrent heat shock protein expression), and the preponderant role of macrophages in myelin destruction. These studies were followed by investigations in the 1990s of upregulated adhesion molecule expression and cytokine (CK)/chemokine release and, in the last few years, T-cell clonality using the polymerase chain reaction (PCR) technique (Hafler and Steinman spearheaded work in this last area). Reactive oxygen species (ROS) and nitrite (NO) have been incriminated as major agents of tissue damage (Hartung). Macrophages serve as the cellular source of these molecules in animals with EAE, and astrocytes appear to be their main source in the MS plaques of human subjects (Brosnan, Trapp).

Repeated attempts to identify a specific causative virus in the central nervous system (CNS) tissue or blood cells of MS patients have failed. In a Russian study performed immediately after World War II, the suspected agent turned out to be rabies virus. Fifty years later, after approximately 20 additional unsubstantiated claims, it remains problematic that any single specific agent is involved. On the other hand, investigation of the epidemic of MS in the Faroe Islands, which took place after the arrival of British troops at the start of World War II, led Kurtzke and Hyllested to the conclusion that the disease is actually caused by a specific infectious agent (1979). Cook and Dowling found evidence that this agent might be the canine distemper virus, closely related to measles.

Geographically and ethnically based studies of prevalence, beginning in the late 1950s, led to the identification of high-prevalence areas in northern Ireland (Millar, 1954), northern Scotland (Sutherland, 1956), and the Shetland and Orkney islands (Poskanzer, 1980) and low-prevalence areas in Australia (Sutherland, 1962), South Africa (Dean, 1967), and Israel (Alter, 1969). This striking "latitude effect" was studied in detail by Kurland in the early 1960s and among US military veterans by Kurtzke (1967). Concurrent socioeconomic studies by the same authors established the greater prevalence of MS in more affluent groups. Kuroiwa, working with Kurland, carried out extensive studies of MS among the Japanese population (low prevalence, definite latitude effect) and Dean showed the near or total absence of MS among African blacks. Later studies showed that there is little or no MS among the Yakuts of central Siberia, the Eskimos (Inuit), and the Hutterites in central Canada. On the other hand, foci of high MS prevalence have been documented in Finland (Wikström), Norway (Nyland), and several other countries.

A study of migrants from northern Europe (Holland, the United Kingdom) to South Africa (Dean, 1966) showed that those migrating before the age of 15 years expressed MS at a prevalence level comparable to that in South Africa, whereas those migrating after the age of 15 years expressed the prevalence of their country of origin, the first clear demonstration that environmental determinants play a significant role in MS expression. In a recent study, Compston related the apparent "transition" in MS susceptibility at about age 15 to the age at which transmission of common viruses (measles, rubella, mumps, EBV) occurs; MS risk increases almost tenfold with age of virus transmission up to 15 years of age. The immunologic (or other) mechanism underlying this "transition" remains unknown. Virus infections were also incriminated as a trigger of MS exacerbations in Sibley's longitudinal studies of a large cohort of patients (1985), confirmed by Paty and later Panitch (1994).

Family and twin studies, begun by McKay and Myrianthopoulos in 1958, were greatly extended during the 1980s by McFarlin and his colleagues, by Compston and others, and especially by Ebers, Sadovnick, Paty, and various collaborators, who worked with a large well-ascertained patient population across Canada. These studies led to the inference, now widely accepted, that susceptibility to MS is genetically determined, with multiple genes being involved. Yet about half of all affected twin pairs are discordant for MS. The conclusion was clear: environmental influences must determine the expression of MS.

Genetic investigations in MS began with Jersild, Svejgaard, and Fog's 1972 study establishing an HLA association for MS susceptibility, confirmed in numerous later studies. An initial emphasis on HLA class I genes (A3 and B7) shifted rapidly to an emphasis on class II (DR-2, -4, and -6, and DQ-w1). A possible association with genes encoding peptide isoforms of the TCR α and β chains was reported first in 1988 (Ciulla et al; Beall et al). There were also reports of an association with gene loci encoding immunoglobulin sequences and elements of the inflammatory process such as alpha-1 antitrypsin. In the 1990s, a broader approach to identification of MS susceptibility genes has been adopted, with the use of pedigreed families, cell and DNA banks, and the rapidly evolving technologies for searching the human genome.

Immunologic investigations of MS, properly speaking, began in 1942 with Kabat's finding of increased globulin in the cerebrospinal fluid (CSF), followed 20 years later by the description of oligoclonal bands (OBs) in CSF IgG (Karcher, Lowenthal 1960). Still later (1974) came Sandberg-Wollheim's identification of B cells in the CSF making IgG, IgM, and IgA; and finally (in the early 1980s) Tourtellotte's demonstration of massive immunoglobulin synthesis in the CNS and CSF compartment. More refined studies of the OBs by Vandvik in the 1970s and the Arnason group and Mehta in the 1980s were in turn followed by the demonstration that the CSF immunoglobulins include antibodies to many viruses (K. Johnson and others) and to CNS myelin constituents such as myelin basic protein (MBP) (e.g., Warren and Catz, 1986).

Studies of blood and CSF T cells began in the 1970s with Antel and Arnason's observation that circulating CD8+ T cells show a loss of nonspecific "suppressor" activity. The same authors (with Reder and other colleagues) later related this loss to decreased expression of CD8 and an increase in surface β-adrenergic receptors. The CSF was found to contain active, cycling cells (Noronha and Arnason, 1980), some reactive with common viruses (Salmi 1983). T-cell clones from the blood and CSF of MS patients and control subjects were shown to include cells specific for MBP (Burns 1983). Olsson and Link (1988) used the enzyme-linked immunosorbent assay (ELISA) spot technique to show the presence in CSF of both T and B cells reactive with a variety of myelin antigens.

In 1990, several laboratory groups (Weiner/Hafler in Boston, McFarland at the NIH, and Wekerle in Munich) independently used T-cell cloning to show that MBP reactivity is limited to a few "immunodominant" epitopes determined by each individual's HLA background. In MS patients, the population of "activated" T cells carrying interleukin (IL)-2 receptors was found to include many cells recognizing MBP, whereas such cells were not present in control patients (Mokhtarian 1990; Zhang and Hafler 1993). As many as 10% of the cycling CSF T cells were MBP or proteolipid protein (PLP) specific. These activated MBP-specific T cells included many mutant cells, as judged by mutations in *hprt* (Allegretta, Sriram 1990) and in pathways governing Ca^{2+} flux (Grimaldi 1994). Since 1990, persistent in vivo "clones" of CD4+ MBP-specific T cells, identified by unique T-cell receptor (TCR) peptide signatures, have been identified by both McFarland's and Hafler's groups, and there appear to be persistent CD8+ clones as well (Monteiro, Gregerson 1995).

Research over the last two decades revealed that abnormalities in immune regulation are characteristic of MS. Antel and Arnason's 1978 finding that circulating CD8+CD28− T cells show a decreased ability to downregulate proliferative and other responses was followed by the demonstration of decreased autologous mixed lymphocyte reaction (AMLR) activity (Hafler, Weiner; Crisp, Greenstein 1985) and decreased "suppressor-inducer" activity (Morimoto, Hafler 1987). Arnason and his colleagues, Reder and Antel, in studies extending over more than a decade, showed that these abnormalities parallel abnormalities of autonomic function and hyperreactivity of the hypothalamic-pituitary axis. Other research demonstrated decreased production of interferon (IFN)-γ in AMLR-stimulated CD8+ T cells (Balashov, Weiner 1995).

The papers on T cells appearing throughout the 1980s and early 1990s were complemented by studies of activated complement components, of CK and CK receptors, and later of adhesion molecules in the blood and CSF of MS patients. The principal players proved to be IL-1, tumor necrosis factor (TNF), IL-2 receptor (R), TNF-R, and intercellular adhesion molecule (ICAM)-1. The possibility that such clinical aspects of MS as fatigue might result from TNF toxicity is currently under investigation.

Other Autoimmune Diseases Dependent Primarily on T Cell–Mediated Immunity

In *postvaccinal encephalomyelitis* (PVE) that develops after rabies vaccination and the *postinfectious encephalomyelitis* (PIE) that follows infection with viruses of the myxovirus, morbilli, pox, and herpesvirus groups, the presence of antibodies against myelin was an early finding (Hurst 1932). Skin tests with MBP (Behan 1968) and in vitro lymphocytic studies with MBP (Lisak, Zweiman 1977; Johnson et al 1984) established the presence of CMI. Griffin and Hemachudha, in more recent studies, showed both strong T-cell reactivity and high-titer antibody against MBP.

Viral models of PIE include *canine distemper*, proposed by Hurst in 1943 as a model for demyelinating diseases in general and studied by Steck and Vandevelde during the 1980s; *JHM virus infection*, producing a subacute demyelinating encephalomyelitis in weanling Lewis rats (Wege, ter Meulen et al 1978); and *neurotropic measles* strains, producing subacute measles encephalomyelitis in mice (Liebert, ter Meulen 1987). In all these models, infection leads to the appearance of circulating MBP-sensitized T cells, capable on transfer of producing typical EAE in syngeneic recipients (Vandevelde 1983; Watanbe, Wege 1983; Liebert, Hashim 1990). In *Semliki Forest virus* infection in mice, studied by Suckling in the late 1970s and by Webb and his colleagues in the 1970s and early 1980s, there is T-cell sensitization to viral antigens and formation of autoantibody reactive with myelin glycolipids (Fazakerly and Webb 1983, 1984). Both elements of the response contribute to lesion formation.

In *Guillain-Barré syndrome* (GBS), also called acute *inflammatory demyelinating polyneuropathy* (AIDP), early observations suggesting a role for antibody (Hirano et al 1971) were followed by evidence for the presence of CMI to peripheral nervous system antigens (Abramsky et al 1975). The disease resembles experimental autoimmune neuritis (EAN) in animals and thus has been thought to be based mainly on CMI. Several investigators demonstrated lymphocytic reactivity against P2, P0, and their peptides and, in some patients, to MBP (Geczy 1985; Burns 1986; Hemachudha, Griffin

1987), whereas others detected antibodies to various myelin glycolipids (Sanders, Koski 1986). In some patients, the disease appeared to be induced by antecedent gastrointestinal infection with *Campylobacter jejuni* strains (Kaldor, Speed 1984). The *acute motor axonal neuropathy* occurring in rural children, in China and Mexico in particular, was also related to infection with specific strains of *C. jejuni* and found to be mediated largely by antibody (McKhann, Griffin et al 1992). *Chronic inflammatory demyelinating polyneuropathy* (CIDP), which is frequently thought of as a peripheral MS equivalent, was investigated somewhat later than AIDP. Lymphocytic reactions against P2, P0, and their peptides were demonstrated here too (Gregson, Hughes 1988), as were antibodies (Koski, Shin 1985).

EAN, which appears to be a good model for AIDP (Waksman, Adams 1955), has been through the full gamut of studies described for EAE, mostly in the 1970s and 1980s. Several investigators implicated P2 and P0 as antigens (Uyemura, Nagai, and Ikuta; Hughes et al 1979, 1987). *Chronic variants of EAN* (models for CIDP) were produced in juvenile animals by repeated immunization or by giving low doses of cyclosporine or cyclophosphamide during immunization (McCombe, Pender 1992). A milder CIDP was produced by immunizing rabbits or rats with galactocerebroside (Saida, Saida 1979) or with sulfated glucuronyl paragleboside (SGPG) (Yu et al 1988, 1991). *Marek's disease* of chickens provided an excellent model for postinfectious AIDP, producing inflammatory lesions like those of EAN and secondary demyelination with axonal sparing (Prineas, Wright 1972). The disease was transferred with spleen cells to normal chickens (Schmahl et al 1975) and associated with both CMI and IgG antibody formation against peripheral nervous system myelin (Stevens and collaborators 1981).

Myasthenia Gravis and Experimental Autoimmune Myasthenia Gravis

Research on myasthenia gravis (MG), the leading example of autoimmune disease mediated primarily by antibody, involved mostly morphologic and immunofluorescence techniques before the discovery of the EAMG model by Patrick and Lindström in 1973. This model was investigated intensively over the ensuing two decades and the same techniques and concepts applied to an almost simultaneous analysis of lesion pathogenesis in the human disease (Table 26-4). EAMG was accepted early as a valid model and antibody was accepted as the principal mediator of disease.

The introduction of T-cell cloning in 1980 led to recognition of the importance of T cells in fueling the anti–acetylcholine receptor (AChR) antibody response and in providing a cell-mediated component to lesion pathogenesis, as suggested by Lennon in her earliest EAMG studies. Immunodominant epitopes, for both T and B cells, were found to be in the α subunit of the AChR. Stefansson has suggested that molecular mimicry, involving microorganisms of the gastrointestinal tract, may be responsible for the pathogenic auto-

immune response. On the other hand, Hohlfeld and Wekerle have recently emphasized the importance of thymic myoid cells bearing AChR as possible initiators of autoimmunization. The thymus plays no role in EAMG, which, in their view, may not provide a correct model for MG pathogenesis.

The study of immune regulation in MG and EAMG was initiated by Pachner and Kantor, who were able to obtain lines of AChR-specific suppressor T cells. Drachman et al adapted some of the newer techniques for inducing tolerance, such as oral administration of antigen, to the EAMG model in the hope of finding new and specific approaches to therapy of the human disease.

Other Autoimmune Diseases Mediated Primarily by Antibody

Investigation of the approximately twenty *paraneoplastic syndromes* began with the systematic studies of the Lambert-Eaton myasthenic syndrome (LEMS) by Newsom-Davis et al starting in 1981, followed by Kornguth's description (in both human subjects and an animal model) of blindness associated with a loss of the large ganglion cells of the retina (1982), and Greenlee and Brashear's first report on progressive cerebellar degeneration (1983). Subsequent studies by these and others, Posner in particular, have concerned humoral antibody as the principal mediator of disease, the identification of target antigens in the nervous system (and corresponding tumor antigens), and the cell function(s) affected by the action of antibody. In LEMS, for example, voltage-gated calcium channels in presynaptic motor nerve terminals were found to serve as the target and apparently identical channel proteins in the responsible tumor, as the immunizing agent (Lang, Newsom-Davis 1985, 1987).

Investigation of the *neuropathic syndromes associated with monoclonal gammopathies* began in the early 1980s. In the best studied of these syndromes, the elevated IgM proved to be a specific antibody binding to carbohydrate epitopes shared by myelin-associated glycoprotein (MAG), several glycoproteins, and two glycolipids known as SGPG and SGLPG (Latov; Quarles; Ilyas; Shy, and others). Yu et al, in the later 1980s, developed rabbit and rat models involving antibody against SGPG-like epitopes expressed in axolemma and nerve terminals and in vascular endothelium. Research on *monoclonal gammopathies with multiple myeloma* demonstrated formation of IgG or IgA with λ as the principal light chain, reactive with endoneurial constituents or chondroitin sulfate. Patients were found to commonly exhibit the *POEMS syndrome* (polyneuropathy, organomegaly, endocrinopathy, myeloma, and skin changes) (Bardwick et al 1980) or *Crow-Fukase syndrome* (Nakanishi et al 1984). Whereas the neuropathologic changes have been thought to be mediated by antibody, the other abnormalities have been tentatively ascribed to neuropeptides/cytokines (e.g., TNF) released from the malignant lymphoid cells (Gherardi et al 1994).

Certain patients with *primary motor neuron disease* (MND) or *amyotrophic lateral sclerosis* (ALS) were

Table 26-4.
Myasthenia Gravis and Experimental Autoimmune Myasthenia Gravis

1949	Castleman, Norris	Lymphoid follicles in the thymus of some cases of MG
1950–70		Light and electron microscopic studies of changes at neuromuscular junction; immunofluorescence studies of antibodies to muscle; myoid cells in the thymus; unsuccessful attempts to produce a myasthenia model with whole muscle as antigen
1968	Goldstein	Autoimmune thymitis (guinea pig): release of peptide Tpo → binding to AChR and MG manifestations
1973	Patrick, Lindström	Production of EAMG in rabbits by immunization with *Torpedo* AChR (purified with α-bungarotoxin from the banded krait)
1973	Fambrough, Drachman	AChR found to be molecular target of MG pathogenesis
1975	Lennon, Lindström	Importance of CMI followed by antibody in EAMG pathogenesis (in rats)
1976	Lindström, Lennon	Circulating antibody to AChR found in 80%–90% of MG patients
1976	Toyka; Lindström	Antibody and cell transfer: animal to animal, human to animal
1976	Fuchs	Genetic basis of EAMG susceptibility
1976, 1978	Engel; Lennon	Mechanisms of receptor loss, contribution of C to damage of neuromuscular junction
1977	Kao, Drachman	Myoid cells in thymus shown to carry AChR
1978	Lindström	Use of AChR subunit peptides to induce EAMG
1979	David	Role of MHC in EAMG susceptibility
1980	Nakao	Additional susceptibility genes in IgH
1982	Thomas, Newsom-Davis	Immunohistochemical and tissue culture studies of thymus changes in MG: CD4+ T cells, B cells/plasma cells, antibody, immune complexes
1984	Hohlfeld	Cloning of AChR-specific T cells from MG patients' thymus
1984, 85	Pachner, Kantor	EAMG in mice: effector T-cell lines and clones, adoptive transfer of disease; suppressor lines
1985	Lennon	Multiple epitopes in AChR: immunodominant epitope in α subunit of AChR: 125–147
1985	Stefansson	Antibodies in MG sera react with GI flora: *Escherichia coli*, *Proteus vulgaris*, *Klebsiella pneumoniae*
1987	Hohlfeld, Toyka	Cloning of AChR-specific T cells from blood and lymph nodes of MG patients
1988	Berrich-Aknin	T-cell epitopes in α subunit of AChR: 125–143, 257–271, 351–368
1992	McIntosh, Drachman	Tolerance in EAMG by injection of AChR coupled to syngeneic cells
1993	Schönbeck et al	Heterotopic transplantation of MG thymus in SCID mice → functioning human thymus tissue and lasting production of antibody vs AChR
1994	Okumura, Drachman	Oral tolerance in EAMG by feeding AChR
1994	Hohlfeld, Wekerle	Fundamental difference between MG (evidence that disease starts in thymus) and EAMG (immune response is entirely peripheral)
1995	Shenoy	Use of TCR V_β knockout mice to determine TCR usage in genesis of EAMG

AChR = acetylcholine receptor; CMI = cell-mediated immunity; C = complement; TCR = T-cell receptor; MHC = major histocompatibility complex; IgH = immunoglobulin heavy chain; SCID = subacute combined immune deficiency.

shown in 1986 to express high titers of IgM associated with plasma cell dyscrasia (Shy, Rowland et al 1986). The principal reactivity of the IgM antibody was found to be directed at unique epitopes (Gal(β1-3)GalNAc and Gal(β1-3)GlcNAc) of gangliosides GM_1 and GD_{1b}. Other patients were reported (Appel 1992) to have antibody against a calcium channel protein in the motor nerve terminal, apparently acting on a different epitope than that affected in LEMS. Engelhardt, working with Appel (1986, 1990), described guinea pig models that he named *experimental autoimmune motor neuron disease*, with degeneration of spinal anterior horn cells and muscle atrophy without inflammation, and *experimental autoimmune gray matter disease*, affecting both upper and lower motor neurons, but with significant accompanying inflammation.

The neurologic complications of *systemic lupus erythematosus* have been shown for the most part to be antibody mediated. Development of standardized batteries of tests for cognitive dysfunction in the late 1970s made it possible to distinguish several strikingly different mechanisms: deposition of immune complexes of

antibody, for example, with DNA, in the choroid plexus, leading to membranous or vascular choroidopathy (Kofe et al 1974; Schwarz, Roberts 1984); antibody against phospholipids with anticoagulant activity, related to microinfarction and dementia (Mueh 1980); and antibody against neuronal constituents producing cognitive dysfunction up to the level of psychosis (Bluestein, Zvaifler 1982; Denburg 1985). Isolated angiitis, in patients with neuropathy, was shown to be an inflammatory, largely monocytic disease that can be mediated by CMI rather than antibody (Lisak 1988). CNS lesions can be studied in lupus-prone strains of mice such as NZB × NZW hybrids or MRL mice.

Other diseases studied in the 1970s and 1980s in which antibody may play a pathogenetic role included Sydenham's chorea, with antibody against neurons of the caudate and subthalamic nuclei (Husby 1976); obsessive-compulsive disorder, with antibody against opiates (Roy et al 1986); major depression, with antibody against both opiates and somatostatin (Roy et al 1988); and the stiff-man syndrome, with antibody against GAD (Solimena 1988).

Neuroimmunologic Diseases Associated with Infection

The modern era in investigation of infectious diseases began with the description of MHC restriction (Zinkernagel and Doherty 1974), which permitted analysis of the respective roles of CD4- and CD8-bearing T cells in immunopathologic reactions of the nervous system, as well as a molecular definition of selective events in the thymus.

Viral Diseases

Viral infections of the nervous system, in humans and animals, can lead to any of several quite distinct immunologic outcomes (Table 26-5). Conditions in which a virus in the nervous system elicits an immunologically mediated inflammatory reaction directed to viral antigens differ sharply from conditions in which viral infection results in autoimmunization, with inflammation and destruction of white matter.

Acute viral encephalitides fall outside the scope of the present review. However, the acute encephalomyelitis produced by Sindbis virus in mice illustrates an important point: The immunologic mechanism underlying lesion production may be distinct from that resulting in viral clearance. The acute disease has the hallmarks of a CMI response to virus while clearance is mediated entirely by antibody, as D. Griffin and her colleagues showed (1972, 1977). Clearance results from the shut off of viral synthesis in infected cells by signals from the viral antigen-antibody complex at the cell surface.

In human T-cell lymphotropic virus type I (HTLV-I)–associated myelopathy/tropical spastic paraparesis (HAM/TSP), the CD4+ T lymphocyte is the principal site of infection. The virus persists in mutated form in blood and spinal fluid cells. Serologic studies began in the late 1970s in Japan, the Caribbean, Africa, and the Seychelle Islands, and were followed by cellular investigations, principally by Jacobson, McFarlin, and their colleagues and by Usuku and Osame et al. Lesions appear to be produced by CD8+ T cells reactive against viral antigens associated with MHC class I on the CD4+ cells. There is no sign of autoimmunization against myelin antigens and no explanation for the CNS localization.

Visna-maedi in sheep is often regarded as a model for HAM/TSP. Its pathogenesis was well worked out by the mid-1970s by Sigurdsson et al in Iceland and later by workers in the United States (Nathanson, Panitch, Haase, Brahic). Narayan et al, in the late 1970s and 1980s, established that virus enters the CNS within monocytes as a so-called Trojan horse, and that the immune response to persistent virus is responsible for the characteristic inflammatory demyelinative lesions and is inhibited by immunosuppressive therapy. Antigenic variation contributes significantly to viral persistence

Table 26-5.
Neuroimmunologic Diseases Associated with Viral Infection*

Human Disorders		Animal Models	
Acute Viral Encephalomyelitis			
—	Viral encephalitis	1955/72/72	Sindbis virus (mice)
Chronic Viral Encephalomyelitis			
1956/79	HAM/TSP	1940/58/77	Visna/maedi (sheep)
		1934/75/76	Theiler's murine encephalitis virus
Acute and Subacute Autoimmune Encephalomyelitis			
1938	ADEM (PIE)	—/1943/76	Canine distemper
		1949/79/83	JHM (coronavirus) (rats)
		1962/87/88	Measles virus (rats, mice)
		1971/78/83	Semliki Forest virus (mice)
Acute, Subacute, and Chronic Autoimmune Neuritis			
1918	AIDP, CIDP	1907/72/75	Marek's disease (chickens)
Chronic Viral Encephalomyelitis, with Failure of Specific Cell-Mediated Responses			
1933/69	SSPE	1936/58/76	Lymphocytic choriomeningitis virus
1975	PRP		
1950	PML	1949/72/—	JHM (coronavirus) (mice)
1985	AIDS dementia	1985	Simian immunodeficiency virus
Chronic "Prion" Encephalomyelitis, with Failure of All Immune Responses			
1920	Spongiform encephalitis	1936/69/—	Scrapie, etc (primates, mice)

*Dates refer to description of disease, identification of virus, and demonstration of major immunologic elements in disease process.
HAM/TSP = human T-cell lymphotropic virus type I–associated myelopathy/tropical spastic paraparesis; ADEM = acute disseminated encephalomyelitis; PIE = postinfectious encephalomyelitis; AIDP = acute inflammatory demyelinating polyneuropathy; CIDP = chronic inflammatory demyelinating polyneuropathy; SSPE = subacute sclerosing panencephalitis; PRP = progressive rubella panencephalitis; PML = progressive multifocal leukoencephalopathy.

and the occurrence of relapses. In a second model, *Theiler's murine encephalitis virus (TMEV)*, the chronic demyelinative phase of infection is eliminated by immunosuppressive therapy, and therefore the disease must be immunologic (Lipton, Dal Canto 1975). Nevertheless, virus persists in CNS glial elements throughout the chronic phase (Brahic et al 1981) and the disease is related to DTH against virus and is MHC class I restricted (Lipton et al; Rodriguez 1985). CD8+ T cells make up the principal reacting population, as with visna and HAM/TSP. The pathogenic immune response has no autoimmune component, as shown by adoptive transfer and reciprocal cross-tolerance experiments involving TMEV and EAE (Miller et al 1987).

As early as 1940, Hurst and King proposed that viral diseases primarily affecting white matter such as canine distemper be considered as models for human demyelinative diseases. This view remains widespread and accounts for continuing interest in these conditions and in new "demyelinating" models. These are listed as "autoimmune" in Table 26-5 and are discussed in the section Other Autoimmune Diseases Dependent Primarily on T Cell–Mediated Immunity.

Failure of the T-cell response (see Table 26-5) may occur because of specific downregulation, as in *subacute sclerosing panencephalitis* (SSPE) and *progressive rubella panencephalitis* (PRP); actual damage or destruction of CD4+ T cells, as in *progressive multifocal leukoencephalopathy* (PML) (in patients with sarcoid, Hodgkin's disease, CLL, or acquired immunodeficiency syndrome (AIDS)) and *AIDS dementia;* or finally the absence of any effective immune response, as in the prion-mediated *spongiform encephalopathies.* SSPE occurs after measles infection in early childhood, and PRP follows congenital or early childhood rubella virus infection. Both show diminished CD8+ T-cell responsiveness to viral antigen (Dhib-Jalbut et al 1988; Wolinsky 1975, 1981). On the other hand, the high antibody titers (Vandvik 1976) imply that Th2 responses are intact or increased. A unique feature of SSPE is that the intracellular virus undergoes progressive loss of viral antigens, M in particular (ter Meulen 1969; Hall, Choppin 1979), and there is decreased expression of virus at the cell surface.

A convincing model of SSPE and PRP is provided by *animals "tolerant" of lymphocytic choriomeningitis virus* (LCMV) after neonatal infection (Traub 1936). Such animals often produce antiviral antibody in later life, accompanied by significant immunopathologic change in the brain. Their tolerance, in current terms, represents a shift from Th1 to Th2, with loss of the ability to clear virus associated with increased help for antibody production. LCMV resembles TMEV in being MHC class I rather than MHC class II restricted (Doherty 1976). CNS disease produced by LCMV in nontolerant mice is actually mediated by CD8+ T cells, and these animals show H-2D–restricted DTH. Virus-specific cytotoxic CD8+ cells clear virus efficiently when transferred to a tolerant infected host.

JHM virus infection in mice may be regarded as an imperfect model of PML. There is actual destruction of T cells in the thymus (Hanaoka 1972), yet there may be a significant antibody response. The lesions, however, as in PML, result from direct viral attack on oligodendroglia (Weiner, Stohlman, Lampert, others). The 15 years of research on *AIDS* and, since 1985, the feline and simian immunodeficiency virus (FIV and SIV) models, have pointed up several separate problems, all relatively new in immunopathology: the mechanism of CD4+ T-cell loss (the principal candidate currently is apoptotic cell death (Ameisen 1992)), the role of a Th1 to Th2 shift in preventing an effective immune response (Sher, Gazzinelli 1992), and the cause of tissue damage expressed as "white matter pallor" (possibly high local production of TNF and other CKs by infected macrophages/microglia (Giulian, Pullian 1991)).

Bacterial and Parasitic Infections

Many bacterial and parasitic infections affecting the nervous system lack credible animal models, and immunologic studies have had to be carried out on human subjects, sometimes in remote sites. In spite of all the difficulties, it is clear that the disease patterns are the same as those observed with viruses: direct infection of the central or peripheral nervous system, associated with an immunologic response to the infectious agent itself; autoimmunization by antigens of the infectious agent and disease production by autoaggressive T cells or autoantibody or both; and chronic disease resulting from infection with failure or "deviation" of the normal immune response.

Lyme disease, produced by *Borrelia burgdorferi,* belongs in the first category. There is in fact considerable similarity between the manifestations of chronic Lyme disease and those of HAM/TSP. Infected individuals form both antibody and T cells specific for the parasite (Pachner 1965). There is, however, an autoimmune component of the response as well (Link et al 1986; Martin 88; Lassmann 1990). *Cerebral toxoplasmosis* (*Toxoplasma gondii*) is another example. Here, fortunately, there is an excellent mouse model, which has been the subject of thorough investigation, mainly since 1990, by Sher and Gazzinelli, and others. The CMI response to the parasite is mediated by specific CD8+ T cells and nonspecific natural killer (NK) cells (with help from CD4+ cells) and macrophages; it involves the successive actions of IL-12 and IL-2 (to turn on the CD8 and NK participants), IFN-γ and TNF-α (to turn on the macrophages), and NO to suppress parasite replication in macrophages and in neurons. In human subjects whose Th1 response fails (e.g., because of AIDS) and in mice with a genetically determined tendency to make a Th2 type of CD8 response (with production of IL-4, IL-10, and transforming growth factor (TGF)-β), the infection can become generalized and overwhelm the host.

An autoimmune response (antibody mediated) was identified by Husby in the late 1970s as the cause of *Sydenham's chorea* (following hemolytic streptococcal infection). The antibody reacted with both streptococcal cell membrane constituents and neurons of the caudate and subthalamic nuclei. In the mid-1980s, it was found that gastrointestinal infections with certain strains of *C. jejuni* may be followed by the demyelinating form of GBS and, a few years later, the same organism was proved to be responsible for the axonal form of GBS and possibly the sensorimotor variant. The evidence for molecular mimicry in these cases is very strong, but the studies so far have been limited to antibody. One should recall here that gram-negative gastrointestinal organisms have also been incriminated as possible causative agents in MG.

American trypanosomiasis or *Chagas' disease*, produced by *Trypanosoma cruzi* and widespread in South and Central America, is characterized by autoimmune responses to multiple components of the nervous system (and also the heart). The neurologic findings include peripheral neuropathy, lymphocytic infiltration, and destruction of parasympathetic ganglia (with secondary effects such as megacolon). Autoantibodies to Schwann cells and the nerve sheath were found by Khoury and by Cossio and others in the 1970s, and to neurons by Wood (1982). A mouse model was described by Eisen and Said in 1985. Since 1990, several autoantigens playing a role in lesion formation have been characterized, mainly by Reed. Notable among these are a cysteinyl proteinase that stimulates both CMI and autoantibody responses, and a neuronal ribosomal phosphoprotein, both cross-reactive with parasite epitopes.

Leprosy is the outstanding example of a microbial infection that induces different neurologic diseases depending on the balance between Th1 and Th2 responses. *Mycobacterium leprae* infects skin and Schwann cells, with production of characteristic skin lesions and neuropathy. Patients with tuberculoid leprosy show a DTH to protein antigens of the organisms and develop well-localized skin and nerve lesions containing few bacteria. At the same time, the cutaneous nerves are invaded and destroyed by a granulomatous reaction containing many giant cells. In patients with lepromatous leprosy, DTH and the lymphocytic reactions of CMI are lacking, titers of antibody are high, the inflammatory response fails, the organisms multiply freely, and the host may die. CD4+ T cells greatly outnumber CD8+ cells in tuberculoid lesions (Kaplan 1982). In lepromatous lesions, in contrast, CD8+ T cells predominate and foamy macrophages full of dividing *M. leprae* occupy the endoneurium and perineurium. Their inability to kill the organisms has been attributed to the absence of IL-2 and IFN-γ. The high levels of antibody neither protect nor contribute to the pathogenesis. Modlin, Bloom, and Sasazuki, starting in 1986, published work suggesting that the failure of CMI in lepromatous leprosy is due to CD8+ suppressor T cells in the lesions, specific for TCR idiotypic determinants of an epitope-specific suppressor-inducer T cell and producing IL-4 (Bloom et al 1982). Since the numbers of mast cells and macrophages are increased in the lesions, they may also serve as sources of the IL-4.

Biologic Aspects of Neuroimmunology

Some biologic aspects of neuroimmunology are presented here in the form of selected highlights, listed in chronologic sequence in a series of tables.

Immune Responses Within the Nervous System

Early studies established that immune reactions differing in mechanism (anaphylactic, immune complex, CMI) maintain their character when they are elicited within the nervous system; "bystander" effects are determined principally by their quantitative aspects and the amount of secondary tissue damage, but may include functional changes as well (Table 26-6). In particular, CKs such as IL-1 and IL-6, IFN-γ, and lymphotoxin or TNF can produce significant changes in adjacent glial and vascular function. With prolonged local antigenic stimulation, as in responses to CNS infection (toxoplasmosis, syphilis) or to tissue autoantigens (MS), such immunologic reactions may evolve to form more or less typical lymphoid tissue within the CNS.

Research after 1980 addressed the problem of identifying the site at which antigen presentation occurs in the central and peripheral nervous systems. Glial elements (astrocytes, Schwann cells) and parenchymal elements (myoblasts) as well as microglia and vascular endothelium were all found to express MHC class II af-

Table 26-6.
Immune Responses within the Nervous System

1941	Jervis; Kopeloff	Bystander effects of anaphylactic and immune complex reactions in CNS
1952, 1953	Poursines; Frick, Lampl; Vollum	Bystander effects of tuberculin reactions in CNS
1962	Silverstein	Congenital toxoplasmosis, syphilis: plasma cells in Virchow-Robin spaces
1979	Prineas	MS: "lymphoid tissue" in Virchow-Robin space
1981	Lampert	Pathologic implications of immunologic reactions in the CNS
1981	Fontana	Astrocytes (interferon-γ): MHC expression, cytokine production, antigen presentation
1986	McCarron, McFarlin	CNS vascular endothelium (interferon-γ): similar findings
1987	Goto; Samuel	Schwann cells (interferon-γ): similar findings
1988	Lassmann; Hickey	Perivascular macrophages are site of antigen presentation in CNS in vivo
1992	Goebels	Myoblasts (interferon-γ): similar findings as in other neural elements

ter stimulation with IFN-γ or TNF and to be capable of acting as antigen-presenting cells in vitro, presenting antigen to specific reactive T cells. However, studies with chimeric animals showed unequivocally that such presentation in vivo is a function of short-lived perivascular monocytes/macrophages.

The Brain as an Immunologically Privileged Site

The prolonged survival of allografts, whether of skin, neural tissue, or purified glial cells, within the CNS (Table 26-7) was long attributed to the absence of lymphatic drainage or the presence of a blood-brain barrier, or both. Only after Cserr's studies did it become clear that there is in fact efficient drainage of antigens by way of both lymphatic channels and the bloodstream. This entire problem was reconsidered after the discovery, by Mossman and Coffman in 1988, of Th1/Th2 relationships and the demonstration that antigen introduced into the brain induces a strong specific Th2 response in the draining lymph nodes and spleen, analogous to the "immune deviation" of responses to antigen introduced into the eye (Streilein). Th2 cells are strongly downregulatory for the characteristic Th1 cells that mediate responses like graft rejection or EAE.

The same considerations (absence of efficient antigen drainage, blood-brain barrier) underlay the early hypothesis that brain antigens are "sequestered" and thus fail to induce thymic or peripheral tolerance (specific T-cell anergy or deletion). It is now clear that myelin and astrocyte antigens, such as MBP and S100-β, are present in the thymus but fail somehow (quantitative reasons? incorrect presentation?) to induce tolerance. When such antigen is purposely injected into the thymus, specific downregulatory cells are generated and immune reactivity mediated by Th1 cells is suppressed. The body's normal state with respect to such antigens appears to be one of "immunologic ignorance," that is,

a failure to react simply because no immunization has occurred.

Autoimmunization by Infectious Agents

The idea of molecular mimicry as the basis for autoimmunization against neural antigens has a long history, but received its first solid experimental support only within the last 20 years (Table 26-8). Examples abound of immunization by viruses, bacteria, parasites, and even tumors, giving rise to either antibody or immune T cells reactive with neuronal cytoplasmic or membrane components or with other elements of neural tissue such as myelin.

As a consequence of the apparent explanatory power of the molecular mimicry hypothesis, however, little attention has been paid to other mechanisms of autoimmunization such as that described by Steck, immunization by host components incorporated in a viral envelope. This process may well underlie the complex pathogenic immune response to Semliki Forest virus, and it requires investigation as a possible mechanism in the genesis of postinfectious forms of ADEM and AIDP, which are usually induced by enveloped viruses.

Psychoneuroimmunology/ Neuroendocrinimmunology

There was a long interval between the first studies suggesting that neurologic "stress" could affect immune responses and that this effect might be mediated by the hypothalamic-pituitary-adrenal axis (HPA) and the first serious modern studies of these relationships (Table 26-9). Functional assessments at the level of the whole organism and of lymphoid cells in culture, begun in the late 1970s, were paralleled by the discovery of close anatomic and molecular interactions among the three systems. Only in the 1990s did it become clear that neurotransmitters, neuropeptide hormones, and certain

Table 26-7.
Suggestion That the Brain Is Immunologically Privileged

1948	Medawar	Allografts of skin to brain are accepted, attributed to blood-brain barrier and absence of lymphatic drainage.
1979	Aguayo	Allografts of nerve to CNS are accepted.
1983	Gumpel	Allografted oligodendrocytes survive in brain.
1986	Le Douarin	Xenograft of spinal cord in chick embryo survives for several months.
1988	Nicholas, Arnason	Allografts of brain in ventricles are long-lived.
1988	Cserr	Drainage of antigens in brain or CSF is via olfactory nerves and cribriform plate to cervical LN and through choroid plexus to blood.
1988	Hochwald, Thorbecke	Antigen in brain or CSF induces Th2 in cervical LN.
1991	Harling-Berg	MBP injection into ventricular CSF induces antibody formation and "tolerance" to EAE.
1962	Waksman	Concept: antigens sequestered in CNS fail to reach thymus and to induce tolerance.
1970	Ellison	MBP injection in thymus induces "tolerance" to EAE.
1992	Campagnoni	MBP homologue is present normally in thymus.
1994	Khoury	MBP injection in thymus induces generation of specific downregulatory cells.
1995	Kojima, Linington	S100-β is also present in thymus.

CSF = cerebrospinal fluid; LN = lymph node; MBP = myelin basic protein.

Table 26-8.
Autoimmunization Induced by Infectious Agents: Some Examples

Molecular Mimicry		
1976	Husby	Sydenham's chorea: cross-immunization between streptococcal cell memnbrane and neurons of subthalamic and caudate nuclei
1983	Fujinami, Oldstone	Cross-immunization between peptides of vaccinia, measles, herpes, and vimentin or keratin
1984	Kaldor	Antibodies in GBS (AIDP) cross-reactive with myelin and specific strains of *Campylobacter jejuni*
1985	Fujinami, Oldstone; Jahnke, Alvord	Sequence homologies between peptides of common viruses and peptides of MBP, P2, etc
1982, 1984, 1986	Latov; Quarles; Ilyas et al	Antibodies in polygammopathies cross-reactive with myelin glycoprotein/glycolipids
1985	Stefansson	Antibodies in MG cross-reactive with *Escherichia coli, Proteus vulgaris, Klebsiella pneumoniae* in gut
1985, 1987	Lang, Newsom-Davis	Antibody against tumor Ca^{2+} channels reactive with channels in motor nerve terminals.
1988	Martin; Lassmann	Anti-*Borrelia* antibodies/T cells include antibodies/T cells vs myelin components, e.g., MOG
1992	Yuki, Miyatake	Antibodies in GBS (AMAN) cross-reactive between axonal glycolipids and *Campylobacter* strains
1992	Reed	*Trypanosoma cruzi*: Cross-reaction between ribosomal phosphoprotein and homologous human protein
1995	Wucherpfennig, Strominger	Viral and bacterial peptides with steric configuration comparable to encephalitogenic peptide of MBP reactive with MBP-specific T cells from MS patients
Other Biologically Significant Mechanisms		
1979	Steck	Host antigen in viral envelope induces both CMI and antibody; vaccinia virus grown in brain → EAE
1981	Fontana; others	Virus infection results in systemic dissemination of interferon-γ, which upregulates MHC expression on macrophages, astrocytes, etc.
1982, 1983, 1985	Nepom, Plotz, Greene	Antibody vs idiotype of antiviral antibody (e.g., anti-reovirus HA) is effectively antibody vs neuronal components (β_2-adrenergic receptor)
1984	Webb	Semliki Forest virus infecting brain induces CMI vs viral proteins but antibody vs brain glycolipids
1993	Kalman, others	Superantigen → relapse of specific autoimmune disease

MBP = myelin basic protein; GBS = Guillain-Barré syndrome; AIDP = acute inflammatory demyelinating polyneuropathy; MG = myasthenia gravis; MDG = myelin oligodendrocyte glycoprotein; AMAN = acute motor axonal neuropathy; MS = multiple sclerosis; CMI = cell-mediated immunity; EAE = experimental autoimmune encephalomyelitis; HA = hemagglutinin.

Table 26-9.
Psychoneuroimmunology/Neuroendocrinimmunology: Some Highlights

Before 1930	Pavlov	Conditioned reflexes are demonstrated.
1936	Selye	Stress acts via HPA axis on immune response.
1938, 1940	Evans; Ingle; Wells and Kendall	HPA hormones (ACTH, cortisone) cause lymphoid involution.
1975	Ader, Cohen	Conditioned reflex can affect immune responses.
1976	Stein	Depression (bereavement) diminishes immune responses.
1977, 1981	Bartrop et al; Keller	Stress reduces nonspecific T-cell responses.
1981	Carroll	Depression augments HPA activity.
1970	Hadden	Immunocytes express receptors for neurotransmitters.
1980	Blalock	Neuropeptide hormones act on lymphocytes and are produced by them in response to immunologic, endocrine, and neurologic stimuli.
1981	Felten; Bulloch, Moore	Autonomic innervation of lymphoid organs is shown.
1988	Chelmicka-Schorr, Arnason	Sympathectomy increases immune responses.
1955	Atkins	Endogenous pyrogen, from stimulated macrophages, acts to stimulate hypothalamic nuclei.
1969	Gery	LAF (now called IL-1), from stimulated macrophages, acts on T cells.
1982	Dinarello	EP and IL-1 are the same molecule.
1982	Fontana	Stimulated astrocytes make IL-1 and other CKs.
1988	Breder, Saper	IL-1, TNF, and other chemokines are made by neurons in hypothalamic and periventricular nuclei, and serve as neurotransmitters for "vegetative" functions.
1992	Breder et al	PGE-secreting cells in organum vasculosum of lamina terminalis (OVLT) mediate between CKs in circulation and neurons secreting CKs.

HPA = hypothalamus-pituitary-adrenal; LAF = lymphocyte-activating factor; IL = interleukin; CK = cytokines; TNF = tumor necrosis factor; PGE = prostaglandin E; IL-1 = interleukin-1; EP = endogenous pyrogen.

cytokines are all produced by and able to act on target cells within each of these systems and that all are involved in patterned responses to exogenous behavioral, neurologic, or immunologic stimuli. The hypothalamic-pituitary-thyroid and -gonadal axes (HPT and HPG) play a role as well.

General References

Blalock JE, ed. Neuroimmunoendocrinology. *Chem Immunol* 1992;52:1–195.

Cohen IR, ed. *Perspectives on Autoimmunity.* Boca Raton: CRC Press, 1988.

Cross AH, Vincent A, Racke MK. *Conference Report: Fourth International Congress of Neuroimmunology.* Amsterdam, 1994. *J Neuroimmunol* 1995;58:117–120.

Davis MM, Buxbaum J. T-Cell Receptor Use in Human Autoimmune Diseases. *Ann New York Acad Sciences* 1995;756:1–464.

Dunnett SB, Richards S-J, eds. Neural Transplantation, from Molecular Basis to Clinical Applications. *Progr Brain Res* 1990;82.

Edelson RL, ed. Antigen and Clone-Specific Immunoregulation. *Ann New York Acad Sciences* 1991;636:1–410.

Gash JM, Sladek JR. Transplantation into the Mammalian CNS. *Progr Brain Res* 1988;78.

Goetzl EJ, Adelman DC, Sreedharan SP. *Neuroimmunology. Adv Immunol* 1990;48:161–190.

Goldstein RA, ed. Neuroimmune disorders. *Immunology and Allergy Clinics of North America* 1988;8:183–348.

Heber-Katz E, Waksman BH. A workshop on Thymus, Clonal Deletion, and Suppressor Systems in Demyelinating Diseases. *J Neuroimmunol* 1992;36:231–238.

Hohlfeld R, Lucas K, eds. Cytokine networks in multiple sclerosis. *Neurology* 1995;45,Suppl 6:S1–S55.

Keane RW, Hickey WF, eds. *Immunology of the Nervous System.* Oxford: Oxford University Press, 1995.

Kies MW, Alvord EC, Jr, eds. *"Allergic" Encephalomyelitis.* Springfield: Charles C Thomas, 1959.

Lassmann H, Waksman BH, Brosnan CF. Mechanisms of vascular and tissue damage in demyelinating diseases. *J Neuroimmunol* 1991;32:83–85.

Lennon V. Cross-talk between nervous and immune systems in response to injury. *Progress in Brain Res* 1994;103:289–292.

Möller G, ed. Chronic Autoimmune Diseases. *Immunol Rev* 1995;144:1–314.

Raine CS, ed. Advances in Neuroimmunology. *Ann New York Acad Sciences* 1988;540:1–745.

Schwartz RS, Rose NR, eds. Autoimmunity: Experimental and Clinical Aspects. *Ann New York Acad Sciences* 1986; 475:1–427.

Silverstein AM. *A History of Immunology.* San Diego: Academic Press, 1989.

Waksman BH, ed. Immunologic Mechanisms in Neurologic and Psychiatric Disease. *Assoc Res Nervous Mental Disease, Res Publs* 1990;68:1–336.

Wilder RL. Neuroendocrine-Immune System Interactions and Autoimmunity. *Ann Rev Immunol* 1995;13:307–338.

Zauderer M. Origin and significance of autoreactive T cells. *Adv Immunol* 1989;45:417–437.

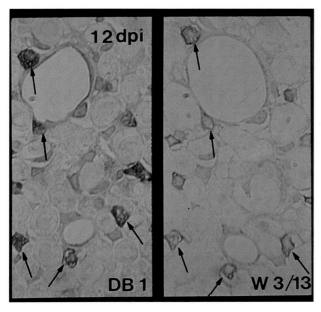

12 dpi

DB 1

W 3/13

Plate I. IFN-γ expression in EAN. Adjacent one micrometer cryosections of ventral root from a Lewis rat with active EAN. Prior to onset of disease, on day 12 after immunization, IFN-γ immunoreactivity (labeling with monoclonal antibody DB-1) can be detected and is mostly associated with invading T lymphocytes recognized by the monoclonal antibody W3/13.

Macrophages   T cells

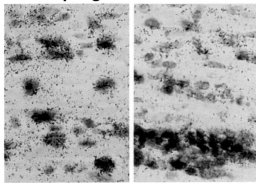

18 d active EAN

Plate II. TGF-β expression in EAN. Coincident with clinical recovery, mRNA for TGF-β1 is upregulated in actively induced EAN in the Lewis rat. Combined immunohistochemistry and in situ hybridization localizes mRNA to both macrophages and T cells.

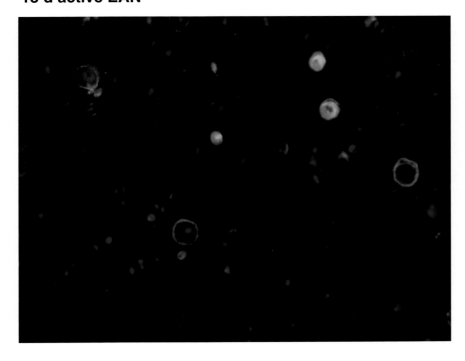

Plate III. Myelin-associated glycoprotein (MAG) expression and localization of IgM deposits in anti-MAG neuropathy. Two-color immunofluorescent light microscopy of a sural nerve biopsy specimen from a patient with anti-MAG neuropathy shows MAG stained red and IgM stained green. This cross-section shows characteristic circular green IgM deposits surrounding some fibers. The colocalization of red and green stains gives a yellow color. There are numerous MAG-positive fibers without any IgM deposits and one circular IgM deposit without MAG staining.

Plate IV. The longitudinal section of the sample used for Plate III shows colocalization of MAG and IgM deposits mostly in association with chevron-like structures that represent Schmidt-Lanterman incisures.

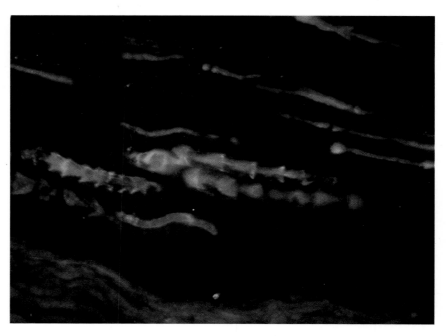

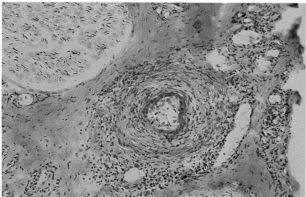

Plate V. Sural nerve biopsy specimen from a patient with nonsystemic vasculitic neuropathy showing perivascular and transmural mononuclear cell infiltration in an epineurial artery producing fibrinoid necrosis of the vessel wall. (Hematoxylin and eosin, ×70.)

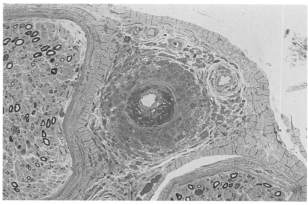

Plate VII. Recent necrosis of an inflamed epineurial vessel in a sural nerve specimen from a patient with polyarteritis nodosa–related vasculitic neuropathy. (Epoxy resin embedded, ×150.)

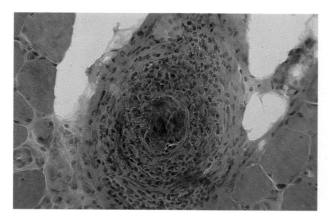

Plate VI. Perimysial artery obtained by peroneus brevis muscle biopsy from a patient with isolated peripheral nerve vasculitis, surrounded and infiltrated by an intense mononuclear cell infiltrate with accompanying vascular necrosis. (Modified Gomori trichrome, ×80.)

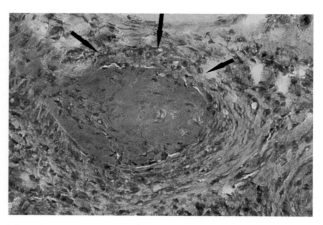

Plate VIII. Later stage of peripheral nerve vasculitis, demonstrating an epineurial artery with focal disruption of the vessel wall (arrows) and luminal obliteration by thrombosis. (Hematoxylin and eosin, ×100.)

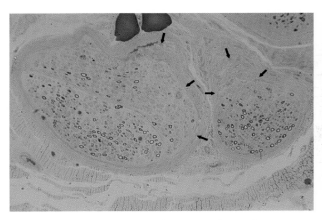

Plate IX. Two adjacent fascicles in a sural nerve biopsy specimen from a patient with rheumatoid vasculitic neuropathy, revealing interfascicular and intrafascicular variation in fiber loss, including two peripheral sectors (arrows) completely devoid of myelinated fibers. (Epoxy resin embedded, ×100.)

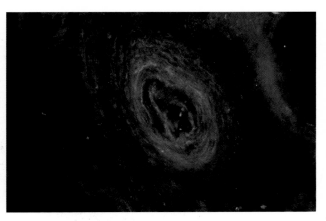

Plate XII. Immunofluorescent staining of sural nerve from a patient with systemic necrotizing vasculitis, showing a single epineurial vessel with transmural deposition of IgM. (Fluorescein-conjugated anti-human IgM, ×125.)

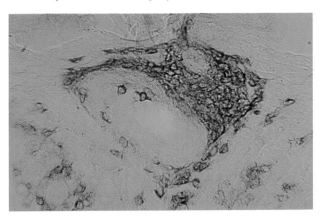

Plate X. Section of superficial peroneal nerve stained for CD2 antigen in a patient with isolated peripheral nerve vasculitis and perineuritis. Two epineurial vessels are surrounded and focally invaded by T cells. (Avidin-biotin-peroxidase, ×100.)

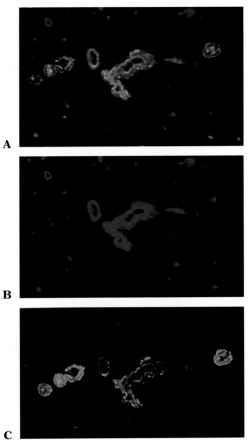

A

B

C

Plate XIII. Endomysial vessels on a transverse section of a fresh-frozen muscle biopsy specimen from a patient with dermatomyositis. The section was immunostained with both *Ulex europaeus* and avidin-rhodamine, which highlights the endothelial cells of the endomysial vessels with a red fluorescence (B), and with antibodies to the C5b-9 membranolytic attack complex (MAC), which highlights the complement deposits with a green fluorescence (C). (A) The double exposure of B and C produces a yellow color from the superimposition of the red fluorescence on the capillary walls and the green fluorescence from the MAC deposits. The presence of MAC deposits on the capillaries implies injury mediated by complement-fixing antibodies. Note that in at least three small blood vessels the MAC has induced severe destruction of the endothelial cell wall, which becomes almost unstainable with *Ulex* (ghost capillaries).

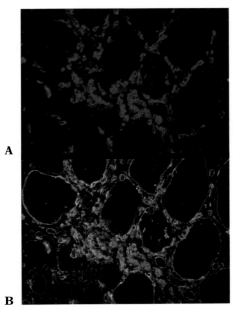

A

B

Plate XI. Cross-sections of muscle biopsy specimens from patients with polymyositis, immunostained for antibodies to CD8 (A) (in red) and MHC class I antigen (in green) dually exposed (B). Note the upregulation of MHC class I on both the infiltrating endomysial cells and the sarcolemma, even in the muscle fibers not surrounded by cells (B).

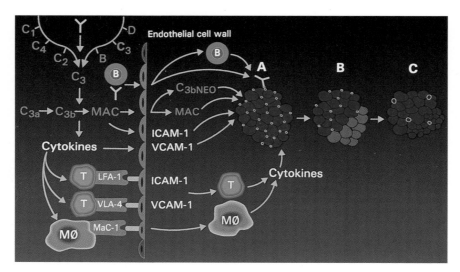

Plate XIV. Sequence of immunopathologic changes in dermatomyositis beginning with activation of complement and formation of C3 through the classic or alternative pathway by antibodies (Y) against endothelial cells. (A) Activated C3 leads to the formation of C3b, C3bNEO, and MAC that transverse across the endothelial cell wall to the endomysial capillaries. (B) Deposition of MAC leads to the destruction and reduced number of capillaries, with ischemia or microinfarcts most prominent in the periphery of the fascicle. (C) Finally, a smaller than normal number of capillaries with dilated diameters remain and perifascicular atrophy ensues. Not only the complement-fixing antibodies (Y) but also B cells, CD8+ T cells, and macrophages traffic to the muscle. The migration of cells from the circulation is facilitated by the vascular cell adhesion molecule (VCAM) and intercellular adhesion molecule (ICAM) whose expression on the endothelial cells is upregulated by the released cytokines. T cells and macrophages through their integrins, very late activation (VLA)-4, leukocyte function–associated antigen (LFA)-1, and Mac-1, bind to the VCAM and ICAM and traffic to the muscle through the endothelial cell wall.

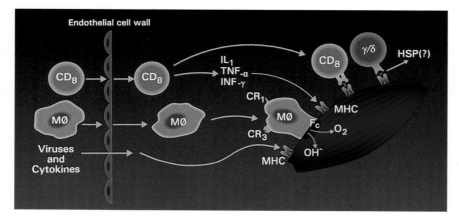

Plate XV. Sequence of events leading to polymyositis. The activated CD8+ cells and macrophages, through their integrins and counterreceptors expressed on the endothelial cells (shown in Plate XIV), traffic to the muscle. The CD8+ cells recognize on the muscle membrane unknown antigen presented in the context of MHC class I expression. Cytokines released in the circulation (possibly by viral infections) facilitate cellular extravasation and upregulation of MHC class I by the muscle fiber. Lymphokines, interleukin (IL)-1, tumor necrosis factor (TNF)-α, and interferon (IFN)-γ secreted by the activated T cells and macrophages enhance the myocytotoxicity and upregulate further the MHC class I expression. Rarely, γ/δ T cells that recognize heat shock protein can be the myocytotoxic cells. Macrophages expressing Fc receptors for IgG and complement are also activated and attach to the muscle fiber (via their Fc receptors), exerting a direct cytotoxic effect.

Brief Dictionary of Immunologic Terms

Accessory signals See Costimulatory signals.

Activation The process by which a resting cell, either a T cell, B cell, or macrophage, becomes stimulated and begins to function in its particular fashion. For T cells, this results in the secretion of cytokines, the production of new proteins, and proliferation. For B cells, this results in the production of cytokines and antibodies, and in antigen processing. For macrophages, this results in increased *phagocytosis* or ingestion of substances, secretion of cytokines, and processing and presentation of antigens.

Adhesion molecule A protein on the surface of white blood cells and endothelial cells that causes the white blood cells to "stick" or bind to the lining of blood vessels. Binding is increased in areas of inflammation. This allows white blood cells to pass through the vessel walls and enter tissues at sites of infection and inflammation.

Allogeneic Having a different genetic background than another member of the same species. Genetically unrelated individuals are allogeneic to one another.

Alpha/beta (α/β) T-cell receptor A *TCR* that is composed of one α and one β chain. More than 90% of T cells in the blood and lymphoid organs have this type of receptor. T cells with α/β receptors can be helper cells, cytotoxic cells, or suppressor cells and can interact with all antigens.

Altered peptide ligand A peptide that is able to bind to the antigen-binding site of the TCR but in so doing is able to only partially stimulate the cascade of intracellular signaling events necessary for full T-cell activation. As a result the T cell becomes incompletely activated and is then unresponsive to subsequent antigenic stimulation by the appropriate peptide ligand.

Anergic Being in a state of anergy.

Anergy An immunologic state in which a T cell or B cell is unable to respond to a particular antigen, even though it once had this capability. Anergy is an active process. It occurs when a T or B cell is exposed to its stimulating antigen in the absence of *costimulatory* signals that are necessary for cell activation. Anergy is a means of regulating immune responses to potentially "dangerous" autologous antigens. It is believed to occur during the development of the normal immune system. If autoimmune cells lose their anergy, they have the potential to cause autoimmune disease.

Antibody Proteins produced by B cells. Unactivated B cells have antibodies only on their surfaces. After activation and differentiation, B cells become specialized antibody-producing cells called *plasma cells*. Antibodies are found in almost all fluids of the body and also on the surfaces of B cells. In contrast to T cells, antibodies can combine with antigen directly, without the need for antigen processing or interaction with additional proteins. Reactions of antibody with antigen can cause the rapid removal of the antigen, can activate a series of enzymes that can kill cells (such as complement), and can result in the release substances (such as histamine) that cause disease (e.g., asthma). Antibodies can also activate macrophages, causing them to ingest or phagocytose foreign materials such as bacteria. There are five classes of antibodies (IgA, IgD, IgG, IgM, and IgE). Each have their own special functions and each are concentrated in different parts of the body.

Antigen Any material that has the capability of stimulating an immune response. Some antigens can be recognized directly by cells of the immune system or by antibodies. Others need to be degraded, processed, and presented in association with proteins of the MHC in order to be recognized by T cells.

Antigen presentation The process by which antigen is processed or catalyzed, combined with other proteins, usually those of the *MHC*, and re-expressed on cell surfaces. Antigen presentation is necessary for T cells to recognize and interact with antigen. It is an active process performed by *antigen-presenting cells*.

Antigen-presenting cell (APC) A cell that has the capacity to ingest, degrade, process, and present an antigen on its surface. The most efficient APCs are macrophages. These are true "professionals." They not only process and present antigen in association with proteins of the MHC but also supply the necessary accessory or costimulatory signals required to activate T cells and B cells. Many cells in the body, including cells in the brain, such as astrocytes, can function as APCs. However, these "nonprofessionals" may not furnish the required costimulation or accessory factors. When antigen presentation occurs in the absence of costimulation, the immune cell may become unresponsive or *anergic*.

Antigen processing The metabolic pathway by which antigen is taken into a cell, degraded by enzymes, and then combined with other proteins in the cell so that it can be presented on the cells surface and be recognizable by T cells. Certain cells, such as macrophages and B cells, are especially efficient in this regard. (See Antigen presentation.)

Anti-idiotypic An immune response directed against the unique antigen-binding site of an antigen-specific receptor. Anti-idiotypic responses can be to the antigen-binding sites of antibodies or TCRs. They have the capability of greatly modifying the immune reactions of these molecules. Anti-idiotypic immune responses to the TCR of cells responsive to *MBP* may modify the course of multiple sclerosis in subpopulations of persons with this illness.

APC See Antigen-presenting cell.

Apoptosis An orderly series of programmed events resulting in the death of a cell. A number of different stimuli result in apoptosis, and it occurs during the normal course of T-lymphocyte maturation and selection in the thymus. Apoptosis is characterized by fragmentation of nuclear chromatin with nuclear membrane and cell wall lysis. For unknown reasons, apoptotic cells do not evoke inflammatory responses.

Astrocyte A cell in the central nervous system that has the capability to participate in immune responses in the central nervous system. Astrocytes can process and present antigen and can secrete immunologically active cytokines. When exposed to interferon-γ, astrocytes are induced to express class

II MHC proteins on their surfaces. Thus, they acquire the capability of stimulating CD4+ lymphocytes. However, astrocytes are not "professional" APCs and are not capable of providing optimal costimulation to T cells. This can result in T cells becoming anergic after contact with antigen-presenting astrocytes.

Autoimmune disease A disease that occurs when the immune system is stimulated by a substance that is a normal constituent of an organisms body. This can result in an immune attack against that substance and the organ that produces it. Examples of autoimmune diseases are certain forms of thyroiditis, type I diabetes, and possibly multiple sclerosis.

Autoimmunity A condition in which the immune system recognizes and responds to an antigen that is a normal constituent of the body. This can occur under normal conditions, for example, during lymphocyte ontogeny, when the immune system recognizes its own MHC proteins. It also can result in disease states.

Autologous Refers to ones own self as opposed to a genetically identical but different individual (syngeneic). Identical twins are syngeneic as are inbred strains of animals.

B Cell An immunocompetent cell that arises in the bone marrow, and then matures or differentiates in the bone marrow or certain other lymphoid tissues (as the spleen and lymph nodes). B cells produce antibody molecules that travel to the cell surface and interact with antigens. This in turn stimulates and activates the B cell to make even more antibody. Each B cell expresses a unique antibody and no two B cells are the same. Some B cells are only activated by antigens when certain T-cell cytokines are present. These responses are called *T cell dependent*. Other B cells recognize antigen directly, without a requirement for costimulation by T cells. These are called *T cell–independent responses*. The main function of B cells is to secrete antibodies. They do so by interacting with antigen and then differentiating to become plasma cells. B cells can also function as APCs. They are very efficient in this regard as they can concentrate particular antigens on their surfaces by virtue of their cell surface antibodies.

Bone marrow The organ present within long bones and vertebral bodies where all immune cells originate. It is also the site where B cells and macrophages differentiate and mature.

CD The abbreviation for *cluster of differentiation*. It is used to categorize the large numbers of proteins on the surfaces of immunocompetent cells. These proteins are given numbers. Some are described here.

CD3 A set of cell surface proteins found only on T cells. They are part of the TCR complex and are necessary for signal transduction from the cell membrane to the cytoplasm once an antigen occupies the antigen-binding site of the TCR.

CD4 A protein found on the surface of a subpopulation of T cells. The CD4 protein binds to class II MHC proteins. T cells with CD4 on their surfaces (CD4+ T cells) recognize antigen in association with class II MHC proteins. This population of T cells is essential for the initiation of many immune responses, including those that produce antibodies and those that produce cytotoxic or "killer" T cells. The CD4 protein on the surfaces of CD4+ T cells interacts with class II MHC proteins and stabilizes the interaction of the TCR and the antigen-MHC complex.

CD8 A protein on the surface of subpopulations of T cells that are usually cytotoxic cells. CD8 interacts with class I MHC proteins. T cells that have CD8 on their surfaces (CD8+ T cells) recognize antigen in association with class I MHC proteins. The CD8 protein interacts with a portion of the class I MHC protein and stabilizes the bond between the TCR and antigen-MHC complex.

Class I MHC proteins A set of proteins on the surface of *almost all* cells of the body. These proteins are recognized by the immune system when a foreign (allogeneic) organ is placed into the body. They induce a very strong immune response that can destroy the transplanted organ. *Autologous* class I proteins are recognized under normal conditions. This occurs during the process of *antigen presentation*. Pieces of processed antigen lodge in the folds or clefts of the class I proteins on the surfaces of APCs. This combination (antigen plus class I protein) is recognized by the CD8+ T cells. Different class I proteins bind different antigens. If an antigen cannot fit into the antigen-binding groove of a class I protein, it will not be recognized by CD8+ T cells. Class I proteins differ among individuals. The genes producing them are inherited. Each person has a mixture of class I genes from their parents and this mixture varies among siblings. Only monozygotic twins have exactly identical class I genes.

Class II MHC proteins A set of proteins on the surface of *some* cells of the body, usually only activated macrophages and B cells and specialized APCs called *dendritic cells*. Other cells, such as astrocytes, can be induced to express class II proteins by exposure to cytokines such as interferon-γ. Class II MHC genes are inherited from both parents. Mixtures of genes will vary among siblings and only identical twins have the same class II MHC genotype. Class II MHC proteins play an essential role in antigen presentation. Pieces of processed antigen lodge in the folds or crevices of class II proteins. The complex of antigen and class II MHC protein is recognized by CD4+ T cells. The antigen-binding clefts of class II proteins vary from protein to protein. Some pieces of processed antigen will not fit into these clefts and therefore will not be recognized by CD4+ T cells. Helper/inducer T cells recognize antigen in association with class II proteins. These cells are required for the initiation and perpetuation of many immune responses. If class II MHC proteins are not present on the surfaces of cells acting as APCs, or are blocked by antibody covering these proteins, CD4+ T cells will not be activated. Antibodies to class II MHC proteins have been used as a means to modulate and suppress immune responses. Certain class II genes are present in a high percentage of patients with autoimmune disease such as multiple sclerosis. This suggests that these genes play a role in determining disease susceptibility.

Clonal deletion A mechanism for removing cells with the potential to react to autologous antigens. By this mechanism T cells that react strongly to autologous antigens or self-antigens are destroyed during their development in the thymus. When lymphocyte clones that have the capacity to produce autoimmune disease are deleted before they mature, the immune system becomes *tolerant* or unresponsive to these autoantigens. If the system fails, and "forbidden" clones are not killed, autoimmune disease may develop. Recent data suggest that clonal deletion is one of several mechanisms for preventing the development of autoimmune disease.

Costimulatory signals Additional signals required to activate T cells after they recognize antigen. If T cells interact with antigen in the absence of these accessory signals, these cells are "turned off" or made *anergic* (see Anergy).

Cytokine A biologically active material secreted by a cell. There are large numbers of cytokines, most of them having effects on the immune system. Examples of cytokines are tumor necrosis factor (TNF), interleukin-2 (IL-2), transforming growth factor (TGF), and interferon-β.

Cytokine receptor The receptor on the surface of a cell to which a particular cytokine binds, and through which it initiates the cascade of intracellular events that define the activity of this agent. Cytokine receptors may be bound to cell surfaces or released (soluble cytokine receptors). Administration of soluble receptors into the circulation can block the cellular effects of cytokines and have been used as treatment for noxious cytokine responses (such as septic shock).

Cytotoxic T cell A T cell that has the capacity to kill other cells after recognizing an antigen on the surface of the target cell. It kills the cell by secreting chemicals that "punch" holes in the targets surface. Most cytotoxic T cells are CD8+, and thus recognize their antigens in association with class I MHC proteins.

Delayed-type hypersensitivity response (DTH response) A pattern of immune responses that results from the activation of T cells, especially CD4+ T cells. This kind of immune response occurs in sensitized individuals about 48 hours after they are rechallenged with the sensitizing antigen. A good example of this is the skin swelling that occurs in purified protein derivative (PPD)–sensitive individuals after intradermal injection of PPD.

Dendritic cell A highly specialized, sessile cell present in skin, lymph nodes, and other organs that is highly efficient as an antigen-processing cell. There are different populations of dendritic cells, with different characteristics and probably different origins. Dendritic cells, especially those in the germinal centers of lymph nodes, may play an important role in immunologic memory by sequestering antigens for prolonged periods of time.

Determinant selection The process by which an MHC protein determines which antigens can be recognized by an organism's immune system. T cells only recognize antigens that have been processed, degraded into pieces or fragments, and then transported to the cell surface nestled in the antigen-binding grooves of MHC proteins. Different MHC proteins have different antigen-binding grooves. Thus, different antigen fragments will fit only in particular MHC antigen-binding clefts. If an antigen cannot be presented in association with an MHC protein, it will not be recognized by a T cell. Therefore, the repertoire of an individual's MHC proteins will determine which antigens can be recognized by that persons T cells. This phenomenon is important in defining which individuals develop certain diseases, particularly autoimmune diseases.

Determinant spreading An immunologic phenomenon in which an immune response is initiated by a particular antigen but then spreads to involve other antigens. It is believed that this occurs as a result of tissue destruction with release of other immunogenic proteins into the circulation.

Experimental autoimmune encephalomyelitis (EAE) An autoimmune disease induced in experimental animals by immunization with myelin or a myelin protein such as MBP or proteolipid protein. There are two forms of EAE, an acute form and a chronic relapsing form. The latter has been used as an animal model of multiple sclerosis. In some ways, EAE is similar to multiple sclerosis. For example, there is a genetic susceptibility with many of the same genes implicated in EAE as in multiple sclerosis (e.g., genes of the MHC and the TCR). However, multiple sclerosis in some animals is not a demyelinating disease. Nevertheless, information learned from EAE has been essential to our understanding of the role of the immune system in an autoimmune disease of the central nervous system. In addition, almost all treatments currently used for multiple sclerosis were first tested in animals with EAE.

Gamma/Delta (γ/δ) T-cell receptor A type of TCR in which the two protein chains making up the receptor are of the γ and δ type. T cells expressing such receptors comprise less than 5% of the total T-cell pool and their exact function in the immune system is not known. They are present in increased numbers in the skin and in mucous membranes. The γ/δ receptor–expressing T cells may be important as a first line of defense against bacterial infection. A very high percentage of these cells respond to heat shock (or stress) proteins.

Gut-associated lymphoid tissues (GALT) Accumulations of lymphoid tissues in the intestine in the form of intra-epithelial lymphocytes and Peyer's patches. There are increased numbers of T cells with γ/δ receptors in the GALT, as well as B cells expressing the IgA class of antibody. When antigens are presented to lymphocytes in the GALT, immune tolerance to these antigens is often produced. This phenomenon is called *oral tolerance*. It is being applied to persons with multiple sclerosis who are fed myelin in an effort to prevent immune responses to central nervous system myelin.

Heat shock proteins (HSPs) Families of proteins that are present within all cells of the body and are essential for the synthesis of new proteins and for degrading altered or denatured proteins. They also called *stress proteins*. Some HSPs are always present in cells; that is, they are *constitutive*. Others are induced by a wide variety of stresses such as heat shock, infection, or exposure to certain toxins. Of great importance is the fact that HSPs are phylogenetically conserved. Thus, HSPs in humans are very similar to HSPs in all other organisms, both mammals and bacteria. Immune responses to HSPs of bacteria have the potential to cause autoimmune responses in humans by virtue of their similarity to human HSPs.

Helper/inducer T cell A subpopulation of T cells involved in initiating and assisting other cells of the immune system. Functions include helping the differentiation of cytotoxic T cells and helping B cells differentiate into antibody-producing cells. Most helper/inducer T cells are CD4+. Thus, they recognize antigens only when complexed to class II MHC proteins.

Homing receptor (see Adhesion molecule) A protein present on the surfaces of endothelial cells that allows circulating lymphocytes and monocytes to "stick" and pass through the vessel wall. In this fashion lymphocytes and monocytes leave the blood and enter parts of the body that are infected or inflamed. A major question in contemporary biology is how these circulating cells know where to go in responding to an infection. A partial answer is that endothelial cells can be induced to express ligands that interact with proteins on the surfaces of lymphocytes and monocytes. These inducible proteins, called *homing receptors*, allow circulating cells to recognize the particular parts of the body in need of immune defense. Homing receptors are generated when endothelial cells are exposed to cytokines such as tumor necrosis factor and interferon-γ. Locally increased concentrations of these materials will lead to an increase in the numbers of inflammatory cells in that region by recruiting them to that site. Antibodies to homing receptors have been used experimentally to prevent the recruitment of cells to sites of inflammation. If there are homing receptors unique to brain capillaries, it may be possible to prevent inflammation in the brain by administering antibodies to these receptors.

Idiotype The unique tertiary structure of the antigen-binding site of an antigen-specific receptor. When antigen-specific receptors such as antibodies and TCRs can be used as antigens, immune responses to the idiotypic regions of these molecules occur. These responses, called *anti-idiotypic* responses, have the capacity to greatly modify the immune reactions of cells or antibodies expressing these idiotypes.

Anti-idiotypic responses to TCRs responding to MBP may ameliorate multiple sclerosis in subpopulations of persons with this disease.

Integrins   A family of receptors expressed on the surfaces of activated T cells. They are involved in lymphocyte homing to sites of tissue infection and inflammation and are required for lymphocyte binding to endothelial cells that express ligands for these receptors.

Interferon-β   A cytokine produced by white blood cells and many other cell types. It has a wide variety of effects on the body in general and on the immune system in particular. It can enhance immune activity as well as suppress cell proliferation. It acts in suppressing viral infections. It increases the killing capacity of cytotoxic T cells and increases the production of antibody by B cells. Many of its actions are the opposite of those of interferon-γ. Recombinant forms of interferon-beta are a therapy for multiple sclerosis.

Interferon-γ   A true lymphokine produced only by activated T cells. It has a wide range of effects that result in both enhancement and suppression of immune function. It also induces cells to produce new proteins. For example, it induces astrocytes to express class II MHC proteins on their surfaces. This in turn allows astrocytes to function as APCs for CD4+ T cells. Since such T cells only recognize antigen when complexed to class II MHC proteins, astrocytes functioning as APCs may contribute to the autoimmune process believed to occur in multiple sclerosis. In one unfortunate yet illuminating clinical trial, injections of interferon-γ increased disease activity in persons with multiple sclerosis.

Interleukin-1 (IL-1)   A cytokine produced by many different cell types but most often by activated macrophages. Activated astrocytes can also produce IL-1. This cytokine has a large number of biologic effects. For the immune system, IL-1 is necessary for the activation and differentiation of T cells. It may also cause astrocytes to multiply and thus may contribute to sclerosis or scar formation in the brains of persons with multiple sclerosis. When IL-1 is injected into the brain, it causes fever and sleep. One theory states that increased amounts of IL-1 in the brains of persons with multiple sclerosis cause the excess fatigue found with this illness.

Interleukin-2 (IL-2)   A cytokine produced by activated T cells, usually helper/inducer cells. IL-2 is necessary for the proliferation of activated T cells. It also contributes to the proliferation of astrocytes and may be involved in the sclerosis or formation of scar tissue in the brains of persons with multiple sclerosis.

Lymphocyte   An immunologically active cell originating in the bone marrow. It is one of the main components of the immune system. There are two large classes of lymphocytes, T cells and B cells. T cells are lymphocytes that migrated to the thymus gland, matured there, and then emigrated. These cells are involved in initiating and amplifying immune responses (see Helper/inducer T cells) and in killing cells (see Cytotoxic T cells). B cells are lymphocytes that matured in the bone marrow and other tissues such as the spleen and lymph nodes. B cells produce antibodies and also serve as APCs for T cells.

Lymphoid organs   Organs composed predominantly of lymphocytes. Lymphoid organs have a rich supply of blood vessels, as they are where lymphocytes enter the circulation and where they return. They are also where antigens are concentrated, processed, and presented to both T cells and B cells. Examples of lymphoid organs are the spleen, lymph nodes, and Peyer's patches. The latter are part of a lymphoid organ system in the intestine called the *gut-associated lymphoid tissue* (GALT). The GALT is especially important because antigens presented to lymphoid cells in this system result in the induction of tolerance.

Lymphokine   A cytokine produced by lymphocytes. An example of a lymphokine is interferon-γ.

Macrophage   A cell originating in the bone marrow that has a wide range of functions. Macrophages can ingest (phagocytose) substances and degrade and destroy them. As such they are able to process and present antigens and are among the most efficient of the APCs. They also produce immunologically active substances such as interleukin-1 and prostaglandins.

Major histocompatibility complex (MHC)   A complex of genes responsible for the production of a series of cell surface proteins called *major histocompatibility complex proteins*. MHC genes are inherited, with each individual receiving a mixture of genes from both parents. Each persons "blend" is relatively unique and constitutes that persons MHC *genotype*. There are two large classes of MHC genes, those that make class I MHC proteins and those that make class II MHC proteins. The two classes are further subdivided into families. In humans there are two families of class I proteins, HLA-A and HLA-B. There are three families of class II proteins, HLA-DR, HLA-DP, and HLA-DQ. Class I and class II proteins are found in different parts of the body. Class I proteins are found on the surface of all cells of the body. These proteins interact with antigens and are recognized by CD8+ T cells. Class II MHC proteins are found mainly on the surfaces of activated macrophages, B cells, and specialized APCs called *dendritic cells*. Certain lymphokines such as interferon-γ induce the expression of class II proteins in cells not usually producing them. Particular genotypes of MHC genes are strongly associated with certain diseases. In multiple sclerosis, there is a strong association between disease and the presence of particular class II MHC genes, especially the HLA-DR genes. This suggests (but does not prove) that MHC proteins are important in determining susceptibility to this illness (see Determinant selection).

MBP   Abbreviation for *myelin basic protein*.

MHC   Abbreviation for *major histocompatibility complex*.

Microglial cell   A cell present in the brain but probably derived from the bone marrow. It is believed to be a monocyte that migrated to the central nervous system and established residence there. It is very important in diseases where the brain becomes infected or inflamed. At such times, microglial cells become activated, look very similar to macrophages, and act as such. That is, they express class II MHC proteins on their cell surfaces, begin to ingest or phagocytose debris, present antigen to T cells, and secrete monokines such as interleukin-1 and prostaglandins.

Molecular mimicry   A phenomenon in which one molecule immunologically "looks" like another molecule. In other words, antigen Z is able to stimulate T cells that also recognize antigen A. This will occur if the two antigens have similar amino acid sequences such that they can interact with the same TCRs and MHC proteins or have a similar tertiary structure. Antigen Z may have entirely different origins yet contain peptides that are the same or similar to those of antigen A. The phenomenon of molecular mimicry can result in disease. This was demonstrated in humans with measles infections of the brain. Many of these individuals developed immune responses to the myelin antigen MBP (see Myelin basic protein). In some instances this was associated with an acute demyelinating disease (acute disseminated encephalomyelitis).

Monocyte   A cell derived from the bone marrow that is found circulating in the blood. Monocytes easily enter all organs of the body. Once a monocyte leaves the circulation, it may remain quiescent. More often it differentiates into a macrophage (see Macrophage).

Monokine   A biologically active substance made by monocytes and macrophages. Interleukin-1 is an example of a monokine.

Myelin basic protein (MBP)   A major protein of central nervous system myelin. When used as an antigen, it induces experimental autoimmune encephalomyelitis (EAE). Normal individuals have lymphocytes that can respond to MBP. Persons with multiple sclerosis have increased numbers of lymphocytes responding to MBP in their blood and spinal fluids. This may represent a *primary* phenomenon, one important for the development of disease. Alternatively it may represent a *secondary* phenomenon, one that occurs because of myelin destruction. When experimental animals are made tolerant to MBP, they do not develop EAE.

Myelin oligodendrocyte protein (MOG)   A myelin-specific protein that is highly encephalitogenic. Immune responses to MOG are present in persons with multiple sclerosis to a much higher extent than in persons with other neurologic diseases. This suggests that immune responses to MOG may be involved in the pathogenesis of multiple sclerosis.

Oral tolerance   The phenomenon whereby ingestion of an antigen results in a loss of immune response to that antigen. This phenomenon is currently being tested as a possible treatment for persons with multiple sclerosis.

PCR   The abbreviation for *polymerase chain reaction.*

Phagocytosis   The process by which a cell ingests or takes in outside material. While many cells can perform this function, some cells are "professionals" in this regard; that is, they have specialized biologic machinery to perform this task. The best example of this is the macrophage.

Plasma cell   A fully differentiated B cell whose main function is to produce antibodies. B cells become plasma cells after they come into contact with their stimulating antigen and after receiving *costimulatory signals* from helper/inducer T cells.

Polymerase chain reaction (PCR)   Molecular biologic technique that results in great amplification of small amounts of RNA and DNA, thus allowing their detection and analysis.

Prostaglandins   A family of proteins produced by macrophages when they become activated. High concentrations of prostaglandins are present at sites of inflammation. They cause changes in blood vessels and damage tissues directly.

Proteolipid protein (PLP)   Another major protein component of myelin. It produces experimental autoimmune encephalomyelitis when used as an antigen. Normal individuals have lymphocytes that respond to PLP. Patients with multiple sclerosis have increased numbers of PLP-responsive lymphocytes in their blood. It is not known whether this represents a *primary* phenomenon, contributing to the disease process, or whether it is a *secondary* response, occurring because of myelin destruction.

Selectins   A family of receptors on the surfaces of activated T cells. These receptors are involved in the homing of lymphocytes to sites of infection and inflammation. They bind to ligands on the surfaces of activated endothelial cells, that is, endothelial cells exposed to inflammatory cytokines such as interferon-γ. Selectin binding is essential for lymphocytes to leave the circulation and enter sites of tissue injury.

Stress proteins   See Heat shock proteins.

Suppressor cell   An immunocompetent cell that can suppress or "downregulate" the immune response of another cell. Suppressor cells can act in an antigen-specific fashion or can be nonspecific suppressors. They can exert their effects in a variety of ways, ranging from interactions with other T cells' TCRs to the secretion of a suppressive cytokine, such as transforming growth factor (TGF)-β. Cells secreting suppressive cytokines will modulate the effects of other T cells in their vicinity. This phenomenon is called *bystander suppression.*

T cell or T lymphocyte   A lymphocyte that originates in the bone marrow, migrates to the thymus gland where it matures and differentiates, and then emigrates. T cells are major components of the immune system. There are numerous populations of T cells. T-cell populations can be defined functionally (helper/inducer, cytotoxic, suppressor). They can be defined on the basis of the antigens they recognize (e.g., anti-MBP T cells). They can be defined on the basis of their T-cell antigen receptors (α/β or γ/δ). Finally, T cells can be defined on the basis of their cell surface proteins (CD4+, CD8+, CD4−/CD8−) and on the basis of the cytokines they secrete when stimulated. Please see definitions for each of these cell populations.

T-cell antigen receptor (TCR)   A protein dimer found only on the surfaces of T cells. It is the antigen-specific receptor of T cells. The TCR is composed of two peptide chains, either an α and a β chain or a γ and a δ chain. Each T cell has a unique TCR and no two T-cell TCRs are the same. Thus, TCRs are *clonally distributed.* The TCR cannot recognize antigen in isolation. It only recognizes an antigen that is processed and complexed to a protein of the MHC. Thus, it is different from an antibody molecule that can combine directly with antigen. Genes coding for TCR proteins are inherited and differ in different individuals. An individuals set of TCR genes determines the "library" of TCRs expressed on that person's T cells. The ability of a person to respond, or *not* to respond, to a particular antigen is determined in part by the library or repertoire of TCRs available for antigen recognition. A recent important observation shows that certain strains of mice respond to a particular antigen with a *very* restricted number of TCRs. In those strains one can prevent an immune response to that antigen by giving the mice antibodies against the TCR that bind to this antigen. This destroys the population of T cells expressing the particular TCR. Some investigators showed that persons with multiple sclerosis respond to MBP with a population of T cells that express a very limited number of TCRs. A preliminary trial in which persons with multiple sclerosis are immunized with these TCR proteins in the hope of selectively destroying the population of T cells responding to MBP is in progress. Results to date indicate that immune responses to TCR peptides can be modified and that therapeutic benefits in some persons with multiple sclerosis may result.

TCR   Abbreviation for *T-cell antigen receptor.*

Th0 cells   A population of cells that secretes patterns of cytokines that overlap with Th1 and Th2 cells. Th0 cells may be precursors of either Th1 or Th2 cells. More likely, Th1 and Th2 cells do not represent discrete populations but are probably the extremes of a continuum, with large numbers of cells producing multiple cytokines with overlapping phenotypes.

Th1 cells   A population of T cells that secretes particular cytokines when stimulated. These are interleukin-2, interferon-γ, and tumor necrosis factor-β. Th1 cells are involved in many delayed-type hypersensitivity reactions. They are involved in the pathogenesis of certain autoimmune diseases such as experimental autoimmune encephalomyelitis and possibly multiple sclerosis.

Th2 cells   A population of cells that secretes particular patterns of cytokines when stimulated. These cytokines are interleukin-2, -4, and -5, among others. Th2 cells are involved in helping B cells to respond to antigens and to differentiate. The actions of Th2 cytokines are frequently antagonistic to those of Th1 cytokines.

Thymus   An organ that is the site of T-cell differentiation and selection. The process of T-cell selection and expansion is a critical one since potentially pathogenic T cells must be eliminated while protective T cells must be selected and allowed to differentiate. The process whereby this occurs is not entirely defined but it involves the destruction of cells that express TCRs with too high or too low an affinity for self MHC and a selection of T cells with sufficient affinity for autologous MHC to allow for antigen recognition. About 90% of cells that enter the thymus die there, by the process of apoptosis. After puberty the thymus begins to involute or degenerate. Most adults have only a fatty tissue remnant of this organ. Under certain disease conditions the thymus can become active again. This occurs in the autoimmune disease myasthenia gravis.

Tolerance A condition in which the immune system is unable to respond to a particular antigen. Tolerance can occur naturally or it can be induced. There are multiple mechanisms for achieving tolerance. Cells responding to a particular antigen can be destroyed (clonal deletion). This occurs normally in the thymus during T-cell development. Cells can encounter antigen in the absence of costimulation, resulting in anergy. Cells can be exposed to cytokines that prevent their responses to antigen (bystander tolerance). Antibodies to TCRs can prevent activation of cells by antigen. Thus, tolerance can be either a negative phenomenon, with loss of immune reactive cells, or an active phenomenon.

Trimolecular complex The complex formed when proteins of the TCR bind to antigen that in turn has complexed to an MHC protein.

Tumor necrosis factor A cytokine produced by activated macrophages, T cells, and many other cells. It has a variety of immunologic functions such as activating T cells, activating B cells to produce antibodies, and activating other macrophages to secrete *prostaglandins*. When injected into the central nervous system, it causes fever and can destroy oligodendrocytes.

Western blot A technique used to determine which antigens bind to an antibody. A mixture of antigens is separated by electrical current. The separated antigens are then mixed with an antibody and the presence of antibody binding is detected using either a dye marker or radioactivity. It is a very sensitive technique and has been useful in detecting instances of molecular mimicry.

Index

Note: Page numbers with an *f* indicate figures; those with a *t* indicate tables; *pl.* indicates color plate numbers.

Acanthamebiasis, 190t
Acetylcholine receptors
    antibodies to, 343, 343f
        characteristics of, 346–347
        monoclonal, 346–347
        pathology of, 344
        synthesis of, 346
    antigen processing and, 351, 352f
    lymphocyte function in, 349t,
        349–351, 350f
    in myasthenia gravis, 342–345, 344f
    in neuromuscular junction, 340–342,
        341f
Acquired immunodeficiency syn-
    drome. *See* AIDS.
Acremoniosis, 190t
ACTH. *See* Adrenocorticotropic hor-
    mone.
Acute disseminated encephalomyelitis
        (ADEM), 107, 116–142, 396,
        399t. *See also* En-
        cephalomyelitis.
    cerebrospinal fluid in, 125–126
    clinical features of, 119–120
    diagnosis of, 125–126
    epidemiology of, 118–119
    Epstein-Barr virus and, 117
    evoked potentials for, 125
    Guillain-Barré syndrome with, 116
    with mass lesions, 138, 139f–141f
    multiple sclerosis after, 131–138, 142
    neuroimaging of, 126–127, 127f–137f
    neuropathology of, 120–122,
        121f–123f
    pathogenesis of, 123–124, 142
    recurrent, 138
    therapies for, 127–131, 142
    trigger for, 117
    after vaccination, 118
Acute hemorrhagic leukoencephalitis
        (AHLE), 116–117
    clinical features of, 118
    corticosteroids for, 129
    diagnosis of, 125
    mass lesion with, 138
    pathology of, 122, 123f
    recurrent, 138
Acute inflammatory demyelinating
        polyradiculoneuropathy. *See*
        Guillain-Barré syndrome.
Acute motor axonal neuropathy
        (AMAN), 294–295

Acute toxic encephalopathy, 138–142
ADC. *See* AIDS dementia complex.
ADCC (antibody-dependent cell-medi-
        ated cytotoxicity), 6, 21, 34, 74
ADEM. *See* Acute disseminated en-
        cephalomyelitis.
Adenohypophysitis, autoimmune, 392t
Adenovirus
    HIV with, 190t
    persistent infection with, 82t
Adhesion molecules. *See also specific
        types.*
    altered expression of, 83–85
    autoimmunity and, 18
    blockade of, 93
    CNS immune response and, 26–28,
        27f
    in glioma, 238–240, 239f
    immune cell recruitment by, 240
    in inflammatory myopathies,
        379–380
Adrenocorticotropic hormone (ACTH)
    HPA axis and, 59
    as immune cell neuropeptide, 59t,
        60t
    in lymphocytes, 62–63, 63f
    in pro-opiomelanocortin gene, 62f
Adult T-cell leukemia (ATL), 206
AHLE. *See* Acute hemorrhagic leuko-
        encephalitis.
AIDS (acquired immunodeficiency
        syndrome). *See also* HIV-1 in-
        fection.
    encephalitis in, 117
    epidemiology of, 189
    immunology of, 191–192
    myositis with, 380–381
    neurologic problems with, 189, 190t
    opportunistic infections in, 190t,
        199–200
    pyomyositis with, 375
    sensory neuropathy with, 388
    wasting syndrome in, 198, 198t
AIDS dementia complex (ADC), 190t,
        192t, 192–197, 193f–197f
    animal model for, 399t, 400
    cerebrospinal fluid in, 197t
    clinical features of, 192, 192t
    management of, 196–197
    pathology of, 192–194, 193f–197f
ALS (amyotrophic lateral sclerosis),
        149t, 162, 172, 397–398

Alveolitis, HTLV with, 207
Alzheimer's disease, 172–182
    clinical features of, 172
    complement proteins in, 176–178,
        176f–178f
    inflammation and, 173–180,
        174f–178f, 175t, 179t
    nongenetic causes of, 173
    pathology of, 172–173
    therapy for, 182, 182f
AMAN (acute motor axonal neuropa-
        thy), 294–295
Amoxicillin, for Lyme disease, 223t,
        224
Amphyphisin antibodies, 151t
Amyloidosis neuropathy, 312
Amyloid plaques
    anti-inflammatory therapy for, 182,
        182f
    complement proteins and, 176–178,
        176f–178f, 180
    microglia and, 178–180, 179t
    neurofibrillary tangles and, 172
Amyotrophic lateral sclerosis (ALS),
        149t, 397–398
    motor neuron dysfunction in, 162
    as neurodegenerative disorder, 172
ANCAs (anti–neutrophil cytoplasmic
        antibodies), 256, 258, 324,
        328f
Anergy
    apoptosis and, 92–93
    immune tolerance and, 14
    induction of, 95
Angiitis. *See also specific types.*
    granulomatous, 325
    immunopathology of, 255t, 256
    isolated, 260
        clinical features of, 262t
        immunopathology of, 255t
    microscopic
        classification of, 317t, 318t
        neuropathy with, 319
Angiography, for vasculitis, 262
Anisomorphic injury, 272
Antibodies. *See also* Monoclonal anti-
        bodies.
    to acetylcholine receptors, 343f,
        343–344
    B-cell secretion of, 3
    to calcium channels, 363–364, 364f
    in central nervous system, 28

Antibodies (*cont.*)
to Fas receptor, 245–246
to gangliosides, 368–370, 370f
in Lambert-Eaton myasthenic syndrome, 364–365, 365f
maturation of, 3
to muscle antigens, 343
for neural cells, 31–32
nonneutralizing, 85
pathogenic role of, 46–49
viral latency and, 83
Antibody-dependent cell-mediated cytotoxicity (ADCC), 6, 21
of CNS viral infection, 74
neural cell injury and, 34
Antiganglioside antibody disorders, 368–370, 370f
Antigen(s)
carcinoembryonic, 238–239
cytoplasmic, 376
differentiation, 233f
glycoconjugate, 42
lipid, 42
melanoma, 233, 233f
in neuromyotonia, 367
onco-neuronal, 150t
peptide alteration in, 236
peripheral nerve, 42–43
processing of, 4, 5, 15
sequestered, 9
specificity of, 2–3
T cell–dependent, 3, 6
transplant, 281–283
tumor, 233, 233f
in glioma, 238
T-cell recognition of, 229–233, 230f–233f
variation in, 80–82
Antigen-presenting cells (APCs), 3
clonal ignorance and, 9
costimulation of, 16, 20
in glioma, 229f–232f, 229–233
microglia and, 28–30, 29f
T-cell interactions with, 239f
transplant grafts and, 282, 283
Antigen-specific immunotherapy, 94–95
Anti-idiotypic responses, 9
Anti–neutrophil cytoplasmic antibodies (ANCAs), 256, 258, 324, 328f
Aortitis, Cogan's syndrome and, 261
APCs. See Antigen-presenting cells.
Apolipoprotein E4, in Alzheimer's disease, 173
Arachidonic acid, neuritis and, 45f, 45–46
Arteritis, 254–265. *See also specific types:* Vasculitis.
giant-cell, 317t, 318t, 322
immunopathology of, 255t
Arthritis
adjuvant, 61
experimental autoimmune, 9
Lyme disease and, 224
MHC linkage in, 13
rheumatoid
circadian rhythms and, 67

methotrexate for, 100
sympathetic nervous system in, 66
vasculitis with, 316, 320
Arthrogryposis multiplex congenita, 346
Aspergillosis, 190t
Asthma, 67–68
Astrocytes
in Alzheimer's disease, 180–182
macrophage chemotactic protein-1 and, 18
neural regeneration and, 271
neurotrophic functions of, 272–276, 274t, 275f
oligodendrocytes and, 274, 275f
Astrocytoma, 228, 237–238
Astroglia
antibodies for, 31–32
cell-mediated immune injury to, 33–37
ciliary neurotrophic factor and, 31, 34
immune reactivity of, 28–30, 29f
cytokines and, 30–31
Asymmetric polyneuropathy, 323
Ataxia
AIDS dementia with, 192t
cerebellar, 131
Miller Fisher syndrome with, 368
neuromyotonia with, 366
paroxysmal, 366
telangiectasia, 58
Autoantibodies. *See also* Antibodies.
in inflammatory myopathies, 376–377
for myasthenia gravis, 342
in vasculitis, 255t, 256
Autoantigens. *See also* Antigen(s).
neuroimmunology and, 17
Autoimmune diabetes disease model, 15
Autoimmune diseases
chemokines in, 18
cytokines in, 19–20
endocrine effects on, 57
experimental, 9, 391, 392t
inclusion-body myositis with, 375
MHC linkage of, 4, 13–14
Th1 cells in, 6
Autoimmunity, 13–22, 86
adhesion ligands in, 18
blood-brain barrier and, 13, 17–18
chemokines in, 18
components of, 14t
cytokines in, 18–20
infectious agents and, 402, 403t
mechanisms of, 20–21, 21f
in myasthenia gravis, 342–344, 343f, 344f
in neuromyotonia, 366–367
regulation of, 20
T-cell activation in, 15–18
tolerance and, 14–15
Autonomic nervous system
immunity and, 55
peripheral immune responses by, 64–65, 65f
Autonomic neuropathy

animal model for, 392t
HIV with, 198t
paraneoplastic, 149t
Autotoxicus, horror, 2
Axons. *See also* Neurons.
degeneration of, 387–389
regeneration of, 271, 385–389
Azathioprine, 97t, 100
for graft rejection, 289
for inflammatory myopathies, 381–382
for vasculitic neuropathy, 330f, 332
for vasculitis, 263–264
AZT (zidovudine), 196
myopathy with, 198t, 199

Bartonella henselae, 190t
B cells, 3
autoimmune tolerance of, 14
differentiation of, 6
follicular exclusion of, 9
maturational arrest of, 9
regulation of, 9
T-cell synergy with, 48f, 50
BCRF1 gene, in Epstein-Barr virus, 237
BDNF (brain-derived neurotrophic factor), 273–274, 274t, 386
Behçet's disease
clinical features of, 262t
HTLV and, 207
interferon-α for, 264
thalidomide for, 333
Bergmann gliosis, 154f
Biopsy
muscle, *pl.* VI–XIII, 376
sural nerve, *pl.* V–XII
Blood-brain barrier (BBB)
autoimmunity and, 13, 17–18
endothelium of, 72
grafts and, 286f–287f
HIV infection and, 194
immune-mediator entry through, 26–28, 27f
immune privilege of, 66–67, 72, 228, 282–283, 402t
Lyme disease and, 222–224
in multiple sclerosis, 105
viral damage to, 73
Borrelia burgdorferi, 218, 400. *See also* Lyme disease.
immunopathogenesis of, 221–222
pyomyositis from, 375
vasculitis with, 261
Brachial neuritis, 149t, 163
Brain
abnormalities of, in multiple sclerosis, 105–107
damage, 55–56
schizophrenia and, 55–56
development of, immunity and, 55–57, 57f
immune privilege of, 66–67, 72, 228, 282–283, 402t
immunologic control by, 55
lesions of, immunity and, 58
Brain-derived neurotrophic factor (BDNF), 273–274, 274t, 386

BRCA1 oncogene, 154
Breast cancer, 160
  neurologic syndromes with, 150t
Büngner's band, 385

Calcitonin gene-related peptide
  (CGRP), 388
Campylobacter jejuni, 124, 368–369,
  401
  Guillain-Barré syndrome after, 296,
    299, 300, 397
Candidiasis
  glioma and, 234
  HIV with, 190t
Canine distemper virus, 399t
  demyelination with, 117
  persistent infection with, 82t
CANOMAD syndrome, 368–369, 370f
Carcinoembryonic antigen (CEA),
  238–239
Carcinoid myopathy, 149t, 150t,
  164–165
  treatment of, 165t
Carcinomatous neuromyopathy, 149t
Castleman's disease, 311–312
CD3 protein complex, 2, 5
CD4+ T cells, 2, 5
  in autoimmune response, 14t
  in dermatomyositis, 164
  in glioma, 229f, 234–235
  in Guillain-Barré syndrome, 295,
    299–300
  in HIV infection, 189, 191–192
  immunosuppression of, 85–86
    corticosteroids for, 97–99
  in inflammatory myopathies, 378
  in leprosy, 401
  in multiple sclerosis, 395
  in paraneoplastic syndromes, 149
  in vasculitis, 257
  viral tropism and, 74
CD8+ T cells, 2, 5
  in autoimmune response, 14t
  in glioma, 229f, 234–235
  in Guillain-Barré syndrome, 295,
    299–300
  in HIV infection, 191–192
  in HTLV infection, 209–210
  in inflammatory myopathies,
    pl. XI–XV, 378–380
  in leprosy, 401
  in multiple sclerosis, 395–396
  in paraneoplastic syndromes, 149,
    166t
  in vasculitis, 257
  viral latency and, 83
  viral tropism and, 74
CEA (carcinoembryonic antigen),
  238–239
Cefotaxime, for Lyme disease, 223t,
  224
Ceftriaxone, 223t, 224
Central nervous system (CNS)
  grafts, 281–289
  HIV infection of, 189, 190t
  humoral immunity in, 28
  immune mediators of, 26–28, 27f,
    34

immune privilege of, 66–67, 72, 228,
    282–283, 402t
immune responses within, 28–31,
    29f, 401t, 401–402
  isolated angiitis of, 255t, 260, 262t
  Lyme disease and, 220t, 220–221
  paraneoplastic disorders of, 148, 149t
  regeneration of, 271–276
  tumors of, 228–246, 229f–233f,
    239f–242f
  vasculature of, 257
  viral infection of, 72, 73
Cerebellum. *See also* Paraneoplastic
    cerebellar degeneration (PCD).
  ataxia and, 131
  Hodgkin's disease and, 153, 153t,
    154–155
Cerebrospinal fluid (CSF)
  in encephalomyelitis, 125–126
  in vasculitis, 262
CGRP (calcitonin gene-related pep-
    tide), 388
Chagas' disease, 401
  HIV with, 190t
Chandipura virus, 117
Chemokines, 5
  across blood-brain barrier, 27f, 28
  in autoimmune diseases, 18
Chlorambucil, 381–382
Chronic inflammatory demyelinating
    polyneuropathy (CIDP), 294,
    300–301, 399t
  dysglobulinemia with, 307
  HIV with, 197–198, 198t
  immune responses in, 300–301
  immunotherapy for, 92
  pathology of, 300
  plasmapheresis for, 100
  steroid therapy for, 99
  treatment for, 301
CIDP. *See* Chronic inflammatory de-
    myelinating polyneuropathy.
Ciliary neurotrophic factor (CNTF),
    273, 274t
  astroglia and, 31, 34
Circadian rhythms, immune response
    and, 55, 67–68
cis-platinum neuropathy, 16
Cladribine, 97t, 100
CLIP (corticotropin-like intermediate
    peptide), 62f
Clonal deletion, 8
Clonal ignorance, 9
Clonal unresponsiveness, 8–9
CMV (cytomegalovirus), 190t, 199, 380
CNS. *See* Central nervous system.
CNTF (ciliary neurotrophic factor), 31,
    34, 273, 274t
Coccidioidosis
  HIV with, 190t
  vasculitis with, 261

Cogan's syndrome, 261
Combinatorial diversity, 232f
Complement
  Alzheimer's disease and, 176–178,
    176f–178f
  amyloid plaques and, 176–178,
    176f–178f
  in autoimmune neuritis, 49–50
  cytotoxicity and, 21
Connective tissue diseases
  inclusion-body myositis with, 375
  vasculitis with, 261, 262t, 318t,
    319–321
Copolymer 1, immunotherapy with,
    94, 110
Cornea, immune privilege of, 67, 282
Coronavirus, demyelination with, 117
Corticosteroids. *See also* Steroids.
  acute disseminated encephalo-
    myelitis (ADEM) and, 128–
    129
  for graft rejection, 288, 289
  for immunosuppression, 97
  for inflammatory myopathies, 381
  pulse therapy for, 101
  side effects of, 99
  for vasculitis, 263, 329–332, 330f
Corticotropin-like intermediate pep-
    tide (CLIP), 62f
Corticotropin-releasing hormone
    (CRH)
  in hypothalamus, 59–61
  as immune cell neuropeptide, 59t,
    60t
Costimulatory molecules, 240f,
    240–241
Coxsackieviruses, 380
CREB proteins, 205–206
C-region genes, 2, 3
CRH (corticotropin-releasing hor-
    mone), 59t, 59–61, 60t
Crow-Fukase syndrome, 163, 311–
    312
  animal model for, 392t, 397
Cryoglobulinemia, essential mixed,
    321–322
  classification of, 317t, 318t
  treatment of, 330f
Cryptococcosis, 190t, 199
Cutaneous leukocytoclastic angiitis,
    317t, 318t
Cyclophosphamide, 97t, 99–100
  for inflammatory myopathies,
    381–382
  for paraneoplastic syndromes, 165t
  pulse therapy for, 101
  side effects of, 100
  for vasculitic neuropathy, 330f, 331
  for vasculitis, 263
Cyclosporine
  for graft rejection, 288, 289
  immunosuppression with, 97t, 100
  for inflammatory myopathies,
    381–382
  for paraneoplastic syndromes, 166t
  for vasculitic neuropathy, 330f, 332
  for vasculitis, 263
Cyproheptadine, 165t

Cytokines, 5–7, 18–20
  anti-inflammatory, 5
  in autoimmune disease, 19–20
  circadian rhythms and, 67
  in CNS viral infections, 77
  glial cell immune regulation of,
      30–31
  in HIV infection, 192, 195, 197f
  in hypothalamus, 34
  in immune response, 14t, 19
  inflammatory, 14t, 19, 326
    astrocytes and, 274–276
    CNS injury and, 272
    myopathy and, 379
    neurotrophic activity of, 272t,
        272–273
  intratumoral delivery of, 244–245
  from macrophages, 4
  neural cell injury by, 33
  neuron regulation by, 58
  neuropeptides and, 58, 59t
  neurotransmitters and, 55
  proinflammatory, pl. I, 5, 44–45
  regulatory, 20
  switch, 20, 21f, 30
  Th2 cells and, 6
  for vasculitis, 264–265
Cytomegalovirus (CMV)
  HIV with, 190t, 199
  pneumonitis with, 380
Cytopathology, 20–21, 21f
Cytotoxicity
  antigen-directed, pl. XI–XV, 378–380
  complement-mediated, 21
  MHC gene expression and, 85
  T-cell, 20–21, 209–210, 210f

ddC (zalcitabine), 196, 198
ddI (didanosine), 196, 198
Dementia
  Alzheimer's disease and, 172
  HIV-related, 190t, 192t, 192–197,
      193f–197f, 197t
    animal model for, 399t, 400
Dendritic cells, 4
  follicular, 6
  immature, 4
Deoxyspergualin, 97t
Depression, antibodies in, 398
Dermatomyositis (DM), 164, 374–382
  clinical features of, 374
  immunopathology of, pl. XIII–XV,
      377–378
  as paraneoplastic syndrome, 149t
  treatment of, 165t, 381–382
Determinant selection, 8
Devic's syndrome, 125
Diabetes mellitus
  MHC linkage in, 13
  rat model for, 15
Didanosine (ddI), 196, 198
Differentiation antigenic peptides,
    233
Diphtheria vaccination, encephalo-
    myelitis after, 116, 118
Distal symmetric polyneuropathy
    (DSPN), 197–198, 198t

Diversity
  combinatorial, 232f
  junctional, 232
DM. See Dermatomyositis.
Dopamine, prolactin secretion and, 64
Down syndrome
  Alzheimer's disease in, 173
  IFN-α/β receptor gene in, 58
Doxycycline, for Lyme disease, 223t,
    224
D-region genes, 2, 3, 232f
DSPN (distal symmetric polyneuropa-
    thy), 197–198, 198t
Dysglobulinemic neuropathies,
    307–312
  IgA/IgG, 311–312
  IgM, pl. III–IV, 307–310
    treatment of, 310–311
Dysphagia, myositis with, 375

EAE. See Experimental autoimmune
    encephalomyelitis.
EAMND (experimental autoimmune
    motor neuron disease), 392t,
    398
EAN. See Experimental autoimmune
    neuritis.
EBV. See Epstein-Barr virus.
EGF (epidermal growth factor), 238
Electroencephalography (EEG), for
    encephalomyelitis, 125
Electromyography (EMG)
  for inflammatory myopathies, 376
  for Lambert-Eaton myasthenic syn-
      drome, 361
  for neuromyotonia, 365–366
Encephalitis, 399t
  ADEM after, 117–118
  herpes simplex, 117– 396
  HIV-related, 190t
  rabies, 118
  subgroups of, 118
  varicella-zoster virus, 117
Encephalomyelitis, 399t. See also spe-
    cific types
  cerebrospinal fluid in, 125–126
  collagen vascular disease versus, 125
  electroencephalography for, 125
  Lyme disease with, 220t, 221, 224
  muscle rigidity with, 160
  paraneoplastic, 156–159, 157f, 158f,
      162
  postinfectious, 116, 396
  postvaccinal, 116, 396
  prion, 399t
Encephalopathy
  HIV, 117, 192, 194f, 197f, 200
  limbic, 157, 165t
  Lyme disease with, 220t, 221
  pathogenesis of, 150t
  in temporal arteritis, 260
  toxic, 138–142
  vasculitis with, 262t
  Wernicke, 150t
Endorphins
  as immune cell neuropeptides, 59t,
      60t

immune effects of, 63
  in pro-opiomelanocortin gene, 62f
End-plate potentials (EPPs), 340–342
  antiganglioside antibodies and, 369,
      370f
  in Lambert-Eaton myasthenic syn-
      drome, 361–362
Enkephalins, 59t
env gene
  in HIV, 190
  in HTLV, 204, 205f
Epidermal growth factor (EGF), 238
EPPs. See End-plate potentials.
Epstein-Barr virus (EBV)
  BCRF1 gene in, 237
  as demyelination trigger, 117, 118
  lymphoma with, 228
  persistent infection with, 82t
  pneumonitis with, 380
  routes of entry, 72–73
Erythema migrans, 218
Essential mixed cryoglobulinemia,
    321–322
  classification of, 317t, 318t
Experimental autoimmune arthritis,
    9
Experimental autoimmune diseases, 2,
    391, 392t
Experimental autoimmune en-
    cephalomyelitis (EAE), 2, 26.
    See also Encephalomyelitis.
  demyelination in, 122f, 123f
  history of, 391–395, 392t–394t
  immune deviation in, 9
  immunoglobulin G in, 21
  macrophage chemotactic protein in,
      18
  monoclonal antibodies for, 96
  as multiple sclerosis model, 92
  myelin basic protein in, 7
  Th1 cells in, 2
  TNF-α and, 8
  triggers for, 123
Experimental autoimmune gray mat-
    ter disease, 398
Experimental autoimmune motor neu-
    ron disease (EAMND), 392t,
    398
Experimental autoimmune myasthenia
    gravis (EAMG), 2, 342–343,
    352–353. See also Myasthenia
    gravis.
  history of, 392t, 397, 398t
  immunogenetics of, 353
Experimental autoimmune neuritis
    (EAN), pl. I–II, 43f, 43–44, 392t
  Guillain-Barré syndrome and, 299,
      300
  ICAM-1 in, 44f
  immunoinflammatory response in,
      pl. II, 46, 46f–47f
  inhibition of, 45f
  macrophages in, 45f, 45–46
  mast cells in, 46
  myelin proteins in, 42
  pathogenic antibodies in, 46–49
  T cells in, pl. I, 43–44

Experimental autoimmune uveitis (EAU), 392t
Eye, immune privilege of, 67, 282

Fas receptor antibodies, 245–246
Fc receptors, 6
    histamine and, 6
    in vasculitis, 256
Fertility
    genes affecting, 57f
    immune effects on, 57
Fibroblast growth factors (FGFs), 273, 274t
Filaments, paired helical, 173
FK 506 (drug), 97t, 288
Follicular exclusion, of B cells, 9

GAD (glutamic acid decarboxylase), 15
gag gene
    in HIV, 190
    in HTLV, 204, 205f
GALT (gut-associated lymphoid tissue), 64
Ganglioneuromas, 159
Ganglioradiculoneuritis, 198t
Gangliosides, antibodies to, 368–370, 370f
Garin-Bujadoux-Bannwarth syndrome, 218, 220
GBS. See Guillain-Barré syndrome.
GCC. See Glucocorticoids.
Giant-cell arteritis, 322
    classification of, 317t, 318t
Glial cells
    immune privilege of, 66
    regulation of, 29f
    γ/δ T cells and, 33
Glial fibrillary acidic protein (GFAP), 28
Glioblastoma, 228, 237–239
Glioma, 241–245, 242f
    immune cell interactions in, 229f–232f, 229–233, 238–240, 239f
    immune response against, 228–229, 229f
    immunosuppression by, 67
    malignant, 242–244
    T-cell responses in, 233–238
    tumor antigens in, 238
Gliosis, Bergmann, 154f
Glucocorticoids (GCC). See also Corticosteroids.
    adjuvant arthritis and, 61
    circadian rhythms and, 67–68
Glucocorticoid receptors
    brain development and, 55–56
    HPA axis and, 57
    vasculitis and, 263
Glutamic acid decarboxylase (GAD), 15
Glycoconjugate antigens, 42
Glycolipids
    antibodies to, 296–299
    structure of, 297t
Goodpasture's syndrome
    autoantibodies in, 256
    plasmapheresis for, 264

Gottron's rash, 374
Gout, nerve damage from, 66
Grafts
    acceptance of, 282–283
    CNS, 281–289
    fetal, 283
        for Parkinson's disease, 281
    genetic disparity with, 283
    rejection of, 282
        immunopathology of, 284–288, 286f–287f
        treatment for, 288–289
    sequential, 289
    tissue trauma with, 283–284
Granulomatous angiitis, 260
Guillain-Barré syndrome (GBS), 198, 198t, 294–300, 399t
    acute disseminated encephalomyelitis with, 116
    after Campylobacter jejuni, 296, 299, 300, 397
    Epstein-Barr virus and, 118
    Fisher-Miller variant of, 124
    history of, 396–397
    Hodgkin's disease and, 164, 166
    immune responses in
        cellular, 299–300
        humoral, 295–299, 297t
    Miller Fisher syndrome and, 368
    myelin proteins in, 42
    as paraneoplastic syndrome, 149t
    pathology of, 294–295
    plasmapheresis for, 97, 100
    treatment of, 300
    varieties of, 294–295
Gut-associated lymphoid tissue (GALT), 64

HAM. See HTLV-I–associated myelopathy.
HCG (human chorionic gonadotropin), 59t
Heat shock proteins, 21, 108
Heberden's nodes, 66
Helical filaments, paired, 173
Henoch-Schönlein purpura, 259
    classification of, 317t, 318t
    vasculitis with, 321
Hepatitis B virus
    polyarteritis nodosa with, 325
    vasculitis with, 330f
Hereditary cerebral hemorrhage with amyloidosis (HCHWA), 173
Herpes simplex virus (HSV)
    encephalitis from, 117–118, 396
    HIV with, 190t, 199–200
    latency of, 83
    persistent infection with, 82t
    routes of entry, 73
Herpesvirus infection
    HIV with, 190t, 199–200
    latency of, 82–83
    multiple sclerosis and, 117
HHV-6 (human herpesvirus-6), 117
Histoplasmosis
    HIV with, 190t
    vasculitis with, 261

HIV-1 (human immunodeficiency virus type 1)
    demyelination with, 117
    discovery of, 189
    immunosuppression with, 85–86
    life cycle of, 190–191
    myositis with, 380–381
    persistent infection with, 82, 82t
    polymyositis and, 378
    routes of entry, 73
    superantigens of, 191
    transmission of, 204
HIV-1 infection, 189–200. See also AIDS.
    blood-brain barrier in, 194
    dementia with, 190t, 192t, 192–197, 193f–197f, 197t
        animal model for, 399t, 400
    dissemination of, 191
    epidemiology of, 189
    immunology of, 191–192
    management of, 196–197
    multinucleated giant cells and, 190, 193
    myopathy with, 198–199
    neoplasms with, 190t, 199
    neurologic problems with, 189, 190t
    neuromuscular disorders with, 197–199, 198t
    opportunistic infections with, 190t, 199–200
    pathogenesis of, 194–195
    virology of, 189–190, 190t
HIV encephalopathy, 117, 192, 194f, 197f, 200
Hodgkin's disease. See also Lymphoma.
    cerebellar dysfunction with, 153, 153t, 154–155
    Guillain-Barré syndrome and, 164, 166
    motor neuron syndrome with, 162
    polyradiculoneuropathy with, 163–164, 165t
    subacute motor neuronopathy with, 150t, 162–163
Horror autotoxicus, 2
HPA. See Hypothalamus-pituitary-adrenal (HPA) axis.
HSV. See Herpes simplex virus.
HTLV-I (human T-cell lymphotropic virus type I), 204–212, 205f, 205t–208t
    demyelination with, 117
    diseases with, 206–210, 208t, 210f
        immunopathogenic model of, 211–212
    genomic structure of, 204, 205f, 205t
    immune response to, 208–209
    myositis with, 380–381
    neural cell injury by, 32–33
    persistent infection with, 82t
    polymyositis and, 378
    routes of entry, 73
    transmission of, 204
HTLV-I–associated myelopathy (HAM), 206, 207t, 399t
    Lyme disease and, 400

HTLV-I–associated myelopathy (HAM)
(*cont.*)
pathology of, 207–209, 208t
T-cell receptor usage in, 210f,
210–211
HTLV-I–specific T-cell cytotoxicity,
209–210, 210f
HTLV-I tax, 204–206, 205t
peptide specificity of, 210, 210f
Hu antibodies, 151t
reactivity of, 156, 157f, 158f
Human chorionic gonadotropin
(HCG), 59t
Human diploid cell strain vaccine
(HDCV), 121
Human herpesvirus-6 (HHV-6), 117.
See also Herpesvirus infection.
Human immunodeficiency virus type
1. *See* HIV-1.
Human T-cell lymphotropic virus type
I. *See* HTLV-I.
6-Hydroxydopamine (6-OHDA), 64
Hypercortisolism, 57
Hypersensitivity vasculitis, 255t,
259–260, 321–322
clinical features of, 262t
Hypothalamus
cytokines in, 34
thermoregulation by, 58
Hypothalamus-pituitary-adrenal (HPA)
axis
circadian rhythms and, 67–68
glucocorticoid receptors and, 57
immune regulation by, 59–63,
61f–63f
in multiple sclerosis, 61
stress response and, 61f, 402–404,
403t

IAC (isolated angiitis of CNS), 255t,
260, 262t
IBM (inclusion-body myositis),
374–382
ICAM-1. *See* Intercellular adhesion
molecule-1.
Idiopathic polymyositis (IPM). *See also*
Polymyositis.
disease monitoring of, 101
immunotherapy for, 92
methotrexate for, 100
steroid therapy for, 99
Idiotypic responses, 9
IE (immediate early) genes, 83
Immune cells
adhesion molecules and, 240
glioma interactions with, 229f–232f,
229–233, 238–240, 239f
neuropeptides from, 59t
Immune complexes
vascular damage by, 327f
in vasculitis, 255t, 256–257
Immune-mediated injury, 31–34, 32f
Immune privilege
of CNS, 66–67, 72, 228, 282–283,
402t
of eyes, 67, 282
of testes, 67

Immune response(s)
adaptive, 5–8
alterations of, 86–88
categories of, 1
cell-mediated, 74–77, 76f
in central nervous system, 26–34
circadian rhythms and, 55
cytokines in, 19
deviation in, 9
evasion of, 80–86, 81f, 82t
genes in, 7–8
against glioma, 228–229, 229f
to HIV, 191–192
to HTLV, 208–209
humoral, 74
within nervous system, 401t,
401–402
in peripheral nervous system, 42
regulation of, 28–31, 29f
to viral infection, 74–77, 76f
Immunity, 17, 26–28, 27f
adaptive, 1–5
autonomic nervous system and, 55
brain development and, 55–57, 57f
brain lesions and, 58
cells of, 1–4
components of, 13, 391, 392t
innate, 1
mate selection and, 57
neural regulation of, 55–68, 385
regulation of, 59–63, 61f–63f
shared neural receptors in, 58–64,
59t–61t, 61f–63f
tumors and, 228–246, 229f–233f,
239f–242f
in vasculitis, 254, 255t
Immunization. *See* Vaccination.
Immunoglobulin(s) (Ig)
B-cell secretion of, 3
classes of, 3
intravenous
for Guillain-Barré syndrome, 300
for inflammatory myopathies,
381–382
for vasculitic neuropathy, 330f
for vasculitis, 264
in Lambert-Eaton myasthenic syndrome, 362–363
for multiple sclerosis, 96
Immunoglobulin A (IgA)
dysglobulinemic neuropathy,
311–312
in Guillain-Barré syndrome, 296
Immunoglobulin G (IgG)
in autoimmune encephalomyelitis,
21
dysglobulinemic neuropathy,
311–312
in Guillain-Barré syndrome, 295–
296
isotypes of, 6
in neuromuscular junction, 344f
in vasculitis, 256
Immunoglobulin M (IgM)
acetylcholine receptor antibodies
and, 347
in amyotrophic lateral sclerosis, 398

dysglobulinemic neuropathy,
pl. III–IV, 307–310
treatment of, 310–311
in Guillain-Barré syndrome, 295–298
MGUS, 163
in vasculitis, 256
Immunologic memory, 6–7
Immunologic tolerance, 14–15
anergy and, 14
induction of, 86
mechanisms of, 8–9
Immunomodulation, non–antigen-
specific, 95–97
Immunosuppression, 85–86
advantages of, 289
factors in, 236–237
for grafts, 284, 288
for inflammatory myopathies,
381–382
non–antigen-specific, 97t, 97–101
opportunistic infections with, 190t,
199–200
for paraneoplastic syndromes, 165t,
165–166, 166t
for vasculitis, 329–332, 330f
Immunotherapy
antigen-specific, 94–95
clinical principles for, 97–101
mechanistic strategies for, 92–94,
93f
for multiple sclerosis, 92, 93f
for paraneoplastic syndromes, 166t
principles of, 92–101
Inclusion-body myositis (IBM),
374–382
clinical features of, 375
immunopathology of, 378–381
treatment of, 381–382
Inflammation
Alzheimer's disease and, 173–180,
174f–178f, 175t, 179t, 182
cells, 7
immunocytochemistry of, 48f
Inflammatory myopathies, 374–382
autoantibodies in, 376–377
clinical features of, 374–376
diagnosis of, 376
immunopathology of, 377–381
treatment of, 381–382
types of, 374
viral infections with, 380–381
Influenza virus
encephalomyelitis after, 118
inflammatory myopathies and, 380
toxic encephalopathy after, 138
Insulin-like growth factor (IGF),
274–275
antisense, 243–244
Intercellular adhesion molecule
(ICAM)-1
in autoimmune neuritis, 44f
in autoimmunity, 18
CNS immune response and, 26, 27f
endothelial cells and, 7
gene regulation of, 85
in glioma, 237–240, 239f
in Guillain-Barré syndrome, 299

in inflammatory myopathies, *pl.* XI–XIV, 378–380
in multiple sclerosis, 106
rhinoviruses and, 73, 85
Schwann cells and, 40, 41f
steroid suppression of, *pl.* XIV–XV, 381
in vasculitic neuropathy, 326f, 326–327
Interferons, trisomy 16 and, 58
Interferon (IFN)-α
in CNS viral infections, 77
role of, 20
for vasculitis, 264
Interferon (IFN)-β
in autoimmune response, 14t
in CNS viral infections, 77
for immunotherapy, 93f, 95–96
for multiple sclerosis, 106
for paraneoplastic syndromes, 166t
Interferon (IFN)-γ
in autoimmune neuritis, *pl.* I, 44–45
in autoimmune response, 14t
in CNS viral infections, 77
endothelial cells and, 7
in inflammatory myopathies, 379
role of, 19
Interleukin (IL)-1
in Alzheimer's disease, 181
immune effects on, 57
Lyme disease and, 223
from macrophages, 4
role of, 19
stress response and, 56
Interleukin (IL)-2
function of, 6
for glioma, 242–243
HTLV and, 205t
in inflammatory myopathies, 379
for multiple sclerosis, 96
Interleukin (IL)-3, 205t
Interleukin (IL)-4
in autoimmune response, 14t
B-cell differentiation and, 6
downregulation by, 20
in inflammatory myopathies, 379
as switch cytokine, 20
transfected tumor cells by, 244–245
Interleukin (IL)-5, 6, 379
Interleukin (IL)-6
HIV and, 191
HTLV and, 205t
Lyme disease and, 223
neural degeneration with, 19
Interleukin (IL)-7, 243
Interleukin (IL)-10
in autoimmune response, 14t
downregulation by, 20
HIV infection and, 191, 192
immunosuppression by, 237
from microglia, 31
Interleukin (IL)-12
HIV infection and, 192
from microglia, 30
Intrathymic clonal deletion, 8
IPM. *See* Idiopathic polymyositis.
Isaacs' syndrome, 149t, 365–368, 367f

Isolated angiitis of CNS (IAC), 255t, 260
clinical features of, 262t
Ixodes ticks, 219–220

Janus kinase enzymes, 95
JC virus
HIV infection with, 200
persistent infection with, 82t
JHM virus infection, 396, 399t, 400
J-region genes, 2, 3, 232f
Junctional folds, 340, 341f

Kaposi's sarcoma, 189, 190t
Kawasaki disease
autoantibodies in, 256
classification of, 317t
immunoglobulin for, 264

Lambert-Eaton myasthenic syndrome (LEMS), 360–365, 364f, 365f
animal models for, 365, 392t
antibodies in, 364–365, 365f
autoantibodies for, 342
clinical features of, 360–361
diagnosis of, 361
lung cancer with, 360
paraneoplastic cerebellar degeneration with, 153t
as paraneoplastic syndrome, 149t, 150t
pathogenesis of, 148
treatment of, 165t, 361
Langerhans' cells, 4, 388
Latency, of viral genes, 82–83
Latency-associated transcript (LATs), 83
Legionella pneumophila, 375
LEMS. *See* Lambert-Eaton myasthenic syndrome.
Lentiviruses, 189–190
Leprosy, 401
Leukemia
hairy cell, 100
HTLV-associated, 206
Leukocyte function–associated antigen (LFA)-1
in immunity, 18
in Guillain-Barré syndrome, 299
Limbic encephalopathy, 157, 165t
Linomide, for multiple sclerosis, 97
Lipotropic hormone (LPH), 62f
Listeriosis, 190t
Lung cancer. *See also* Small-cell lung cancer (SCLC).
neurologic syndromes with, 150t
Lupus. *See also* Systemic lupus erythematosus (SLE).
murine, 16
vasculitis with, 261
Luteinizing hormone (LH), 59t, 60t
Lyme disease, 218–225, 400
clinical features of, 219–221, 220t
diagnosis of, 219, 219t
history of, 218–219
immunopathogenesis of, 221–223
optic neuritis with, 116

pathophysiology of, 221
pyomyositis with, 375
treatment of, 223t, 223–224
vaccine development for, 224
vasculitis with, 261
Lymphocyte function–associated antigen (LFA), 238–239
Lymphocytes, 1–3. *See also specific types.*
circulation of, 7
costimulation of, 16, 20
in myasthenia gravis, 349t, 349–351, 350f
in nerve fiber degeneration, 388
trafficking of, 96
Lymphocytic choriomeningitis virus (LCMV)
animal model for, 399t, 400
immunosuppression with, 85–86
persistent infection by, 80, 81f
T-cell response and, 15
Lymphoma. *See also specific types.*
Epstein-Barr virus and, 228
HIV with, 190t
HTLV with, 206
motor neuron syndrome with, 162
neuropathy with, 198t
paraneoplastic syndrome with, 155–156
polyradiculoneuropathy with, 163–164
subacute motor neuronopathy with, 150t, 162–163
Lymphomatoid granulomatosis
clinical features of, 262t
immunopathology of, 255t

Macrophage chemotactic protein (MCP)-1, 18
Macrophages, 14
in autoimmune neuritis, 45f, 45–46
in central nervous system, 34
MHC proteins and, 3–4
nerve degeneration and, 387–388
nerve regeneration and, 389
MAG. *See* Myelin-associated glycoprotein.
Major depressive disorder, antibodies in, 398
Major histocompatibility complex (MHC) proteins, 4–5
in Alzheimer's disease, 174–175, 175t
antigen-presenting cells and, 3
autoimmune diseases and, 13–14
classes of, 4–5, 57f
genes of, 57f
in glioma, 229, 229f
HTLV and, 205t
immune response and, 27f, 27–28
macrophages and, 3–4
peptide binding to, 8
polymorphism of, 4
roles of, 4
superantigens to, 87
suppression of, 85
transplant antigens and, 281–283
viral resistance and, 77–80, 78f, 79f

MAP kinase, 95
Marek's disease, 399t
Mate selection, immune effects on, 57
MBP. *See* Myelin basic protein.
Measles virus, 399t
  encephalomyelitis after, 116, 118,
    396
  persistent infection with, 82t, 83
  in subacute sclerosing panencephali-
    tis, 83, 84f
Melanocyte-stimulating hormone
    (MSH)
  as immune cell neuropeptide, 59t,
    60t
  immune effects of, 63
  in pro-opiomelanocortin gene, 62f
Melanoma
  antigens, 233, 233f
  neurologic syndrome with, 150t
Memory T cells, 7
Meningitis
  HIV-related, 190t
  from Lyme disease, 220, 220t, 224
MEPPs. *See* Miniature end-plate po-
    tentials.
Methotrexate
  immunosuppression with, 97t, 100
  for inflammatory myopathies,
    381–382
  for vasculitic neuropathy, 330f, 332
Methylprednisolone
  for multiple sclerosis, 99
  for optic neuritis, 135
  for vasculitic neuropathy, 330f, 331
MFS (Miller Fisher syndrome), 368
MGUS (monoclonal gammopathy of
    unknown significance), 163,
    307
MHC. *See* Major histocompatibility
    complex (MHC) proteins.
MHV (mouse hepatitis virus), 77, 82t
Microglia
  activated, 27f
  in Alzheimer's disease, 174f, 180–182
  amyloid plaques and, 178–180, 179t
  antibodies for, 31–32
  antigens expressed on, 175t, 175–176
  cell-mediated immune injury to,
    33–37
  immune reactivity of, 29f, 29–31
  perivascular, 28
  as phagocytes, 72
  proliferation of, 28
Microscopic polyangiitis, 317t, 318t,
    319
Migration inhibitory protein (MIP)-1,
    18
Miller Fisher syndrome (MFS), 368
Miniature end-plate potentials
    (MEPPs), 340–342
  antiganglioside antibodies and, 369,
    370f
  in Lambert-Eaton myasthenic syn-
    drome, 361–362
Mitochondrial myopathy, 198t
Mitoxantrone, 97t
MMN (multifocal motor neuropathy),
    369

MMTV (mouse mammary tumor
    virus), 87–88
MND. *See* Motor neuron disease.
MOG (myelin-oligodendrocyte glyco-
    protein), 123
Molecular mimicry, 17, 86–87
Monoclonal antibodies
  to acetylcholine receptors, 346–347
  for multiple sclerosis, 2–3, 96
  against myelin-associated glycopro-
    tein, 307
  peripheral tolerance and, 16–17
  for vasculitis, 264, 333
Monoclonal gammopathy of unknown
    significance (MGUS), 163, 307
Monocytes, 14
  across blood-brain barrier, 27f
  microglia and, 28
Mononeuritis multiplex
  HIV infection with, 198t
  Lyme disease with, 220t
Motor neuron disease (MND), 150t,
    162–163, 397–398
  antiganglioside antibodies and,
    368–370, 370f
  experimental autoimmune, 398
  paraneoplastic, 149t, 162–163
    encephalomyelitis with, 162
Mouse hepatitis virus (MHV)
  cytokines and, 77
  persistent infection with, 82t
Mouse mammary tumor virus
    (MMTV), 87–88
Mucormycosis
  HIV with, 190t
  vasculitis with, 261
Multifocal motor neuropathy (MMN),
    369
Multiple sclerosis (MS)
  after acute disseminated encephalo-
    myelitis, 131–138, 142
  animal models for, 92
  chemokines in, 18
  corticosteroids for, 97–99
  denervation supersensitivity in,
    65–66
  disease monitoring of, 101
  environmental factors in, 109
  experimental drugs for, 96–97
  genetic factors in, 108–109
  heat shock proteins in, 108
  history of, 395–396
  HPA axis in, 61
  HTLV-associated myelopathy and,
    206, 207t
  human herpesvirus-6 and, 117
  IFN-γ in, 19
  immunology of, 105–110
  immunosuppressants for, 97t,
    97–101
  immunotherapy for, 92, 93f
  interferon-β for, 20
  MHC linkage in, 13
  monoclonal antibodies for, 2–3
  myelin basic protein in, 2, 7–8, 19
  as neurodegenerative disorder, 172
  neuropathology of, 105–107
  optic neuritis in, 99, 132, 134

sympathetic nervous system in,
    65–66
  Th1 cells in, 6
  transverse myelopathy and, 138
  treatments for, 109–110
Mumps
  encephalomyelitis after, 118
  myositis after, 380
Muscle biopsy, for vasculitis,
    pl. VI–XIII, 376
Muscular dystrophy, 379
Myasthenia gravis (MG), 340–354
  autoantibodies for, 342
  autoimmunity in, 342–344, 343f,
    344f, 360
  clinical features of, 342
  immunogenetics of, 344–346, 345t
  immunotherapy for, 92
  lymphocytes in, 349t, 349–351, 350f
  neonatal, 346
  neuromuscular junction in, 343–344,
    344f
  ocular, 344–345, 345t
  onset of, 345–346
  as paraneoplastic syndrome, 149t
  plasmapheresis for, 97, 100
  seronegative, 351–352, 352f
  steroid therapy for, 99
  target autoantigen in, 87
  thymectomy for, 97, 99, 100, 342
  thymoma with, 148, 150t, 346–349,
    349t
  thymus in, 347, 348f
  treatment of, 165t, 342
Mycobacterium infections
  glioma and, 234
  HIV with, 190t
  leprosy from, 401
myc oncogene, 159
Mycoplasma infections
  myelitis with, 116
  superantigen of, 87
Myelin
  composition of, 42
  regeneration of, 271
Myelin-associated glycoprotein (MAG)
  antibodies to, 163, 308–310
  dysglobulinemic neuropathy with,
    pl. III–IV, 307–310
    treatment of, 310–311
  expression of, 310
  in peripheral nervous system, 42–43
Myelin basic protein (MBP), 7
  in autoimmune encephalomyelitis,
    7
  copolymer 1 of, 94, 110
  microglia and, 29
  in multiple sclerosis, 2, 7–8, 110
Myelinoclastic diffuse sclerosis, 138
Myelin-oligodendrocyte glycoprotein
    (MOG), 123
Myelitis. *See also* Encephalomyelitis.
  paraneoplastic, 149t
  transverse, 134f, 136f–137f
    after vaccination, 131–132
Myeloma
  neuropathy in, 311
  osteolytic multiple, 163

osteosclerotic, 163
   treatment of, 166t
Myelopathy
   HTLV-associated, 206, 207t
   necrotizing
      HIV with, 197–199, 198t
      paraneoplastic, 149t, 164
      vacuolar, HIV-related, 190t
      vasculitis with, 262t
Myoclonus, spinal, 160
Myopathy. *See also specific types.*
   cachetic, 149t, 150t
   carcinoid, 149t, 150t, 164–165
      treatment of, 165t
   HIV with, 197–199, 198t
   necrotizing, 149t, 164
   toxic noninflammatory, 375
   vasculitis with, 262t
Myositis
   animal model for, 392t
   postviral, 380–381

Narcolepsy, 56–57, 57f
   animal model for, 392t
Natural killer (NK) cells, 3
   CNS viral infection and, 76f
   in inflammatory myopathies, *pl.* XI,
      378–380
   in innate immune system, 1
   neural cell injury by, 33
   transforming growth factor-β and,
      236
NCAM (neural cellular adhesion molecule), 238–239
Necrotizing myopathy
   HIV with, 197–199, 198t
   paraneoplastic, 149t, 164
Necrotizing vasculitis. *See also* Vasculitis.
   classification of, 318t, 318–321
   HIV infection with, 198t
   polyarteritis nodosa as, 258
Nemaline myopathy, 197–199, 198t
Neonatal myasthenia gravis, 346. *See
   also* Myasthenia gravis (MG).
Nerve growth factor (NGF), 273–274,
      274t
   HTLV and, 205t
   as immune cell neuropeptide, 59t, 61t
   immune response and, 58, 64
   macrophages and, 389
   in wallerian degeneration, 386
Nervous system
   autonomic, 55, 64–65, 65f
      dysfunction of, 149t, 198t, 392t
   central. *See* Central nervous system
      (CNS).
   immune responses within, 401t,
      401–402
   paraneoplastic disorders of, 148
   peripheral. *See* Peripheral nervous
      system.
   shared immune receptors in, 58–64,
      59t–61t, 61f–63f
   sympathetic. *See* Sympathetic ner-
      vous system.
Neural cells
   immune effects on, 57, 385

immune-mediated injury to, 31–34,
      32f
Neural cellular adhesion molecule
      (NCAM), 238–239
Neuritis. *See also specific types.*
   autoimmune, 399t
   brachial, 149t, 163
   optic. *See* Optic neuritis.
Neuroblastoma, 150t
Neuroendocrinimmunology, 402–404,
      403t
Neurofibrillary tangles (NFTs), 172,
      173
Neuromuscular junction (NMJ),
      340–342, 341f
   acetylcholine receptor, 340–342, 341f
   as archetypal synapse, 340
   in myasthenia gravis, 343–344, 344f
   serum factors and, 342
Neuromyotonia (NMT)
   acquired, 365–368, 367f
      clinical features of, 366
      pathogenesis of, 366–368, 367f
      treatment of, 366
   paraneoplastic, 149t
Neurons
   AIDS dementia and, 192–193
   antibodies for, 31–32
   degeneration of, 387–389
   motor, 150t, 162–163, 341f
      calcium channel antibodies and,
         364
   regeneration of, 271, 385–389
   Theiler's murine encephalomyelitis
      virus in, 75f
   transforming growth factor and, 58
Neuropathy. *See also specific types.*
   in amyloidosis, 312
   dysglobulinemic, 307–312
   in IgG dysglobulinemia, 311
   in myeloma, 311
   paraneoplastic, 149t
Neuropeptides
   cytokines and, 58, 59t
   from immune cells, 59t
   schizophrenia and, 56
Neurosyphilis, 218
   encephalomyelitis versus, 125
   HIV with, 190t
   vasculitis from, 261, 318t
Neurotrophin-3 (NT-3), 273–274, 274t
Neurotropic viruses, 72–74, 75f
NFTs (neurofibrillary tangles), 172, 173
NGF. *See* Nerve growth factor.
Nitric oxide, in autoimmune response,
      14t
NK cells. *See* Natural killer (NK) cells.
N-methyl-D-aspartate (NMDA)
   as excitotoxin, 273
   in HIV infection, 194–195
   neuron injury and, 33
   neurotoxicity of, 180–182
NMJ. *See* Neuromuscular junction.
NMT. *See* Neuromyotonia.
N-myc oncogene, 159
Nocardiosis, 190t
Non-Hodgkin's lymphoma. *See* Lym-
   phoma.

Nonneutralizing antibodies, 85
Nonsteroidal anti-inflammatory drugs
      (NSAIDs), 264
Noradrenergic innervation, of spleen,
      65f
Nova gene, 155
N-region genes, 2, 3

Obsessive-compulsive disorder (OCD),
      398
Ocular myasthenia gravis, 344–345,
      345t
Oligodendrocytes
   astrocytes and, 274, 275f
   regeneration of, 271
Oligodendroglia, 32–33
Oncogenes
   BRCA1, 154
   N-*myc*, 159
   transfection of, 244
   tumor antigens of, 233f
Onco-neuronal antigens, 150t
Opportunistic infections, in AIDS,
      190t, 199–200
Opsoclonus-myoclonus, 149t–151t, 159
Optic neuritis
   bilateral simultaneous, 137–138
   cerebrospinal fluid in, 126
   Lyme disease and, 116
   multiple sclerosis and, 99, 132, 134
   treatment of, 135
   after vaccination, 116, 131–132
Oral tolerance, 95, 110
Osteolytic multiple myeloma, 163
Osteoporosis, corticosteroids and,
      332–333
Osteosclerotic myeloma, 163
   treatment of, 166t
Ovarian cancer
   neurologic syndromes with, 150t
   Yo antibodies in, 153–154
Oxytocin, 59t, 60t

P0/P2 proteins
   Guillain-Barré syndrome and, 299
   in PNS myelin, 42
PAN. *See* Polyarteritis nodosa.
Papovaviruses. *See also specific types.*
   HIV with, 190t, 200
   persistent infection with, 82t
Paramyxovirus, 118, 380
Paraneoplastic cerebellar degeneration
      (PCD), 149t, 150t, 153t,
      153–156, 154f–156f
   diagnosis of, 153
   Hodgkin's disease with, 154–155
   pathogenesis of, 148
   Ri antibodies in, 155, 156f
   small-cell lung cancer with, 153t,
      155–156
   treatment of, 166t
   Yo antibodies with, 153–154, 154f,
      155f
Paraneoplastic encephalomyelitis
      (PEM), 149, 149t, 150t,
      156–159, 157f, 158f. *See also*
      Encephalomyelitis.
   motor neuron dysfunction with, 162

Paraneoplastic encephalomyelitis (*cont.*)
neurologic symptoms with, 158f
treatment of, 165t
Paraneoplastic motor neuron dysfunction, 162–163
Paraneoplastic neurologic disorders, 148–166
antibodies with, 151t
diagnosis of, 149–152, 150t–152t
pathogenesis of, 148–149, 150t
treatment of, 165t, 165–166, 166t
Paraneoplastic opsoclonus-myoclonus, 149t–151t, 159
treatment of, 165t
Paraneoplastic retinopathy, 151t, 160
Paraneoplastic sensory neuronopathy (PSN), 149, 149t, 160–162, 161f
neurologic symptoms with, 158f
toxic neuropathies versus, 162
treatment of, 166t
Parkinson's disease
fetal allografts for, 281
as neurodegenerative disorder, 172
PCD. *See* Paraneoplastic cerebellar degeneration.
PEM. *See* Paraneoplastic encephalomyelitis.
Penicillin, for Lyme disease, 223t, 224
Periarteritis nodosa. *See* Polyarteritis nodosa (PAN).
Peripheral clonal unresponsiveness, 8–9
Peripheral nerve antigens, 42–43
Peripheral nervous system
HIV-related infections of, 190t
immune responses in, 49f, 64–65, 65f
immunoinflammatory disorders of, 42, 107–108
isolated vasculitis of, 260
local immune responses in, 40–50
nerve fiber regeneration in, 386–387
paraneoplastic syndromes of, 148, 149t, 160–165, 161f
viral infection of, 73
Peripheral neuropathy
with HIV infection, 197–198, 198t
with Lyme disease, 220t, 220–221, 224
Miller Fisher syndrome and, 368
myeloma with, 311
sulfate glucuronyl paragleboside and, 392t
of unknown etiology, 307
vasculitis with, *pl.* V–VI, 262t, 318t, 322–323, 323t
Waldenström's macroglobulinemia with, 307–308
Peripheral tolerance, 16–17
Pertussis vaccine
encephalomyelitis after, 118
encephalopathy after, 139–140
PIE (postinfectious encephalomyelitis), 116, 396, 399t
Plasma cells, 6–7

Plasma cell dyscrasias, 149t, 163
Plasmapheresis
for encephalomyelitis, 129–130
indications for, 97, 100, 264
for inflammatory myopathies, 381–382
for paraneoplastic syndromes, 165t, 166t
for vasculitic neuropathy, 332
for vasculitis, 264
PLP (proteolipid protein), 123
PM. *See* Polymyositis.
PML (progressive multifocal leukoencephalopathy), 200, 399t, 400
Pneumocystis carinii, 189
Pneumonitis, viral, 380
POEMS syndrome, 163, 311–312
animal model for, 392t, 397
pol gene
in HIV, 190
in HTLV, 204, 205f
Polio vaccination, encephalomyelitis after, 116, 118
Poliovirus, cell tropism of, 73–74
Polyangiitis, microscopic
classification of, 317t, 318t
neuropathy with, 319
Polyangiitis overlap syndrome, 318t, 319
Polyarteritis nodosa (PAN), 258–259
classification of, 317t, 318t
clinical features of, 262t
epidemiology of, 316
hepatitis B and, 325
immunopathology of, 255t
neuropathy with, 319
plasmapheresis for, 264
vaso-occlusion with, 257, 332
Polymorphonuclear leukocytes
in innate immune system, 1
in nerve fiber degeneration, 388
Polymyalgia rheumatica, 260
Polymyositis (PM), 164, 374–382. *See also* Idiopathic polymyositis (IPM).
clinical features of, 374–375
HIV with, 198–199
HTLV with, 207
immunopathology of, *pl.* XI–XV, 378–381
as paraneoplastic syndrome, 149t
parasitic, 375
treatment of, 381–382
Polyneuropathy, asymmetric, 323
Polyradiculoneuropathy. *See also* Guillain-Barré syndrome (GBS).
HIV with, 197–198, 198t
paraneoplastic, 163–164
POMC (pro-opiomelanocortin) gene, 62, 62f
Postinfectious encephalomyelitis (PIE), 116, 396, 399t. *See also* Encephalomyelitis.
Postvaccinal encephalomyelitis (PVE), 116, 118, 124, 391, 396
Prednisolone
for multiple sclerosis, 99
for optic neuritis, 135

Prednisone
for inflammatory myopathies, 381
for vasculitic neuropathy, 330f, 331
for vasculitis, 263
Progressive multifocal leukoencephalopathy (PML), 200, 399t, 400
Progressive rubella panencephalitis (PRP), 399t, 400
Prolactin
dopamine and, 64
as immune cell neuropeptide, 59t, 60t
immune regulation by, 63–64
Pro-opiomelanocortin (POMC) gene, 62, 62f
Prostaglandin E₁, vasculitis and, 264
Prostaglandins, from macrophages, 4
Proteolipid protein (PLP), 123
Prothymocytes, 1
PRP (progressive rubella panencephalitis), 399t, 400
Pseudomyotonia, 366
PSN. *See* Paraneoplastic sensory neuronopathy.
Psoralen ultraviolet light treatment, 96–97
Psychoneuroimmunology, 402–404, 403t
Psychosis, AIDS dementia with, 192t
PVE (postvaccinal encephalomyelitis), 116, 118, 124, 391, 396
Pyomyositis, 375

Rabies vaccine
encephalomyelitis from, 116, 124, 391
types of, 121
Rabies virus
encephalitis from, 118
persistent infection with, 82t
Ramified cells, 28
Rapamycin, 288
Reactive oxygen intermediates, 181
Rejection. *See under* Grafts.
Reovirus, 82t
Retinal ganglion cell blindness, 392t
Retinopathy
cancer-associated, 149t
paraneoplastic, 151t, 160
Retroviruses
inflammatory myopathies and, 380–381
open reading frames of, 204
Reye's syndrome, 138–139
Rheumatoid arthritis. *See* Arthritis, rheumatoid.
Rhinoviruses, 73, 85
Rhizopus infection, 190t
Ri antibodies, in paraneoplastic syndromes, 155, 156f
Ross River virus, 82t
Rubella, encephalomyelitis after, 116, 118

Scarlet fever, encephalomyelitis after, 118
Schilder's disease, 138

Schizophrenia, brain damage in, 55–56
Schwann cells, 340, 341f
  in peripheral nervous system, 40–42, 41f
  in wallerian degeneration, 385–386
SCLC. *See* Small-cell lung cancer.
Sclerosis
  dermatomyositis with, 374
  neuropathy with, 321
Scrapie, 399t
Seizures
  AIDS dementia with, 192t
  vasculitis with, 262t
Selectins
  in autoimmunity, 18
  in HIV infection, 194
  leukocyte migration and, 26–27
Semliki Forest virus, 117, 396
  animal model for, 399t
  persistent infection with, 82t
Serum sickness, 321
Severe combined immunodeficient mice, 353
SGPG (sulfate glucuronyl paragleboside), 392t
Shawl sign, 374
Sinbis virus, 399t
Sjögren's syndrome
  HTLV and, 207
  neuropathy with, 161–162, 320
  symptoms of, 161–162
  vasculitis with, 261–262
SLE. *See* Systemic lupus erythematosus.
Small-cell lung cancer (SCLC), 150t
  Lambert-Eaton myasthenic syndrome with, 360
  neurologic syndromes with, 150t
  paraneoplastic syndromes with, 153t, 155–157
  sensory neuronopathy with, 148
  vasculitic neuropathy with, 164
Smallpox, encephalomyelitis after, 116, 118, 396
Somatostatin, 59t, 60t
Spinal myoclonus, 160
Spleen, noradrenergic innervation of, 65f
Spongiform encephalitis, 399t
SSPE (subacute sclerosing panencephalitis), 83, 84f, 117, 399t, 400
Staphylococcus aureus
  HIV with, 190t
  polymyositis from, 375
  superantigen of, 87
Steroids, 165t, 165–166, 166t. *See also* Corticosteroids; Glucocorticoids (GCC).
Steroid-sparing effect, 381
Stiff-man syndrome
  antibodies in, 398
  clinical features of, 160
  paraneoplastic, 149t, 150t
Streptococcus polymyositis, 375
Stress response, HPA axis and, 61f, 402–404, 403t
Stroke, vasculitis with, 262t

Strongyloidiasis, 190t
Subacute motor neuronopathy, 150t, 162–163
Subacute sclerosing panencephalitis (SSPE), 117, 399t, 400
  measles virus and, 83, 84f
Subarachnoid hemorrhage, vasculitis with, 262t
Substance P, 59t, 60t, 66
  role of, 57
Sulfasalazine, 97t
Sulfate glucuronyl paragleboside (SGPG), 392t
Superantigens, 87–88
  HIV-encoded, 191
Sural nerve biopsy, *pl.* V–XII
Sydenham's chorea, 398, 400–401
Sympathetic nervous system
  in arthritis, 66
  immunity and, 58
  in multiple sclerosis, 65–66
  neuropeptides of, 66
Syphilis, 218
  encephalomyelitis versus, 125
  HIV with, 190t
  vasculitis with, 261, 318t
Systemic lupus erythematosus (SLE)
  animal model for, 392t
  autoantibodies in, 398
  neuropathy with, 320
  vasculitis with, 261

Takayasu's arteritis
  classification of, 317t, 318t
  clinical features of, 262t
  immunopathology of, 255t
tat gene, 190
Tau protein, 173
Taxol neuropathy, 16
TCC (terminal complement complex), 46, 49–50
T cells. *See also* Lymphocytes; *specific types.*
  activation of, 231f
    autoimmune, 15–18
    costimulation for, 16, 20
  in adaptive immune system, 1–3
  α/β
    in cell-mediated immune injury, 32–33
    in multiple sclerosis, 105, 395
  antigen-presenting cell interactions with, 239f
  anti-idiotypic, 94
  in autoimmune neuritis, 43–44
  autoimmune tolerance of, 14–15
  B-cell synergy with, 48f, 50
  circulation of, 7
  cytotoxic, 20–21
    in inflammatory myopathies, *pl.* XI, XV, 378–380
  γ/δ, 21
    in cell-mediated immune injury, 33
    in inflammatory myopathies, 378
    in multiple sclerosis, 105–106, 395
  memory, 7
  regulation of, 8–9
  selection process of, 2, 4, 5

  superantigen stimulation of, 87–88
  surface proteins of, 2, 255f
  tissue entry by, 17–18
T cell–dependent antigens, 3, 6
T-cell receptors (TCRs)
  antigenic specificity of, 2–3
  in autoimmune neuritis, 43–44
  blockade of, 93
  costimulatory molecule of, 240f, 240–241
  genes of, 2
  in glioma, 229f, 233–238
  in HTLV-associated myelopathy, 210f, 210–211
  in inflammatory myopathies, 378–379
  molecular analysis of, 237–238
  regulatory networks of, 9
  tumor antigens and, 229–233, 230f–233f
  types of, 2
  "vaccination" of, 2–3
T-cell receptor therapy, 94–95
T-cell vaccination, 94–95
TCRs. *See* T-cell receptors.
Temporal arteritis, 260
  classification of, 317t, 318t
  clinical features of, 262t
  immunopathology of, 255t
Terminal complement complex (TCC), 46, 49–50
Testes, immune privilege of, 67
Tetanus vaccination, encephalomyelitis after, 116, 118
Theiler's murine encephalomyelitis virus (TMEV), 399t, 400
  cell tropism of, 74, 75f
  demyelination with, 117
  MHC regulation in, 77–80, 78f, 79f
  persistent infection with, 82t
Th1/Th2 cells, 6
  for immunotherapy, 94
  as switch cytokines, 20
Thymectomy, for myasthenia gravis, 97, 99, 100, 342
Thymoma
  acetylcholine receptor antibodies in, 343f
  myasthenia gravis with, 148, 150t, 346–349, 349t
Thymus
  antigen presentation in, 15
  clonal deletion in, 8
  dendritic cells in, 3
  function of, 1–2
  in myasthenia gravis, 342, 345t, 347, 348f
  selection processes in, 14–15
Thyroid-stimulating hormone (TSH), 59t, 60t
TLI (total lymphoid irradiation), 96, 97t, 100, 382
TMEV. *See* Theiler's murine encephalomyelitis virus.
TNF. *See* Tumor necrosis factor.
Tolerance
  anergy and, 14
  autoimmune, 14–15

Tolerance (*cont.*)
mechanisms of, 8–9
oral, 95, 110
peripheral, 16–17
Total lymphoid irradiation (TLI), 96, 97t, 100, 382
Toxic encephalopathy, 138–142
Toxic neuropathies, 162
Toxoplasmosis, 400
HIV infection with, 190t, 199
polymyositis with, 375
vasculitis with, 261
Transforming growth factor (TGF)-α, 272t, 272–273
neurons and, 58
Transforming growth factor (TGF)-β
in autoimmune neuritis, *pl.* II
in autoimmune response, 14t
downregulation by, 20
from glia cells, 31
for glioma, 244, 245
HIV and, 194
HTLV and, 194
immunosuppression by, 236–237
in inflammatory myopathies, 379
for multiple sclerosis, 96
neurons and, 58
Th2 cells and, 6
Transplants
CNS, 281–289
donors for, 289
immunologic issues with, 288–289
Transverse myelitis, 134f
spinal cord in, 136f–137f
after vaccination, 131–132
Transverse myelopathy, 138
Treponema pallidum. See also Syphilis.
HIV with, 190t
Lyme disease versus, 218
Trimolecular complex, 58
Trisomy 16, interferon and, 58
Tropical spastic paraparesis (TSP), 206, 207t, 399t
Lyme disease and, 400
pathology of, 207–209, 208t
T-cell receptor usage in, 210f, 210–211
Tropism, viral, 73–74, 75f
Trypanosoma cruzi, 190t, 401
TSTAs (tumor-specific transplantation antigens), 233, 233f
d-Tubocurarine, 352
Tumor cells
gene transfer into, 242f
vaccines for, 241–245
Tumor necrosis factor (TNF)-α
autoimmune encephalomyelitis and, 8
in autoimmune response, 14t
HIV and, 191, 194, 197f, 197t
HTLV and, 205t
in inflammatory myopathies, 379
Lyme disease and, 223
from macrophages, 4
MHC-linked genes of, 14
for multiple sclerosis, 96
neural cell injury by, 33
neural degeneration with, 19–20

neuron injury and, 272–273, 276
production of, 19
Tumor necrosis factor (TNF)-β
HTLV and, 205t
as lymphotoxin, 19
neural cell injury by, 33
Tumor necrosis factor (TNF)-γ, 33
Tumor-specific transplantation antigens (TSTAs), 233, 233f

Uveitis
experimental autoimmune, 392t
HTLV infection with, 206–207

Vaccination
encephalomyelitis after, 116, 118, 124, 391, 396
immunologic memory and, 6–7
Lyme disease and, 224
T-cell, 94–95
for tumor cells, 241–245, 242f
Vacuolar myelopathy, 190t
van der Waals reactions, 4
Varicella-zoster virus (VZV)
encephalomyelitis, 116, 117
HIV with, 199–200, 190t
myelitis with, 116
persistent infection with, 82t
toxic encephalopathy after, 138
Vascular cell adhesion molecule (VCAM)-1
in autoimmunity, 18
CNS immune response and, 26–27, 27f
endothelial cells and, 7
in glioma, 237–240, 239f
in Guillain-Barré syndrome, 299
in HIV infection, 194
in inflammatory myopathies, *pl.* XIV, 379–380
in multiple sclerosis, 106
in vasculitis, 326, 326f
Vasculitic neuropathy, 164, 261, 316–333
clinical features of, 323–324
diagnosis of, *pl.* VII–XII, 262t, 324–325
HIV infection with, 198t
as paraneoplastic syndrome, 149t
pathogenesis of, 325–329, 326f–328f
sural nerve biopsy and, *pl.* V–XII
treatment of, 329–333, 330f
Vasculitis, 254–265, 316–333
autoantibodies in, 255t, 256
from *Borrelia burgdorferi,* 222–223
cell-mediated cytotoxicity in, 328f
classification of, 316–317, 317t, 318t
clinical features of, 254
diagnosis of, 262, 262t
encephalomyelitis versus, 125
endothelial interactions in, 254–256, 255f
epidemiology of, 316
HIV-related, 190t, 198t
hypersensitivity, 255t, 259–260, 321–322
clinical features of, 262t

immunopathology of, 254–258, 255f, 255t
from infections, 317–318, 318t
lupus, 261
monoclonal antibodies for, 333
necrotizing, 198t, 258
classification of, 318t, 318–321
systemic, 318t
neuroimaging for, 262
nonsystemic, *pl.* V–VI, 322–323, 323t
paraneoplastic, 164
treatment of, 166t
rheumatoid, 316, 320
secondary, 261–262, 319–320
treatment of, 262–265
Vasoactive intestinal peptide (VIP), 59t, 60t, 66
Vaso-occlusive disease
treatment of, 332
vasculitis with, 257
VCAM-1. *See* Vascular cell adhesion molecule-1.
Venezuelan equine encephalomyelitis virus, 117
Very late activation antigen (VLA)-4
in autoimmune neuritis, 44
in autoimmunity, 18
CNS immune response and, 26
in Guillain-Barré syndrome, 299
in multiple sclerosis, 106
in vasculitic neuropathy, 326, 326f
Vesicular stomatitis virus, 117
VGCCs. *See* Voltage-gated calcium channels.
VGPC (voltage-gated potassium channel), 366–368, 367f
VIP (vasoactive intestinal peptide), 59t, 60t, 66
Viral-immune interactions, 72–88
Viral infections, 399t, 399–400
cytokines in, 77
host immune response to, 74–77, 76f
inflammatory myopathies with, 380–381
persistent, 80–86, 81f, 82t
Viremia, 73
Viruses. *See also specific types.*
cell tropism of, 73–74, 75f
latency of, 82–83
neurotropic, 72–74, 75f
Virus-induced demyelination, 117–118
Visna virus, 82t, 399t
Vitamin B$_{12}$ deficiency, 125
VLA. *See* Very late activation antigen.
Voltage-gated calcium channels (VGCCs), 150t, 360, 361f
antibodies to, 151t, 363–364, 364f
in Lambert-Eaton myasthenic syndrome, 362–363
paraneoplastic cerebellar degeneration with, 153t
small-cell lung cancer and, 148
Voltage-gated potassium channel (VGPC), 366–368, 367f
V-region genes, 2, 3, 232f
V sign, in dermatomyositis, 374
VZV. *See* Varicella-zoster virus.

Waldenström's macroglobulinemia, 150t, 163
  peripheral neuropathy with, 307–308
  treatment of, 311
Wallerian degeneration, 385–386
Wasting syndrome, AIDS, 198, 198t
Wegener's granulomatosis, 260
  classification of, 317t, 318t
  clinical features of, 262t

immunopathology of, 255t
  neuropathy with, 319
Wernicke encephalopathy, 150t
Western blot, for Lyme disease, 219, 219t

Xenopus assay, 368

Yo antibodies, 151t

in ovarian cancer, 153–154
  with paraneoplastic cerebellar degeneration, 153–154, 154f, 155f

Zalcitabine (ddC), 196, 198
Zeitgebers, 67
Zidovudine (AZT), 196
  myopathy with, 198t, 199